HUGH—Human Gene Nomenclature
HVAC—Heating, Ventilation, and Air Conditioning
I/S—Information Systems
IADL—Instrumental Activities of Daily Living
ICD 9 CM—International Classification of Diseases, 9th Version, Clinical Modification
ICD—International Classification of Diseases
ICD-10—International Classification of Diseases, 10th Revision
ICD-10-PCS—International Classification of Diseases, 10th Revision, Procedural Coding System
ICD-9—International Classification of Diseases, 9th Revision
ICD-O-3—International Classification of Disease for Oncology, Third Edition
ICD-O—International Classification of Disease-Oncology
ICF—Intermediate Care Facility
IDDM—Insulin Dependent Diabetes Mellitus
IDS—Integrated Delivery System
IEC—International Electrotechnical Commission
IEEE 1073—Institute of Electrical and Electronic Engineers 1073
IEEE—Institute of Electrical and Electronics Engineers
IETF—Internet Engineering Task Force
IHS—Indian Health Service
IIHI—Individually Identifiable Health Information
IOM—Institute of Medicine
IPA—Independent Practice Association
IR—Incidence Rate
IRB—Institutional Review Board
IRCA—Immigration Reform and Control Act
IRS—Internal Revenue Service
IS/SI—Intensity of Service/Severity of Illness
ISO—International Standardization of Organization
IT—Information Technology
JAD—Joint Application Development
JCAHO—Joint Commission on Accreditation of Healthcare Organizations
JVM—Java Virtual Machine
LAN—Local Area Network
LHR—Legal Health Record
LIP—Licensed Independent Practitioner
LOINC—Logical Observation Identifiers Names and Codes
LPN—Licensed Practical Nurse
LVN—Licensed Vocational Nurse
MBHO—Managed Behavioral Healthcare Organization
MBO—Management by Objectives
MCO—Managed Care Organization
MD—Medical Doctor
MDS—Minimum Data Set
MeSH—Medical Subject Headings
MFD—Multifunctional Device
MIB—Medical Information Bureau
MIS—Management Information Systems
MMA—Medicare Modernization Act
MPI—Master Patient Index
MSO—Medical Staff Organization
MUMPS—Massachusetts General Hospital Utility Multi-Programming System
NAHDO—National Association of Health Data Organizations
NAHIT—National Alliance for Health Information Technology
NANDA—North American Nursing Diagnosis Association
NCCAM—National Center for Complementary and Alternative Medicine
NCHS—National Center for Health Statistics
NCI—National Cancer Institute
NCPDP—National Council of Prescription Drug Programs

NCQA—National Committee for Quality Assurance
NCRA—National Cancer Registrars Association, Inc.
NCVHS—National Committee on Vital and Health Statistics
NDC—National Drug Codes
NDF-RT—National Drug File Reference Terminology
NEDSS—National Electronic Disease Surveillance System
NGT—Nominal Group Technique
NHII—National Health Information Infrastructure
NHIN—Nationwide Health Information Network
NIC—Nursing Interventions Classification
NIDDM—Non-Insulin-Dependent Diabetes Mellitus
NIH—National Institutes of Health
NI—Nosocomial Infections
NIOSH—National Institute for Occupational Safety and Health
NIST—National Institute of Standards and Technology
NLM—National Library of Medicine
NLNAC—National League for Nursing Accrediting Commission, Inc.
NLN—National League for Nursing
NLRA—National Labor Relations Act
NLRB—National Labor Relations Board
NMDS—Nursing Minimum Data Set
NMMDS—Nursing Management Minimum Data Set
NOC—Nursing Outcomes Classification
NP—Nurse Practitioner
NPDB—National Practitioner Data Bank
NPI—National Provider Identifier
NPPES—National Plan and Provider Enumeration System
NQF—National Quality Forum
NRC—National Resource Center
NTDB—National Trauma Data Bank
OASIS—Outcome and Assessment Information Set
OCR—Optical Character Recognition
OFCCP—Office of Federal Contract Compliance Program
OIG—Office of the Inspector General
OMB—Office of Management and Budget's Office
ONCHIT—Office of the Coordinator of Health Information Technology
ONC—Office of the National Coordinator of Health Information Technology
OPTM—Organ Procurement and Transplantation Network
ORHP—Office of Rural Health Policy
OSHA—Occupational Safety and Health Administration Act
P2P—Peer-to-Peer
P4P—Pay for Performance
PA—Physician Assistant
PACS—Picture Archiving and Communication System
PCAOB—Public Company Accounting Oversight Board
PCE—Potentially Compensable Event
PC—Personal Computer (microsystem or minicomputer)
PCS—Procedural Coding System
PDA—Personal Digital Assistant
PDCA—Plan, Do, Check, Act
PHI—Personal Health Information
PHI—Personally-identifiable Health Information
PHI—Protected Health Information
PHR—Personal Health Record
PHS—Public Health Service
PMB—Pharmacy Benefits Manager
PMRI—Patient Medical Record Information
PNDS—Perioperative Nursing Data Set
POMR—Problem-Oriented Medical Record
POS—Point of Service
PPI—Pixels Per Inch
PPO—Preferred Provider Organization
PPS—Prospective Payment System

PSI—
QIC—
QI—Quality Improvement
QWL—Quality of Work Life
r—Correlation Coefficent
RAI—Resident Assessment Instrument
RAID—Redundant Array of Independent Disks
RBAC—Role Based Access Control
RBRVS—Resource-Based Relative Value Scale
RCI—Rapid Cycle Improvement
RELMA—Regenstrief LOINC Mapping Assistant
RFID—Radio Frequency Identification Device
RFI—Request for Information
RFP—Request for Proposal
RHIA—Registered Health Information Administrator
RHIO—Regional Health Information Organizations
RHIT—Registered Health Information Technician
ROI—Return on Investment
ROI—Release of Information
RRL—Registered Record Librarian
RR—Relative Risk
RSI—Repetitive Stress (or Strain) Injury
RVU—Relative Value Unit
SAN—Storage Area Network
SAS—Statistical Analysis System
SDO—Standards Development Organization
SEER—Surveillance, Epidemiology, and End Results
SEIU—Service Employees International Union
SGML—Standardized Generalized Markup Language
S-HTTP—Secure Hypertext Transfer Protocol
SIP—Surgical Infection Prevention
SMR—Standardized Mortality Ratio
SNODENT—Systematized Nomenclature of Dentistry
SNOMED CT—Systematized Nomenclature of Human and Veterinary Medicine
SNOP—Systematized Nomenclature of Pathology
SNO—Sub Network Organization
SOAP—Subjective, Objective, Assessment, Plan
SOW—Statement of Work
SPC—Statistical Process Control
SPSS—Statistical Package for Social Sciences
SQC—Statistical Quality Control
SQL—Standard Query Language
SSA—Social Security Administration
SSL—Secure Socket Layer
SSN—Social Security Number
TCP/IP—Transmission Control Protocol/Internet Protocol
TEFRA—Tax Equity and Fiscal Responsibility Act
TNM—Tumor, Lymph Node, and Metastases
TN—True Negatives
TP—True Positives
TQM—Total Quality Management
UACDS—Uniform Ambulatory Care Data Set
UB-04—Uniform Billing Code of 2004
UHDDS—Uniform Hospital Discharge Data Set
UM—Utilization Management
UMLS—Unified Medical Language
UNOS—United Network for Organ Sharing
UPIN—Unique Personal/Physician Identification Number
UPS—Uninterruptable Power Supply
URAC—Utilization Review Accreditation Commission
VAMC—Veterans Administration Medical Center
VA—Veterans Administration
VPN—Virtual Private Network
W3—World Wide Web Consortium
WAN—Wide Area Network
WEP—Wired Equivalent Privacy
WHO—World Health Organization
WORM—Write Once Read Many
WPA—Wi-Fi Protected Access
WWW—World Wide Web
XML—Extensible Markup Language

ELSEVIER

evolve

HEALTH INFORMATION:
Management of a Strategic Resource

THIRD EDITION

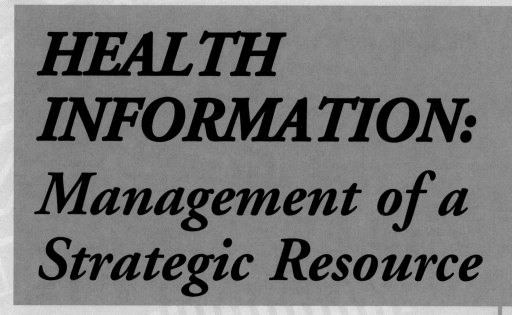

HEALTH INFORMATION:
Management of a Strategic Resource

MERVAT ABDELHAK, PhD, RHIA, FAHIMA
Managing Editor
Department Chair and Associate Professor Health
Information Management
School of Health and Rehabilitation Sciences
University of Pittsburgh, Pennsylvania

SARA GROSTICK, MA, RHIA, FAHIMA
Director
Health Information Management Program
and Associate Professor
School of Health Professions
University of Alabama at Birmingham
Birmingham, Alabama

MARY ALICE HANKEN, PhD, CHP, RHIA
Independent Consultant; Senior Lecturer
Health Information Administration Program
School of Public Health and Community
Medicine
University of Washington
Seattle, Washington

ELLEN JACOBS, MEd, RHIA
Director and Associate Professor
Health Information Management Programs
College of Saint Mary
Omaha, Nebraska

SAUNDERS

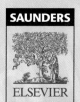

ELSEVIER

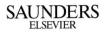

11830 Westline Industrial Drive
St. Louis, Missouri 63146

HEALTH INFORMATION: MANAGEMENT OF A
STRATEGIC RESOURCE, THIRD EDITION

ISBN-13: 978-1-4160-3002-7
ISBN-10: 1-4160-3002-6

Notice

Neither the Publisher nor the Editors assume any responsibility for any loss or injury and/or damage to persons or property arising out of or related to any use of the material contained in this book. It is the responsibility of the treating practitioner, relying on independent expertise and knowledge of the patient, to determine the best treatment and method of application for the patient.

The Publisher

Library of Congress Cataloging-in-Publication Data

Health information : management of a strategic resource/by Mervat Abdelhak ... [et al.].
   —3rd ed.
      p. cm.
   Includes bibliographical references (p.   ).
   ISBN-13: 978-1-4160-3002-7   ISBN-10: 1-4160-3002-6
      1. Medical informatics. 2. Information resources management. I. Abdelhak, Mervat.

R858.H35 2007
610.285—dc22

2006051295

ISBN-13: 978-1-4160-3002-7
ISBN-10: 1-4160-3002-6

Acquisitions Editor: Susan Cole
Developmental Editor: Colin Odell
Publishing Services Manager: Patricia Tannian
Project Manager: Claire Kramer
Design Direction: Steven Stave

Printed in the United States of America

Last digit is the print number: 9 8 7 6 5 4 3

I dedicate this work to my parents, who, even though they are miles and miles away, continue to be my inspiration; to my sons, Jonathan and Matthew, who are my life; to my administrative assistant, Patti Grofic, who made it all happen and happen on time; to my colleagues at the University of Pittsburgh, who have stimulated me; and to my coeditors—it has been a joyous experience that I will treasure forever. Thank you all.

Mervat Abdelhak

I dedicate this book to Alan, Laura, and Charles, who make life memorable; the Health Information Management students at UAB, past and present, who make teaching a rewarding career; and Ellen, Mervat, and Mary Alice, who make editing a book an adventure and an extraordinary experience.

Sara Grostick

This labor of love and professional commitment is dedicated to my many colleagues, students, and friends in health information management. I do this work for you. Thanks to my husband, Jim, and children, Kathy, Jamie, and Paul, who have been a part of various health information management activities; to Mervat, Sara, and Ellen, who are great teammates; and to the Elsevier staff, who bring their publishing expertise to this project.

Mary Alice Hanken

I dedicate my contributions to this work to the health information management students and professionals. They keep me grounded in reality while opening my sights to possibilities. I further dedicate this work to my children, Danny and Becky, for giving me the most instructive life lessons of hope, peace, and creativity; to the contributors to this work for their willingness to share their expertise; and to Mervat, Sara and Mary Alice for their patience, support, and gift of friendship.

Ellen Jacobs

Contributors

Marion J. Ball, EdD
Fellow, IBM Global Leadership Initiative
Business Consulting Services
Professor, Johns Hopkins University School of
Nursing
Vice President, Healthlink
Baltimore, Maryland
Chapter 19 *Viewpoints*

Meryl Bloomrosen, MBA, RHIA
Associate Vice President, American Medical Informatics Association
Washington, District of Columbia
Chapter 3 *Health Information Infrastructure and Systems*

Melanie S. Brodnik, PhD, RHIA
Director & Associate Professor, Health Information Management &
Systems Division
School of Allied Medical Professions
The Ohio State University
Columbus, Ohio
Chapter 2 *The Health Informatics and Information Management
Profession*

Jean S. Clark, RHIA
Service Line Director, Health Information Management
Services
Roper Saint Francis Healthcare
Charleston, South Carolina
Chapter 19 *Viewpoints*

Jill Callahan Dennis, JD, RHIA
Principal, Health Risk Advantage
Parker, Colorado
Chapter 15 *Privacy and Health Law*

Don E. Detmer, MD, MA
President and Chief Executive Officer, American Medical Informatics
Association
Bethesda, Maryland
Professor of Medical Education, Department of Public Health
Services
School of Medicine
University of Virginia
Charlottesville, Virginia
Chapter 19 *Viewpoints*

Bill G. Felkey, MS
Professor of Pharmacy Care Systems
Auburn University
Auburn, Alabama
Chapter 19 *Viewpoints*

Jennifer Garvin, PhD, RHIA, CPHQ, CCS, CTR, FAHIMA
Postdoctoral Fellow, Center for Health Equity Research and
Promotion
Philadelphia Veterans Administration Medical Center
Philadelphia, Pennsylvania
Chapter 14 *Data Analysis and Use*

Gail Graham, RHIA
Director, Health Data and Informations
VHA Office of Information
Department of Veterans Affairs
Washington, District of Columbia
Chapter 6 *Classification Systems, Clinical Vocabularies, and
Terminology*

Michael D. Gray, MIE
President, Starfish Healthcare Consulting, Inc.
Auburn, Alabama
Chapter 19 *Viewpoints*

Stanley P. Greenberg, BA, RHIT
President, Greenberg & Associates, Inc.
Skokie, Illinois
Chapter 7 *Data Access and Retention*

Darice Grzybowski, MA, RHIA, FAHIMA
President, HIMentors, LLC
LaGrange Park, Illinois
Chapter 7 *Data Access and Retention*

Mary Alice Hanken, PhD, CHP, RHIA
Independent Consultant; Senior Lecturer
Health Information Administration Program
School of Public Health and Community Medicine
University of Washington
Seattle, Washington
Chapters 9, 10, and 19 *Information Systems Life Cycle and Project
Management; Managing Electronic Health Record Systems:
Collaboration and Implementation; Viewpoints*

Anita Hazelwood, MLS, RHIA, FAHIMA
Professor, Health Information Management
University of Louisiana at Lafayette
Lafayette, Louisiana
Chapter 17 *Operational Management*

Susan Helbig, MA, RHIA
Director and Privacy Officer, Health Information Management
VA Puget Sound Health Care System
Seattle, Washington
Lecturer, Health Information Administration
School of Public Health and Community Medicine
University of Washington
Seattle, Washington
Chapter 5 *Electronic Health Record Systems*

—

Bryant Karras, MD
Assistant Professor, Health Services
School of Public Health and Community Medicine
Biomedical and Health Informatics School of Medicine
Co-director, Clinical Informatics Research Group
Founding Faculty, Center for Public Health Informatics
University of Washington
Seattle, Washington
Chapter 19 *Viewpoints*

Linda L. Kloss, MA, RHIA, FAHIMA
Executive Vice President/Chief Executive Officer, American Health
Information Management Association
Chicago, Illinois
Chapter 19 *Viewpoints*

Gretchen F. Murphy, MEd, RHIA, FAHIMA
Director, Health Information Administration
School of Public Health & Community Medicine
University of Washington
Seattle, Washington
Chapters 5, 9, and 10 *Electronic Health Record Systems; Information
Systems Life Cycle and Project Management; Managing Electronic
Health Record Systems: Collaboration and Implementation*

Bryon D. Pickard, MBA, RHIA
Director of Operations, Vanderbilt Medical Group Business Office
Vanderbilt University Medical Center
Nashville, Tennessee
Chapter 18 *Revenue Cycle and Financial Management*

Midge Noel Ray, MSN, RN, CCS
Associate Professor, Department of Health Services Administration
School of Health Professions
University of Alabama at Birmingham
Birmingham, Alabama
Chapter 1 *Health Care Systems*

Wesley M. Rohrer III, PhD, MBA
Assistant Chair, Health Management Education
Associate Director, MHA and MPH Programs
Assistant Professor, Health Policy and Management
Graduate School of Public Health
University of Pittsburgh
President, Parent Board of Directors
UCP of Pittsburgh, Inc.
Pittsburgh, Pennsylvania
Chapter 16 *Human Resource Management*

Elaine Rubinstein, PhD
Adjunct Professor, Department of Health Information Management
Research Specialist, Office of Measurement and Evaluation of Teaching
University of Pittsburgh
Pittsburgh, Pennsylvania
Chapter 11 *Statistics*

Melissa Saul, MS
Director, Clinical Research Informatics Service
Schools of the Health Sciences
University of Pittsburgh
Adjunct Associate Professor, Health Information Management
Department of Medicine
University of Pittsburgh
Pittsburgh, Pennsylvania
Chapter 8 *Technology, Applications, and Security*

Donna J. Slovensky, PhD, RHIA, FAHIMA
Professor and Director, BS in Health Sciences Program
Health Services Administration
School of Health Professions
University of Alabama at Birmingham
Birmingham, Alabama
Chapter 13 *Performance Management and Patient Safety*

Patrice Spath, BA, RHIT
Assistant Professor, Health Services Administration
University of Alabama at Birmingham
Birmingham, Alabama
Health Care Quality Specialist, Brown-Spath & Associates
Forest Grove, Oregon
Chapter 13 *Performance Management and Patient Safety*

Kathleen Strouse, MS, CPHIMS
President, Cooper Thomas, LLC
Washington, District of Columbia
Chapter 6 *Classification Systems, Clinical Vocabularies, and
Terminology*

Mary Spivey Teslow, MLIS, RHIA
Assistant Professor, Department of Health Sciences
Health Information Administration
Western Carolina University
Cullowhee, North Carolina
Chapter 4 *Health Data Concepts*

Carol A. Venable, MPH, RHIA, FAHIMA
Professor and Department Head, Health Information Management
The University of Louisiana at Lafayette
Lafayette, Louisiana
Chapter 17 *Operational Management*

Valerie J.M. Watzlaf, PhD, RHIA, FAHIMA
Associate Professor, Department of Health Information Management
School of Health and Rehabilitation Sciences
University of Pittsburgh
Pittsburgh, Pennsylvania
Chapters 11 and 12 *Statistics; Research and Epidemiology*

Jeffrey J. Williamson
Vice President of Education, American Medical Informatics
Association
Bethesda, Maryland
Chapter 19 *Viewpoints*

Foreword

Health information management (HIM) professionals are facing an unprecedented opportunity to help shape the future, not only of health information management, but also of health care delivery. As with any profession, and certainly true for the practice of medicine, managing information effectively is essential to producing high-quality results. The amount of information generated about patients and the volumes of literature published each year are daunting. Yet, only by having the most up-to-date patient information, knowledge, and information management tools can health care professionals make the right decision at the right time. As the country adopts electronic health record systems more broadly, HIM professionals should be equal participants on that journey.

The third edition of this book contains foundational knowledge necessary to fully participate in the transformation of health care delivery through effective management of health information and proactive clinical decision support. Mastering the concepts in this book will equip HIM professionals to lead the transition from paper to electronic records. HIM professionals have an in-depth knowledge of coding and classification systems and their proper use to characterize clinical content in the medical record. Accurate coding of clinical content drives computerized clinical decision support for providers and supports patient safety and quality improvement. In short, without proper structuring of health information, medical records will simply not keep pace with the information demands of health care. Standardized coding systems need to keep up with changes in medical knowledge. HIM professionals must champion these changes and ensure that policy makers adopt contemporary coding systems in a timely manner. Despite the importance of codes, however, there will always

be a place for text, which must be properly managed for efficient entry and retrieval.

The next profound transformation in health care delivery involves engaging patients as active participants on their health care team. This implies more than just providers speaking of "patient-centered care"; it *is* the *patient's* care. To fully participate in their own care, patients must have access to their health data, relevant knowledge, and tools to maintain or change their health behaviors. Personal health records (PHRs) will provide patients with this access. HIM professionals will have a central role in protecting patient privacy and ensuring the accuracy of data in the PHR. Many, if not most, of the HIM principles that apply to maintaining a medical record apply to the PHR, especially if the data are to be used in medical decision making. HIM professionals have always been patient advocates on matters concerning health information in the patients' medical records; increasing the use of PHRs broadens the scope of information under the professional's purview.

This is an exciting time to be an HIM professional. It is a time when leaders in the field can help define how information is organized, managed, used, shared, and acted on—by all members of the health care team, including the patient. Dealing with the transformational aspects of electronic health information will require more than updates to existing policies and processes; it will require new thinking and new approaches to managing that information. The material in this textbook provides an excellent foundation. Mastering its content will help us create a new health care system.

Paul C. Tang, MD, MS

Preface

INTENDED AUDIENCE

Health Information: Management of a Strategic Resource and a set of integrated tools, the ancillaries, in its third edition, are developed for health information management (HIM) students and practitioners who are interested in today's reliable systems and tomorrow's future direction to guide and influence practice, education, and research. The purpose of this book is to develop and support health information professionals who believe that their profession is crucial to the success and efficacy of the health care system. *Health Information: Management of a Strategic Resource* helps practitioners and students alike to realize the broader perspective of the scope and domains of HIM practice and to understand the expanded boundaries and roles that exist today and the opportunities that lie within our reach to influence professional advancement and tomorrow's practice. It is also hoped that this book will aid HIM professionals in viewing their profession with confidence, pride, and excitement.

Health Information: Management of a Strategic Resource will also serve as a valuable tool to others who are changing the health care system from a paper to an electronic environment. Finally, the book may realize its greatest value in expanding the expectations and understanding of health professionals—administrators, information systems professionals, researchers, policy developers, and others—about the role(s) of HIM professionals and the contributions they make to the quality of health care.

In today's fast-changing health care system, HIM professionals must lead the efforts in changing to an electronic health record and thus must adapt faster; expand their scope and domains of practice; use data, information, and technology in a new way; and assess their performance. HIM professionals must update their knowledge constantly and approach their expanded roles and functions with a new mind-set. This book presents a fresh insight and a new approach in addressing the fundamentals and important issues within the field of HIM. Today's most reliable and workable systems are presented by an impressive list of contributors. Viewpoints toward tomorrow's challenges should stimulate discussion and future action.

CONCEPTUAL FRAMEWORK AND ORGANIZATION

The editors designed the book based on a conceptual framework with an agreed-on set of assumptions instead of presenting a series of chapters with isolated information on tasks, tools, and functions. The following are the underlying assumptions on which chapter outlines were developed and contributors were selected:

1. Health information is indeed a strategic resource crucial to the health of individual patients and the population, as well as to the success of the health care institution or enterprise.
2. Health care must be patient centered.
3. Health care consumers are becoming more engaged and responsible for their own health. The development and use of a personal health record (PHR) will continue to be encouraged and supported.
4. Changing from a paper to an electronic health record is a given.
5. Health information professionals are leaders in the transformation to electronic health records, aiding in the design, management, and use of health care data and health information systems.
6. Health care data are to be viewed as a continuum beginning with patient-specific data (clinical data), moving to aggregate data (such as performance data, utilization review, and risk management data), to knowledge-based data (used in planning and decision support), and then to comparative, community-wide data (used in policy development) external to the enterprise or institution.
7. The quality of data and the data-to-information transformation are paramount to the efficacy of any information system; thus emphasis is on the use of information that has value in decision making, evaluation, planning, marketing, and policy development.
8. The integration and assimilation of technology in the health information manager's daily functions will be a reality in the next generation of practice, if not a reality already.
9. The transition to the electronic health record is an excellent opportunity, and its success depends on the

scope and domain of practice of health information management professionals.

10. The quality of health care depends on a functioning information infrastructure with quality health care data.

Health Information: Management of a Strategic Resource is organized into five major sections and is composed of 19 chapters by more then 30 contributors. Each chapter includes a chapter outline, key words, and defined abbreviations. An exclusive Web site for our readers, as well as other relevant Web sites, is included to guide readers to additional information. The glossary provides a comprehensive listing of all the key words.

Section One: Foundations of Health Information Management begins with an overview of health care systems. Chapter 1 (Health Care Systems) includes topics on e-health, evidence-based medicine, and consumer centric health care, and it is followed by Chapter 2 (The Health Informatics and Information Management Profession), which is a review of the HIM professions with a focus on HIM and its development, structure, goals, and roles from the mid-1800s to today.

Section Two: Health Care Data and Information Systems begins with Chapter 3 (Health Information Infrastructure and Systems), which discusses the private and public initiatives toward the development of a Nationwide Health Information Network (NHIN) and Regional Health Information Organizations (RHIOs). Chapter 4 (Health Data Concepts) presents a variety of data elements required or collected and maintained in the health care industry. The chapter also addresses the users of data systems and the role of HIM professionals in data collection. Chapter 5 (Electronic Health Record Systems) addresses the fundamentals of an electronic health record (EHR) and the transition process from a paper medical record to the electronic health record. The definition of a legal medical record is also presented. Chapter 6 (Classification Systems, Clinical Vocabularies, and Terminology) addresses clinical terminologies, vocabularies, and data standards. Chapter 7 (Data Access and Retention) compares and contrasts systems for numbering, storing, and retrieving while applying today's newest technologies to access and storage problems.

Section Three: Health Care Informatics begins with Chapter 8 (Technology, Applications, and Security), which covers various information technologies and their use in health care environments. Data quality and security and the role of HIM in these areas are a focus of this chapter. Chapter 9 (Information Systems Life Cycle and Project Management) addresses the analysis, design, implementation, and evaluation of health information systems with discussion of the tools and aids used in these phases. Chapter 10 (Managing Electronic Health Record Systems: Collaboration and Implementation) addresses how best to bring the user perspective to working with information systems technology staff to achieve an EHR system.

Section Four: Data Management and Use emphasizes the data-to-information transformation and focuses on the use of quality information to improve the decision-making abilities of the enterprise and the quality of health care. Chapter 11 (Statistics) provides the foundation for understanding statistics and its use and for organizing and displaying results. Chapter 12 (Research and Epidemiology) helps the reader in designing research studies and understanding epidemiology with applications specific to health information management. Chapter 13 (Performance Management and Patient Safety) describes the various methods for assessing and improving the quality of care and services rendered in today's health care systems, while emphasizing the crucial role of health information management professionals in that area. Chapter 14 (Data Analysis and Use) provides a pragmatic view of how data are used in health care, from registries to reimbursement to clinical outcomes. Chapter 15 (Privacy and Health Law) addresses the legal issues pertinent to the practice of health information management and today's health care system.

Section Five: Management begins with Chapter 16 (Human Resource Management), which explores the societal, legislative, organizational, functional, and personal objectives and activities of human resource management. Performance evaluation, employment law, multicultural workforce, and career planning are some of the topics addressed. Chapter 17 (Operational Management) addresses standards and methods of improvement, with systems analysis, ergonomics, and design process. Reengineering and project management methods and activities are also addressed. Chapter 18 (Revenue Cycle and Financial Management) addresses financial planning and financial accounting methods, while emphasizing the role of the HIM professional in revenue management. Chapter 19 (Viewpoints) presents the views of various leaders within the health care industry about today's and tomorrow's issues and challenges in health care.

SUPPLEMENTAL AND INSTRUCTIONAL RESOURCES

- *Evolve Resources:* The companion Evolve Web site provides Internet-based course management tools that instructors can use to reinforce and expand on the concepts they deliver in class. Instructors can use the Evolve site to publish their class syllabus, outline, and lecture notes; to set up "virtual office hours" and e-mail communication; to share important dates and information through the online class calendar; and to encourage student participation through chat rooms and discussion boards. For students, there are links to Web sites with related material and an additional question bank to accompany the study guide.
- *The Study Guide:* This contains integrated tools available to students, educators, and practitioners, including pretest

and chapter review questions and assignments, such as case studies, group exercises, field experience activities, and thought questions.

- *The Instructor's Resource Manual and CD:* This includes answers to the study guide assignments, educational hints, and lists of instructor resources; a PowerPoint "image library" of figures and tables from the textbook; and a test bank with more than 1000 questions and answers in electronic form to assist in test construction, scoring, and the generation of grades and test statistics.

We would like to thank the contributors for their willingness to take part in this endeavor and share their expertise. Their insights, suggestions, and questions have greatly strengthened the book and ancillaries, bringing our vision to life.

We shall be grateful to readers who have suggestions for additions or revisions or who are interested in sharing their experiences in using the book and its ancillaries with us. We hope that *Health Information: Management of a Strategic Resource,* third edition, and its ancillaries will be a valuable resource as we move into the twenty-first century and address the challenges that touch all of us.

Mervat Abdelhak, Managing Editor
Sara Grostick
Mary Alice Hanken
Ellen Jacobs

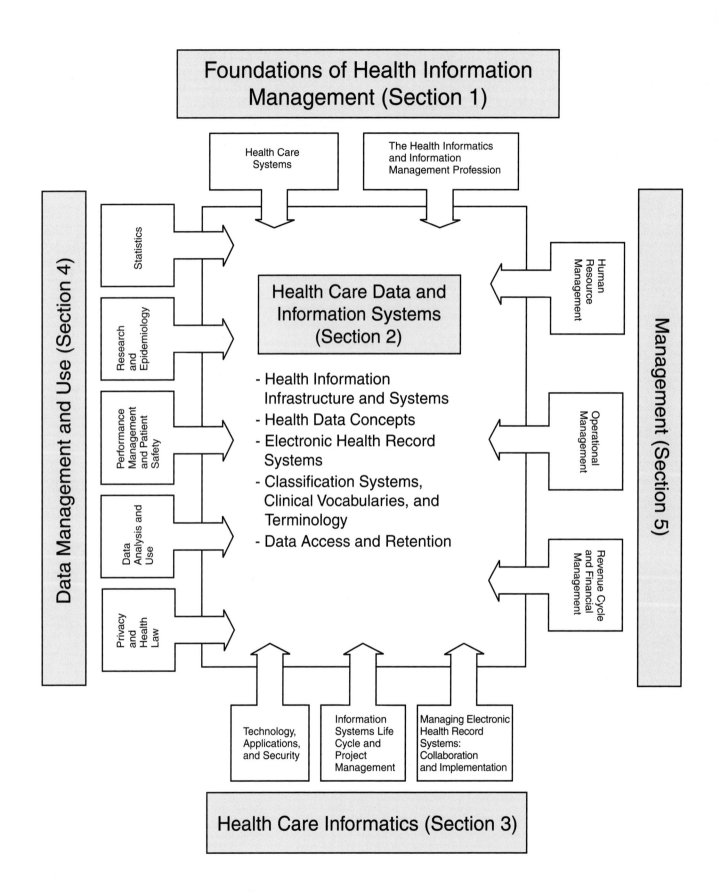

Foundations of Health Information Management (Section 1)

Health Care Systems

The Health Informatics and Information Management Profession

Data Management and Use (Section 4)

Statistics

Research and Epidemiology

Performance Management and Patient Safety

Data Analysis and Use

Privacy and Health Law

Health Care Data and Information Systems (Section 2)

- Health Information Infrastructure and Systems
- Health Data Concepts
- Electronic Health Record Systems
- Classification Systems, Clinical Vocabularies, and Terminology
- Data Access and Retention

Human Resource Management

Operational Management

Revenue Cycle and Financial Management

Management (Section 5)

Technology, Applications, and Security

Information Systems Life Cycle and Project Management

Managing Electronic Health Record Systems: Collaboration and Implementation

Health Care Informatics (Section 3)

Contents

section **1**

**FOUNDATIONS OF HEALTH
INFORMATION MANAGEMENT** 1

chapter 1
HEALTH CARE SYSTEMS 2

Evolution of Health Care Systems in the United States 5

Health Care in the Nineteenth Century 5
Twentieth-Century Reforms 6
Health Care in the Twenty-First Century 8
Healthy People 2010 9

Regulatory Agencies and Organizations 9
Federal Government as Regulator 9
The Role of States 12
State Health Departments 12
Legislation 13
Accreditation 14
Regulatory Mechanisms of Health Occupations 15

Health Care Delivery Systems 16
Continuum of Care 16
Ambulatory Care 17
Hospitals 18
Subacute Care 27
Home Care (Home Health Care) 27
Long-Term Care Facilities 28
Hospice Care 28
Respite Care 29
Complementary and Alternative Medicine 29
E-Health 29
Adult Day Care Services 29
Mobile Diagnostic Services 29
Contract Services 29
Integrated Delivery Systems 30

Health Care Professionals 30
Health Care Team 30

Financing Health Care 34
Reimbursement 34
Managed Care 35
Utilization Management 36
Government's Role as Payer 36

Technology in Health Information 38
Point-of-Care Clinical Information Systems 38
Electronic Data Exchange 38

Decision Support Systems 39
Electronic Health Record 39
National Health Information Infrastructure 39
Institute of Medicine 39
Future Issues 39

chapter 2
**THE HEALTH INFORMATICS AND
INFORMATION MANAGEMENT
PROFESSION** 42

**Health Information Management—A Profession in
Transformation** 44
**The Patient Record—Source of Health Data and
Information** 44
Evolution of the Patient Record 45
Early History 45
Influential Forces 46
Evolution of the Health Information Management Profession 49
Early History 49
1990s Forward 49
Formation of Education Programs 51
Professional Certification 52
Maintenance of Certification and Lifelong Learning 54
Fellowship Program 55
**American Health Information Management
Association Today** 56
*American Health Information Management
Association Communications* 57
**Foundation of Research and Education in
Health Information Management** 58
The Professional Code of Ethics 58
Looking to the Future 59

section **2**

**HEALTH CARE DATA AND
INFORMATION SYSTEMS** 63

chapter 3
**HEALTH INFORMATION
INFRASTRUCTURE AND SYSTEMS** 64

Health Information Technology in Health Care 66
Background 66
Federal Involvement in Health Information Technology 67
Congress 73

Role of the Private Sector 73

Compelling Reasons to Implement Health
Information Technology 73

Obstacles to Health Information Technology
Adoption 79

Emerging Health Information Networks 81

Organization and Governance Issues 84

Technical Issues 84

Financial Issues 87

Privacy, Security and Confidentiality Issues 87

Role of Health Information Management 88

chapter 4

HEALTH DATA CONCEPTS 92

Health Data Users and Decision Making 95

Users and Uses of Health Data 95

Decision Making 96

Overview of the Patient Record 97

The Unique Roles of the Patient Health Record 97

Definitions 97

Data Collection Standards 98

Governmental 98

Overview of Information and Data Sets 99

Core Health Data Elements 100

Nongovernmental 100

Basic Principles of Data Collection 102

User Needs 102

Documentation Responsibilities 102

General Documentation Forms and Views 102

Documentation Guidelines 113

Format Types 114

Design and Control of Paper Forms and Computer
Views and Templates 115

Forms or Views Team 115

General Design Principles 116

Other Display Features 121

General Control Principles 121

Forms/Views Summary 122

Health Record Flow and Processing 122

Medical Transcription 122

Methods to Ensure Data Quality 122

Record Content Review and Retrospective Completion 124

Data Quality Monitoring Methods and Solutions 126

Quality Assessment and Improvement Study
of Patient Record Documentation 126

Special Concerns of Alternative Care Settings 127

Clinical Staff Activities Related to Data Quality 128

Facility Structure That Encourages Data Quality 128

Data Needs Across the Health Care Continuum 129

Minimum Data Sets 129

Acute Care 129

Rehabilitation 137

Home Health Care 137

Hospice 141

Behavioral Health 142

Electronic Health Record Initiatives 143

Characteristics of Data Quality 143

ASTM Standards Development 145

ASTM E1384 Content Guide for the
Electronic Health Record 146

ASTM E1384 Major Segments 146

Summary and Management Issues 149

chapter 5

ELECTRONIC HEALTH RECORD
SYSTEMS 152

Electronic Health Records: The Case for
Quality and Change 154

The Patient Record 154

What Are Electronic Health Records and
Electronic Health Record Systems and What Are
Their Functions? 155

Electronic Health Records 155

Electronic Health Record Systems and Their Functions 156

Standards Development and the Electronic Health
Record 156

Legal Health Record 157

Designated Record Set 162

Electronic Health Record System Functions and
Patient Record Development 163

Why Do Current Industry Forces Advance the Case for
Electronic Health Record Systems
Successfully Today? 165

Industry Forces That Advance Electronic
Health Record Adoption 165

Patient Safety and Data 165

National Focus on Improving Health
Information and Technology 166

Paper Record Drawbacks 167

Cost Containment and Return on Investment 168

How Do Technical Infrastructure, Data Requirements,
and Operations Workflow Fit in Electronic
Health Record Systems? 168

Technical Infrastructure and Data Requirements 168

Data Requirements for the Electronic Health Record 168

Clinical Data Repositories 169

Vocabularies and the Electronic Health Record 170

How Do Issues and Barriers Affect Electronic
Health Record Planning and Implementation? 171

Selected Issues and Barriers 171

Cost Issues 171

Infrastructure Requirements 171

Laws and Progress 172

Confidentiality and Security 172

Health Care Information Standards and Interoperability 172

When Are Electronic Health Record Systems Part
of Migration Paths in Health Care
Organizations? 173

Organizational Migration Benchmarks 173

Who Offers Relevant Benchmark Data About
the Electronic Health Record Experience? 176

How Do Health Information Management
Business Processes Change in the Electronic
Health Record Environment? 177

What Management Questions/Topics Need to Be Discussed
  as We Move to the Virtual Health Information
  Department?   177
Introduction   177
Documentation Principles   177
The Physical Past   178
The Emerging Present   179
The Future Now   185
How Are Organizational Policies and Business Rules
  Changing to Guide Electronic Health Record
  Users and Systems?   186
Virtual Health Information Management
  Department   190
Challenge to Health Information Professionals   190
Summary   195

chapter 6
CLASSIFICATION SYSTEMS, CLINICAL VOCABULARIES, AND TERMINOLOGY   198

Terms About Terms   200
Administrative Terminologies   201
International Classification of Diseases   201
Derivations of the International Classification of Diseases   202
Current Procedural Terminology   203
Healthcare Common Procedure Coding System   203
Diagnosis Related Groups   203
Adaptation of Administrative Terminologies   203
Clinical Terminologies   204
Systematized Nomenclature of Medicine   204
Logical Observation Identifiers Names and Codes   205
Drug Terminologies   207
Nursing Terminologies   207
The Role of the Unified Medical Language System   208
Terminology Characteristics   208
Health Data Standards   211
Consolidated Health Informatics   212
National Committee on Vital and Health Statistics   213
Interoperability: The Lingua Franca of the
  Electronic Health Record World   213
Development and Selection of Health Data
  Standards   214
Electronic Health Record Functional Model   215
A National Network for Health Information
  Exchange   215
Benefits of a National Network   216

chapter 7
DATA ACCESS AND RETENTION   218

Access and Retention of Paper-Based Records   220
Record Identification   220
Filing Equipment   221
Space Management   223
Filing Methods   223
Master Patient Index   226
Records Management Issues   234
Record Tracking   237

Record Retention   240
The Legal Health Record Definition   242
Disaster Recovery   242
Computer Technology in Automated Data
  Access and Retention   243
Hardware   243
Input, Output, and Storage Devices   243
Terminals and Workstations   244
Pen-Based Devices   244
Radiofrequency Identification   245
Document Imaging Devices   245
Voice Recognition   245
Computer-Assisted Coding Tools   245
Communications   246
Client Server Technology   246
Access and Retention of Image-Based Records   247
Micrographics   247
Electronic Document Management   255

section 3
HEALTH CARE INFORMATICS   267

chapter 8
TECHNOLOGY, APPLICATIONS, AND SECURITY   268

Health Information Infrastructure, Technology,
  and Applications   270
Scope of Health Information Systems   271
Computers in Health Care—Past and Present   271
Computer Fundamentals   273
Software   275
Designing the User Interface   280
User Interface Team   281
General Design Principles   282
Computer Applications   283
Administrative Applications   283
Clinical Applications   284
Emerging Technologies   287
Bar Coding   287
Radiofrequency Identification Device   288
Internet and Web Services   288
Telemedicine   292
Fundamentals   292
Implementation   292
Computer Security   293
Authentication Tools   294
Reporting Capabilities   296
Physical Security   296
External Controls   296
Data Management Technology   299
Data Mart   299
Data Modeling   301

c h a p t e r   9

INFORMATION SYSTEMS LIFE CYCLE
AND PROJECT MANAGEMENT ... 304

Introduction ... 306
   System Analysis, Design, and Implementation ... 306
The Players ... 307
   *Role of the Health Information Management
     Professional* ... 308
Project Management ... 308
System Life Cycles ... 310
   General System Life Cycle ... 310
   Information System Life Cycles ... 310
   Information System Life Cycles in the Organization ... 311
   *Aggregate Information Life Cycle of the
     Organization* ... 312
   System Obsolescence ... 312
Information System Development Life Cycle ... 313
   Principles for System Development ... 313
   Problem Analysis Basics ... 313
Analysis ... 314
   Tools and Aids for System Analysis ... 314
   *Investigative Strategies for Analysis of
     Requirements* ... 324
   Analysis Document ... 330
   System Design ... 331
   Design Principles ... 332
Role of Prototyping in System Development ... 334
System Implementation ... 335
   User Preparation and Training ... 335
   Site Preparation ... 336
   System Testing and Conversion ... 336
   Startup ... 337
System Evaluation and Benefits Realization ... 337
   Benefits Realization ... 338
   Cost-Benefit Analysis ... 339
   Cost-Effectiveness Analysis ... 341
   Other Evaluation Methods and Techniques ... 342
Purchasing Process: Request for Proposal ... 343
   Request for Information ... 343
   Planning Steps Before Request for Proposal Preparation ... 344
   Analyzing System Requirements ... 344
   Development of System Specifications ... 344
   Development and Distribution of the Request for Proposal ... 344
   Evaluation Criteria ... 349
   Demonstrations and Site Visits ... 351
   System Selection and Contract Negotiation ... 352

c h a p t e r   1 0

MANAGING ELECTRONIC HEALTH RECORD
SYSTEMS: COLLABORATION AND
IMPLEMENTATION ... 354

Value of User Perspective ... 356
   A Natural Dependence ... 356
Environmental Basics (Required for True Collaboration) ... 356
   Four Shared Environmental Basics ... 357
   Four Unshared Environmental Basics ... 359

The Tide Turns ... 362
Process Modeling ... 362
Database Design ... 363
Implementation Readiness ... 363
   User Processes and Procedures ... 363
   Plan Transition ... 364
   Training ... 364
   Prepare User Manual(s) ... 365
   Data Migration ... 365
   System Testing ... 365
   "Go Live" ... 365
System and Project Evaluation ... 366

s e c t i o n 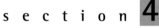 4

DATA MANAGEMENT AND USE ... 369

c h a p t e r   1 1

STATISTICS ... 370

Overview of Statistics and Data Presentation ... 372
   Role of the Health Information Management Professional ... 372
Health Care Statistics ... 372
   Vital Statistics ... 372
   Rates, Ratios, Proportions, and Percentages ... 373
   Mortality Rates ... 373
   Autopsy Rates ... 378
   Morbidity Rates ... 379
   Census Statistics ... 382
Organizing and Displaying the Data ... 384
   Types of Data ... 384
   Types of Data Display ... 385
Statistical Measures and Tests ... 388
   Descriptive Statistics ... 388
   Inferential Statistics ... 392

c h a p t e r   1 2

RESEARCH AND EPIDEMIOLOGY ... 402

Overview of Research and Epidemiology ... 404
Role of the Health Information Management Professional ... 404
Designing the Research Proposal ... 406
   Hypothesis and Research Questions ... 406
   Review of Literature ... 406
   Methodology (Draft) ... 408
   Research Plan ... 408
Validity and Reliability ... 411
   Validity ... 411
   Sensitivity and Specificity ... 412
   Reliability ... 412
Biases ... 414
   Confounding Variables ... 414
   Sampling Variability ... 414
   Ascertainment or Selection Bias ... 414
   Diagnosis Bias ... 414
   Nonresponse Bias ... 414

Survival Bias   414
Recall Bias   414
Interviewer Bias   414
Prevarication Bias   415
Epidemiologic/Research Study Designs   415
Descriptive Study   415
Analytic Study Design   421
Experimental Epidemiology   426
Use of Computer Software in Research   429
Outcome Studies and Epidemiology   430
Study Procedures   431
Data Analysis   431

chapter 13
PERFORMANCE MANAGEMENT
AND PATIENT SAFETY   436
The Big Picture and Key Players   438
Federal Oversight Agencies   438
Accrediting Bodies   439
National Quality Awards   439
Purchasers   439
Consumers   440
National Health Care Quality Measurement Priorities   440
Performance Measurement   441
Structure, Process, and Outcome Measures   441
Structure Measures   442
Process Measures   442
Outcome Measures   442
Developing Performance Measures   443
Collecting Measurement Data   444
Performance Assessment   444
Reports for Analysis   445
Performance Goals and Targets   446
Use of Comparative Data   446
Performance Improvement   447
Performance Improvement Models   447
Process Improvement Tools   450
Patient Safety   454
Safety Measurement   455
Patient Safety Databases   456
Safety Improvement   458
Root Cause Analysis   459
Proactive Risk Assessment   459
Risk Management   460
Loss Prevention and Reduction   461
Claims Management   461
Utilization Management   462
External Requirements   462
Program Components   463
Plan and Program Structure   465
Credentialing   466
External Requirements   467
Credentialing Program Components   467
Role of Managers   468

chapter 14
DATA ANALYSIS AND USE   472
Data Uses   474
Registries Overview   474
Case Definition and Eligibility   474
Case Finding   474
Abstracting   475
Registry Quality Control   475
Confidentiality of Registry Information   475
Cancer Registries   475
Hospital Cancer Registries   476
Population-Based Cancer Registries   476
Cancer Registry Abstracting   477
Cancer Registry Coding   477
Cancer Registry Staging   477
Quality Management of the Cancer Program
    and Registry Data   478
Use of Cancer Registry Data   479
The Cancer Registrar Profession   479
Birth Defects Registries   479
Birth Defects Case Definition and Coding   481
Quality Control of Birth Defects Registry Data   481
Use of Birth Defects Registry Data   481
Death Registries   481
Diabetes Registries   482
Diabetes Registry Case Finding   482
Implant Registries   482
Immunization Registries   483
Immunization Registry Case Finding and Data Use   483
Organ Transplant Registries   483
Transplant Case Registration and Data Use   484
Trauma Registries   484
Trauma Registry Case Finding and Data Use   484
Research and Use of Data   485
Health Services Research   485
Medical Research   485
Role of a Data Broker in Research   485
Public Health   486
Planning and Assessment   486
Data and Health   486
Performance Management   486
Outcomes   487
Outcomes Data and Information Systems   488
Outcomes Data Use   488
Outcomes and the Electronic Health Record   488
Outcome Indicators   489
Outcomes and Coding Issues   490
Desirable Outcome Systems   491
Clinical Decision Support   494
Data Dictionary   495
Data Dictionary Definitions   495
Purpose of the Data Dictionary   496
Scope of the Data Dictionary   496
Meta-Content of the Data Dictionary   496
Building the Data Dictionary   497

Criteria for Data Element Inclusion 497
Cataloging Standards 497

c h a p t e r   1 5
PRIVACY AND HEALTH LAW 502

Why Are Legal Issues Important to Health Information
   Management Professionals? 504
Fundamentals of the Legal System 504
Sources of Law 504
The Legal System 506
The Court System 506
Cases That Involve Health Care Facilities and Providers 507
Legal Obligations and Risks of Health Care Facilities
   and Individual Health Care Providers 511
Duties to Patients, in General 511
Duty to Maintain Health Information 511
Duty to Retain Health Information and Other
   Key Documents and to Keep Them Secure 512
Duty to Maintain Confidentiality 515
Internal Uses and External Disclosures of
   Health Information 517
General Principles Regarding Access and
   Disclosure Policies 517
Duty to Provide Care That Meets Professional Standards 529
Duty to Obtain Informed Consent to Treatment 531
Duty to Provide a Safe Environment for Patients
   and Visitors 532
Duty to Supervise the Actions of Employees
   and the Professional Staff 533
Contract Liability Issues and the Health Information
   Management Department 536
Legal Resources for Health Information
   Management Professionals 537

s e c t i o n   **5**
MANAGEMENT 541

c h a p t e r   1 6
HUMAN RESOURCE MANAGEMENT 542

Human Resource Management 544
Navigating Through Turbulent Times 544
Broad Environmental Forces 544
Forces Transforming Health Care 545
Challenges for Health Information Management
   Professionals 545
Systems Perspective on Human Resource Management 552
Systems Approach Applied to Health Information Services 555
Systems Perspective Applied to Human
   Resource Management 556
Environmental Influences and Human
   Resource Management 557
Legal and Regulatory Requirements Affecting
   Human Resource Management 561
Internal Environment of the Health Care Organization 569
Future Issues 601

c h a p t e r   1 7
OPERATIONAL MANAGEMENT 604

Introduction 606
Individual Work Processes (Micro Level) 606
Organizing Work 606
Work Distribution Chart 606
Productivity 611
Work Simplification or Methods Improvement 614
Systems and Organizational Level (Midlevel) 623
Systems Analysis and Design 623
Organizational Structure 626
Organization-Wide Level 627
Change Management 627
Strategic Management 627
Situational Analysis 627
Strategy Formulation 628
Strategic Implementation 629
Strategic Control 629
Project Management 629
Information Technology Applications 634
Re-Enginnering 636
Design and Management of Space in Health
   Information Services 637
Work Space Design 637
Design of the Workstation 641

c h a p t e r   1 8
REVENUE CYCLE AND
FINANCIAL MANAGEMENT 648

Historical Perspective 650
Payment for Health Care Services 650
Managing the Revenue Cycle 652
Front-end Activities 653
Back-end Activities 656
Financial Aspects of Fraud and Abuse Compliance 660
Setting Priorities for Financial Decisions 661
Management Accounting 661
Mission 662
Goals 662
Objectives 662
The Budget and Business Plan 662
Budgets 662
Who Participates in Budget Development? 663
Budget Periods and Types 663
Budgeting for Staff 664
Using the Budget as a Control 664
Preparing a Business Plan 664
Identifying Trends 665
Staffing Information 666
Program and Automation Assessments 666
The Four M's 666
Developing the Business Plan and Budget 667
Cost Allocations 668
Why Does Allocation Occur? 668
Allocation Methods 668

*Why Is Cost Allocation Methodology Important
for the HIM Professional?* 668

Financial Accounting 669
Fundamental Accounting Principles and Concepts 669
Financial Management Duties 671
Cash and Accrual Systems 671
Fiscal Periods 672

**Using Financial Reports to Provide Management
Information** 672

Using Ratios to Evaluate Financial Data 674
Liquidity Ratio 674
Turnover Ratio or Activity Ratio 674
Performance Ratio 675
Capitalization Ratio 675

Capital Expense and Investment Decisions 675
Capital Expenditures 675
Capital Request Evaluation Process 676
Time Value of Money 676
Compounding 676
Discounting 676
Net Present Value 678
Accounting Rate of Return 679
Payback Method 680
Arguments Pro and Con for Evaluation Methods 680

Other Phases of Financial Management 680
Implementing 680
Seeking Alternatives 680
Role of the HIM Professional in Financial Management 680

chapter 19
VIEWPOINTS 682

Transforming Health Information Management 684
The Case for a Wired Health Care System 684
A Compelling Vision 684
A Health Information Management Profession in Transition 685
Milestones for Change 685

**Health Professionals for Translational, Clinical,
and Public Health/Population Informatics** 686
Biomedical/Health Informatics 686
Workforce Needs 687
AMIA's 10 × 10 Program 687
Other Education Initiatives 687

Collaborating for Change 688

Technology and Change 688
Two Case Studies 688
Lessons Learned 689
Collaboration 689
Nursing 689
Health Information Management 690
Technology as Enabler 690

International Health Information Management 690
*International Federation of Health Records
Organizations* 690
The Electronic Health Record 690
Clinical Data Management 691
*Privacy, Security, and Confidentiality of
Personal Health Information* 691
Education 691
Needs of Developing Countries 691
The Joint Commission 692
International Opportunities 692

Public Health Information: A Strategic Resource 692
Public Health and Medical Care 692
Population-Based Data 692
Information Needs and Core Public Health Functions 693
Public Health Programs 694
Health Problems and Costs 695
Improving Health 695
Integrating the Information System 695
Legal Context 696
Cooperation 696

**A Vision of Digital Information Convergence:
"How Connected Do You Want to Be?"** 699
Closed-Loop Solutions (On-line and Real Time) 699
Telecommuting Oversight 699
Self-Care Management 700
Integration for Patient Safety 700
Digital Dashboards 700
Multidisciplinary Collaboration 701
Therapeutic Outcomes Monitoring 701
Digital Information Convergence 701
Priorities and Trends 702

Glossary 705

Index 733

section 1

Foundations of Health Information Management

chapter 1

Health Care Systems

Midge Noel Ray

 Additional content,
http://evolve.elsevier.com/Abdelhak/

 Review exercises can be found
in the Study Guide

Chapter Contents

Evolution of Health Care Systems in the United States
Health Care in the Nineteenth Century
Twentieth Century Reforms
Health Care in the Twenty-First Century
Healthy People 2010
Regulatory Agencies and Organizations
Federal Government as Regulator
    Department of Health and Human Services
    Social Security Administration
    Occupational Safety and Health Administration
The Role of States
State Health Departments
    Licensure of Health Care Facilities
Legislation
Accreditation
    The Joint Commission
    American Osteopathic Association
    Commission on Accreditation of Rehabilitation Facilities
    Community Health Accreditation Program
    National Committee for Quality Assurance
Regulatory Mechanisms of Health Occupations
    American Medical Association
    American Osteopathic Association Bureau of Professional
      Education
    Commission on Accreditation of Allied Health Education
      Programs
    Commission on Accreditation for Health Informatics and
      Information Management Education
    National League for Nursing Accrediting Commission, Inc.
    State Licensure of Practitioners
Health Care Delivery Systems
Continuum of Care
Ambulatory Care
    Physician Practices
    Community Health Centers

Key Words

Accreditation	Coinsurance	Evidence-based medicine
Acute care	Complementary and alternative	Ex officio
Advance directive	medicine	Fee-for-service
Alternative medicine	Conditions of participation	Fiscal intermediary
Ambulatory care	Continuum of care	Gatekeeper
Ancillary services	Contracted amount	Governing body
Assisted living	Copayment	Health
Bed size (bed count)	Critical access hospital	Health care services
Behavioral health	Deductible	Home health care
Beneficiaries	Deemed status	Horizontal integration
Benefit period	Direct pay	Hospice
Capitation	Durable medical equipment	Hospital
Case management	E-health	Hospital ambulatory care
Catchment area	Electronic health record	Hospital formulary
Certification	Electronic medical record	Hospital inpatient
Claim	Emergency department	Hospital patient
Client	Encounter	Indigent
Clinical privileges	Episode of care	Inpatient

Community-Based Care
   Surgicenters and Urgent Care Centers
   Hospital Ambulatory Care
Hospitals
   Ownership
   Bed Size (Bed Count)
   Length of Stay
   Clinical Classification
   Hospital Patients
   Organization
   Composition and Structure
   Leadership
   Medical Staff (Professional Staff Organization)
   Essential Services
   Health Information Management
Subacute Care
Home Care (Home Health Care)
Long-Term Care Facilities
Hospice Care
Respite Care
Complementary and Alternative Medicine
E-Health
Adult Day Care Services
Mobile Diagnostic Services
Contract Services
Integrated Delivery Systems

Health Care Professionals
Health Care Team
   Physicians
   Physician Assistant
   Nursing
   Nursing Care Models
   Allied Health Professionals

Financing Health Care
Reimbursement

Managed Care
   Health Maintenance Organizations
   Preferred Provider Organizations
   Case Management
   Point-of-Service Plan
Utilization Management
Government's Role as Payer
   Medicare
   Medicaid
   State Children's Health Insurance Program
   Tricare
   Workers' Compensation
Technology in Health Information
Point-of-Care Clinical Information Systems
Electronic Data Interchange
Decision Support Systems
Electronic Health Record
National Health Information Infrastructure
Institute of Medicine
Future Issues

Abbreviations

ACF—Administration for Children and Families
ACS—American Cancer Society/American College of Surgeons
AHA—American Hospital Association
AHIMA—American Health Information Management Association
AHRQ—Agency for Healthcare Research and Quality
AMA—American Medical Association
ANA—American Nurses Association
AOA—American Osteopathic Association

Continued

Insurance
Integrated delivery system
Licensure
Life care centers
Long-term care
Managed care
Medicaid
Medically indigent
Medicare
Morbidity
Mortality
Nursing facility
Observation patient
Osteopathic medicine
Out-of-pocket costs
Outpatient
Outsourcing
Palliative care
Participating physicians

Patient
Patient assessment
Patient centered care
Payer
Personal health record
Point of service
Practice act
Pre-existing condition
Preferred provider organization
Premium
Primary care
Proprietary
Prospective payment system
Provider
Rehabilitation
Reimbursement formula
Resident
Respite care
Retrospective payment system

Satellite clinic
Secondary care
Self-pay
Sliding scale fee
Solo practice
Swing beds
Telehealth
Tertiary care
The Joint Commission
Third party payer
Trauma center
Triage
Tricare
Usual, customary, and reasonable
   charges
Utilization review
Vertical integration

AoA—Administration on Aging

ASCP—American Society of Clinical Pathologists

BCBS—Blue Cross and Blue Shield

CAAHEP—Commission on Accreditation of Allied Health Education Programs

CAH—Critical Access Hospital

CAHIIM—Commission on Accreditation of Health Informatics and Information Management Education

CAM—Complementary and Alternative Medicine

CARF—Commission on Accreditation of Rehabilitation Facilities

CDC—Centers for Disease Control and Prevention

CDSS—Clinical Decision Support System

CEO—Chief Executive Officer

CFO—Chief Financial Officer

CHAMPUS—Civilian Health and Medical Program for the Uniformed Services

CHAP—Community Health Accreditation Program

CHC—Community Health Center

CIO—Chief Information Officer

CMS—Centers for Medicare and Medicaid Services

CNA—Certified Nursing Assistant

COBRA—Consolidated Omnibus Reconciliation Act

COO—Chief Operating Officer

COP—(Medicare) Conditions of Participation

CRNA—Certified Registered Nurse Anesthetist

DHHS—Department of Health and Human Services

DME—Durable Medical Equipment

DO—Doctor of Osteopathy

DRG—Diagnosis Related Group

DSS—Decision Support Systems

ED—Emergency Department

EHR—Electronic Health Record

EMR—Electronic Medical Record

EMTALA—Emergency Medical Treatment and Active Labor Act

ESRD—End Stage Renal Disease

FDA—Food and Drug Administration

FI—Fiscal Intermediary

FLEX—Federation Licensing Exam

GDP—Gross Domestic Product

HCFA—Health Care Financing Administration (now CMS)

HIPAA—Health Insurance Portability and Accountability Act

HCO—Health Care Organization

HIM—Health Information Management

HMO—Health Maintenance Organization

HRSA—Health Resources Services Administration

IDS—Integrated Delivery System

IPA—Independent Practice Association

IHS—Indian Health Service

IOM—Institute of Medicine

JCAHO—Joint Commission on Accreditation of Healthcare Organizations (now The Joint Commission)

LPN—Licensed Practical Nurse

LTC—Long-Term Care

MCAT—Medical College Admission Test

MCO—Managed Care Organization

MD—Medical Doctor

MMA—Medicare Modernization Act

NCCAM—National Center for Complimentary and Alternative Medicine

NCQA—National Committee For Quality Assurance

NHII—National Health Information Infrastructure

NHIN—National Health Information Network

NIH—National Institutes of Health

NLN—National League for Nursing

NLNAC—National League for Nursing Accrediting Commission, Inc.

NP—Nurse Practitioner

OIG—Office of Inspector General

OSHA—Occupational Safety and Health Administration

PA—Physician Assistant

PHR—Personal Health Record

PHS—Public Health Service

POS—Point of Service

PPO—Preferred Provider Organization

PPS—Prospective Payment System

QIO—Quality Improvement Organization

RN—Registered Nurse

SCHIP—State Children's Health Program

SSA—Social Security Administration

TEFRA—Tax Equity and Fiscal Responsibility Act

VA—Veterans Administration

Objectives

- Define key words.
- Describe the evolution of the United States health care system beginning with health care in the nineteenth century through *Healthy People 2010*.
- Identify and describe the regulators of health care, including government and nongovernment entities.
- Outline the role of the federal, state, and local governments in the provision of health care.
- Identify legislation that affects or regulates health care in the United States.
- Distinguish between the various health care organizations responsible for providing health care.
- Describe the classification of acute health care facilities, including bed size, ownership and control, population served, and services offered.
- Describe the organizational structures of the hospital as discussed within this chapter.
- Describe the role and responsibilities of the governing body and administrative heads employed in the health care organizations.
- Outline the organizational structure of the professional staff, including the membership, clinical privileges, services, committees, and bylaws.

- Identify and define the scope of the ancillary and support services and departments in health care facilities.
- Describe categories of the health workforce and address education, licensing and certification requirements, and areas of expertise.
- State current mechanisms of financing health care.
- Describe specific information technologies and how they affect the health care systems.

Health information management (HIM) is a vital component of the health care delivery system. Therefore it is crucial for health information professionals to understand the structure of that system. This chapter introduces the reader to the health care system, including what the system is like and how it functions and identifies its components. Topics include the history, influencing factors, payers, regulatory agencies, structure, operation, and workforce of health care systems in the United States.

EVOLUTION OF HEALTH CARE SYSTEMS IN THE UNITED STATES

From its inception hundreds of years ago to the present, the health care system has been continually evolving. In the United States, virtually every person is in some way a patient or a consumer of health care at some point. Most people are born either in a hospital or outside the hospital with the assistance of a health care professional. Other people come in contact with the health care system in a variety of ways, including physical examination, immunizations, employee physicals, school vision and hearing screens, emergency care, and public health service announcements.

Before proceeding, see Box 1-1 for key definitions.

Health Care in the Nineteenth Century

The nineteenth century saw the development and organization of professional education and health-related associations. The first school in the United States dedicated to training physicians was founded in 1765 in Philadelphia. Before this time, the only training an American physician received was by way of apprenticeship with an older physician. As the population in the United States grew and moved westward, the demand for more hospitals and physicians increased. To meet the growing need for more physicians, a large number of new medical schools were opened, most of which were profit oriented. By the end of the nineteenth century, there were no fewer than 400 medical schools in the United States, most of questionable quality.[2]

In 1847 a group of physicians formed the American Medical Association (AMA) for the primary purpose of establishing and supporting a code of ethics for physicians in

Box 1-1 KEY DEFINITIONS

Health—Health is best defined by the World Health Organization as a state of complete physical, mental, and social well-being and not merely the absence of disease or infirmity.[1]

Care—Care is the management of, responsibility for, or attention to the safety and well-being of another person or other persons.[3]

Health care services—Health care services are the processes that contribute to the health and well-being of the person. Services may be provided in a variety of health care settings, such as the hospital, ambulatory, or home setting, and include nursing, medical, surgical, or other health-related services.[3]

Patient—A patient is an individual, including one who is deceased, who is receiving or using or who has received health care services.[3]

Client—A person who receives professional services; a patient in the behavioral health setting, adult day care, or home health care may be referred to as a client.

Inpatient—Inpatient refers to a patient who is receiving health care services and is provided room, board, and continuous nursing service in a unit or area of the hospital.[3]

Outpatient—Outpatient is a patient who is receiving health care services at a hospital without being hospitalized, institutionalized, or admitted as an inpatient.

Resident—A patient who resides in a long-term care facility.

Payer—A payer is an organization or individual who provides the money to pay for health care services.

Provider—Any entity that provides health care services to patients, including health care organizations (hospitals, clinics) and health care professionals.

their duties to their patients and the profession. The AMA initially examined the poor quality of medical education and the questionable ethics of practicing physicians. Today, membership in the AMA is open to any physician in good standing and includes local, city, and state medical societies. The AMA is dedicated to promoting the science and art of medicine, improving public health, making health care policy, and servicing the professional needs of its members.[4]

The American Hospital Association (AHA) was founded in 1848 for the purpose of promoting public welfare by providing better health care in the hospitals. The AHA funds and conducts research and educational programs, maintains data on hospital profiles, and represents hospital interests in legal and legislative matters, all of which are directed at improving the nation's health care system.[5]

In the late nineteenth century, states became involved in health care when mental health reformers pushed for an innovation, that insanity be managed as a medical or mental disorder. State governments established mental institutions for the confinement of the mentally ill rather than housing them in the poorhouses and prisons. However, because of inadequate funding, mental institutions soon became overcrowded and living conditions were deplorable.

In the mid-1800s there is evidence of the earliest forms of managed care. Plantation owners in Hawaii; mining companies in Pennsylvania and Minnesota; and lumber companies in Washington, Wisconsin, and Michigan tried to attract and keep immigrant workers by offering medical care for their workers. The companies contracted with local physicians and hospitals for a set number of beds. Some of the companies even built medical clinics and hospitals. Physicians who agreed to contract with these companies were ostracized from the local medical societies and were even threatened with revocation of their medical licenses.[6]

Twentieth-Century Reforms

In the early 1900s, most hospitals were viewed as boardinghouses for the poor and sick; physicians did not take histories and perform physical examinations on admission, and seldom did they document assessments or diagnoses. The private sector, however, showed little interest in serving the population as a whole; the assumption was that local government would pay for health care for the poor.[7]

Between the 1870s and 1920s, the number of U.S. hospitals increased from fewer than 200 to more than 6000. Private benevolence was responsible for establishing hundreds of new hospitals that were not interested in serving the poor. By 1910, there were as many hospitals per 1000 population as there are today, and, as is still true today, part of the population was not being served.

In 1910, Abraham Flexner conducted a study on the quality of medical education in the United States. The famous Flexner Report identified serious problems and inconsistencies that existed in medical education. As a result, many of the profit-oriented schools were closed and those that remained open underwent significant curriculum revision. In addition, the AMA initiated an accreditation process that ranked schools according to their performance. The Flexner Report established a model for medical education that is still used in many medical schools today.

In 1913, the American College of Surgeons (ACS) was founded. One of its purposes was to develop a system of hospital standardization that would improve patient care and recognize hospitals that had the highest ideals. To establish the standards, the ACS began collecting data from health records. At this time, the ACS realized that health record documentation was inadequate. In 1917, the ACS founded the Hospital Standardization Program, which laid the groundwork for establishing standards of care. The first ACS report revealed that, of the 692 hospitals surveyed, only 89 met minimum standards and some of the most prestigious hospitals did not meet approval. After issuing this report, the ACS adopted the *Minimum Standards,* which identified the essential standards for proper care and treatment of hospital patients. They included specifications that established an organized medical staff and required that certain diagnostic and therapeutic facilities be available and that a health record be written for every patient. The standards specified, among other things, that the record be complete, accurate, and accessible.[7] In fact, the standards for health care in use today continue to encompass the documentation requirements identified in 1919 (Box 1-2).

Although hospital admissions increased dramatically from 1935 to the end of World War II in 1945, the unemployed, disabled, elderly, and others who could not pay were excluded. The economy was growing, and technological advances continued in the medical field. The need for more hospitals and high-quality health care accessible to all Americans increased. In 1946, Senators Lister Hill and Harold H. Burton sponsored the Hospital Survey and Construction Act. This legislation, known as the Hill-Burton Act, provided funding for the construction of hospitals and other health care facilities on the basis of state need. For the next 25 years, as a result of this program, hospital construction and expansion flourished.

In the early 1950s, the ACS Hospital Standardization Program was overburdened by the huge increase in the numbers of hospitals, nonsurgical specialties, and the

---

Box 1-2 MEDICAL RECORD SPECIFICATIONS IDENTIFIED IN THE *MINIMUM STANDARDS* BY THE AMERICAN COLLEGE OF SURGEONS, 1919

A complete case record should be developed, including the following:
- Patient identification data
- Complaint
- Personal and family history
- History of current illness
- Physical examination
- Special examinations (consultations, radiography, clinical laboratory)
- Provisional or working diagnosis
- Medical and surgical treatments
- Progress notes
- Gross and microscopic findings
- Final diagnosis
- Condition on discharge
- Follow-up
- Autopsy findings in the event of death

Adapted from American College of Surgeons: Minimum standards, 1919, *Bull Am Coll Surg* 8:4, 1924.

perception that medial care was becoming more sophisticated. As a result, the Joint Commission on Accreditation of Hospitals (JCAH) was founded in 1952 and adopted the Hospital Standardization Program from the ACS.[7]

In the 1950s, Americans began to want more technology that would be accessible to all people at an affordable cost. As advances were made in the medical field, the demand for health care services and the cost to provide those services grew. The attitude became "more is better." In addition, medical advances extended life expectancy, resulting in an increase in the elderly population. With the growing elderly population came a growth in the incidence of chronic diseases. As hospital care became more expensive, those who were uninsured or underinsured—primarily the poor and the elderly—could not access the health care system. Up to this point, the federal and state governments did little to control hospital costs. However, in 1965 Congress amended the Social Security Act of 1935, Public Law 89-97, establishing both Title XVIII, *Health Insurance for the Aged* (now called Medicare), and Title XIX, which extended the Kerr-Mills Medical Assistance Program (now called **Medicaid**). **Medicare** is a federally funded program that provides health insurance for elderly people and certain other groups, and **Medicaid** supports the states in paying for health care for the indigent.[8] An **indigent** is one who is without the means for subsistence—poor or impoverished. At this time, the federal government became a significant player in the health care delivery system because it not only funded and operated the Medicare program but also assisted the states with the Medicaid program. These programs are discussed further in the section on financing health care later in this chapter. In response to the federal government's establishing and regulating the Medicare and Medicaid programs, states began writing more and, in some cases, their first regulatory codes.

In the 1960s, there was a proliferation of various health care facilities, including long-term care, psychiatric and substance abuse facilities, and programs for the developmentally disabled. The JCAH not only redefined the standards to be the optimal achievable, as opposed to minimum standards, but also began developing standards for the various types of health care facilities.[7] During the late 1980s, the JCAH reflected its broader scope by changing its name to the Joint Commission on Accreditation of Healthcare Organizations (JCAHO) (Box 1-3). It is now known as The Joint Commisson.

Toward the turn of the century there were not only concerns for the cost of health care and quality but also for increased awareness for patient safety. In 1999 the Institute

---

Box 1-3 HISTORICAL LANDMARKS AFFECTING HEALTH CARE SYSTEMS

1910

Flexner Report, published by Abraham Flexner, revealed serious problems that existed in medical education. The report served as an impetus to establishing the accreditation of medical schools by the AMA.

1913

ACS was founded for the purposes of establishing standards of care and recognizing those hospitals that have high ideals.

1917

American College of Surgeons (ACS) established the Hospital Standardization Program, which began testing basic standards of care.

1919

ACS adopted the *Minimum Standards*, which identified factors that are essential to proper care and treatment of hospital patients.

1935

Social Security Act was passed, which provided grants for old age assistance and benefits, unemployment compensation, and aid to dependent children, maternal and child welfare, and other groups. It also established social security.

1946

Hospital Survey and Construction Act (Hill-Burton Act) was passed, which provided funding for the construction of health care facilities and equipment on the basis of state need.

1952

Joint Commission on Accreditation of Hospitals was founded, which adopted the Hospital Standardization Program from the ACS; in the late 1980s, JCAH changed the name to the Joint Commission on Accreditation of Healthcare Organizations.

1953

Department of Health, Education, and Welfare (HEW) was formed for the purpose of addressing issues related to the health, education, and welfare of the people of the United States.

1961

The Community Health Services and Facilities Act provided grants for the establishment of voluntary health planning agencies at the local level; it resulted in community health centers to serve low-income areas.

1965

Title III of the Older Americans Act established funding for transportation and for chore, homemaker, and home health aides for the elderly.

1965

Congress amended the Social Security Act of 1935 (PL 89-97), which established Title XVIII, Health Insurance for the Aged (Medicare), and Title XIVX, Medical Assistance Program (Medicaid).

Continued

Box 1-3 HISTORICAL LANDMARKS AFFECTING HEALTH CARE SYSTEMS—cont'd

1970

The Occupational Safety and Health Act was passed, which mandated employers to provide a safe and healthy work environment and therefore resulted in the development of standards.

1977

The Committee on Allied Health Education and Accreditation was founded by the AMA for the purpose of accrediting allied health programs; it disbanded in 1994.

1980

HEW was reorganized into the Department of Health and Human Services (DHHS), a federal cabinet-level department responsible for health issues, including health care and costs, welfare of various populations, occupational safety, and income security plans.

1982

The Tax Equity and Fiscal Responsibility Act (TEFRA), PL97-248, established a mechanism for controlling the cost of the Medicare program; this act set a limit on reimbursement and required the development of the prospective payment system (later to be known as diagnosis-related groups).

1985

Consolidated Omnibus Budget Reconciliation Act (COBRA) established Emergency Medical Treatment and Active Labor Act (EMTALA), which is known as the "Patient Antidumping Law." It established criteria for the transfer and discharge of Medicare and Medicaid patients between two acute-care hospitals.

1987

The Nursing Home Reform Act, effective in 1990, required nursing facilities (long-term care facilities) to employ sufficient nursing personnel, 24 hours per day, to provide care to each resident according to the care plan.

1989

The Omnibus Budget Reconciliation Act brought attention and support to the production and dissemination of scientific and policy-relevant information that improves quality, reduces cost, and enhances effectiveness of health care and established the Agency for Health Care Research and Quality (AHRQ).

1990

The Patient Self-Determination Act resulted from the *Cruzan v. Missouri* (1990) case in which the court upheld patient wishes at the end of life. The Act increased the public's awareness of state laws governing patient options and rights and advance directives.

1991

DHHS commissioned the Workgroup on Electronic Data Interchange to identify ways of increasing the number of claims processed electronically, which would reduce administrative costs.

1992

The Computer-Based Patient Record Institute was created for the purpose of developing strategy that supports the development and adoption of the computer-based patient record.

1996 (implemented in 1998)

Health Insurance Portability and Accountability Act (HIPAA) is directed at improving access, affordability, and adequacy of health insurance; established fraud and abuse detection program for health plans. It includes provision for administrative simplification that addresses privacy and security of personal health information and uniform definitions for transactions and code sets.

---

of Medicine (IOM) published *To Err Is Human,* which reported that between 44,000 and 98,000 deaths per year are attributable to medical errors at a cost of about $17 and $29 billion, respectively.[2] Medical errors include adverse drug events, mismatched blood types, and surgery on wrong patient or limb. With this report has come increasing attention to patient safety and bringing more information to the point of care with the use of technology.[9] In 2004, the World Health Organization began supporting dialogue among health leaders, consumers, and health ministers to discuss patient safety.

Health Care in the Twenty-First Century

The health care system in the United States has evolved into a complex system composed of multiple types of facilities, providers, payers, and regulators and consumers who are demanding more and better health care. There is a proliferation of sophisticated technology for both medical practice and information management. The technology available in financial, administrative, and clinical information systems affects the quality, cost, and efficiency of

health care systems. The technological advances in medicine support prevention, early diagnosis, shorter hospital stays, patient safety, and increased outpatient services and home health care.

In 2003 health spending slowed for the first time since 1996 and still U.S. health care costs are about 15.3% of the U.S. gross domestic product (GDP).[10] The total national health care expenditures in the United States increased to $1.7 trillion,[11] yet millions of people were uninsured or could not access the system. Those without insurance either cannot afford it or cannot find an insurance company that is willing to sell them a policy at any price. Insurance companies often cancel contracts with patients who have expensive (catastrophic costs) health care needs, as is the case with chronic conditions such as cancer, kidney disease, and heart disease. Those who cannot access the health care system may live in areas where little or no health care is available or do not have transportation.

Advances in technology and scientific developments have supported a healthier lifestyle and a longer life expectancy. For women, life expectancy increased from 49.1 years in 1900 to 80.1 years in 2003, and for men, from 49.1 years to

74.8 years.[11] And with the longer life expectancy has come tremendous growth in the need for home health and long-term care (LTC).

Health care continues to be costly and not accessible to all citizens, yet consumers continued to demand more and better care. As a result, there has been tremendous pressure to reform the manner in which health care is delivered to contain the cost and still provide high-quality care to all.[12] The sources of the pressure are numerous. They include the federal government, which is concerned with the cost of health care and its accessibility; the consumers, who have become more educated and are demanding more and better quality; the providers, who want to maintain their market share, cut their costs, and realize a profit; and the taxpayers, who are underinsured or uninsured or who feel overburdened with taxation that finances health care. The changes that are occurring are evidenced by the shift from inpatient care to outpatient care, increased legislation on patient rights, and the increase in alternative health care systems. The result is a health care system that is evolving into a more patient-/consumer-centric culture. **Patient centered** care allows patients to have more control over their care and access to their health care information. Evidence of patient-centric care includes the following:

- Making cost and quality data on hospitals and providers available to the consumer, such as the "Quality Check" function on The Joint Commission Web site where consumers can check on the accreditation findings of health care organizations (HCOs).
- Supporting patients in setting up their own **personal health records** (PHRs) through making provider records accessible to patients through web portals and other methods.[13]
- Protecting the patient's privacy and security of health information by legislation.
- Increasing communication between patient and provider by email or voice mail.

AHIMA has defined a PHR as:

The personal health record (PHR) is an electronic, lifelong resource of health information needed by individuals to make health decisions. Individuals own and manage the information in the PHR, which comes from healthcare providers and the individual. The PHR is maintained in a secure and private environment, with the individual determining rights of access. The PHR does not replace the legal record of any provider.[13]

With such problems as the escalating cost of health care, the number of uninsured, and the existence of underserved rural areas where medical care is not available, there continues to be a great impetus to reform the manner in which health care is delivered in the United States. Various plans for health care reform have been developed by different professional organizations, members of Congress, state governments, and the federal government. Most of the plans for health care reform address such issues as universal coverage, meaning health care for every citizen; health care costs; and the quality and safety of the health care provided.

Healthy People 2010

The U.S. Department of Health and Human Services (DHHS) has established goals that promote health and prevention of disease. One of the DHHS reports is Healthy People 2000, which used data systems to identify national opportunities for health improvement. Some of the national data systems used to formulate the goals that would lead to a better quality of life include data on adult use of tobacco, a continuing survey of individual food intake, a national crime survey, and birth and infant death data. *Healthy Communities 2000: Model Standards, Guidelines for Community Attainment of Year 2000 Objectives* was developed to provide assistance to state and local governments in reaching their goals.[14] This report was updated as *Healthy People 2010*, which identified national objectives for disease prevention and health promotion. Although the *Healthy People 2010* objectives are disease and indicator specific, the primary goals are to increase the quality and years of healthy life and to eliminate health disparities.[15]

REGULATORY AGENCIES AND ORGANIZATIONS

External forces that regulate the health care industry include, but are not limited to, the DHHS, The Joint Commission, the American Osteopathic Association, the Community Health Accreditation Program (CHAP) of the National League for Nursing, the Commission on Accreditation of Rehabilitation Facilities (CARF), and the state departments of public health. The regulatory activities of health care facilities are primarily directed at quality, utilization, and cost of care, whereas the regulatory activities that affect educational programs and the health care workforce are directed at quality and supply of manpower.

Federal Government as Regulator

The federal government has been involved in the regulation of the health care systems since the early part of the century, primarily in the consumer's interest. In 1906, the Pure Food and Drug Act was passed because of the unsanitary conditions that prevailed in the food production industry, and in 1938 the Food, Drug, and Cosmetic Act was passed to regulate the food, drug, and cosmetic industry. This act mandated that manufacturers prove safety, specify composition and method of manufacture, and provide labeling and package inserts. Interestingly, it was not until 1962 that manufacturers were required to prove efficacy (i.e., how effective a product is).

Department of Health and Human Services

The branch of the federal government that is primarily responsible for the numerous regulatory programs that affect the health industry is the DHHS, formerly the Department of Health, Education, and Welfare (HEW). HEW, created in 1953, underwent numerous reorganizations that led to the creation of the DHHS in 1980. The organization of the DHHS is quite complex and includes numerous administrations, divisions, offices, centers, and

agencies; the highest ranking official is the secretary of the DHHS, who advises the president of the United States on issues regarding health, welfare, income security plans, and programs and projects of the DHHS. The DHHS has regional offices that work with the states and communities in carrying out various programs.

Organization of DHHS. The organizational structure of the DHHS encompasses various agencies, centers, and offices, some of which are discussed in the following section and identified in the DHHS organizational chart illustrated in Figure 1-1.

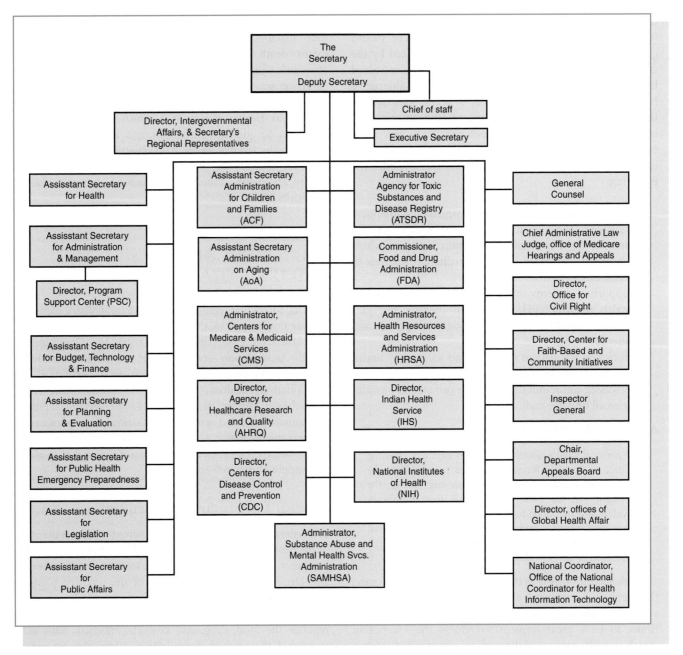

Figure 1-1 Organizational structure of the U.S. Department of Health and Human Services. (From U.S. Department of Health and Human Services: http://www.hhs.gov/about/orgchart.html. Accessed March 10, 2006.)

Office of Inspector General. The responsibility of conducting and monitoring audits, inspections, and investigations regarding programs or projects sponsored by the DHHS is delegated to the Office of Inspector General (OIG). For example, this office investigates cases of alleged fraud and abuse that occur in Medicare and Medicaid programs and recommends corrective action in such cases.

Administration for Children and Families. The Administration for Children and Families is committed to the development of children, youth, and families and to supporting activities that improve and enrich these groups. This agency administers and funds state grants regarding such issues as adoption, runaway and homeless youth, prevention and treatment of child abuse, and child welfare services.

Administration on Aging. The Administration on Aging (AoA) was created in response to the Amendment to the Older American Act of 1965. It supports a range of programs that offer services and opportunities for older Americans. The AoA is an advocate for older persons; it works to increase awareness of the contribution that older Americans make and alerts the public regarding the needs of older people.

Agency for Healthcare Research and Quality. The Agency for Healthcare Research and Quality (AHRQ) was established by the Omnibus Budget Reconciliation Act of 1989, which placed greater emphasis on health services research. The primary focus is to produce and disseminate scientific and policy-relevant information that improves the quality, reduces the cost, and enhances the effectiveness of health care.

Agency for Toxic Substances and Disease Registry. The Agency for Toxic Substances and Disease Registry is committed to protecting both workers and the public from exposure to and the adverse effects of hazardous substances. The agency, among other functions, collects, analyzes, and disseminates information regarding mortality rates, disease, and hazardous substances; establishes registries for long-term follow-up; and develops programs for public response to health emergencies.

Centers for Disease Control and Prevention. The Centers for Disease Control and Prevention (CDC) is concerned with communicable diseases, environmental health, and foreign quarantine activities. The CDC also works with state and local agencies regarding these matters and provides consultation, education, and training. For example, the CDC has established recommendations (standards) called "Universal Precautions" that are guidelines for health care workers to minimize the spread of infectious substances.

Food and Drug Administration. The Food and Drug Administration (FDA) is responsible for the safety of foods, drugs, medical devices, cosmetics, and radiation-emitting equipment. Responsibilities include proper labeling, product information, safety, and efficacy.

Substance Abuse and Mental Health Services Administration. The Substance Abuse and Mental Health Services Administration is concerned with the effective prevention and treatment of addictive and mental disorders. The administration emphasizes state-of-the-art practice that is based on science, high quality, and access to health care for these disorders.

Health Resources and Services Administration. The Health Resources and Services Administration (HRSA) is primarily involved in the distribution of major grant funding to state governments and the private sector.

National Institutes of Health. The National Institutes of Health (NIH) is a major medical research center composed of numerous institutes and centers (e.g., National Institute on Aging, National Center for Nursing Research, National Cancer Institute). It is a major source of funding for health-related research (e.g., aging, cancer, women's health issues, obesity, nutrition).

Surgeon General. The surgeon general reports to the Assistant Secretary for Health and is appointed by the President of the United States to serve a 4-year term. The primary role of the surgeon general is to provide leadership and management for the Public Health Service (PHS) Commissioned Corps and to serve as advisor on public health and scientific issues, including current and long-term health issues, emergency preparedness and response, protection and enhancement of the health of the nation, and provision of leadership on health initiatives such as prevention of spread of infectious diseases and tobacco cessation.[16]

Indian Health Service. The Indian Health Service (IHS) is responsible for providing health care through a network of hospitals, health centers, health stations, and school health centers and through contracts with private providers to eligible Native Americans.

Centers for Medicare and Medicaid Services. The Centers for Medicare and Medicaid Services (CMS), formerly Health Care Financing Administration (HCFA), is responsible for the Medicare program and the federal government's role in the Medicaid programs, with special emphasis on quality and utilization control. Through its programs, CMS is involved in the health care of the elderly, disabled, and poor.

The CMS establishes rules and regulations that govern the Medicare program. To be eligible for Medicare and Medicaid reimbursement, providers must demonstrate compliance with the *Conditions of Participation* (COP), which were originally published in Regulation Number 5, Federal Health Insurance for the Aged. Revisions to the COP are published in the *Federal Register*. Compliance with the COP is regulated by the states. The review of HCOs to determine compliance with the COP is the responsibility of the states. However, Title XVIII, the Medicare Act, specifies that the facilities accredited by The Joint Commission and AOA be deemed in compliance with the Medicare Conditions of Participation for Hospitals[7]; those accredited are said to have **deemed status.**

Meeting the requirements of the COP is referred to as being certified. However, the term **certification** is also used to refer to the process by which government and nongovernment organizations evaluate educational programs, health care facilities, and individuals as having met predetermined standards. To ensure high-quality care, the CMS established a national network of Quality Improvement Organizations (QIOs) for each U.S. state and territory and for the District of Columbia. The QIOs work with health care providers and consumers to promote a high quality of care and to investigate complaints about care. The QIOs, discussed in further detail in Chapter 13, also work to protect the Medicare trust fund and ensure that payments are made for only medically necessary services.

Social Security Administration

Before 1995, the Social Security Administration (SSA) was within the organizational structure of the DHHS. However, in 1995 it became an independent agency. The Social Security Administration manages the social security program for elderly, disabled, and blind people and for survivors (dependents). The social security program is financed by contributions from employees, employers, and self-employed people, which are placed in a fund. When earnings stop or are reduced because of retirement, death, or disability, the fund pays monthly cash amounts to supplement the loss of income.

Occupational Safety and Health Administration

In 1970, Congress passed the Occupational Safety and Health Act, which mandated that employers provide a safe and healthy work environment. The Occupational Safety and Health Administration (OSHA) is responsible for developing standards and regulations and conducting inspections and investigations to determine compliance, and it proposes corrective actions for noncompliance in matters related to occupational safety and health. Other agencies involved in establishing standards for occupational safety and health include government agencies, such as the CDC, and professional organizations, such as the ACS. The guidelines, recommendations, and standards are directed at protecting employees from occupational health hazards, such as minimizing the risk of contracting disease from asbestos in old buildings, contracting acquired immunodeficiency syndrome (AIDS) in health care facilities and developing repetitive motion injuries such carpal tunnel syndrome.

The Role of States

State governments have regulatory involvement in the health care systems through state-owned and state-operated facilities, the funding of medical education and teaching hospitals, the certification of health care facilities according to the Medicare COP, maintenance of public health departments, and licensing of health care facilities and health occupations. Hospital ownership, medical education, certification, and licensing of health occupations are discussed in other sections; therefore, only the states' roles in public health departments and in licensing health care facilities are addressed in this section.

State Health Departments

The organization of state health departments varies from state to state but is a joint venture between the state and the local communities. The health care provided is usually directed toward maternal and child health care, communicable diseases, and chronic diseases. The maternal and child care services usually provide obstetric care, family planning, well-baby checkups, vaccinations, and other services. Health care for communicable diseases involves teaching the patient and community about transmission and prevention of certain diseases, diagnosing and treating communicable diseases such as measles and gonorrhea, and tracking the source of the communicable disease. Some of the chronic diseases that the public health department might manage are mental illness, substance abuse, hypertension, and diabetes. HIM professionals need to be knowledgeable about the organization of the state health department in the state where they reside or practice; information is usually available through the county health department.

State and local health departments have important roles in collecting information through vital statistics and communicable disease reporting, in ensuring safe drinking water and environment, and in bioterrorism.

Public health is a general term that refers to a wide array of activities directed at promoting the health of populations. Activities include efforts directed at prevention and early detection of disease and promotion of health in the general and in special populations. Many of the programs/activities are conducted by the states and funded by state and federal monies. The programs and activities include, among other activities, immunizations, behavior modification through education, health screenings and periodic examinations, and therapeutic interventions. For example, to reduce tobacco use, numerous state and federal initiatives are directed at educating the public about the risk of tobacco use, advice about how to quit, funding for counseling/advising patients on smoking cessation, and a hotline for consumers desiring to quit.

Licensure of Health Care Facilities

Licensure gives legal approval for a facility to operate or for a person to practice within his or her profession (Table 1-1). Virtually every state requires that hospitals, nursing homes,

Table 1-1 REGULATION OF HEALTH CARE PROVIDERS

	State Government	National Nongovernmental
Health care professionals	Licensure	Registration/ certification
Health care facilities	Licensure	Accreditation

and pharmacies be licensed to operate, although the requirements and standards for licensure may differ from state to state. State licensure is mandatory. Federal facilities such as those of the Department of Veterans Affairs do not require state licensure.

Although licensure requirements vary, health care facilities must meet certain basic criteria that are determined by state regulatory agencies. The standards address such concerns as adequacy of staffing, personnel employed to provide services, physical aspects of the facility (equipment, buildings), and services provided, including health records. Survey for licensure is typically performed annually, and the standards are usually considered t o be minimally acceptable for operation. Some states also accept Joint Commission Accreditation as proof of meeting licensure requirements.

Legislation

Following is a brief discussion of selected legislation that has had a major impact on health care delivery in the United States.

The Consolidated Omnibus Budget Reconciliation Act (COBRA) of 1985 was written out of a concern for the management of indigent patients. COBRA established the Emergency Medical Treatment and Labor Act (EMTALA), which is known as the "Patient Antidumping Law." EMTALA established criteria for Medicare-certified facilities and physicians responsible for the transfer and discharge of patients. The law requires that every patient, regardless of ability to pay, who arrives at an emergency department with an emergency medical condition, including active labor, be provided a medical screening examination and stabilizing medical care. If the facility is unable to provide stabilizing treatment or if the patient requests, a transfer to an appropriate facility should be done.[17]

In 1989, the Omnibus Budget Reconciliation Act was passed, which emphasizes the production and dissemination of scientific and policy-relevant information that improves the quality, reduces the cost, and enhances the effectiveness of health care. This act promoted the development of outcome measures (criteria) for health care quality.

The Patient Self Determination Act of 1990 was a result of the Supreme Court's ruling in *Cruzan v. Missouri* (1990) that upheld patient wishes although the decision meant inevitable death for the patient. The act is intended to increase the public's awareness of the respective state laws governing patient options for health care, patient rights, and advance directives. An **advance directive** is a legal, written document that specifies patient preferences regarding future health care or specifies another person to make medical decisions in the event the patient has an incurable or irreversible condition and is unable to communicate his or her wishes; the patient must be competent at the time the document is prepared and signed. The advance directive guides the health care team in making decisions about life-sustaining treatment and organ donation and usually designates a person to assume authority for the patient. The statute requires providers to develop written policies and procedures on self-determination and to document in each health record regardless of whether an advance directive has been signed.[12] The HIM or risk management department is responsible for ensuring that the proper documentation is in each health record. (See Chapter 15, Privacy and Health Law, for further information.)

Today, some medical conditions can be extremely costly to treat, and that cost represents a major expense to the business community, insurance companies, managed-care organizations (MCOs), and other health care payers. The result has been the dropping of coverage of high-cost patients or even dropping of the businesses that employ them by these major payers. The individual is then unable to secure health insurance and incurs health care costs that are financially devastating. As a result, in 1996 Congress passed the Health Insurance Portability and Accountability Act (HIPAA), which is a comprehensive law dealing with a variety of health care issues mainly directed at improving access, affordability, and adequacy of health insurance.[18]

One of the main provisions of HIPAA was to provide for the portability of group health insurance when a person changes employers. Before the enactment of HIPAA, employees often had to wait for coverage themselves or for one of their dependents because of pre-existing conditions such as asthma or high blood pressure. This potential loss of health insurance coverage kept individuals from changing jobs and advancing in their careers. HIPAA allowed for continuous coverage when a person changed from one group insurance plan to another. The act also established tax breaks for purchasers of long-term care insurance and self-employed purchasers of health insurance and created a fraud and abuse program for health plans.[18]

HIPAA included many other provisions that affected operation of HCOs. Some that had the greatest affect on HIM can be found in the administrative simplification section. The Privacy and Security Rules are included in this section. The Privacy Rule applies to protected health information in any format created and or used by health care providers, health care plans, and health care clearinghouses. The HIPAA security rule is concerned with the protection of the electronic health information. The advent of HIPAA has brought about expanded roles and responsibilities for HIM professionals—that is, protecting privacy and maintaining the security of electronic health care transactions and records. The federal regulations standardize the privacy and security practices in the health care industry throughout the United Stated. Before HIPAA, laws differed among states. Privacy is discussed in further detail in Chapter 15 and security in Chapter 8.

Accreditation

The process by which a private nongovernmental organization or agency performs an external review and grants recognition to a program of study or institution that meets certain predetermined standards is called **accreditation.** The review process and the standards are devised and regulated by professional organizations such as The Joint Commission and the AOA. Although the process is voluntary, there are financial and legal incentives for HCOs to attain accreditation. Advantages of accreditation are numerous and include the following:

- Required for reimbursement for certain patient groups
- Validates the quality of health care institutions, programs, and services
- Provides a competitive edge over nonaccredited facilities

The HIM department plays a crucial role in accreditation because the review of health information data is a major part of the accreditation process. The HIM professionals should have access to and be familiar with the standards contained in the most current accreditation manual for the type of HCO in which they are employed.

The Joint Commission

The Joint Commission is a private, nonprofit organization that establishes guidelines and standards for the operation and management of health care facilities with emphasis on the health care functions crucial to patient care. The mission of The Joint Commission is "To continuously improve the safety and quality of care provided to the public through the provision of health care accreditation and related services that support performance improvement in health care organizations."[19]

The standards are based on HCOs being responsible for providing a high quality of health care to the people they serve while efficiently using resources. Currently, when an organization is found to be in substantial compliance with The Joint Commission standards, accreditation may be awarded for up to 3 years. However, at the time of writing of this publication, The Joint Commission is shifting the accreditation process from the triennial survey to a continuing collection of monitors and unannounced surveys with emphasis on the safety and quality of care, treatment, and services.

The Joint Commission accredits numerous types of HCOs. Some examples of the HCOs for which standards are developed include hospitals, behavioral health care organizations, long-term care organizations, home care organizations, ambulatory care organizations, pathology and clinical laboratory services, office-based surgery practices, and MCOs.[19] As mentioned earlier, The Joint Commission has information available on its Web site for consumers to check on the accreditation status of health care facilities.

American Osteopathic Association

Much like The Joint Commission, the American Osteopathic Association (AOA) has a voluntary program that accredits osteopathic medical colleges and health care facilities. Their mission is to promote osteopathic medicine through education, research, and delivery of quality health care that is cost-effective. **Osteopathic medicine** is based on the theory that all body systems are interconnected and therefore the focus of health care is directed at the whole person.[20] Because two thirds of the body is composed of muscle and bone, osteopathic medicine places a great deal of emphasis on the musculoskeletal system. The hospitals that are accredited are recognized by the DHHS as having "deemed status," and therefore they are eligible to receive Medicare funds.

Commission on Accreditation of Rehabilitation Facilities

Founded in 1966, CARF is an independent accrediting agency for rehabilitation facilities. **Rehabilitation** is the processes of treatment and education that leads the disabled person to the achievement of maximum independence and function and a personal sense of well-being. The mission of CARF is to promote the delivery of quality services to people with disabilities. As a result of this mission, CARF sets and maintains standards directed at improving quality of care, shares aggregate data, identifies competent organizations that provide rehabilitative services, and provides an organized forum in which people served, providers, and others can participate in quality improvement.[21]

Community Health Accreditation Program

The independent, nonprofit organization that accredits community-based HCOs, including home health and hospice agencies, is the Community Health Accreditation Program (CHAP). Unlike those of other accrediting bodies, CHAP standards are consumer oriented, with more emphasis on the patient perspective than on the clinical aspect of care. Like The Joint Commission, HCOs accredited by CHAP are deemed to have met the Medicare COP.

National Committee for Quality Assurance

The National Committee for Quality Assurance (NCQA) is a nonprofit, independent accrediting agency for MCOs that originated in 1989. Its mission is to improve the quality of patient care and health plan performance in conjunction with managed-care plans, purchasers, consumers, and the public. One component of quality improvement plan is the Health Plan Employer Data and Information Set, which is a standardized set of performance measures designed to allow purchasers and consumers to compare the performance of managed-care plans.[22]

Regulatory Mechanisms of Health Occupations

Numerous agencies, organizations, and pieces of legislation regulate the education and practice of the various health occupations. The regulatory activities include state licensure of practitioners, accreditation of educational programs, certification of practitioners, and legislation that governs practice. A few of these activities are discussed here. Licensure, like that of HCOs, is required to practice the profession, whereas registration and certification are voluntary processes and not required by law to practice that profession. Individual HCOs may require certification or registration as a condition of employment.

American Medical Association

The AMA is a professional organization for physicians that is involved in the accreditation of medical schools, residency programs, and certain allied health programs.

American Osteopathic Association Bureau of Professional Education

This bureau is the only accrediting agency for osteopathic medical education in the United States. Programs that are accredited meet or exceed the standards for educational quality that have been established by the association. The AOA has certifying boards that offer certification for numerous specialties and procedures that the osteopathic physician may pursue (e.g., nuclear medicine, gynecology, proctology, blood-banking and transfusion medicine, sports medicine, angiography). It also regulates its membership by requiring a minimum number of continuing education credits to retain membership.[20]

Commission on Accreditation of Allied Health Education Programs

The Commission on Accreditation of Allied Health Education Programs (CAAHEP) accredits 20 different health science occupations, more than 2000 programs, and is recognized as the largest accreditor in health sciences. CAAHEP works with professional organizations in the accreditation process.[23] For example, CAAHEP works with American Association of Respiratory Care in accrediting respiratory therapy educational programs.

Commission on Accreditation for Health Informatics and Information Management Education

The Commission on Accreditation for Health Informatics and Information Management Education (CAHIIM) is the accrediting organization for degree-granting programs in health informatics and information management. CAHIIM accreditation means that an educational program has voluntarily undergone a rigorous review process and has been determined to meet or exceed the standards set by the sponsoring professional organization, the American Health Information Management Association (AHIMA) in cooperation with the Commission.[24] This process is discussed further in Chapter 2.

National League for Nursing Accrediting Commission, Inc.

The accrediting body for schools of nursing that offer diplomas or associate, bachelor's, master's, and doctoral degrees in nursing is the National League for Nursing Accrediting Commission, Inc. (NLNAC). The NLNAC establishes standards for the nursing curriculum, including programs for registered nurses and licensed practical nurses. The NLNAC accreditation process is tied to the individual state nursing examinations and licensure and is accountable to the National League for Nursing, which is the professional organization for nurses.[25]

In addition, many health care professions provide for the accreditation of their educational program and certification or registration of the members of their profession through their own and affiliations of their professional association.

State Licensure of Practitioners

In the licensing of practitioners, states have the right to control the entry into certain professions through licensure and the right to revoke the license. The license itself is a permit issued by the state that authorizes a person to practice in a specified area; without this permission, such practice is illegal.

Each state establishes its own licensing requirements and restricts certain activities to those who are licensed by that state. Licensure requirements involve completion of a program of study and examination by the state. Restrictions are specific for the license.[12] For example, prescribing and dispensing medications were at one time restricted to licensed physicians. Today, however, many states have given prescriptive authority to nurse practitioners (NPs) and others. The health occupations that require licensure to practice include medicine, osteopathy, nursing, nursing home administration, dentistry, podiatry, and numerous others, depending on the state. Some professions, such as occupational therapy, are both licensed and certified.

The state law that defines the rights and scope of practice of each profession and the requirements to attain a license is often called the **Practice Act.** In the case of nursing, it is called the Nursing Practice Act. Because these laws and regulations define the scope of practice, they are often an area of contention between professions when the scopes overlap. The Practice Acts also define the conditions for endorsement (reciprocity) between states. Although endorsement varies from state to state, most states require a current and active license from another state graduation from an approved educational program, and a minimum number of years of practice.

HEALTH CARE DELIVERY SYSTEMS

Continuum of Care

The **continuum of care** is the full range of health care services provided, moving from the least acute and least intensive to the most acute and most intensive, or vice versa. Note that The Joint Commission defines the continuum of care as matching the level and type of health care with the continuing needs of the individual.[19] Table 1-2 identifies the components of the continuum of health care services.

Primary care is most often considered the care provided at the point of first contact (**encounter**) with the health care provider in an ambulatory care setting; the care is continuous and comprehensive and may involve **episodes of care** for a specific condition during a period of relatively continuous care. The provider, usually a physician, coordinates and manages all aspects of the patient's health care, including the preventive care and use of consultants and community resources as appropriate. Primary care encompasses preventive care (comprehensive care) and acute care. Health care services directed at preventing disease or injury, minimizing the consequences of existing conditions, and promoting health are the major objectives of preventive care. Annual physical examinations, immuni-

zations, family planning, vision and hearing screens, health education, and early detection of disease are examples of preventive medicine. **Acute care,** on the other hand, implies the treatment of common illnesses and injuries, such as nausea, vomiting, and abrasions. Providers of primary care are family practitioners, internists, pediatricians, obstetricians, gynecologists, physician assistants, and NPs; the care is commonly provided in one of many ambulatory care settings. Primary care providers often serve as gatekeepers. A **gatekeeper** refers to the primary care physician who participates in a comprehensive managed-care plan and who is responsible for coordinating all care provided to the managed-care enrollee (patient). The focus of care is on prevention through regular physical examinations and other primary care services (education, immunization, family planning, emergency care). If a patient needs to see a specialist, the gatekeeper must make the referral and thereby controls the access to all other care.

Secondary care, a term not as widely used as primary or tertiary care, implies care by a specialist, usually through referral from the primary care physician. **Tertiary care** is a term used for the care provided at facilities with advanced technologies and specialized intensive care units, such as teaching institutions and university medical centers. The institutions that are recognized as providers of tertiary care are often involved in biomedical research. The providers are specialists who are widely recognized for their expertise in

Table 1-2   CONTINUUM OF HEALTH CARE SERVICES

Health Care Service	Description	Examples of Setting
Preventive care	Care directed at preventing injury or condition. Examples: immunizations, genetic testing, use of safety belts	Physician office, public health departments, clinics
Primary care	Care provided at point of first contact, includes preventive care, acute care, early detection, and intervention	Physician office, public health departments, clinics
Specialist care	Care directed at specific body organ or system or specific disease	Specialists such as gastroenterologists, cardiologists, and psychiatrists
Long-term care	Medical and nonmedical care provided for chronic, debilitating conditions such as Alzheimer's disease, chronic obstructive pulmonary disease, quadriplegia	Home health care, long-term care facilities
Rehabilitative care	Care directed at restoring disabled person to maximum physical, mental, and vocational health; goal is independence and productivity	Inpatient and outpatient rehabilitation facilities, home health care, and rehabilitation departments of hospitals and long-term care
Respite care	Short-term care in which care is provided to patient for purpose of providing caregiver with time off/rest	Patient/family home; adult day care; long-term care facilities
End-of-life care	Hospice care provided to patients in last 6 months of life; includes the palliative and supportive care of terminally ill patients and their families	Patient or family home care, skilled nursing home

specific areas of medicine and include specialists such as endocrinologists, hematologists, oncologists, thoracic surgeons, and neurosurgeons.

Ambulatory Care

Ambulatory care is a comprehensive term for all types of health care provided in an outpatient setting; the patient travels to and from the facility on the same day and is not hospitalized, institutionalized, or admitted as an inpatient. For example, a resident of a nursing home may be transported to the outpatient department at the hospital for a mammogram (radiograph of the breast) and then returned to the nursing home later the same day. This person is a resident (inpatient) of the nursing home but an outpatient of the hospital.

There are two major types of ambulatory (or outpatient) care:

- Care provided in free-standing medical centers. Examples of free-standing medical centers include physicians' solo, partnership, or group practices; public health department; community health centers (CHCs); and urgent care centers.
- Care provided in organized settings that function independently of the physicians providing the care. The settings for this type of ambulatory care include hospital-owned clinics, outpatient departments, ambulatory treatment units, emergency departments, ancillary services, staff health maintenance organizations (HMOs), and urgent care centers. Note that urgent care centers and others may be in either type of setting, depending on ownership of the facility. The physician may be an employee of the urgent care facility or may be the owner and provider.

Physician Practices

Physician practices have historically been private practices; however, with health care reform, physicians are collaborating, networking, and forming alliances with other providers, including managed-care programs, and hospitals, all of which are described in the section on financing of health care.

Private Practice. The term private practice usually refers to physicians or other health care providers who are established in an independent practice that is for profit. Although providers of health care include numerous professionals (dentists, podiatrists, chiropractors) who can by law practice independently, this discussion focuses on the physician as the provider. The primary mode by which physicians provide health care is within their private medical office (practice), although this is changing.

Some physicians are self-employed and legally the sole owners of their practices; these **solo practices** are on the decline. Most physicians in solo practices have an informal arrangement with other physicians to "take call" when they are not available. "Take call" refers to the practice of one physician managing care for another physician's patients, which allows the physician to take time away from work.

A partnership is a legal agreement between two or more physicians to share certain expenses and profits. The term partnership may apply to group practice (three or more physicians) if the group has entered a legal agreement to share certain assets and liabilities as determined by the agreement. The agreement specifies that the physicians are employees of the practice, with all monies generated and expenses from the practice to be pooled and redistributed to the physicians according to the agreement. The size, composition, organizational structure, and financial arrangements of the groups are highly varied. Some group practices may have arrangements that involve sharing certain central services and still maintaining the physicians' individual practices. For example, each physician has his or her own office but may purchase office equipment and supplies or contract with a medical transcription service as a group. This concept allows the physician to remain independent and be competitive in the marketplace.

The group practice may be composed of many physicians of the same specialty or may be a multispecialty group. An example of a same-specialty practice is a group of obstetricians and gynecologists or a group of ophthalmologists. The group shares office space, equipment, nursing and support staff, and patient call (providing care 24 hours a day). The multispecialty group offers services in at least two specialty areas. A women's center is a good example of a multispecialty group practice; the providers at a women's center may include pediatricians, obstetricians, gynecologists, infertility specialists, and gerontologists. Many of the larger groups have their own ancillary services, such as a clinical laboratory and radiology units.

Community Health Centers

In 1961, the Community Health Services and Facilities Act provided grants for the establishment of voluntary health planning agencies at the local level. These demonstration projects were developed to serve low-income areas. Community health centers (CHCs) were designed to provide comprehensive care in a catchment area that has limited or nonexistent health services for certain populations or special health needs. A **catchment area** is a defined geographic area that is served by a health care program, project, or facility such as a hospital or mental health center. Services provided are usually directed at population groups and range from immunizations, diagnostic testing, and screening to nutrition counseling and family planning.

Funding for CHCs comes from a variety of sources, including monies from private, state, and federal grants; federal funds from the Public Health Service and the Bureau of Community Health Services of DHHS; and funds from local or state health departments. Care at the centers may be provided at no charge or the cost may be based on the patient's ability to pay, which is referred to as a **sliding scale fee.**[3]

Community-Based Care

The term community-based care refers to the delivery of services that go beyond an institutional setting and reach out into the community. These services may include adult day care centers, clinics at public schools, visits by medical staff to homeless shelters, house calls to the homebound and elderly, meal services provided to elderly who are in need (Meals on Wheels Association of America), and mobile vans to provide testing and screening. Community-based programs are financed by a combination of funding that includes Medicare, Medicaid, other federal and state moneys, private donations, and other sources. In 1965, Title III of the Older Americans Act established funding for transportation and for chore, homemaker, and home health aides for the elderly, all of which are forms of community-based care.

Surgicenters and Urgent Care Centers

Free-standing surgical facilities in which surgical procedures can be safely performed on the day of admission or on an outpatient basis are called surgicenters or ambulatory surgery centers. Many hospitals offer outpatient surgery. Patients need to be well enough to withstand the surgery and go home afterward. Urgent care, medical walk-in, and convenience care centers are for patients who need routine care or who have minor but urgent health problems. The facilities are usually open at least 12 hours a day, 7 days a week, and do not require appointments. The patient population is composed of those who do not have an established relationship with a physician in the area, those who are not established with any physician, and those whose physician is not accessible at the time of need.

Hospital Ambulatory Care

Hospital ambulatory care is "hospital-directed" health care that is provided to patients who are not admitted as inpatients and for which the hospital is responsible, regardless of the location of the health care. Hospital ambulatory care services include satellite clinics, observation units, outpatient departments, ancillary services, and other specialty clinics.

Satellite Clinics. Hospitals may own and operate one or more ambulatory care facilities called **satellite clinics** that are not located on the campus of the main hospital. Satellite clinics are established in areas that are convenient to the patients,[3] such as places of employment, or in areas that are closer to a specific patient population.

Observation Unit. The observation unit of the hospital is a unit, department, or beds for the **observation patient** who needs assessment, evaluation, or monitoring because of a significant degree of instability or disability that does not require admission to the hospital as an inpatient. For the Medicare patient, CMS suggests that the physician use 24 hours as a benchmark; that is, if the patient is expected to require hospital care for 24 or more hours and or meets the inpatient criteria for hospital admission, the physician should admit the patient as an inpatient as opposed to an observation patient. The observation period should not exceed 36 to 48 hours.

Outpatient Departments. In outpatient departments or clinics of a hospital, primary care or specialized medical care is provided to patients who are not admitted. In addition to primary care, outpatient departments diagnose and treat conditions that are not emergent in nature and yet require intervention within a short period of time, such as earaches, nausea, vomiting, diarrhea, muscle sprains, dizziness, headaches, and conjunctivitis. The specialty clinics that many hospitals operate include preadmission testing, pediatrics, obstetrics, gynecology, orthopedics, and surgery; the larger tertiary hospitals may offer clinics for such specialties as low-birth-weight neonatal care, high-risk pregnancy, sports medicine, and cancer.

Outpatient surgery departments include units within the hospital as well as satellite surgery centers that perform surgery for which admission is not required.

Ancillary Services (Professional Service Departments). **Ancillary services** departments provide diagnostic and therapeutic services at the request of a physician to both inpatients and outpatients; the departments include radiology (medical imaging), clinical laboratory, physical therapy, occupational therapy, respiratory therapy, cardiographics, pharmacy, and so on. For example, physicians who are not equipped or trained to perform certain diagnostic procedures such as colonoscopy would refer the patient to the appropriate ancillary department for the procedure. Ancillary services differ from other areas of the hospital because the hospital is able to charge patients or third parties directly and, therefore, generate revenue for the hospital. They are under the direction of physicians.

Hospitals

There is no single definition of the word hospital, and the hospital of the present is undergoing tremendous change because of pressures to contain cost and support a continuum of care that is of high quality and accessible to all. The hospital description provided in this section characterizes the traditional, stand-alone hospital.

The AHA defines a **hospital** as a health care facility that has an organized medical and professional staff, inpatient beds available 24 hours a day and the primary function of providing inpatient medical, nursing, and other health-related services for surgical and nonsurgical conditions and usually provides some outpatient services, especially emergency care.[5]

Hospitals may be classified in numerous ways, including the following:

- Ownership
- Number of beds

- Length of stay
- Clinical classification
- Patients
- Organization

Recently, the **critical access hospital** (CAH) has evolved to meet the needs of a population that does not have adequate acute care facilities. A CAH is certified by the state as being necessary to the residents in the community or no hospital or other CAH is within 35 miles of the CAH. The CAH provides acute inpatient care, has no more than 25 beds, and has an annual average length of stay of 96 hours.[5]

Ownership

Hospitals are either government owned (federal, state, or local) or nongovernment owned (Figure 1-2). Government-owned hospitals are not for profit, whereas non-government-owned hospitals may be for profit or not for profit. Federally owned hospitals receive funding and administrative direction from the branch of the government that owns them. The federal government finances health care services and facilities for active and retired military

personnel, their dependents, veterans, merchant marines, Native Americans, Native Alaskans, and other groups. For some of these groups—for example, the merchant marines—the health care provided is contracted out, whereas other groups, such as the American Indians, have their own government-funded and operated health care facilities.

The Department of Veterans Affairs (VA) medical centers are federally owned health care facilities that provide health benefits to people who have served in the U.S. military. Eligibility for hospital care requires that the person have a service-related condition or disability or be unable to pay for health care. Currently the VA owns and operates 157 hospitals and more than 1300 sites that provide care including ambulatory care and community-based outpatient clinics, nursing homes, and rehabilitation treatment programs. The VA is organized into 21 Veterans Integrated Service Networks that oversee and manage the various VA health care facilities. The Department of Defense provides health care for active and retired military personnel and their dependents. The facilities owned and operated by the department include the Army, Navy, Air Force, and Marine Corps, all of which offer comprehensive health care either on military bases or in regional centers.[26]

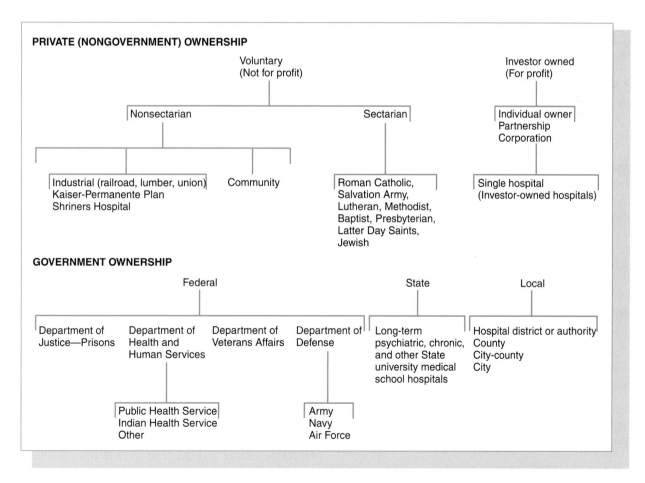

Figure 1-2 Classification of hospitals. (From Longest B Jr, Rakich JS, Darr K: *Managing health services organizations,* ed 4, Baltimore, 2000, Health Professions Press. Used by permission.)

Much like federally owned hospitals, state, county, and city hospitals are guided by the respective government, depending on the needs of the population served. State hospitals include facilities for mental illness, the developmentally disabled, chronic disease, and medical education. County, district, and city hospitals are usually established to meet the health care needs of their communities. These facilities are governed by locally elected officials.

Non-Government-Owned Hospitals. The two types of non-government-owned hospitals are as follows:

- For profit
- Not for profit

The for-profit hospitals, also called **proprietary,** private, or investor-owned hospitals, are governed by the individual, partnership, or corporation that owns them. The larger corporations may own numerous hospitals or hospital chains and offer stock that is publicly traded.

The not-for-profit (voluntary) hospitals include those that are owned by churches and religious orders (e.g., Catholic, Protestant) and those that are owned by industries, unions, and fraternal organizations or just community hospitals as on the Figure 1-2. The faith-based hospitals may incorporate aspects of the religion in their philosophy about care and leadership of the hospital. For example, Catholic hospitals may prohibit sterilization procedures performed for the purpose of birth control.

Bed Size (Bed Count)

The total number of inpatient beds with which the facility is equipped and staffed for patient admissions is its **bed size.** A facility is licensed by the state for a specific number of beds.

Length of Stay

The average length of stay for a hospital determines whether the hospital is classified as a short-term (acute) care facility or long-term care facility. If the average length of stay is less than 30 days, the hospital is classified as a short-term (or acute) care facility; if the average length of stay is 30 or more days, the hospital is classified as a long-term care facility.

Clinical Classification

According to the AHA, there are four major types of hospitals[5]:

- General
- Special
- Rehabilitation and chronic disease
- Psychiatric

Note that some references and literature classify rehabilitation and chronic disease hospitals and psychiatric hospitals as specialty hospitals.

General Hospital. The general hospital provides patient services, diagnostic and therapeutic, for various medical conditions. These services include the following[5]:

- Radiographic services
- Clinical laboratory services
- Operating room services

Specialty Hospital. The specialty hospital provides diagnostic and therapeutic services for patients with a specific medical condition. Many hospitals provide health care for specific groups of people, such as children (pediatric hospitals) or women (women's hospitals). In addition, specialty hospitals provide care for specific conditions or diseases, such as mental illness (psychiatric hospitals), cancer (cancer hospitals), or burns (burn hospitals).

Rehabilitation and Chronic Disease Hospital. The rehabilitation and chronic disease facility provides diagnostic and therapeutic services to patients who are disabled or handicapped and require restorative and adjustive services. Of vital importance in these facilities are the physical therapy, occupational therapy, speech therapy, and psychological and social work services that are provided.

Psychiatric Hospital. The primary purpose of the psychiatric hospital is to provide diagnostic and therapeutic services for patients with a mental illness or a psychiatric-related illness. The primary focus of the health care is to provide **behavioral health** services, which includes psychiatric, psychological, and social work services to the patient.

Hospital Patients

People who are receiving or using health care services for which the hospital is liable or held accountable are considered to be **hospital patients.** Hospital patients include inpatients, observation patients, ambulatory care patients, emergency patients, and newborn inpatients. To be considered a **hospital inpatient,** the patient generally stays overnight and is provided room, board, and nursing service in a unit or area of the hospital. All other types of hospital patients are discussed under the appropriate service areas.

Organization

The following discussion is typical of the traditional hospital setting for a general acute care facility. However, with health care reform, hospitals are undergoing quantum changes, including the formation of joint ventures and alliances and partnering with MCOs, physicians, and other HCOs. Hospitals operate under numerous organizational schemes; a few of these are described in this section.

Historically, most hospitals have been organized in a hierarchical form in which the individuals at the top have authority that passes downward through a chain of command (Figure 1-3). This vertical operation gives the governing body the ultimate authority, followed by the chief executive officer (CEO). The organization includes a governing body, administration, medical staff, department heads or directors, supervisors, and numerous subordinates down to the staff and line workers. Communication is fairly

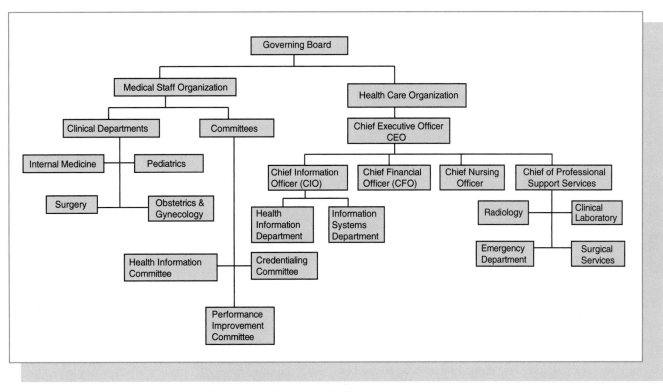

Figure 1-3 Health care facility organization chart.

restricted to the vertical. Physicians do not fall within the chain of command because they are not employees of the hospital.

The matrix organization is increasing in popularity because it is flexible and supports multidimensional organization. The matrix organization supports general managers who focus on managing people and processes as opposed to strategy and structure. As the health care system has grown to be very complex, it has become increasingly difficult for one person (i.e., CEO) to manage the organization effectively, so the matrix organization will have talented leaders who are focused on certain processes. The matrix organization gives way to horizontal, informal communications that embrace individual capabilities. Employees have dual responsibilities and may have two or more supervisors, but they have a shared vision that supports the organization as a whole.[27]

Another type of organizational scheme is product line management. With this model, the hospital may be organized around product line categories, such as obstetric, rehabilitation, and cardiology units, as opposed to departments, such as nursing, pharmacy, and respiratory therapy.

Composition and Structure

Although most hospitals today are forming alliances with other health care providers or are part of multihospital systems, the discussion of the organization is specific to the free-standing hospital. The organizational chart of a typical traditional hospital is shown in Figure 1-3.

The **governing body** or board, often called the board of trustees, board of governors, or board of directors, is a group of individuals who have the ultimate legal authority and responsibility for the operation of the hospital, including the quality and cost of care. The governing body of a voluntary (not-for-profit) hospital is usually composed of about 6 (for smaller hospitals) to 25 (for larger hospitals) board members who are not paid. Board membership is usually made up of influential business and community leaders who have a vested interest in their community and perhaps a skill that would be of value to the board. For example, a business executive can provide support for the business aspect, and an attorney would have a better understanding of the legal issues. The medical staff has the right to be represented on the governing board. The CEO, medical staff, and other insiders may be members of the governing board but may or may not have voting privileges; the nonvoting members are often referred to as **ex officio** members.

According to the The Joint Commission standards,[19] the hospital is required to do the following:

- Identify how it is governed and the key individuals involved
- Establish policy and promote performance improvement
- Provide for management and planning for the institution
- Adopt bylaws addressing legal accountability and responsibilities to patients served
- Provide for appropriate medical staff (see Chapter 13)

- Establish a criteria-based process for selecting a qualified and competent CEO
- Provide for compliance with applicable laws and regulations
- Provide for collaboration of leaders in developing, reviewing, and revising policies and procedures
- Provide for conflict resolution

The governing board functions according to bylaws established by the board, has regular meetings with documented minutes of the meetings, and has subcommittees that assist in the responsibilities of the governing board. The bylaws delineate the purposes of the organization, the composition and responsibilities of the board, meeting requirements, duties and responsibilities of officers and committees, selection of board members and officers, and revisions and amendments of the bylaws.

The governing board has standing committees and special committees. Standing committees may include the executive committee (conducts interim business), finance committee, medical staff, nominating committee, personnel, physician recruitment, and long-range planning. Special committees or task forces are created for specific projects or tasks and are disbanded on completion of the project or task.

The governing board has the ultimate responsibility for the quality of patient care and it depends on the HIM department to provide documentation to assist in and support decision making and long-range planning for the hospital. The JCAHO has identified numerous information processes for which the governing body and organizational leaders are responsible, including obtaining, managing, and using information to improve patient care, governance, management, and support processes.[19] The governing body and administration depend on the HIM department not only to perform these processes in a timely, accurate manner but also to ensure the accessibility, security, confidentiality, and integrity of the data in compliance with internal and external regulations.

Leadership

The makeup of the leadership differs from hospital to hospital, depending on the hospital's size and organizational scheme. The Joint Commission states that the primary role of the leadership is planning, directing, coordinating, providing, and improving health care that responds to community and patient needs and improves health care outcomes. Leadership may be composed of a wide variety of organizational leaders or only a few, some of whom are briefly described here.

Chief Executive Officer. The CEO, also called hospital administrator or president, is recruited and selected by the governing board. This person is the principal administrative official of the hospital or other health care facility. At one time, the CEO was responsible for the day-to-day operation of the hospital. Today, however, the CEO is not only concerned with the daily operations but must work closely with department heads, project managers, committees, and others to support the mission and achieve the goals of the health care facility.

The CEO serves as a liaison between the governing board and the medical staff. The Joint Commission standards stipulate that effective leadership of the hospital does the following[19]:

- Develops a strategic plan that supports the organization's mission, vision, and values
- Communicates the mission, vision, and plan throughout the organization
- Provides the framework to accomplish the goals that fulfill the vision

At least annually, the plan for providing patient care should be reviewed to determine whether it meets identified patient needs and is consistent with the hospital mission; the plan should be revised as appropriate. The HIM department is involved in the preparation of much of the documentation, especially the following[23]:

- Clinical information
- Accreditation standards
- Risk management
- Utilization review
- Quality of patient care

Chief Operating Officer. Large hospitals often have several chief operating officers (COOs), also called executive vice president, vice president, or associate administrator, who report directly to the CEO. The COO provides leadership, direction, and administration of operations in compliance with the mission and strategic plan of the organization. He or she oversees the operation of specific departments. For example, the COO may be responsible for coordinating hospital activities, such as ancillary or support services and other functional areas.

Chief Information Officer. The chief information officer holds an executive position with primary responsibility for information resources management in the organization. He or she is involved in strategic planning, management, design, integration, and implementation of health information systems. Health information systems embrace the financial, administrative, and clinical information needs of the health care facility or organization. In hospitals, the usual departments that report to the chief information officer are information systems, telecommunications, HIM, and management engineering.

Chief Financial Officer. The financial operations of a health care institution are under the direction of the chief financial officer (CFO), who is sometimes called director of finance or fiscal affairs director. Although the title may vary, this person is often a director or hospital vice president who reports directly to the CEO or some other level in the administration. The CEO and the CFO also report to a finance committee within the governing body of the hospital. The finance committee is an advisory group within the board that is responsible for reviewing the hospital's financial position and making fiscally related decisions. According to The Joint Commision, the board and the CEO are responsible for the control and use of all financial resources.[19] The daily financial operation, however, is usually delegated to the CFO.

The financial department of a health care institution, under the direction of the CFO, is responsible for functions such as accounting, inventory control, payroll, accounts payable and receivable, cash management, billing, credit and collections, budgeting, cost accounting, fund accounting, and internal control. The functions within the finance arena involve the recording and reporting of financial information, the management of cash and other hospital assets, and planning and control. The CFO has overall responsibility for these areas and acts as an adviser to the CEO and the governing board on both daily operational issues and plans for the future.

Medical Staff (Professional Staff Organization)

The medical staff is a formally organized staff of licensed physicians and other licensed providers as permitted by law (e.g., dentists, podiatrists, chiropractors) with the authority and responsibility to maintain proper standards of medical care. The medical staff is governed by its own bylaws, rules, and regulations, which must be approved by the hospital's governing board. The Joint Commission standards state that the primary responsibility of the medical staff is the quality of the professional services provided by the members with clinical privileges and the responsibility of being accountable to the governing body. **Clinical privileges** refer to the permission granted by the appropriate authority (governing board) to practitioners to provide well-defined patient care services in the granting institution on the basis of licensure, education, training, experience, competence, health status, and judgment. Each member of the medical staff has delineated clinical privileges that identify the specific patient care services the member may provide or perform independently in the hospital.[19]

The medical staff responsibilities include recommending to the governing board staff appointments and reappointments, credentialing, which is delineating clinical privileges (see Chapter 13), continuing medical education, and maintaining a high quality of patient care.

The organizational scheme of the medical staff includes officers, committees, and clinical services. The Joint Commission requires that there be an executive committee that is empowered to conduct medical staff business between staff meetings and that is responsible to the governing body. In smaller hospitals, the medical staff as a whole serves as the executive committee. The executive committee is composed of members of the medical staff and an ex officio member from administration, usually the CEO or the CEO's designee.

The members of the medical staff are organized into areas of clinical services and departments that are usually representative of the medical specialties. Each service or department has an appointed director, department head, or chairperson. The services that are common to most hospitals are internal medicine, surgery, anesthesiology, pediatrics, obstetrics and gynecology, psychiatry, neurology, radiology and diagnostic imaging, and pathology. These are briefly defined in Table 1-3.

Table 1-3   MEDICAL SPECIALTIES

Specialty	Description/Examples of Diagnoses and Procedures
Anesthesiology	Study and art of anesthesia administration, with and without loss of consciousness: epidural anesthesia, spinal anesthesia, inhalation of ether, analgesia maintenance
Cardiology	Study of cardiovascular system and treatment of its diseases: rheumatic heart disease, coronary artery disease, myocardial infarction, congestive heart failure
Cardiovascular surgery	Surgical specialty of the heart and blood vessels: coronary artery bypass graft, coronary arthrectomy, cardiac catheterization, coronary angioplasty
Dermatology	Study and treatment of skin and diseases/conditions of skin: basal cell carcinoma, exfoliative dermatitis, pityriasis rosea, biopsies/excisions of lesions, cellulitis, acne vulgaris
Endocrinology	Study and treatment of the endocrine glands: diabetes mellitus (types I and II), thyroiditis, Addison's disease, adrenal virilism
Family medicine	Medical specialty that provides continuing, comprehensive health care for individuals and families. It is a specialty in breadth that integrates the biological, clinical, and behavioral sciences. Scope of family medicine encompasses all ages, both sexes, each organ system, and every disease entity.
Gastroenterology	Study of digestive system and treatment of its disorders, including esophagus, stomach, intestines, liver, pancreas, and gallbladder, and ulcers, gastroenteritis, pylorospasm, gastritis, Crohn's disease

Continued

Table 1-3 MEDICAL SPECIALTIES—cont'd

Specialty	Description/Examples of Diagnoses and Procedures
Gynecology	Surgical specialty concerned with study of female reproductive and urinary systems and treatment of disorders: endometriosis, cystitis, herpes genitalia, mastitis, uterine prolapse, infertility
Hematology	Study and treatment of blood, blood-forming tissues, and blood disorders: anemias, leukemia, hemophilia, thrombocytopenic purpura, bone marrow biopsy
Infectious disease	Study and treatment of diseases caused by pathogenic micro-organisms, including contagious and noncontagious infections: AIDS, syphilis, tuberculosis, hepatitis, wound infections
Internal medicine	Study and treatment of disease of internal organs with nonsurgical therapy: hypertension, rheumatoid arthritis, meningitis
Nephrology	Study and treatment of kidney and its diseases: acute and chronic kidney failure, polycystic kidney disease, nephrolithiasis, pyelonephritis, glomerulonephritis
Neurology	Study and treatment of nervous system and its diseases: cerebral palsy, brain abscess, cerebrovascular attack, Alzheimer's disease, Parkinson's disease
Neurosurgery	Surgical specialty involving study of nervous system and treatment of disorders: hydrocephalus, meningomyelocele, brain abscess, carpal tunnel syndrome
Obstetrics	Surgical specialty concerned with management of pregnancy, including prenatal, perinatal, and postnatal stages: normal pregnancy, placenta previa, eclampsia, ectopic pregnancy, gestational diabetes
Oncology	Study and treatment of cancer, including benign and malignant: melanoma, squamous cell carcinoma, multiple myeloma, Hodgkin's disease, leukemia
Ophthalmology	Surgical specialty concerned with study of eye and treatment of visual problems: cataracts, corneal transplant, diabetic retinopathy, visual acuity, optic nerve damage
Orthopedics	Surgical specialty dealing with musculoskeletal system, including prevention of disorders and restoration of function: arthritis, fractures, scoliosis, joint replacements, osteomyelitis
Otorhinolaryngology	Surgical specialty dealing with study and treatment of disorders of ears, nose, and throat: acute tracheitis, tonsillectomy and adenoidectomy, sinusitis, otitis media, deviated nasal septum
Pediatrics	Study and care of children, including normal growth and development: chickenpox, cystic fibrosis, pneumonia, immunizations, diarrhea, gastritis, mumps
Plastic and reconstructive surgery	Surgical specialty concerned with repair, restoration, and reconstruction of body structures: blepharoplasty, scar revision, liposuction, breast reduction and reconstruction, dermabrasion
Psychiatry	Study, diagnosis, and treatment of mental illness: anorexia nervosa, clinical depression, alcohol withdrawal syndrome, senile dementia
Pulmonary medicine	Study, diagnosis, and treatment of lung disorders: pneumonia, chronic obstructive pulmonary disease, asthma, cystic fibrosis, bronchiectasis, respiratory failure
Radiology	Use of radiant energy in study, diagnosis, and treatment of disease: computed tomography, radiography, echocardiography, magnetic resonance imaging, radiation therapy
Thoracic surgery	Surgical specialty dealing with study and treatment of thorax and its disorders: pneumonectomy, diaphragmatic hernia, lung abscess, thoracotomy, bronchial lavage
Urology	Surgical specialty concerned with study and treatment of male genitourinary system and female urinary system: vasectomy, nephrolithiasis, benign prostatic hyperplasia, transurethral resection of prostate

Essential Services

The Joint Commission identifies hospital services that must be provided on a regular basis and that are necessary for patient assessment and care. **Patient assessment** is the process of obtaining appropriate and necessary information about each individual seeking entry into a health care setting or service. The following services are essential to this function.[19]

Nursing Care. The nursing service is usually organized under the direction of a nurse executive (director, vice president), with nursing supervisors, department heads, charge nurses, and staff nurses. The nurse executive has the responsibility and authority to establish nursing standards, policies, and procedures that are in compliance with state law and professional standards.[28]

Within an HCO, there are different levels of nursing, including staff nurse, nurse manager, clinical nurse specialist, and private duty nurse. The staff nurse provides direct patient care in a specific unit with assigned patients. For example, a registered nurse (RN) or a licensed practical nurse (LPN) may be the staff nurse assigned to five patients in the well-baby nursery during the evening shift. The nurse manager may be a head nurse, nursing supervisor, or department head who is responsible for certain units or staff. This person makes patient assignments and staffing decisions and is responsible for the quality of care provided by the nursing staff. The clinical nurse specialist is considered an expert in a specialized area, such as neonatology or pain management. This person is an RN with advanced education or experience in the area of expertise. The clinical nurse specialist also works in research, education, administration, and consultation.[20] The private duty nurse is an RN or LPN who is employed by an external agency or individual to provide direct patient care to one patient for 8 to 12 hours over a period of time.

Some facilities may employ nursing assistants who, depending on the work environment, are known by many different names, including certified nursing assistants (CNAs), patient care technicians, nurses aides, orderlies, and home health aides. The nursing assistants are eligible for certification that involves approximately 2 weeks of training and clinical experience and, on completion and examination, they become certified nursing assistants.[29] Nursing assistants work under the supervision of a nurse and they provide basic patient care, such as assisting the patient with bathing, dressing, and eating and obtaining vital signs.

Nursing care is based on a process that involves assessment, diagnosis, outcomes and planning, implementation, and evaluation of patient care, and the documentation in the health record must reflect this process. The HIM department often collaborates with the nursing service in collecting, analyzing, and disseminating data; in developing reports; and in addressing issues related to the health record. Issues of critical importance are the authenticity, completeness, timeliness, integrity, and security of both the paper and the electronic health record.

Diagnostic Radiology Services. The diagnostic radiology department (medical imaging department) functions in the diagnosing of diseases and conditions by using ionizing radiation (e.g., radiography, computed tomography, radioactive isotopes), ultrasonography, and magnetic resonance imaging. The Joint Commission requires health care facilities to provide diagnostic testing, including imaging, that is relevant both to determining the patient's health care needs and to the treatment of the patient.[19] An example of a diagnostic radiology procedure is mammography (breast radiography), which maybe performed for the purpose of diagnosing breast cancers; an example of a therapeutic procedure is radiation therapy, which is performed for the purpose of treating malignant neoplasms (cancers).

The radiology department is headed by a radiologist (a physician), who may be called the chief or director of radiology. Under the direction of the radiologist is the technical staff, which includes physicians (radiation therapists, radiation physicists), radiology technologists, and radiation therapy technologists. Radiation therapy is often a separate department as well.

Nuclear Medicine. Nuclear medicine may be considered part of the radiology department or it may be a separate department. It is distinguished from radiology, however, because the procedures involve the use of radioisotopes (radionuclides) for diagnosing and treating the patient. Unlike that in radiography, the image created in nuclear medicine gives information not only about the structure but also about the function of the organ or tissue under study. Examples of diagnostic procedures performed in nuclear medicine are nuclear scans of the thyroid, heart, and liver and radioimmunoassays, which are used to detect hormones and drugs in blood samples.

The staff in nuclear medicine, which is under the direction of a physician who specializes in nuclear medicine, includes nuclear medicine technicians or staff from the radiology department.

Dietary (Nutrition) Services. The dietetic service considers all nutritional aspects of the patient and patient care and provides high-quality nutrition to every patient. According to The Joint Commission, nutritional care must be provided in a timely and effective manner. Such care consists of nutritional assessment; nutritional therapy; diet preparation, distribution, or administration; nutritional education; and monitoring of the nutritional care of patients.[19]

Nutritional care is interdisciplinary and, therefore, involves not only dietetic services but also other members of the health care team, such as physicians and nurses. Dietetic services employ clinical dietitians, who are responsible for the therapeutic care of patients. Additional dietary staff is employed to assist with the preparation, serving, and delivery of food and the maintenance of dining services for the staff and visitors.

Pathology and Clinical Laboratory Services. This ancillary area assists in the prevention, diagnosis, and treatment of disease by examination and study of tissue specimens, blood and body secretions, and wound scrapings and drainage. The pathology and clinical laboratory department functions in serology, histology, cytology, bacteriology, hematology, blood bank, organ bank, biochemistry, and tissue preparation. These departments are commonly subunits of the pathology department.

Pathology and clinical laboratory services employ a variety of health professionals—medical laboratory technologist, medical laboratory technician, histotechnologist, and cytotechnologist—all of whom work under the direction of a pathologist.

Emergency Services. Emergency care service is a vital component of the acute care facility that provides care around the clock to patients that present with conditions that are urgent, life-threatening, or potentially disabling. The **emergency department** (ED) functional areas include a trauma area, a casting room, examination rooms, and observation beds. A patient in the ED can be managed in one of the following ways: treated and discharged to home, treated and admitted for observation, treated and admitted to an inpatient unit, assessed and sent to surgery, stabilized and transferred to another facility, or, in the event of death, transferred to the morgue. Emergency services are primarily provided by physicians and RNs who specialize in emergency medicine.

In the ED, the patient has usually had the acute onset of a serious condition, such as a myocardial infarction (heart attack) or closed head injury, or has a complication of a chronic condition, such as ketoacidosis, which may occur with diabetes mellitus. When the patient arrives, the ED staff performs triage. The term triage is a French word originating from care on battlefields, where quick decisions had to be made regarding who could wait for care, who needed immediate care, and who was beyond benefiting from care. In the ED, **triage** is the process of sorting out for the purpose of early assessment to determine the urgency and priority for care and to determine the appropriate source of care. Triage promotes efficiency and effectiveness in the management of the diverse patient group arriving in the ED.[30]

In the United States, emergency patients are a diverse group because the need for care may range from relatively minor to serious, urgent, or life threatening. People who do not have access to health care often use the ED for nonemergency problems. The inability to access health care may be due to numerous factors, such as an inability to pay, being either underinsured or uninsured, or not having a health care provider available in the area or at the time of need. In some areas urgent care centers are not available and patients use the ED for minor health problems.

In the United States, trauma is the leading cause of death in the 34 years or younger age group, and many of those deaths occur in EDs that are not recognized as trauma centers. To minimize the morbidity and mortality rate related to trauma, trauma centers were developed. **Morbidity** refers to the extent of illness, injury, or disability in a given population, and **mortality** means the death rate in a given population. A **trauma center** is an emergency care center that is specially staffed and equipped to handle trauma patients; most trauma centers are equipped with an air transport system. EDs are accredited by the American College of Surgeons and accredited EDs are determined to meet the Standards for Trauma Center Accreditation according to the level of emergency care, I through IV, that they are capable of providing. The designated level of care is crucial to the decision making of emergency personnel (paramedics, emergency medical technicians) in determining which facility is best suited to handle the health care needs of the transported patient. The assigned level of care is based on the center's hours of operation; availability of physicians, nurses, and other trained staff; and access to laboratory, radiology, surgery, anesthesia, equipment, and drugs. Emergency centers ranked as level I offer the most comprehensive emergency care 24 hours a day, with at least one emergency care physician on duty and access to various specialists. Level II and level III emergency services are also staffed 24 hours a day but have more lenient requirements for the availability of specialty physicians and nurses. Level IV centers are not required to operate all hours of the day but must be prepared to render life-saving care and make referrals to appropriate centers for additional medical services. EDs that are accredited to provide level I or II care are recognized as trauma centers.[30]

Pharmaceutical Service. The pharmaceutical service is responsible for maintaining an adequate supply of medications, providing nursing units with floor stock, and preparing and dispensing medications with appropriate documentation. The pharmacist also prepares the intravenous fluids with any necessary additives and monitors adverse effects of drugs. Floor stock is an inventory of drugs that is maintained on each nursing unit; the stock varies in each unit, depending on the type of unit (e.g., cardiac intensive care versus a pediatric unit). The pharmaceutical service will maintain a **hospital formulary** that provides information on drugs that are approved and maintained by the HCO. The hospital formulary contains information on drugs including, but not limited to, names, dosages and strengths, packaging, characteristics, and clinical usage.

The pharmaceutical service is under the direction of a state-licensed pharmacist, who is assisted by pharmaceutical technicians.

Physical Rehabilitation Services. The diagnosis and treatment of certain musculoskeletal and neuromuscular diseases and conditions are responsibilities of physical medicine and rehabilitation. This area covers physical therapy, occupational therapy, speech therapy, and audiology. Physical therapists are state licensed and trained to use light, heat, cold, water, ultrasound, electricity, and manual manipulation to improve or correct a musculoskeletal or neuromuscular problem. They often teach the patient exercises that will help to strengthen specific muscle groups or assist the patient to ambulate (walk) with an artificial limb. Occupational therapists work with the patient to minimize disability and teach the patient to compensate for the disability. For example, a patient who is permanently confined to a wheelchair and needs to resume housekeeping responsibilities may be taught how to shop for groceries or how to prepare a meal. Speech pathologists are concerned with human communication; they teach the patient how to compensate for difficulty with speech or the inability to speak. For example, a patient who stutters is taught speech exercises to help control or minimize the stuttering. Audiology is the science of hearing, and an audiologist would examine, evaluate, and prescribe therapy to patients with a hearing deficit.

Respiratory Care Services. Respiratory care services encompass diagnostic and therapeutic procedures for a wide variety of patients. The service is responsible for assisting with the provision of care for patients with various acute and chronic lung conditions. Responsibilities include administering oxygen, performing pulmonary function studies, administering inhalants such as bronchodilators, performing chest physiotherapy, obtaining and analyzing arterial blood gases, setting up and maintaining mechanical ventilators, and assisting in cardiopulmonary resuscitation. These therapists work under the direct order of a physician and provide respiratory care in all patient care areas of the hospital, as necessary.

Social Services. The department of social services is staffed by medical and psychiatric social workers who work with the patient and family members to help them understand the social, economic, and emotional factors related to therapy and recovery; identify and coordinate necessary community and medical care resources; and collaborate with and educate the hospital staff regarding social service concerns. Social workers are often responsible for discharge planning, thereby supporting the continuum of care.

Other Services. Information on additional hospital services, such as pastoral care, ethics, patient representatives, patient escort, plant technology and safety management, and central supply, may be obtained by surveying area health care facilities.

Health Information Management

Although this book is devoted to HIM, a brief discussion is included to round out the functions of the hospital. The HIM department, or medical records department, is primarily responsible for the management of all paper and electronic patient information. It must develop and maintain an information system that is consistent with the mission of the health care facility and in compliance with regulatory and accrediting agencies. The department is responsible for the organization, maintenance, production, and dissemination of information, including privacy, data security, integrity, and access. Some of the functions of the department include clinical data management, transcription of medical and surgical notes, coding of diagnoses and surgical procedures, disclosing health information to authorized users, and retrieving and storing medical information. With the technological advances in information management, the increased demands for patient data, and

the push for cost containment, efficiency, and accessibility of health care, the area of HIM is rapidly evolving and growing. As we move toward the electronic health record, new opportunities and challenges will evolve and many of the roles and functions will change. HIM is discussed in detail in Chapter 2.

Subacute Care

Subacute care is a transitional level of care that may be necessary immediately after the initial phase of an acute illness. It is more commonly used with patients who have been hospitalized and are not yet ready for return to the long-term care facility or to home care. The patient does require more advanced or specialized nursing care than is normally provided in the nursing facility or in home health programs. The location of subacute care may be a designated area of either the hospital or a nursing facility or may be provided by a home health agency.

Home Care (Home Health Care)

Home health care is the provision of medical and non-medical care in the home or place of residence to promote, maintain, or restore health or to minimize the effect of disease or disability.[3] With the exception of hospice, the location of the health care services distinguishes home health from other types of care facilities and programs. Home care services mainly provide care for rehabilitation therapies and postacute care. Home health services are a medical adjunct to acute care, which extends the continuum of care from the inpatient to the home setting.

The patient population for home health care is dominated by elderly people, although nonelderly adults and children use the service. Home health care for the elderly population is viewed as achieving cost savings compared with longer hospital stays or long-term care. It is also life enriching because it enables patients to remain in the comfort of their homes.

Home health has grown rapidly since 1965, when the Medicare program was established and allowed reimbursement for home care. The Medicare definition of home health care stipulates that the needed nursing care, physical therapy, or speech therapy must be skilled intermittent care provided under a physician's written direction and plan of care in the residence of the homebound client.[31] Simply put, Medicare requires that the home care provided be physician directed and that it involve regularly scheduled home visits. For example, a home care patient who is receiving oxygen therapy may be initially visited four times a week for 1 week by an RN. One of the goals of therapy is to have the patient or family assume responsibility for care, with visits by the RN being reduced to once or twice a week. On the other hand, if the patient is living alone and needs assistance with self-care, then a nurse's aide, in addition to the RN, may visit every other day to assist with personal care.

Long-Term Care Facilities

Long-term care is health care that is provided over a long period of time (30 or more days) to patients who have chronic diseases or disabilities. The facilities providing the long-term care are considered to be nonacute care facilities. The type of care a patient can receive is highly variable and ranges from personal care and social, recreational, and dietary services to skilled nursing or rehabilitation care.[5] Patients admitted to long-term care facilities are usually called residents because the patient resides in the facility. The term nursing home is a layperson's term for any and all long-term care facilities; the appropriate term is skilled **nursing facility.**

Skilled nursing facilities are required by law to employ sufficient nursing personnel on a 24-hour basis to provide care to each resident according to the care plan.[5] Among other things, nursing facilities are required to provide skilled nursing care and related services for patients who require medical, nursing, or rehabilitative care. Examples of skilled nursing facility care include wound care, intravenous injections, and physical or speech therapy. The need for custodial care (i.e., assistance with bathing, eating, and dressing) does not qualify the patient for Medicare coverage in a skilled nursing facility. However, Medicare will cover these services along with the activities of daily living for patients requiring skilled nursing care or rehabilitative services.[32]

To be certified as a Medicare or Medicaid provider, a nursing facility must comply with the *Conditions of Participation.* A long-term care facility is licensed by the state to provide a designated level of care, which may simply be personal care or room and board or may require skilled nursing. A facility may be licensed to provide different levels of care; if so, the number of beds for each level of care is designated.

The patient population in long-term care facilities is primarily elderly people who are unable to live independently, but it also includes people of all ages who are convalescing or being rehabilitated or who have a chronic condition that requires long-term health care services (e.g., Alzheimer's disease, senile dementia).

There are several types of long-term care facilities.

Assisted Living. An **assisted living** facility typically offers housing and board with a broad range of personal and supportive care services.

Domiciliary or Custodial (Residential). Supervision, room, and board are provided for people who are unable to live independently. Most residents need assistance with activities of daily living (e.g., bathing, eating, dressing).

Independent Living Facility. An independent living facility is composed of apartments and condominiums that allow residents to live independently; assistance (e.g., dietary, health care, social services) is available as needed by residents.

Life Care Centers. Also called retirement communities, **life care centers** provide living accommodations and meals for a monthly fee. They offer a variety of services, including housekeeping, recreation, health care, laundry, and exercise programs.

Nursing Facility. This is a comprehensive term for a long-term care facility that provides nursing care and related services for residents who require medical, nursing, or rehabilitative care. A sufficient number of skilled nursing personnel must be employed on a 24-hour basis to provide care to residents according to the care plan.

Swing Beds. Hospital **swing beds** are designated beds that have the flexibility of serving as acute care or postacute long-term beds. Certain small, rural hospitals or CAHs that are Medicare certified are allowed to have swing beds for acute or skilled nursing facility health care. Among other things, the patient using the swing bed for postacute care must have been an inpatient in an acute care facility for 3 consecutive days and on discharge is admitted to the swing bed hospital for posthospital extended care. The costs for the posthospital extended care are covered by Medicare Part A. The concept of swing beds was established by the Social Security Act.

Hospice Care

The concept of hospice, meaning "given to hospitality," dates back to the medieval period, when weary travelers were provided a place for shelter and rest. Today, a **hospice** is a multidisciplinary health care program that is responsible for the palliative and supportive care of terminally ill patients and their families, with consideration for their physical, spiritual, social, and economic needs. **Palliative care** consists of health care services that relieve or alleviate patient symptoms and discomforts, such as pain and nausea; it is not curative. The primary goal of a hospice is to allow patients to die with dignity in their homes or a homelike environment. Most hospice patients have cancer, but many hospices accept other terminally ill patients, such as those with AIDS or end-stage kidney, heart, or lung disease.[12]

The type of program that is suitable often depends on the patient's condition and the support available in the patient's home (Table 1-4). For the patient who remains in the home, most hospices require that a primary caregiver be identified who will assist with care; the primary caregiver may be a spouse, family member, friend, or live-in companion. Other hospice programs, such as skilled nursing facilities, may have units or beds for hospice patients who are unable to remain in their homes. Hospice patients may require hospitalization for acute symptom management (pain, vomiting, infection) or when the primary care person needs a respite or break.

Hospice programs are physician directed and multidisciplinary in that numerous caregivers are involved in providing care. Caregivers for hospice include nurses, social workers, nurse's aides, clergy, dietitians, and trained volunteers,

Table 1-4   MODELS OF HOSPICE CARE

Type	Description
Home health agency–based	Owned and operated by private, free-standing home health agencies; care provided in home
Hospital-based	Owned and operated by hospital: rooms/departments allotted for hospice care; care provided in facility or home
Independent community-based	Usually nonprofit; governed by community board, independent; care provided in home
Nursing facility–based	Owned and operated by a nursing facility; rooms/units allotted for hospice care; care provided in facility
Other models	Owned by religious orders, HMOs, combinations of the above models

who run errands, mow grass, do housekeeping chores, cook, and perform other necessary jobs that allow the patient to remain in the home.

Reimbursement for hospice care comes from Medicare, Medicaid, private pay, third-party payers, community funds, and other sources.

Respite Care

Respite care is a type of short-term care in which the focus of care is on giving caregivers time off and yet continue the care of the patient. This may involve someone spending the day with the patient in the home, admitting the patient to an adult or child day care, or providing temporary institutionalization. Respite care is often provided to caregivers of terminally ill patients or severely disabled children or adults.

Complementary and Alternative Medicine

Complementary and alternative medicine (CAM) refers to therapies (usually not included in Western medicine) that may or may not have been proven to be effective. Complementary medicine includes those practices that could be used along with conventional therapies. For example, aromatherapy might be used to relax a patient after a surgical procedure, whereas **alternative medicine** consists of those practices that would be used in lieu of conventional medicine. For example, patients may choose to use dietary supplements of soy protein to lower blood cholesterol as opposed to the cholesterol-lowering medications whose efficacies have been proven. The CAM therapies include

herbal remedies, massage therapy, natural food diets, acupuncture, and biofeedback. The National Institutes of Health established the National Center for Complementary and Alternative Medicine to explore the science, train researchers, and disseminate authoritative information to the public and professionals regarding CAM.[33]

E-Health

E-health is the use of emerging information and communication technology, especially the Internet, to improve or enable health and health care. The field of e-health includes a range of functions and capabilities such as specialized search engines focused on various kinds of health care; provider and payer Web sites, some of which give consumers access to their own information or the ability to communicate with the provider, make appointments, or renew prescriptions; support groups; Web-based physician consultations; self-care or monitoring systems; telemedicine; and disease management. As with other Internet-related sectors, the status of the e-health arena is extremely fluid and characterized by rapid developments in the commercial and noncommercial sectors.

Adult Day Care Services

An adult day care service is a health care program that provides supervision, medical and psychological care, and social activities for older adults (referred to as **clients**) who reside at home. These clients either cannot stay alone or prefer the social interaction during the day. Services provided may include intake assessment, health monitoring, occupational therapy, personal care, activities, transportation, and meals.[5]

Mobile Diagnostic Services

A growing trend is to transport health care services to the patient, especially in the area of diagnostic procedures and preventive services. Mammography and magnetic resonance imaging require expensive equipment that may not be available in small communities and rural areas. Mobile units from larger health care facilities are now transporting this advanced equipment and staff to these areas. Preventive services such as immunizations, blood pressure measurement, and cholesterol screening are easily provided from mobile units, which may even be staffed by volunteer health professionals.

Contract Services

The use of contract services, also called **outsourcing,** by HCOs is increasing. Contract services may include food, laundry, housekeeping, medical waste disposal, release of information services, transcription, coding, collections, and clinical services such as physical therapy, emergency care, and speech pathology. With the increase in the use of contract services, providers are expecting improved quality with cost containment.

Integrated Delivery Systems

In recent years **integrated delivery systems** (IDS), which involve various ownerships and linkages among hospitals, physicians, and insurers, have evolved. An IDS is a **vertical integration** of HCOs, defined as a network of health care organizations that provide or arrange to provide a continuum of services to a population; the network assumes the clinical and fiscal responsibility for the outcomes and health status of the population.[12] The IDS may include an acute care facility, a subacute care facility, a long-term care facility, a pediatric hospital, a rehabilitation facility, a psychiatric hospital, and numerous physicians and may provide mobile diagnostic services. The IDS is formed for the purpose of (1) providing more cost-effective care than an array of HCOs, (2) contracting with providers who take responsibility for the quality of care and provide the care in a cost-effective manner, and (3) protecting the autonomy of participating providers. By participating in an IDS, providers have input into how the IDS is run and get more patient referrals.

Although the IDS is a vertical integration, a merging of HCOs offering services at the same point on the continuum of care is a **horizontal integration**.[12] For example, an acute care hospital may join with another hospital that provides similar services but to a different population and/or at a different location.

HEALTH CARE PROFESSIONALS

The health care systems in the United States are labor intensive, using large numbers of highly skilled health care professionals and practitioners. There are more than 200 different health occupations in the United States. The places of employment are just as varied, including hospitals, medical offices, insurance companies, nursing facilities, pharmacies, MCOs, schools, correctional facilities, and pharmaceutical and medical supply companies.

Wilson and Neuhauser[34] define health care professionals as having the following attributes:

- Certification or licensure is required for membership in the profession.
- A national or regional professional association exists.
- A defined body of scientific knowledge and certain technical skills are required for practice.
- A code of ethics exists.
- Members of the profession practice with a degree of authority and have expertise for decision making in their area of competence.

Health Care Team

Almost all health care is provided by a multidisciplinary team of professionals. Being a member of the health care team requires that each person be responsible for his or her area of expertise with consideration for the contributions of other team members. The ultimate goal is comprehensive care for the patient as a whole. The health care team is composed of individuals who work either directly or indirectly to accomplish the goals of patient care. A physician directs the health care team by determining the plan of care, with team members complementing and supplementing each other's contributions. The makeup of the team depends on the patient's needs, the setting for health care, and the physician. For example, the health care team for a patient who is a resident in a long-term care facility consists of a primary care physician (perhaps a gerontologist), nursing staff (RN, LPN), a dietitian, a physical therapist, a recreation therapist, a nursing assistant, and a pharmacist. A patient in this setting is not likely to need a nurse anesthetist or surgeon.

Terms such as technologist, technician, therapist, paraprofessional, assistant, and aide are often used to describe certain health care providers. Technologist and therapist imply education at or above the bachelor degree level; technician and assistant indicate education or training at or above the associate degree level; and assistant and aide refer to on-the-job training.

Most health care occupations can be classified into one of the following categories:

- Independent practitioner
- Dependent practitioner
- Supporting staff

The independent practitioner category includes those who by law may provide a range of services without the consent or approval of a third party. The dependent practitioner category includes those who by law may deliver a limited range of services (often specified by law) under the supervision or authorization of the independent practitioner. Some health occupations may move from one category to another, depending on state law; for example, nurse practitioner and nurse midwife may be in either the dependent or the independent category on the basis of responsibilities and place of employment. The term midlevel practitioner refers to individuals, other than physicians, dentists, or podiatrists, who can dispense controlled substances within their professional practice. The midlevel practitioner is a dependent practitioner who may be a nurse midwife, nurse anesthetist, or physician assistant, among others. The third category is the supporting staff, who function under the supervision or authorization of independent or dependent practitioners.[7] A fourth category that must be identified is the noncaregiving group, which includes all people who have no direct patient contact yet make significant contributions to the healthcare systems. Examples of the various groups are shown in Table 1-5.

Table 1–5 EXAMPLES OF HEALTH CARE PROFESSIONALS

Health Professional and Credentialing Process/Examples	Brief Description
Cytotechnologist Certification: CT (ASCP)	Assists pathologists in microscopic examination of cellular samples to diagnose infectious disease, cancers, and other conditions and identify micro-organisms; employed in pathology departments of hospitals, private or research laboratories
Emergency Medical Technician–Paramedic National Registration and in some states, licensure: NREMT-P	Works under direction of physician, providing basic and advanced life support to patients including emergency drug administration, intravenous fluid therapy, electrocardiogram interpretation, and assisted ventilation; employed in fire and police departments, ambulance services, hospitals, emergency clinics
Medical Assistant Certification: CMA, CMA-C, CMA-A	Multiskilled person who assists in clinical or administrative areas of ambulatory care; works under supervision of physician
Medical Laboratory Technician or Clinical Laboratory Technician Certification by American Society of Clinical Pathologists or National Certifying Agency: MLT (ASCP), CLT (NCA)	Performs laboratory procedures on blood and other specimens for diagnostic and therapeutic purposes; works in hospital laboratories, physician offices, and reference/independent laboratories
Health Information Administrator Registration: RHIA	Designs and maintains health information systems to collect, assess, and disseminate health care data; employed in management/administrative positions in HCOs
Medical Technologist or Clinical Laboratory Scientist Certification or registration: MT (ASCP), CLS (NCA)	Responsible for analyzing body fluids, tissues, cells and other specimens to assist in detection, diagnosis, and management of disease; employed in hospital laboratories, physician offices, and reference/independent laboratories
Nuclear Medicine Technologist Certification and/or registration: CNMT, RT (N)	Performs imaging procedures using radionuclides for diagnostic, therapeutic, and investigative purposes; works in hospitals, public health, research laboratories, manufacturing companies
Occupational Therapy Assistant Certification and in some states, licensure: COTA	Works under direction of occupational therapist; assists with assessment and treatment of patients with physical, developmental, or psychological deficits; employed in hospitals, clinics, rehabilitation and long-term care facilities
Occupational Therapist Certification and in some states, licensure: OTR-L	Provides assessment and intervention to minimize physical, developmental, or psychological deficits that restrict activities of daily living and employment; employed in hospitals, rehabilitation and long-term care facilities, clinics
Physical therapist Licensure: RPT	Uses heat, cold, exercises, electricity, manipulation, and ultraviolet radiation in restoration of function, prevention of disability, and management of musculoskeletal pain after injury or disease; works in hospitals, private offices, nursing homes and community health centers
Radiographer Registration: RT(R)	Produces and processes x-ray films, including specialized procedures such as angiography and mammography used in prevention, diagnosis, and management of disease, injury, or anomaly; employed in hospitals, ambulatory care, independent/ reference laboratories

Physicians

The primary leader of the traditional health care team is most often the physician; some exceptions to this are the independent practices of nurse practitioners, podiatrists, chiropractors, optometrists, and nurse midwives. A physician is qualified by formal education and legal authority through licensure to practice medicine. Typically, physicians have practiced medicine by using clinical guidelines and policies that were primarily derived from expert opinion and clinical judgment. Today there is a trend toward physicians using **evidence-based medicine** to make medical decisions, which means that the guidelines or medical decision making is supported by research.[3]

Types. There are two types of physicians: Doctor of Medicine (MD) and Doctor of Osteopathic Medicine (DO). Both types of physicians are licensed by each state as medical practitioners who may diagnose, provide treatment, perform surgery, and prescribe medication. They both complete 4 years of medical education, a supervised internship/ residency program, and state licensing examinations. The DO practices comprehensive medicine that uses manipulative therapy along with more traditional forms of therapy.

Medical Education and Training. The framework for medical education as we know it today dates back to 1910, when Abraham Flexner published a report that identified numerous serious deficiencies and inconsistencies in medical education. As a result of this report, most medical schools follow the Flexner model.

Today, admission to medical school requires 3 to 4 years of undergraduate work in the sciences and a competitive score on the Medical College Admission Test (MCAT). Medical school (undergraduate medical education) consists of medical science courses and clinical experience. The medical degree is awarded on completion of medical school. However, a person must still pass an examination to obtain a state license to practice medicine.

Licensure. The Federation Licensing Examination (FLEX) is a standardized licensure test developed by the Federation of State Medical Boards of the United States in 1968. The scores for successful completion vary from state to state.

An alternative to the FLEX is an examination developed by the National Board of Medical Examiners. The Board is dedicated to preparing and administering high-quality examinations for state licensure, collaborating with the state licensing boards in achieving goals of quality, supporting quality in medical education, and developing and evaluating testing methods, medical knowledge, and competence. The three-part NBME examination allows the student to be tested at intervals during training. After passing the NBME or the FLEX examination and completing 1 year of residency, a medical physician may apply for state licensure, which authorizes him or her to practice medicine.

After graduation from medical school, the physician may complete a residency that consists of several years of training in a teaching hospital; during residency, the physician works under the supervision of licensed physicians. The residency program is considered to be graduate medical education. Depending on the chosen specialty, the residency may vary from 3 to 7 years. Because of the large numbers of physicians who require a residency program, a National Residency Matching Program was established to match applicants with hospital preferences, much like a clearinghouse for the residency program. The hospital residency programs are accredited by the Accreditation Council on Graduate Medical Education, which is composed of representatives from the public, residents, federal government, and professional organi-zations, including the AMA, AHA, and American Board of Medical Specialties.

Although there is an increasing demand for generalists (i.e., family practitioners, internists), many physicians seek certification in a specialty area. There are many specialties and subspecialties in the practice of medicine, such as neurology, hematology, oncology, cardiology, and pediatrics. Examples of surgical specialties and subspecialties are orthopedics, obstetrics, gynecology, and neurosurgery. To become board certified, the physician must meet certain requirements established by the Board of Certification, which is under the jurisdiction of the specialty. For example, to become board certified, surgeons must demonstrate additional training time and proven competence and complete rigorous examination. In addition, physicians who are accepted for a fellowship at a specialty college are highly respected by the medical profession in their area of expertise.

Physician Assistant

The physician assistant (PA) is a midlevel practitioner trained to assist the physician in various capacities, including evaluating, monitoring, and diagnosing patients. In addition, PAs may perform routine therapeutic procedures, counsel, and refer patients as necessary. Some states grant the PA prescriptive authority. Most PAs are employed in primary care and have proved to be cost-effective.

A surgeon assistant is a PA who has specialized in surgery. In addition to assisting the surgeon during operative procedures, the surgeon assistant performs other health care services including physical assessments and patient education.

Nursing

In the United States, nursing is the single largest health care profession; as of 2003, there were more than 2.6 million RNs employed in the United States.[28] They are employed in a wide variety of facilities, including hospitals, physician offices, patient homes, schools, camps, occupational and industrial settings, public health facilities, and private practice. Therefore, it is important for the HIM professional to have a good understanding of the roles and respon-sibilities of the nurse in health care systems.

Professional nursing is defined by the American Nurses Association (ANA) as having the follow six elements[28]:

- Facilitating health and healing through a caring relationship
- Attention to the human experiences and responses to health and illness
- Integrating objective data with knowledge gained from the patient or group's subjective experience
- Applying scientific knowledge to the processes of diagnosis and treatment
- Advancing professional nursing knowledge through scholarly inquiry and
- Influencing social and public policy to promote social justice.

Nursing practice includes but is not limited to clinical practice, administration, education, research, consultation, and management. Nursing care standards have been developed by professional organizations, such as the ANA; the standards address policies, procedures, and written mechanisms. Although nursing care is integrated and provided throughout various settings, nursing practice itself is regulated by the individual states as stipulated by the Nurse Practice Act of each state.

Nursing Care Models

Nursing care may be provided by different models, including primary nursing, patient-focused care, and team nursing. The term primary implies that one nurse is responsible for the management of care for each assigned patient. With primary nursing, the RN is responsible for the entire patient stay, 24 hours a day. The RN develops a written plan of care for each patient assignment. All other nurses who are providing care to this patient follow, update, and revise the plan of care as necessary.

Types and Education. The major types of nursing are registered nursing and licensed practical nursing (sometimes called licensed vocational nursing). Table 1-6 outlines the education and training of nurses and their various roles and responsibilities. To practice as an RN, one must graduate from a state-approved school of nursing and pass a state licensing examination.

Specialties. In addition to the various educational levels of nursing, many specialties and subspecialties are available, including the following:

- Certified nurse midwife—An RN who has completed advanced training in a program accredited by the American College of Nurse-Midwives and who is certified as a nurse midwife. The primary focus of health care is on well-woman gynecologic and low-risk obstetric care, including prenatal, labor and delivery, and postpartum care.[35]
- Certified registered nurse anesthetist—An RN with specialized training in the administration and control of anesthesia and in the evaluation and management of a patient's physiology during the preoperative, operative, and postoperative periods. Requirements for practice include completion of a master's degree in a nurse anesthetist program accredited by the American Association of Nurse Anesthetists and successful completion of a national certification examination.[36]
- Nurse Practitioner (NP)—An RN who is prepared to provide primary and preventive health care services. NPs practice in all types of health care settings, such as clinics, hospitals, schools, and private practice. They usually specialize in a specific area, such as family practice, pediatrics, public health, geriatrics, or maternal-infant care. Certification for nurse practitioners is offered by professional organizations such as the National Board of Pediatric Nurse Practitioners.[35]

Allied Health Professionals

The federal government has defined an allied health professional (PL 102-408, the Health Professions Education Amendment of 1991) as a health professional other than an RN or a PA who (1) has received a certificate; an associate, bachelor's, master's, or doctoral degree, or postdoctoral training in a science relating to health care and (2) shares in the responsibility for the delivery of health care services or related services, including the following:

- Identification, evaluation, and prevention of diseases and disorders
- Dietary and nutritional services

Table 1-6 EDUCATION FOR PROFESSIONAL NURSES

Degree/Level Attained	Years of College	Examples of Roles and Responsibilities
Doctor of Science in Nursing (DNS) or Doctor of Philosophy (PhD)	3-5 years graduate work (postbaccalaureate) with clinical	Researcher, educator, administrator, clinician, director of nursing
Master of Science in Nursing (MSN)	5-6 academic years with clinical	Nurse practitioner, clinical nurse specialist, administrator, director of nursing, supervisor, nurse manager
Baccalaureate degree (BSN)	4 full years with clinical	Nursing supervisor, head nurse, charge nurse, nurse manager
Associate degree	2 years with clinical	Charge nurse, nurse manager, staff nurse
Diploma	27-36 months with clinical	Charge nurse, nurse manager, staff nurse
Licensed practical nurse (LPN)/licensed vocational nurse (LVN)	1 year with clinical	Staff nurse, nurse manager; works under the supervision of RN, physician, or some other professional authorized by state law

- Health promotion services
- Rehabilitation services
- Health systems management services
- Those meeting the federal government's definition, such as HIM professionals

Allied health professionals are involved in every facet of care, including diagnostic and therapeutic procedures, education, counseling, and evaluation and management of care, all of which are directed at assisting the physician with patient care. Many allied health professionals are employed in an ancillary department of the hospital. As health care delivery has advanced in sophisticated technology and specialization, the area of allied health has grown tremendously. There are hundreds of health care occupations in the United States, some of which are found in HIM, medical technology, respiratory therapy, occupational therapy, physical therapy, and nutritional therapy.

Although not true for HIM professionals, most allied health personnel function by order of physicians. In hospitals that are organized by departments, allied health professionals are employed in a specific department; in hospitals that are organized by function, allied health professionals may be cross-trained in several areas and employed in units that provide patient-focused care. Allied health professionals were discussed in the section on the organization of hospitals.

FINANCING HEALTH CARE

Paying for health care services in the United States is a complex system that involves multiple payers and numerous mechanisms of payment. Payment methods may be direct pay or indirect pay. Payment by the patient to the provider and is referred to as **self-pay, out-of-pocket** pay, or **direct pay.** Indirect pay involves payment by a third party on behalf of the patient. Indirect payers may be the government, insurance companies, managed-care programs, or self-insured companies.

Insurance is a purchased contract (policy) in which the purchaser (insured) is protected from loss by the insurer's agreeing to reimburse for such loss. When the patient contracts with a health insurance company to provide health care coverage, payments for health care are considered indirect; in **coinsurance,** the insured is partially liable for the debt. Many people are employed by companies that offer health care insurance at a group rate; the company may finance its own insurance company (self-insured companies) or contract with an insurance company to provide coverage. Some employers (purchasers) may pay for the insurance in its entirety, some share the cost of premiums, and others merely negotiate the group rate and the employee bears the entire cost. Some health care providers are beginning to contract directly with employers to provide health care, eliminating the insurance carriers; this direct contracting reduces costs. Despite the expense, some individuals purchase their own health insurance because group insurance is not available to them.

One of the largest nonprofit insurance companies in the United States is Blue Cross and Blue Shield of America (BCBS). BCBS is composed of Blue Cross, which is insurance that covers certain hospital services, and Blue Shield, which is insurance that covers certain physician services and other health care services. Like other insurance companies, BCBS negotiates numerous health care contracts with employers, professional organizations or associations, schools, and individuals. The coverage, benefits, costs, deductibles, grace periods, and other policy specifications vary from group to group (Box 1-4).

Reimbursement

Reimbursement is critical to the livelihood of every health care facility and provider. In the United States, reimbursement for health care is a function of multiple payers, some of which are discussed in this section. The agreement between the third-party payers and the providers concerning what will be paid for and how much will be paid to the provider is called the **reimbursement formula.** These formulas are quite complicated and differ according to what was negotiated between the provider and the third-party payer. These are often referred to as the **contracted amount.**

Historically, payment for health care services has been by the **retrospective payment system.** With this payment method, the charges for the health care services is determined after the health care was provided. The actual amount paid may be based on fee-for-service or on the usual, customary, and reasonable charges. **Fee-for-service** is a reimbursement method in which the cost is based on the provider's charge for each service (e.g., charges for each x-ray test, laboratory test). Hospitals are paid on the basis of the number of days the patient needed care and the resources used during the course of treatment, such as medications, laboratory tests, and medical supplies. The **usual, customary, and reasonable charges** are based on the physician's usual charge for the service, the amount that physicians in the area usually charge for the same service, and whether the amount charged is reasonable for the service provided. In low-income community or public health programs, the cost for care may be based on the patient's ability to pay, referred to as a **sliding scale fee.**

Another form of reimbursement, the capitation method, is common in managed-care programs. In the **capitation** method, a prepaid, fixed amount is paid to the provider for each person (per capita) served, regardless of how much or how often the patient receives health care services.[3]

Box 1-4 TERMINOLOGY COMMON TO HEALTH INSURANCE POLICIES

Benefit
Amount of money paid for specific health care services or, in managed care, the health care services that will be provided or for which the provider will be paid

Beneficiary
One who is eligible to receive or is receiving benefits from an insurance policy or a managed-care program

Benefit period
Time frame in which the insurance benefits are covered, varies from insurance policy to policy

Claim
Request for payment by the insured or the provider for services covered

Copayment
Type of cost sharing in which the insured (subscriber) pays out-of-pocket a fixed amount for health care service

Coverage
Types of diseases, conditions, and diagnostic and therapeutic procedures for which the insurance policy will pay

Deductible
Amount of cost that the beneficiary must incur before the insurance will assume liability for the remaining cost

Exclusion
Specific conditions or hazards for which a health care policy will not grant benefit payments; often includes pre-existing conditions and experimental therapy

Fiscal intermediary
Contractor that manages the health care claims

Insurance
Purchased contract (policy) in which the purchaser (insured) is protected from loss by the insurer's agreeing to reimburse for such loss

Out-of-pocket costs
Monies that the patient pays directly to the health care provider

Payer
Party who is financially responsible for reimbursement of health care cost

Premium
Payment required to maintain policy coverage; usually paid periodically

Pre-existing condition
Disease, injury, or condition identified as having occurred before a specific date

Reimbursement
Payment by a third party to a provider of health care

Rider
Policy amendment that either increases or decreases benefits

Policy
Written contract between insurance company and subscriber (insured) that specifies the coverage, benefits, exclusions, copayments, deductibles, benefit period, and so on

Subscriber
Person who elects to enroll or participate in managed care or purchase health care insurance

Third-party payer
Party (insurance company, state or federal government, other) that is responsible for paying the provider on behalf of the insured (subscriber, patient, member) for health care services rendered

Managed Care

The HIM professional needs to develop an understanding of managed care because it greatly affects the health care field' and has unique information needs. **Managed care** is a generic term for a health care reimbursement system that is designed to minimize use of services and contain costs while ensuring the quality of care. The term managed care encompasses a continuum of practice arrangements, including HMOs, **preferred provider organizations** (PPOs), and other alternative delivery systems. The characteristics of the various managed-care programs are highly varied; some are discussed here.

MCOs contract with employers, unions, individuals, and other purchasers to provide comprehensive health care to people who voluntarily enroll in the plan. On the basis of the arrangement, the MCO provides the health care services or arranges for services while still controlling the cost and use of those services With this in mind, one can see that some models integrate health insurance, delivery, and payment within one organization and exercise control over utilization.[12] Providers who agree to participate in the managed-care plans may be salaried employees, paid fee-for-service or by capitation, or may negotiate a unique financial arrangement.

Health Maintenance Organizations

The oldest of the managed-care plans is the HMO, which integrates health care delivery with insurance for health care. The HMO was actually in existence before the concept of managed care. The health care services may be provided directly or by contract with other providers. The concept of prepaying a fixed amount per person (capitation) for health care services dates back to 1906, when a group of physicians offered health care services to a lumber company. The Western Clinic of Tacoma, Washington, offered the lumber company health care services for a fixed amount per capita. One of the largest and best known of the HMOs is Kaiser Permanente in California; a nonprofit HMO that is hospital based, employs full-time physicians, and provides comprehensive care.

The HMO models feature the following characteristics:

- Subscribers voluntarily enroll in the plan.
- Providers voluntarily agree to participate in the plan.
- An explicit contractual responsibility for providing health care services is assumed by the HMO.
- A prefixed periodic payment or **capitation** is made by the HMO to the provider regardless of how much or how often the patient uses the services.
- The financial risk is borne by the HMO and the provider.
- Patients receive no coverage when using providers outside of the HMO network or receive care from a provider without a referral from a primary care physician.

The three types of HMOs are the following:

- Staff model—An organization in which salaried physicians are employed by the HMO to provide care only for HMO subscribers; providers practice within the same facility. The HMO owns and operates ambulatory-care facilities that include ancillary services and physician offices. Inpatient care is usually under contract with local health care facilities.
- Group model—HMO contracts with group practices and hospitals to provide comprehensive health care services to subscribers. The groups of physicians are usually multispecialty.
- Network type—HMO contracts with a variety of providers to provide health care to subscribers; a physician's patient population may include not only the HMO's patients but also other HMO and non-HMO patients.

The independent practice association (IPA) is a group of physicians organized into a health care provider organization that furnishes services to patients who have signed up for a prepayment plan in which the physician services are supplied by the independent practice association. The patient population of the physician participating in such an association includes both HMO and non-HMO patients.[3]

Preferred Provider Organizations

A PPO is a network of physicians and/or health care organizations who enter into an agreement with payers or employers to provide health care services on a discounted fee schedule in return for increased patient volume. Patients are encouraged to use these providers by having a lower deductible, copayment, and coinsurance for services given by these providers. Patients are discouraged from using nonparticipating providers by paying higher nonnegotiated fees for their copays and deductibles. However, they would receive some coverage.

Case Management

Case management is an aspect of health care that refers to all activities including assessment, treatment planning, referral, and follow-up that ensures the provision of comprehensive and continuous services and the coordination of payment and reimbursement of care.[5] The individual responsible for coordinating all the care is designated the case manager (gatekeeper, primary care provider). This concept becomes crucial when the MCO is managing the care of patients with complex conditions such as cancer, AIDS, or chronic obstructive pulmonary disease. In these complex cases, the MCO (or providers) may employ case managers who coordinate and monitor the secondary and tertiary care that is needed.[12] The case manager would be an experienced health care professional who is knowledgeable about the clinical aspect of the patient's condition and the available resources.

Point-of-Service Plan

The **point-of-service** (POS) plan may be integrated in a number of different managed-care plans, including the HMO. The POS plan merely requires the enrollee (patient) to select a provider at the time, and each time, care is provided. The managed-care plan may be a POS plan or may offer POS as an option. The selected provider may or may not be a participant in the MCO. If enrollees are required to select a provider at the time they are enrolled in the managed-care plan, it is called a point-of-enrollment plan.

Utilization Management

In an attempt to control the cost of health care, many payers require some form of utilization review. **Utilization review** is the process of evaluating the efficiency and appropriateness of health care services according to predetermined criteria. A full discussion of utilization review is found in Chapter 13.

Government's Role as Payer

The bulk of the government's spending on health care goes to the Medicare and Medicaid programs. In 1965, the federal government spent $5.5 billion on health, whereas in 2005 the net federal spending on Medicare alone was $265 billion.[9] As a result of the spiraling costs, the federal government is pressing for changes to contain health care costs. Because both Medicare and Medicaid are modeled after private insurance companies, so much of the terminology is common to many insurance policies.

Medicare

Eligibility, Coverage, and Benefits The Medicare program is designed to help pay health care costs for those aged

65 years and older, and for other groups, including people with permanent kidney damage (referred to as end-stage renal disease or ESRD) and those receiving disability benefits for a minimum of 24 months. The specific requirements for Medicare eligibility are published in the annual Medicare handbook available on the Medicare Web site. People who are enrolled in Medicare or Medicaid programs are called **beneficiaries.**[32]

The Medicare program consists of Parts A B, C, and D, which cover different medical costs and are governed by different rules.

Hospital insurance, called Part A, helps to pay for inpatient hospital care, inpatient care in a nursing facility, home health care, and hospice care. Part A pays for the hospital costs that include a semiprivate room, meals, nursing service, medications, laboratory tests and radiology, intensive care, operating and recovery room, medical supplies, rehabilitation services, and preparatory services related to kidney transplantation. The physician's fees are not covered by Part A, although the beneficiary is hospitalized and receiving physician services.[32]

Medicare medical insurance, Part B, is a voluntary insurance program designed to supplement the cost of inpatient and outpatient care that is not covered under Part A. Part B coverage includes the physician's fee for services such as diagnostic tests, medical and surgical services, radiography, **durable medical equipment** (DME), ambulance service, home health, radiation therapy, and other outpatient services.[32] Durable medical equipment is equipment such as wheelchairs, oxygen equipment, walkers, and other devices prescribed by the physician for use in the home.

Medicare Part C, also known as Medicare Advantage, is available to beneficiaries that are enrolled in Medicare Parts A and B. Medicare Part C offers various managed-care plans, including HMO, POS, and PPO plans, among others, and private fee-for-service plans previously discussed. Depending on the type of plan selected, services may include preventive care and drug benefits and may have additional monthly premiums because of the extra benefits.[32]

The Medicare Prescription Drug, Improvement, and Modernization Act of 2003, commonly known as the Medicare Modernization Act (MMA), expanded Medicare coverage. The law provides for outpatient prescription drug coverage, expanded health plan options, improved access to health care for rural Americans, and covers preventive care services, such as flu shots and mammograms.

Medicare Part D, also known as the Medicare Prescription Drug Plan, is an insurance that covers the cost of prescription drugs. There are numerous plans and the coverage and cost depends on the plan selected. Some plans have higher deductibles but may cover more expensive drugs. The beneficiary pays a monthly premium and a deductible and a part of the drug cost. Medicare prescription drug coverage is available through either Medicare Part C or Part D.[32]

Reimbursement Under Medicare. Hospitals, physicians, and other health care providers are reimbursed for services delivered to a Medicare beneficiary through a **fiscal intermediary** (FI).[31] The intermediary is an organization that has contracted to manage the processing of claims and payments to the providers for Medicare Part A, according to federal regulations. The federal government assigns local insurance companies or BCBS plans to act as intermediaries and operate under contract to process Medicare claims. The fiscal intermediaries vary within states or regional areas. From 1966 to 1983, hospitals were paid by the retrospective payment system. Charges for inpatient services were submitted directly to the Medicare Part A fiscal intermediary and were paid on the basis of the reasonable cost of providing the care.

Financing of Medicare. The Medicare program is administered by the CMS of the DHHS. Financing of Part A is primarily by payroll tax, unless the beneficiary does not qualify for federal retirement benefits (Social Security); Part B is financed by federal appropriations with monthly premiums paid by the Medicare beneficiary.

The Medicare beneficiary is required to pay deductibles and **copayments** for health care services covered by Part A. In addition, the beneficiary pays monthly premiums, the deductible, and a percentage of the charges for Medicare Part B. A **deductible** is the cost that must be incurred by the patient beneficiary before the insurer assumes liability for the remaining charges. Copays and deductibles are also required for prescription drug coverage under Medicare Part D.[32]

In 1982, Congress passed the Tax Equity and Fiscal Responsibility Act (TEFRA), Public Law 97-248, which mandated the development of a mechanism for controlling the cost of the Medicare program and created the **prospective payment system** (PPS), a reimbursement method where the amount of payment is determined in advance of services rendered. Rates are established annually by the CMS. Under this system, the reimbursement for hospital inpatient care of Medicare patients is determined by a classification scheme called diagnosis-related groups (DRG), and reimbursement for physician services is based on the resource-based relative value scale (RBRVS). If a particular inpatient case requires more than the average number of days in the hospital or consumes expensive hospital resources, the hospital may lose money on that patient. Conversely, patients who require fewer resources save the hospital money. Providers have to maintain quality and yet be careful not to order excessive tests or extend treatment beyond what is considered medically necessary by the CMS. Prospective reimbursement systems are used in all types of organizations along the continuum of care, including out-hospital ambulatory care, skilled nursing facilities, and home health care. The prospective payment systems are discussed in more details in Chapter 18.

Medicaid

Originally called the Medical Assistance Program, Medicaid was established by Title XIX of the Social Security Act. **Medicaid** is a joint program between the state and the federal governments to provide health care to welfare recipients in the different states. Like other government programs, Medicaid has changed somewhat since its inception in 1965. This discussion is restricted to the program as it exists at time of publication.

Eligibility for coverage is determined by the individual states but must provide for welfare recipients, poor children younger than 5 years of age, certain low-income pregnant women, and medically indigent people. The **medically indigent** are those whose incomes are above what would normally qualify for Medicaid but whose medical expenses are high enough to bring their adjusted income to the poverty level. A great deal of variability exists from state to state. Each state sets its own limits regarding income that is considered to be at poverty level. Although the states vary in coverage and eligibility, they must comply with the federal guidelines.

The federal government identifies certain essential services that Medicaid must provide. They are inpatient and outpatient hospital care, physician services, laboratory and radiology services, skilled nursing care for those over age 21 years, home health care, family planning services, and early and periodic screening, diagnosis, and treatment of individuals under age 21 years. Each state can choose to provide additional health care benefits, such as medical care services by licensed practitioners other than medical doctors, dental care, physical therapy, eyeglasses, and prescription drugs.

The federal government shares in the cost of the Medicaid program with each state. The percentage of cost sharing varies on the basis of the per capita (per person) income of the state. In addition, the states can set copayments and deductibles for the medically indigent and for the optional services for welfare recipients.

Medicaid Reimbursement. Each state sets its own terms for Medicaid reimbursement to hospitals and health care providers. In some areas of the country, Medicaid recipients are encouraged to join managed-care plans.

Because of the variation in coverage and the fact that there is still a population that does not qualify for Medicaid yet cannot afford or access health care, the program is under scrutiny. The federal government is pushing for universal health care coverage, and some states are looking at mandatory insurance benefits by employers.

State Children's Health Insurance Program

The Balanced Budget Act of 1997 created the State Children's Health Insurance Program (SCHIP). This state-administered program offers health insurance for uninsured children up to the age of 19 years. It is designed to provide health insurance to families that may not be eligible for Medicaid because of their income. Each state establishes its own guidelines for enrollment, eligibility, and services. The basic services include hospitalizations, physician visits, immunizations, and emergency department visits.

Tricare

The Department of Defense provides health care for active and retired military personnel and their dependents. Health care for active duty and retired military personnel and their families and survivors is currently covered by **Tricare,** formerly the Civilian Health and Medical Program for the Uniformed Services (CHAMPUS).[37]

Workers' Compensation

Each state has workers' compensation insurance laws. This insurance pays for medical expenses and lost income, protection against lost occupational skills, and capacity and death benefits for survivors for workers who were injured or became ills as a result of work. Workers' compensation is funded by employer insurance programs. Most workers' compensation programs will pay lost wages and health care costs.

TECHNOLOGY IN HEALTH INFORMATION

Point-of-Care Clinical Information Systems

Point-of-care clinical information systems (point-of-service information systems) allow caregivers to capture and input data where health care service is provided and may be at the time of patient care. A point-of-care system can collect data directly from monitoring devices such as those in intensive care units. Many systems for point-of-care documentation are moving to wireless systems, giving clinicians more flexibility and accurate, timely reporting and patient-focused care.

Electronic Data Exchange

Electronic data exchange provides the ability to edit, submit, and pay health care claims by way of electronic transfer. In 1991, the Workgroup on Electronic Data Interchange was commissioned by the secretary of DHHS to reduce the cost of health care administration by increasing the number of claims processed electronically. The goal was to identify ways to increase electronic exchange quickly and effectively. Electronic data exchange requires a level of standardization in the way the data are formatted, making it easier for different computer systems to exchange data.[38] The Transaction and Code Set Regulations of the section of the HIPAA Administrative Simplification Rules address the standardization of the transactions between providers and payers.

Decision Support Systems

A decision support system (DSS) is a computerized system that gathers information from various sources and uses analytical models to assist providers in clinical decision making regarding administrative, clinical, and cost issues. For example, a clinical decision support system (CDSS) called Quick Medical Reference provides information about signs, symptoms, diagnosis, and treatment of more than 700 diseases. Other clinical decision support systems provide reminders or make recommendations on the basis of clinical guidelines.

Electronic Health Record

Transitioning from the paper medical record to the electronic health record continues to bring about numerous challenges that include privacy, data security, technology, policy, people, and processes; it is discussed in detail in Chapter 5. The most commonly used standards for developing electronic clinical and administrative datasets were established by the Health Level Seven (HL7) of the American National Standards Institute (ANSI). The standards are focused on the exchange, management, and integration of electronic health care information for health care organizations.

Electronic patient records that are developed by individual health care providers/organizations are **electronic medical records** (EMRs) that are composed of whole files as opposed to individual data elements. There are hundreds of different types of information systems that make up the EMR. The EMR is primarily used by a specific entity. The data from the EMR is the source of data for the **electronic health record** (EHR). The EHR represents the ability to easily share medical information by way of interfaces among stakeholders including patients, providers, payers/insurers, and government agencies. Wherever the patient seeks health care, the information should follow and be accessible. Among other things, data sharing by EHR is very important to forming health care policy, public health reporting, aggregating data for research, billing, and managing patient accounts.

National Health Information Infrastructure

The challenges of medical errors, inconsistent quality, and escalating health care costs has prompted the need for a National Health Information Infrastructure or Network (NHII or NHIN) that encompasses an EHR system for all providers and the ability to communicate electronically so that a complete EHR is assembled at the point of care. The

Institute of Medicine (IOM) has released numerous reports that call for the need to develop the NHII. The NHII will be a network of local health information structures that allow for the exchange of health information within the community including clinician information systems, consumer health information, ancillary health systems, decision support systems, educational components, and communication/networking systems that allow for integration of information across sites.[9] Although the project is to be developed and operated by the private sector, the DHHS has taken the lead in trying to move the initiative forward by convening stakeholder meetseminating the vision.

Institute of Medicine

The IOM of the National Academy of Science is a nonprofit organization that serves as an advisor to the nation on issues related to improving health. The IOM has addressed issues such as the number of uninsured Americans, immunization safety, autism, health literacy, childhood obesity, privacy of personal health care data, and the disclosure to the public of cost and quality information about institutions and clinicians.[9]

A report from the General Accounting Office identified the following ways in which the EHR can improve health care delivery:

- Provides data that are more accessible, of better quality, versatile for display, and easier to retrieve—all of which support decision making
- Enhances outcomes research by capturing clinical data from large databases
- Improves hospitals' efficiency by reducing cost and enhancing staff productivity

The integration of clinical data management into a common database allows the HCOs to develop strategies that support quality, control cost, and examine processes to improve efficiency. The integration further supports the collaboration and coordination of efforts by all health care professionals.

Clinical information systems are critical to address the changing health care environment needs for containing costs, improving quality, and providing accessible health care, all of which are vital components of health care reform.

FUTURE ISSUES

Up until recently the primary stakeholders in health care were the HCOs, providers, and payers. Today and more so in the future, the health care industry will have a greater awareness and recognition of the consumer as an important stakeholder. Consumers are more informed, participating in health care decision-making and taking more responsibility for their health care. In addition, in an arena that is balancing the business of health care, technology, and social welfare goals, there continues to be concern for quality, cost, and access to care.

With the evolution of the EHR there continue to be serious concerns about data security and confidentiality. HIM professionals will have numerous opportunities to affect the direction of health care by addressing issues of security and integrity of the EHR, practice standards, regulatory issues, and documentation that improves patient care quality and facilitating the development and use of the personal health record. The continued growth in ambulatory care, long-term care, and home health care has brought to the forefront the information needs in these areas. HIM professionals are and will continue to be of vital importance to the information needs of every component of health care systems but particularly the innovative programs that are emerging and the needs that the EHR movement has brought about.

Key Concepts

- Health care delivery systems in the areas of ambulatory care, home health care, and long-term care are rapidly growing and there is increasing need for the HIM professional to assist with the information needs of these areas.
- Increased regulations, with focus on cost containment, accessibility, and quality, have the potential to create a very complex health care delivery system resulting in new opportunities for HIM professionals.
- The technological advances in information management, the increased demands for patient data, and the push for cost containment, efficiency, and accessibility of health care have resulted in new challenges for the HIM professional.
- To function as an effective health care professional, the HIM professional must develop a good understanding of the organization and structure of the health care industry as a whole and the health care facilities constituting the industry.
- The information needs that are created by the EHR and other technologies present unique opportunities and challenges for HIM, such as regulatory issues, privacy, standards, data security, integrity, and ownership.

REFERENCES

1. World Health Organization: About the WHO (2003): http://www.who.int/about/en/.
2. Ackerknecht EH: Medicine of ancient civilization. In Ackerknecht EH, editor: A short history of medicine, ed 4, Baltimore, 1982, Johns Hopkins Press pp 21-26.
3. AHIMA: Pocket glossary health information management and technology, Chicago, 2006, American Health Information Management Association.
4. American Medical Association http://www.ama-assn.org/.
5. American Hospital Association: AHA guide to the health care field, Chicago, 2006, American Hospital Association.
6. Knight W: What is managed care? In Managed care: What it is and how it works, Gaithersburg, MD, 1998, Aspen Publishers, 1998, pp 19-43.
7. Roberts JS, Coale JG, Redman RR: A history of the Joint Commission on Accreditation of Hospitals, JAMA 258:936-940, 1987.
8. Sultz HA, Young KM: Financing health care. In Health care USA—Understanding its organization and delivery, ed 4, Gaithersburg, MD, 2004, Aspen Publishers.
9. Institute of Medicine: To err is human: Building a safer health system: National Academy Press (2000): www.nap.edu/books/0309068371/html/.
10. Smith C, Cowan C, Sensenig A, Catlin A, Health Accounts Team: Health spending slows in 2003, Health Affairs 24:185-194, 2005.
11. National Center for Health Statistics: Preliminary data for 2003, vol 53, No. 15, 2005, National Center for Health Statistics.
12. Shi L, Singh DA: Delivering health care in America—A systems approach, Gaithersburg, MD, 2004, Aspen Publishers.
13. AHIMA e-HIM Personal Health Record Work Group: The role of the personal health record in the EHR, J AHIMA 76:64A-64D, 2005.
14. U.S. Department of Health and Human Services: Healthy people 2000: National health promotion and disease prevention objectives, publication No. PHS 91-50212, Washington, DC, 1991, Public Health Service.
15. U.S. Department of Health and Human Services: Healthy people 2010: Understanding and improving health, ed 2, Washington, DC, 2000, U.S. Government Printing Office.
16. Office of the Surgeon General. http://www.surgeongeneral.gov/aboutoffice.html.
17. Centers for Medicare and Medicaid Services, EMTALA Overview. http://www.cms.hhs.gov/providers/emtala/default.asp.
18. Health Insurance Portability and Accountability Act of 1996: http://aspe.hhs.gov/admnsimp/pl104191.htm.
19. Joint Commission on Accreditation of Healthcare Organizations: Comprehensive accreditation manual for hospitals, Chicago, 2005, Joint Commission on Accreditation of Healthcare Organizations.
20. American Osteopathic Association: About osteopathic medicine: http://www.osteopathic.org. Updated 2006.
21. CARF mission, vision, core values and purpose (2005): http://www.carf.org/consumer.aspx?content=content/About/mission.htm.
22. About NCQA (2004): http://www.ncqa.org/about/about.htm.
23. CAAHEP: What is CAAHEP, Clearwater, FL, CAAHEP (2005): http:www.caahep.org.
24. Commission on Accreditation of Health Informatics and Information Management Education (CAHIIM). The CAHIIM mission 2006. http://www.cahiim.org.
25. National League for Nursing Accrediting Commission, Inc: www.nlnac.org. 2002.
26. Veterans Administration Office of Human Resources and Administration: VA organization briefing book (2005): http://www.va.gov/about_va/.
27. Bartlett CA, Ghoshal S: Matrix management: not a 22. structure, a frame of mind, Business Review July/August:138-145, 1990.
28. American Nurses Association: Nursing facts: registered nurses: today's registered nurse—numbers and demographics, Washington, DC, 2003, American Nurses Association.
29. Certified nursing assistants, devoted to nursing assistant. What is a CNA (2004): http://nursingassistantcentral.homestead.com.
30. Read S: Do formal controls always achieve control? The case of triage in accident and emergency departments, Health Serv Manage Res 7:31-41, 1994.
31. Centers for Medicare and Medicaid Services: Medicare fact sheet, 2005, Centers for Medicare and Medicaid Services.
32. U.S. Department of Health and Human Services: National Medicare handbook: Medicare and you 2006, Publication No. CMS 10050, Baltimore, 2006, Center for Medicare and Medicaid Services.

33. National Center for Complementary and Alternative Medicine: Get the facts—what is complementary and alternative medicine:http://www.nccam.hih.gov/health/whatiscam. Updated October 2005.

34. Wilson FA, Neuhauser D: Health manpower. In *Health services in the United States*, ed 2, Cambridge, MA, 1987, Ballinger, p 61.

35. American Nurses Association Nursing World: Nursing facts: advanced practice nursing: a new age in health care. http://www.nursingworld.org/readrom/fsadvprc.htm. Updated 2006.

36. American Association of Nurse Anesthetists: *Nurse anesthetists at a glance*, updated February 2006, http://www.aana.com/aboutaana.asp.

37. Department of Defense TRICARE fact sheet: http://www.tricare.osd.mil/Factsheets/viewfactsheet.cfm?id=174.

38. Slee VN, Slee DA, Schmidt HJ: *Slee's health care terms*, St. Paul, 2001, Tringa Press, p. 356.

chapter 2

The Health Informatics and Information Management Profession

Melanie S. Brodnik

Additional content,
http://evolve.elsevier.com/Abdelhak/

Review exercises can be found
in the Study Guide

Chapter Contents

Health Information Management—A Profession in
 Transformation
The Patient Record—Source of Health Data and
 Information
Evolution of the Patient Record
 Early History
 Influential Forces
  Accreditation
  Licensing of Health Care Facilities
  Paying for Health Care
  Technology
Evolution of the Health Information Management
 Profession
 Early History
 1990s Forward
 Formation of Education Programs
  Accreditation of Educational Programs
 Professional Certification
  Registered Health Information Administrator and Registered
   Health Information Technologist
  Certified Coding Associate, Certified Coding Specialist,
   Certified Coding Specialist–Physician Based
  Certified in Healthcare Privacy, Certified in Healthcare
   Security, Certified in Healthcare Privacy and Security
  Importance of Professional Certification
  Other Relevant Credentials
Maintenance of Certification and Lifelong Learning
Fellowship Program

Key Words

Accreditation
Accredited record technician
Ambulatory payment classification
 system
Certification
Certified coding assistant
Certified coding specialist
Certified coding specialist–physician
 based
Certified in Healthcare Privacy
Certified in Healthcare Privacy and
 Security
Certified in Healthcare Security
Certified record librarian
Code of ethics
Commission on Accreditation of
 Health Informatics and Information
 Management
Communities of Practice
Conditions of participation
Council on Accreditation
Council on Certification

Credential
Data
Diagnosis related group
Electronic health
Electronic health information
 management
Electronic health record
Electronic medical record
Fee-for-service
Fellow American Health Information
 Management Association
Foundation of Research and Education
Health Insurance Portability and
 Accountability Act
Hybrid record
Information
Knowledge
Licensure
Longitudinal record
Managed care
Medicaid
Medicare

National health information
 infrastructure
Office of the National Coordinator for
 Health Information Technology
Patient record
Profession
Prospective payment
Record
Regional health information
 organizations
Registered health information
 administrator
Registered health information
 technician
Registered record librarian
Registration
Standardization movement
Tax Equity and Fiscal Responsibility
 Act
The Joint Commission (formerly
 JCAHO)

American Health Information Management Association Today
  American Health Information Management Association Communications
Foundation of Research and Education in Health Information Management
The Professional Code of Ethics
Looking to the Future

Abbreviations

AAMRL—American Association Medical Record Librarians

ACP—American College of Physicians

ACS—American College of Surgeons

AHA—American Hospital Association

AHIMA—American Health Information Management Association

AMA—American Medical Association

AMRA—American Medical Record Association

APC—Ambulatory payment classification

ARLNA—Association of Record Librarians of North America

ART—Accredited record technician

CAAHEP—Commission on the Accreditation of Allied Health Education Programs

CAHIIM—Commission on Accreditation of Health Informatics and Information Management

CCA—Certified coding assistant

CCS—Certified coding specialist

CCS-P—Certified coding specialist-physician-based

CHP—Certified in Healthcare Privacy

CHPS—Certified in Healthcare Privacy and Security

CHS—Certified in Healthcare Security

COA—Council on Accreditation

COC—Council on Certification

CPRI—Computer-based Patient Record Institute

E-HEALTH—Electronic health

E-HIM—Electronic Health Information Management

EHR—Electronic Health Record

EMR—Electronic Medical Record

FAHIMA—Fellow of the American Health Information Management Association

DRG—Diagnosis related group

FORE—Foundation of Research and Education

HIM—Health information management

HIT—Health information technology

HIPAA—Health Insurance Portability and Accountability Act of 1996

JCAHO—Joint Commission on Accreditation of Healthcare Organizations (now The Joint Commission)

NHII—National Health Information Infrastructure

ONC—Office of the National Coordinator for Health Information Technology

RHIO—Regional Health Information Organizations

RHIA—Registered health information administrator

RHIT—Registered health information technician

RRL—Registered record librarian

TEFRA—Tax Equity and Fiscal Responsibility Act

Objectives

After reading this chapter, the reader will be able to do the following:

- Define the key words.
- Discuss the patient record as a source of health data and information.
- Trace the early evolution of patient records in health care.
- Describe key forces that have influenced the evolution of the patient record.
- Discuss how technology has influenced the demand for electronic health records and a national health information infrastructure.
- Trace the early evolution of the health information management profession.
- Describe the impact of information technology on the health information management profession and the issues the profession faces in an electronic health care environment.
- Discuss the requirements for initial and continuing certification within the health information management profession and the profession's commitment to lifelong learning.
- Describe the benefits of seeking and maintaining professional certification.
- Identify the governance and volunteer structure of American Health Information Management Association and what membership has to offer the professional.
- Discuss the principles found within the American Health Information Management Association Code of Ethics and how they apply in today's health care environment.

This chapter traces the evolution of the patient record and the health information management (HIM) profession in the United States to its current status. The primary professional association for HIM professionals in the United States is the American Health Information Management Association (AHIMA). Its mission and role in accreditation of educational programs, credentialing of professionals, support of professional development opportunities, code of ethics, and key initiatives to move the profession forward are discussed. The history of the profession is intricately linked to the development of landmark changes in the health care system. The roles of HIM professionals are diverse and the variety of opportunities has increased in ways the early founders of the profession could never have imagined. However, one main thread continues to bind the past to the future—the goal of supporting quality health care through quality information.

HEALTH INFORMATION MANAGEMENT—A PROFESSION IN TRANSFORMATION

The HIM profession and the health care industry in general are experiencing a fundamental change in the way health care data and information are collected, processed, communicated, and managed as a result of advances in information and communication technology. The paper-based patient record environment is transitioning to an electronic health record (EHR) environment to support patient safety, improve patient care, control health care costs, and provide better public health surveillance. The changing nature of the data and information system infrastructure within the health care industry is driving a transformation in the roles and functions of HIM practice. Although this change is occurring, the fundamental values of the profession remain intact. The profession's focus from its inception has been on improving patient care through better documentation and ensuring the privacy, confidentiality, and security of patient information. Today, HIM professionals articulate the same values while working collaboratively with others to establish a health care information infrastructure that provides quality data to support quality health care while balancing the consumers' right to privacy of their health care information with the legitimate uses of this information for administrative, financial, clinical, research, and public health purposes.

THE PATIENT RECORD—SOURCE OF HEALTH DATA AND INFORMATION

The patient record is a primary source of health data and information for the health care industry. Data refer to raw facts, characters, or symbols that, when organized and processed to produce meaning, result in information. Knowledge is derived from information once information is organized, analyzed, and synthesized by the user. A record is a body of known or recorded facts regarding someone or something. When an individual seeks care or treatment from a health care provider, a record of that care or treatment is generated. The data collected from and on the patient are stored in the patient record. The record maybe called a patient record, medical record, health record, clinical record, resident record, client record, and so forth, depending on the nature and philosophy of the health care setting where the record was generated. In any case, the patient record is created as a direct result of the health care delivered in that setting. It is the legal documentation of care provided to an individual by the medical or health care professionals who practice in the setting. The data, information, or record may have the term "clinical" preceding it to denote that the data, information, or record relates specifically to the care and treatment of a patient.

The data and information documented in the record and the record in total are used for the following purposes:

- Documenting health care services provided to an individual to support continuing communication and decision making among health care providers
- Establishing a record of health care services provided to an individual that can be used as evidence in legal proceedings
- Assessing the efficiency and effectiveness of the health care services provided
- Documenting health care services provided to support reimbursement claims that are submitted to payers
- Supplying data and information that support the strategic planning, administrative decision making, public health surveillance, and research activities and support the public policy development related to health care, such as regulations, legislation, and accreditation standards.

The use of data contained in the patient record has increased with the growing complexity of health care decision making and the increasing complexity of the health care delivery system. Whether patients receive treatment in a hospital, long-term care facility, or physician office, the patients are likely to encounter a variety of health care providers working collaboratively to provide the most effective treatment or care for these patients. This situation creates a heightened reliance by care providers on the patient record as a means of communication and as a source of data for decision making.

Documentation within the patient record is the basis for health care billing and reimbursement. Third-party payers such as insurance companies and the federal government through programs such as Medicare and Medicaid use the data documented in the record as proof of the care delivered to the patient. Without appropriate documentation to support the care given, the health care setting or provider will not be reimbursed for services rendered.

The data and information in the patient record are used to substantiate whether the patient received quality care or treatment in the most effective and efficient way possible. Because the cost of health care represents a large portion of the United State's gross national product, efforts to control spiraling health care costs while providing quality health care place extra importance on the patient record.

Not only are the data and information within the patient record used to substantiate the care given for reimbursement and quality proposes, it is also a legal document that confirms whether treatment was delivered in a manner appropriate for the given health problem. The record is used to show proof in a court of law of what transpired during the course of a patient's illness and treatment. As a legal document, the patient record is defined as a record that is "generated at or for a healthcare organization as its business record and is the record that would be released upon request."[1]

The patient record is a valuable source of data for research, program evaluation, education, and public health studies. Data from the record is aggregated for these purposes. Published data on acquired immunodeficiency syndrome, sexually transmitted diseases, diseases caused by certain infections, and outbreaks of illness such as severe acute respiratory syndrome or the avian flu rely on careful documentation in the patient record or source document. Hospital mortality rates are published as are performance reports on health care organizations. Some health plans also provide performance information to consumers, sometimes referred to as "report cards," to help the consumers evaluate and select the health plan they wish to participate in.[2] All this is made possible by the data generated from patient care.

EVOLUTION OF THE PATIENT RECORD

We are aware of the importance patient records play in today's health care environment. However, how did patient records evolve as a primary source of health care data and information, and what forces influenced this evolution? In addition, what are the milestones in the history of this evolution that have brought us to today's need for EHR systems and a national health information infrastructure?

Early History

The value of recording patient information has been recognized since prehistoric times. The methods used to record early attempts to treat disease were primitive and differ markedly from the electronic information systems now in use. Prehistoric cave paintings are thought to be the earliest accounts of treating the sick. The paintings depict skull trephination and the amputation of fingers and other parts of the extremities. As civilizations developed, stone carvings were made in addition to drawings, and eventually pen and paper became the mode for recording words and thoughts.[3]

Methods for maintaining patient records were slow to develop, and the earliest institutions used some abbreviated form. Many hospitals appear to have used a ledger to record at least minimum information about a patient—for example, name, address, date of birth, and major health problem. The use of ledgers for record keeping was popular in other businesses as well. They were used by banks, hotels, and other commercial enterprises. Many pioneer record keepers, such as Thomas Jefferson, George Washington, and Benjamin Franklin, used ledger-style recordings, so it is not surprising that the health care field initially adopted a similar system.

The New York Hospital, established in 1771, did not begin recording patient clinical information until around 1790. Early medical records at Pennsylvania Hospital, established in Philadelphia in 1792 as a result of the leadership of Benjamin Franklin, included entries of the patient's name, address, and ailment. A number of entries were made in Franklin's handwriting. Charity Hospital in New Orleans entered its first medical records in large ledgers. Many of its earliest patients were seamen, and the terminology used reflects this nautical influence. Massachusetts General Hospital, established in 1821, maintained patient records from its beginning. These records were sufficiently comprehensive to enable the cataloging of diseases and operations.[4] One Virginia hospital, established in 1911, maintained its first clinical records in leather-bound volumes that contained between 50 and 100 patient records per volume. Each volume was labeled in gold leaf lettering.

The ledger style of recording patient care was most popular in these early hospitals. As the record-keeping process became more detailed and interest in learning from treatment experience increased, the minimal ledger entry was no longer sufficient. Early record keepers in hospitals looked beyond ledgers to find ways of making patient records more accessible and useful by moving from ledgers to individual patient records. These records were organized into systems that allowed easier retrieval of a patient's record and the data within the document.

In the early hospitals, only a small circle of health care providers had access to the patient records. The records were brief and contained carefully handwritten entries. In time the information recorded in the patient record was organized into various types of reports such as patient history and physical examination, operative report, progress report, nursing notes, laboratory findings, and so on. Some hospitals filed the records of similar diseases or treatments together to help in the learning process. Others set up indexes to identify diseases and treatments and associate them with particular patient records. When the typewriter was invented in 1874 early hospitals adopted this new form of "information technology" to process their health care data. They began typing the lengthy handwritten documents within the patient record such as operative reports and history and physical examinations. Over time, patient records came to contain scores of documents in a wide variety of formats and media accessed by a wide variety of legitimate users for multiple reasons. For the most part the patient record has remained paper based; however, the paper form of the record no longer meets the demands placed on it. The paper record can be in only one place at one time, and the data, once entered into the paper record, cannot be manipulated to show trends or relationships among data as may be uniquely required by an individual user of the record. Many forces have influenced the importance of patient records and the need to move the paper-based record to an electronic format.

Influential Forces

Accreditation

By the turn of the twentieth century hospitals were viewed as boardinghouses for the poor and sick, and issues related to the shortcomings of medical education and the quality of documentation in patient records surfaced. To address these issues, voluntary organizations and state and federal governments began efforts to standardize and regulate the delivery of health care. The American Medical Association (AMA) and American Hospital Association (AHA) were already 50 years old by the turn of the century. However, the organization that was most aware of the need for quality patient records was the American College of Surgeons (ACS). The ACS brought to the forefront the realization that, to assess the quality of physician education and the resulting treatment provided to patients, those performing the assessment needed data and the primary source of these data was the patient record.

To elevate the quality of surgery being performed in hospitals, the ACS established minimum standards that included specifications for the content of the patient's record and required that certain activities be documented within a specified time frame. In 1918, the ACS began to survey hospitals to see whether the standards were being met and found that "only 89 of the 692 hospitals of 100 or more beds surveyed met the minimum standards."[5] The ACS provided leadership and funding for the accreditation activity and also helped form the professional organization now known as AHIMA, which will be discussed later in this chapter.

The other voluntary organizations of the AMA, AHA, American College of Physicians, and the Canadian Hospital Association joined the ACS to support the early accreditation body. The Canadian Hospital Association eventually withdrew from the body and formed its own accreditation program in Canada. In 1952 the remaining voluntary member organizations formed the Joint Commission on the Accreditation of Hospitals (JCAH) to carry on with the hospital accreditation program. The JCAH expanded its accreditation activity to incorporate all types of health care organizations, all of whom must maintain patient records (sometimes called resident, client, or medical records). The JCAH now provides accreditation standards for 11 health care organizations. It added *organizations* to its name to become the Joint Commission on the Accreditation of Healthcare Organizations (JCAHO) to denote that it now accredits more than just hospitals, and it is now known as The Joint Commission. Throughout the years The Joint Commission has set expectations for quality patient care with the patient record as the primary source of data to substantiate this care. Specific standards related to the content of patient records and the processes for storing, retrieving, and protecting patient data and records were identified and now make up one chapter within the accreditation manuals devoted specifically to information management.[6]

Licensing of Health Care Facilities

Running parallel to the accreditation programs offered by the early voluntary organizations and later The Joint Commission, states began programs to license facilities. Although many of the state licensing codes focused heavily on the physical facility to ensure safe surroundings, they also included sections on the basic requirements for a patient record and patient record system. State licensing boards, or in some cases registration boards, required that health care facilities accredited by The Joint Commission must also meet the state licensing requirements to be authorized to provide health care services. As standards and regulations evolved, health care facilities were required to adhere to whichever standard or regulation was more stringent. This occurred because generally the voluntary Joint Commission accreditation review involves standards that are a level or a step up from the state-mandated minimum requirements. However, at times the state licensing requirements are more specific than Joint Commission standards. For example, states may require a specific retention period for patient records, whereas The Joint Commission standard for record retention may simply require that the organization have a retention policy for patient records.

Paying for Health Care

In time, as the U.S. population grew and more hospitals were built to meet the need for health care services, various methods for funding the services emerged. Private health insurance appeared in the first half of the century and federal programs for insuring selected segments of the population appeared in 1965. Both these third-party payer sources have significantly contributed to the demand for health care data, as found in the patient record. Also, these third-party payers have heavily influenced methods for documenting in the patient record and fast and accurate retrieval of this documentation for reimbursement purposes.

Employers began to add benefits to workers' compensation packages in the form of health insurance as early as

1929. Major expansion of health insurance benefits and programs occurred in the 1950s and 1960s, followed by another major thrust for funding health care through managed-care plans. Over the years, insurance companies and managed-care organizations have increased the quantity and specificity of the documentation from the patient record required to support each claim for health care services that is submitted for payment. Likewise state and federal governments have done the same through Medicare and Medicaid programs.[7]

In 1965, Congress added provisions to the Social Security Act that created Medicare and Medicaid (see Chapter 1). This significant event resulted in the addition of regulations at the federal and state levels for patient records. Many of the basic Joint Commission standards were incorporated in the regulations of these programs. Now, instead of voluntary standards, the regulations were part of the federal Conditions of Participation.[8] The Conditions of Participation spelled out for health care providers the regulations they must follow to be reimbursed for the health care given to patients when using Medicare and Medicaid as their payment source. One regulation required that each admission of a patient to the hospital was subject to review and potential denial of payment if the admission was judged, after the fact, to be unnecessary. The federal government set up a monitoring system for Medicare patients that reviewed the appropriate use of hospital resources and the quality of patient care. Much of the review focused on the patient record as the primary source of information. The phrase "if it isn't documented, it wasn't done" became a mantra during this time in an attempt to communicate the increasing importance of proper documentation in the patient record under the Medicare review program.

The Medicare and Medicaid programs were essentially a fee-for-service style of reimbursement. If a service was provided that the programs had agreed to cover, a payment would be received at a discounted rate. The system encouraged more services to generate more payment. Spiraling health care costs over the next 15 years led Congress to search for ways to control these costs. One solution was to move from a fee-for-service style of reimbursement to a prospective payment method. The prospective payment method compared with the fee-for-service method of reimbursement is based on payment rates that are established in advance and that reflect an average of what a service should cost. Thus, between 1980 and 2002 Congress moved to a prospective payment system method of reimbursing health care for seven health care services: ambulatory surgery centers (1980), inpatient acute-care hospitals (1983), skilled nursing facilities (1998), home health agencies (2000), outpatient hospital services (2001), inpatient rehabilitation facilities (2002), and long-term care hospitals (2002).[7] The patient record is the primary source for the data that justifies each claim submitted for the above prospective payment systems. Thus, the need to improve methods of collecting, processing, communicating, and managing data from patient records is paramount in meeting the demands for increased information and quality patient care.

Technology

Throughout the twentieth and into the twenty-first centuries innovation and adoption of technology has increasingly been used as a tool to support diagnostic, therapeutic, monitoring, and educational activities associated with direct patient care. The results produced through the application of technology in patient care were reported in the primary patient record; however, the actual scan or image produced by the application was stored in another location. As information technology matured over the years and the demand for more information increased, new approaches to the patient record have emerged. Data may become part of the record without forcing the data to appear on paper; that is, data from images, voice, and sound can be an integral part of a primary patient record that is electronic in format.

In the 1980s a significant breakthrough in the processing of data and information occurred when personal computers and data communication technologies entered the marketplace and became more affordable. These technologies enabled hospitals and other health care providers to increase their reliance on health information technology (HIT) as a means of staying competitive in an increasingly information-intensive industry. The challenge was to move the paper-based patient record to an electronic format in total. In such a format the patient record can be composed of electronic databases (or repositories of data) that contain the health care information generated on the patient while treated in a given health care facility. The data within the database can be accessed and arranged in multiple ways such as a longitudinal record from birth to death of a patient, an in-depth view of a single, current health problem of how one individual is being managed, or the records (data) of many individuals merged to provide information on the outcome of particular treatments across a population of patients.

To address this challenge, in 1989 the Institute of Medicine undertook a study to improve patient records through the use of information technology. The Institute of Medicine convened a committee of industry experts who reported in 1991 that health care professionals and organizations should be encouraged to adopt computer-based patient records as a standard for all records related to patient care. They defined the patient record of the future as one that "will reside in a system specifically designed to support users by providing accessibility to complete and accurate data, alerts, reminders, clinical support systems, links to medical knowledge and other aids."[9] If the patient record was computerized, it could allow multiple users to access data at the same time. Researchers could also access the data in aggregate form if they were looking for data on a certain type of treatment but did not need to identify an individual patient. One recommendation of this study was that the "public and private sectors join in establishing a Computer-based Patient Record Institute to promote and facilitate development, implementation, and dissemination of the CPR."[9] The institute was formed and functioned throughout the 1990s as a supporter of efforts toward computerizing patient records.

During the 1990s there was continuous growth of information and communication technologies, including the Internet, Web-based applications, wireless communication, and telephony in regard to patient care and treatment. As a result, the concept of electronic health or "e-health" emerged. E-health denotes the following:

> … health services and information delivered or enhanced through the Internet and related technologies. In a broader sense, the term characterizes not only a technical development, but also a state-of-mind, a way of thinking, an attitude, and a commitment for networked, global thinking, to improve health care locally, regionally, and worldwide by using information and communication technology.[10]

By the end of the 1990s we saw a growing reliance on e-health in all phases and aspects of health care and life. The need for public health preparedness and disease surveillance systems to address terrorism and other public health concerns on a national and global basis emerged. There was a growing emphasis on bringing the consumer of health care into the picture as a way to improve care and control costs. The concept of consumers taking charge of their health care by keeping their own personal health record and linking the care giver and consumer through HIT was seen as important to the future of health care delivery.

Up to this time the patient record was adapting to the HIT applications used by a given care provider such as hospitals or physician office practices. Providers were adopting applications to electronically capture, process, and retrieve data from all or parts of the patient record. As a result, patient records in some instances became a combination of paper, digitized information, and imaged documents. We begin to see patient records and patient record systems in some organizations change from strictly paper-based documents to what is now termed a hybrid record. A hybrid record refers to a record that includes both paper and electronic documents and uses both manual and electronic processes to store and retrieve the documents.[11] A complete EHR was not yet the norm of practice for a variety of reasons, including a lack of data standards and interoperability, investment costs, acceptance of HIT by staff, and availability of staff to implement EHR systems. To address these barriers, the federal government and a number of public-private organizations began investigating ways to speed up the adoption of EHRs as a means to improve the quality, safety, efficiency, and cost of health care.[12]

In January 2004, President George W. Bush highlighted the importance of information technology in health care in his State of the Union Address. He stated, "By computerizing health records, we can avoid dangerous medical mistakes, reduce costs, and improve care."[13] The following April President Bush issued an executive order that called for widespread adoption of interoperable EHRs within 10 years and established the position of the National Coordinator for Health Information Technology.[14] Subsequently, in June 2004, the President's Information Technology Advisory Committee (PITAC) published a report that suggested to reduce health care costs, control medical and medication errors, reduce needless duplication of diagnostic tests, and monitor public health and bioterrorism concerns the government should enable ways to develop a twenty-first century EHR system.[12]

The PITAC proposed a framework for a health care information infrastructure that would be composed of four elements: EHRs for all Americans; computer-assisted clinical decision support; computerized provider order entry and secure, private, interoperable, electronic health information exchange.[12] The PITAC report was followed by a progress report from the Office of the National Coordinator for Health Information Technology (ONC) which laid out strategic action to achieve a vision of consumer-centric and information-rich health care. To achieve this vision, the ONC would support efforts to implement EHRs and regional health information organizations to support an overall national health information infrastructure.[14] Since these documents were published the federal government has taken an action-oriented role in facilitating the adoption of HIT and EHR systems, which will be discussed in more detail later in the book. In addition, a number of grants have been funded,[15] and proposed legislation has been introduced to support the ONC efforts. In 2006, during his State of the Union address President Bush once again reaffirmed the government's commitment to interoperable EHRs and a national health care information infrastructure.

Today, when asked what constitutes a patient record, one has to look beyond a hard copy paper-based document to a broader view of an electronic record that fulfills several purposes as well as serving as the core for a national health information infrastructure. Over time, the patient record has mirrored the changes in health care. As health care has become more complex, the patient record has evolved to address these complexities. It has emerged from prehistoric cave drawings to paper records to hybrid records and now to electronic records. In an electronic format attention has been paid to patient records that are generated and reside within a health care delivery organization or records that become part of regional health networks or other information exchange entities. The changes in the patient record have given rise to the establishment and evolution of the HIM professional who now functions as a key leader in transitioning the health care industry from paper-based patient records to EHR systems.

EVOLUTION OF THE HEALTH INFORMATION MANAGEMENT PROFESSION

Early History

The early efforts by the medical profession to upgrade the education of physicians and to evaluate the quality of care provided to patients have a direct link to the beginning of the HIM profession in the United States. The HIM profession evolved from the need for accurate and complete records regarding the care and treatment of patients as one means of improving and standardizing health care. The ACS's standardization program was the catalyst for organizing and educating a group of people who could assist hospitals in meeting the informational needs of accrediting bodies and medical educators. Hospital medical record departments were forming and a knowledgeable workforce was needed to implement and manage methods of collecting, storing, and retrieving patient data and records. In 1928, Dr. Malcolm MacEachern, director of hospital activities at the ACS and an important leader in the hospital standardization movement, recognized that more was needed to bring about change in the quality of patient records.[16] He invited medical record workers from the United States and Canada to attend a meeting of the Clinical Congress of the ACS. The meeting program and exhibits were devoted to medical record documentation and standard-setting efforts of the ACS. The meeting resulted in the medical record workers organizing to form the Association of Record Librarians of North America (ARLNA). Grace Whiting Myers, Librarian Emeritus of Massachusetts General Hospital, was elected the first president of the association.[16]

The following year the ARLNA held its first annual meeting, in Chicago. Fifty-three charter members adopted the association's constitution and bylaws and identified ways to communicate and educate a medical record workforce. At the close of the meeting, the members decided to communicate through the publication of a quarterly journal, *Bulletin of the Association of Record Librarians of North America*. In addition, a committee was formed to develop a course of study for medical record librarians. This course of study laid the groundwork for the profession's development of education programs at the associate, baccalaureate, and master's degree levels.[17] The efforts of this committee are discussed in more detail below under the section on *Formation of Education Programs*.

Along with the development of standardized educational curriculum, the ARLNA determined that it needed to set standards for its members and formed a Board of Registration in 1933. The board developed rules and regulations for registering members as a registered record librarian (RRL). The rules and regulations set by the board in essence "certified" that the individual met certain criteria

or standards that entitled him or her to bear the credential RRL.[18] Additional certifications that have been added over the years are discussed below.

By 1939 the young association revised its bylaws to allow for state associations to become affiliates of the national association. The Canadian members of the association eventually broke away and formed their own association in 1944.[19] The ARLNA subsequently changed its name to the American Association of Medical Record Librarians and opened its first executive office in Chicago with the help of the AHA and moved to its own headquarters in 1946.[20] Over the next 30 years the association moved forward with activities that built a body of knowledge that supported academic program growth, program accreditation, professional certification, and continuing education. In 1970 the association changed its name to the American Medical Record Association and changed its name once again in 1991 to the American Health Information Management Association.[21]

1990s Forward

Each change in the association's name was to accommodate the changing roles and responsibilities of its members as a result of changes in the health care industry. The 1991 name change reflected the profession's look toward the future where paper-based patient records would be replaced with EHRs and HIM practice would move into an electronic age of information management. The AHIMA Vision 2000 outlined how HIM practice was likely to evolve in the 1990s. In 1996 Vision 2006 was published to project what roles health information managers may assume in an electronic health care environment.[22] As the decade of the 1990s closed, it was evident that e-health had permeated the health care landscape and that many of the skills HIM professionals used to manage paper medical record systems could easily transfer to an e-health organization.[23] The AHIMA e-health Task Force reported in 2002 that:

> The knowledge and expertise of managing the handwritten medical records containing source patient data has evolved from independent management of paper medical records in settings across the continuum of care to scanning the paper documents for multiple user access, to entering data into automated systems that generate electronic patient data, to integrated delivery systems that electronically manage the patient across the continuum of care, to network integration and e-health information management.[23]

The task force also suggested additional roles HIM professionals were suited to perform as the profession transitions into an e-health information management (e-HIM) environment.

The AHIMA subsequently focused on e-HIM as one of its major initiatives for 2003 and convened a task force of industry experts to develop a vision statement of HIM practice in 2010. An update to the 2010 vision statement of

American College of Surgeons

health information was offered by Bloomrosen in 2005 and now reads as: *The future state of health information is electronic, consumer-centered, comprehensive, longitudinal, accessible, credible, and secure. Ownership of health information is a shared responsibility between the consumer and provider.*[24] The vision statement moves health information out of a paper environment into an electronic environment. In turn, the practice of HIM in 2010 was defined as:

> Health information management is the body of knowledge and practice that ensures the availability of health information to facilitate real-time health care delivery and critical health-related decision making for multiple purposes across diverse organizations, settings, and disciplines.[25]

Certainly this definition of HIM practice will continue to evolve, as have previous definitions. The e-HIM task force suggested roles and competencies that HIM professionals will provide as HIM practice transitions to an electronic environment (Box 2-1).

The ultimate role and job responsibilities of the HIM professional will depend on the individuals' education, experience, and work setting. Important recommendations from the report have continued to guide AHIMA activities related to a number of initiatives such as workforce development, industry partnerships and collaborations, professional self development, education reform, research, and grantsmanship.

As paper-based medical record systems are increasingly converted to EHR systems, one area of practice that is undergoing significant change is the HIM department, whether in a hospital, long-term care, or other type of health care provider organization or agency. The movement is

---

Box 2-1 HIM PROFESSIONAL ROLES AND COMPETENCIES IN AN E-HIM ENVIRONMENT

HIM Professional Roles
- Business process engineer
- Clinical research protocol designer and manager
- Clinical trials manager
- Clinical vocabulary manager
- Consumer advocate
- Data analyst
- Data facilitator
- Data/information broker
- Data/information presenter
- Data sets, nomenclature, and classification standards developer
- Data miner
- Data navigator
- Data quality and integrity manager
- Data resource manager
- Data security, privacy, confidentiality manager
- Data translator
- Information systems designer
- Work and data flow analyst

Competencies in e-HIM
- Establishing and guiding national, local, and state health information policy development and implementation
- Establishing and implementing policies, practices, and procedures governing all aspects of HIM
- Establishing and implementing standards for privacy, security, and confidentiality of health information
- Establishing and implementing policies and standards for monitoring of data integrity, accuracy, validity, authenticity, and version control
- Developing health information format and content standards to ensure the collection of complete, accurate, timely, and complete health information
- Facilitating communication of health information across organizational health care teams and among different entities
- Facilitating the concurrent use of health information for multiple purposes (such as for direct patient care, outcomes measurement and evaluation, wellness and prevention, research, public health and policy development)
- Managing compliance, regulatory, accreditation, licensure, and (re)certification programs and activities
- Analyzing and synthesizing qualitative and quantitative health information for various and diverse needs and audiences
- Developing, designing, and implementing clinical vocabularies
- Translating and interpreting health information for consumers and their caregivers
- Helping consumers to access and obtain diverse and often complex health information
- Informing and educating consumers about health information issues
- Providing the context to understand, analyze, and interpret health information
- Helping providers understand data flow and reporting requirements within the context of dynamic rules, regulations, and guidelines
- Leading business process redesign efforts

Source: A vision of the e-HIM future: a report from the AHIMA e-HIM Task Force, *J Am Health Inform Manage Assoc:* http://library.ahima.org/xpedio/groups/public/documents/ahima/bok1_020835.hcsp?dDocName-bok1_020835. Accessed August 7, 2006.

toward a virtual department; thus, each function within the department must be re-engineered, such as release of information, and in some cases eliminated, such as pulling records for clinic visits, as the processes for EHRs change. HIM professionals are engaged in a wide variety of leadership, management, and specialized technical activities as this transformation takes place. HIM professionals may find themselves in positions with responsibility for setting standards and policies governing how health care data are collected, maintained, and disseminated. They are data quality experts and advocates for and trainers of the users of health care information. They also act as expert advisors on the appropriate uses of and interpretation of health care data and the privacy and security of the data. Some HIM professionals are partners with HIT professionals and health information users in the planning, design, and implementation of EHR systems and regional or national information networks.[25,26]

Today, members of the HIM profession work in a wide variety of health care settings, government agencies, and industry. They work wherever health data are collected, organized, and analyzed, including accounting and consulting firms, insurance companies, and research centers. An increasing number of professionals are involved in software development, marketing, and implementation as members of the information system staff within health care organizations or within software vendor environments. Regional and national health information networks provide another opportunity to HIM professionals. Many members are engaged in entrepreneurial business ventures that demonstrate their ability to blend business knowledge with the professional discipline. The knowledge and skills of HIM professionals are found in the roles they assume in more than 40 different types of job settings with more than 200 different job titles. The need for HIM professionals continues to grow as emerging technologies require qualified individuals to help others access information to support clinical decision making, research, financial management, and personal health management.[26] The AHIMA's efforts have been key in advancing the roles of HIM professionals through supporting cutting-edge academic programs, offering certification and professional development opportunities, and engaging in key initiatives that support HIM practice.

Formation of Education Programs

Education has been a building block of the HIM profession since 1928 when at its annual meeting ARLNA members formed a committee to develop a curriculum for the education of medical record librarians. The curriculum was finalized in 1932 and was used to establish academic programs for medical record librarians. The first schools for the education of medical record librarians were provisionally approved in 1934.[21] Early programs were in hospitals and required from 2 to 4 years of college, with some requiring graduation from an approved nursing school. As programs were established, it became apparent

that uniform standards for all medical record programs were needed; thus, the "Essentials of an Acceptable School for Medical Record Librarians" were developed by the ARLNA in 1943.[21] This document became the foundation for the association's accreditation program described below.

By 1952, 19 schools offered formal educational programs for medical record librarians.[21] Although these formal educational programs were established in a number of sites, the number of professionals graduating did not meet the needs of the hospitals. This led to the decision to train another level of personnel to aid the medical record librarian. In 1953, six schools for training medical record technicians were approved. These programs were 9 to 12 months in length and located in hospitals; no formal academic credit was granted. After completion of the technician program, the graduate was eligible to write a certification examination. On successful completion of the examination, the individual was granted the credential Accredited Record Technician (ART).[27] During the 1960s and 1970s, education programs at both the medical record librarian and medical record technician levels transitioned to 2- and 4-year college or university settings. This transition occurred as the profession's body of knowledge grew, and expanded skills in the work setting were required of program graduates.

In addition to the formal education programs found in universities and colleges, the professional association developed a correspondence course in 1961 to train more support staff at the technician level. Hospital-based technician programs were not producing enough graduates at the time to fill the workforce needs. Over time, the course was revised, and additional college requirements were added to the program in an effort to make the educational preparation of its graduates relatively comparable to that of graduates of the 2-year associate degree program.[28] In 1991, when the professional association changed its name to the AHIMA, the college and university programs also changed their program names to HIM. The correspondence course followed suit and was retitled the Independent Study Program for the Health Information Technician (ISP for HITs). By 1998, at was determined that the ISP for HITs was no longer needed because there were 165 community or technical college technician programs in existence. The ISP was discontinued, with all enrolled students required to complete the program by December 31, 2001.

As of this writing, there are 233 educational programs in HIM. Some offer the baccalaureate degree level (46) and others offer the associate degree level (187) with program numbers continuing to expand. Many baccalaureate degree programs also offer a postbaccalaureate degree option for those individuals who already possess a baccalaureate or advanced degree but wish to pursue the HIM degree. The curriculum in associate and baccalaureate degree programs has evolved over time to accommodate the increased demands for health care data and information.

The most significant changes in curriculum occurred in the mid 1990s, when curriculum models were developed for associate, baccalaureate, and master's degree programs in HIM. The models reflected the content and competencies required of HIM professionals in the twenty-first century.[29-31] These models were developed as part of a continuing discussion of the profession's future. The discussion identified the need for graduate education in HIM as a natural progression in the development of the HIM discipline. The content domains of the curriculum models were subsequently integrated into the *Standards for Health Information Management Education (Baccalaureate Degree and Associate Degree Programs)*.[32, 33] These standards are the basis for HIM program accreditation.

The curriculum models and content domains for the baccalaureate degree and associate degree HIM programs were updated in 2005, and the model for graduate education was updated in 2006. In addition, in 2004 the AHIMA Education Strategy Committee developed a framework for HIM education, which provided a general descriptor for graduates of each of the academic program levels. The descriptors emphasize the roles of HIM graduates in both a paper and electronic work environment. A brief synopsis of the descriptors follows:

Associate Degree HIM—Possesses technical expertise in health data collection, analysis, monitoring, maintenance, and reporting activities in accordance with established data quality principles, legal and regulatory standards, and professional best practice guidelines. These functions encompass, among other areas, processing and using health data for billing, compliance, and surveillance purposes.

Baccalaureate Degree HIM—Possesses expertise to develop, implement, or manage individual, aggregate, and public health care data collection and reporting systems. These systems ensure quality, integrity, availability, and preservation of health care data in support of patient safety and privacy, confidentiality, and security of health information.

Master's Degree HIM—Engages in executive level, enterprise-wide, administrative, research, or applied health informatics activities. Focus is on evolving strategic and operational relevance and robustness of clinical information resources in health care industry and public health sector. Performs research to advance body of knowledge and standards associated with the management of health information.[34]

Accreditation of Educational Programs

Because of close ties to the AMA and ACS and their accreditation program for medical schools, the AHIMA (formally ARLNA) developed an accreditation program for medical record librarian programs in 1943. Accreditation is defined as a voluntary, nongovernmental process that educational programs elect to participate in as a means of demonstrating to the public that a program meets or exceeds stated standards of educational quality. The program

accreditation for medical record librarians began in 1943, as noted above, and in 1953 the 2-year medical record technician degree programs were added to the accreditation agenda. The *Essentials of an Acceptable School for Medical Record Librarians* became the *Standards for Health Information Management Education (Baccalaureate Degree and Associate Degree Programs)*.[29,30] These standards represent the minimum requirements an education program must follow to achieve program accreditation. The standards indicate that the program curriculum must meet or exceed course content as published in the AHIMA Model Curriculum Entry-Level Competencies and Knowledge Clusters for 2- and 4-year education programs.[35-38]

From 1943 to 1994, the association collaborated with the AMA's Council on Allied Health Education and Accreditation to accredit the HIM associate and baccalaureate degree programs at colleges and universities in the United States and U.S. territories. In 1994, the council split from the AMA and became the Council on Accreditation of Allied Health Educational Programs (CAAHEP). The CAAHEP and AHIMA worked together to accredit education programs until 2004, when AHIMA moved to establish its own accrediting body for education programs: the Commission on Accreditation for Health Informatics and Information Management Education (CAHIIM).[39] Undergraduate HIM programs previously accredited by CAAHEP are now accredited under CAHIIM. The CAHIIM also offers an approval process for master's degree programs in HIM, which will convert to an accreditation process in the future.[31] Two other approval programs are offered by AHIMA, but they do not fall under the responsibility of CAHIIM. There are approval programs for Coding and for Transcription that are administered by the AHIMA Approval Committee for Certificate Programs.

Professional Certification

The focus of accreditation is on demonstrating to the public that a program or organization meets or exceeds stated standards of quality. An individual can also demonstrate to the public that he or she meets or exceeds stated standards of competence by obtaining professional certification. Licensure, certification, or registration are used by government and nongovernment agencies as a means of protecting the public from individuals who have not met the standards of practice prescribed by a given state or profession. Individuals who do meet these standards are given the right to use specific credentials that denote they have demonstrated a level of competence in their field of practice. Individuals who obtain credentials are required to maintain their credential over time by meeting continuing education requirements as defined by the agency or organization that supports the credential.

Licensure occurs at the state level and is overseen by a state licensing board or agency. An individual must meet eligibility requirements defined by the state before the individual is granted a license to practice. Demonstration of eligibility is usually through successful completion of an education program and passing of a licensing examination. Most health professionals that treat or touch patients in some way are required to be licensed by the state in which they practice. For example, occupational therapists, physical therapists, and respiratory therapists must complete certain educational requirements and take state licensing examinations before they are allowed to practice in a state. Demonstrated success of these two requirements enables these practitioners to use the credential "Licensed (L)" in their occupational title, such as Licensed Occupational Therapist (L/OT). Some health care professionals, such occupational therapists, possess both a license and a certification credential, Registered Occupational Therapist (R/OT).

How do certification and registration differ from licensure? Certification refers to "the process by which a non-governmental agency or association grants recognition of competence to an individual who has met predetermined qualifications specified by that agency or association."[40] Registration entails entering on an official list an individual who has been certified as eligible by set qualifications of an organization or agency. In regard to HIM, professional certification began in 1933 when the AHIMA (formally ARLNA) formed a Board of Registration to set standards for its members. One standard set by this new certifying body was that an individual had to be 21 years of age and in good moral and ethical character.[41] No formal examination of the candidate was required at that time. The credential bestowed on the individual who met these early standards was RRL.

By 1952, an examination component was added to the eligibility requirements and remains so today. Certification examinations are constructed from detailed job analysis studies of individuals working in the field. The analyses are updated every 3 to 5 years by the examination body. The job analysis study verifies the tasks performed by practitioners, which is then used to develop the test specifications and questions for a given certification examination. Over the years the profession's certification process has expanded to reflect the education and responsibilities of HIM professionals practicing in a variety of roles.

The AHIMA's certifying body is the Council on Certification (COC). The COC is responsible for "creating and maintaining certification and recertification processes whereby the public can be assured that certified individuals have met or maintain a level of competency required to deliver quality health information."[40] The AHIMA offered eight credentials until 2007, at which time two of the credentials were combined into one credential. Each of the credentials is discussed below:

- Registered Health Information Administrator (RHIA)
- Registered Health Information Technician (RHIT)
- Certified Coding Associate (CCA)
- Certified Coding Specialist (CCS)
- Certified Coding Specialist-Physician Based (CCS-P)
- Certified in Healthcare Privacy (CHP)

- Certified in Healthcare Security (CHS)
- Certified in Healthcare Privacy and Security (CHPS)

Registered Health Information Administrator and Registered Health Information Technologist

RHIA and RHIT credentials (formally RRL and ART, respectively) focus on HIM at an entry level of practice. Both credentials require that an individual pass a certification examination and be a graduate of a HIM education program that meets at least one of the following criteria:

- Accredited by the CAHIIM, or
- Qualifications of such a program at the candidate's graduation must have met the requirements of the designated accrediting authority for an accredited program, or
- Foreign educational institution that has reciprocity with AHIMA.

An individual wishing to take the RHIA examination must have successfully met the academic requirements of a CAHIIM-accredited HIM program at the baccalaureate degree level or have a certificate of completion from a CAHIIM-accredited HIM program, plus a baccalaureate degree from a regionally accredited college or university. An individual wishing to take the RHIT examination must have successfully met the academic requirements of a CAHIIM-accredited HIM program at the associate degree level. In addition, an individual who successfully completed the AHIMA Independent Study program, which no longer is offered, was eligible for the RHIT examination. The RHIA functions in the managerial areas of health services and information systems and the uses of health-related data for planning, delivering, and evaluating health care. The RHIT typically functions in the technical areas of health data collection, analysis, and monitoring and often specializes in coding diagnoses and procedures for reimbursement and research purposes.[42]

Certified Coding Associate, Certified Coding Specialist, Certified Coding Specialist-Physician Based

In 1992, AHIMA moved into specialty certification as it recognized the need to offer credentials in a specific area of practice: medical diagnostic and procedural coding. Coders are technical specialists who are a part of the health information services team in a health care organization. Their primary function is to assign diagnosis and procedure codes to clinical data on the basis of their review of the documentation in the patient record and the application of national, and facility-specific, coding guidelines. Accuracy in coding is extremely important for research, revenue, and reimbursement purposes, as discussed earlier in the section on the evolving patient record. To address the increasing need for coders who possessed the necessary competence to engage in quality coding, AHIMA implemented both entry-level and advanced coding credentials. Coding is also a knowledge and skill component in the entry-level credentialing examinations for RHITs and RHIAs.

Three coding certification options are available. The education eligibility requirements for these three credentials include a high school diploma from a U.S. high school or equivalent educational background. Experience is not required but is strongly recommended in the areas of hospital or ambulatory care patient record coding. The CCA, an entry-level credential, was implemented in 2002. The recommended amount of experience for this credential is 6 months or completion of an AHIMA-approved coding certificate program or other formal training program.[43] The CCS credential was implemented in 1992, and in 1997 the CCS-P was established. The CCS examination focuses on inpatient coding systems, whereas the CCS-P examination focuses on ambulatory care coding. Both the CCS and CCS-P credentials are for the more experienced coder. It is suggested that an individual have at least 3 or more years of coding experience to be successful on these examinations.[44]

Certified in Healthcare Privacy, Certified in Healthcare Security, Certified in Healthcare Privacy and Security

A third category of credentials offered by the AHIMA relates to health care privacy and security. In 1996, the Health Insurance Portability and Accountability Act (HIPAA) required that health care providers, payers, and plans appoint privacy and security officials to carry out mandatory duties as prescribed in the HIPAA regulations. The regulations asked for privacy officers who would be responsible for the development and implementation of privacy-related policies and procedures and security officials whose duties would be the management and supervision of security measures to protect personal patient information.[45] In 2002 the AHIMA implemented and sponsored the CHP credential, subsequently the CHS credentials.

The CHP credential validates an individual's expertise in designing, implementing, and administering comprehensive privacy protection programs in all types of health care settings. The CHS credential validates the expertise of an individual who holds advanced competency in the design, implementation, and administration of comprehensive security protection programs. The certification exams for these two credentials were combined into one certification exam in 2007. Successful completion of the combined exam results in the credential CHPS. Eligibility for the CHPS exam requires that an individual must have either a baccalaureate degree and a minimum of 4 years of experience in health care management or an advanced graduate degree (e.g., JD, MD, PhD) and 2 years of experience in health care management. A third option is a prior credential such as an RHIA or an RHIT with a baccalaureate or advanced graduate degree and a minimum of 2 years of experience in health care management.[45]

Importance of Professional Certification

The importance of certification should not be underestimated. Research indicates that individuals who are certified tend to promote quality work outcomes.[46] In addition, in 2005 AHIMA surveyed employers seeking their opinion on the value of industry credentials. Survey results revealed that, overall, employers think favorably of industry credentials. Credentialed employees help reduce exposure to fraud and abuse and improve the delivery of quality health care. Employers tend to hire individuals with a credential over those without one and prefer credentials when promoting employees. Credentialed employees tend to earn more than uncredentialed employees. Employers also reported that the credential tells them the individual has met certain education requirements, possesses a certain competency level as proven by examination, and must stay informed through continuing education requirements.[47] Thus, the importance of obtaining certification and maintaining the credential(s) cannot be overemphasized. A credential can be key to professional success and future opportunities in the marketplace.

Other Relevant Credentials

There are a number of other specialty credentials that HIM professionals may consider, depending on personal interests and their current AHIMA credentials. Each credential has its own set of eligibility requirements and in some cases continuing education requirements. A few of the more common credentials and their sponsoring organizations are listed below:

- **CPER**—Certified Professional in Electronic Health Records, offered by the Health IT Certification, *http://www.healthitcertification.com/*
- **CPHIT**—Certified Professional in Health Information Technology, offered by the Health IT Certification, *http://www.healthitcertification.com/*
- **CPHIMS**—Certified Professional in Health Information Management Systems, offered by the Health Information and Management System Society, *http://www.himss.org/ASP/index.asp*
- **CPHQ**—Certified Professional Health Quality, offered by the Health Care Quality Board, *http://www.cphq.org/*
- **CMT**—Certified Medical Transcriptionist, offered by the American Association of Medical Transcriptionists, *http://www.aamt.org/ScriptContent/Index.cfm*
- **CPC**—Certified Coding Professional, offered by the American Academy of Professional Coders, *http://www.aapc.com/certification/certification.html*
- **CTR**—Certified Tumor Registrar, offered by the National Cancer Registrars Association, *http://www.ncra-usa.org/certification/*

Maintenance of Certification and Lifelong Learning

Once a person receives a credential through the AHIMA's certification process, that person is required to maintain the credential by engaging in continuing education activity. Early in the profession's history it was recognized that the astonishing rate of change in medical science and the delivery of health care would require continuing learning on the part of HIM professionals to stay current in the field. The AHIMA was an early proponent of lifelong learning, offering its first formal continuing education institute in 1939.[21] In 1973, AHIMA adopted a formal maintenance of certification program that required the acquisition of a certain number of continuing education units (CEUs) on the basis of the credential. Standards for maintaining certification were defined along with CEU-qualifying activities.

The maintenance of the certification program is continually updated to reflect changes in the field and the addition of new credentials to the program. CEUs must be obtained in a 2-year cycle. The number of CEUs that must be obtained will depend on the type and number of AHIMA credentials held.[48] Overall, 80% of all CEUs must be earned in the domain of HIM. Basically, the HIM domain encompasses the following content areas where CEUs may be obtained:

- **Technology**: existing and emerging technologies for the collection of clinical data, the transformation of clinical data to useful health information, and the communication and protection of information.
- **Management development**: organizational management theory and practices and human resource management techniques to improve departmental adaptability, innovation, service quality, and operational efficiency.
- **Clinical data management**: data analysis of quality and clinical resources appropriate to the clinical setting including database management, coding compliance using coding or payment systems to ensure cost-effectiveness of services rendered.
- **Performance improvement**: quality processes to ensure quality data are generating consistent, timely

quality information; to develop systems that are flexible and adaptable in a constantly changing health care environment.

- **External forces**: regulatory requirements and appropriate compliance initiatives (policies, procedures, protocols, and technology) for hospitals and others including required practices for accrediting bodies and federal and state rules and regulations.
- **Clinical foundations**: understanding of human anatomy and physiology, the nature of disease processes, protocols of diagnosis and treatment of major diseases including drugs, laboratory and other tests; to apply to reading, coding, and abstracting of medical information to support quality care and associated databases.
- **Privacy and Security**: current health care regulations that promote protection of medical information and electronic transmission of health information; patient advocacy related to privacy rights.[48]

Although individuals who hold an AHIMA credential are required to maintain their certifications through continuing education activities, there is overall support among AHIMA members for the concept of lifelong learning. Lifelong learning is the responsibility of every individual who wishes to enter and survive in a work environment that continually faces global, economic, and technological changes. The AHIMA members affirmation of lifelong learning is delineated in the 2004 resolution *Lifelong Learning: The Guiding Principles for Professional Development*[49] (Box 2-2).

Fellowship Program

In 1999, the AHIMA implemented a fellowship program that is open to any individual who is an active, honorary, or senior member of AHIMA. The program is designed to recognize AHIMA members who have made significant and

---

Box 2-2 EMBRACING LIFELONG LEARNING: THE GUIDING PRINCIPLES FOR PROFESSIONAL DEVELOPMENT

Whereas, the health care and technology environment will continually change the HIM professionals' role;

Whereas, data show that individuals who continually advance their educational standings are rewarded with the highest compensation;

Whereas, the most sought-after professionals are flexible and can demonstrate their knowledge and skills;

Whereas, HIM professionals' skills and competencies are a valuable and integral part of the health care arena; and

Whereas, ultimate success depends on the willingness of individual members to take responsibility for preparing for new roles by acquiring new knowledge and skills; therefore, be it

Resolved, that AHIMA make available the new knowledge and skills that will enhance members' value in the marketplace;

Resolved, that AHIMA members commit to mentoring and helping others to advance HIM practice; and

Resolved, that AHIMA members make the commitment to lifelong learning and professional development so that HIM professionals continue to be vital players in ensuring quality health care through quality information.

Whereas, ultimate success depends on the willingness of individual members to take responsibility for preparing for new roles by acquiring new knowledge and skills; therefore, be it

Resolved, that AHIMA make available the new knowledge and skills that will enhance members' value in the marketplace;

Resolved, that AHIMA members commit to mentoring and helping others to advance HIM practice; and

Resolved, that AHIMA members make the commitment to lifelong learning and professional development so that HIM professionals continue to be vital players in ensuring quality health care through quality information.

Source: Text of the lifelong learning resolution (2004 convention wrap-up), *J AHIMA* 75:64, 2004.

sustained contributions to the profession over time. Contributions can be made in any one or all of the following areas: innovation and knowledge sharing, meritorious service, and excellence in practice or education. The fellowship program is designed to bring together senior HIM professionals as an organizational resource and to provide an incentive to members to contribute to the advancement of the profession.[50]

Eligibility for fellowship requires that an individual have a minimum of 10 years of full-time professional experience in HIM or a related field, 10 years of continuous AHIMA membership, evidence of sustained and substantial professional achievement, and a minimum of a master's degree. The fellowship program also offers a candidacy provision for those individuals who do not meet the criteria but wish to work toward fellowship over time. The process for fellowship designation requires that an individual complete an application that is reviewed for approval by the AHIMA Fellowship Committee. On approval by this committee, fellow status is conferred and the individual may use the credential Fellow of the American Health Information Management Association. It is a lifetime recognition that is subject to continuing AHIMA membership and compliance with the AHIMA Code of Ethics.[50]

AMERICAN HEALTH INFORMATION MANAGEMENT ASSOCIATION TODAY

The AHIMA has enjoyed a long history of accomplishments, many of which have been discussed earlier in the chapter. It has organized and reorganized itself throughout its history to meet the needs of its members and the changing dynamics of the HIM profession. Today, the AHIMA is more than 75 years old. Its membership is over 50,000 and it continues to grow at a rate of 5% per year. Members are classified as either active, student, new graduate, or senior; thus, its membership structure allows anyone interested in HIM to join the association[51] (Box 2-3).

The benefits of AHIMA membership are numerous. The AHIMA is a member-centered organization (Figure 2-1) that provides members with key resources to assist with all aspects of HIM practice. Most important, the AHIMA champions and represents the profession in advocacy matters and key professional alliances, which keeps the profession in the forefront of issues related to its members and their professional domain of practice.

The AHIMA is headquartered in Chicago and also supports a satellite office in Washington, DC. It is a federation made up of 52 component state associations (CSAs), including the District of Columbia and Puerto Rico. The CSAs are affiliated with AHIMA and agree to support and carry out certain member benefits and activities that support the overall goal of the national association. The work of the AHIMA is carried out through a volunteer and staff structure.

The volunteer structure of the association is responsible for setting the policies of the organization and for providing direction to a wide variety of essential AHIMA activities. The AHIMA governs itself through a national Board of Directors (BOD) that is elected by the membership. The Board is comprised of a President, President-Elect, Past President Director, and nine directors. The chief executive officer of the association is an ex officio member of the Board and is hired by the BOD. An important function of the BOD is overseeing the strategic direction of the association and its assets both intellectual and financial. The BOD is aided by a House of Delegates (HOD).

The HOD is composed of members who are elected leaders from their respective CSAs. The number of delegates from each state varies depending on the number of active members in the state, up to a maximum of five delegates per any one state. The HOD serves as the association's legislative body. For example, it has the power to approve the standards related to maintenance of certification and HIM educational programs. It also advises the BOD in the development and modification of the association's strategic direction and plans. There is a strong collaborative working relationship between the BOD and the HOD because both groups work in tandem to strategically move the profession

---

Box 2-3   AHIMA MEMBERSHIP CATEGORIES

- Active
  For AHIMA-credentialed professionals, this membership entitles you to the entire breadth of member products and services.
- Student
  Students formally enrolled in an AHIMA-accredited or AHIMA-approved HIM program, including programs pending accreditation or approval, or AHIMA's Coding Basics, who do not already have an AHIMA credential are eligible to apply for student membership. Eligibility is verified with the program director. Special benefits for student members: AHIMA Mentor Program, Student Community of Practice and Student Connection e-news.

- New Graduate
  New Graduate membership is for AHIMA Student Members only. After graduation from an AHIMA accredited HIT, HIA, approved Coding, or Masters program, AHIMA Student Members may join as a New Graduate Member at a reduced annual dues rate. This is limited to 1 year.
- Senior
  In recognition of service to the profession, current AHIMA members 65 years old and over are eligible for this member type.

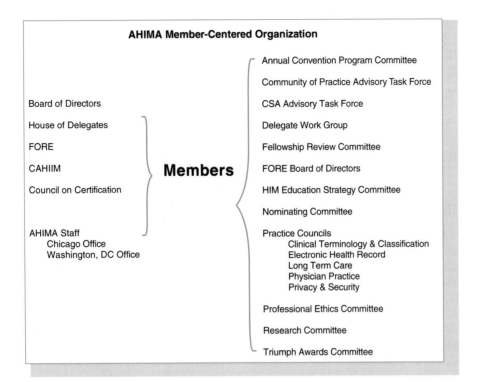

Figure 2-1 AHIMA is a member-centered organization, with support resources for its members.

forward and to provide industry leadership in matters related to HIM.

In addition to the BOD and HOD, the volunteer structure consists of the COC and CAHIIM, whose functions were discussed above, as well as committees, practice councils, and task forces. Members on the COC and CAHIIM are elected through national balloting while membership on the committees, practice councils, and task forces are by appointment. In 2006 there were 17 volunteer groups at the national level excluding the COC and CAHIIM. The number varies by year on the basis of the strategic direction and need of the association. Collectively, more than 1000 members serve the AHIMA and CSAs in a volunteer capacity. Volunteerism has been at the heart of the association's activities for more than 75 years and continues to serve as a driving force in moving the profession forward.

Working in tandem with the volunteer structure are some 100+ association employees. The AHIMA staff is responsible for carrying out the day-to-day operation of the association. The staff works collaboratively with the volunteer structure to support the association's vision, mission, and values. In addition, the staff works with the volunteer structure to carry out the strategic priorities set each year by the association leadership. In the last several years these priorities have focused on HIT issues encompassing, EHRs, privacy and security, standards for data interchange and systems interoperability, and a national health care information infrastructure.[52] In addition, priorities have called for improvements in the way medical and surgical information is coded for reimbursement and research purposes. This entails using the newest edition of the *International Classification of Disease*, 10th edition, and other various forms of the classification system.[52] The AHIMA is an industry leader in many of the activities just mentioned. It has formed alliances with numerous organizations and agencies such as the American Medical Informatics Association to accomplish its priorities and serve its members.[52]

American Health Information Management Association Communications

Communication is fundamental to supporting an association's members. The AHIMA communicates with its members though a variety of publications such as newsletters, practice briefs, electronic alerts, and professional journals—*Journal of the American Health Information Management Association*[53] and *Perspective in Health Information Management*.[54] The latter is an on-line peer reviewed research journal that was implemented in 2003 to foster the professions commitment to research and scholarship. In addition, AHIMA recognized that association members with like issues and concerns would benefit from a way to network with others in similar areas of practice or with similar concerns. Given the availability of the Internet and the advantages of the World Wide Web, AHIMA sought to support member professional development through the implementation of a Web-based communication capability called Communities of Practice (CoP). The AHIMA CoP is an on-line tool for connecting association members. The CoP provides up-to-date news and links to resources such as the associations on-line library—Book of Knowledge. It helps to keep members informed on the latest trends in HIM, helps the member solve problems, to network, career build, and much more.[55] Currently, there are more than 135 CoPs that a member can chose to join.

FOUNDATION OF RESEARCH AND EDUCATION IN HEALTH INFORMATION MANAGEMENT

An important indicator of the AHIMA growth as a professional association and its contribution to the profession is evident in the Foundation of Research and Education in Health Information Management (FORE). The FORE is a separately incorporated affiliate organization that actively promotes education and research in the HIM field. The foundation's role is to provide financial and intellectual resources that support innovation and advancement in HIM for the betterment of the profession, health care, and the public.[56] The FORE functions with its own Board of Directors who are appointed by the AHIMA BOD. The FORE offers grants-in-aid to support research activities and professional self-development opportunities, scholarships, professional recognition awards, and more. An example of some of the programs initiated through FORE funding include benchmarking and best practices research, study of the HIM workforce, and curriculum and faculty support.[56]

THE PROFESSIONAL CODE OF ETHICS

A code of ethics guides the practice of individuals who choose a given profession. It sets forth the values and principles defined by the profession as acceptable behavior within a practice setting. The HIM profession enacted its first set of ethical principles in 1957 and has since revised the code four times (1977, 1988, 1998, and 2004). Revisions of the code over the years demonstrate the importance that AHIMA places on making sure the code is relevant to all members irrespective of credential, membership status, practice functions, or work settings. The code is kept up to date and in line with the changing practice patterns and responsibilities of the HIM professional. The most recent revision of the code occurred in 2004. Eleven ethical principles were defined and a set of guidelines were developed to help interpret the vode and to further delineate behaviors and situations to help clarify a principle.[57]

The principles of the code are fundamental to the role of a HIM professional in the work environment. HIM professionals are in positions of responsibility where they must ensure that the processes followed keep the organization in compliance with its various licensing, accrediting, and legal obligations. In addition, they are in positions in which confidential information is entrusted to them. HIM professionals extend this trust by serving as an advocate for the protection and monitoring of such information. The code also speaks to the profession's fundamental duty to engage in lifelong learning and activities that will guide future development of systems to meet the changing needs of the health care industry (Box 2-4).

Box 2-4 AHIMA CODE OF ETHICS 2004

Ethical Principles: The following ethical principles are based on the core values of the American Health Information Management Association and apply to all health information management professionals.

Health information management professionals:

I. Advocate, uphold, and defend the individual's right to privacy and the doctrine of confidentiality in the use and disclosure of information.

II. Put service and the health and welfare of persons before self-interest and conduct themselves in the practice of the profession so as to bring honor to themselves, their peers, and to the health information management profession.

III. Preserve, protect, and secure personal health information in any form or medium and hold in the highest regard the contents of the records and other information of a confidential nature, taking into account the applicable statutes and regulations.

IV. Refuse to participate in or conceal unethical practices or procedures.

V. Advance health information management knowledge and practice through continuing education, research, publications, and presentations.

VI. Recruit and mentor students, peers, and colleagues to develop and strengthen the professional workforce.

VII. Represent the profession accurately to the public.

VIII. Perform honorably health information management association responsibilities, either appointed or elected, and preserve the confidentiality of any privileged information made known in any official capacity.

IX. State truthfully and accurately their credentials, professional education, and experiences.

X. Facilitate interdisciplinary collaboration in situations supporting health information practice.

XI. Respect the inherent dignity and worth of every person.

Used with permission from American Health Information Management Association, Chicago, Illinois.

LOOKING TO THE FUTURE

Health information technology is allowing the transfer and linkage of data well beyond the walls of a health care facility. This technology is supporting the conversion of patient records to EHRs and EHR systems. Such a conversion cannot be successful unless the data to be transferred, manipulated, and aggregated are well defined, valid, and reliable.

As more data become available in electronic form, more potential uses and users will emerge. The capabilities of technology must be tempered with expertise related to appropriate uses of the data and legitimate users. The pioneering HIM professionals used the resources of the day to help create accurate records that documented patient care. Today's professionals have the same responsibilities but many more challenges, as the value and volume of health information increases and the growing number of users and uses of the information also increases. As HIM professional roles and responsibilities change to accommodate the demands of the health care industry, it is important that the profession maintain leadership in the management of patient data, information, and EHRs and systems. The AHIMA and all its members will continue to play a key role in the future of health care and the complex, integrated information system needed to support the delivery of efficient, quality care in an expanding and transforming health care system.

Key Concepts

- The importance of recording clinical information is recognized from patient records maintained in early civilizations. The first U.S. hospitals used patient records notable for their brevity compared with the amount and variety of clinical data collected today. Diagnostic and treatment methods have been greatly expanded by new technologies, resulting in an increase in the volume and complexity of information in the patient record.
- The American College of Surgeons influenced health records through its Hospital Standardization Movement in the early 1900s. The College recognized the value of medical records in assessing the quality of physician education and treatment. Subsequently, The Joint Commission continued to expand and shape the content of the patient record and systems for managing health care information through voluntary accreditation.
- Development of the patient record and development of health care in the United States have been concurrent as physicians, hospitals, early medical record professionals, and early regulatory agencies recognized the importance

of the patient record in evaluating patient care and developing reimbursement sources and payment systems.
- The initiation of federally funded Medicare and Medicaid programs in the mid 1960s led to the involvement of federal governmental agencies in patient record issues. In 1983, the Tax Equity and Fiscal Responsibility Act became law, bringing prospective pricing to health care, and enhanced the value of the patient record because it became the key document for supporting and determining reimbursement to hospitals.
- In 1996, the Health Insurance Portability and Accessibility Act (HIPAA) was enacted, which enhanced the federal government's involvement in the development of standards that are required for electronic capture and transmission of clinical information. The HIPAA legislation also invigorated the government's efforts to ensure that health care organizations are complying with reimbursement regulations and coding guidelines associated with the submission of claims for services rendered to federally funded patients. Both these aspects of the HIPAA legislation have served to focus attention on the accessibility of the patient record, the quality of the documentation in the patient record, and the integrity of the processes associated with the uses of the data within the patient record.
- The beginning of the medical record profession and the founding of its professional association, now known as AHIMA, are important for linking the profession to HIM as it is practiced in the twenty-first century. The profession's focus from early times has been on the enhancement of patient care through better documentation. The educational efforts of the association are significant as they demonstrate a continuing concern for quality preparation of health information professionals for the workforce. The concept and importance of lifelong learning is recognized as a main contributor to the profession's ability to adapt to changing practices patterns and demands. The association established standards early on for its education accreditation program and for certifying the competence of practitioners through its certification program. Because the profession's body of knowledge focuses on management, information systems, and clinical medicine, HIM professionals are employable in a wide variety of settings with a wide variety of job titles.
- Numerous factors have contributed to the demand for patient data and the information contained with a patient's record. Advances in technology have made it possible for this information to be shared by many users in many different locations. The health care industry was somewhat slow in adapting HIT to address its information needs. However, the industry is now in a dramatic push to implement EHRs and the systems used to collect, store, and disseminate the data and information within such records as a way to control health care costs and improve the quality of patient care. The federal

government has supported this push through establishing the Office of the National Coordinator for Health Information Technology, and other public-private groups have been engaged in numerous activities to bring about a national health information infrastructure. As a result, the HIM profession is moving rapidly to an e-HIM environment. Such an environment requires a rethinking of how patient records are managed and what skills the HIM professional needs to support a changing practice environment.

- The AHIMA has assumed leadership in moving the profession forward through active collaboration and partnerships with other organizations committed to an electronic health care environment. The AHIMA is involved in initiatives to advance the role of HIM professionals related to standards for data interchange and system interoperability, privacy and security, EHR implementation, and the national health information infrastructure.

REFERENCES

1. e-HIM Work Group on Defining the Legal Health Record: The legal process and electronic health records, *J Am Health Inform Manage Assoc* 76:96A-96D, 2005.
2. National Healthcare Quality Report, Agency for Healthcare Research and Quality 2005. Retrieved from http://www.qualitytools.ahrq.gov/. Accessed August 7, 2006.
3. Bettman CC: *Pictorial history of medicine*, Springfield, IL, 1979, Charles C Thomas, p. 16.
4. Huffman EK: *Health information management*, ed 10, Berwyn, IL, 1994, Physicians' Record, p. 3.
5. American Medical Record Association: The years of growth and development, *Med Record News* 50(1):66, 1978.
6. Joint Commission Resources Manuals. Retrieved from http://www.jcrinc.com/publications.asp?durki=50(1):77. Accessed August 7, 2006.
7. Casto AB, Layman E: *Principles of healthcare reimbursement*, Chicago, 2006, American Health Information Management Association.
8. Conditions of Coverage and Conditions of Participation, Center for Medicare and Medicaid Services. Retrieved from http://new.cms.hhs.gov/CFCsAndCoPs/01_Overview.asp#TopOfPage. Accessed August 7, 2006.
9. Institute of Medicine: *The computer-based patient record: An essential technology for health care*, rev ed, Washington, DC, 1997, National Academy Press.
10. Eysenbach G: What is e-health? *J Medical Internet Res* (June 18)3(2):e20, 2001.
11. American Health Information Management Association: *Complete medical record in a hybrid EHR environment, I: Managing the transition*, Practice brief, 2003, Chicago, American Health Information Management Association.
12. Revolutionizing health care through information technology: President's Information Technology Advisory Committee, National Coordination Office for Information Technology Research and Development, 2004. Retrieved from http://www.nitrd.gov. Accessed August 7, 2006.
13. Bush GW: Executive order 13335: Incentives for the use of health information technology and establishing the position of the National Health Information Technology Coordinator; 2004. Retrieved from http://www.whitehouse.gov/news/releases/2004/04/20040427-4.html. Accessed August 7, 2006.
14. Office for the National Coordinator for Health Information Technology: The decade of health information technology: Delivering consumer-centric and information-rich health care, Washington, DC, July 21, 2004. Retrieved from http://www.hhs.gov/healthit/documents/hitframework.pdf. Accessed August 7, 2006.
15. National Resource Center for Health Information Technology, Electronic Medical/Health Records, Agency for Health Research and Quality. Retrieved from http://healthit.ahrq.gov/portal/server.pt?open=514&objID=5554&mode=2&holderDisplayURL=http://prodportallb.ahrq.gov:7087/publishedcontent/publish/communities/k_o/knowledge_library/key_topics/health_briefing_01232006114616/electronic_medical_health_records.html. Accessed August 7, 2006.
16. American Medical Records Association: The years of growth and development, *Med Record News* 50(1):66, 1978.
17. *Bull Assoc Record Librarians North Am* 1(1), 1930.
18. *Bull Assoc Record Librarians North Am* 12(4):102, 1941.
19. *Bull Assoc Record Librarians North Am* 14, p. 14, 1939.
20. American Medical Record Association: The years of growth and development, *Med Record News* 49(5):84-90, 1978.
21. American Medical Record Association: The years of growth and development, *Med Record News* 49(5):84-90, 1978.
22. AHIMA: *Evolving careers*, Chicago: American Health Information Management Association, 1998.
23. E-health Task Force: Your job in the e-health era, *J Am Health Inform Manage Assoc* 73:32-35, 2002.
24. Bloomrosen M: e-HIM: From vision to reality, *J Am Health Inform Manage Assoc* 76(9):36-41, October 2005. Available at: http:// library.ahima.org/xpedio/groups/public/documents/ahima/bok1_028133.hcsp?dDocName=bok1_028133. Accessed August 7, 2006.
25. A vision of the e-HIM future: a report from the AHIMA e-HIM Task Force, *J Am Health Inform Mange Assoc:* http://library.ahima.org/xpedio/groups/public/documents/ahima/bok1_020835.hcsp?dDocName=bok1_020835. Accessed August 7, 2006.
26. Embracing the future: New times, new opportunities for health information managers, summary findings from the HIM Workforce Study, 2005, American Health Information Management Association, Foundation for Research and Education in Health Information Management, Chicago. Available at: http://library.ahima.org/xpedio/-idcplg?IdcService=GET_HIGHLIGHT_INFO&QueryText=%28Embracing+the+future%29%3cand%3e%28xPublishSite%3csubstring%3e%60BoK%60%29&SortField=xPubDate&SortOrder=Desc&dDocName=bok1_027397&HighlightType=HtmlHighlight&dWebExtension=hcsp.
27. *J Am Assoc Medical Record Librarians* 49(5):79, 1953.
28. American Medical Record Association: The years of growth and development, *Med Record News* 50:83, 1979.
29. American Health Information Management Association: Curriculum model associate degree education in health information management framework for HIM education (2005). Retrieved from http://library.ahima.org/xpedio/groups/public/documents/ahima/bok1_026333.pdf. Accessed August 7, 2006.
30. American Health Information Management Association: Curriculum model baccalaureate degree education in health information management framework for HIM education (2005). Retrieved from http://library.ahima.org/xpedio/groups/public/documents/ahima/bok1_026332.pdf. Accessed August 7, 2006.
31. American Health Information Management Association: *Program approval manual for health information management applied health informatics graduate degree levels*, 2006, Chicago, American Health Information Management Association.
32. Commission on Accreditation for Health Informatics and Information Management: Standards for health information management education—Baccalaureate degree, (2005). Retrieved from http://www.cahiim.org/standards/. Accessed August 7 2006.
33. Commission on Accreditation for Health Informatics and Information Management: Standards for health information management education—Associate degree (2005). Retrieved from http://www.cahiim.org/standards/. Accessed August 7, 2006.

34. Russell L, Patena K: Preparing tomorrow's professionals: A new framework for HIM education, *J Am Health Inform Manage Assoc* 75: 23-26, 2004.

35. American Health Information Management Association: HIM baccalaureate degree entry-level competencies domains, subdomains, and tasks, for 2005 and beyond (2004). Retrieved from http://www.ahimanet.org/COP/AssemblyonEducation/Resources/Attachment.fusion?AttachmentID=11130. Accessed August 7, 2006.

36. American Health Information Management Association: HIM baccalaureate degree knowledge cluster content and competency levels (2005). Retrieved from http://library.ahima.org/xpedio/groups/-public/documents/ahima/bok1_025411.doc. Accessed August 7, 2006.

37. American Health Information Management Association: HIM associate degree entry-level competencies domains, subdomains, and tasks, for 2006 and beyond (2004). Retrieved from http://www.-ahimanet.org/COP/AssemblyonEducation/Resources/Attachment.fusion?AttachmentID=11131. Accessed August 7, 2006.

38. American Health Information Management Association: HIM associate degree level knowledge cluster content and competency levels (2005). Retrieved from http://library.ahima.org/xpedio/groups/-public/documents/ahima/bok1_025380.doc. Accessed August 7, 2006.

39. American Health Information Management Association: Commission on Accreditation of Health Informatics and Information Management Education. Retrieved from http://www.cahiim.org/. Accessed August 7, 2006.

40. American Health Information Management Association: About certification. Retrieved from http://www.ahima.org/certification/-about.asp. Accessed August 7, 2006.

41. *Bull Am Assoc Med Record Librarians* 12(4):102, 1941.

42. American Health Information Management Association: Candidate handbook Registered Health Record Administrator (RHIA), Registered Health Record Technician (RHIT) (2006). Retrieved from http://www.ahima.org/certification/documents/2006/06-RHIA-RHIT-final_hndbk.pdf. Accessed August 7, 2006.

43. American Health Information Management Association: Candidate handbook Certified Coding Assistant (2006). Retrieved from http://www.ahima.org/certification/documents/2006/06-CCAhandbook.pdf. Accessed August 7, 2006.

44. American Health Information Management Association: Candidate handbook Certified Coding Specialist, Certified Coding Specialist-Physician Based (2006). Retrieved from http://www.ahima.org/-certification/documents/05-CCS_CCSPhndbk.pdf. Accessed August 7, 2006.

45. American Health Information Management Association: Candidate handbook Certified in Healthcare Privacy (2006). Retrieved from http://www.ahima.org/certification/documents/2006/2006-CHP-hndbook.pdf. Accessed August 7, 2006.

46. Parker W, Smith G: Certification as a predictor of quality performance. Presented at the National Organization for Competency Assurance 2004 Annual Educational Conference, Miami, FL. Retrieved from http://irecusa.org/articles/static/1/binaries/CertificationasaPredictorNOCA1104.pdf?PHPSESSID=e7921d19cfeacf6b707bf0a3c55b6766. Accessed August 7, 2006.

47. American Health Information Management Association: Employers value credentials in healthcare—An AHIMA survey (2005). Retrieved from http://www.ahima.org/hitweek/EmployeeValuesurvey.pdf#page-%3D2. Accessed August 7, 2006.

48. American Health Information Management Association: Standards for maintenance of continuing education units in certification HIM domain. Retrieved from http://www.ahima.org/certification/-documents/HIMDomain.pdf. Accessed August 7, 2006.

49. Text of the lifelong learning resolution (2004 convention wrap-up), *J Am Health Inform Manage Assoc* 76:64, 2005.

50. American Health Information Management Association: Fellowship program. Retrieved from http://www.ahima.org/fellow/. Accessed August 7, 2006.

51. American Health Information Management Association: Membership. Retrieved from http://www.ahima.org/membership/membership-_types.asp. Accessed August 7, 2006.

52. American Health Information Management Association: Facts. Retrieved from http://www.ahima.org/about/about.asp. Accessed August 7, 2006.

53. Journal of the American Health Information Management Association. Retrieved from http://www.ahima.org/journal.

54. Perspectives in health information management. Retrieved from http://www.ahima.org/perspectives/. Accessed August 7, 2006.

55. Lane L: Communities of practice: Harnessing the power of knowledge, *J Am Health Inform Manage Assoc* 73: 24-27, 2002.

56. About FORE (2006). Retrieved from http://www.ahima.org/fore/-about.asp. Accessed August 7, 2006.

57. AHIMA Code of ethics, 1957, 1977, 1988, and 1998: Revised and adopted by AHIMA House of Delegates—July 1, 2004. Retrieved from http://library.ahima.org/xpedio/groups/public/documents/ahima/bok1_024277.hcsp?dDocName=bok1_024277. Accessed August 7, 2006.

Health Care Data and Information Systems

chapter 3

Health Information Infrastructure and Systems

Meryl Bloomrosen

Additional content,
http:evolve.elsevier.com/Abdelhak/

Review exercises can be found
in the Study Guide

Chapter Contents

Health Information Technology in Health Care
Background
Federal Involvement in Health Information Technology
  Congress
Role of the Private Sector
Compelling Reasons to Implement Health Information Technology
Obstacles to Health Information Technology Adoption
Emerging Health Information Networks
  Organization and Governance Issues
  Technical Issues
  Financial Issues
  Privacy, Security, and Confidentiality Issues
Role of Health Information Management

Key Words

Health information technology
EHR systems
National Health Information
  Network
Regional Health Information
  Organization

Abbreviations

ADE—Adverse Drug Event
AHRQ—Agency for Healthcare Quality and Research
AHIC—American Health Information Community
AHIP—America's Health Insurance Plan
AQA—Ambulatory Quality Alliance
CAP—College of American Pathologists
CMS—Centers for Medicare and Medicaid Services
CDS—Clinical Decision Support
CCBH—Connecting Communities for Better Health
CCHIT—Commission on the Certification for Health Information Technology
CITL—Center for Information Technology Leadership
CPOE—Computerized Physician Order Entry
CHI—Consolidated Health Informatics Standards
CHT—Center for Health Transformation
DHHS—Department of Health and Human Services
DICOM—Digital Imaging Communications in Medicine
DOQ-IT—Doctors' Office Quality Information Technology
DSS—Decision Support System
EHRs—Electronic Health Records
EMR—Electronic Medical Record
ERX—Electronic Prescribing
FDA—Food and Drug Administration
GAO—General Accounting Office
GPO—Government Printing Office
HIE—Health Information Exchange
HIT—Health Information Technology
HISPC—Health Information Security and Privacy Collaboration
HIPAA—Health Insurance Portability and Accountability Act
HISSB—Health Information and Surveillance Systems Board
HL7—Health Level 7
HRSA—Health Resources and Services Administration

HUGH—Human Gene Nomenclature

IOM—Institute of Medicine

IEEE 1073—Institute of Electrical and Electronics Engineers 1073

LOINC—Laboratory Logical Observation Identifier Name Codes

NCPCP—National Council on Prescription Drug Programs

NCVHS—National Center for Vital and Health Statistics

NDF-RT—National Drug File Reference Terminology

NHII—National Health Information Infrastructure

NHIN—Nationwide Health Information Network

NRC—National Resource Center

OMB—Office of Management and Budget's Office

ONC—Office of the National Coordinator for Health Information Technology

ORHP—Office of Rural Health Policy

P2P—Peer-to-peer

PHI—Personal Health Information

PHR—Personal Health Record

QIO—Quality Improvement Organization

RFI—Request for Information

RHIOs—Regional Health Information Organizations

RIO—Return on Investments

SNO—Sub Network Organization

SNOMED CT—Systemized Nomenclature of Medicine Clinical Terms

SDOS—Standards Development Organizations

Objectives

After reading this chapter, the reader will be able to do the following:

- Define the key words.
- Identify public and private sector initiatives and organizations in health information technology and health information exchange.
- Illustrate and understand the role of health information management in designing, developing, and implementing electronic health information technology and exchange policies and processes across organizations and multiple stakeholders.
- Understand the complex political, technical, legal, logistical, privacy-security, and clinical workflow factors contributing to the discussions of health information technology and exchange among and across multiple data sources and users.
- Identify potential management issues facing health care and information management professionals resulting from the migration and implementation of health information technology and systems.
- Understand the role and importance of (administrative and clinical) data content and messaging standards in achieving the goals of transforming the health care system.

HEALTH INFORMATION TECHNOLOGY IN HEALTH CARE

Every aspect of the health care industry is highly fragmented, which has led to untenable levels of administrative complexity and compromises to quality of care. One of the top-ranking challenges faced by most providers is the timeliness and efficiency of access to patient information. Patient data are most frequently recorded and stored in paper-based systems and shared across organizations every day through low-technology modes such as fax, mail, and courier, costing unnecessarily high labor and nonlabor expenses. Patients are misdiagnosed and mistreated because of a lack of timely and easily available information at the point of care.*†[1]

The earliest activities devoted to health information technology (HIT) implementation focused first on the automation of administrative functions. Subsequently, attention has moved to address improvements in patient safety and clinical care. Most recently, activities are addressing how to provide for the exchange of clinical and administrative information and to facilitate industry use of more standardized electronic communications across organizations.

Efforts to date have largely operated independent of each other. Today, there are numerous efforts underway to coordinate and integrate activities and to leverage lessons learned from one activity to another.[2] For example, over the last decade we have seen the implementation of nationwide efforts toward administrative simplification under the Health Insurance Portability and Accountability Act of 1996 (HIPAA) and the related rise in electronic claims processing.

It has long been recognized that providers need data to treat their patients and to choose among treatment modalities: payers require data to verify eligibility for treatment and to determine medical necessity for care, researchers need data for various outcomes measurement projects, and regulators and policy makers require data to make prudent and cost-effective decisions that will ensure the public health and well-being of our country's citizens. The national policy agenda for HIT, health information exchange (HIE), and electronic health records (EHR) in the public and private sectors has been developing rapidly and is seen as a top priority.[3] These policy discussions have concluded that health care data and information should be universally digitized. Improving patient safety and increasing the quality of health care are primary motivating factors in most public and private sector efforts. Increasingly multiple and previously diverse activities are being coordinated and leveraged together so that ideally we can all yield the economic and social benefits that are optimistically promised.

This peak in activity seemed to be propelled with the President's State of the Union Address in 2004 followed by the creation of the Department of Health and Human Services (DHHS) Office of the National Coordinator for HIT (ONC) and the Release of the Strategic Framework, the federal funding of HIT projects by several agencies of the DHHS, and the numerous bills introduced in Congress that address various aspects of HIT and HIE. The National Health Information Infrastructure concept envisions providing electronically the information necessary for decision making at the time it is needed, in the place where it is needed, and to the people who need it. It would connect physicians, hospitals, health care purchasers and payers, researchers, public health professionals, and consumers. It is a comprehensive knowledge-based network of interoperable systems of clinical, public health, and personal health information.[4] Early attention to the importance of improving access to health information led to increasing efforts for the creation of a National Health Information Infrastructure Network (NHIN), an endeavor working toward a vision of an effective, efficient, high-quality health care system that harnesses the power of shared data to improve the health of all Americans. Subsequently, the concept of the NHIN was defined by DHHS as an Internet-based architecture that links disparate health care information systems together to allow patients, physicians, hospitals, community health centers, and public health agencies across the country to share clinical information securely.[5]

BACKGROUND

For decades, the need for an improved HIT infrastructure has been a recurring theme in Institute of Medicine (IOM) reports, recommendations by the National Committee on Vital and Health Statistics, and innumerable testimonies before congressional committees.

In the IOM's report, "Crossing the Quality Chasm"[5a] the members of the institute, among other things, recommended the following:

> Recommendation 19: Congress, the executive branch, leaders of health care organizations, public and private sector purchasers, and health informatics associations and vendors should make a renewed national commitment to building an information infrastructure to support health care delivery, consumer health, quality measurement and improvement, public accountability, clinical and health services research, and clinical education. This commitment should lead to the elimination of most handwritten clinical data by the end of the decade.

---

*Health information technology is broadly defined as the use of information and communication technology in health care.
†EHR systems are defined by the Institute of Medicine's letter report on the key capabilities of an electronic Health Record System.1 EHR systems will include the ability to collect longitudinal data for and about a person in an electronic format; immediate electronic access to person and population level information by authorized users; provision of knowledge and decision-support tools that enhance the safety, quality and efficiency of health care; and support of efficient processes for health care delivery.

In particular, HIT was identified as a critical environmental force that would significantly improve health care quality. Numerous activities in both the public and private sectors were quickly expanded.[6,7] Some of the more notable recent events are described below.

In July 2003, the DHHS Agency for Healthcare Research and Quality (AHRQ) convened a diverse group of approximately 50 experts who helped the agency to identify gaps in knowledge relating to the use of HIT and provided recommendations on important thematic areas. Among the panel's many recommendations were the need for more research on the impact of HIT on important health-related outcomes; more research on HIT in diverse health care settings; the need to support local and regional HIT collaborative projects that would lead to standards-based data sharing across health care delivery sites; the need to demonstrate the value of HIT in improving patient safety and quality of care, including direct/indirect and tangible/intangible benefits; the need to study incentives and disincentives to the adoption and use of HIT; the need for technical assistance to providers, organizations, and communities to implement HIT successfully in their environment; and the need to develop and disseminate evidence-based, executable knowledge content and decision-support tools to support clinical decision making. The panel also encouraged collaboration between AHRQ and other federal agencies, such as the Office for Rural Health Policy and the Office for the Advancement of Telehealth at the Health Resources and Services Administration and the Center for Medicare and Medicaid Services (CMS), to leverage the resources, expertise, and experiences of these diverse federal agencies and increase the program's success. Finally, the panel stressed the need for developing collaborative partnerships and HIT programs that are viable and sustainable.[8]

The IOM released several reports such as "Crossing the Quality Chasm" that detail these needs, and various other organizations have focused industry attention on electronic health information and information technology.[9-14]

Many different components of the federal government touch on health care, and increasingly, federal leadership in HIT is more focused and coordinated. Although there is some integration of these efforts, until recently there has been neither a single voice for this effort nor a holistic set of goals for change. The ONC has been given the responsibility for coordinating HIT efforts throughout the federal government. As part of the outreach effort, the programs, projects, and policies that involve HIT are being compiled.

FEDERAL INVOLVEMENT IN HEALTH INFORMATION TECHNOLOGY

The DHHS's involvement in HIT and health information standards has been long standing. The goal is to develop and implement a nationwide interoperable HIT infrastructure, improve the quality and efficiency of health care, and help consumers manage their care and safety. For many years the federal government has supported research into medical informatics and the use of computers in clinical practice with the objective to increase the use of computers in health care. Most recently, a number of initiatives have gained considerable momentum to establish messaging and data content standards. Table 3-1 provides an overview of these activities.[15]

DHHS agencies such as the AHRQ, the Food and Drug Administration, the Health Resources and Services Administration, the CMS, and others have made adoption of technologies a priority (Figure 3-1). In a general sense these efforts have the following purpose:

- Provide funding for HIT to improve the quality, safety, and efficiency of the nation's health care system

Table 3-1   SELECTED HIT/HIE FEDERAL INITIATIVES

Consolidated Health Informatics Initiative The CHI is one of several projects launched as part of the president's e-Government initiative, which aims to improve government efficiency, effectiveness, and responsiveness to citizens while making it easier for citizens to obtain services and interact with the federal government. The CHI involves all federal agencies relating to health care, including the Department of Defense, Department of Veterans' Affairs, the CMS, the Centers for Disease Control and Prevention, and the National Institutes for Health. This project will provide the basis for a simplified and unified system for sharing and revising medical information among government agencies and their private health care providers and insurers, ultimately leading to a single mechanism for making records accessible.	DHHS
Health Alert Network The network is a project being developed at the CDC as part of its Public Health Emergency Preparedness and Response Program. The project is intended to ensure communications capacity at all local and state health departments through full Internet connectivity and training. That capacity will ensure the ability to broadcast and receive health alerts at every level of the public health system.	CDC

CDC, Centers for Disease Control and Prevention; *NIP*, National Immunization Program.

Continued

Table 3-1   SELECTED HIT/HIE FEDERAL INITIATIVES—cont'd

National Electronic Disease Surveillance System The system is an initiative that promotes the use of data and information system standards to advance the development of efficient, integrated, and interoperable surveillance systems at federal, state, and local levels. This broad initiative is designed to facilitate the electronic transfer of appropriate information from clinical information systems in the health care industry to public health departments, reduce provider burden in the provision of information, and enhance both the timeliness and quality of information provided.	CDC
National Immunization Program The program is committed to promoting the development and maintenance of state- and community-based computerized registries that capture immunization information on all children. Working with the National Vaccine Advisory Committee, NIP has identified minimum core immunization data elements that enable consistent data collection by immunization registry systems.	CDC

CDC, Centers for Disease Control and Prevention; *NIP*, National Immunization Program.

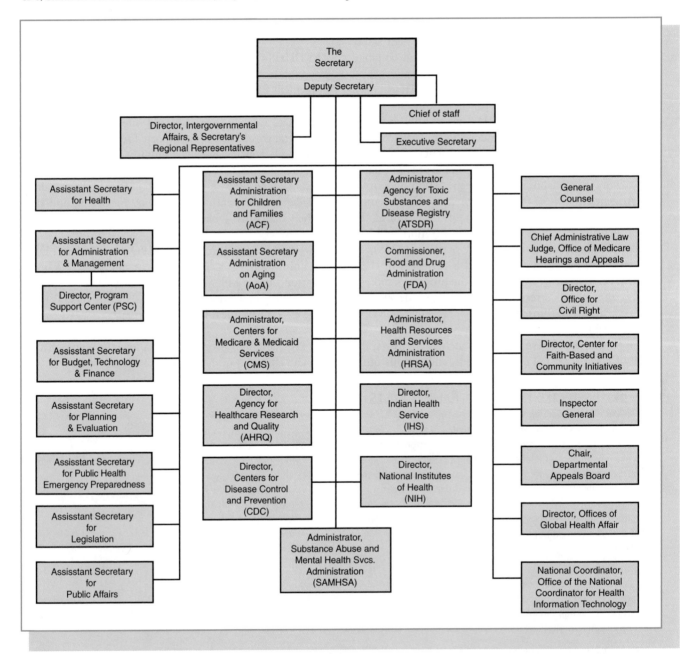

Figure 3-1   Organizational chart of the Department of Health and Human Services. (From U.S. Department of Health and Human Services: http://www.hhs.gov/about/orgchart.html. Accessed March 10, 2006.)

- Have health care practitioners use information technology to assist in the delivery of patient care and to document that care
- Establish standard ways to exchange data electronically for health care delivery, research, public health, and payment
- Make investments to identify and speed the adoption of new technologies throughout the health care system
- Foster the development of data standards
- Advance the use of EHRs and accelerate secure sharing of health information among providers

The DHHS has played a leadership role in fostering the development of data standards. Efforts to date include the Consolidated Health Informatics Initiative and support for the National Health Information Infrastructure. Both activities have resulted in the adoption of standards for federal programs. The Consolidated Health Informatics (CHI) initiative is one of the Office of Management and Budget's eGov initiatives. CHI is a collaborative effort to adopt health information interoperability standards, particularly health vocabulary and messaging standards, for implementation in federal government systems. About 20 department/agencies including the DHHS, the Department of Defense, and the Department of Veteran's Affairs are active in the CHI governance process.

CHI adopted 20 uniform standards for electronic exchange of clinical information to be used across the federal health enterprise. On March 21, 2003, the DHHS and the Departments of Defense and Veterans Affairs announced the first set of uniform standards for the electronic exchange of clinical health information to be adopted across the federal government. The standards all federal agencies will adopt are as follows:

- Health Level 7 (HL7) messaging standards to ensure that each federal agency can share information that will improve coordinated care for patients, such as entries of orders, scheduling appointments and tests, and better coordination of the admittance, discharge, and transfer of patients.
- National Council on Prescription Drug Programs standards for ordering drugs from retail pharmacies to standardize information between health care providers and the pharmacies. These standards already have been adopted under HIPAA (1996) and ensures that parts of the three federal departments that aren't covered by HIPAA will also use the same standards.
- Institute of Electrical and Electronics Engineers 1073 series of standards allow for health care providers to plug medical devices into information and computer systems that allow health care providers to monitor information from an intensive care unit or through telehealth services on Indian reservations and in other circumstances.
- Digital Imaging Communications in Medicine standards enable images and associated diagnostic information to be retrieved and transferred from various manufacturers' devices and from medical staff work stations.
- Laboratory Logical Observation Identifier Name Codes standardize the electronic exchange of clinical laboratory results.

On May 6, 2004, the DHHS and the Departments of Defense and Veterans Affairs announced the adoption of 15 additional standards agreed to by the CHI initiative to allow for electronic exchange of clinical information across the federal government. The 15 new standards build on the existing set of five standards adopted by the DHHS in March 2003. The new standards agreed to by federal agencies will be used as agencies develop and implement new information technology systems.

The specific new standards are as follows:

- HL7 vocabulary standards for demographic information, units of measure, immunizations, and clinical encounters, and HL7's Clinical Document Architecture standard for text-based reports (five standards)
- The College of American Pathologists Systematized Nomenclature of Medicine Clinical Terms for laboratory result contents, nonlaboratory interventions and procedures, anatomy, diagnosis and problems, and nursing. The DHHS is making this available for use in the United States at no charge to users. (five standards)
- Laboratory Logical Observation Identifier Name Codes to standardize the electronic exchange of laboratory test orders and drug label section headers (one standard)
- HIPAA transactions and code sets for electronic exchange of health-related information to perform billing or administrative functions. These are the same standards now required under HIPAA for health plans, health care clearinghouses, and those health care providers who engage in certain electronic transactions. (one standard)
- A set of federal terminologies related to medications, including the Food and Drug Administration's names and codes for ingredients, manufactured dosage forms, drug products, and medication packages; the National Library of Medicine's RxNORM for describing clinical drugs; and the Veterans Administration's National Drug File Reference Terminology for specific drug classifications (one standard)
- The Human Gene Nomenclature for exchanging information regarding the role of genes in biomedical research in the federal health sector (one standard)
- The Environmental Protection Agency's Substance Registry System for nonmedicinal chemicals of importance to health care (one standard)

In July 2003, DHHS asked the IOM and HL7 to design a functional model and standard for the EHR. DHHS also announced that the department has signed an agreement with the College of American Pathologists to license the college's standardized medical vocabulary system and make it available without charge throughout the United States. The IOM issued its report, entitled "Key Capabilities of an Electronic Health Record System," on July 31, 2003. In October 2003, the General Accounting Office released a report called, "Information Technology. Benefits Realized for Selected Health Care Functions."

In September 2004, the AHRQ awarded $139 million in contracts and grants to promote the use of HIT through the development of networks for sharing clinical data and projects for planning, implementing, and demonstrating the value of HIT. The goals of these research projects are as follows:

- Improve patient safety by reducing medical errors.
- Increase health information sharing among providers, laboratories, pharmacies, and patients.
- Help patients transition between health care settings.
- Reduce duplicative and unnecessary testing.
- Increase our knowledge and understanding of the clinical, safety, quality, financial, and organizational value and benefits of HIT.

In July 2004, DHHS released the "Framework for Strategic Action, The Decade of Health Information Technology: Delivering Consumer-Centric and Information-Rich Health Care." The goals of this 10-year plan are to transform the delivery of health care by building a new health information infrastructure, including EHRs, and a new network to link health records nationwide. The plan established three interrelated core strategies:

- Promoting EHR adoption by clinicians
- Supporting the creation of regional health care information organizations (RHIO)
- Facilitating interoperability on a national scale

AHRQ's HIT Portfolio (research initiative) on HIT is critical to the nation's 10-year strategy to bring health care into the twenty-first century by advancing the use of information technology. The AHRQ initiative includes $139 million in grants and contracts in 40 states to support and stimulate investment in HIT, especially in rural and underserved areas. Through these and other projects, AHRQ and its partners will identify challenges to HIT adoption and use, solutions and best practices for making HIT work, and tools that will help hospitals and clinicians successfully incorporate new information technology. The portfolio includes grants to more than 100 health care stakeholders who are at various levels of HIT adoption and contracts to five states to launch health information exchange networks.

The AHRQ National Resource Center for Health Information Technology (the National Resource Center [NRC]), which was launched in September 2004, is playing a pivotal role in achieving the goals of DHHS to modernize health care through the best and most effective use of information technology. The NRC will encourage adoption of HIT by sharing the knowledge and findings that result from the real-world laboratory created in AHRQ's HIT initiative, as well as from other resources. The NRC supports the work of the HIT projects funded by AHRQ and other federal partners and will provide direct technical assistance and consulting services to individual projects during all phases of the work to develop and use HIT. Particular focus is placed on providing services to support challenges facing HIT implementation in rural settings.

The Commission on Systemic Interoperability, which was authorized by the Medicare Modernization Act, held its first meeting in January 2005. The commission is developing a strategy to make health care information instantly accessible at all times by consumers and their health care providers. The final report was released in October 2005.[16]

In May 2005, DHHS Secretary Mike Leavitt issued a report citing investment in information technology as an essential high priority for the American health care system and the U.S. economy. The report is entitled "Health Information Technology Leadership Panel: Final Report." The panel identified three key imperatives for HIT[17]:

- Widespread adoption of interoperable HIT should be a top priority for the U.S. health care system.
- The federal government should use its leverage as the nation's largest health care payer and provider to drive adoption of HIT.
- Private sector purchasers and health care organizations can and should collaborate alongside the federal government to drive adoption of HIT.

In June 2005, DHHS Secretary Mike Leavitt announced the formation of a national collaboration, the American Health Information Community (AHIC), to advance efforts to reach President Bush's call for most Americans to have EHRs within 10 years. The AHIC will help nationwide transition to EHRs—including common standards and interoperability—in a smooth, market-led way. The AHIC, formed under the auspices of the Federal Advisory Committee Act, will provide input and recommendations to the DHHS on how to make health records digital and interoperable and ensure that the privacy and security of those records are protected.[18]

The implementation by the CMS of the many HIT-related provisions of the Medicare Modernization Act, including those related to Doctor's Office Quality Information Technology, electronic prescribing standards, demonstration programs that include incentives for HIT, and long-term care demonstrations that will leverage information technology.

Under the direction of CMS, the Quality Improvement Organization (QIO) Program consists of a national network of 53 QIOs, responsible for each U.S. state, territory, and the District of Columbia. QIOs work with consumers and physicians, hospitals, and other caregivers to refine care delivery systems to make sure patients get the right care at the right time, particularly patients from underserved populations. The program also safeguards the integrity of the Medicare Trust Fund by ensuring that payment is made only for medically necessary services and investigates beneficiary complaints about quality of care. The Doctor's Office Quality Information Technology initiative promoted the adoption of EHRs and information technology in small- to medium-sized physician offices nationwide. The program aimed to help physicians increase access to patient information, decision support, and reference data and to improve patient-clinician communications. QIOs are currently transitioning from the seventh Scope of Work (SOW) to the eighth SOW, which began in August 2005 and runs through 2008. One of the areas new to the statement of work is HIT. Beginning in 2005, QIO assistance to physicians expands from a broad focus on improving preventive and chronic care to helping groups of practices in each state—particularly small and medium-sized practices—adopt and use HIT, address the needs of underserved populations, and improve prescribing. Using information technology, QIOs will work with 5% of adult primary care physician practices in every state to help them adopt and use HIT to improve the quality and efficiency of care—including e-prescribing, registries, e-labs, and deployment of full EHR systems. QIOs will help physicians select HIT products, reorganize workflow and care processes, and undertake quality improvement projects to realize the benefits of HIT.[19]

DHHS regulations require electronic prescriptions for Medicare concurrent with the prescription drug benefit (January 2006). The e-prescribing regulations adopt standards for the following:

- Transactions between prescribers and dispensers for new prescriptions, prescription refill request and response, prescription change request and response, prescription cancellation request and response, and related messaging and administrative transactions; eligibility and benefits inquires and responses between drug prescribers and prescription drug plans
- Eligibility and benefits inquiries and responses between dispensers and Part D sponsors
- Formulary and benefit coverage i formation, including information on the availability of lower cost, therapeutically appropriate alternative drugs, if certain characteristics are met

Table 3-2 depicts various DHHS activities. An organizational chart of the DHHS is included as Figure 3-1. ONC is responsible for coordinating federal activities relating to HIT.

In the fall of 2005, DHHS awarded three multimillion dollar contracts to public-private groups to accelerate the adoption of HIT and the secure portability of health infor-

Table 3-2 SELECTED ACTIVITIES BY ORGANIZATION

Selected DHHS Agencies/Organizations	Representative HIT/HIE Related Activities
AHRQ DHHS agency	In September 2004, awarded $139 million in contracts and grants to more than 100 communities, hospitals, providers, and health care systems in 40 states to develop statewide and regional networks, promote access to HIT, and encourage adoption of HIT. Awarded contracts totaling $25 million to the states of Colorado, Indiana, Rhode Island, Tennessee, and Utah to develop statewide and regional networks allowing health care providers, laboratories, major purchasers of health care, public and private payers, hospitals, ambulatory care facilities, home health care providers, and long-term care providers to use HIT to communicate and share information. Awarded a multiyear contract to establish and operate the NRC. The NRC will encourage adoption of HIT by sharing the knowledge and findings that result from the real-world laboratory created within AHRQ's HIT initiative.
AHIC Advisory body	On September 13, 2005, DHHS Secretary Mike Leavitt announced the membership for the AHIC, which is being formed to help advance efforts to reach President Bush's call for most Americans to have EHRs within 10 years. AHIC is a federally chartered commission and will provide input and recommendations to DHHS on how to make health records digital and interoperable and ensure that the privacy and security of those records are protected, in a smooth, market-led way.
CMS DHHS agency	Electronic prescribing, or "e-prescribing," enables a physician to transmit a prescription electronically to the patient's choice of pharmacy. It also enables physicians and pharmacies to obtain information about the patient's eligibility and medication history from drug plans. Having better access to patient information at the point of care makes writing, filling and receiving prescriptions quicker and easier. E-prescribing can also help reduce prescription errors from hard-to-read physician handwriting and by automating the process of checking for drug interactions and allergies.

Continued

Table 3-2 SELECTED ACTIVITIES BY ORGANIZATION—cont'd

Selected DHHS Agencies/Organizations	Representative HIT/HIE Related Activities
	New regulations that support adoption of e-prescribing and EHRs were announced on October 5, 2005, by DHHS Secretary Mike Leavitt. These proposals will speed adoption of HITs by hospitals, physicians, and other health care providers to improve quality and safety for Medicare beneficiaries and all Americans. Taken together, they represent a major step forward in meeting President Bush's goal of widespread adoption of EHR. CMS and the DHHS Office of Inspector General proposed rules announced on October 5, 2005, represent a unified effort to advance the goal of improving the health care of Medicare beneficiaries and all Americans through the use of e-prescribing and EHR systems. CMS has issued a final rule contracting the "foundation standards" for e-prescribing that all Medicare prescription drug plans must support.
CDC DHHS agency	The CDC is one of the 13 major operating components of the DHHS, which is the principal agency in the U.S. government for protecting the health and safety of all Americans and for providing essential human services, especially for those people who are least able to help themselves. The PHIN is CDC's vision for advancing fully capable and interoperable information systems in the many organizations that participate in public health. PHIN is a national initiative to implement a multiorganizational business and technical architecture for public health information systems.
Commission on Systemic Interoperability Advisory body	The Commission on Systemic Interoperability, authorized by the Medicare Modernization Act, held its first meeting on January 10, 2005. Congress created the commission as part of the Medicare Modernization Act of 2003 and charged the commission with developing recommendations, priorities, and a timeline for implementing an electronic HIE network. On October 25, 2005, the commission released its report, entitled "Ending the Document Game: Connecting and Transforming Your Healthcare Through Information Technology.
HRSA, Office for the Advancement of Telehealth DHHS agency	The office within the HRSA is a standards supporting and promoting organization. It was established to be the focal point for the HRSA's telehealth activities and a catalyst for the wider adoption of advanced technologies in the provision of health care services and education. Telehealth is defined as the use of electronic information and telecommunications technologies to support long-distance clinical health care, patient and professional health-related education, public health, and health administration
NCVHS Advisory body	The NCVHS is the advisory body to DHHS and Congress on health information policy. NCVHS has taken a critical leadership role in driving the creation of a NHIN, including the creation of the report "Information for Health: A Strategy for Building a National Health Information Network," which was published in November 2001.
NIH DHHS agency	The NIH today is one of the world's foremost medical research centers and the federal focal point for medical research in the United States. The NIH, comprising 27 separate institutes and centers, is one of eight health agencies of the Public Health Service which, in turn, is part of the DHHS. Simply described, the goal of NIH research is to acquire new knowledge to help prevent, detect, diagnose, and treat disease and disability. The National Cancer Institute is currently developing the cancer Biomedical Informatics Grid (caBIG). It is an open-source, open-access, voluntary information network that will enable cancer researchers to share tools, standards, data, applications, and technologies according to agreed-on common standards and needs.
ONC DHHS agency	Serves as the Secretary's principal advisor on the development, application, and use of HIT; coordinates DHHS HIT programs; ensures that DHHS health information technology policy and programs are coordinated with those of other relevant executive branch agencies; and to the extent permitted by law, develops, maintains, and directs the implementation of a strategic plan to guide the nationwide implementation of interoperable HIT in both the public and private health care sectors that will reduce medical errors, improve quality, and produce greater value for health care expenditures, and coordinates outreach and consultation by the relevant executive branch agencies with the public and private sectors. Awarded (in December 2005) contracts totaling

Table 3-2 SELECTED ACTIVITIES BY ORGANIZATION—cont'd

Selected DHHS Agencies/Organizations	Representative HIT/HIE Related Activities
	$18.6 million to four groups of health care and HIT organizations to develop prototypes for an NHIN architecture.* Awarded three contracts totaling $17.5 million to public-private groups that will accelerate the adoption of HIT and the secure portability of health information across the United States.
	Sponsored a project to look at how automated coding software and a nationwide interoperable HIT infrastructure can address healthcare fraud issues. The project was conducted through a contract with the Foundation of Research and Education of the American Health Information Management Association. The contract focused on two main tasks. Task One was a descriptive study of the issues and the steps in the development and use of automated coding software that will enhance healthcare antifraud activities. Task Two identified best practices to enhance the capabilities of a nationwide interoperable HIT infrastructure to assist in health care fraud prevention, detection, and prosecution.

NRC, National Resource Center; *CDC*, Centers for Disease Control and Prevention; *PHIN*, Public Health Information Network; *HRSA*, Health Resources and Services Administration; *NCVHS*, National Committee on Vital and Health Statistics; *NIH*, National Institutes of Health.

mation across the United States. These groups have strategic partnerships to develop the building blocks necessary for achieving the president's goal of widespread adoption of interoperable EHRs within 10 years.

The HIT partnerships will do the following:

- Create and evaluate processes for harmonizing health information standards
- Develop criteria to certify and evaluate HIT products
- Develop solutions to address variations in business policies and state laws that affect privacy and security practices that may pose challenges to the secure communication of health information

As part of the contracts, these partnerships will deliver reports to the AHIC.

These three partnerships were established through contracts between private, nonprofit entities and the DHHS.

Table 3-3 describes some of the contracts that have been awarded.

Congress

Congress is also playing a significant leadership role—bipartisan support of the use of HIT to improve health care has snowballed recently. Multiple bills have been introduced by both parties that include significant components related to HIT and HIE.

ROLE OF THE PRIVATE SECTOR

The private sector has also demonstrated significant leadership with the emergence of several initiatives and programs designed to improve health care through infor-

mation technology. Examples of such activities and organizations are shown in Table 3-4.

The private sector has also been very active in conferences and programs, including the eHealth Initiative's Connecting Communities for Better Health Program providing seed funding and technical support to states, regions, and communities involved in HIE and Connecting for Health, a public-private collaborative launched and funded by the Markle Foundation, with additional support from the Robert Wood Johnson Foundation, getting consensus among multiple stakeholders on a Roadmap for Electronic Connectivity, and several large employers and health plans conducting "market experiments" involving incentives to practicing clinicians, hospitals, and other providers for improving quality using HIT (e.g., Bridges to Excellence).

COMPELLING REASONS TO IMPLEMENT HEALTH INFORMATION TECHNOLOGY

Several key reasons for accelerated implementation of HIT for administrative and clinical data exchange have been identified and reported. It is important to note that, generally, these benefits are often unique to the specific setting and are not necessarily applicable to other settings. Nevertheless, providers have and continue to implement a wide range of clinical and administrative applications within their organizations, integrated delivery systems, office practices, and health plans. The literature describes various and diverse methods to develop systems.[20-26]

In an effort to provide high-quality care in a more cost-effective manner, health care providers have implemented various systems. Frequently noted applications and infor-

Table 3-3 SELECTED ONC CONTRACTS

Standards Harmonization Process
Harmonization of data standards is fundamental to the success of widespread interoperability—the seamless and secure exchange of patient information electronically. Today, there are many standards for HIE, but there are variations and gaps that hinder interoperability and the widespread adoption of HIT. DHHS awarded a contract to the American National Standards Institute, a nonprofit organization that administers and coordinates the U.S. voluntary standardization activities, to convene the HITSP. The HITSP will bring together U.S. standards development organizations and other stakeholders. The HITSP will develop, prototype, and evaluate a harmonization process for achieving a widely accepted and useful set of HIT standards that will support interoperability among health care software applications, particularly EHRs.

Compliance Certification Process
More then 200 EHR products are on the market, but there are no criteria for objectively evaluating product capabilities. This limits widespread investment in, and uptake of, these tools and hinders informed purchasing decisions. There are also no criteria by which communication architectures can be standardized in a way that would allow two different EHRs to communicate with each other. DHHS awarded a contract to the CCHIT to develop criteria and evaluation processes for certifying EHRs and the infrastructure or network components through which they interoperate. CCHIT is a private, nonprofit organization established to develop an efficient, credible, and sustainable mechanism for certifying health care information technology products. CCHIT is responsible to develop ambulatory EHR certification criteria. Criteria will include the capabilities of EHRs to protect health information, standards by which EHRs can share health information, and clinical features that improve patient outcomes.

Privacy and Security Solutions
Regulations promulgated pursuant to HIPAA established baseline health care privacy requirements for protected health information and established security requirements for electronically protected health information. Many states have adopted policies that go beyond HIPAA. The manner in which hospitals, physicians, and other health care organizations implement required security and privacy policies varies and is tailored to meet their individual organizations' needs. These variations in policies present challenges for widespread electronic HIE. The HISPC is a partnership consisting of a multidisciplinary team of experts and the National Governor's Association. The HISPC will work with approximately 40 states or territorial governments to assess and develop plans to address variations in organization-level business policies and state laws that affect privacy and security practices that may pose challenges to interoperable HIE.

HITSP, Health Information Technology Standards Panel; *CCHIT*, Certification Commission for Health Information Technology; *HISPC*, Health Information Security and Privacy Collaboration.

Table 3-4 REPRESENTATIVE PRIVATE SECTOR ACTIVITIES AND ORGANIZATIONS

AcademyHealth
AcademyHealth is the professional home for health services researchers, policy analysts, and practitioners and a leading nonpartisan resource for the best in health research and policy. The organization promotes the use of objective research and analysis to inform health policy and practice. With a diverse membership that includes more than 3700 individuals and 125 affiliate organizations, AcademyHealth fosters networking and professional growth and development for those working to improve health and health care.

All Kids Count
This project, funded by the Robert Wood Johnson Foundation, started in 1992 with the development and implementation of immunization registries. The current phase is one of communication and integration to foster integration/linkage of child health information systems, specifically including immunization registries and other systems that have both clinical and public health importance. One of its major activities is All Kids Count Connections, a collaboration of state and local health departments moving toward integration of health information systems such as immunization registries and screening initiatives for certain childhood problems.

Ambulatory Care Quality Alliance
The Ambulatory Care Quality Alliance—the American Academy of Family Physicians, the American College of Physicians, America's Health Insurance Plans, and AHRQ—consists of a large body of stakeholders that represents clinicians, consumers, purchasers, health plans, and others. In May 2005 the alliance announced having reached consensus on a uniform starter set of 26 clinical performance measures.

American Health Information Management Association
AHIMA is the premier association of HIM professionals. AHIMA's 50,000 members are dedicated to the effective management of personal health information needed to deliver quality health care to the public. Founded in 1928 to improve the quality of medical records, AHIMA is committed to advancing the HIM profession in an increasingly electronic and global environment through leadership in advocacy, education, certification, and lifelong learning. One of AHIMA's areas of strategic focus is electronic HIM (e-HIM). Their goals are to:

- Promote the migration from paper to an EMR information infrastructure
- Reinvent how institutional and personal health information and medical records are managed
- Deliver measurable cost and quality results from improved information management.

Table 3-4   REPRESENTATIVE PRIVATE SECTOR ACTIVITIES AND ORGANIZATIONS—cont'd

American Medical Informatics Association

The AMIA has a membership of individuals, institutions, and corporations dedicated to developing and using information technologies to improve health care. AMIA was formed in 1990 by the merger of three organizations: the American Association for Medical Systems and Informatics, the American College of Medical Informatics, and the Symposium on Computer Applications in Medical Care. The 3200 members of AMIA include physicians, nurses, computer and information scientists, biomedical engineers, medical librarians, and academic researchers and educators. AMIA is the official U.S. representative organization to the International Medical Informatics Association.

American Nursing Informatics Association

The organization provides a forum and networking opportunities for nurses working in health care informatics, facilitating the integration of data and knowledge to support care of patients and decision making for nurses and other providers. The group focuses on integrating nursing science, computer science and information science to manage and communicate data and information in nursing practice.

Association of Medical Directors of Information Systems

AMDIS is a forum for growth and development of chief medical information officers and other physicians entering positions of responsibility in medical informatics and information technology. AMDIS presents lessons learned from leaders in the field today, provides a body of information needed to be effective information systems leaders, and acts as a vehicle to forge important industry connections.

Bridges to Excellence

A group of employers, physicians, health plans, and patients have come together to create Bridges to Excellence. Guided by three principles, its purpose is to create programs that will realign everyone's incentives around higher quality:

- Reengineering care processes to reduce mistakes will require investments, for which purchasers should create incentives
- Significant reductions in defects (misuse, underuse, overuse) will reduce the waste and inefficiencies in the health care system today
- Increased accountability and quality improvements will be encouraged by the release of comparative provider performance data, delivered to consumers in a compelling way

California HealthCare Foundation

The California HealthCare Foundation is an independent philanthropy committed to improving the way health care is delivered and financed in California and helping consumers make informed health care and coverage decisions. Formed in 1996, the goal is to ensure that all Californians have access to affordable, quality health care. The foundation commissions research and analysis, publishes and disseminates information, convenes stakeholders, and funds development of programs and models aimed at improving the health care delivery and financing systems.

Center for Health Information Technology

The center, a division of the American Academy of Family Physicians, promotes and facilitates adoption and optimal use of HIT among academy members and other office-based clinicians. Initial work is focused on overcoming barriers of high cost, complexity, and lack of standardization, all of which stand in the way of small medical practices attempting to acquire and effectively use information technology in their offices.

Center for Health Transformation

The Center for Health Transformation is a collaboration dedicated to the creation of a twenty-first century intelligent health system in which knowledge saves lives and saves money for all Americans. The membership comprises health care providers, government leaders, large employers, small businesses, research institutions, universities, professional and industry associations, solution providers, patient and disease advocacy groups, and others.

College of Healthcare Information Management Executives

CHIME's aims are to serve the professional needs of health care chief information officers and to advance the strategic application of information technology in innovative ways that improve the effectiveness of health care delivery. CHIME provides networking, education, and career development while also supporting easy access to current information technology trends, research, and information pertaining to the use of information technology in health care.

Connecting for Health

Connecting for Health is a public-private collaborative of the Markle Foundation that will advance an interconnected, electronic national health information infrastructure by focusing on adopting national clinical data standards for interoperability, ensuring secure and private transmission of medical information, and working to understand consumers' needs and expectations from an interconnected health information system.

Continued

Table 3-4 REPRESENTATIVE PRIVATE SECTOR ACTIVITIES AND ORGANIZATIONS—cont'd

eHealth Initiative
The eHealth Initiative and its foundation are independent, nonprofit affiliated organizations whose missions are the same: to drive improvement in the quality, safety, and efficiency of health care through information and information technology. The eHealth Initiative represents the multiple and diverse stakeholders in health care who want to improve health and health care through information and information technology, including consumer and patient groups, employers and purchasers, health plans, HIT suppliers, hospitals, laboratories, medical and pharmaceutical device manufacturers, practicing clinicians, public health agencies, quality improvement/standards organizations, and state, regional, and community-based health information organizations. In addition, the eHealth Initiative Foundation works closely with leaders in the public sector through its various public-private sector partnerships.

Healthcare Information and Management Systems Society
The association is focused on providing leadership for the optimal use of health care information technology and management systems by framing public policy and industry practices through initiatives in advocacy, education, and professional development. Among the initiatives are a series of new programs to support and accelerate health care standards development, definition of an electronic medical record, and involvement of the health care information technology vendor community in building a minimum set of functions and features into information technology software products.

InformationLinks
Connecting Public Health with Health Information Exchanges is a program that will provide grants to support the participation of state and local public health agencies in health information exchanges. The program will make funds available to public health agencies for activities in support of population-based public health services, as opposed to direct provision of health care (e.g., safety-net provider services). The program is designed as a one-time, short-term stimulus to catalyze and facilitate greater participation by public health agencies in HIEs. State and local health departments and nonprofit organizations, such as public health institutes, specifically designated by a state or local health department to receive funds on their behalf, are eligible to apply.

Leapfrog Group
The Leapfrog Group is a voluntary program created to help save lives and reduce preventable medical mistakes by mobilizing employer purchasing power to initiate breakthrough improvements in the safety of health care and by giving consumers information to make more informed hospital choices. The Leapfrog Group was founded by The Business Roundtable, a national association of Fortune 500 chief executive officers and consists of more than 140 public and private organizations that provide health care benefits.

Michigan Electronic Medical Record Initiative
The goal of the initiative is to establish a statewide, standards-based, patient-centered EMR system linking disparate computerized patient record systems across independent providers. It will demonstrate a distributed, longitudinal patient record from fragments held in disparate databases owned by independent entities, using a system architecture based on Web services and grid computing. The system aims to show that "political" barriers to data sharing among institutions can be overcome given a technological architecture and a business approach that does not devalue institutional data holdings. Projected benefits of the system include cost reductions, enhancements in quality, and better emergency preparedness.

National Alliance for Health Information Technology
This alliance is a diverse partnership of leaders from all health care sectors working to advance the adoption and implementation of health care information technology to achieve measurable improvements in patient safety, quality of care, and operating performance. The alliance collaborates with health care and government leaders to accelerate the implementation of world-class, standards-based information technology aimed at creating the most effective, safe, unified, and inclusive health system possible.

National Association of Health Data Organizations
The association is a membership organization dedicated to strengthening the nation's health information system. It serves as a broker of expertise for the development and enhancement of statewide and national health information systems and brings together a network of state, federal, and private sector technical and policy leaders and consultants to expand health systems development and shape responsible health information policies.

National Committee for Quality Assurance
The National Committee for Quality Assurance is the leading independent organization providing information that allows employers and consumers of health care to distinguish among health plans and physicians on the basis of quality of care. The committee has developed Physician Practice Connections to assess office practices' performance in the areas of clinical information systems, patient education and support, and care management. Physician Practice Connections is the performance assessment program for the Bridges to Excellence rewards program, Physician Office Link.

National Center for Emergency Medicine Informatics
The not-for-profit center is focused on advancement of emergency medicine through the application of information technology. The organization is driven by the belief that the greatest advances in medicine over the next two decades will result from the application of the tools and principles of information science to the problems of clinical medicine. New developments in informatics will drive advances in clinical care, medical administration, medical research, and medical education.

Table 3-4   REPRESENTATIVE PRIVATE SECTOR ACTIVITIES AND ORGANIZATIONS—cont'd

Patient Safety Institute

The Patient Safety Institute is a not-for-profit collaborative and voluntary initiative that combines the power of technology and the strength of patient-provider relationships to improve care and lower the costs of health care. It functions to reduce medical errors, lower costs of health care, and strengthen privacy and security.

Public Health Data Standards Consortium

The goal of this voluntary confederation is to develop, promote, and implement data standards for population health practice and research. The confederation is composed of federal, state, and local health agencies; national and local professional associations; and public- and private-sector organizations and individuals. The consortium recognizes that, although clinical data forms the core of a national health information network, such a network also needs environmental, sociocultural and economic data to support the health care decision process and provide timely response to a public health threat.

Public Health Informatics Institute

The Public Health Informatics Institute is a program of the Robert Wood Johnson Foundation, whose goal is to foster collaboration among public health agencies in the conception, design, acquisition, and deployment of software tools to eliminate redundant efforts, speed up development processes, and reduce costs.

Public Health Information Network

The network is a framework for crosscutting and unifying data streams for the early detection of public health issues and emergencies. It is composed of five key components: detection and monitoring, data analysis, knowledge management, alerting, and response. Through defined data and vocabulary standards and strong collaborative relationships, the Public Health Information Network will enable consistent exchange of response, health and disease tracking data among public health partners. The association represents the community of professionals engaged in HIM, providing support to members and strengthening the industry and profession. It represents more than 45,000 specially educated health information management professionals who work throughout the health care industry. These professionals serve the health care industry and the public by managing, analyzing, and using data vital for patient care—and making it accessible to health care providers when needed to diagnose, treat, and care for patients.

Public Health Information Network

The network is a framework for crosscutting and unifying data streams for the early detection of public health issues and emergencies. It is composed of five key components: detection and monitoring, data analysis, knowledge management, alerting, and response. Through defined data and vocabulary standards and strong collaborative relationships, the Public Health Information Network will enable consistent exchange of response, health and disease tracking data among public health partners. The association represents the community of professionals engaged in HIM, providing support to members and strengthening the industry and profession. It represents more than 45,000 specially educated health information management professionals who work throughout the health care industry. These professionals serve the health care industry and the public by managing, analyzing, and using data vital for patient care—and making it accessible to health care providers when needed to diagnose, treat, and care for patients.

Robert Wood Johnson Foundation

As the nation's largest philanthropy devoted exclusively to improving the health and health care of all Americans, the RWJ Foundation works with a diverse group of organizations and individuals to identify solutions and achieve comprehensive, meaningful, and timely change. The RWJ Foundation seeks to improve the health and health care of all Americans. RWJ supports training, education, research (excluding biomedical research), and projects that demonstrate the effective delivery of health care services. In December 2005, RWJ announced new grants to support the participation of state and local public health agencies in HIEs. The new program, InformationLinks, is designed to accelerate the innovative and effective use of information technology by state and local public health agencies. Twenty-one grants of up to $100,000 were awarded to state and local health departments and public health institutes for 12-month projects. The grantee sites are working with health care providers to improve the use of regional data-sharing networks or HIEs.

AHIMA, American Health Information Management Association; *AMIA*, American Medical Informatics Association; *AMDIS*, Association of Medical Directors of Information Systems; *CHIME*, College of Healthcare Information Management Executives; *RWJ*, Robert Wood Johnson.

mation technology–enabled processes are depicted in Table 3-5.

Implementers generally believe that HIT implementations offer benefits. Although the specific benefits may vary and often relate to the unique features and levels of system functionality, the literature overwhelmingly notes the benefits of HIT applications. Some have been well documented, such as improved quality of care, better patient access, improved patient satisfaction, and increased system efficiencies. Case

studies and articles describe numerous examples of how HIT is being used in many initiatives, having been successfully implemented over many years. Generally, there is widespread agreement that HIT has had and will continue to have an enormously positive impact on health care practice and delivery, enhanced patient safety, and ultimately lower costs.[27,28]

Increasingly, research is demonstrating the great potential for HIT applications such as EHRa, e-prescribing, com-

Table 3-5 REPRESENTATIVE APPLICATIONS AND INFORMATION TECHNOLOGY–ENABLED PROCESSES

Administrative and Financial	Clinical Care
• Accreditation and licensure reporting • Appointment scheduling • Bar coding • Billing • Claims submission, reconciliation, and adjudication • Claims processing • Communications • Customer service • E-mail (communications between providers and patients) • Enrollment and eligibility verification • Financial management • HEDIS data collection • Internet/Intranet and Web applications • Internet access for patient and provider communications • Patient identity management • Patient registration • Prevention outreach • Public health reporting (i.e., immunization, newborn screening, lead poisoning) • Scanning documents • Syndrome and disease surveillance	• Automated clinical guidelines and protocols • Case management • Clinical alerts and reminders • Clinical data warehousing and data mining • CPOE • DSS • Digital imaging, capture, and transmission • Disease management • Disease registries • EHRs • Electronic monitoring systems • eRX • Immunizations tracking • Infectious disease management programs • Imaging • Medication history • Order entry, management, and results reporting • Patient reminders • Personal health records • Physician alerts • Picture archiving and communications systems • Results routing and reporting • Speech recognition and transcription • Telemedicine, telehealth, and teleradiology

puterized physician order entry (CPOE), and clinical decision support to improvements in nearly all areas related to improving population health. Rapid diffusion and adoption of evidence-based HIT innovation promises to revolutionize health in the United States by reducing medical errors, improving the quality of care delivered, controlling health care costs, empowering individuals to understand and address their health care needs, and supporting public health surveillance. The federal AHRQ identified five goals for the adoption of health information technology[29]:

- Improve patient safety by reducing medical errors
- Increase health information sharing between providers, laboratories, pharmacies, and patients
- Help patients transition between health care settings
- Reduce duplicative and unnecessary testing
- Increase our knowledge and understanding of the clinical safety, quality, financial and organizational value, and benefits of HIT

Beyond provider adoption of HIT, real population-level gains from these systems will occur when standardization allows for a basic level of interoperability and data sharing across systems, providers, communities, and regions. An example, the American Society for Testing and Materials, a standards development organization, has designed and adopted a health informatics standard titled "Specification for Continuity of Care (E2369-05)" in support of the AHRQ goal of helping patients transition between health care settings. The continuity of care document has specific data items that have been agreed on and are supported by the American Academy of Family Physicians, the American Academy of Pediatrics, the Massachusetts Medical Society, the American Medical Association, the Healthcare Management and Systems Society, the Patient Safety Institute, the American Health Care Association, the National Association for the Support of Long-Term Care, the Mobile Healthcare Alliance, the Medical Group Management Association, and the American College of Osteopathic Physicians as useful in transitioning patients between health care settings and providers. The standard uses XML to identify the data components.

Examples of potential identified benefits of using HIT are noted in Table 3-6.

The value of HIT and HIE may differ depending on the stakeholder and specific application(s) (Table 3-7).[30]

Examples of quantifiable benefits indicate that methods to measure benefits vary widely. Some report performing formal return on investment or cost-benefit analyses before investing in HIT resources. Others describe measuring the financial outcomes in the sense of quantifiable improvements in operating expenses and new revenue for their health systems.[31-37]

Generally, measures of success vary widely and include formal and informal analyses of financial impact results. Some use a return-on-investment method to assess the financial impact of service-related operating expenses compared with revenue gains from improved service delivery. In some instances, the measurable financial improvements attributed to or facilitated by an information system have included the ability to control or reduce operating expenses (such as those related to personnel, printing, or storage costs) or to expand the services offered by the health care organization. It is generally reported that successful HIT implementations require significant investments of time and therefore a system's financial return should also be measured over time; benefits are not immediate.[38-40]

Table 3-6 POTENTIAL BENEFITS FOR USING HEALTH INFORMATION TECHNOLOGY

Clinical Related	Administrative, Financial, and Organizational Related
Reduced medication and other medical errors	Increased staff productivity
Fewer and avoided adverse events	Reductions in staff time spent handling test results
Improved quality of care	Decrease in telephone calls requesting patient information
Ability to respond more quickly to patient needs	Decrease in mailing and faxing patient information
Enhanced customer/patient service	Streamlined administrative processes
Better communication between patients and clinicians	Improved data quality for research and clinical trials
More accurate and complete clinical care documentation	More accurate and complete clinical care documentation
Better communication with referring physicians	More timely public health reporting
Integrating patient data with clinical decision support	Less redundant data entry
databases, pharmacy and laboratory data, and emergency	Significant job enhancement for nurses
systems	Better compliance with regulatory requirements
Developing networked CPOE	More accurate, legible, and timely clinical documentation
Helping identify and prevent adverse drug events	Increased access to data
Developing chronic disease treatment systems, including	Increased job satisfaction
diabetes patient registries	Improved work flow
Creating clinical DSSs	Enhanced communication across care team
Improve patient transitions between health care facilities and	Better communication between patients and clinicians
home	Better communication with referring physicians
Enable clinicians to assess patient information at the point of	More timely, complete, and accurate capture of codes and charges
care	Fewer rejected claims
More timely and comprehensive infection control processes	Improvements in electronic claims processing
Increased time for hands-on patient care	Increased operating efficiencies
Improved patient confidence in care	Economies of scale
Better information for clinical decisions and treatment options	Decreased costs associated with staffing and paper storage
Reduced practice variation	Enhanced recruitment of qualified clinicians
Improved patient satisfaction	Fewer duplicative tests
Reduce medical errors and improve overall patient safety	Decreased operating costs
Increase the identification and reporting of medical errors and	Reduced storage and transcription costs
adverse events	Reduced per claim processing costs
Decrease in the number of actual errors and adverse events	Reduced supply costs
Decreased patient waiting times	More timely payment and reimbursement
Better patient compliance with treatment plans	Reduction in duplicate tests and diagnostic procedures
Streamlined disease and case management	Fewer inpatient hospitalizations
	Fewer emergency department admissions
	Shorter hospital stays

Others measure benefits in more qualitative terms, such as attaining business objectives, maintaining operational viability, and retaining critical staff. For instance, one benefit to implementing patient access to personal health records, patient-physician electronic messaging, and automated appointment scheduling is better communication, less hassle, and improved patient satisfaction. HIT also enhances continuity of patient care through better communication between and among practitioners, providers, and patients.

OBSTACLES TO HEALTH INFORMATION TECHNOLOGY ADOPTION

Despite the promise of information technology, physicians and hospitals are not adopting clinical information systems at a very rapid rate. There are three primary reasons for this slow rate of adoption. First, although these systems have been shown to provide financial benefits, little, if any, of these benefits (including avoiding office visits, reduction in acute care, and improved compliance with medications) accrue to the small office providers who pay for the systems. Instead, the benefits are enjoyed by other organizations, including health plans and employers. Second, provider organizations that implement new information technology systems often must make difficult modifications to their existing clinical workflow and decision-making processes. Not surprisingly, clinicians who work in these organizations are often reluctant to make such changes, particularly in the absence of any perceived benefits to the organization. Finally, there are barriers to connecting these systems to allow for information sharing among disparate organizations through regional and national interoperability. These barriers include perceived legal limitations on such

Table 3-7 VALUE BY STAKEHOLDER PERSPECTIVE

Stakeholder Perspective	Overall Benefit/Value
Providers and clinicians	Timely access to data for improved decision making
	Rapid access to data at point of care
	Reduced clerical and administrative costs
	More efficient and appropriate patient referrals
	Increased safety in prescribing/monitoring medication compliance
	Timely alerts to contraindications
	Improved coordination of care
	Enhanced revenue through decrease in rejected claims
Payers	Improved customer service
	Improved disease and care management
	Improved information to support research, audit, and policy development
	Reduced costs
Public health agencies	More comprehensive and timely data
	Enhanced physician participation
	Easier integration of data from disparate sources
	Earlier detection of disease outbreaks
	More timely detection of cases that suggest a local epidemic
	Enhanced outcomes analysis
	Better bioterrorism preparedness
	Enhanced and unified syndrome surveillance
Patients and consumers	Improved quality of care
	Better coordination of care
	Safer care
	Decreased costs of care
	Informed consumer choice
	Fewer redundant tests
Data providers (i.e., commercial laboratories, pharmacies, PBMS)	Enhanced public relations
	Decreased write offs from unnecessary/duplicative tests
	Decreased EDI costs
	Increased data processing efficiencies
	Reduced administrative costs
	Increased patient compliance

PBMS, Pharmaceutical benefits management systems; *EDI*, electronic data interchange.

information sharing and the limited capacity of health care organizations to organize regionally.[41]

According to studies by the RAND Corporation, the U.S. health care system could save lives and $162 billion annually with widespread use of HIT. The study examined HIT's potential health and financial benefits. Cost savings stem from several sources, including CPOE, increased efficiency in hospitals and physician practices, reduced length of hospital stay and administrative costs, and optimized drug use.[42,43]

There are also several issues related to attaining implementation of HIT. Although there has been significant progress on articulating and working toward this vision, significant obstacles to HIT adoption exist. A recent study finds financial benefits in the use and implementation of CPOE.[44] A survey of members of the American Academy of Family Physicians found that slightly less than one fourth of respondents use an EHR.[45] The report cites a number of barriers to more widespread adoption of this technology

(including financial, leadership, and knowledge barriers). HIT implementation is complex and costly, requiring detailed knowledge of health care financing issues, clinical processes, patients' and providers' perspectives, and expectations, organizational management, technical applications, and important legal issues.

In another study RAND specifically looked at CPOE systems and found that the following:

- Electronic prescribing systems may greatly reduce medication errors, thereby maximizing patient safety and health.
- Menus that aid in selecting appropriate medication doses and other specific features are important for achieving these goals.
- Currently used electronic prescribing systems vary widely in their features and capabilities and may not produce the best results for patient safety and health, but it should be possible to implement about two thirds of the guidelines in the next 3 years.[46,47]

Another report compares health care with the use of information technology in other industries. It estimates potential savings and costs of widespread adoption of electronic medical record (EMR) systems, models important health and safety benefits, and concludes that effective EMR implementation and networking could eventually save more than $81 billion annually—by improving health care efficiency and safety—and that HIT-enabled prevention and management of chronic disease could eventually double those savings while increasing health and other social benefits. However, this is unlikely to be realized without related changes to the health care system.[48]

In addition, financial returns associated with HIT implementation are sometimes viewed as too diffuse to justify investment from individual health system actors. Because of these obstacles, in part, health sector lags almost every other field in the application of information technology. Where elements of such technology exist in health care settings today, too often they are not interoperable, which greatly reduces their effectiveness.

Health care is delivered by various providers across multiple settings. Clinical information is complex and there are few incentives in place for information sharing across settings. Organizational and change management issues are also challenging in a clinical environment. Some of these challenges are listed in Table 3-8.

EMERGING HEALTH INFORMATION NETWORKS

There is widespread recognition of the need for HIT and exchange/interoperability at the national level, and many

Table 3-8 POTENTIAL CHALLENGES

Technology costs	There are high costs for HIT software, hardware, upgrades, and maintenance. Systems and products are costly and practically unaffordable. Providers do not have ready access to the upfront operating capital required for HIT investment. Providers agree that, regardless of the application or the vendor, HIT requires significant upfront investment. Providers face competing priorities for limited resources.
Legacy systems	Systems that were implemented in the earlier decades were often installed as stand-alone systems and the costs to replace or to integrate these systems are significant, as are costs for continuing systems maintenance and upkeep. Many legacy and stand-alone systems exist. There are significant costs to integrate these different, isolated, and fragmented systems. HIT is expensive and it has been difficult to generate the significant capital needed for the initial and continuing HIT investments.
Implementation costs	HIT implementation requires significant resources in terms of capital, time, and staffing; level of access to this capital varies.
Developing and maintaining system interoperability	There are a wide range of available systems and applications, further complicating the ability to convey information from one system to another without costly custom interfaces. Health care is complex and no two providers or institutions are identical. A successful solution in one setting is not necessarily transferable to another. Vendors vary greatly in terms of their stability, the levels of their system capabilities and functionality, and their ability to successfully implement and support their proposed solutions. Systems are often not compatible or interoperable—they cannot talk to one another. Electronic connections must exist among all providers and institutions. Currently there is fragmented use of technology with minimal interoperability and the continued existence of many legacy systems. Providers cannot easily communicate with each other because systems cannot exchange information. Providers have merged into or formed larger delivery systems, often resulting in numerous disparate and sometimes duplicative systems. The EHR as envisioned by many implies total consolidation of all patient data from before birth to the present, accessible by those with a need to know, and available at all points of care. This will require full interoperability within and among all health care organizations. Additionally, vendor and technology neutrality is essential.
Ensuring authorized access to and privacy of personal health information	Can data be exchanged so that patient privacy is ensured? Maintaining confidential personal information is essential, especially with the implementation of increasingly advanced technology. Balancing national privacy requirements with state level regulations is challenging. Developing and implementing agreements to facilitate HIE but governing data access and protecting patient privacy are critical.

Continued

Table 3-8 POTENTIAL CHALLENGES—cont'd

Developing and implementing standards	This lack of data content and transmittal and messaging standards prevents interoperability and sharing of data. Although ASTM and HI7 have developed content and messaging standards during the last 10 years, their work has not been fully integrated into the workplace. Standards are developed by voluntary private groups and ratified as national standards by the American National Standards Institute. The fact that a standard has been approved does not mean that it is adopted by the health care or health information vendor community. ASTM did initial work in standards related to privacy and confidentiality before HIPAA. These reference standards are still available for use as organizations and vendors continue to address continued concerns about privacy and confidentiality—balancing the needs for public access to information with the need for patient privacy and systems security.
Identifying the business case and value proposition	Providers that invest/implement HIT absorb the full cost of system acquisition and implementation, but the benefits accrue to many others (insurers, benefit managers, employers, regulators). Those who stand to benefit the most from provider HIT implementation are typically not the ones who pay for it. Efforts to create incentives for HIT adoption and to reduce the risk of technology investments.
Connecting providers and clinicians	To help streamline quality and health status reporting and monitoring and to reduce redundant data collection and reporting. Motivating clinicians to adopt technologies (such as EHRs) remains difficult because of business and clinical process and work flow disruptions during initial implementation. Additionally, the upfront technology investments and costs are high and the financial benefits of HIT often accrue to others.

ASTM, American Society for Testing and Materials.

local, state, and regional health information networks already exist or are in developmental stages. The creation of an NHIN also offers the opportunity to increase information exchange between the clinical care community and the clinical and biomedical research communities.[49] Studies have shown that clinical applications must interconnect if small and medium-size physician practices are to achieve the majority of the clinical decision benefit of an EHR. Such interconnectivity provides sufficient sources of data for patient information and it supports vital functionality, including advanced decision-support systems. To connect clinical applications, however, the health care industry must deploy a common technical framework based on open standards, built on the Internet as a network of networks, and health care organizations must work together to share information.[50]

Numerous RHIOs that facilitate HIE have emerged in many states throughout the country. Many states have one or more regional or community-based health information technology projects or prototype HIEs that have received federal or private sector funding. These efforts include the design, planning, development, implementation, and evaluation of the exchange and linkage of data among and across multiple stakeholders.[51] In addition to regional or state level organizations and entities, subnetwork organizations (SNO) have been proposed by some as critical to the success of efforts to establish nationwide interoperability. Each region or subnetwork needs an entity (SNO) to oversee its health information environment. Regional subnetworks have a public interest responsibility to address the needs of the

entire population and all health information providers. Some subnetworks will be geographically based and others will be functional or organizational, crossing geographical boundaries. Some of these enterprise or private subnetworks (e.g., a large health system or research network) may not be subject to the same public interest governance and policy obligations. The responsibilities of the SNOs include the following[52]:

- Establishing a multistakeholder governance structure that includes the representation of patients and consumers and safety net providers. The governance structure should be formalized and address the corporate and tax status of the SNO, its business plan and budget, intellectual property ownership and management, the entity's statement of purpose and objectives, its decision making model, and its long-term strategic plan. Various types of governance model are acceptable.
- Defining and meeting the particular information access needs of the region or subnetwork while addressing the needs of patient populations that cross multiple communities nationwide or are contiguous but cross state lines.
- Organizing the creation of "Articles of Federation" and other user agreements. A common set of multilateral policies, procedures, and standards to facilitate reliable, efficient sharing of health data among authorized users is required. The participating members of the health network must belong to and comply with agreements of a federation. Formal federation with clear agreements

allows participants to access information that they have been authorized to share.

- Supervising uniform adoption of information sharing policies or Articles of Federation by participating entities and mechanisms for their enforcement (e.g., sanctions).
- Developing policies to address the need for retention and persistence of data.
- Addressing conflicts among relevant stakeholders in a timely way.
- Building, maintaining, and managing the regional record locator services and other subnetwork systems and services.
- Ensuring that subnetwork systems and the end-point systems of their members (including the record locator service) adhere to the common framework.
- Providing support to participants in the federation.
- Establishing the financial sustainability models for the entity; responsibilities include the following:
- Working with community payers, purchasers, and providers to discuss participation, incentives, and appropriate funding models.
- Monitoring relevant stakeholder participation regarding conformance with the common framework and adoption incentives.
- Ensuring that all the information capabilities that define the HIE (including public health reporting and surveillance, research, and improving health care quality) can be met over time.

There is no standard definition or single model at this time, but a framework for appropriate functions and organizational models is emerging.[53,54] Health care delivery is delivered by various providers across multiple settings. Because patients receive care from multiple providers over an increasingly dispersed geographical area, the challenge in collecting, coordinating, and accessing relevant, meaningful, and timely information has been and continues to be challenging. Further, little is known about the benefits, challenges, and experiences associated with sharing or exchanging information at the community level between and among providers, institutions, and other organizations. However, the more widespread use of the Internet, and the continued refinement of communications and telecommunications technologies and the adoption of content and messaging standards, provides an additional opportunity to address the current fragmentation of clinical information among multiple providers and across sites of care.

There is an increasing number of community based efforts at health information exchange. Table 3-9 depicts a number of characteristics of these emerging and operational efforts.[51]

The eHealth Foundation depicted the phases or stages of these efforts according to a variety of criteria. According to eHealth Initiative's 2005 survey, there were more than 103 HIE initiatives and organizations in the United States. RHIOs offer promising models and potential building blocks for a nationwide health information network. In

Table 3-9 SELECTED CHARACTERISTICS OF HEALTH INFORMATION EXCHANGES

Goals	Functionality	Data Exchanged
• Reduce costs • Provide economies of scale • Offer extensive cost-recovering health-related services to providers, related agencies, and consumers • Support a fully integrated, longitudinal health record • Provide services to multiple stakeholders • Allow competitors to collaborate to share information • Provide technology-based information services to help maintain optimal health for all residents of community • Move administrative transactions between health care purchasers, payers, and providers • Improve the completeness and accuracy of health information	• Results retrieval • Clinical messaging/document delivery • Data entry • Reporting • Clinical decision support • Public health: • Case detection (electronic laboratory reporting) • Cancer research (supported by National Cancer Institute) • Showing outcome results • Prompting physicians to screen • Immunization registry • Syndromic surveillance by emergency department chief complaint • Secure exchange of confidential information • Secure encryption of e-mail • Digital signature of e-mail • Digital signature for other documents • Laboratory reporting	• Emergency department and outpatient visits • Inpatient laboratory results • Hospitalization discharge summaries • Radiology reports • Tumor registry data • Anatomical pathology reports • Immunizations • Ambulatory notes • Vital signs • Visit reasons and diagnoses • Medication profile • Cardiac testing (echocardiograms, catheterizations, etc.) • Radiology images • Gastroenterology reports • Problem lists/diagnoses • Laboratory results • Medications • Allergies • Immunizations • Patient identification data • Facility and practitioner identification data

Continued

Table 3-9 SELECTED CHARACTERISTICS OF HEALTH INFORMATION EXCHANGES—cont'd

Goals	Functionality	Data Exchanged
• Promote the adoption of data standards and implement electronic data exchange • Encourage stakeholders to share the information needed to make good health care decisions, monitor patient populations, and support value-based purchasing • Improve inefficient information systems and provide for the open, secure exchange of information among trading partners • Protect the privacy and confidentiality of individuals while balancing the need to monitor health care performance and quality	• Laboratory reporting • Birth reports • Death reports from funeral homes • Reportable events • Disease registries • Trauma registries • Scheduling • Local and national laboratory e-mail • Billing data access for physician offices • Local and national laboratory electronic access • Identity correlation service—correlates multiple patient identities across disparate systems. • Information locator service—identifies where clinical data resides on a correlated patient and accesses requested records for an authorized user • Access control service—supports HIPPA compliance by enabling user-defined security rules, including role-based access and logging of all data access events • Clinician and consumer portals—gives clinician end users the ability to perform customized patient searches and locate clinical results while using a browser-based user interface. The consumer/patient portal gives views of the same information and is managed by the patient's caregiver.	• Emergency department facility identification, emergency department practitioner type • Emergency department payment data • Emergency department arrival and first assessment data • Chief complaint, triage acuity, mode of arrival, vitals signs • Emergency department history and physical examination data • Coded cause of injury ICD-9-E codes • Emergency department procedure and results data • Emergency department disposition and diagnosis data • Emergency department disposition, ICD-9-CM coded diagnoses • Laboratory results • Radiology results (images, voices, file/dictation, reports) • Pharmacy results (medication history) • Medical record transcription • Administrative data (eligibility, referrals, authorizations)

ICD-9-CM, International Classification of Diseases, ninth revision, Clinical Modification.

2004, AHRQ awarded contracts to develop state-wide networks allowing major purchasers of health care, public and private payers, hospitals, ambulatory care facilities, home health care providers, and long-term care providers to use HIT to communicate and share information. Table 3-10 depicts selected operational efforts at community health information exchange.

In 2005, the Robert Wood Johnson Foundation awarded grants as part of its InformationLinks program. The grants support the participation of state and local public health agencies in HIEs.[21] Awardees are listed in Table 3-11.

Issues and questions that need resolution include the following.[5,55]

Organization and Governance Issues

- How will the project/entity be organized? Governed? Managed?
- What is the organization's scope and mission?
- What is the organization's legal and tax status?
- How will practicing clinicians be engaged?
- Which organizations will participate in the project? What are the terms and conditions of participation?
- How will participants communicate?
- Who will participate? What will the legal structure be? Who will have control?
- How will stakeholders be convinced to adopt and implement HIT and participate in HIE?
- How to prepare clinicians for changes in clinical and business processes

Technical Issues

- How will the technical issues, including those related to architecture, applications, data content, and messaging standards be dealt with?
- How does information get to the point of care when needed?

Table 3-10   SELECTED STATE AND REGIONAL PROJECTS IN HEALTH INFORMATION TECHNOLOGY AND HEALTH INFORMATION EXCHANGE

Colorado Connecting Communities: Health Information Collaborative
Implements statewide information and communications technologies to enable clinicians to access patient information from other clinical data repositories at the point of care. University of Colorado Health Sciences Center; Aurora, Colorado

Delaware Health Information Network
Created in July 1997 as a public instrumentality of the state to advance the creation of a statewide health information and electronic data interchange network for public and private use. It functions under the direction and control of the Health Care Commission. It addresses Delaware's needs for timely, reliable, and relevant health care information. Delaware Health Information Network, Dover, Delaware

Indiana University, Regenstrief Institute: An Evolving Statewide Indiana Information Infrastructure
www.regenstrief.org
Develops and implements HIE using an established technical infrastructure and interconnects local health information infrastructures; also implements a statewide public health surveillance network that links all hospitals to share emergency department data.

Indiana University School of Medicine, Indianapolis, Indiana
Inland Northwest Health Services: Spokane, Washington
http://www.inhs.org/newsite/about/html/about.html
Makes extensive use of HIT. Thirty-two facilities are connected through a private network and use a standard information system. All patient records for facilities are stored by use of a unique Master Patient Index. The integrated database contains all data associated with hospital inpatient and emergency department visits, including physician orders, medication information, laboratory data, and radiological images.

MA-SHARE
http://www.mahealthdata.org/index.html
The Massachusetts Health Data Consortium initiated MA-SHARE in March 2003 with the goal of establishing a network for community clinical connectivity. The Massachusetts Health Data Consortium is a public/private organization of that serves as a neutral entity in the collection and dissemination of health care–related data and a forum for the exchange of ideas between health care organizations. The group is funded by membership fees from government agencies, private companies, the eHealth Initiative, and grants from member health care organizations.

North Carolina Healthcare Information and Communications Alliance
www.nchica.org
Begun in 1994. In 1997, a project called PAiRS (Provider Access to Immunization Registry Securely) was initiated to prove that secure access to an aggregated data set could be done with use of the Internet. Childhood immunizations were selected because there was a recognized need for providing access to the records, the records were relatively harmless should any breaches of security take place, and the state immunization registry staff were anxious to provide access and to begin the process of developing a statewide system with full input and retrieval capabilities. A number of public and private forces came together to build the demonstration capability.

Rhode Island: State and Regional Demonstrations in Health Information Technology
Plans, develops, implements, and evaluates a master patient index to facilitate interoperability and sharing patient data between public and private health care sectors. State of Rhode Island, Providence, Rhode Island

Santa Barbara County Care Data Exchange
http://ccbh.ehealthinitiative.org/profiles/SBCCDE.mspx;
http://www.chcf.org/documents/ihealth/SantaBarbaraFSWeb.pdf
http://www.chcf.org/documents/ihealth/SBCCDEInterimReport.pdf
Run as a partnership between public and private health care organizations within Santa Barbara County, California, and CareScience, a national provider of on-line care management services to hospitals, health systems, and pharmaceutical and biotechnology companies. These parties include providers, payers, hospitals, clinics, laboratories, pharmacies, and the University of California–Santa Barbara.

Taconic Health Information Network and Community
http://ccbh.ehealthinitiative.org/Awardee_Taconic.mspx
http://www.taconicipa.com/info/press.cfm
An HIE connecting community physicians, hospitals, reference laboratories, pharmacies, payers, employers, and consumers within New York's Hudson Valley. A unique part is support and user training provided to clinicians and their staffs. These aids encourage adoption of HIT.

Continued

Table 3-10 SELECTED STATE AND REGIONAL PROJECTS IN HEALTH INFORMATION TECHNOLOGY AND HEALTH INFORMATION EXCHANGE—cont'd

Tennessee-Volunteer eHealth Initiative
Plans, implements, and evaluates a state-based regional data sharing and interoperability service interconnecting the health care entities in three counties including needs assessment for health care improvement and reforming TennCare. Vanderbilt University Medical Center; Nashville, Tennessee

Utah Health Information Network
Clinical Improving Communication Between Health Care Providers by a State-wide Infrastructure
Expands and enhances current statewide network for the electronic exchange of patient administrative and clinical data and supports the adoption of EMRs. Utah Health Information Network, Murray, Utah

Table 3-11 ROBERT WOOD JOHNSON FOUNDATION INFORMATION LINKS GRANTS

California–Mendocino County Department of Public Health, Ukiah, California
This community-based effort will expand Mendocino Securing Health Access and Records Exchange, or SHARE, a nationally recognized HIE demonstration project, from its safety net clinic roots into a full HIE that can operate across the entire regional health care sector.

California–County of Santa Cruz, Santa Cruz, California
This project will bring together information technology experts, convened by the health department, to plan a community-wide health information exchange.

California–Imperial County, El Centro, California
The Integrating Information—Improving the Exchange Project will work with existing data exchanges for communicable disease, laboratory result reporting, immunization registry, access to health care, and human immunodeficiency virus/acquired immune deficiency syndrome to improve HIE between local, state, and national partners.

Colorado–Mesa County Health Department, Grand Junction, Colorado
The Mesa County Public Health Information Exchange Project will work with the existing Quality Health Network electronic HIE to establish a filter to automatically notify Mesa County Health Department when a reportable condition has been diagnosed or treated.

Colorado–State of Colorado Department of Public Health and Environment
This project will identify barriers and solutions to sharing newborn screening results in a statewide information exchange.

Colorado–Denver Health and Hospital Authority, Denver, Colorado
This project will leverage the experience, momentum, and collaborative Colorado Health Information Exchange environment to define an atmosphere where public health surveillance systems are a natural product of HIT investments.

Indiana–State of Indiana, Indiana State Department of Health
The Indiana State Department of Health will develop a model health exchange network that identifies the components, resources and personnel needed in the state and local community to establish an information exchange.

Kansas–State of Kansas Department of Health and Environment
This project will initiate a public-private partnership between the Kansas Immunization Registry and an electronic community health record managed by the employer-driven, nonprofit Kansas City Health Exchange to enable a two-way flow of immunization registry data.

Louisiana–Louisiana Public Health Institute, Baton Rouge, Louisiana
The Louisiana Health Information Exchange project will develop shared disease control protocols between public health and health care to support rapid and coordinated diagnosis, treatment and prevention of human immunodeficiency virus infection, sexually transmitted disease, tuberculosis, and hepatitis C.

Maine–Maine Center for Public Health, Augusta, Maine
Connecting Maine will strengthen the relationship between public health and health care informatics by joining two innovative data integration efforts—Maine's Integrated Public Health Information System and Maine's nascent HIE, the Maine Health Information Network Technology project.

Michigan–County of Ingham, Mason, Michigan
This project will support a multistaged research and development process to embed public health surveillance, epidemiological, and health promotion capabilities in a regional health information organization.

Minnesota–State of Minnesota Department of Public Health
This project will implement strategic policy actions to establish governance for exchange of information between public health systems and clinical practice settings.

Table 3-11 ROBERT WOOD JOHNSON FOUNDATION INFORMATION LINKS GRANTS—cont'd

New York City–New York City Department of Health and Mental Hygiene, New York, New York
The overall objective of the Primary Care Health Information Technology Strategy project is to help small and mid-sized primary care providers, especially community health centers, in adopting public health–focused HIT solutions (including EHRs and eRX).

New York–Research Foundation of State University of New York
The Public Health Institute at the State University of New York, Stony Brook, in partnership with the Suffolk County Department of Health Services, will develop a regional public health information organization for Suffolk County, New York.

Ohio–Hamilton County General Health District, Cincinnati, Ohio
The Greater Cincinnati Public Health InformationLinks Project will strengthen the existing collaboration between public health authorities and HealthBridge, a fully funded and operational regional health information organization serving southwest Ohio and northern Kentucky.

Puerto Rico–Commonwealth of Puerto Rico Department of Health
This project will help create an HIE by developing a PublicHealth Statistical System, with the purpose of tracking health trends in Puerto Rico for 15 main areas of public health and sharing information with constituents in the health community.

Rhode Island–State of Rhode Island Department of Health
This project will help accelerate adoption of electronic data standards for use in the HIE and convert laboratory and child health data to facilitate data flow between the department and the HIE.

Tennessee–State of Tennessee Department of Finance and Administration
The Tennessee Health Network project will leverage relationships with three existing regional health information organizations to facilitate public/private health data sharing.

Texas–City of Austin Health and Human Services Department, Austin, Texas
This project will create a plan to improve the exchange of immunization information between the health department, safety net providers, and community stakeholders (such as school district nurses and private providers).

Utah–State of Utah, Utah Department of Health
This project will develop a business plan for continuing statewide public health participation in electronic exchange of clinical data through an existing network and assess new opportunities for public health participation in HIE.

Wisconsin–State of Wisconsin Department of Health and Family Services
This project will define the public health role in the Wisconsin's Public Health Information Network and help encourage public health participation.

- Will data be stored in a central repository or will it stay with the sources and be accessed by others from the outside?
- How will technological standards be selected?
- How will semantic interoperability be ensured (all participants must be using the same words to describe the same things)?
- How will data be transferred?
- How will patient, provider, and system user identity be ensured?
- Who has the authority to see what data?
- How will the accuracy and validity of the data be ensured?
- What functions or services will be provided?
- What data are published from the data sources to the data exchange?
- How are the data accessed? Stored? Compiled? Managed? Reported? Published?

Financial Issues

- How much will this cost? Who will pay? How much?
- How will upfront and continuing funding and sustainable business models be addressed?
- What is the business case for exchanging data?

Privacy, Security, and Confidentiality Issues

- How will legal issues such as fraud and abuse, antitrust concerns, and HIPAA compliance be dealt with?
- How will patient, provider, and user identification issues be handled?
- How will privacy, security, and confidentiality of data be handled? Secure connectivity and transport?
- How and when will data be accessed? By whom?
- What data content and quality control processes will be established?
- How will decisions be made? Conflicts resolved?
- How will compliance with state and federal requirements be ensured?

In this era of rapidly changing technologies and innovation and the impact of various environmental, political, and societal factors on the delivery of health care, we need more than ever to understand the evolution of successful HIE and the potential of HIE to address these issues. Identifying the factors critical to success and the impediments to moving forward are essential to realizing the full potential of HIE. Regionally based collaborative efforts are seen as an increasing critical element to advance the broader adoption and use of HIT.

Today's proponents of HIE still have high hopes for improving care and cutting costs by sharing information among providers, payers, and purchasers. The Center for Information Technology Leadership announced research findings demonstrating that standardized health care information exchange among health care information technology systems would deliver national savings of $86.8 billion annually after full implementation and would result in significant direct financial benefits for providers and other stakeholders. The report on HIE examines in detail the impact of the electronic flow of health care information and its role in improving patient safety and the quality of care. It measures the importance of seamless interoperability among vital sectors of the U.S. health care delivery system.[56,57]

Communities need to assess their readiness for local and regional data sharing by conducting a rigorous review of the technical, clinical, and organizational capacity and capabilities and the level of community commitment and the availability of local leadership to spearhead the effort. Communities also need to address the various policy and regulatory changes, and security and privacy, medical malpractice, and practice transformation.[58]

ROLE OF HEALTH INFORMATION MANAGEMENT

HIT and HIE offer enormous opportunity for the U.S. health care system. It is becoming increasingly apparent that investments in HIT and HIE provide significant returns across a variety of metrics. HIT provides increased delivery system efficiencies and cost savings, contributes to greater patient safety and better patient care, and achieves clinical and business process improvements. Patients benefit from the comprehensive adoption of HIT and the ability to share data within and across sites of care and among clinicians. Ultimately, other stakeholders such as employers, payers, policy makers, public health officials, and regulators will benefit from the ability to share and exchange data.[59-63]

The ability to exchange information quickly and accurately within and across systems is paramount in health care delivery. But to realize the true potential, much more work must be undertaken. Over the last several years, health system leaders and the federal government have recognized the potential for electronic health information to transform the quality and efficiency of care delivery. There is growing interest in adopting EHRs, computerized order entry, and other technology-enabled automation components that compose an EHR system. There is a flurry of activity associated with development and implementation of community, state, and regional health information exchange.[63,64] Establishment of standards for content and message delivery and receipt are in various stages of agreement and execution.

HIM professionals' contribution to determining how the meanings of clinical and administrative terms are defined and represented is essential.

Health information management skills can help address and resolve the health information management (HIM) challenges likely to be encountered, including those related to the activities listed in Table 3-12.

Key Concepts

Across the health care industry, stakeholders are committed to improved quality of care and better patient safety. Many envision a twenty-first century health care system that is:

- Integrated and linked by information technology,
- Consumer centered, and
- Using new drugs, technologies, and medical procedures to perform medical miracles.

This vision requires that health care be delivered efficiently and cost effectively. Key players in the industry are mobilizing around their collective interests in facilitating HIT and are supporting activities to further the adoption and deployment of HIT. We are seeing a rapid acceleration of continuing activities to help ensure the success of current efforts building on numerous efforts undertaken earlier.[65-71]

HIT has been identified as essential in transforming the U.S. health care system—making it safer and more efficient and improving the quality of care for patients overall. HIT applications and systems such as EHRs, electronic prescribing (eRX), bedside bar coding, CPOE, and decision support systems (DSS) are widely seen as central to reducing errors and improving quality.

In their quest to improve the quality of patient care, many health care providers continue to take advantage of information and communications technology. Unfortunately, their growing difficulty in investing scarce resources into increasingly expensive HIT, as well as the current lack of standards for HIT systems, have hampered the widespread adoption and implementation of these technologies.

The ability to capture, manage, and take advantage of computerized data and information is also essential to continuously improving excellence in health services research and public policy. A consensus has emerged that the nation's medical system must replace its outdated and frequently error-plagued paper-based approach to information management. More recently, efforts are underway to plan, develop, and implement a national approach to collecting and sharing information among and across health care providers, payers, patients, and policy makers to achieve the national vision of improved health care for all citizens. The role of HIM in these efforts is essential to their success.

Health care decisions rely on ready access to clear, concise, and up-to-date information—information that is

Table 3-12 HEALTH INFORMATION MANAGEMENT ACTIVITIES

- Adopting and implementing EHRs
- Assessing and establishing organizational and community readiness
- Assessing workflow analysis and redesign
- Ensuring and facilitating patient identity management
- Ensuring clinician adoption and use
- Ensuring compliance and regulation
- Ensuring data content and quality
- Complying with accreditation and licensing requirements
- Convening stakeholders for HIE efforts
- Defining organizational goals and program focus
- Defining the legal medical record
- Demonstrating value and benefit
- Determining data definitions and representation
- Determining user authentication verification processes and policies
- Developing agreements to facilitate HIE
- Developing and conducting user training and orientation
- Developing and testing features and functions
- Developing the vision for secured access to EHRs
- Developing the vision for secured access to personal health information
- Developing, implementing, and overseeing data access and sharing strategies, policies, and procedures
- Encouraging use and adoption of HIT
- Ensuring secure transactions
- Establishing confidentiality, privacy, and security policies and procedures
- Establishing consensus on data standards
- Establishing data and record ownership and control
- Facilitating collaboration among participating stakeholders
- Facilitating negotiation and data collection from data sources
- Implementing access and authentication policies and procedures
- Implementing data and transmission standards
- Implementing stakeholder and participant agreements
- Integrating the personal health record
- Maintaining and managing the legal medical record
- Managing and overseeing access and authentication functions and activities
- Managing data publishing in an HIE
- Participating in technology selection, implementation, and deployment
- Participating in various standards-setting organizations
- Participating in business process reengineering of clinical and administrative practices
- Planning for backup and contingency
- Promoting HIT and HIE as a priority
- Protecting the patient and public interests
- Revamping procedures, processes, and workflow
- Setting and establishing HIM policies and procedures
- Training and educating participants
- Transitioning from legacy systems

increasingly complex and highly dynamic. Yet the health care industry continues to face challenging issues. The industry grapples with high and increasing levels of competition, heavy legislative and regulatory burdens, and competing demands for better quality, lower costs, and increased access to services.

HIT solutions have long been and continue to be touted as the industry's solution to these problems. HIT has been around for decades, but the industry is still a long way from full implementation. Its is increasingly apparent that HIT will provide costs and savings, contribute to greater patient safety and better patient care, allow for increased delivery systems efficiencies, and achieve clinical and business process improvements. Ultimately, the industry will benefit greatly from the comprehensive automation of health care and related processes.

HIT can drive across-the-board positive changes and enhance value in care delivery. In particular, applications such as EHRs, eRX, and bedside bar coding have been identified and promoted as necessary to facilitate a safer and more efficient health care system. However, there has been limited adoption and implementation of these new technologies. Ultimately, more widespread adoption of HIT will eliminate or reduce/diminish duplicative information gathering and will ensure delivery of health care based on timely, relevant, and complete information.

The U.S. health care industry is currently poised on the brink of a revolution that holds the promise of improved quality and efficiency, after years of halting progress, missteps, and a few striking but isolated successes in the application of HIT to the delivery of health care. Recently, national leaders in government and industry have recognized anew the critical importance of rapidly motivating, facilitating, and achieving the vision of a unified NHIN based on locally implemented information technology.

Great challenges remain, however.[72-77] Among others, these challenges include developing standards for capturing and sharing data, dealing with privacy and confidentiality concerns, achieving widespread adoption throughout the industry across diverse providers, demonstrating a convincing case that HIT investments improve quality of care and represent sound business decisions, ensuring project sustainability, and developing and maintaining a trained workforce skilled in HIT and HIM.

These technologies are readily available for commercial adoption by providers, including physicians, health plans, and hospitals. Evidence demonstrates the efficacy of these tools in addressing health status problems that result from process failures. However, clinical information technology adoption has been slow to date, and studies predict varying rates of EHR adoption in the future.

HIT offers enormous potential, but it remains slowed by challenges and barriers—full implementation is still far off.

With regard to the opportunities presented by HIT, it is becoming increasingly apparent that HIT will provide savings, contribute to greater patient safety, enhance patient care, allow for increased delivery systems efficiencies, and achieve clinical and business process improvements. As such, HIT can drive across-the-board positive changes and enhance value in care delivery. In particular, applications such as EMRs, eRX, and bedside bar coding have been identified and promoted as necessary to facilitate a safer and more efficient health care system. Patients will benefit from the comprehensive adoption of HIT and the ability to share data within and across sites of care and among clinicians. Ultimately, other stakeholders such as employers, payers, and regulators will benefit from the ability to share and exchange data.

REFERENCES

1. Institute of Medicine: Letter report on the key capabilities of an electronic health record system: http://www.iom.edu/report.asp?id=-14391. Accessed January 2, 2007.
2. http://www.hhs.gov/healthit/mission.html. Accessed February 2006.
3. Starr P: Smart technology, stunted policy: Developing health information networks, *Health Affairs* 16:91-105, 1997.
4. National Health Information Infrastructure: http://aspe.hhs.gov/sp/-NHII/. Accessed August 14, 2006.
5. *State and regional experience in health information collection, sharing and reporting: A review of national and regional demonstration projects resources innovations and opportunities*, 2005, Wisconsin Public Health and Health Policy Institute, Department of Population Health Sciences, University of Wisconsin Medical School, Madison.
5a. Committee on Quality of Health Care in America, Institute of America: *Crossing the quality chasm: a new health system for the 21st century*, 2001, Washington, DC, National Academies Press.
6. Office of the National Coordinator for Health Information Technology: Health IT strategic framework: Executive summary (July 2004). http://www.dhhs.gov/healthit/executivesummary.html. Accessed August 14, 2006.
7. Summary of Nationwide Health Information Network (NHIN) Request for Information (RFI) responses June 2005, Washington, DC, 2005, U.S. Department of Health and Human Services Office of the National Coordinator for Health Information Technology.
8. Agency for Healthcare Quality and Research: A summary of the proceedings:http://www.ahrq.gov/data/hitmeet.htm. Accessed August 14, 2006.
9. Institute of Medicine: Fostering rapid advances in health care: Learning from system demonstrations. In Corrigan JM, Greiner A, Erickson SM, editors. *Health care finance and delivery systems*, Washington, DC, 2002, Committee on Rapid Advance Demonstration Projects.
10. Institute of Medicine: *The future of the public's health in the 21st century*, Washington, D.C., 2002, Committee on Assuring the Health of the Public in the 21st Century.
11. Institute of Medicine: *Who will keep the public healthy: Educating public health professionals for the 21st century*, Washington, D.C., 2002, Committee on Educating Public Health Professionals for the 21st Century.
12. Institute of Medicine: *Key capabilities of an electronic health record system*, Washington, DC, 2003, Committee on Data Standards for Patient Safety Institute of Medicine.
13. Aspden P, Corrigan JM, Wolcott J et al, editors, Committee on Data Standards for Patient Safety *Patient safety: Achieving a new standard of care*, Washington, DC, 2003, Institute of Medicine.
14. Adams K, Corrigan JM, editors, Committee on Identifying Priority Areas for Quality Improvement: *Priority areas for national action: Transforming healthcare quality*, Washington, DC, 2003, Institute of Medicine.
15. The White House Office of Management and Budget: http://www.whitehouse.gov/omb/egov/c-3-6-chi.html. Accessed September 1, 2006.
16. Commission on Systemic Interoperability: http://www.nlm.nih.gov/csi/csi_home.html. Accessed January 2, 2007.
17. http://www.hhs.gov/healthit/sechitlp.html. Accessed February 2006.
18. http://www.hhs.gov/healthit/ahic/workgroups.html. Accessed January 2, 2007.
19. American Health Quality Association: http://www.ahqa.org/pub/189_817_5174.cfm. Accessed August 14, 2006.
20. National Committee on Vital and Health Statistics: *Information for health: A strategy for building the national health information infrastructure*, Washington, DC, 2001, National Committee on Vital and Health Statistics.
21. General Accounting Office: *Information technology: Benefits realized for selected health care functions*, publication No. GAO-04-224, 2003, General Accounting Office, Washington, DC.
22. Agency for Health Care Quality and Research: Case study finds computerized ICU information system care can significantly reduce time spent by nurses on documentation, press release, October 10, 2003.
23. Ball M, Garets DE, Handler T: Leveraging IT to improve patient safety, 2003, Yearbook of Medical Informatics of the International Medical Informatics Association, Heidelberg, Germany.
24. Bates DW, GawandeAA: Improving patient safety with information technology, *N Engl J Med* 348:2526-2534, 2003.
25. Vogel LH: Finding value from IT investments: exploring the elusive ROI in healthcare, *J Healthcare Information Manage* 17:20-28, 2003.
26. Newell L, Christensen D: Who's counting now? ROI for patient safety initiatives, *J Healthc Inf Manag* 17:29-35, 2003.
27. Hillestad R, Bigelow J, Bower A et al: Can electronic medical record systems transform health care? Potential health benefits, savings and costs, *Health Affairs* 24:1103-1117. 2005.
28. Cutler DM, Feldman NE, Horwitz JR: U.S. adoption of computerized physician order entry systems, *Health Affairs* 24:1654-1663, 2005.
29. Agency for Healthcare Research and Quality: *Health IT to advance excellence in health care*, publication No. 05-M021 Rockville, MD, 2005, Agency for Healthcare Research and Quality: http://healthit.ahrq.gov. Accessed August 14, 2006.
30. Frisse M: Lessons learned from state and RHIOs: organizational, technical and financial aspects. Presented at the Third Annual Connecting Communities Learning Forum and Exhibition: http://ccbh.ehealthinitiative.org/ccbhconference/. Accessed January 2, 2007.
31. Health information technology, *Health Affairs* 24(5):1148-1366, September/October 2005.
32. Working Group on Financial, Organizational, and Legal Sustainability of Health Information Exchange: financial, legal and organizational approaches to achieving electronic connectivity in healthcare, *Connecting for Health*: www.connectingforhealth.org. Accessed September 1, 2006.
33. Lee J: Computerized physician order entry (CPOE) systems, Research Synthesis, AcademyHealth (2002): http://www.academyhealth.org/syntheses/cpoe.htm. Accessed December 28, 2005.
34. Coye MJ, Bernstein WS: Perspective: Improving America's health care system by investing in information technology, *Health Affairs* 22:56-58, 2003.
35. Bates DW, Leape LL, Cullen DJ et al: Effect of computerized physician order entry and a team intervention on prevention of serious medication errors, *JAMA* 280:1311-1316, 1998.
36. Bates DW, Spell N, Cullen DJ et al: The costs of adverse drug events in hospitalized patients, *JAMA* 277:307-311, 1997.
37. Classen DC, Pestotnik SL, Evans RS et al: Adverse drug events in hospitalized patients: Excess length of stay, extra costs, and attributable mortality, *JAMA* 277: 301-306, 1997.

38. Leape LL, Bates DW, Cullen DJ: Systems analysis of adverse drug events, *JAMA* 274:34-43, 1995.

39. Leapfrog Group: Computerized physician order entry (CPOE): Fact sheet: Washington, DC (2000). Accessed August 11, 2002.

40. Hillestad R, Bigelow J, Bower A et al: Can electronic medical record systems transform health care? Potential health benefits, savings, and costs, *Health Affairs* 24:1103-1117, 2005.

41. Frisse ME: State and community-based efforts to foster interoperability, *Health Affairs (Millwood)* 24:1190-1196, 2005.

42. Fonkych K, Taylor R: The state and pattern of health information technology adoption: http://www.rand.org/pubs/monographs/-MG409/index.html. Accessed February 2006.

43. Girosi F, Meili R, Scoville R: Extrapolating evidence of health information technology savings and costs:http://www.rand.org/-pubs/monographs/MG410/. Accessed February 2006.

44. Kaushal R, Jha AK, Franz C et al: Return on investment for a computerized physician order entry system, *J Am Med Informatics Assoc* 13:261-266, 2006.

45. Center for Health Information Technology: http://www. centerforhit. org/x1655.xml. Accessed February 2006.

46. Bower AG: The diffusion and value of healthcare information technology: http://www.rand.org/pubs/monographs/MG272-1/. Accessed September 1, 2006.

47. Bell D, Marken RS, Meili R et al.: Electronic prescribing systems: Making it safer to take your medicine? http://www.rand.org/pubs/-research_briefs/RB9052/. Accessed September 1, 2006.

48. Hillestad R, Bigelow J, Bower A et al: Can electronic medical record systems transform health care? Potential health benefits, savings and costs, *Health Affairs* 24:1103-1117, 2005.

49. Accelerating research through the National Health Information Network. Presented January 7, 2005, Washington, DC, FasterCures and the Markle Foundation

50. Working Group on Financial, Organizational, and Legal Sustainability of Health Information Exchange: financial, legal and organizational approaches to achieving electronic connectivity in healthcare, *Connecting for Health*: www.connectingforhealth.org. Accessed September 1, 2006.

51. Frisse M, Marchibroda J, Welebob E: HIE takes shape in the states, *J AHIMA* 76:24-8, 30, 2005.

52. Connecting for Health: http://www.connectingforhealth.org/-resources/collaborative_response/hie_overall_structure/2.php. Accessed January 2, 2006.

53. Qual-IT United Hospital Fund: www.uhfnyc.org. Accessed September 2, 2006.

54. Goldsmith J, Blumenthal D,Rishel W: Federal health information policy: A case of arrested development, *Health Affairs* 22:44-55, 2003.

55. Robert Wood Johnson Foundation: http://www.rwjf.org/newsroom/newsreleasesdetail.jsp?id=10386. Accessed January 2, 2006.

56. Results from the Research into the Financial Value of Healthcare Information Exchange and Interoperability HIMSS annual conference, presented February 23, 2004, Orlando, Florida.

57. Center for Information Technology Leadership: Healthcare information exchange and interoperability: www.himss.org. Accessed August 14, 2006.

58. MacDonald K, Metzger J: Connecting communities: strategies for physician portals and regional data sharing—including results from a recent survey by the College of Healthcare Information Management Executives, 2004: www.cio-chime.org. Accessed September 2, 2006.

59. Lorenzi NM: Strategies for creating successful local health information infrastructure initiatives, 2003 Contract No. 03EASPE00722: http://aspe.hhs.gov/sp/nhii/LHII-Lorenzi-12.16.03.pdf. Accessed January 2, 2007.

60. Beauchamp N, Eng TR: Sustaining eHealth in challenging times Summary report at the Third Annual eHealth Developers Summit, November 6-8, 2002, Tempe, AZ, eHealth Institute.

61. Community Health Information Networks, SunHealth Alliance and First Consulting Group, *Healthcare Information Management* 2:15-20, 1995.

62. Rybowski L, Rubin R: *Building an infrastructure for community health information: Lessons from the frontier*, 1998, Seattle, WA, Foundation for Health Care Quality.

63. Frisse M: State and community-based efforts to foster interoperability, *Health Affairs* 24:1190-1196, 2005.

64. McDonald CJ, Overhage JM, Barnes M et al: The Indiana network for patient care: a working local health information infrastructure. An example of a working infrastructure collaboration that links data from five health systems and hundreds of millions of entries, *Health Aff (Millwood)* 24:1214-1220, 2005.

65. Gottlieb LK, Stone EM, Stone D et al: Regulatory and policy barriers to effective clinical data exchange: lessons learned from MedsInfo-ED. This pilot project can obtain the medication history for a majority of five million covered patients from only six data sources, *Health Aff (Millwood)* 24:1197-1204, 2005.

66. Agency for Healthcare Research and Quality: *Healthcare informatics standards activities of selected federal agencies (a compendium)*, Rockville, MD: 1999, Agency for Healthcare Research and Quality.

67. Agency for Healthcare Research and Quality: *Summary report: Current healthcare informatics standards activities of federal agencies*, Rockville, MD, 1999, Agency for Healthcare Research and Quality.

68. Agency for Healthcare Research and Quality: *Patient safety reporting systems and research in HHS: Fact sheet*, Rockville, MD, 2001, Agency for Healthcare Research and Quality.

69. Agency for Healthcare Research and Quality: *Bioterrorism preparedness and response: Use of information technologies and decision support systems*, Summary, Evidence Report/Technology Assessment, publication No., Rockville, MD, 2002, Agency for Healthcare Research and Quality.

70. Agency for Healthcare Research and Quality: *Medical informatics for better and safer health care*, Summary, Research in Action, publication No. 02-0031, Rockville, MD, 2002, Agency for Healthcare Research and Quality: http://www.ahrq.gov/data/informatics/informatria.htm. Accessed August 14, 2006.

71. Agency for Healthcare Research and Quality: Case study finds computerized ICU information system care can significantly reduce time spent by nurses on documentation, press release, October 10, Rockville, MD, 2003, Agency for Healthcare Research and Quality.

72. Agency for Healthcare Research and Quality: *Expert panel meeting: health information technology*, Rockville, MD, 2003, Agency for Healthcare Research and Quality.

73. Jeffries J: New e-HIM initiative will reinvent HIM practice, support infrastructure, *J AHIMA* 74:70, 2003.

74. Bloomrosen M: e-HIM: From vision to reality, *J AHIMA* 76:36-41, 2005: [expanded online version]. Accessed September 1, 2006.

75. Wing P, Langelier MH: The future of HIM: Employer insights into the coming decade of rapid change, *J AHIMA* 75:28-32, 2004.

76. American Health Information Management Association and American Medical Informatics Association: Building the work force for health information transformation: http://www.ahima.org/-emerging_issues/Workforce_web.pdf. Accessed September 1, 2006.

77. Yasnoff WA, Humphreys BL, Overhage JM et al: A consensus action agenda for achieving the national health information infrastructure, *J Am Med Inform Assoc* 11:332-338, 2004.

78. Detmer DE: Building the national health information infrastructure for personal health, health care services, public health, and research, *BMC Med Inform Decision Making* 3:1, 2003. Published on-line January 6, 2003. Accessed September 1, 2006.

chapter 4

Health Data Concepts

Mary Spivey Teslow

 Additional content,
http://evolve.elsevier.com/Abdelhak/

 Review exercises can be found
in the Study Guide

Key Words

Abbreviation list
Abstracting
Advocacy
Aggregate data
Authentication
Bar code reader
Chart order
Continuing record review
Data
Database
Data set
Demographics
Electronic data interchange
Encounter
Information
Legal analysis
Licensed independent practitioner
Longitudinal patient record
Optical character readers
Patient health record
Personal health record
Practitioner
Primary patient record
Promulgated
Provider
Public health
Qualitative analysis
Quantitative analysis
Secondary patient record
Stakeholders
Statistical analysis
Third-party payer
Unique identifier
View

Chapter Contents

Health Data Users and Decision Making
  Users and Uses of Health Data
    Patients
    Health Care Practitioners
    Health Care Providers and Administrators
    Third-Party Payers
    Utilization and Case Managers
    Quality of Care Committees
    Accrediting, Licensing, and Certifying Agencies
    Governmental Agencies and Public Health
    Employers
    Attorneys and the Courts in the Judicial Process
    Planners and Policy Developers
    Educators and Trainers
    Researchers and Epidemiologists
    Media Reporters
  Decision Making
Overview of the Patient Record
  The Unique Roles of the Patient Health Record
  Definitions
    Data
    Patient Health Record
Data Collection Standards
  Governmental
    Department of Health and Human Services
  Overview of Information and Data Sets
  Core Health Data Elements
    Centers for Disease Control and Prevention
  Nongovernmental
    Accrediting Organizations
    Professional Organizations
    Researchers and Other Groups
Basic Principles of Data Collection
  User Needs
  Documentation Responsibilities
  General Documentation Forms and Views
    Patient Identification
    Administrative Forms
    Clinical Forms
    Operative Forms
    Obstetrical Data
    Neonatal Data
    Nursing Forms
    Ancillary Forms
  Documentation Guidelines
    General
    Abbreviations and Symbols
    Paper-Based Records
    Authentication
  Format Types
    Source-Oriented Medical Record
    Problem-Oriented Medical Record
    Integrated Record
Design and Control of Paper Forms and Computer Views and Templates
  Forms or Views Team
  General Design Principles
    Needs of Users

Purpose of the Form or View
Selection and Sequencing of Items
Standard Terminology, Abbreviations, and Format
Instructions
Simplification
Paper Forms Design and Production
Computer View/Screen Format Design
On-Line System Interface
Other Display Features
General Control Principles
Forms/View Summary

Health Record Flow and Processing
Medical Transcription

Methods to Ensure Data Quality
Record Content Review and Retrospective Completion

Data Quality Monitoring Methods and Solutions
Quality Assessment and Improvement Study of Patient
Record Documentation
Quantitative Analysis
Qualitative Analysis
Legal Analysis
Special Concerns of Alternative Care Settings
Clinical Staff Activities Related to Data Quality
Medical Record Committee
Continuing Record Reviews
Facility Structure That Encourages Data Quality
The Joint Commission Information Management Standards
Information Resources Management Committee

Data Needs Across the Health Care Continuum
Minimum Data Sets
Acute Care
Data Needs
Uniform Hospital Discharge Data Set
Special Forms and Views
Issues in Data Collection
Ambulatory Care
Data Needs
Uniform Ambulatory Care Data Set
Data Elements for Emergency Department Systems
Special Forms and Views
Issues in Data Collection and Data Quality
Long-Term Care
Data Needs
MDS 2.0: Minimum Data Set for Nursing Home Resident
Assessment and Care Screening
Special Forms and Views
Issues in Data Collection and Quality
Rehabilitation
Issues in Data Collection
Home Health Care
Data Needs
Outcome and Assessment Information Set
Special Forms and Views
Issues in Data Collection and Quality
Hospice
Special Forms
Issues in Data Collection and Quality
Behavioral Health
Data Needs
Special Forms and Views
Issues in Data Collection and Quality

Electronic Patient Record Initiatives
Characteristics of Data Quality
Definition
Accuracy
Accessibility
Comprehensiveness
Consistency
Currency
Data Definition
Granularity
Integrity
Precision
Relevance
Timeliness
ASTM Standards Development
ASTM E1384 Content Guide for the Electronic Patient
Record
ASTM E1384 Major Segments

Summary and Management Issues

Appendixes (Found on the Evolve site)
Appendix A: Core Health Data Elements
Appendix B: Sample Health Record Reports
Appendix C: Recommended Joint Commission
Documentation Review Criteria
Appendix D: MDS 2.0—Minimum Data Set for Nursing
Home Resident Assessment and Care Screening
Appendix E: Outcome and Assessment Information Set

Abbreviations

ADL—activities of daily living

AHIMA—American Health Information Management Association

ANSI—American National Standards Institute

ASTM—American Society for Testing and Materials

CARF—Commission on Accreditation of Rehabilitation Facilities

CMS—Centers for Medicare and Medicaid Services

DEEDS—Data Elements for Emergency Department Systems

DHHS—Department of Health and Human Services

DQM—Data quality management

EDI—electronic data interchange

EHR—electronic health record

FI—fiscal intermediary

H&P—History and physical

HEDIS—Health Plan Employer Data and Information Set

HIPAA—Health Insurance Portability and Accountability Act

IADL—instrumental activities of daily living

IOM—Institute of Medicine

LIP—licensed independent practitioner

JCAHO—Joint Commission on Accreditation of Healthcare
Organizations (now The Joint Commission)

MCO—managed care organization

MDS—Minimum Data Set

NAHDO—National Association of Health Data Organizations

NCHS—National Center for Health Statistics

Continued

NCVHS—National Committee on Vital and Health Statistics

NEDSS—National Electronic Disease Surveillance System

NMDS—Nursing Minimum Data Set

NMMDS—Nursing Management Minimum Data Set

NPPES—National Plan and Provider Enumeration System

OASIS—Outcome and Assessment Information Set

PHI—personally-identifiable health information

PHR—personal health record

POMR—problem-oriented medical record

QI—quality improvement

RAI—resident assessment instrument

SOAP—subjective, objective, assessment, plan

SSN—social security number

UACDS—Uniform Ambulatory Care Data Set

UHDDS—Uniform Hospital Discharge Data Set

UPIN—unique personal/physician identification number

Objectives ●

After reading this chapter, the reader will be able to do the following:

- Define key words.
- Define, compare, and contrast data and information.
- Describe the five unique roles of the health record.
- Discuss the importance of data in the care of the patient.
- Describe the major users of health care data and the importance of addressing the needs of each.

- Identify the steps in the management decision-making process with particular attention to step 2, the collection of data.
- Evaluate and apply principles of forms and computer view design.
- Describe the importance of quality data and the mechanisms and controls used to ensure quality.
- Define the characteristics of data quality.
- Identify concerns related to data and the protection of patient confidentiality.
- Discuss the importance of consistency and comparability in data collection both within an institution and across the health care delivery system.
- Describe the concept and importance of a personal identification number.
- Identify the major information and data sets, their scope, and special features.
- Identify the values and uses of uniform data sets.
- Identify the basic forms and format of the paper-based health record.
- Describe the purposes and techniques related to record analysis, including quantitative, qualitative, and legal.
- Describe the purposes and techniques related to clinical record reviews.
- Compare and contrast the records for ambulatory care, acute care, long-term care and rehabilitation, home care, hospice, and behavioral health care.
- Evaluate and apply principles of forms design.
- Explain ASTM E1384 and its relationship to the electronic health record and data collection.
- Describe the role of the health information manager in data collection and in determining the content of the clinical record.

The health care delivery system continues to evolve in both size and complexity, representing more than 15% of the gross domestic product of the United States in the early twenty-first century. The system is an elaborate and dynamic mosaic composed of consumers with diverse needs and an increasing array of providers in multiple types of facilities and locations, as well as an intricate management system monitored by payers, regulators, and accrediting bodies. Working together, their goal is to provide consumers with high-quality care that is accessible and cost-effective.

The patient record is the information centerpiece of the health care decision-making process, both for individual patient treatment and for its potential to collect or **aggregate data** (which does not identify any specific patients) for research and other purposes. In either electronic or paper form, it contains the essential data and information to answer the key questions related to the who, what, when, where, why, and how of patient care (Box 4-1).

Box 4-1   ESSENTIAL HEALTH DATA AND INFORMATION QUESTIONS

Who?
Who are the patient, the provider, and the payer?

What?
What services were provided and at what cost?

When?
When were the services provided?

Where?
Where were the services provided?

Why?
Why were the services provided, or what was the justification for the services?

How?
How effective were the services, or what was the outcome?

HEALTH DATA USERS AND DECISION MAKING

Users and Uses of Health Data

There are many users—both individuals and groups—who rely on health data and who demand quality in the data collected, analyzed, interpreted, and reported, including those described below. Figure 4-1 illustrates this environment and the numerous external forces that influence the patient's care and its documentation.

Patients

Patients use their medical data to understand their health care and to become more active participants in maintaining or improving their health. Data can also be used in monitoring care when additional treatment is necessary. For example, patients with diabetes or hypertension can make a difference by actively participating in controlling and monitoring their condition. Data are also used by patients to document the services received, to serve as proof of identity or disability, and to verify billed services. The American Health Information Management Association (AHIMA) has taken an **advocacy** position in promoting understanding of the **personal health record** (PHR) through their MyPHR consumer education programs and a related Web site (*www.myPHR.com*).

Health Care Practitioners

Physicians, nurses, and other clinicians who are treating the patient use the record as a primary means of communication among themselves. **Practitioners** at the follow-up facility or agency to which the patient is transferred after discharge rely on the data for continuing care. In a residential facility nursing staff review and evaluate the data to develop care plans outlining important nursing interventions. Health care practitioners in every setting use the clinical record as a resource.

Health Care Providers and Administrators

The term health care **provider** is broad based. It includes organizations that deliver health care services, such as hospitals, outpatient clinics, long-term care facilities, home care agencies, and hospices. Providers also can be individual practitioners. The health record collects the data that document the provision of services. Providers use these data to evaluate care, monitor the use of resources, and receive payment for services rendered. Administrators analyze financial and patient case mix information for business planning and marketing activities.

Third-Party Payers

Data are the basis of claims processing to pay for the health care services provided. **Third-party payers** include private insurance companies, managed-care organizations (MCOs), and fiscal intermediaries (FIs) who process claims for Medicare and Medicaid. Because the purpose of health data is to document the steps taken to prevent illness and promote wellness and the course of illness and treatment, the data become the basis for determining the appropriate payment to be made. Although capitated care may change the current billing systems, payers still want to know the services provided for the dollars spent. Even if transaction-based bills as we know them today disappear, data will be needed to document services provided. Billing data are currently the basis for reporting and managing costs of care. Payers for government insurance plans (i.e., Medicare and

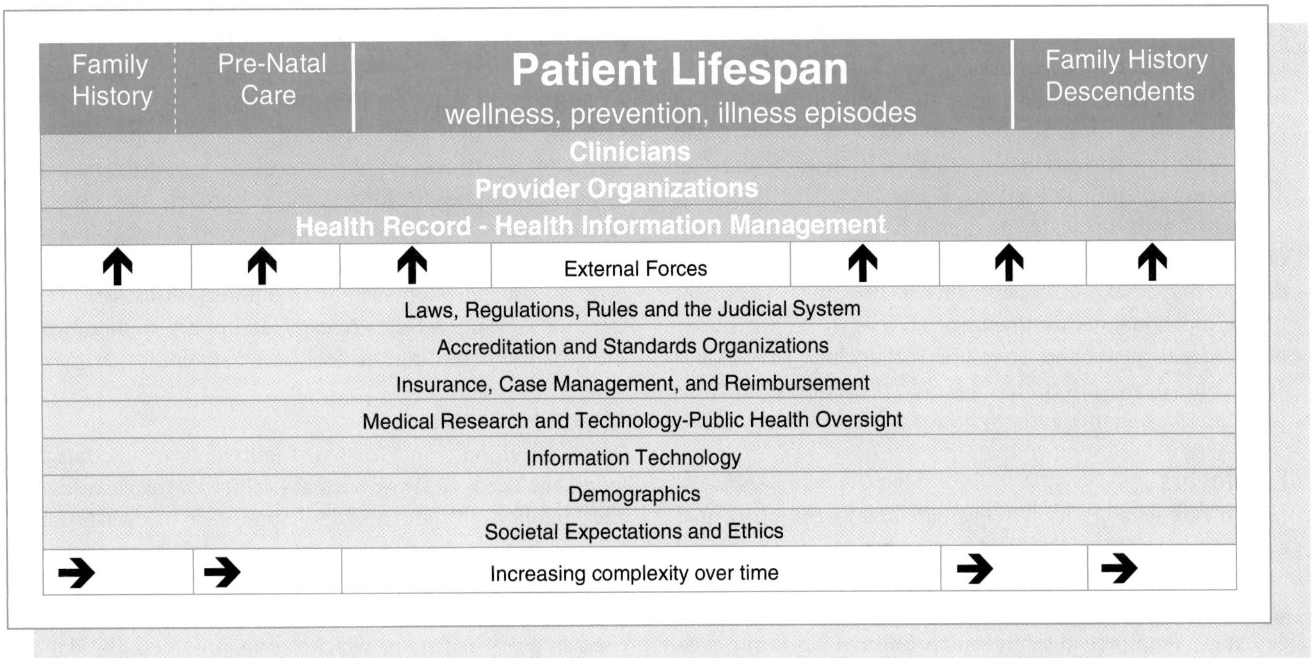

Figure 4-1 The influence of the health care environment on patient care and its documentation.

Medicaid) also actively monitor the appropriateness of the care and services given to a patient.

Utilization and Case Managers

Health care data include descriptions of care given and the justification for services. All organizational resources, including supplies, equipment, services, and providers, can be taken into consideration in a utilization review. Case management seeks to coordinate care so that the patient is cared for in the most clinically cost-effective manner. The emphasis is on disease management, especially for patients with chronic problems. Criteria are available for some facets of the case management process, such as admission, continued stay, and discharge from an inpatient facility and day-to-day management of specific chronic problems.

Quality of Care Committees

It is essential that the delivery of health care be monitored continuously; both concurrently and retrospectively. The basis for these reviews and the performance of quality assessment is the data recorded at the time care is given. Quality assessment and improvement committees use the information as a basis for analysis, study, and evaluation of the quality of care given to the patient. Recent studies by the Institutes of Medicine (IOM) on patient safety have increased the focus on these efforts. The National Physician Data Bank uses secondary health care data to ensure that only qualified physicians practice medicine.

Accrediting, Licensing, and Certifying Agencies

Accrediting, licensing, and certifying agencies review patient records to provide public assurance that quality health care is being provided. The data serve as evidence in assessing compliance with standards of care and in accrediting various health care organizations.

Governmental Agencies and Public Health

Governmental agencies at the local, state, and federal levels use health care data to determine the appropriate use of governmental financial resources for health care facilities and educational and correctional institutions. Reviews are done on a continuing and retrospective basis. **Public health** is concerned with threats to the overall health of a community on the basis of population-based health data analysis in contrast to medical health care, which focuses on the treatment of the individual. Governments at all levels establish public health departments and programs that include surveillance and control of infectious disease, prevention such as vaccination programs, and promotion of healthy behaviors.

Employers

Health care data are used to evaluate and assess job-related conditions and injuries and to determine occupational hazards that may impede effective performance in the workplace. Employers also use the data to determine the extent of employee disabilities, to improve working conditions, and to manage employee benefit programs. Health care benefits have continued to rise in cost to both employers and employees. Health data are used to select health insurance companies, evaluate quality, and manage costs.

Attorneys and the Courts in the Judicial Process

Attorneys and the courts use the records as documentary evidence of a patient's course of treatment to protect the legal interests of the patient, health care providers, treating facility, and the public. Health care data are often the basis of evidence for the adjudication of both civil and criminal cases. The documentation may support the claims made by the individuals in a case, and it is often the only evidence available. In addition, data may aid in determining the need for admission of the mentally ill for treatment.

Planners and Policy Developers

State health departments use information related to vital statistics, disease incidence and prevalence, reports of child and elder abuse, and so on to provide aggregate data for public policy development and for intervention in individual situations as needed. Data are the basis for supporting the continuing need for services and the addition of new services by a health care organization. Health care delivery is a dynamic process that requires the evaluation of current needs and future demands for the individual provider and the community in general.

Educators and Trainers

Within the health care setting there are many individuals who are learning the skills of quality health care service delivery. Data documentation assists these people in tying the theory learned in the classroom to the practical aspects of care. Conferences and presentations about care already delivered are useful in training health care personnel. Data from the patient record are the basis for many continuing education programs and conferences that review treatment outcomes.

Researchers and Epidemiologists

Clinical research is a significant aspect of the improvement of care and assessment of the effectiveness of treatment and improved methods for future care. Researchers may also study the cost-effectiveness of patient care, review patient outcomes, and assess the use of technology. Epidemiologists help with early disease detection such as an outbreak of *Escherichia coli* infections. Health services research and policy studies provide information regarding the health care system.

Media Reporters

Radio, television, and Web-based journalists report data that the public needs to know, such as health hazards, diseases that affect public health, and new developments in medical research.

Decision Making

Used in every setting in which care is provided, the data in the patient record are the essential resource for clinical and administrative decisions. Effective decision making proceeds through the following steps:

1. Problem identification
2. Data collection
3. Development of alternatives
4. Selection of the best alternative
5. Action
6. Follow-up and evaluation

Data collection is not an isolated function. It has a significant impact on both the efficiency and the effectiveness of the decision-making process. Well-defined and accurately collected data enhance the likelihood of an effective decision but do not guarantee it.

Overseeing the use of patient data in planning, management, and research has long been the purview of health information managers. To be efficient, health information management (HIM) professionals must carefully consider the purposes for data collection and gather sufficient data items, but no more than required. Significant costs are associated with data collection, including staff time for entry, review, and management and computer time and storage. Cost-effectiveness requires resistance to the "more-is-better" philosophy. The only reason to collect data is to satisfy an identified need for the retention, retrieval, and use of data and to generate meaningful information. Once the essential data items are identified, it is generally agreed that data should be captured only once and used by all portions of the system that require access to that particular data item. Health care documentation is often done in narrative form, which requires extraction of key pieces of data. As we standardize health data and as systems become more astute at automating the data extraction process, clinical data will be more available.

The wide variety of uses for the data in the patient record provide the HIM manager with the challenge of collecting the necessary data to support and promote the efficiency and effectiveness on behalf of the patient, the provider, the facility, as well as public health. Each of these constituencies benefits from the reliability and validity promoted by consistent definitions of data elements. Such definitions aid in facilitating data exchange and reducing misunderstandings. Standards are at the heart of a consistent data collection plan that supports the needs of individuals, organizations, and the health care delivery system at large.

OVERVIEW OF THE PATIENT RECORD

The Unique Roles of the Patient Health Record

A patient's health record plays five unique roles[1]:

1. It represents that patient's health history; that is, it is a record of the patient's health status and the health services provided over time.

2. It provides a method for clinical communication and care planning among the individual health care practitioners serving the patient.
3. It serves as the legal document describing the health care services provided.
4. It is a source of data for clinical, health services, and outcomes research.
5. It serves as a major resource for health care practitioner education.

Definitions

Data

Data are a collection of elements on a given subject; the raw facts and figures expressed in text, numbers, symbols, and images; facts, ideas, or concepts that can be captured, communicated, and processed either manually or electronically. The word data is plural and is used whenever more than one data element is described. Datum appropriately describes a single data element.

Information. Information is data that have been processed into meaningful form—either manually or by computer—to make them valuable to the user. Data and information are not synonymous. **Information** adds to a representation and tells the recipient something that was not known before. For example, graphing blood sugar levels over time reveals a trend not apparent from individual values. What is information for one person may not be information for another.

Patient Health Record

The **patient health record** collects the data and information and generates reports—either on paper or electronically. It is the primary legal record documenting the health care services provided to a person in any aspect of the health care system. The term includes routine clinical or office records, records of care in any health-related setting, preventive care, lifestyle evaluation, research protocols, and various clinical databases. This repository of information about a single patient is generated by health care practitioners as a direct result of interaction with a patient or with individuals who have personal knowledge of the patient (or with both). The record contains information about the patient and other individuals as they relate to the health of the patient. The term patient health record is generally synonymous with medical record, health record, patient care record, primary patient record, client record, and resident record. It should be noted that health record is a more comprehensive term that includes prevention and screening data where medical record more typically refers to encounters related to illness.

Primary Patient Record. The **primary patient record** is the record that is used by health care practitioners while providing patient care services to review patient data or document their own observations, actions, or instructions.

Secondary Patient Record. The **secondary patient record** is a subset that is derived from the primary record and contains selected data elements. Such secondary records or databases aid both clinicians and nonclinical individuals (that is, those not involved in direct patient care) in supporting, evaluating, and advancing patient care. Patient care support refers to administration, regulation, and payment functions. Patient care evaluation refers to quality assurance, utilization review, and medical or legal audits. Patient care advancement refers to research.

Longitudinal Patient Record. The **longitudinal patient record** is a comprehensive patient record compiled and accessible over the individual's life span from birth to death. It is a valuable resource for clinical decision making that provides easy access to medical history, reduces repeated diagnostic testing and treatments, and promotes patient safety through medical alerts and information on allergies, drug reactions, and interactions.

Paper-based records have been unable to achieve the advantages of longitudinal records because of their lack of standardization, difficulty in organizing, and limited access. One of the substantial advantages of moving to an electronic health record (EHR), or linkage of records, is the opportunity to create longitudinal patient records. The Veteran's Administration has led the way in creating longitudinal electronic patient records to serve their patient population.

DATA COLLECTION STANDARDS

The patient health record is currently a combination of discrete data elements and narrative in various media, including paper, electronic, voice, images, and waveforms. A variety of organizations and agencies in the public and private sectors are engaged in extensive efforts to standardize the record, including the development of data content and collection standards.

Governmental

Efforts to standardize health care data have existed since early efforts to record mortality and then morbidity data. Beginning in the 1990s, striking changes occurred in health and health care and in health data and information systems. Both the national environment for health information systems and the nature of the information systems have changed dramatically. The new electronic information environment is raising new privacy issues and magnifying the importance of ensuring that current policies are appropriate for new technologies.

One must keep in mind that, while various agencies, committees, organizations and individuals are working to develop new standards, others are currently collecting data at an accelerating rate. Multiple governmental, professional, and private groups are working toward a consensus on standards for both record content and electronic data transfer. It behooves all **stakeholders** to be aware of the goals, mandates, and activities

of the others and to maintain effective communication within the health information community. The AHIMA works diligently representing its membership in these areas.

Department of Health and Human Services

Collection, analysis, and dissemination of health-related information are crucial aspects of the responsibilities of the Department of Health and Human Services (DHHS). The DHHS also plays a national leadership role in health data standards and health information privacy policy and is charged with the responsibility for implementation of the administrative simplification provisions of the Health Insurance Portability and Accountability Act of 1996 (HIPAA). In addition, the DHHS engages in cooperative efforts with standards organizations, professional organizations, state and local governments, other countries, and the international community to foster health data standards, comparability, and cross-national research. Figure 4-2 illustrates the scope of the federal government's involvement in health data standard activities.

Health and Human Services Data Council. The DHHS Data Council coordinates all health and nonhealth data collection and analysis activities of the department, including an integrated health data collection strategy, coordination of health data standards, and health information and privacy policy issues, including the implementation of the administrative simplification provisions of HIPAA.

National Committee on Vital and Health Statistics. The National Committee on Vital and Health Statistics (NCVHS) is the statutory public advisory body to DHHS on health data, statistics, and national health information policy. This committee serves as a national forum for the collaboration of interested parties to accelerate the evolution of public and private health information systems toward more uniform, shared data standards within a framework protecting privacy and security. The NCVHS encourages the evolution of a shared, public-private national health information infrastructure that will promote the availability of valid, credible, timely, and comparable health data. With sensitivity to policy considerations and priorities, the NCVHS provides scientific and technical advice and guidance regarding the design and operation of health statistics and information systems and services and coordination of health data requirements. It also assists and advises DHHS on HIPAA implementation and informs decision making about data policy by DHHS, states, local governments, and the private sector.

National Center for Health Statistics. To clarify the names and acronyms, mention is made here of the National Center for Health Statistics (NCHS), which may easily be confused with the NCVHS. The NCHS is a part of the Centers for Disease Control and Prevention (CDC) of the DHHS and it is the federal government's principal vital and health statistics agency. The NCHS provides a wide variety of data with which to monitor the nation's health. Although the data provided by the NCHS are used by policymakers in Congress and the

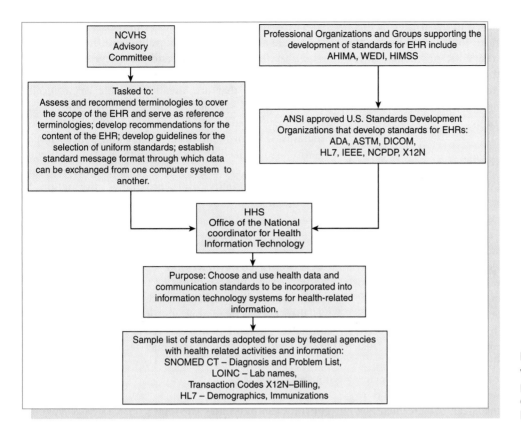

Figure 4-2 Federal and private sector activities that support the development and use of standards for electronic health record systems.

administration, by medical researchers, and by others in the health community, the NCHS should not be mistaken for the NCVHS, which is a public policy advisory board. The role of the NCHS is discussed in other chapters.

Overview of Information and Data Sets

The NCVHS has been the leading government agency in the area of standardization of health information, primarily through uniform **data sets,** since its initial charter in the 1950s. It addresses the need for uniform, comparable standards across geographic areas, populations, systems,

institutions, and sites of care to maximize the effectiveness of health promotion and care and minimize the burden on those responsible for generating the data. To this end, the NCVHS has advised the DHHS on such matters as federal-state relationships, nomenclatures and classification systems, core data sets, and access and confidentiality issues.

The data sets **promulgated** by the NCVHS have become de facto standards in their areas for data collection by federal and state agencies and by public and private data abstracting organizations. They have influenced both the *Conditions of Participation* and claim forms on which Medicare and Medicaid data sets are based. Table 4-1 identifies the existing

Table 4-1 FEDERAL INFORMATION AND DATA SETS

Acronym	Name	Purpose
DEEDS	Data Elements for Emergency Department Systems	Uniform specifications for data entered into hospital ED records
MDS	Minimum Data Set for Long-Term Care	Comprehensive functional assessment of long-term care patients
OASIS	Outcome and Assessment Information Set	Core items of comprehensive assessment for adult home care patients; forms basis for measuring patient outcomes
UACDS	Uniform Ambulatory Care Data Set	Improve ability to compare data in ambulatory care settings
UHDDS	Uniform Hospital Discharge Data Set	Uniform collection of data on inpatients; used by federal and state agencies

federal data sets, which are discussed in detail later in this chapter. These data sets are intended to describe significant minimal data about patients, residents, or clients. It is important to remember, however, that, although these data are essential to the patient record and patient care, additional data are necessary for a comprehensive record that supports the delivery of that care.

Core Health Data Elements

The achievements of the NCVHS regarding minimum data sets have been significant. However, the ever-expanding sites of care, combined with the increasing use of electronic data, have made it imperative that all health data collection activities, when possible, use standardized data elements and definitions. Standardized data elements are also vitally important in the managed care field, in which there is a need to follow individuals through a continuum of care and at multiple sites. Performance monitoring and outcomes research are two additional areas that are currently hampered by the inability to link data sets from various sources because of varying data elements and definitions.

In 1996, the NCVHS completed a 2-year project to review the current state of health-related core data sets and to promote consensus by identifying areas of agreement on core health data elements and definitions. The goal has been to develop a set of data elements with agreed-on standardized definitions, not to specify a data set for mandated external reporting. The list of recommended data elements is by no means exhaustive and, unlike the result of earlier activities, is not a "data set" to be used in a specific setting.[2]

The 42 data elements are listed in Table 4-2. They contain the elements selected for the first phase of this process and apply to persons seen in both ambulatory and inpatient settings unless otherwise specified. Consensus has been reached on definitions for the majority of these elements; for others, definitions must still be finalized; and for a third group, additional study and testing are needed. The rationale and discussion sections provide valuable insight into the issues of data standardization. For the first 12 elements, with the exception of a unique identifier, information may not have to be collected at each encounter. Standard electronic formats are recommended to the extent that they have been developed. A column has been added to provide comparison with the American Society for Testing and Materials (ASTM) standard ASTM E1384, which is described in more detail later in this chapter.

Centers for Disease Control and Prevention.

The implementation of data sets and the core data elements have provided additional opportunities for research, reporting, and prevention. The CDC has developed the National Electronic Disease Surveillance System (NEDSS). NEDSS is an initiative that promotes the use of data and information standards to advance the development of efficient, integrated, and interoperable public health surveillance systems at the federal, state, and local levels. A primary goal of NEDSS is the continuing, automatic capture and analysis of data that are already available electronically. This Web-based strategy is intended to monitor and assess disease trends, guide prevention and intervention programs, inform public health policy and policy makers, identify issues needing public health research, provide information for community and program planning, and protect confidentiality while providing information to those who need to know.

Nongovernmental

Accrediting Organizations

A wide variety of accrediting organizations set voluntary standards regarding health record data. Although it is voluntary, there are several reasons why organizations choose to be accredited. Accreditation may reduce reviews by the state and federal government and may facilitate payment for services and assure consumers and payers that a high quality of care is provided.

The Joint Commission. The Joint Commission is by far the oldest and best known organizational accrediting body. It has developed accreditation standards across many settings in the health care continuum. Standards for each of the settings address information management. Specifics are covered later in this chapter (*www.jointcommission.org*).

National Committee on Quality Assurance. The National Committee on Quality Assurance (NCQA) is the source for information about the quality of the nation's managed care plans, which is used by consumers and employers in making health care choices. NCQA uses the Health Plan Employer Data and Information Set (HEDIS) to measure performance (*www.ncqa.org*).

Other Accrediting Bodies. Various other specialty accrediting bodies exist, such as the American Osteopathic Association (AOA), the Commission on Accreditation of Rehabilitation Facilities (CARF), and the American Association of Ambulatory Health Care (AAAHC).

Professional Organizations

The quality of health care data relies on the excellence of data collection at the time of service, the information system model design and implementation, data monitoring and evaluation, and the services provided by or under the direction of the HIM professional. In addition to continuing assessment of the quality of health data, continuous monitoring and evaluation of the quality of HIM services (based on practice standards) must be essential activities in all health care or non-health-care organizations that have these services.

Table 4-2 COMPARISON OF CORE HEALTH DATA ELEMENTS

National Committee on Vital and Health Statistics*	ASTM1384-02a†
Personal/Enrollment Data	X
01. Personal/unique identifier (b)	X
02. Date of birth	X
03. Sex	X
04. Race and ethnicity	X
05. Residence	X
06. Marital status	X
07. Living/residential arrangement (a)	X
08. Self-reported health status (b)	X
09. Functional status (b)	X
10. Years of schooling	X
11. Patient's relationship to subscriber/person eligible for entitlement	X
12. Current or most recent occupation and industry (b)	X
Encounter Data	
13. Type of encounter (b)	X
14. Admission date (inpatient)	X
15. Discharge date (inpatient)	X
16. Date of encounter (outpatient and physician services)	X
17. Facility identification (a)	X
18. Type of facility/place of encounter (a)	X
19. Health care practitioner identification (outpatient) (a)	X
20. Provider location or address of encounter (outpatient)	X
21. Attending physician identification (inpatient) (a)	X
22. Operating clinician identification (a)	X
23. Health care practitioner specialty (a)	X
24. Principal diagnosis (inpatient)	Problem
25. Primary diagnosis (inpatient)	Problem
26. Other diagnoses (inpatient)	Problem
27. Qualifier for other diagnoses (inpatient)	Problem
28. Patient's stated reason for visit or chief complaint (outpatient) (a)	Problem
29. Diagnosis chiefly responsible for services provided (outpatient)	Problem
30. Other diagnoses (outpatient)	Problem
31. External cause of injury	Problem
32. Birth weight of neonate	X
33. Principal procedure (inpatient)	X
34. Other procedures (inpatient)	X
35. Dates of procedures (inpatient)	X
36. Procedures and services (outpatient)	X
37. Medications prescribed	
38. Disposition of patient (inpatient) (a)	
39. Disposition (outpatient)	
40. Patient's expected sources of payment (a)	X
41. Injury related to employment	X
42. Total billed charges (a)	X

*NCVHS footnotes: as of August 1996. (a) Element for which substantial agreement has been reached but for which some amount of additional work is needed; (b) element which has been recognized as significant but for which considerable work remains to be undertaken. A lack of footnote indicates that these elements are ready for implementation.
†ASTM E1384 is described in more detail later in this chapter.

Professional organizations take leadership positions and are advocates for their segment of the industry. They promote education and life-long learning by providing resources, including publications, seminars, and on-line learning as well as opportunities for certification. Membership in professional organizations provides access to resources and colleagues that support maintaining a high level of professional competence. Three important examples follow.

The American Health Information Management Association. AHIMA is dedicated to the effective management of personal health information needed to deliver quality health care to the public (see *www.ahima.org*). Of particular importance are professional practice guidelines called "Practice Briefs." They present best practices and are excellent for personal continuing education and evaluation of present organizational practices.

Healthcare Information and Management Systems Society. The Healthcare Information and Management Systems Society (HIMSS) focuses on the optimal use of health care information technology and management systems for the betterment of human health (see *www.himss.org*).

American Medical Informatics Association. The American Medical Informatics Association (AMIA) provides leadership in the development and implementation of information systems to improve patient care (see *www.amia.org*).

American Association for Medical Transcription. The American Association for Medical Transcription (AAMT) is committed to the creation of quality health record reports from dictation produced by medical language specialists as well as the evolution of the medical transcription industry (see *www.aamt.org*).

Researchers and Other Groups

A variety of informatics researchers and specialty groups are developing and testing data sets. An example is the work done at the University of Iowa on a Nursing Management Minimum Data Set (NMMDS), which is a research-based management data set that includes 17 across-settings elements. NMMDS is designed to meet the nurse executive need for a specific nursing management data capture system that will produce accurate, reliable, and useful data for decision making. Additional projects explore the usefulness of large data repositories with three minimum data sets, including: NMMDS, the Nursing Minimum Data Set (NMDS), and the Uniform Hospital Discharge Data Set (UHDDS), as well as the American Nurses Association Quality Indicators that support effectiveness research. It is reasonable to anticipate significant growth in this research.

BASIC PRINCIPLES OF DATA COLLECTION

User Needs

Understanding standards, rules, and regulations is a solid foundation for developing a quality health record. However, before one can be confident that a fully functioning record has been designed, it is essential to consider the specialized needs of all the users of the record, including the organization as an entity and all internal and external users. Discussion takes place in committees, including those described in The Joint Commission standards, and in other groups within the facility as well as with department heads and may include special interests from research to marketing. Understanding the flow of data and information throughout the health care facility and larger health system ensures that computer views (or screens) and paper forms are designed to facilitate the collection of data elements as care is provided. Training and practice in the design of computer views and paper forms and computer-based data capture techniques make the HIM professional a valuable management resource.

Documentation Responsibilities

It is the responsibility of the health care organization to identify who may provide care and then document that care in the patient record. The foundation for these decisions is state licensure laws, which specify the legal scope of practice for health care providers. State laws vary and current laws must be consulted. For example, Washington State allows advanced registered nurse practitioners (ARNPs) to practice independently and prescribe medications. ARNPs are required to have a physician resource identified in case they need assistance or consultation. Other clinicians, such as nurse midwives and physician assistants, have varying levels of independent practice, which may require supervision and a countersignature on documentation. Additional consideration should be given to reimbursement issues, including Medicare and Medicaid.

The organization's decisions are specified in policies and procedures and, where there is an organized medical staff, in the medical staff bylaws, rules, and regulations. The Joint Commission defines a **licensed independent practitioner** (LIP) as "any individual permitted by law and by the organization to provide care, treatment, and services without direction or supervision." The process of credentialing, including the scope of privileges, is discussed in more detail in another chapter.

General Documentation Forms and Views

Although there are various data collection standards, accrediting and regulatory bodies and professional organizations do not require or recommend particular forms or views for documenting patient care. While facilities are responsible for creating their own tools, it is not necessary to start from scratch. There are books, journals, newsletters, and vendor catalogs that offer examples. Local professional organizations and networking with colleagues can also lead to valuable suggestions on what has worked well and what has not. Some acute-care samples are provided as an appendix to this chapter, and others can be found in the accompanying study guide.

To provide a starting point, forms commonly included in the paper health record are listed in Table 4-3 and described in the next section. Some examples are provided in the Study Guide and on the Web site (Evolve).

Table 4-3 OVERVIEW OF COMMON HEALTH RECORD FORMS AND VIEWS BY FREQUENCY AND MAJOR SITES OF CARE

Form	Acute Care	Ambulatory Care	Long-Term Care	Home Health Care	Hospice Care	Behavioral Health Care
Administrative Forms						
Registration record	F	F	F	F	F	F
Consent to treatment	F	F	F	F	F	F
Acknowledgment of HIPAA privacy notice	F	F	F	F	F	F
Consent to release information	F	F	F	F	F	F
Acknowledgment of patient's rights	O	R	F	O	O	F
Advance directives	F	F	F	F	F	F
Consent to special procedures	F	O	O	R	R	O
Patient's legal status	R	M	O	M	M	F
Property/valuables list	F	R	F	R	O	O
Service agreement	M	M	M	F	F	M
Transfer/referral form	F	M	F	M	F	R
Birth certificate	F	O	M	O	R	R
Death certificate	O	O	F	O	F	R
Clinical Forms						
Registration record	F	F	F	F	F	F
Emergency record	O	F	M	M	M	M
Problem list	M	F	M	O	R	R
Medical history/review of systems	F	F	F	F	F	F
Psychiatric/psychological history	R	R	R	R	R	F
Physical examination	F	F	F	F	F	F
Encounter record	M	F	M	M	M	F
Interdisciplinary patient care plan	R	R	F	F	O	F
Physician's orders	F	F	F	F	F	F
Progress notes	F	F	F	F	F	F
Consultation report	F	O	R	R	R	O
Discharge/interval summary	F	F	F	F	F	F
Operative Forms						
Anesthesia report	F	O	R	M	M	M
Recovery room report	F	O	R	M	M	M
Operative report	F	O	R	M	M	M
Pathology report	F	O	O	O	O	O
Obstetrical Data						
Antepartum record	F	O	M	M	M	M
Labor and delivery record	F	O	M	M	M	M
Postpartum record	F	O	M	M	M	M
Neonatal Data						
Birth history	F	O	M	M	M	M
Neonatal identification	F	O	M	M	M	M
Neonatal physical examination	F	O	M	M	M	M
Neonatal progress notes	F	O	M	M	M	M
Nursing Forms						
Nursing notes	F	O	F	F	F	F
Graphic sheet	F	R	F	R	F	F
Medication sheet	F	R	F	R	F	F
Special care units	F	M	M	M	M	M

F, Frequent; *O,* occasionally; *R,* rarely; *M,* may never be seen in this record.

Continued

Table 4-3 OVERVIEW OF COMMON HEALTH RECORD FORMS AND VIEWS BY FREQUENCY AND MAJOR SITES OF CARE—cont'd

Form	Acute Care	Ambulatory Care	Long-Term Care	Home Health Care	Hospice Care	Behavioral Health Care
Ancillary Forms						
Electrocardiograph	F	F	F	F	F	O
Laboratory reports	F	F	F	F	F	F
Radiology/imaging reports	F	F	O	O	O	O
Radiation therapy	R	R	R	R	R	M
Therapeutic services (e.g., physical therapy, respiratory therapy)	F	F	F	F	R	O
Case management/social services	F	F	F	F	F	F
Patient or family teaching and participation	F	O	O	O	O	F
Discharge or follow-up plan	F	R	O	F	M	F

F, Frequent; *O,* occasionally; *R,* rarely; *M,* may never be seen in this record.

Any differences in application are discussed under the appropriate care setting. Hospitals tend to be the most complex care setting and may have the widest variety of forms. Views meet the same needs but through their smaller, more flexible logical structure. A more complete understanding of the role of each form or view will develop through the balance of this chapter, related topics in other chapters, and through continuing professional education and experience.

Patient Identification

All forms and views must identify the patient, including all sides and segments of multipart paper forms and all screens of computer views. In most settings, a **unique identifier** number is assigned to link the patient to their record. This number is used on all record forms and views to collect all patient data in the correct record or to be accessed by computer database query. The patient name and number are contained in a database called the **master patient index** (MPI). It is the most essential tool for any health information department that numbers its records because it is the link between the patient's name and number. The MPI is discussed in other chapters as it relates to access and retention of the clinical record and as one of the building blocks in an EHR system.

Administrative Forms

Registration Record. Basic **demographic,** or patient identification data, and financial data are routinely collected for every patient in every care setting unless the patient or the patient's representative is unable to provide these data. The data are collected before care is rendered and include sufficient items to identify the patient positively, such as name, address, date of birth, next of kin, payment arrangements, and a patient identification number. Basic clinical data are also supplied on this form. The registration record is one of the most commonly computerized forms. It may

also be called an identification sheet, face or summary sheet, or admission-discharge record.

Consent to Treatment. All care settings must receive a consent for treatment from the patient or guardian. Special legal considerations exist in emergency situations. The body of the form contains a statement indicating that the patient agrees to receive basic, routine services, diagnostic procedures, and medical care. An additional statement explains that treatment outcomes cannot be guaranteed.

Acknowledgment of Health Information Portability and Accountability Act Privacy Notice. As part of the HIPAA privacy rule, covered entities are required to provide patients with a Notice of Privacy Practices and update as needed. They are also required to make a good faith effort to obtain a written acknowledgment of receipt of the notice, except in emergency situations. If there are changes in privacy practices, an updated copy should be signed and dated.

Consent to Release Information. The patient's signature authorizes the exchange of personally identifiable health information between the provider and other organizations. Most commonly, this specifies release of health information compiled during the episode of care to third-party payers. It may also permit the provider to request relevant health information from previous providers. This form is particularly appropriate to have translated into other languages. Verbal translation may also be necessary. It is generally understood that the provider has permission to release medical information for continuation of care. Confidentiality and legal considerations must be followed carefully in designing this form.

Acknowledgment of Patient Rights. This form lists the patient's rights while the patient is under care. A patient must be informed of his or her rights at the initiation of care, and there should be written evidence of this. One method of obtaining the evidence is to have the patient sign a copy and place it in the record as proof of the patient's being informed. If there are any changes in these rights, an updated copy should be signed and dated by the patient or guardian and added to the record.

Advance Directives. Advance directives give instructions regarding the patient's or guardian's wishes in special medical situations. The Patient Self-Determination Act (PSDA), effective December 1991, requires that all patients older than 18 years be given written information about their rights under state laws so that they can make decisions concerning medical care, including their right to refuse or accept medical or surgical treatment. Also covered under the law is information regarding a patient's right to formulate advance directives, such as living wills and durable powers of attorney for health care. Although the law requires that patients be informed, it does not require that the advance directives be included in the chart. Patients are increasingly considering these options, discussing them with their family and personal advisers such as clergy and attorneys, and then executing the appropriate documents and including appropriate information in the record.

Consent to Special Procedures. A special consent is required to authorize any nonroutine diagnostic or therapeutic procedure before it is performed on the patient. For special consents to be valid, the physician must explain in lay terms the procedure named, the risks of having or refusing the procedure, available alternative procedures, and the likely outcome. Again, no guarantees are given. Signature by the patient or guardian confirms that the explanation has been given and understood and that the procedure has been agreed to. This form is particularly appropriate to have translated into other languages. Verbal translation may also be necessary. Both the *Conditions of Participation* and The Joint Commission require that the medical staff bylaws, rules, and regulations address informed consent, including which procedures are covered. Consent must always be obtained, with the properly executed form on the chart before surgery. In emergencies, when consent is unavailable, the reason should be documented.

Property and Valuables List. An inventory of property and valuables brought by the patient should be created if the care involves an admission. Any items secured on the patient's behalf should be noted. Items such as visual aids, dentures, mobility devices, and prostheses are included, and the list is signed by the patient or a representative of the patient and a representative of the facility. Patients should be discouraged from retaining expensive, nonmedical items in their rooms.

Birth and Death Certificates. State laws require the filing of vital records, including birth and death certificates. The forms and procedures vary by state; frequently, copies are kept in the patient record.

Clinical Forms

Registration Record. In a hospital setting the registration record, discussed earlier, may also contain the attending physician's statement of diagnoses, intended procedures, and any allergies or sensitivities. In a clinic setting the registration record may contain a chief complaint and allergies as stated by the patient. Although not required, the inclusion of clinical data has many benefits. Any necessary third-party authorization for services can be obtained, appropriate unit or room assignment can be made, and nursing care can begin. Standard terminology should be used and abbreviations and symbols avoided. The acute care registration/admission-discharge paper record may also contain data on consultations and the disposition of the patient, including whether an autopsy was performed on a deceased patient. If the organization places the data into a database, then all "registration related" data could be present and used as appropriate.

History and Physical Examination. The medical history and physical examination (H&P) is a single report with the two segments as described below. In acute care, The Joint Commission requires a report of a comprehensive H&P be completed and available within 24 hours, or sooner if surgery is to be performed. The Joint Commission permits an interval history and physical examination when a patient is admitted within 30 days for the same condition. In this circumstance, the H&P is updated as needed. This key document is typically dictated and transcribed. A written note is provided in the chart while the report is being prepared.

Medical History and Review of Systems. The medical history, including a review of systems, forms the foundation for establishing a provisional diagnosis and developing a treatment plan. If the patient cannot reliably provide this important information, it should be obtained from the most knowledgeable available source. The source should be identified. As with other forms or views, standardization is important. An outline of the sequence of data items may be printed on the form or represented as fields to be completed on one or more views. Computerization, with the options of alerts and alarms, makes it easier to ensure that all essential data items have been captured. Whichever technology is used, the tone should be impartial and reflect the patient's statements.

The components of the medical history consist of the chief complaint or a description of the symptoms that caused the patient to seek medical attention, the history of the current illness, medical history, family history, social history including health maintenance, and a review of systems (Table 4-4). The Joint Commission also requires that a developmental age evaluation and educational needs assessment be included when the patient is a child or adolescent. All symptoms (positive data) should be documented, and the term "normal" (or negative data)

Table 4-4 MEDICAL HISTORY—TYPICAL SEGMENTS AND CONTENT

Purpose: The medical history is a conversation to gather information from the patient, to establish a trusting and supportive relationship, and to offer information and counseling. The scope and focus of the health history vary according to the clinical setting, the patient's agenda and problem, and the clinician's goals. The following is a classic representation, though there are variations.

Segments	Complaints and Symptoms
CC: Chief complaint	Concise and succinct description of why patient is seeking medical attention in his or her own words. Complaints or goals
HPI: History of present illness	Detailed chronological account of development of patient's illness, from appearance of first symptom to present situation. Includes pertinent negatives. A helpful mnemonic: OPQRST—onset, provocation, quality (what is it like?), radiation (does it travel?), severity (-0 to 10), time (interval? now? before?) Current medications. A helpful mnemonic is PORCH: prescription, over-the-counter, recreational, compliance, herbal
PMH: Past medical history	Summary of childhood and adult illnesses and conditions, such as infectious diseases, pregnancies, accidents, and hospitalizations Allergies and drug sensitivities or no known allergies (NKA) Past surgical history: previous operations
FH: Family history	Age and health or cause of death of each immediate family member. Diseases among relatives in which heredity or contact might play a role, such as allergies, cancer, and infectious, psychiatric, metabolic, endocrine, cardiovascular, and renal diseases. May include a diagram.
SH: Social history	Daily routine: dietary, sleep, and exercise patterns; use of caffeine, tobacco, alcohol, and other drugs and related substances, etc. Education and occupation, home environment and significant others, important experiences, leisure activities, religious affiliations and beliefs Health maintenance: immunizations, screening tests, safe sex, safety measures such as seatbelts, bicycle helmets, smoke alarms, etc.
ROS: Review of systems	Systematic inventory designed to uncover current or past subjective symptoms that includes the following types of data:
General:	Usual weight, recent weight changes, fever, weakness, fatigue
Skin:	Rashes, lumps, sores, itching, dryness, color change, changes in hair or nails, eruptions, dryness, cyanosis, jaundice; changes in skin, hair, and nails
Head:	Headache (duration, severity, character, location) head injury, dizziness, lightheadedness
Eyes:	Glasses or contact lenses, last eye examination, change in vision, glaucoma, cataracts, pain, redness, dry eyes, excessive tearing, double vision, blurred vision, spots, specks, flashing lights
Ears:	Hearing, discharge, tinnitus, dizziness, pain, vertigo, earaches, infection, discharge, use or nonuse of hearing aids
Nose:	Head colds, epistaxis, discharges, obstruction, postnasal drip, sinus pain, itching, hay fever
Mouth and throat:	Condition of teeth and gums, bleeding gums, last dental examination, sores or soreness, redness, hoarseness, difficulty in swallowing, dentures, dry mouth
Neck:	Lumps, "swollen glands," goiter, pain, or stiffness
Breasts:	Lumps, pain or discomfort, nipple discharge, self-examination, last mammogram
Respiratory system:	Chest pain, wheezing, cough, dyspnea, sputum (color and quantity), hemoptysis, asthma, bronchitis, emphysema, pneumonia, tuberculosis, pleurisy, last chest x-ray
Cardiovascular system:	Heart trouble, high blood pressure, chest pain, palpitations, rheumatic fever, heart murmur, dyspnea, orthopnea, paroxysmal nocturnal dyspnea, edema, tachycardia, vertigo, faintness, past ECG or other test results
Gastrointestinal system:	Appetite, thirst, indigestion, food intolerance, nausea, vomiting, anorexia, bulimia, hematemesis, rectal bleeding, change in bowel habits, diarrhea, constipation, flatus, hemorrhoids, jaundice, liver or gallbladder trouble, frequency of bowel movements
Urinary system:	Frequent or painful urination, nocturia, hematuria, incontinence, urinary infection, urgency, stones

Table 4-4 MEDICAL HISTORY—TYPICAL SEGMENTS AND CONTENT—cont'd

Purpose: The medical history is a conversation to gather information from the patient, to establish a trusting and supportive relationship, and to offer information and counseling. The scope and focus of the health history vary according to the clinical setting, the patient's agenda and problem, and the clinician's goals. The following is a classic representation, though there are variations.

Segments	Complaints and Symptoms
Genitoreproductive system:	General: birth control, sexually transmitted diseases, exposure to HIV, sexual preference, interest, satisfaction Male: sores, discharge from penis, hernias, testicular pain or masses, erectile dysfunction, perineal numbness Female: age at menarche, regularity, frequency and duration of menstruation, dysmenorrhea, menorrhagia, bleeding between periods or after intercourse, tampon use, pregnancies, births, symptoms of menopause
Peripheral vascular and extremities:	Intermittent claudication, leg cramps, varicose veins, past clots, thrombophlebitis
Musculoskeletal system:	Joint pain or stiffness, arthritis, gout, backache, muscle pain, cramps, swelling, redness, limitation in motor activity, previous fractures and other injuries
Neurological system:	Fainting, blackouts, seizures, paralysis, tingling, tremors, memory loss
Hematologic system:	Anemia, easy bruising or bleeding, past transfusions and any reactions
Endocrine system:	Thyroid disease; heat and cold intolerance; excessive sweating, thirst, hunger, or urination
Psychiatric disorders:	Nervousness, tension, mood including depression, memory, insomnia, headache, nightmares, personality disorders, anxiety disorders, mood disorders, suicidal ideation, obsessive-compulsive disorder, flashbacks

Adapted from Bickley LS, Szilagyi PG: *Bates' guide to physical examination and history taking*, ed 8, Philadelphia, 2002, JB Lippincott.

should be discouraged except in summary statements. (See the activity on the personal family history.)

Physical Examination. The physical examination adds objective data to the subjective data provided by the patient in the history. Together, they provide the foundation from which the practitioner can establish a diagnosis and begin to develop a treatment plan. The examination should include all body systems (Table 4-5) and consider the patient's age, sex, and symptoms. Any existing diagnostic data or physical findings are also included. A definitive diagnosis may not be possible, in which event a provisional (tentative) diagnosis may be used. If several diagnoses potentially fit the patient's clinical presentation, this list of alternatives is called a differential diagnosis. In addition, a clinical impression and an intended course of action are required.

Interdisciplinary Patient Care Plan. Most care sites are required to have an interdisciplinary patient care plan. Exceptions are the physician's office or clinic and the acute-care hospital, where the physician plan and other practitioners' plans are documented separately. The care plan is the foundation around which patient care is organized because it contains input from the unique perspective of each discipline involved. It includes an assessment, statement of goals, identification of specific activities or strategies to achieve those goals, and periodic assessment of goal attainment. The care plan is initiated when a patient is admitted or begins care, and it is periodically updated. The

discipline responsible for implementing each part of the plan is identified. The plan is reviewed and revised as often as the organization, regulatory agencies, and accrediting bodies require, when goals are achieved, or as the circumstances of the patient change. Changes in the care plan can easily be summarized at discharge. Because of its central role in planning and providing care, the care plan is a valuable tool in evaluating both individual patient care and overall organizational patient care performance.

Physician/Practitioner's Orders. LIPs, as identified in the organization's policies and procedures and medical staff bylaws, rules, and regulations, communicate their plans for the patient by giving written or verbal orders or directions to the nursing staff and other practitioners. Orders are needed for any type of treatment or diagnostic procedure. Standing orders are a set of routine orders used for patients with a particular diagnosis or to prepare for or follow up a procedure. This type of order is discouraged, particularly with managed care, because the actions may not all be medically necessary for all patients. However, treatment guidelines and protocols that incorporate best practices for treating particular problems are being used. Orders based on these protocols provide a basic set of orders modified to address an individual patient's situation. Because they initiate actions, it is particularly important that all orders are dated and signed by the LIP giving the order. The Joint Commission requires that verbal orders or telephone orders for the exchange of critical test results be verified through a

Table 4-5 PHYSICAL EXAMINATION—TYPICAL SEGMENTS AND CONTENT

Purpose: Guided by the subjective information obtained from the review of systems in the medical history, the clinician seeks objective information through the physical examination. The following is a classic "head-to-toe" sequence, although there are variations. How complete various segments are will vary by setting and the patient's complaint.

Segments	Content
General condition	Apparent state of health, signs of distress, posture, weight, height, skin color, dress and personal hygiene, reactions to persons and things, facial expression, manner, orientation, mood, state of awareness, speech
Vital signs	Temperature, pulse, respiration, blood pressure, pain
Skin	Color, vascularity, lesions, edema, moisture, temperature, texture, thickness, mobility and turgor, hands and nails
Head	Hair, scalp, skull, face
Eyes	Visual acuity and fields; position and alignment of the eyes, eyebrows, eyelids; tearing; conjunctivae; sclerae; corneas; irises; size, shape, equality, reaction to light and accommodation of pupils; extraocular movements, ophthalmoscopic examination
Ears	Auditory acuity, auricles, canals, tympanic membranes, discharge
Nose and sinuses	External nose, airways, mucosa, septum, sinus tenderness, discharge, bleeding, smell
Mouth and throat	Lips, oral mucosa, gums, teeth, tongue, palate, tonsils, pharynx, palate, uvula, postnasal drip, sores, lesions
Neck	Stiffness, thyroid, trachea, vessels, lymph nodes, salivary glands, jugular venous distention
Thorax and lungs	Anterior and posterior, shape, symmetry, retractions, percussion Breath sounds: adventitious sounds, fremitus, breath sounds, friction, spoken voice, whispered voice
Breasts, axillae	Symmetrical, tenderness, dimpling, masses, scars, discharge from nipples, axillary nodes
Cardiovascular system	Location and quality of apical impulse, thrill, pulsation, rhythm, sounds, murmurs, friction rub, jugular venous pressure and pulse, carotid artery pulse
Abdomen	Contour, peristalsis, scars, rigidity, rebound, tenderness, spasm, masses, distention, fluid, hernia, bowel sounds and bruits, palpable organs
Genitourinary system	Male: scars, lesions, discharge, penis, scrotum, epididymis, varicocele, hydrocele, rectal examination Female: external genitalia, Skene's glands and Bartholin's glands, vagina, cervix, uterus, adnexa, rectal examination, Papanicolaou smear
Musculoskeletal system	Spine and extremities, deformities, swelling, redness, tenderness, range of motion, muscle tone, weakness
Lymphatics	Palpable cervical, axillary, inguinal nodes; location; size; consistency; mobility and tenderness
Blood vessels	Pulses, color, temperature, vessel walls, veins
Neurological system	Cranial nerves, coordination, reflexes, biceps, triceps, patellar, Achilles, abdominal, Babinski, Romberg, gait, compare right and left, distal and proximal; Sensory: pain, temperature, touch, position, vibration
Mental Status	If not done during the examination: mood, thought processes and content, abnormal perceptions, insight and judgment, memory and attention, information and vocabulary, calculating abilities, abstract thinking, dementia screening
Diagnosis(es)	Impression: single diagnosis, provisional diagnosis, or differential diagnosis

Adapted from Bickley LS, Szilagyi PG: *Bates' guide to physical examination and history taking,* ed 8, Philadelphia, 2002, JB Lippincott.

"read back" procedure. In addition, these orders must be authenticated within the time specified by state or federal law and regulations as well as the medical staff bylaws, rules, and regulations, if the organization has an organized medical staff. With the exception of office visits, orders are needed for admission and discharge from facilities and for treatments such as radiation therapy. An admission order is written at the initiation of care, and a discharge order should be written for every patient when the physician determines that release is appropriate. Lack of a discharge order may indicate that the patient left against medical advice (AMA). If this situation occurs, the circumstances should be documented in the progress notes and discharge summary. Some variations on physicians' orders can be encountered in special settings, such as residential and behavioral health. For example, in ambulatory behavioral health a team may prepare a treatment plan that includes the services to be provided. The treatment plan then contains "orders" for treatment and may be signed by one or more of the clinicians involved in the client's treatment.

Progress Notes. Progress notes are interval statements that document the patient's illness and response to treatment as specifically as possible. Which practitioners write progress notes varies with the health care setting. For example, physicians write the majority of progress notes in their offices, and these notes are the focal point when patients are admitted for care. Because nurses coordinate and provide most of the patient care in home health, their notes are most prominent. In mental health, progress notes feature the primary clinician's documentation of counseling. Progress notes may be integrated, with all providers writing sequentially on the same sheets, or they may be separated, with physicians, nurses, and other providers writing separately, perhaps on custom-designed forms or views. The computer views can be organized by date, type, author, or some other variable.

Regardless of where the progress notes are located, any practitioner who writes such notes is responsible for recording observations about the patient's progress and response to treatment from the perspective of his or her profession. For example, physician progress notes for admitted patients should include an admission note, subsequent notes, and a final note. The admission note provides an overview of the patient at admission and adds any relevant information that is not included in the history and physical examination. The frequency of subsequent progress notes depends on the patient's condition and the site of care and its medical staff bylaws, rules, and regulations. Acute care notes are written daily, whereas long-term care notes may appropriately be written monthly. All treatments provided and the patient's response to each are to be included, as are any complications the patient may have. When care of the patient is transferred from one physician to another, the physician releasing the patient should write a summary of the patient's course to that point. At the end of the admission, along with the discharge order, a final note is written stating the patient's general condition and instructions for the patient's activity, diet, medications, and any follow-up appointments. If the patient dies during the admission, the final notes describe the circumstances regarding the death, the findings, the cause of death, and whether an autopsy was performed.

Consultation Report. A consultation report contains an opinion about a patient's condition by a practitioner other than the attending physician. Opinions may be sought from pharmacists, dietitians, physical and occupational therapists, dentists, other physicians, and so on. The opinion is based on a review of the patient record, an examination of the patient, and a conference with the attending physician. Many facilities, particularly in acute care, combine the request section, where the attending physician states the reason for consultation, with a space for the response, where the consultant details his or her findings and recommendations. Each signs his or her respective section.

The *Conditions of Participation* for hospitals require that the medical staff bylaws, rules, and regulations address the status of consultants. To be considered a consultant, a practitioner must be well qualified by training, experience, and competence to give an opinion in the specialty in which the advice is sought. It is the responsibility of the attending physician to request a consultation. The categories of patients for which consultations must be requested are as follows:

- Patients who are not good medical or surgical risks
- Patients whose diagnoses are obscure
- Patients whose physicians have doubts about the best therapeutic measure(s) to be taken
- Patients who are involved in situations in which there is a question of criminal activity

In emergencies, exceptions may be made. The *Conditions* also state that routine procedures, such as radiologic studies, electrocardiograms, tissue examinations, and proctoscopic and cystoscopic procedures, are not normally considered consultations.

Discharge and Interval Summary. The discharge and interval summary, or clinical résumé, concisely reviews the patient's course. It is typically associated with admissions, but it may be provided in other care settings. The summary begins with the reason for admission and includes chronological descriptions of significant findings from examinations and tests and procedures and therapies performed along with the patient's response. Details regarding discharge are also recorded, including the condition on discharge related to the condition on admission and follow-up instructions specifying medications, level of physical activity, diet, follow-up care, and patient teaching. Because the discharge summary is referred to frequently, standard terminology is essential and abbreviations and ambiguous terms such as "improved" should be diligently avoided. All relevant diagnoses established by the time of discharge and all operative procedures performed should be recorded in standard terminology that indicates topography and etiology as necessary. When final diagnoses and procedures are listed on more than one form, attention must be paid to their agreement. In special cases, a final progress note may substitute for a discharge summary. Patients admitted for less than 48 hours with minor problems, uncomplicated deliveries, and normal neonates are examples. The discharge summary should be written or dictated immediately after discharge and authenticated.

Operative Forms

Data from each operative event are collected by using a set of forms or views that are considered a unit. The consent for surgery and the pathology report are added to the forms described next.

Anesthesia Report. Procedures that require more than a local anesthetic also require an anesthesia report. Preoperative medication is recorded with time, concentration, and effect. The anesthetic agent is then documented, including the amount, route of administration, effect, and duration. The patient's condition throughout the procedure is described, including vital signs, blood loss, transfusions, and intravenous fluids given. The report should also describe any surgical manipulation that may affect anesthesia care, any complications during anesthesia, and any treatments that are unlikely to be documented elsewhere. The practitioner administering the anesthesia (either a nurse anesthetist or an anesthesiologist) records the data and signs the report.

Special anesthesia-specific notes are also required before and after surgery. The preanesthesia note, usually found in the progress notes, describes the planned procedure, the choice of anesthetic, and an examination of the patient. Also discussed are laboratory results, any drug history, any past or potential problems, and preanesthesia medications. The postanesthesia note may be in the progress notes, the recovery room record, or the anesthesia report. It documents the patient's condition, specifying the nature and extent of any complications. The postanesthesia note should be completed within 24 hours after surgery. Both notes are signed by the practitioner responsible for administering the anesthesia. The Joint Commission requires at least one postanesthesia visit that describes the presence or absence of anesthesia-related complications. A visit is usually considered to occur apart from the operative or recovery area. Notes must specify time and date, with one visit occurring soon after surgery and another after the patient has completely recovered. The patient's condition may require additional visits. Although it is preferable that these notes be made by a physician or oral surgeon, any practitioner with pertinent comments regarding the patient's anesthesia care may add notes. If anesthesia personnel are unavailable to provide the documentation, the physician or dentist discharging the patient may complete the notes.

Recovery Room Record. The recovery room is designed to care for patients immediately after surgery or anesthesia. A separate form is typically used to record complete observation from the time the patient arrives in the recovery room until departure for the nursing unit or other destination. The Joint Commission requires that this form include the patient's condition and level of consciousness when entering and leaving the unit; vital signs; status reports of infusions, surgical dressings, tubes, catheters, or drains; and any treatment provided in the unit. The postanesthesia note may be documented on this form and, depending on its design, may be signed by a physician, nurse, or both.

Operative Report. All patients who undergo surgery must have an operative report included in their records. The top portion provides identifying data, including the names of the surgeon and any assistants, and the date, duration, and name of the procedure. A postoperative diagnosis is required. A preoperative diagnosis, which should be entered in the progress notes before surgery, is also desirable for easy comparison. The body of the report contains a full description of the surgical approach, normal and abnormal findings, organs explored, procedures, implants, ligatures, sutures, and the number of packs, drains, and sponges used, and the condition of the patient at the conclusion of surgery. The report should be written or dictated immediately after surgery, included in the record as soon as possible, and signed by the surgeon. If this is not possible, continuity of care can still be maintained by writing a timely and detailed operative note in the record.

Pathology Report. A pathology report documents tissue examinations that may be microscopic in addition to being macroscopic (gross). The tissue may have been removed from the patient during a specialized procedure, such as a biopsy, or during surgery. It may have been expelled, such as in an abortion, or be the entire body, as when an autopsy is performed. Occasionally, objects such as coins are submitted as well. As in a consultation, the tissue or object is identified, a clinical diagnosis provided, and an opinion requested. The pathologist examines the specimen and, at a minimum, writes a report describing its gross diagnostic features. A policy decision needs to be made regarding which specimens require only a gross examination and diagnosis. This decision may vary, depending on how and where the pathologist practices, but involves the medical staff in acute care. When a microscopic examination is performed, it is the basis for the diagnosis. The pathologist dictates and signs the transcribed report, and the original is included in the patient's record. When the report documents an autopsy, the pathologist summarizes the patient's illness and treatment, followed by a detailed report of gross findings and an anatomic diagnosis at autopsy. An autopsy is a lengthy procedure, and as many as 60 days may pass before reports are completed. A provisional autopsy diagnosis should be recorded in the patient's record within 3 days. Both reports are also signed by the pathologist.

Obstetrical Data

Another set of forms or views is collected for obstetrical care. Again, any appropriate consent for surgery or associated pathology report is added to the forms described next. The American College of Obstetricians and Gynecologists identifies the recommended content for these forms in its *Standards for Obstetric-Gynecologic Services.*

Antepartum Record. The antepartum or prenatal record begins in the office or clinic of the obstetrician or nurse midwife. Ideally started early in the pregnancy, the record includes a comprehensive history and physical examination as described previously, with particular attention to menstrual history, reproductive history including live births and abortions, a risk assessment, and attendance at any childbirth classes. Beyond routine laboratory tests, the blood group and Rh factor, rubella status, cervical cytological examination, and a syphilis screen should be checked. Women may choose to have their children at home, in a birthing center, or in a hospital. Whichever site is selected, a copy or abstract of current prenatal information should be available at the birthing site by at least the estimated thirty-sixth week of pregnancy. Arrangements should also be made for access to this information and to hospital care in case of an emergency in a birthing center or at home.

Labor and Delivery Record. This record tracks the patient from admission through delivery to the postpartum period. The antepartum record should be reviewed with attention to the special items already described. An evaluation is then made by the physician or nurse midwife, including an updated history or a complete history if there is no antepartum record, noting data on contractions, status of membranes, presence of significant bleeding, time and content of the patient's last intake of food or fluid, drug intake and allergies, choice of anesthesia, and plans to breast-feed or bottle feed. The mother is monitored frequently, as is the child, with a fetal monitor. In the normal case, this is done by a nurse. At delivery, details regarding the mother are recorded, similar to those of a surgery. The neonate is also described, including his or her Apgar score (an infant rating system at 1 and 5 minutes after birth), sex, weight, length, onset of respiration, abnormalities, and treatment to the eyes. Any fetal monitoring strips are identified and annotated with relevant data; they become part of the patient record.

Postpartum Record. Postpartum data include information about the condition of the mother after delivery. The record may be a special form or it may be included in the progress notes. In either case, attention is paid to assessing the lochia and condition of the breasts, fundus, and perineum as well as the usual postoperative status. Nursing staff continue this documentation as long as it is relevant.

Neonatal Data

As a live birth takes place, this new person is given his or her own record. The neonatal record includes the regular history, physical examination, and progress notes, with the addition of special identification data. The record for healthy neonates is usually brief.

Birth History. The birth history record may be shared with the mother's record, including pertinent history regarding pregnancy, any diseases, and delivery. The Apgar score, any prematurity or anomalies, and any problems that occur

before transfer to the nursery are noted. Nurses or physicians sign the appropriate sections.

Neonatal Identification. While the neonate is still in the delivery room, two identical bands are prepared noting the mother's number and the neonate's sex and time of birth. One band is placed on the mother and the other is placed on the neonate. A band number and identification form about the mother and neonate are also prepared. Both bands and forms should be checked by two responsible practitioners before the neonate leaves the delivery room. Footprinting and fingerprinting, if done, also require special forms. The nurse in charge of the delivery room is responsible for the identification process and signs the sheets along with any participating obstetrician.

Neonatal Physical Examination. The neonatal physical examination repeats the birth data and concentrates on a detailed description of the neonate's appearance. The attending physician should examine the apparently healthy neonate as soon as possible and before discharge. If the infant should remain in the hospital for additional days, additional notes are made. These notes are added to the infant's record and signed by the physician.

Neonate Progress Notes. Neonates who remain in the hospital have progress notes added to the chart as well as other forms as needed. The American Academy of Pediatrics recommends frequent recording of vital signs until the neonate is stable (usually within 12 hours after birth). The Joint Commission particularly requires that neonates who receive oxygen therapy should have the concentration recorded at intervals as written in the policies and procedures of the facility's nursery.

Nursing Forms

Although nurses document on many forms within the record, the following forms are used exclusively by the nursing staff. Nurses typically perform an assessment that is used to develop a nursing plan of care. Nurses should write their conclusions as nursing diagnoses.

Nursing Notes. Nurses may write nurses' notes or contribute to integrated progress notes. Regardless of the form, these notes describe the patient and his or her condition in objective, behavioral terms. Quantitative data are encouraged. The documentation begins with an admission note, including notification of the physician of the admission. Subsequent notes are written as needed and include nursing interventions and the patient's response. The documentation ends with a discharge note. If the patient should die, a death note is written, including notification of the physician.

Graphic Sheet. A graphic sheet is used to plot the patient's vital signs (temperature, pulse and respiratory rates, and blood pressure). Additional information may be noted, including weight and intake and output of fluids and solids. The frequency of entries depends on the patient's condition. One form usually provides space for six entries a day for several days, and additional sheets are added as needed. Nurses typically sign the form once and thereafter initial their entries.

Medication Sheet. The medication sheet provides a detailed record of the medicines given orally, topically, or by injection, inhalation, and infusion. The date, time, name of drug, dose, and route of administration are included. If it is not possible to administer a scheduled dose, this is also noted and an explanation given in the nurses' notes. The practitioner giving the dose initials the entry.

Special Care Units. Special units such as the intensive care unit and coronary care unit often have forms to suit their particular patient populations.

Ancillary Forms

Ancillary data are typically collected by practitioners other than physicians and nurses, with the exception of patient and family teaching and case and staff conferences in which a wide variety of clinicians may participate.

Electrocardiographic Reports. The electrocardiograph records the electrical activity of the heart. The normal recording shows five waves, with the P wave indicating contraction of the atria followed by Q, R, S, and T waves, which relate to the contraction of the ventricles. Surface electrodes placed on the patient transmit impulses to the electrocardiograph. The electrocardiogram is the graphic tracing produced by plotting these waves against time on a continuous paper roll or as a computer view. The report contains the cardiologist's signed interpretation and may include the tracing. When tracings are not provided, they are stored in the laboratory for reference.

Laboratory Reports. Laboratory reports detail analysis or examination of blood, urine, stool, and other body substances. The medical laboratory may be within the facility or one that is used on a contractual basis. The laboratory usually provides the results of urinalysis and blood chemistry and hematology, microbiology, and serology reports. Tests should be completed and reported promptly. A report identifies the date, time, test, results, and the reference values for the test's normal range. Reports are usually computer generated and may be printed on standard-sized pages or on small slips designed to be taped on mounting sheets. Cumulative reports may be provided, which reduce the bulk of the chart. In an electronic view laboratory results can be profiled over time and presented in graphic format. When blood banking is done, the American Association of Blood Banks has particular requirements detailed in its *Technical Manual.*

Radiology and Imaging Reports. Radiology reports describe diagnostic or therapeutic services. Diagnostic procedures include modalities such as radiography, nuclear medicine, computed tomography, magnetic resonance imaging, and ultrasonography, which create an image that can be visualized. On a form similar to that used for the consultation, the upper portion notes the attending physician's request for the study and specifies the area to be examined. A physician, usually a radiologist, dictates or writes a description of the image and adds an impression at the bottom of the form. Both physicians sign their respective sections. In a computerized view the image can be viewed on-line and a portion of the image can be enlarged if needed for detailed visualization. Films and computer images are stored in the department that produced them.

Radiation Therapy. Therapeutic radiology services more closely resemble the consultation process. They are major procedures that require a special consent. A treatment plan is written; each treatment is reported, including the amount of radiation given for each dose, and a summary is provided. The therapeutic radiologist signs each report.

Therapeutic Services. Therapies (e.g., physical, occupational, respiratory, speech, dietary) include assessment and treatment plans designed to restore patient function. The therapist documents the services, including the patient's response, and signs the report or progress notes. Care plans are updated as needed, and a summary may be completed at the end of the episode of care. Notes are objective and goal oriented. The Joint Commission has documentation requirements for each of these services, particularly as they relate to rehabilitative care.

Case Management and Social Service Record. Case management records contain data on the patient's background, social information, and problems identified by the patient, family, and case manager. The case manager has access to a great deal of sensitive personal information in addition to private medical information. The formal record includes a plan of action, progress notes, and a discharge note.

Patient and Family Teaching and Participation. Evidence of patient and family teaching and understanding has become increasingly important as more treatments become available for patients and families to implement at home. Lifestyle changes are also appropriate topics for teaching. A wide variety of practitioners engage in patient and family teaching along the continuum of care. Regardless of the profession or the setting, the teaching and the re-demonstration of understanding should be described. If any preprinted material is provided, it should also be noted and a copy kept on file in the HIM department if it should be needed to interpret the record. Some segments of health care require documentation of family participation in planning, goal setting, and carrying out of lifestyle changes, therapies, or other activities.

Discharge and Follow-Up Plan. A discharge plan is begun at the time of admission or initiation of services; it gives a general assessment of plans to maintain continuity after this episode of care. This may represent transfer from acute care to long-term care, initiation of home health care, or provision of one or several available community services. Any agencies to be used should be identified. Social service often coordinates the plan, which includes both medical and financial arrangements and considers the family's needs as well as those of the patient.

Documentation Guidelines

Although practitioners are trained to document patient care during their education, organizations should provide training in their specific policies, procedures, and systems. These efforts support communication, continuity of care, and overall high-quality patient care. In addition, because the patient record is also the facility's business record, such efforts will support compliance with federal and state regulations and accreditation, professional practice, and legal standards. It is often said, "If it isn't documented, it wasn't done." Ultimately, the individual practitioners are responsible for the quality of their entries, including authentication.

Paper forms and computer views provide the structure for the documentation of patient care activities. Although they support a complete and quality record, they do not guarantee it. The system and the individuals who document in the clinical record contribute to the quality of the content of the record. If the health record is to fulfill its unique roles for the patient, providers, as a legal record, for researchers and education, the content must be of high quality. Table 4-6 presents some essential entry guidelines.

General

The patient's name and other key identifying data must be on all pages of the record and on a computer view. The author's identity can be authenticated as described below and must include credentials to indicate his or her role in the patient's care. Authors must only document their own interactions for the patient and avoid charting for others because they are legally responsible for both their care and their entries. In some care environments one individual may be designated to draft the treatment plan that is based on the input of several team members. One or more team members may sign the plan. Using the appropriate form or view facilitates others' finding the information in the record. Forms and views also help remind practitioners of care elements and essential documentation.

Entries should include the date and time and should be charted as close to the time of care as possible. Notes should never be written in anticipation of care being provided

Table 4-6 HEALTH RECORD ENTRY DOCUMENTATION

General Guidelines
- **Identify the patient:** name and number on all new pages added to the chart
- **Identify the author:** signed with an initial, last name, and credentials
- **Documents only the author's care:** never anyone else's.
- **Uses the proper form or view:** it aids communication by structuring the chart
- **Complete all items:** to ensure completion of all content.
- **Includes date and time:** to relate observations/activities to each other.
- **Are timely:** recorded shortly after, and never before, completing patient care
- **Are specific:** record patient behavior and complaints in specific terms.
- **Are exact:** noting time, effect, and results of all procedures, avoiding ditto marks
- **Are concise:** recording all necessary information and nothing else. Avoids meaningless phrases, the word "patient" and complete sentences
- **Spell correctly, use standard terms and symbols**
- **Abbreviations:** use only approved and safe abbreviations

Paper-Based Records
- **Are legible:** ensuring that other members of the care team can read the entries.
- **Use black ink:** ensures the best photocopies, faxes, and document imaging.
- **Leave no blank lines:** draw a line through the center of an empty line to present charting by someone else in the area signed
- **Chart omissions as a new entry:** never backdate or add to prior entries
- **Never obscure entries:** draw a line though any mistake and write "error" or "mistaken entry" above it. Erasures, white out, and heavy mark outs create doubt when the record is needed by other users.

because other events may intervene, creating errors in the sequence of events. Descriptions are best understood when they are specific and exact and include the use of standard terms spelled correctly. Although accuracy and clarity are essential, notes do not require complete sentences. In most care settings, notes are written in a concise style. The word "patient" is not routinely required because it is understood to be the patient's chart.

Abbreviations and Symbols

The use of abbreviations, acronyms (terms created from the first letter of several words), and symbols save substantial time for practitioners. They also pose significant risks of being misunderstood either through poor handwriting or the fact that many have more than one meaning. Health care organizations should establish policies and maintain an official **abbreviation list** approved by the organization and, if appropriate, its medical staff for use in patient care documentation. When more than one definition exists, only one should be approved, with the preferred approach being to avoid the abbreviation entirely. Research by the IOM published in 2000 focused the attention of the public and health professionals on a variety of patient safety issues. In response, the Joint Commission has established national patient safety goals, which include prohibiting the use of "dangerous" abbreviations, acronyms, and symbols in patient records. These abbreviations, acronyms, and symbols have caused confusion or problems in their handwritten form. The minimum "do not use" list includes such items as avoiding "U" for unit, which can be mistaken for 0, 4, or cc. Spelling out "unit" is preferred.

Paper-Based Records

Several historic charting challenges, such as legibility and author identification, are substantially resolved by the use of EHRs. Where paper records are still used, practitioners should be encouraged to write legibly and to use black ink, which promotes good quality photocopying, faxing, and document imaging. No blank lines should remain between entries, where others can chart. Any omissions should be charted as new entries and marked as such. When errors occur, corrections should be made with a single line so as not to obscure the entry. A notation such as "mistaken entry" or "error" should be added and initialed and the corrected documentation entered. See further discussion of corrections and amendments in the chapter on legal aspects.

Authentication

Authentication identifies the author of an entry in the patient record and that the entry has been verified or validated by the author. Only the author can sign an entry. Countersignatures may also be required according to organizational policy. If any of the information is in disagreement, additions or corrections should be made before authentication. The Joint Commission requires that a minimum of the following four documents be authenticated: H&Ps, operative reports, consultations, and discharge summaries. There are several methods for authentication. Medical staff bylaws, rules, and regulations as well as federal and state laws should be consulted regarding their use. Practitioners may sign with their first initials, last names, and credentials or disciplines, with full names being preferred if similar names exist. Initials may be used when there is a legend available in the record providing the full signature and the related initials. The use of signature stamps typically requires the owner to sign a statement that only they will use the stamp. Because of their high potential for abuse, signature stamps should be discouraged. Electronic signatures may include an e-mail signature, digitized image of a signature, a unique logon and PIN (personal identification number), unique biometric identifier (such as a fingerprint), or digital signature using encryption. These technologies are discussed further in later chapters.

Format Types

The organization of the paper-based health record is referred to as its format. As with forms in general, there are no directives on which format to use. Facilities are free to design their own as long as the format chosen is standardized. The reference that defines the facility's standard sequence of pages to be followed in each record is called a **chart order.** There may be a different order for records during care and after discharge. As part of its responsibility to ensure communication among practitioners, the medical staff participates with representatives of other departments on the organization's information management or medical record committee. This committee should approve forms to be used in the clinical record as well as the organizing format. There are three common formats: source oriented, problem oriented, and integrated.

Source-Oriented Medical Record

The most common paper-based health record format is source oriented, meaning that the record is organized into sections according to the practitioners who are the source of both the treatment and the data collection. Within each section, sheets are arranged in chronological order, perhaps with some divisions by episodes of care. During admissions, the current episode is typically kept at the nursing unit in reverse chronological order with the most recent materials on the top. The trend is to keep the record in this order rather than commit the staff time to reversing the chart. If a record is kept in the same order during care and after care it may also be referred to as "universal" chart order. With implementation of the EHR, the order of the paper will cease to be an issue; however, there will be times when the content of the EHR will be printed out and will need an organizing format. An advantage of standardized source-oriented records is the speed with which an individual sheet can be located. The major disadvantage is lack of a clear picture of the patient's problems and how each department is contributing to their resolution.

Problem-Oriented Medical Record

The problem-oriented medical record (POMR) was developed by Dr. Lawrence L. Weed in the 1960s in response to the major deficiency in the source-oriented format—lack of a clear picture of the patient's problems. The POMR system focuses on the documentation of a logical, organized plan of clinical thought by practitioners. The system has four parts: a database, problem list, initial plan, and progress notes. The database was an early minimum data set (MDS) similar to those in place today. The problem list is a dynamic document showing titles, numbers, and dates of problems and it serves as a table of contents of the record. The problem is stated at the level of the physician's current understanding and modified as further data accumulate. Problems may be initial symptoms or well-defined diagnoses. The problems are past and present and social, financial, and demographic as well as medical. The initial

Table 4-7 PROGRESS NOTE ELEMENTS
PROBLEM-ORIENTED MEDICAL RECORD

S =	subjective, which records what the patient states is the problem
O =	objective, which records what the practitioner identifies through the history, physical examination, and diagnostic tests
A =	assessment, which combines the subjective and objective into a conclusion
P =	plan, or what approach is going to be taken to resolve the problem

plans describe what will be done to investigate or treat each problem. Plans refer to the problem number and can be of three types: the need to collect more decision-making information, therapy (e.g., medications, treatments), and patient education. Progress notes are written in a distinctive style according to the acronym SOAP, translated as shown in Table 4-7. SOAP notes are also numbered to correspond to the problems. The discharge summary is considered a special progress note.

Weed suggested that forms be designed to support the numbering and tracking of problems. He was also an early advocate of a team approach, encouraging all practitioners participating in the patient's care to document sequentially in the progress notes. Each practitioner would contribute as appropriate to his or her training, licensure, and understanding of the problem. The major advantage of the POMR is that it creates a holistic picture of the patient and his or her care. Although it does not guarantee quality care, it provides an excellent communication and evaluation tool that highlights the thinking process. The major disadvantage is the time and commitment needed on the part of the practitioners to implement and maintain the system. With the exception of the SOAP style of progress notes and the problem list, the full system has not been widely accepted for use with the paper-based health record. Components of the system, such as the problem list and SOAP notes, are often used in ambulatory settings. Behavioral health transformed the problem list into a list of goals and objectives that serves the same function as a problem list. Behavioral health may use a modification of SOAP notes that combines the "S" and "O' into "Data" resulting in DAP—Data, Assessment, and Plan to structure progress notes. The POMR is finding renewed support in the EHR model because of its logical approach to organizing data.

Integrated Medical Record

The integrated record is strictly chronological without any divisions by source. This format keeps the episode of care clearly defined by date, which is an advantage when the flow of care is being considered. The major disadvantage is that information from the same source, such as laboratory data, is not easily compared. Some chart order arrangements integrate selected types of forms, such as progress notes, while keeping others, such as radiology reports, by source. Integrated progress notes resemble the team approach of the POMR, which provides a more holistic view of the patient. If progress notes are integrated, paper forms can be designed to easily find/track the notes of a particular category of practitioner.

DESIGN AND CONTROL OF PAPER FORMS AND COMPUTER VIEWS AND TEMPLATES

When forms or computer **views** (information on screens) and templates are well designed and controlled, they enhance technology by providing a smooth link in the communication process. They permit recording of varying data without recopying constant information. This reduces clerical work, decreases the number of errors, and increases efficiency. When they are well designed, they assist in actual direct patient care. Many of the principles of design of forms or views apply to both paper and computer forms. Templates and some specific guidelines for computer formats are also discussed in Chapters 5 and 8.

As with data collection and technology, form or view design should emphasize the needs of users. It is the responsibility of each health care facility to develop its own forms or views. Accrediting and regulatory bodies such as The Joint Commission and the Centers for Medicare and Medicaid Services (CMS) and standards organizations such as ASTM do not recommend particular forms or views with which to collect their required data elements, nor do professional organizations such as the American Hospital Association (AHA) and AHIMA. When developing forms or views, the designer can refer to health information books, journals, and newsletters, including those noted in the chapter references, and can consult professional colleagues in similar facilities for ideas. In some geographical areas, several facilities have formally joined together and adopted basic health record forms and views that are acceptable to the medical staffs of each facility. This saves the time of health care providers who practice at more than one site and facilitates the paper or electronic interchange necessary to care for patients and carry out the business of each facility. It also permits administrative cost savings through bulk purchasing and reduced programming charges. Such strategies are also common in corporate facilities, where core forms or views are designed for all the facilities, and local facilities design their own additions according to guidelines that have been provided.

With the transition from the paper-based record to the electronic record, paper forms will decline. However, there are other business purposes for which good form designs are helpful and HIM professionals should be prepared to guide their design and production.

Forms or Views Team

The management of forms or views is a collaborative process. Members of the forms or views team include representatives from the following services:

- HIM
- Information systems
- Materials management
- Patient care services
- Quality improvement
- Others as needed

The HIM professional plays a leadership role by providing knowledge of rules and regulations related to health record content, medical science, computer applications, the flow of data throughout the facility, and the information needs of the health care delivery system. The forms or views design and control process also benefits from the involvement of an information systems manager who is responsible for computer input and output, a materials or purchasing manager who is responsible for inventory and ordering paper forms, a patient care professional who represents clinical needs, a quality improvement professional to provide input regarding forms or views created to address quality issues, and others as needed. The team's charge may be to work on administrative and patient information applications and to become involved in the selection of data collection technology. The team forwards its patient-related recommendations to the clinical information committee for approval, and its administrative recommendations follow the organizational chain of command.

General Design Principles

Needs of Users

The needs of both internal and external users must be considered when designing forms or views. It is important to remember that users are not only the patient and providers but also the administrative, financial, and legal staff of the facility. External users collect data from many locations, and the data are combined or aggregated. These may be local, state, and federal agencies and other planning and research groups. Collecting enough of the right type of data to satisfy this range of users means clearly defining the purpose of the form or view.

Purpose of the Form or View

Patient record forms serve many purposes. They standardize, identify and instruct, facilitate documentation and decision making, and promote consistency in data collection, reporting, and interpretation. Forms identify patients and practitioners and instruct them step by step in what data items to gather, where to obtain them, and how to record them. Good instructions, when followed, facilitate complete and accurate documentation, which is the foundation of effective decision making.

History and physical forms provide good examples of these purposes. When standardized, all elements of the history, review of systems, and physical examination (as listed in the ASTM standard) are collected. Both the patient and the practitioner are identified with names and unique numbers either electronically or manually. The patient may follow a set of instructions on paper or computer to provide his or her medical history. The provider then follows a set of instructions when performing the review of systems and proceeding with the physical examination. The documentation thus collected is the foundation on which the patient and practitioner can make decisions and take action regarding lifestyle changes, diagnostic testing, medications, or other treatments. At the close of an encounter a return appointment is frequently scheduled, which assigns responsibility to both the patient and the practitioner for follow-up. Thus, the history and physical form or view has structured the majority of the communication between the patient and the practitioner and continues to communicate with other users as the need arises.

Selection and Sequencing of Items

When the purpose of the form or view is established, the next step is to construct a list or grid of required data to ensure the collection of all essential items and the elimination of unnecessary or redundant items. Effective and efficient sequencing of the form or view should follow the traditional pattern—from left to right and top to bottom—permitting a continuous operation whether reading, writing, or entering data on the computer. The flow should be logical and take into consideration the order of data collection or transfer. In addition, numbering items makes references to both items and written instructions on completion of forms faster and easier.

Standard Terminology, Abbreviations, and Format

Often, large numbers of people use each form or view within an organization, and with the expansion of the EHR this number increases. Effective communication, therefore, depends on the use of terminology that is understood by all. Use of standard terminology, when available, is recommended. For example, standard definitions for commonly collected data items published by ASTM are described later in this chapter. When standard definitions are not available, the form or view should supply the definition. Standard definitions are particularly important when linked databases are used.

Words, numbers, and abbreviations should be standardized as well. For example, users need to know whether hyphens should be included when entering social security numbers. They also need instructions on how many digits to use for patient record numbers and how to enter coded data. Abbreviations have great appeal for health care providers because they save both reading time and entry time. Their major liability is misunderstanding. Caregivers depend on understanding the record to provide quality care. Administrative, legal, licensure, accreditation, and personal uses also depend on a clear understanding of the record. As mentioned earlier, any abbreviations permitted in the patient record must be understood by all.

Another aspect of form or view design that promotes consistency is the development of a master format or template. The placement of data in the same sequence on similar forms or views with similar layouts facilitates rapid entry and retrieval. Consistent location of patient identification and unique identification number are an example.

Instructions

Instructions should briefly identify who should complete the data items and should provide any additional guidance that is necessary. Computer views typically provide this information on introductory screens and as needed throughout data entry. Paper forms usually separate the instructions from the data entry spaces and place them at the top. The identification and distribution of copies also need to be specified. If the instructions need to be more extensive, they can be printed on the back, on a separate sheet, or in an administrative manual. If any of these alternatives are used, reference to the location of instructions should be made on the face of the form.

Simplification

With such a host of users, purposes, technologies, terms, and formats, it is easy to feel overwhelmed by the complexity. The last general consideration is to attempt to keep forms or views simple. Forms or views should be created only when there is an established need that is not being adequately handled by an existing form or view or when revision is impractical. The purpose of a form or view management program is to ensure that each tool has a desired purpose, that only necessary forms or views are maintained, and that all forms or views are documented and available. Simplification provides considerable savings in time, effort, and materials.

Paper Forms Design and Production

When the health care facility uses paper forms for data collection, discussion with a printer can provide basic information and help avoid costly mistakes. The development of a standardized guide, such as the example shown in Figure 4-3 developed by one health care facility, also helps to ensure satisfactory results. The major segments of a paper form are the header and footer, introduction and instructions, and body and close. A guide, called a chart order, is also necessary to standardize the assembly sequence of various documents within the paper health record.

Header and Footer. The title and subtitle (if any) identify the form and are typically positioned at the top as a header. In facilities that bind their records at the top, it is easier to locate the title if it appears at the bottom. Form titles should appear in the same font and font size on each form. Forms

for external use should include the facility name, address, phone number, and perhaps a logo. Any code that is required for scanning technology should appear as part of the header. The footer contains information about the form, such as the control number, edition date, and page numbers or letters, usually at the left. This location enables reference information to be visible in most types of bindings and makes it easier to locate forms in the stockroom. Forms that have multiple pages or that are printed on both sides should carry a footer on each page. This assists printing, completion, and insertion in the patient record. The edition date is particularly important in ensuring that only the current version of the form is used and that obsolete versions are destroyed. Also included in the header or footer is a place to imprint the patient's name and health record number. There should be a place to imprint the patient's name and number on all pages of a multipage form or on each side of double-sided forms.

Introduction and Instructions. The introduction should explain the purpose of the form. The title is often sufficient, but occasionally patients and others outside the organization may need a subtitle and an additional explanation to understand the form's intent to complete it appropriately. The history form to be completed by the patient is an example.

Body and Close. The body contains the main content of the form, and the close provides the space for authenticating or approving signatures. The documentation method and the data item to be completed should determine the appropriate size of entry space to be drawn on the form. The amount of information a form can contain is significantly affected by spacing. For example, computer-printed or typewritten words require $1/_{16}$ inch vertical height, whereas handwritten words require $1/_3$ inch. When multiple-copy forms, such as carbon or no-carbon-required (NCR) packs are used, more space may be needed for handwritten material because of the need to increase handwriting pressure, which frequently results in larger handwriting size.

Fonts. Type styles should be well chosen and contribute to readability. Items of similar importance should be equal in size and type, and the overall number of different fonts used should be low. Italics and boldface characters should be used to maintain the effect of emphasis only. Style considerations may include the requirement to use a specified font type that is identified with the name and logo of the organization.

Rules and Lines. Rules are vertical or horizontal lines that structure the form. They may vary in style but serve to divide the form into logical sections and to direct data entry length and location. If several people have areas to complete, the data sets each person is to document should be presented in the order of completion. Heavy lines can help to separate sections of the form visually. Horizontal lines on forms are desirable for long sections of the forms that are handwritten.

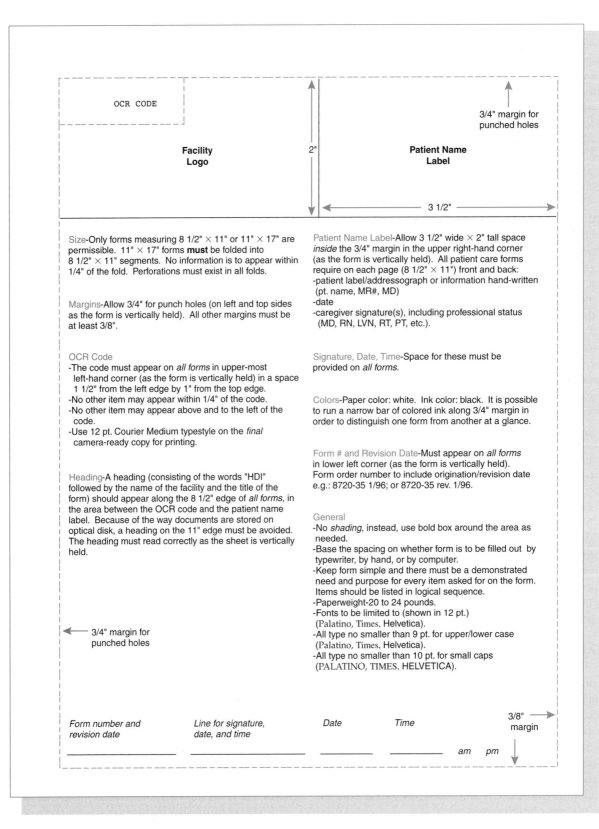

Figure 4–3 Vertical forms guide.

OCR CODE

**Facility
Logo**

2"

**Patient Name
Label**

3/4" margin for
punched holes

3 1/2"

Size-Only forms measuring 8 1/2" × 11" or 11" × 17" are permissible. 11" × 17" forms **must** be folded into 8 1/2" × 11" segments. No information is to appear within 1/4" of the fold. Perforations must exist in all folds.

Margins-Allow 3/4" for punch holes (on left and top sides as the form is vertically held). All other margins must be at least 3/8".

OCR Code
-The code must appear on *all forms* in upper-most left-hand corner (as the form is vertically held) in a space 1 1/2" from the left edge by 1" from the top edge.
-No other item may appear within 1/4" of the code.
-No other item may appear above and to the left of the code.
-Use 12 pt. Courier Medium typestyle on the *final* camera-ready copy for printing.

Heading-A heading (consisting of the words "HDI" followed by the name of the facility and the title of the form) should appear along the 8 1/2" edge of *all forms*, in the area between the OCR code and the patient name label. Because of the way documents are stored on optical disk, a heading on the 11" edge must be avoided. The heading must read correctly as the sheet is vertically held.

3/4" margin for
punched holes

Patient Name Label-Allow 3 1/2" wide × 2" tall space *inside* the 3/4" margin in the upper right-hand corner (as the form is vertically held). All patient care forms require on each page (8 1/2" × 11") front and back:
-patient label/addressograph or information hand-written (pt. name, MR#, MD)
-date
-caregiver signature(s), including professional status (MD, RN, LVN, RT, PT, etc.).

Signature, Date, Time-Space for these must be provided on *all forms.*

Colors-Paper color: white. Ink color: black. It is possible to run a narrow bar of colored ink along 3/4" margin in order to distinguish one form from another at a glance.

Form # and Revision Date-Must appear on *all forms* in lower left corner (as the form is vertically held). Form order number to include origination/revision date e.g.: 8720-35 1/96; or 8720-35 rev. 1/96.

General
-No *shading*, instead, use bold box around the area as needed.
-Base the spacing on whether form is to be filled out by typewriter, by hand, or by computer.
-Keep form simple and there must be a demonstrated need and purpose for every item asked for on the form. Items should be listed in logical sequence.
-Paperweight-20 to 24 pounds.
-Fonts to be limited to (shown in 12 pt.) (Palatino, Times, Helvetica).
-All type no smaller than 9 pt. for upper/lower case (Palatino, Times, Helvetica).
-All type no smaller than 10 pt. for small caps (PALATINO, TIMES, HELVETICA).

Form number and
revision date

Line for signature,
date, and time

Date

Time

3/8"
margin

am   pm

Examples are forms for handwritten progress notes and physicians' orders. Rules are often used to create smaller sections or boxes for data on a form, such as the top section of the admission/discharge Record (face sheet). Vertical and horizontal rules should be aligned as much as possible to make the form less "busy" visually. Box titles or captions should be located to the upper left of the boxes in small font sizes. Check boxes or lines (sometimes called ballot boxes) are other time savers that conserve space and improve legibility. When check boxes or lines are used, there should be consistency throughout the form whether the boxes or lines are to the immediate left or immediate right of the caption. These should be aligned vertically when appropriate. The box or line to check should be very close to the caption so that the person performing the documentation checks the correct line or box.

Borders. Rules that frame a section are called borders. Borders are preferable to screening or shading, which often causes indistinct electronic copies and transmissions. Some sections may be intentionally obscured or blacked out when, for confidentiality, data items are not desired on every copy of a form. Borders around an entire form create a margin. Margins provide visual appeal as well as being important for printing. For example, a space of $^3/_4$ inch may be necessary for punched holes, and allowances may be needed for printing equipment. Forms that are to be typed should have at least a $^1/_2$-inch margin at the bottom to avoid paper slippage in the platen when typing near the bottom of the page.

Production Considerations. If data are to be entered on a computer screen or view and then printed on a preprinted paper form (e.g., billing form, patient care plan form), refer to the vendor or machine specifications for correct data placement. If the form is not designed appropriately, data will not be printed in the exact locations required on the form. If data entry on a form is to be done by typewriter, the spacing and alignments should be carefully designed to avoid constant readjustment of the forms in the machine while typing. Discussing such specifications with a printer or the purchasing department is important in all aspects of form design.

Beyond design guidelines, paper forms require some production considerations. The master is the original from which copies are produced. Masters may be designed and produced internally by desktop publishing software or advanced word processing techniques and a high-resolution laser printer. This approach is quick, easy, and cost-effective, particularly when photocopying is the method of duplication. When more elaborate and formal printing is needed, the master should be created by a professional typesetter. In either case, the master should be carefully proofread before reproduction.

Physical building of the form refers to its size and special properties. Using standard-sized paper, such as $8^1/_2 \times 11$ inches, keeps costs low and facilitates copying and filing. Use of double-sided forms is discouraged because of the need to turn them over when photocopying, microfilming, or computer scanning. Oversized forms involve similar special copying considerations because they require reduction or other special handling. Undersized forms that are to be pasted, in a shingled manner, onto health record forms should be avoided because of extra time needed for chart preparation when photocopying, scanning, or filming.

Multipart forms require planning to provide sufficient copies and construction with carbon sheets, carbon spots, or NCR paper. This packet of pages creates a forms set that is precollated and prefastened with a perforated stub. The advantages of multipart forms include standardization; having to write data only once, which reduces mistakes; and being able to provide quick, inexpensive copies. The disadvantages include the limited number of copies that these forms can create. Although copies in carbon packs are easier to read and more copies can be made per original than NCR copies, the carbon paper between the copies must be removed, which creates waste. Ink smears on copies and hands frequently result when tearing the carbon sets apart. NCR copies, although cleaner, are difficult to read, especially the copies beyond two or three in the set, and the ink can fade with time. Photocopies of NCR copies are nearly impossible to read. Extra copies that are created and not used in multipart forms diminish any original savings and produce additional waste.

Forms may be produced as individual form sets or as a continuous-feed strip. Forms may also be prepared as unit sets consisting of single forms glued along one edge to create a pad. Paper has many features, including weight grade, grain, and finish. These aspects combine to affect the form's suitability, durability, and permanence. Suitability reflects how easy the paper is to read and write on (e.g., does the ink smear because it is too grainy?); durability concerns how well a form stands up to handling; permanence reflects how long the paper lasts in hard copy. It is extremely important that the paper's weight is suitable for use with copiers, facsimile machines, and scanning equipment. A weight of 20 to 24 pounds is recommended for health records. For electronic, environmental, and cost reasons, white paper is recommended. If color is necessary, a tinted border may be used. The ink should be a standard black because this type reproduces best and should meet scanning specifications. The use of additional text colors should be limited because it adds to the cost of the form.

Duplicating methods include in-house preparation and commercial printing. In-house preparation entails the creation of the master and reproduction, most commonly by photocopying. Because this method is expensive, it is most suitable for a trial period or when only a small quantity of forms is needed. The same in-house master can be used for offset printing and is more cost-effective for very large quantities. The commercial printer is also best for providing value-added features, such as hole punching, perforating, collating, carbonizing, and prenumbering, which can be done in conjunction with the printing process. (See the forms design activity in the supplements.)

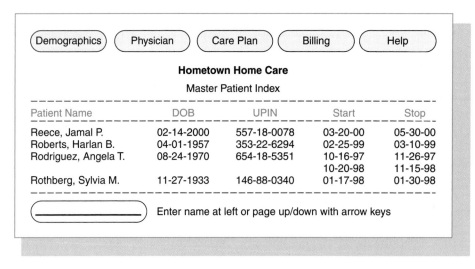

Figure 4-4 Sample master patient index view.

Computer View/Screen Format Design

Computer views share the following general design features with paper forms:

- Needs of user
- Purpose of view
- Selection and sequencing of essential data items
- Standardization of terminology, abbreviations, and formats
- Provision of instructions
- Attention to simplification

There are profound differences as well. The computer view refers to the screen format for both data entry and monitor output. Figure 4-4 illustrates a sample master patient index computer view. The power of database management systems allows tremendous flexibility in which views are created for data capture and data displays, including still and moving images and sound as well as text and graphs—all in living color. Computer views require menus of alternatives to be developed and screen or window formats that may include spots to touch with a finger or light pen. It is helpful to remember that standards such as those of ASTM are only a foundation from which to begin the process of selecting data items. Once captured, the data elements may be retrieved in new configurations to meet the needs of many different user groups. For example, a physician may want to view graphs that show the trends of laboratory data along with a menu of therapy options with costs, supported by a reference from a linked database. A social worker developing a discharge plan may select a summary of the patient's functional level, living arrangements, and insurance benefits to compare with services provided and prices charged by local home health care providers. This flexibility lends to both the promise and the problems of designing computer views.

On-Line System Interface

A person entering or viewing data encounters computer logic at the boundary where users and computers meet on line—the system interface. Good interface designs help make this interaction user friendly while reducing errors. Windows is the most common interface format, in which each window can show information drawn from a different source or database table. In some situations, systems can run separate applications in independent windows. Figure 4-5 shows such a **graphical user interface** (GUI), with three windows overlaid one on top of the other and the icons and tool bar at the top. Well-designed screen views or forms for data entry make it possible to

- Organize the data entry fields in logical format
- Include field edits
- Include passwords to add, delete, or modify data
- Allow simultaneous entry or updating in many tables at one time
- Include brief instructions on the screens or provide more lengthy help screens
- Make the screens attractive through the use of color, lines, borders, and so on
- Use default values in a field to eliminate the need to key repeated data between entries (e.g., the date field could be automatically set up to add today's date without the need to key the characters)
- Allow automatic sequential numbering (e.g., accession register numbers)
- Show data on the screen from a different table when the key field is entered (e.g., for the MPI screen form, when the doctor's number is entered, the doctor's name, address, and so on can automatically appear on the screen)
- Develop or customize menus or submenus to add, delete, or change data

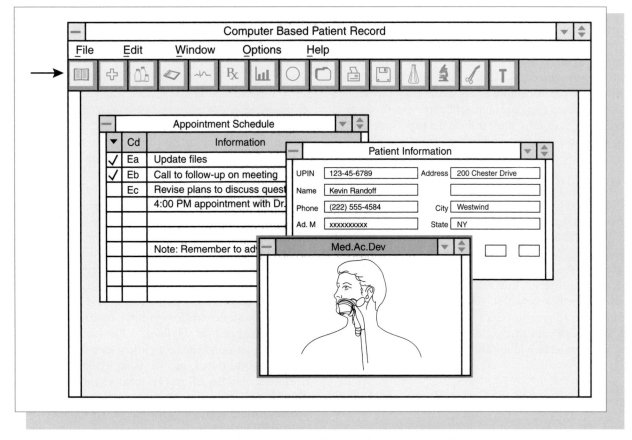

Figure 4-5 Graphical user guide. Arrow is pointing to tool bar.

Windows-style interfaces provide menus that pull down from choices shown on a tool bar at the top of the screen. A menu is an important component of a computer view because it is central to ease of navigation. Therefore, a carefully constructed sequence of menus is part of a comprehensive design. Windows interfaces are used not only on PCs but also on mainframe and minicomputer systems.

Other Display Features

In comparison with an $8\frac{1}{2} \times 11$–inch sheet of paper, the computer page or view is the size of a 12-inch television screen. The number of characters per line and number of lines per view vary among terminals and software, some of which allow the user to change the size of the view. Typically, users can view the equivalent of one third of a page at a time, requiring that more views be created to collect an equivalent amount of data. The advantages are that segments of a paper form completed by different practitioners can be separated for individual attention. The fact that the EHR completes part of the view with stored data is also a major advantage. Text displays can be customized with different background and font colors. Color coding text and menus can be helpful in distinguishing special features, such as instructions.

Blinking may be added to characters or words to attract the user's attention, and scrolling moves the screen up or down a line or page at a time. As with paper forms, special features should be kept to a minimum to enhance their emphasis and simplify the view.

General Control Principles

View identification is key to control. If the view does not have a name or number, reference to that view is subject to a great deal of misunderstanding. As mentioned, paper forms should contain a control number on each page, and computer views should be identified on the screen or in the system's written documentation. Users should not develop or customize their own data entry views without approval of their supervisors or form or view management team. Although substantial advantages of view customization are flexibility and the related user satisfaction, it is not without its disadvantages. The need to ensure that all data elements are collected, that an audit trail of views is available for legal purposes, and that confidentiality is maintained requires that standardization programs, procedural guidelines, and input and output controls be developed.

Computer systems also involve cost considerations. The paper output from the EHR system can vary from a simple printout of data entered to volumes of daily and summary reports. In all, the volume can easily exceed that generated in a paper health record environment. The output can be programmed to happen automatically or can be requested by use of report generators, and it can easily become overwhelming. To control output as well as information overload and its associated costs and confidentiality risks, the form or view management team must include the paper output in its scope of concerns.

Forms/Views Summary

Well-designed forms or views facilitate work by guiding the user through data entry, interpretation, and validation. They also contribute to the quantity and quality of work performed. A continuing process of review and revision maximizes the benefits by clarifying ambiguities and collecting only necessary data items, which allows time to be devoted to other activities. Other chapters of this text explore the range of issues related to data analysis, evaluation, use, and access. (See the activities on forms design and evaluation in the Study Guide.)

HEALTH RECORD FLOW AND PROCESSING

The patient health record begins with the patient's arrival at admission and is developed with the forms and documentation guidelines described previously. Figure 4-6 illustrates the model flow of the inpatient record in both the document-based and database environments. Currently a wide variety of hybrid versions of record systems exists. After admission, the MPI is queried for the patient's unique personal identifier number. The MPI is the most essential HIM tool in an organization that numbers its records because it is the bridge between the patient and the record number. Extensive guidance is given by AHIMA in the development and maintenance of the MPI. During and after patient care, key reports such as the H&P are dictated, transcribed, and added to the patient chart. These reports and other documentation are completed and authenticated. After patient discharge, the paper record is forwarded to the HIM department for retrospective completion. Assembly is the arrangement of the chart in the designated chart order. Quantitative and qualitative analysis are described below. Diagnoses and procedures are coded and abstracted for reimbursement and statistics. When complete, the chart is archived in the permanent file. Migration to a database model for the EHR and for record processing will provide numerous advantages, including facilitating the provision of records from previous episodes of care, more rapid inclusion of dictated and transcribed reports, promotion of authentication at the time of care, and more rapid completion and abstracting. Chapter 5 provides additional insight into the advantages of the electronic health record.

Medical Transcription

Several of the key reports in the health record are routinely dictated by the provider, including the H&P, operative report, consultation, and discharge summary in acute care. Other dictated reports may include pathology, radiology, and diagnostic imaging reports and progress notes. After providers dictate the report, the content is retrieved by medical transcriptionists who use word processing software to create the completed document for authentication and inclusion in the original health record. As organizations move increasingly toward the EHR, providers should be encouraged to dictate reports and use voice recognition technology to facilitate timely electronic access. The format of reports is included in the responsibilities of the forms/views/templates design team.

Transcription is a core function in the flow of health record information and requires specific management attention. As we've seen in the previous discussion, several important reports have accreditation and regulatory time frames for completion (for example, availability of the H&P on the chart within 24 hours). Providers depend on a prompt turnaround time for patient care. The next section addresses additional record completion requirements. Because a backlog of reports compromises record completion and may compromise compliance, management processes must be put in place and closely monitored.

Transcriptionists are medical language specialists who bring important skills to the HIM team. Certification is available through the American Association for Medical Transcription (AAMT) (www.aamt.org), which also provides resources for management. Staffing may be provided internally with employees on site or at home, through contract services, or by outsourcing. Transcription systems must be purchased and interfaced with other computer systems. Dictation is increasingly digital and may include voice recognition software. Transcription is accomplished by use of word processing software including special references. These management and technology issues are discussed in other chapters.

METHODS TO ENSURE DATA QUALITY

HIM professionals have always been concerned about the quality of information in both primary and secondary health records and have used various methods to help ensure the accuracy and completeness of these records. Data quality activities are a priority for the HIM professional because of the many users and uses of the data; these functions have a sharper focus with the advent of the EHR because the model changes from ensuring data quality through documentation audits and retrospective completion of missing reports to designing systems that ensure data quality at the point of service and then monitoring the effectiveness of these systems. The Joint Commission's current approach to

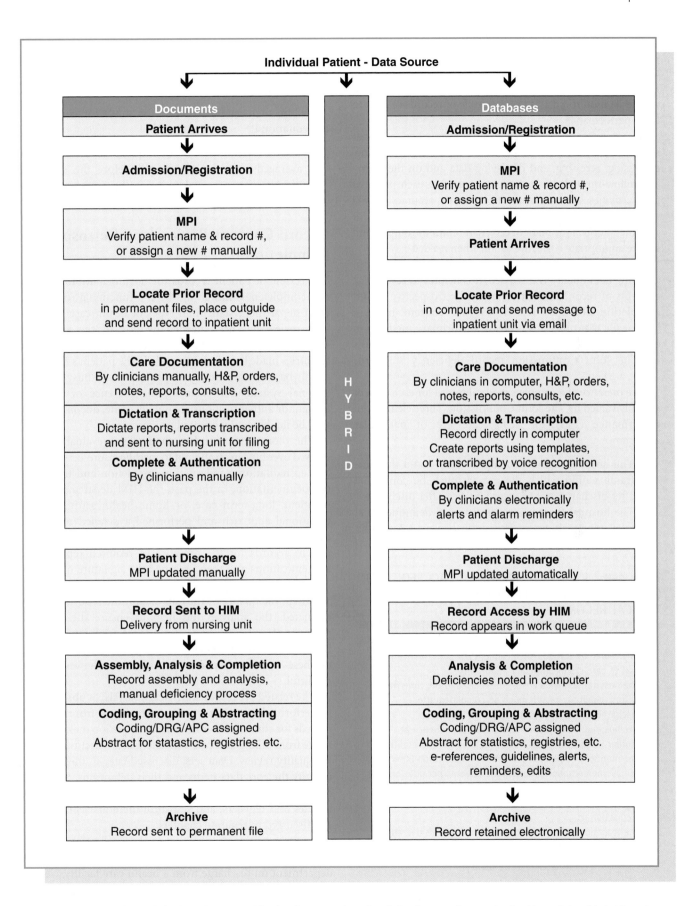

Figure 4-6 Model flow of the inpatient record in the document-based and database environments. A wide variety of hybrid versions may exist that combine documents and databases.

continuing record review is consistent with the philosophy of expecting data to be recorded concurrent with the patient care event and monitoring to see that it happens. In The Joint Commission model, the facility determines what should be monitored and uses a sample of records or data to track performance.

The accuracy of data depends on the manual or computer information system design for collecting, recording, storing, processing, accessing, and displaying data and on the ability and follow-through of the people involved in each phase of these activities. One crucial way to ensure the accuracy of data is to develop systems that ensure accuracy and timeliness of documentation at the point of care, to monitor the output, and to take appropriate corrective action when needed.

Before the quality improvement study approach to assessing data quality is discussed, it is helpful to review the concepts of record content review and retrospective record completion activities related to that content because historically that process was one of the primary methods to obtain missing data and authentications. It was also the basis for The Joint Commission record deficiency standards (Table 4-8).

The presence of a complete medical record for each patient is highly valued by The Joint Commission. Three elements of performance (EPs) for acute care are of particular importance.

- The hospital defines a complete record and the time frame within which the record much be completed after discharge, not to exceed 30 days after discharge
- The hospital measures medical record delinquency at regular intervals, no less frequently than every 3 months.

Table 4-8   JOINT COMMISSION FOR ACCREDITATION OF HEALTHCARE ORGANIZATIONS AND DELINQUENT MEDICAL RECORDS

The presence of a complete medical record for each patient is highly valued by JCAHO. Three elements of performance (EPs) for acute care are of particular importance.
- The hospital defines a complete record and the time frame within which the record much be completed after discharge, not to exceed 30 days after discharge
- The hospital measures medical record delinquency at regular intervals, no less frequently than every 3 months.
- The number of delinquent records is greater than 50% of the average number of discharged patients per quarter, over the previous 12 months.

Failure to meet the criteria is grounds for Conditional Accreditation if:
- The total number of delinquent medical records averaged over the 12 months before survey is greater than or equal to twice the average monthly patient discharge rate.

From Joint Commission on Accreditation of Healthcare Organizations: *Comprehensive accreditation manual for hospitals (CAMH), scoring guidelines,* Chicago, 2005, Joint Commission for Accreditation of Healthcare Organizations.

- If the number of delinquent records is greater than 50% of the average number of discharged patients per quarter over the previous 12 months, verify the context.

Failure to meet the criteria is grounds for conditional accreditation if

- The total number of delinquent medical records averaged over the 12 months before the survey is greater than or equal to twice the average monthly patient discharge rate.[3]

Record Content Review and Retrospective Completion

The review of patient records for documentation accuracy and completeness has always been a functional role of the HIM department staff in all types of health care facilities. This review has been needed because of the variety of sources of patient record information and the large number of entries made by different people in the patient's record on a daily basis. If the health care provider has a busy day or if internal systems for ensuring the presence of required content or authentications are not adequate, documentation may be inadvertently omitted or inaccurate.

The thoroughness and method of this evaluation have evolved over time in an attempt to meet licensure, certification, and accreditation standards for completion and timeliness of documentation. In the past, the HIM department in an inpatient, long-term care, or home health setting used a traditional approach and performed a detailed review, or **quantitative analysis,** of all predischarge or postdischarge patient records for the presence of required reports and authentications and then obtained the signature or reports retrospectively, often weeks or months after the event. Although the quality of the data within the reports was not evaluated, the analyses did help to ensure the eventual presence of authentications and categories of data required by standard-setting agencies. The usefulness and legal value of these very late reports and signatures, however, were doubtful.

The related process of **statistical analysis,** or **abstracting,** is performed to select specific data items from medical records for clinical and administrative decision making. Uses range from billing and case-mix analysis to selection of cases for quality review. Data sets, discussed later in this chapter, identify the core data items and their definitions. Statistical analysis also uses nomenclatures and classification systems, indexes and registers, and statistical methods. These topics are discussed in separate chapters.

In the traditional retrospective data collection process, after the patient's paper record has been received in the HIM department on discharge from a health care facility, clerical staff assemble the record forms in a prescribed order (or leave the recording the "universal" order) and then review all records for missing authentications and reports. Although categories of information reviewed vary with each facility, those typically checked include the following:

- Listings of principal and secondary diagnoses on discharge
- Presence of discharge summaries, history, physical reports, and operative or procedure reports

In addition, forms are checked to see whether there is correct patient identification on every page (front and back) and if all physician reports, progress notes, and orders are authenticated by the appropriate resident or attending physician. Some facilities may review for the presence of other reports and authorizations. Documentation review may be performed at the nursing unit while the patient is still active. If the record is incomplete, a deficiency slip is prepared by the analyst that itemizes missing documentation or signatures (Figure 4-7).[4] Pages are flagged with colored tabs at the location of missing signatures, and appropriate HIM department procedures are followed to obtain these from the physician or other providers.

The method used to assist physicians in record completion after patient discharge varies by facility and includes either a manual or a computer system of physician notification, record location tracking, and administrative reporting. One copy of the deficiency slip is usually attached

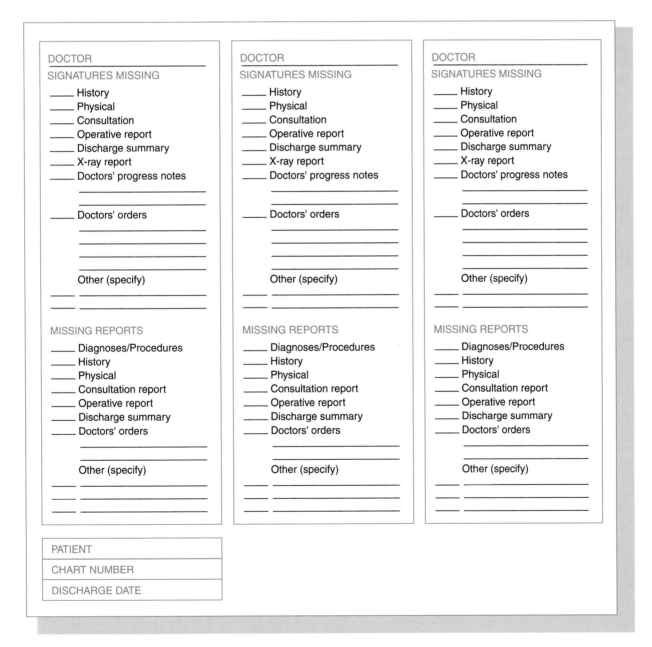

Figure 4-7 Deficiency slip.

to the record. The incomplete record is either placed in a designated record completion area or interfiled in the main record storage area.

If the retrospective completion process is in use at the facility, it usually has a requirement that providers complete reports and records according to the time frame specified in organization policies and procedures and/or the medical staff bylaws. The requirements in policies and procedures are based on good professional practice, laws and regulations, and accreditation standards. When an incomplete record has not been finished within the time specified, it is termed a **delinquent record.** Most hospitals have some type of physician sanction when delinquent records exist. Some may impose fines on the basis of the number of delinquent records. Others may temporarily place a physician on a suspension or no-admissions list until delinquent records are completed. In this instance, physicians may not admit patients or arrange surgery for unscheduled patients unless authorization is received from the chief of staff or designated hospital administrator.

Because of the seriousness of the sanctions for both the physician and the hospital, and the amount of resources used in a paper environment, it is extremely important that the detailed retrospective completion process be reviewed to determine whether it should continue. The HIM professional should take the lead in encouraging the facility to evaluate this process because this is not a value-added activity related to quality data, and it is an expensive activity for the facility. If the medical staff, hospital administration, and legal counsel deem it important to continue detailed deficiency analysis in a paper-based environment, then policies and procedures need to be specific. For example, if the procedure for obtaining signatures retrospectively is to continue, then the review should be done on a predischarge basis to obtain the signatures as close to data entry as possible. Only orders that the medical staff consider potentially hazardous to the patient as outlined in the medical staff's rules and regulations should be checked for authentication. Only key reports should be monitored to determine whether they are present with follow-up as appropriate. They include the H&P, operative reports, pathology reports, radiology reports, and discharge summary. Although these reports may be received after patient discharge and are of questionable value to the hospital at that point, they are still helpful to follow-up facilities that are treating the patient, which rely on the data in these reports. The reports would be more valuable, however, if they were sent to them at the time of patient transfer to the facility or organization. (See the activity on delinquent record statistics in the Study Guide.)

DATA QUALITY MONITORING METHODS AND SOLUTIONS

If the database system is developed to allow data quality capture and reporting and if point-of-care systems are designed to capture data correctly, the next step is to monitor data in patient records and secondary reporting systems to determine possible quality problems so that corrective action can be taken when necessary.

Quality Assessment and Improvement Study of Patient Record Documentation

One method to evaluate data quality is to do a quality improvement (QI) study of a sample of paper or computerized patient records that assesses the presence of reports and authentications and the quality of the information documented in the entries. The purpose is not to obtain data retrospectively but to monitor the adequacy of current systems and to make changes in the information system when needed.

Quantitative Analysis

Performing a quantitative analysis means ensuring the following:

- Patient identification on every paper form (front and back) and screen is correct.
- All necessary authorizations or consents are present and signed or authenticated by the patient or legal representative, including those for general agreement, specific procedures, photographs, experimental treatment, advance directives, and autopsy.
- Documented principal diagnosis on discharge, secondary diagnoses, and procedures are present in the appropriate form or location within the record. This information is completed and authenticated by the physician or authorized clinician.
- Discharge summary is present, when required, and authenticated.
- H&P are present, documented within the time frame required by appropriate regulations, and authenticated as appropriate.
- Consultation report is present and authenticated when a consultation request appears in the listing of physician or practitioner orders.
- All diagnostic tests ordered by the physician or practitioner are present and authenticated by comparing physician orders, financial bill, and the test reports documented in the patient's health record.
- An admitting progress note, a discharge progress note, and an appropriate number of notes (frequency depends on the type of case or health care agency) documented by physicians or clinicians throughout the patient's care process are present.
- Each physician or practitioner order entered into the record is authenticated. An admitting and a discharge physician or practitioner order are present. Orders are present for all consultations, diagnostic tests, and procedures when these reports are found in the record.

- Operative, procedure, or therapy reports are present and authenticated when orders, consent forms, or other documentation in the record indicates that they were performed.
- A pathology report is present and authenticated when the operative report indicates that tissue was removed.
- Preoperative, operative, and postoperative anesthesia reports are present and authenticated.
- Nursing or ancillary health professionals' reports and notes are present and authenticated.
- Reports required for patients treated in specialized units, such as those for patients receiving care in the obstetrics unit, neonatal nursery, or mental health or rehabilitation units, are present and authenticated.
- Preliminary and final autopsy reports on patients who have died at the facility are present and authenticated.

The amount of detailed checking varies by facility according to the nature of the QI study, type of health care agency, and facility policy.

Qualitative Analysis

A **qualitative analysis** involves the following checks:

- Review for obvious documentation inconsistencies related to diagnoses found on admission forms, physical examination, operative and pathology reports, care plans, and discharge summary.
- Analyze the record to determine whether documentation written by various health care providers for one patient reflects consistency.
- Compare the patient's pharmacy drug profile with the medication administration record to determine consistency.
- Review an inpatient record to determine whether it reflects the general location of the patient at all times or whether serious time gaps exist. Times noted on nursing documentation indicating when the patient left the unit and returned to it can be used as the reference point for this type of study.
- Determine whether the patient record reflects the progression of care, including the symptoms, diagnoses, tests, treatments, reasons for the treatments, results, patient education, location of patient after discharge, and follow-up plans.
- Interview the patient or family. Review recorded patient demographic information and medical history with the patient several hours or days after admission to determine completeness and accuracy. A patient may be too physically ill or mentally confused at admission or the family may be too preoccupied with the patient to provide valid data.
- Compare written instructions to the patient that are documented in the record with the patient's or family's understanding of those instructions. Ask the patient or family to repeat instructions to verify consistency.
- Review for other documentation as determined by the individual facility.

The results are presented to the appropriate medical or clinical staff committee for appropriate follow-up.

Legal Analysis

A **legal analysis** consists of checking for the following:

- Entries are documented in ink if a paper record or recorded on other legally recognized media, such as microfilm or a disk. The entries are legible and timely.
- If gaps in documentation appear on handwritten pages, such as progress notes, orders, or nurses' notes, a line is drawn through this area to prevent future tampering.
- Entries are authenticated by the person who made the observation or who conducted the test or treatment.
- If regulations, standards, or hospital policy requires an attending physician to complete a report and if the report is written by a resident, the report should reflect authentication by both persons. Examples are physical examinations, consultations, and operative reports.
- Errors in documentation are corrected in a legal manner. Amendments include alteration of the health information by modification, correction, addition, or deletion or by documentation in the wrong record. All amendments should be made in an explicit and timely manner. For paper records, a single line is drawn through the error, the phrase "error in entry" or synonymous words are written, the new information is inserted, and the corrected entry is dated and authenticated by the person making the change. This process leaves the change in view whether it is a modification, a correction, or a deletion. Amended entries should be readily identifiable to readers, with the original entry retained and linked to the amendment. For computerized records, policies and procedures must be established to track the process accurately from error identification or request for amendment through the completion of the amendment or its possible denial. ASTM Standard 2017-99 addresses amendments in a computerized health information system. See Chapter 5 for additional discussion of amendments in an EHR.
- No misfiled documents are present.

Special Concerns of Alternative Care Settings

The HIM professional needs to design a flexible approach in ensuring data quality that considers the type of health care facility, its data requirements, level of technology available, type of health care providers who are the major sources of documentation, types of common documentation problems, and results related to missing documentation (e.g., loss of revenue). Whether retrospective documentation should occur is a decision to be made by the facility administrator, medical staff or medical director, and legal counsel with advice from the HIM professional. However, accuracy of documentation at the point of care should be emphasized and quality studies of samples of clinical records are appropriate.

Clinical Staff Activities Related to Data Quality

Medical Record Committee

Responsibility for the timeliness and accuracy of patient records is shared by the clinicians providing care and the organization's staff who design and support the record system. The committee is often composed of representatives of the medical staff, administration, HIM department, nursing, and other departments or services. Together they develop policies related to analysis of patient records for documentation deficiencies, including items to review, frequency, and types of penalties for incomplete reports. The committee also coordinates activities with clinical staff departments and other medical staff groups related to clinical documentation, such as QI committees and credentialing committees. If no separate medical record committee exists, these functions are carried out by other committees. For example, in a hospital setting with an open medical staff, relevant documentation policies developed by the medical record committee, such as loss of admitting privileges for incomplete records, are adopted by the medical staff as a whole and incorporated in medical staff regulations.

Continuing Record Reviews

Hospital medical records should be reviewed on a continuing basis at the point of care and based on organization-defined indicators that addresses the presence, timeliness, readability (whether handwritten or printed), quality, consistency clarity, accuracy, completeness, and authentication of data and information contained within the record.[3]

In describing the process at her hospital, Lewis[5] indicates that a review for documentation refers to the "completeness, adequacy, appropriateness, accuracy, and quality of documentation rather than to the quality of clinical care." A detailed documentation review of a representative sample (5%) of the health records is completed by her hospital's HIM staff, physician reviewers, and nursing staff. HIM personnel review the record for the presence of specified content in reports. For example, the operative report for each surgery is reviewed to determine the presence of a description of the findings, technical approach used, specimens removed, preoperative diagnosis, postoperative diagnosis, surgical indications, estimated blood loss, and detailed description of the procedure performed. Other reports in the record that are reviewed for the presence of content by the HIM staff include the H&P, anesthesia report,

discharge summary, consultations, and progress notes. (See the activity on the evaluation of content in the Study Guide.)

Lewis[5] further describes the review by the physicians, which relates to the quality of specified content. For example, the physician reads and indicates whether the H&P is adequate to meet requirements, whether the discharge summary has adequate medical information to provide continuity of care, whether progress notes adequately reflect the patient's course in the hospital and are sufficient to permit continuity of care, and so on. Nursing staff review the adequacy of nursing documentation.

Simple check-off review forms have been developed for record analysis. The completed evaluation forms are reviewed by the HIM professional, summarized in report format, and presented to the medical record committee for review and action.

The ability to perform accurate health record reviews for the quality of patient care is affected by the accuracy and completeness of the documentation describing the patient's health history, diagnostic and therapeutic care, examination and test results, and status. For example, The Joint Commission and its ORXY initiative[3] are moving the accreditation process from a "snapshot" once every 3 years to a continuous quality improvement process. It includes the use of core measures (limited to hospitals in 2005) to focus the accreditation process on key patient care, treatment, and service issues. Examples of current measures include community-acquired pneumonia and heart failure. The more recent tracer method, which applies to all accredited facilities, places increased emphasis on open medical record review at the point of care. The HIM director must be familiar with the requirements for all documentation indicators. The Joint Commission continually updates its approach to quality reviews. For the most current information, check The Joint Commission Web site at *jointcommission.org*. The Joint Commission and other initiatives are discussed in the chapter on quality improvement.

The success of these systems depends on the presence of required information in the health record. Careful planning is needed to develop data systems to meet these requirements. It is crucial that staff who perform QI studies and those who report results of core measures work jointly with the HIM professional to design the data collection processes and refer documentation problems to the appropriate medical staff committee or other committee and the HIM professional for resolution.

Facility Structure That Encourages Data Quality

The Joint Commission Information Management Standards

The Joint Commission in its *Comprehensive Accreditation Manual for Hospitals* (CAMH) recognizes the need to combine information management requirements into one chapter in an effort to promote coordination of activities that relate to the acquisition, analysis, and reporting of information within the health care facility.

The Joint Commission standards require the following:

- Institution-wide planning and design of information management processes
- Confidentiality, security, and integrity of information
- Uniform data definitions and methods of data capture
- Education and training in principles of information management by decision makers as well as those who generate, collect, and analyze data and information
- Timely, accurate transmission of data in standardized formats when possible
- Integration and reporting of data with linkages of patient care and non-patient-care data across departments and care modes over time

Detailed list of patient-specific data

- Aggregate data from the entire institution
- Incorporation of knowledge-based information, including the library, formulary, and poison control information, in the information management systems plan
- Contributions to and use of external reference databases

The AHIMA actively participated in the development of this Joint Commission standard.

Information Resources Management Committee

Although many health care facilities have an information resources management committee (also called management information system committee, health information systems committee, or data quality council) to coordinate automation activities, not all are truly successful because of the lack of adequate leadership, competition between departments, lack of a mission, and so on. The Joint Commission requires coordination of activities, and its information management standard can help to focus more centralized planning within a facility. The HIM and information system departments must work closely together to meet The Joint Commission information management standards. A chief information officer (CIO) and a chief technology officer (CTO) are management positions in some health care organizations. The information resources management committee, with the assistance of the CIO and CTO, assist with hardware and software selections, approve systems to ensure the quality of computer data input activities, ensure the inventory of facility databases and the preparation of data dictionaries, approve the frequency and distribution of computer reports, and approve systems to ensure report accuracy.

DATA NEEDS ACROSS THE HEALTH CARE CONTINUUM

Having explored the general concepts of data collection, we now investigate the specific applications along the health care continuum. As the health care delivery system has diversified, the number of providers and locations with which a patient will interact over a lifetime has multiplied. The following major areas of care are typically identified:

- Acute care
- Ambulatory care
- Long-term care (including rehabilitation)
- Home care (including hospice)
- Behavioral health care

Efforts such as those by the NCVHS have taken on the challenge of establishing standard definitions for data elements to enhance the effectiveness and efficiency of **electronic data interchange** (EDI). Initiatives have been intentionally designed to incorporate the requirements of various previously existing content directives, such as The Joint Commission standards; government regulations, including the *Conditions of Participation* for Medicare; and MDSs.

Minimum Data Sets

The purpose of all MDSs, as with the core health data elements, is to promote comparability and compatibility of data by using standard data items with uniform definitions. Although the data items are recommended as a common core, they do not constitute a complete record. In light of the data item definitions provided earlier, their presentation in the following sections has been abbreviated, and only special areas of interest have been highlighted. When any standard or data set is applied, it is important to refer to the most recent edition. MDSs exist for ambulatory care, acute care, long-term care, and home care. In situations in which an MDS is not available, such as behavioral health, it is appropriate to use core data elements and other data sets as guides.

Acute Care

Acute care, which is provided to hospital inpatients, has the longest history of regulation and accreditation. Hospitals may be small rural community facilities, large urban tertiary care centers, or designed to address the needs of specific patient populations. Acute care was the focus of the early phases of the prospective payment system, which provided incentives to reduce the lengths of stay and contain costs. This mandate has been successful in achieving its goal, with inpatient acute care admissions continuing to decline. As a result, ambulatory care, long-term care, and home health care have all been substantially affected. Because of the resulting change in how patients receive their care, the severity of illness and the intensity of service in acute care hospitals have increased. Because the length of stay in acute care sites is reduced, sicker patients are also being treated in long-term care and home health programs. Although acute care is facing many challenges, it has the advantage of being centralized, with a staff that is sophisticated and well controlled and that has the longest history of documenting patient care.

Data Needs

Acute care hospitals function for three shifts, 7 days a week, every week of the year (sometimes referred to as 24/7/365), and they collect a great deal of highly technical data. The federal *Conditions of Participation* detail the content of the inpatient record expected in hospitals that serve Medicare and Medicaid patients, as does The Joint Commission CAMH and state licensing regulations. Most of the basic forms/data described are included in the inpatient record. The MDS that applies in the inpatient hospital segment of the delivery system is the UHDDS. (See the UHDDS activity.)

Uniform Hospital Discharge Data Set

The UHDDS was promulgated by the secretary of the Department of Health, Education, and Welfare in 1974 as a minimum, common core of data on individual hospital discharges in the Medicare and Medicaid programs.[6] As with other MDSs, the purpose was to improve uniformity and comparability of data. The UHDDS has undergone several revisions and is under the direction of the NCVHS of the DHHS. The UHDDS contains the following 20 items and is not segmented. Again, details are limited and the most current edition should be consulted.

01. Personal identification
02. Date of birth (month, day, and year)
03. Sex
04. Race and ethnicity
05. Residence (usual residence, full address, and zip code [nine-digit zip code, if available])
06. Hospital identification number (Three options are given for this institutional number, with the Medicare provider number as the recommended choice. The federal tax identification number or the AHA number is preferred to creating a new number.)
07. Admission date (month, day, and year)
08. Type of admission (scheduled or unscheduled)
09. Discharge date (month, day, and year)
10. Attending physician identification (UPIN)
11. Operating physician identification (UPIN)
12. Principal diagnosis (The condition established after study to be chiefly responsible for occasioning the admission of the patient to the hospital for care.)
13. Other diagnoses (All conditions that coexist at the time of admission or that develop subsequently that affect the treatment received or the length of stay. Diagnoses that relate to an earlier episode and have no bearing on the current hospital stay are excluded.)
14. Qualifier for other diagnoses (A qualifier is given for each diagnosis coded under "other diagnoses" to indicate whether the onset of the diagnosis preceded or followed admission to the hospital. The option "uncertain" is permitted.)
15. External cause-of-injury code (Hospitals should complete this item whenever there is a diagnosis of an injury, poisoning, or adverse effect.)
16. Birth weight of neonate
17. Procedures and dates
    a. All significant procedures are to be reported. A significant procedure is one that (1) is surgical in nature, (2) carries a procedural risk, (3) carries an anesthetic risk, or (4) requires specialized training.
    b. The date of each significant procedure must be reported.
    c. When multiple procedures are reported, the principal procedure is designated. The principal procedure is one that was performed for definitive treatment rather than one performed for diagnostic or exploratory purposes or was necessary to take care of a complication. If two procedures appear to be principal, then the one most related to the principal diagnosis is selected as the principal procedure.
    d. The UPIN of the person performing the principal procedure must be reported.
18. Disposition of the patient
    a. Discharged home (not to home health service)
    b. Discharged to acute care hospital
    c. Discharged to nursing facility
    d. Discharged to home to be under the care of a home health service
    e. Discharged to other health care facility
    f. Left AMA
    g. Alive, other, or alive, not stated
    h. Died
19. Patient's expected source of payment
    a. Primary source
    b. Other source
20. Total charges (List all charges billed by the hospital for this hospitalization. Professional charges for individual patient care by physicians are excluded.)

Special Forms and Views

Most acute-care forms have been described previously, although, as mentioned, they are typically more elaborate than those for other sites of care. Of particular note are time frames related to the history and physical examination.

History and Physical Examination. If a history and physical examination have been performed within a week before admission, such as in the office of a physician staff member, then a durable, legible copy of this report may be added to the record with any interval changes documented. When the patient is readmitted within 30 days for the same or a related problem, an interval history and physical examination may be completed if the original is readily available.

Issues in Data Collection

Acute care has the advantage of a long history of improving documentation and data collection. Emphasis on data collection has increased since the implementation of the prospective payment system. Mandates to decrease lengths of stay have required that more data be collected before admission and that data be readily available to expedite treatment. Trends toward ambulatory and home care have resulted in admissions being limited to the most severely ill patients receiving the most intensive services.

Ambulatory Care

Four major trends since the mid 1980s have contributed to the shift away from acute inpatient care toward ambulatory care:

- Technology has provided the opportunity for many diagnostic tests, therapies, and surgeries to be done in the outpatient setting. Predictions for the year 2000 included expectations that 80% of all surgical procedures would be done in ambulatory surgical centers.
- Government, third-party payers, and business have provided reimbursement incentives, including prospective payment, to encourage the use of this more cost-effective segment of the delivery system. Another prediction is that 80% to 90% of hospital revenues will come from ambulatory care.
- Managed care focuses on the primary care physician as the coordinator (or gatekeeper) of the patient's care, selecting other providers and care sites according to the patient's needs. Use of outpatient services is emphasized and often required to achieve the cost-saving objectives of managed care.
- Consumerism, which has increased since the mid 1960s, has also encouraged the expansion of this alternative to inpatient treatment primarily because of accessibility and convenience.

Ambulatory care, or outpatient care, has emerged as the centerpiece of the U.S. health care delivery system. Physicians' offices and clinics are the most frequently used and most familiar care sites. Patients may be referred to other sites, including urgent care centers, diagnostic centers, free-standing surgery centers, and specialty care centers, for dialysis, physical therapy, and radiation therapy. Hospitals, in addition to providing acute inpatient care, offer the following types of ambulatory care:

- Ancillary services, such as laboratory and diagnostic imaging
- An organized outpatient department, which may include both primary care and specialty clinics
- Ambulatory surgery
- Emergency department (ED)

Multiple delivery sites and entry points for ambulatory care create unique operational challenges for hospitals. In addition, the definition of ambulatory care within a given facility is continually evolving as hospitals expand these services to keep pace with technologic advances.

Data Needs

As noted in the NCVHS core health data elements and as we will see in the EHR, the patient record is designed around a core header or demographic segment collected at the outset of care and updated as needed. This re-emphasizes the centrality of ambulatory care to both the data collection and patient care processes. The Joint Commission *Comprehensive Accreditation Manual for Ambulatory Care* (CAMAC) details the content of the outpatient record. In addition to the *Conditions of Participation* and The Joint Commission requirements, it is important to investigate other accrediting bodies such as the NCQA and the AAAHC as well as any state regulations that specify record content. The MDS that applies in this segment of the delivery system is the Uniform Ambulatory Care Data Set (UACDS). A more recent addition is the Data Elements for Emergency Departments (DEEDS).

Uniform Ambulatory Care Data Set

The NCVHS approved the UACDS in 1989.[6] This data set was the product of collaboration between its Subcommittee on Ambulatory Care Statistics and the Interagency Task Force of the DHHS. The task force was charged with surveying the data needs of the DHHS agencies, and the subcommittee considered the applicability of the data set to the wider health care delivery system, including other agencies; private providers, practitioners, and payers; and researchers. Providers are encouraged to record all items in the individual patient's record, although some may be located in billing records. When this is the case, the ability to link data from separate sources is an important requirement. The data set includes segments that describe the patient, the provider, and the encounter. Most items are required; some are optional. Detail of items is limited, given the core health data elements definitions stated previously. As with all MDSs, the most current edition should be consulted.

SEGMENT 1: PATIENT DATA ITEMS

01. Personal identification (including name and number)
02. Residence (usual residence, full address, and zip code)
03. Date of birth (month, day, and year)
04. Sex
05. Race and ethnic background
06. Living arrangement and marital status (optional)
    Living Arrangement
    a. Alone
    b. With spouse (alternate: with spouse or unrelated partner)
    c. With children
    d. With parent or guardian
    e. With relative other than spouse, children, or parents
    f. With nonrelatives
    g. Unknown
    Multiple responses can be made to this item because of living arrangements that are a combination of spouse, children, parents, and nonrelatives. Longitudinal studies will have the opportunity to study transitions from one type of living arrangement or marital status to another.

SEGMENT 2: PROVIDER DATA ITEMS

An individual provider has been defined as a health care professional who delivers services or is professionally responsible for services delivered to a patient, who is exercising independent judgment in the care of the patient, and who is not under the immediate supervision of another health care professional. An encounter is defined as a professional contact between a patient and a provider during which services are delivered.

The following characteristics should be collected for the provider of record for each encounter. The user may decide to collect the additional provider data element, discussed earlier under definitions, for the provider who initiated the encounter (if different from the provider who delivered or was responsible for the services delivered). If such a decision is made, consideration will also have to be given to the necessary identification elements required for this item.

07. Provider identification (name and UPIN)
08. Location or address
09. Profession
    This is the profession in which the provider is currently engaged and includes physicians (physicians and osteopaths), dentists (doctors of dental surgery [DDS] and dental medicine [DMDs]), other licensed or certified health care professionals, and other health care providers. The specialty should be listed.

SEGMENT 3: ENCOUNTER DATA ITEMS

10. Date, place or site, and address of encounter, if different from item 08.
    a. Date of encounter: month, day, and year
    b. Place or site of encounter (a list of 29 places of encounter are provided; examples include office, home, and hospital outpatient)
    c. Address of facility where services were rendered when different from item 08
11. Patient's reason for encounter (optional)
    Describe all conditions that require evaluation or treatment or management at the time of the encounter as designated by the provider. It is recommended that the standard coding convention for this purpose should be the widely used *International Classification of Diseases* and, in the United States, its clinical modification (i.e., ICD-9-CM or ICD-10-CM), with all codes available for use. This approach should accommodate the coding of symptoms, ill-defined conditions, and the problems when a firm diagnosis has not been established.

    The condition that should be listed first is the diagnosis, problem, symptom, or reason for encounter shown in the patient record to be chiefly responsible for the ambulatory care services provided during the encounter. List additional codes that describe any coexisting conditions. Do not code diagnoses documented as "probable," "suspected," or "questionable," or "rule out" as if they were established. Rather, code the condition or symptom to the highest degree of certainty for that encounter.

12. Services
    Describe all diagnostic services of any type, including history, physical examination, laboratory, radiography, and others performed that are pertinent to the patient's reasons for the encounter; all therapeutic services performed at the time of the encounter; and all preventive services and procedures performed at the time of the encounter. Also, describe to the extent possible the provision to the patient of drugs and biologicals, supplies, appliances, and equipment.

    The diagnostic, therapeutic, and preventive services rendered in connection with the encounter should be captured where they are provided. The CMS's Healthcare Common Procedure Coding System (HCPCS), which is based on the Current Procedural Terminology (CPT) for physician services and has been augmented for non-physician services, is the most inclusive coding system for fostering uniformity in reporting these services.

13. Disposition
    This is the provider's statement of the next step in the care of the patient. As many categories as apply should be reported. At a minimum, the following classification is suggested:
    a. No follow-up planned
    b. Follow-up planned
       (01) Return anticipated as necessary but not scheduled
       (02) Return to the current provider at a specific date
       (03) Telephone follow-up
       (04) Returned to referring provider
       (05) Referred to other individual provider
       (06) Referred to other provider for consultation
       (07) Referred to an adjunctive provider agency
       (08) Transferred to other individual provider
       (09) Admit to acute care hospital
       (10) Admit to residential health care facility
       (11) Other
14. Patient's expected sources of payment
    Related to E1384, Segment 3, Financial. Eleven source categories are provided—for example, self-insured, insurance companies, workers' compensation, and government programs, including Medicare, Medicaid, and others.
    a. Primary source
    b. Secondary source
    c. Other sources
    d. Payment mechanism (related to this service)
       (01) Fee-for-service
       (02) Health maintenance organization/prepaid plan
       (03) Unknown or unidentified
15. Total charges
    List all charges for procedures and services rendered to the patient during this encounter. This includes a technical component or facility fee when billed separately from the professional component.

Data Elements for Emergency Department Systems

The National Center for Injury Prevention and Control (NCIPC) is coordinating a national effort to develop uniform specifications for data entered in ED patient records. The initial product is DEEDS. These recommendations are intended for use by individuals and organizations responsible for maintaining record systems in 24-hour, hospital-based EDs throughout the United States. If the data definitions, coding conventions, and other recommended specifications are widely adopted, then incompatibilities in ED records can be substantially reduced. Further, because the recommendations incorporate national standards for electronic data interchange, implementation of DEEDS in EHR systems can facilitate communication and integration with other automated information systems. NCIPC plans to coordinate a multidisciplinary evaluation of DEEDS after its initial release seeking to improve this first set of recommendations. DEEDS is composed of eight sections:

Section 1: Patient Identification Data
Section 2: Facility and Practitioner Identification Data
Section 3: ED Payment Data
Section 4: ED Arrival and First Assessment Data
Section 5: ED History and Physical Examination Data
Section 6: ED Procedure and Results Data
Section 7: ED Medication Data
Section 8: ED Disposition and Diagnosis Data

Special Forms and Views

Problem List. Ambulatory care is the one setting in which the problem list from the POMR has become a standard requirement. Symptoms and diagnoses are listed as Dr. Weed designed, with allergies, medications, significant surgeries, and perhaps any durable medical equipment that the provider has supplied.

Encounter Record. As defined in E1384 (ASTM), an encounter is a professional contact between a patient and a provider during which services are delivered. The recording of ambulatory care encounters, with the exception of emergency care, is often done on a single form with minimum structure and used by all medical providers. Rubber stamps or stickers may be used to prompt for data items or serve as alerts. The *Conditions of Participation* for hospitals note the following standard when describing outpatient documentation: Enough information about the patient must be included to ensure continuity of care, including the following:

• Medical history
• Physical findings
• Laboratory and diagnostic test results
• Diagnosis
• Treatment record

The Joint Commission has the following requirements:

• Identification
• Relevant history of the illness or injury and physical findings
• Diagnostic and therapeutic orders
• Clinical observations, including results of treatment
• Reports of procedures, tests, and results
• Diagnostic impression
• Patient disposition and any pertinent instructions given for follow-up care
• Immunization record
• Allergy history
• Growth charts for pediatric patients
• Referral information to and from agencies

In addition, procedures and outpatient surgeries must be documented in a manner similar to that described under General Forms and Views.

Emergency Record. No form benefits more from efficient design than the emergency record. Data collection may begin with an ambulance service picking up the patient in the community. Vital signs, history of the current illness, monitoring of the patient's condition, and any procedures performed are documented. If the problem resolves or the patient dies, this is the complete record of care. If the patient is transferred to a hospital emergency department, a copy of this record may be attached or necessary information abstracted onto the hospital form. The *Conditions of Participation* for hospitals require the following data items:

• Identification
• History of the disease or injury
• Physical findings
• Laboratory and radiology reports, if needed
• Diagnosis
• Treatment
• Disposition of the case

The responsible physician signs the record. The Joint Commission specifies that the following items be included:

• Identification
• Time and means of arrival
• History of current illness or injury
• Physical findings and vital signs
• Emergency care given before arrival
• Diagnostic and therapeutic orders
• Reports of procedures, tests, and results
• Clinical observations, including results of treatment
• Diagnostic impression
• Conclusion at the termination of treatment, including final disposition, patient's condition at discharge, and any instructions given to the patient or family for follow-up care
• Patient leaving AMA

Items are usually recorded on a single form divided into appropriate segments. A form is completed for each emergency encounter, with the original kept by the provider. A copy may be sent to the patient's physician. If you need additional resources in the area of emergency and trauma information, there are additional resources that deal with emergency transport data in ASTM standards, the DEEDS data work, and in trauma registry efforts.

Issues in Data Collection and Data Quality

Maintaining continuity of care across multiple providers and practitioners delivering a wide scope of services is one of the most challenging aspects of ambulatory care. The potential for the EHR to transform this exchange of information into a truly dynamic process will have profound advantages for providers, practitioners, and, particularly, patients. Because the record may develop over a long period of time, organization is important so that essential data can be located easily and not overlooked. All encounters, including those over the telephone or perhaps on-line, must be documented. Specificity is often a problem inherent to ambulatory care when diagnoses are in the process of being clarified. Change in ambulatory care reimbursement to a prospective payment system has required increasing detail in encounter records. Surgical reports have often omitted such items as length and size of lesions excised and wounds repaired; a description of the layers of fascia, muscle, and skin involved in a repair; wound debridement for major infections or contaminations; and complications encountered during or after a service.

An outpatient clinic or a physician's office has data requirements and documentation practices for records similar to but different from those of an acute care hospital. A continuous QI approach for documentation review may be more appropriate than would a continuing daily record review on all patient visits. The Ambulatory Care Section of AHIMA provides an excellent discussion related to this process in the outpatient setting and has a sample QI form that could be used[7] (Figure 4-8). Many outpatient surgical centers use the same manual or automated systems to monitor data quality as do acute inpatient facilities.

Stopwatch studies of physician outpatient clinic activities have shown that 50% of the physician's day is spent on direct patient care activities related to patient interviews, examinations, and procedures and the other half of the time is spent on "housekeeping" activities including reviewing records, documenting records, dictating reports, and reviewing x-ray films. To allow more patient appointments to occur during the day, an important revenue consideration, it is crucial for the HIM professional to evaluate current practices of the physician, review the clinic office system and organizational structure, and modify the information system to help improve physician efficiency.

For example, a clinic may find that if a physician documented in the visit note what he or she planned to do at the patient's next visit, the nurses or medical assistants could review the record the day before the next appointment and would know how to prepare the examination or treatment room for that visit and which supplies were needed for that encounter. Encouraging the physician to document orders rather than give verbal orders decreases the chance for error by the office staff. Physicians may resort to verbal orders because documentation time may be excessive. The HIM professional should identify the nature of the problem, evaluate the current system, and find solutions to the problem. Improved efficiency of documentation of orders might be accomplished by using simple check-off paper forms or by having physicians input data directly into the computer with a mouse, keyboard, touch screen, or handheld or pen-based device.

Surveys and focused interviews with physicians and the clinic staff can determine their satisfaction with the current system, their ideas, their needs, how they would like to use computers in their practice, the type of computer training they would like, and their satisfaction with transcription and other systems.

Long-Term Care

Integral to cost containment is the concern over the effect of the tremendous growth in the elderly population. The Bureau of the Census has projected a doubling of the 65-years-or-older age group between 1980 and 2020 with an even more rapid increase in the 85-years-or-older age group. The reimbursement incentives that cause shorter lengths of stay in acute care facilities result in the discharge of patients with more complex problems to long-term care facilities.

Data Needs

Lengths of stay in long-term care facilities may extend from months through years. A great deal of routine data is collected, which typically accumulates into multiple volumes. The *Conditions of Participation* detail the content of the long-term care record, as does The Joint Commission's *Comprehensive Accreditation Manual for Long Term Care* (CAMLTC). The MDS that applies to this segment of the delivery system is the Minimum Data Set for Nursing Home Resident Assessment and Care Screening Version 2.0.[8] As with all MDSs, the most current edition should be consulted.

MDS 2.0: Minimum Data Set for Nursing Home Resident Assessment and Care Screening

This MDS is under the direction of the NCVHS and shares the purpose of increasing uniformity and comparability of data. The MDS was originally developed in 1980, with Version 2.0 being implemented in the late 1990s. As with other MDSs, the current edition should be consulted. The MDS 2.0 is divided into alphabetic sections provided here. Additional detail is provided in Appendix D along with the Basic Assessment Tracking Form and Background (face sheet) information at admission. The items that follow represent the Full Assessment Form. There is also a follow-up assessment version.

Deficiency Analysis

Medical Record Number_____

Primary Care Physician _____

	Present	Absent	Not Applicable	Specify
General Documentation Requirements				
The medical record contains patient identification data.				
Significant diagnosis/symptom/surgeries are entered on the summary list.				
Current and past medications are entered on the medication sheet.				
Medical record entries are dated and signed by practitioner name and profession.				
Medical record entries are legible to clinical personnel.				
Presence or absence of allergies is documented in a prominent and uniform location.				
Every patient visit includes documentation of: -chief complaint/purpose of visit -history and physical consistent with chief complaint -diagnosis or impression -treatment -patient disposition, referral, instructions -signature of practitioner				
Immunization record includes: -date -vaccine manufacturer name and lot number				
Diagnostic Reports				
Test results are filed in sequential order. All test results initialed and dated by practitioner.				
The medical record contains evidence of informed consent prior to performance of any invasive procedure.				
Preanesthesia Evaluation				
The preanesthesia evaluation is recorded prior to surgery.				
The preanesthesia evaluation includes documentation of: -review of patient's medical history -previous anesthetic experiences -current medications -date and signature of anesthesiologist				

Figure 4-8 Ambulatory deficiency analysis. (From Feste LK: *Ambulatory care documentation*, Chicago, 1989, American Medical Record Association.)

Section A: Identification and Background Information
Section B: Cognitive Patterns
Section C: Communication/Hearing Patterns
Section D: Vision Patterns
Section E: Mood and Behavior Patterns
Section F: Psychosocial Well-Being

Section G: Physical Functioning and Structural Problems
Section H: Continence in Past 14 Days
Section I: Disease Diagnoses
Section J: Health Conditions
Section K: Oral/Nutritional Status
Section L: Oral Dental Status

Section M: Skin Condition
Section N: Activity Pursuit Patterns
Section O: Medications
Section P: Special Treatments and Procedures
Section Q: Discharge Potential and Overall Status
Section R Assessment Information
Section S: State-Required Data
Section T: Therapy Supplement for Medicare PPS
Section U: Medications Case Mix Demo
Section V: Resident Assessment Protocol Summary (RAP),
including signatures and dates

Special Forms and Views

The long-term residential care record is similar to the acute care record in that it is also a record of an admission to a facility. Differences include a longer record, which typically needs to be thinned during the length of stay, and the emphasis on nursing care. Details of functional capacity, bowel and bladder habits, and medication interactions also take on prominence.

Pharmacy Consultation. Because most elderly people take multiple medications, a pharmacy consultation is required to review for potential drug interactions, discrepancies in medications ordered versus those given, and any recommended changes. The consultation may appear on the physician's order sheet, in the progress notes, or on its own sheet and it should be documented monthly.

Transfer or Referral Form. When a resident is admitted to a facility, a transfer form provided by the hospital, physician, or other facility should accompany the patient or follow immediately. The form facilitates the continuity of care and should include the following:

- Reason for admission
- Diagnosis
- Current medical information
- Rehabilitative potential

The physician should certify the level of care required and the anticipated length of stay. The form should also contain the following administrative data:

- Identification (resident's UPIN)
- Names of the transferring and receiving institutions
- Date of transfer
- Diagnoses
- Physician's and any nurse's report

When patients are routinely transferred between facilities, it is common to have a transfer agreement signed by both institutions. This formalizes and facilitates the continuing exchange of information whenever patients move between the institutions. Transfers between long-term care facilities are also possible.

Issues in Data Collection and Quality

Long-term care facilities have had to adjust to the extensive MDS. Many have computerized these data and have benefited from the alerts and alarms and the automatic generation of the patient care plan. The update intervals are also automatically identified. One particular difficulty in documenting long-term care is that the patient's status may change more slowly or in smaller increments. Practitioners need to be encouraged to be continuously attentive to even small changes in patient status and reflect them in the patient's record.

Long-term care records are created for patients or residents who stay at a nursing facility for months or years. Because documentation requirements vary significantly from those for acute inpatient settings, many of the traditional acute care inpatient record documentation review systems need to be modified to meet the needs of the long-term care industry. Quantitative and qualitative reviews are usually done within 1 to 2 days after admission and then periodically at least every 30 to 60 days and again at discharge. Quality assessment and assurance worksheet forms can also be developed to check documentation for specific topics. See criteria developed by Noe for QI documentation reviews (Tables 4-9 and 4-10).

Table 4-9 CRITERIA FOR DOCUMENTATION OF RESIDENTS WITH SKIN AT RISK FOR PRESSURE SORES

1. Assessment present on admission
2. Skin assessment completed
3. Problem on problem list
4. Problem on care plan
5. If developed in the facility, has physician been notified?
6. Are there physician orders for treatment?
7. Are treatments administered at specified intervals?
8. Are weekly assessments and progress documented?

Criteria developed by Marilyn Noe, RHIA, Long-term Care Consultant, North Pacific Data Service, Bellevue, Washington.

Table 4-10 CRITERIA FOR DOCUMENTATION OF WEIGHTS OF RESIDENTS

1. Problem and goal on care plan
2. Weighing frequency on care plan
3. Weighing frequency on nursing assistant care flow sheets
4. Weights recorded according to schedule
5. Discrepancies in weights and unplanned gain or loss have evidence of follow-up
6. Physician notified, when necessary; documented in progress notes
7. Consultation with dietician

Criteria developed by Marilyn Noe, RHIA, Long-term Care Consultant, North Pacific Data Service, Bellevue, Washington.

Rehabilitation

Rehabilitation facilities vary widely in type from infant development to spinal cord injury, from chronic pain management to vocational evaluation. The range of services is equally extensive, from prosthetics to patient advocacy, from activities of daily living (ADLs) to audiology. Matching the patient's needs to the type of facility and its services is an important case management function. When the facility has been selected, the patient is registered or admitted and oriented. During this screening process, the patient is assessed and the interdisciplinary patient care plan developed. Any services that need to be referred are arranged.

The Commission on Accreditation of Rehabilitation Facilities (CARF) has developed standards requiring that a single record be maintained for any patient and that it include the following:

- Identification data
- Pertinent history
- Diagnosis of disability
- Rehabilitation problems, goals, and prognosis
- Reports of assessments and individual program planning
- Reports from referring sources and service referrals
- Reports from outside consultations and laboratory, radiology, orthotic, and prosthetic services
- Designation of a manager for the patient's program
- Evidence of the patient's or family's participation in decision making
- Evaluation reports from each service
- Reports of staff conferences
- Patient's total program plan
- Plans from each service
- Signed and dated service and progress reports
- Correspondence pertinent to the patient
- Release forms
- Discharge report
- Follow-up reports

Issues in Data Collection

In rehabilitation, it is common for departments to keep raw patient data, such as attendance, which are summarized for the record. Maintaining a comprehensive unit record must therefore be closely monitored for compliance with standards.

Home Health Care

Home health care describes services provided to the patient in his or her place of residence. Like ambulatory care, home health has been the recipient of both increased patient volume and regulatory attention as incentives have been provided to find alternatives to acute care. Advances in technology have added momentum to the home care

movement with the availability of infusion for antibiotic therapy and chemotherapy, total parenteral nutrition, respiratory care (including ventilators), and other high-technology treatments. A nurse manager typically co-ordinates a case on the basis of the attending physician's orders. Health care analysts predict that home care will become the hospital of the twenty-first century, which should see an increase in the number, regulation, and sophistication of home care agencies.

Regulations for home health care are more limited than for acute or long-term care and substantially follow the *Conditions of Participation* for Medicare-certified home health agencies. The focus is on collecting the following data to complete the standard CMS forms:

- Home health certification and plan of treatment
- Medical update and patient information
- Plan of treatment
- Medical update and patient information addendum
- Home health agency intermediary medical information report

To be Medicare certified, an agency must provide skilled nursing care and at least one of the following therapeutic services: physical, speech, or occupational therapy; medical social services; or home health aide services. The CMS classifies home health agencies into the following categories:

- Hospital or provider based
- Proprietary
- Private nonprofit
- Government (state or local health and welfare departments)
- Voluntary nonprofit (Visiting Nurses Association)

Data Needs

The Joint Commission *Comprehensive Accreditation Manual for Home Care* (CAHMHC) provides standards for both home care and hospice. In addition, the National League for Nursing (NLN) has an accreditation program. The National Homecare Council represents and accredits agencies that provide homemaker and home health aid services and includes some record-keeping guidelines.

Outcome and Assessment Information Set

In January 1999, final regulations were published implementing a data set for home health care, titled the Outcome and Assessment Information Set (OASIS).[9] It was an outcome of the Omnibus Budget Reconciliation Act of 1987, which mandated that Medicare monitor the quality of home health care and services with a standardized, reproducible assessment instrument. There are versions for start of care, transfer, follow-up, and discharge. A standard definition of a home care visit or length of stay has yet to be developed. For the purpose of Medicare reimbursement, each encounter with a health care practitioner is a visit; for example, if the nurse and the respiratory therapist both see the patient on the same day, two visits are counted. The MDS that follows represents the start-of-care version. The main segments are presented here and in Appendix E. As with the other data sets, there is additional detail and the current version should be consulted.

- Clinical record items
- Demographics and patient history
- Living arrangements
- Sensory status
- Integumentary status
- Respiratory status
- Elimination status
- Neuro/emotional/behavioral status
- ADLs/instrumental ADLs (IADLs)
- Medications
- Equipment management

Special Forms and Views

The central coordinating tool in the home care record is the interdisciplinary patient care plan. A summary should be provided for the attending physician at least every 60 days. When the patient is discharged from a particular service, a service summary is written, followed by an overall discharge summary at the termination of care. Most of the documentation is done by nurses and therapists. If the care is provided through a hospital, the home care record should be combined with the inpatient unit record.

Service Agreement. The patient or guardian should sign a service agreement that outlines the services to be provided, the times services are to be provided, the charges, and the parties responsible for payment.

Issues in Data Collection and Quality

One of the major challenges in home care is that a significant part of the record may remain in the home for documentation by practitioners representing various disciplines who provide care at intervals. Returning these portions of the record to the agency needs attention as one aspect of coordinating a team diverse in specialty and location. The record in the home should also contain the name of the agency, the people to contact along with their telephone numbers, patient or family instructions for care, a list of medications with potential adverse effects, and emergency instructions. The presence of this information in the home should be documented in the agency record. Training in patient record practices may also need special attention. Because the staff is not centralized, well-designed policies and procedures and initial orientation and follow-up sessions are important. Homemakers, companions, and family members may need to be instructed on how to record data.

Home health records pose special problems related to record documentation systems. Laptops and other computerized systems are being implemented, but although some of these records remain paper-based, these problems will continue because the patient is not located at the health care facility when treatment is rendered. Figure 4-9 shows a flow chart of documentation received concerning home health patients at a typical agency. Initial referring information is obtained by telephone or facsimile (fax) from the transferring health care facility or physician. Copies of the referring facility's history and physical report, discharge summary, and transfer form are critical at this point. A clinician is assigned to the patient, and the referring information must be available to the nurse or therapist before the first home visit. The clinician verifies demographic and reimbursement information with the patient on the first visit, and signed patient consent-for-care forms are obtained. Subsequent information is recorded in the patient's home, clinician's car or home, agency office, or other location by the clinician. The documentation includes the following:

- Assessments
- Plans of treatment
- Progress notes (one note per visit is required)
- Clinician discharge summary

This information is brought to the agency's HIM department at a later time (often several days later) for incorporation in the patient record. The original patient record must not leave the office to avoid the possibility of tampering or loss and so that it is available for others who need access to the record, such as other clinicians involved in the case and clinical supervisors. Therefore, the nurse or therapist relies on copies of original records that are maintained at home or in the car, preferably in a locked briefcase when not stored at the clinician's office desk. The nurse or therapist may not visit the office every day, which may create problems in terms of record access and updating of the original record by the clinician. Paper record systems in home health agencies not only pose systems problems but also have the potential to create major problems related to loss of confidentiality.

Designing a method of documentation review for a paper record system is difficult at best. Abraham[10] has written an excellent discussion of client record review guidelines and procedures. The first review should be done within 10 days of patient admission to the home health agency. The record should be reviewed for the following:

- Receipt of information from transferring facilities (correct and complete referral information)
- Presence and authentication of assessment documents by all professional disciplines involved in the case
- Plans of treatment and other reports
- Signed consent-for-care forms from the patient
- Every 30 to 60 days while the patient is still active and again at discharge, the record should be reviewed to make sure the following are present:
- Team case conference notes

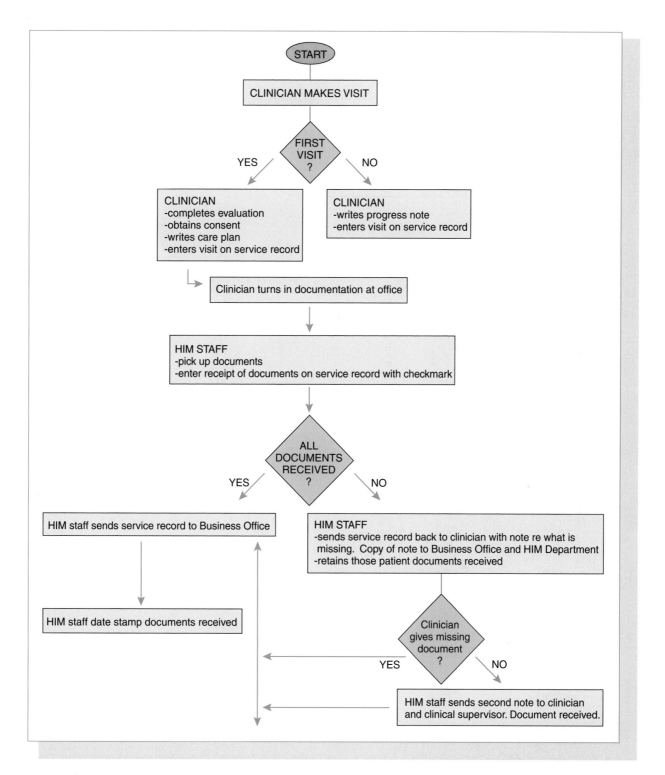

Figure 4-9 Home health care documentation flowchart, manual system. (From Feste LK: *Ambulatory care documentation,* Chicago, 1989, American Medical Record Association.)

Continued

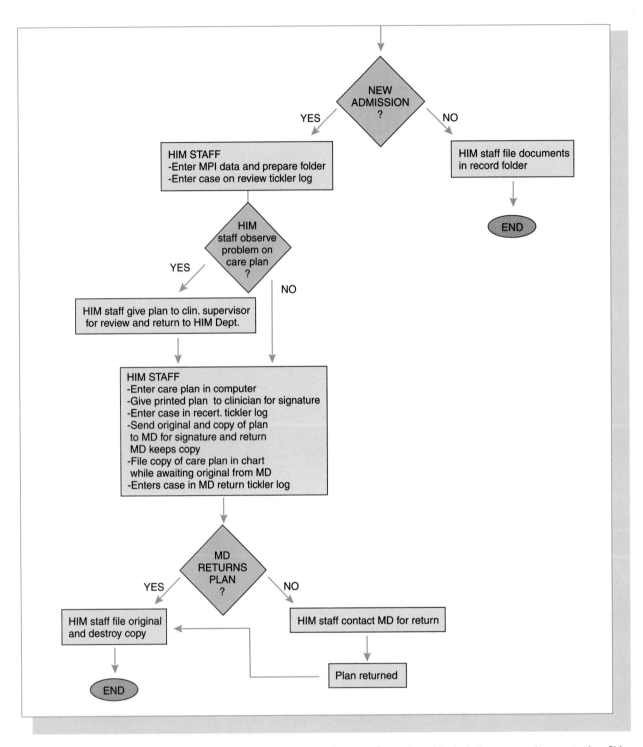

Figure 4-9, cont'd Home health care documentation flowchart, manual system. (From Feste LK: *Ambulatory care documentation,* Chicago, 1989, American Medical Record Association.)

- Updated and signed plans of treatment and orders from physicians
- Home health aide supervisory visit notes by a nurse or therapist
- Clinician discharge summary and other reports
- Authenticated progress notes for each visit made by the clinician

Third-party payers require a progress note for each visit billed. If the note is not present, the agency could lose revenue for that visit. This last item is difficult to review because the patient is usually not visited every day. Therefore, a method needs to be devised to match the date of each billed visit with the presence of a progress note. In many agencies, this is a complex problem because thousands of patient visits may be made each month. Many agencies have daily or weekly individual employee service records, sometimes referred to as "itineraries," on which the clinician documents each patient visit (Figure 4-10). This form is sent to the business office, which uses it as the data source for billing third-party payers and as an employee time card. Many agencies require that the clinician attach the individual progress notes to these handwritten service records and bring them to the HIM department. The HIM department staff records the receipt of these progress notes by comparing them with each visit noted on the service record. They follow through on missing documentation with the clinician before the final monthly bill is submitted to the third-party payer by the business office. Other agencies bill directly from the progress notes and do no further checking. Some agencies perform random review only, comparing bills with patient records to assess accuracy. A paper clinical record system is cumbersome for home health agencies, not only for the clinicians but also for the HIM department staff. To ensure data quality, it is imperative that the HIM professional understand and evaluate the agency's current system of data collection and make changes as necessary.

Hospice

Hospice care provides supportive services for terminally ill patients, their families, and significant others. Psychosocial support and spiritual support are central to this type of care, and only palliative medical attention is provided. In addition to the interdisciplinary team of health care providers, volunteers contribute in important ways to patient care. Hospice services are frequently provided in the home. A primary caregiver, who may be a relative or friend, is identified. Home care or an inpatient admission may occur

Patients visited	Travel Time	Visit Time	Type of Visit	Miles

Employee: _____ Date: _____

HOURS			TIME CARD	
Visits			Regular hours	
Travel			Overtime hours	
Patient office time			Holiday	
Meetings			Vacation	
Other (specify)			Sick leave	
TOTAL			Mileage	
			Parking/Toll	
			Pager	

Employee Signature _____

Supervisor Signature _____

Date _____

Figure 4-10 Employee service record.

for symptomatic management, but no life-prolonging measures are undertaken. Hospice is a philosophy of care more than a location. A unique feature of hospice care is that not only the patient but also the family or significant other are provided services. The family or significant other may receive after care for as long as 1 year after the death, depending on the need.

The following data are required by The Joint Commission hospice standards:

- Identification
- All pertinent diagnoses
- Prognosis
- Designation of an attending physician
- Designation of the family member or person to be notified in the event of an emergency or death

An interdisciplinary patient care plan is the foundation of the record. Both a physical and a psychosocial assessment are required. The physical assessment describes functional capacity, acute or chronic pain, and other physical symptoms and their management. The psychosocial assessment of the patient and the family includes spiritual needs. As in other care settings, updating of the care plan is continual. A review of the care plan is required every 30 days and must be documented. A summary of care is prepared and should include information on the coordination of transfer from the hospital to home care and when the patient dies. The Medicare *Conditions of Participation* closely follow The Joint Commission standards. A specific addition relates to following the hospice patient care plan even when inpatient services are provided. Medicare reimburses hospices at four levels: routine home care, continuous home care, inpatient respite care, and general inpatient care. Data collected should justify the level of care provided. The National Hospice Organization is a resource for data collection guidelines.

Hospice is more specific in defining its episodes than home care is. The first episode of care begins with the patient's or family's admission to the hospice program and ends when the patient is transferred or is discharged or dies. This episode includes all services provided, regardless of the setting. The second episode of care begins with the patient's death and the transition of the family or significant other on the next day into bereavement care and ends when the survivors are discharged, perhaps as much as 1 year later.

Special Forms

If the hospice care is provided by a hospital or home care agency, the completed record should be filed with other records of the patient. Forms documenting spiritual needs and responses, pain assessment and management, and bereavement are particularly important in the hospice setting.

Issues in Data Collection and Quality

Like home care, hospice employs a diverse team of people in various locations. Coordination and training are among the most important concerns. Hospice records usually reflect the characteristics of the facility or agency that maintains the hospice program. The hospice program often uses forms that are the same as or similar to those of the facility as a whole, and it uses many of the same record completion review procedures. Many hospices are affiliated with home health agencies or long-term care facilities and their records reflect those systems. Abraham provides forms, record content requirements, and procedures unique to hospice programs.[10]

Behavioral Health

Behavioral health provides services in a variety of settings to individuals who have an array of problems from mental health to chemical dependency. The individuals served may be developmentally disabled, elderly, children, homeless, in prison, or working and struggling with emotional issues. It is estimated that at any given time more than 45% of adults and youth in the United States have problems that would benefit from behavioral health services.[11] Behavioral health services are traditionally not recognized by payers as equal to physical health problems, although a number of states have begun to require that health insurance cover behavioral health care. This coverage is usually limited to certain diagnoses or to a limited number of visits per year. Some individuals are treated for their behavioral health problem by their medical provider; others are treated by specialists in the mental health or chemical dependency services. Behavioral health services work closely with primary care medical providers. Two unique features of behavioral health are close monitoring of the patient's legal status and additional attention to confidentiality. Legal requirements must be carefully reviewed when planning and managing patient information. Organizations may provide inpatient or outpatient care and adult, child, and adolescent care.

Data Needs

Behavioral health programs are regulated by various state and federal requirements, the *Conditions of Participation* and by The Joint Commission in the *Comprehensive Accreditation Manual for Behavioral Health Care* (CAMBHC). In addition, CARF has extended its accreditation efforts from medical rehabilitation to behavioral health with its *Behavioral Health Standards Manual*. There is currently no MDS, but data collection resembles patterns previously described for inpatient or outpatient care. A preliminary treatment plan is required on admission, with an initial plan, based on a comprehensive assessment, completed within 72 hours if an individual is admitted to a psychiatric hospital or detoxification facility. Physical examinations are also required in inpatient and residential programs. A detailed initial assessment or intake is completed on an individual who registers for outpatient treatment in a behavioral health organization.

Special Forms and Views

The previously explained forms and views apply to behavioral health care, with some additions. The interdisciplinary patient care plan is reviewed during case conferences. Incident and accident reports are of particular importance. Issues of patients' rights receive particular attention in behavioral health care because of its potentially restrictive nature. Patients and guardians must be informed of their rights, and whenever a patient's rights are denied, justification must be documented. When the reason for the denial is no longer present, rights must be restored.

Comprehensive Initial Assessment. In addition to basic assessment features, the patient's legal status is assessed, and social, recreational, and vocational assessments are included.

Psychiatric History and Diagnosis Report. In addition to the detailed initial assessment, a psychiatrist evaluates the individual on admission to an inpatient facility. Outpatient organizations also determine the need for a psychiatrist's evaluation or consultation.

Special Assessments. When there is concern about suicide, a lethality assessment is performed. Additional assessments such as a cultural assessment are useful and performed as appropriate. Although physical health is not the primary focus, behavioral health may recommend that a client get a physical examination, a nutritional assessment, or a dental examination. When treatments such as seclusion, restraint, or electroconvulsive therapy are considered in an inpatient or residential setting, an additional assessment is required. Seclusion, restraint, and electroconvulsive therapy must be very closely monitored because of the risk to the individual involved.

Restraint and Seclusion. When a client is disruptive, the least restrictive attempts at control are attempted first. In a behavioral health environment, staff are trained in de-escalation techniques. If the client continues to disrupt the inpatient or residential therapeutic environment, seclusion may be considered. If this is unsuccessful, restraint is a further action that may be taken. Restraint and seclusion should be used only to protect the client and others and to avoid damage to the facility. In an outpatient environment staff seldom use restraint, tending more toward a de-escalation model. However, if a client's behavior is endangering himself or herself or others, staff may call the police. If either restraint or seclusion is chosen as a treatment procedure, the assessment with justification, implementation, monitoring, and termination of restraint or seclusion must be carefully documented. As mentioned, a physician must assess the client and provide a clinical justification and attempt to manage the client by use of less-restrictive measures. An order is then written that is to last no longer than 24 hours. Staff are to monitor the client every 15 minutes. If restraint or seclusion should be required in an emergency, trained staff may proceed, with a phone order from the physician for continuation. In any event, when restraint or seclusion is considered necessary for longer than 24 hours,

the head of the professional staff should be informed and the case reviewed.

Electroconvulsive and Other Therapy. Electroconvulsive therapy, psychosurgery, behavior modification using painful stimuli, and experimental treatment are other areas of behavioral health treatment in which extreme care must be exercised and documentation meticulously recorded. Special consents must be signed by the client or guardian. Other therapies that may be used include therapeutic passes and behavior modification contracts. If either of these is used, any agreements with and response from the client should be included in the record.

Issues in Data Collection and Quality

Historically, behavioral health care has been difficult to quantify, and records have relied almost exclusively on narrative description, with the exception of diagnoses, procedures, services, and medications ordered. The need for quantifiable measures has been addressed through behavioral severity scales and global assessment of function scales to assess clients. As in other care settings, it remains important that practitioners document as clearly and objectively as possible.

ELECTRONIC HEALTH RECORD INITIATIVES

As patient records are migrating from paper-based to the EHR systems, the characteristics of data quality continue to be refined.

Characteristics of Data Quality

Definition

The term "quality" has several meanings according to the dictionary. The following definitions are especially pertinent to the HIM professional:

- A degree of excellence of a thing
- A required character or property that belongs to a thing's essential nature

The expression "data quality" suggests the correctness of data. When reference is made to the "qualities of data," however, the characteristics or attributes that make up data or factual information are implied (Table 4-11). Both concepts are integral in the development of health information systems and the subsequent monitoring of data to ensure that the information produced is accurate and dependable.

The quality of data is the outcome of data quality management (DQM). DQM skills and roles are not new to HIM professionals. To illustrate them, the AHIMA published "Practice Brief: Data Quality Management Model in 1998."[12] The DQM functions involve continuous data

Table 4–11 CHARACTERISTICS OF DATA QUALITY

Accuracy: Data are the correct values and are valid.

Accessibility: Data items should be easily obtainable and legal to collect.

Comprehensiveness: All required data items are included. Ensure that the entire scope of the data is collected and document intentional limitations.

Consistency: The value of the data should be reliable and the same across applications.

Currency: The data should be up to date. A datum value is up to date if it is current for a specific point in time. It is outdated if it was current at some preceding time yet incorrect at a later time.

Definition: Clear definitions should be provided so that current and future data users will know what the data mean. Each data element should have clear meaning and acceptable values.

Granularity: The attributes and values of data should be defined at the correct level of detail.

Integrity: Data are true to the source and have not been altered or destroyed.

Precision: Data values should be just large enough to support the application or process.

Relevancy: The data are meaningful to the performance of the process or application for which they are collected.

Timeliness: Timeliness is determined by how the data are being used and their context.

quality improvement throughout the enterprise and include data application, collection, analysis, and warehousing. The practice brief includes a graphic of the DQM domains as they relate to the characteristics of data integrity and examples of each characteristic within each domain. The model is generic and adaptable to any care setting and for any application. It is a tool or model for HIM professionals to make the transition into organization or entity-wide DQM roles. For the purpose of this chapter, the characteristics and their relationship to data collection are provided. The full practice brief should be consulted for further details.

Accuracy

Data are the correct values and they are valid. In data collection, ensuring accuracy involves appropriate education and training and timely and appropriate communication of data definitions to those who collect data. The data represent what was intended or defined by their official source, are objective or unbiased, and comply with known standards. For example, data accuracy helps ensure that if a patient's sex is female, it is accurately recorded as female and not male.

Accessibility

Data items should be easily obtainable and legal to collect. When the data collection instrument is developed, methods to obtain needed data and ensure that the best, least costly method is selected should be used. The amount of accessible data may be increased through system interfaces and integration of systems. For example, the best and easiest method to obtain demographic information may be to obtain it from an existing system. Another method may be to assign data collection by the expertise of each team member. For example, the admission staff collects demographic data, the nursing staff collects symptoms, and the HIM staff assigns codes. Team members should be assigned accordingly.

Comprehensiveness

All required data items are included. Ensure that the entire scope of the data is collected and document intentional limitations. Cost-effective comprehensive data collection may be achieved by interface with or download from other automated systems. Data definition and data precision affect comprehensive data collection (see these characteristics in the following).

Consistency

The value of the data should be reliable and the same across applications. In data collection, the use of data definitions, extensive training, standardized data collection (procedures, rules, edits, and process), and integrated or interfaced systems facilitates consistency.

Currency

The data should be up to date. A datum is up to date if it is current for a specific point in time. It is outdated if it was current at some preceding time yet incorrect at a later time. Data definitions change or are modified over time. These should be documented so that current and future users know what the data mean. These changes should be communicated in a timely manner to those collecting data and to the end users.

Data Definition

Clear definitions should be provided so that current and future data users know what the data mean. Each data element should have clear meaning and acceptable values. Clear, concise data definitions facilitate accurate data collection. For example, the definition of patient disposition may be "the patient's anticipated location or status after release or discharge." Acceptable values for this data element should be defined. The instrument of collection should include data definitions and ensure that data integrity characteristics are managed.

Granularity

The attributes and values of data should be defined at the correct level of detail. Collect data at the appropriate level of detail or granularity. For example, the temperature of 100° F may be recorded. The granularity for recording outdoor temperatures is different from that for recording patient temperatures. If patient Jane Doe's temperature is 100° F, does that mean 99.6° F or 100.4° F? Appropriate granularity for this application dictates that the data need to be recorded to the first decimal point, whereas appropriate granularity for recording outdoor temperatures may not require it.

Integrity

Integrity is the property that data are true to the source and have not been altered or destroyed in an unauthorized manner or by unauthorized users, the extent to which data are complete, accurate, consistent, and timely.

It is a security principle that protects information from being modified or otherwise corrupted either maliciously or accidentally. In addition, data are identically maintained during any operation, such as transfer, storage, and retrieval. For example, integrity can be threatened by hardware problems, power outages, and disk crashes, but most often integrity is threatened by application software or viruses. In a database program, data integrity can be threatened if two users are allowed to update the same item or record at the same time. Record or file locking, where only a single user is allowed access to a given record at any one point in time, is one method of ensuring data integrity. In a paper-based system the integrity of the clinical record system could be at risk when an organization has individuals or departments that keep a "shadow record" or a record at their location in addition to the legal record of the organization. The data from the shadow record may not be incorporated into the legal record of the organization.

Precision

Data values should be just large enough to support the application or process. To collect data precise enough for the application, acceptable values or value ranges for each data item must be defined. For example, values for sex should be limited to male, female, and unknown or information should be collected by age ranges.

Relevance

Relevance means that the data are meaningful to the performance of the process or application for which they are collected. To better ensure relevance, a pilot of the data collection instrument should be completed to validate its use. A "parallel" test may also be appropriate, completing the new or revised instrument and the current process simultaneously. Results should be communicated to those collecting data and to the end users. Changes should be facilitated or negotiated as needed across disciplines or users.

Timeliness

Timeliness is determined by how the data are being used and their context. Timely data collection is a function of the process and collection instrument.

ASTM Standards Development

The AHIMA has published guides on the content of patient records and professional practice standards for a number of clinical settings. It has also supported the formal development of voluntary standards for EHRs by working with the ASTM, a national standards development body. The ASTM was formed more than 90 years ago to develop industrial standards. More recently, a section of ASTM has developed in health care informatics. Committees are formed and revised as this effort evolves. Examples include E1762 Standard Guide for Authentication of Healthcare Information, E1714-00 Standard Guide for Properties of a Universal Healthcare Identifier (UHID), and E1284 Standard Guide for Construction of a Clinical Nomenclature for Support of Electronic Health Records.

An ASTM standard is a published guide that defines and describes how business processes or data are to be managed consistently. The standard may specify how a computer application should be designed or how data elements are to be defined. Standards are also written as guides—for example, a guide for a software development process. Standards offer models for adoption and, in some cases, a specific blueprint to be followed.

The data elements contained in the standard E1384-02a, Content and Structure of the Electronic Health Record,[1] are based on research on the common data sets of interest in health care (e.g., UHDDS, UACDS) and on new or missing elements needed to fully describe the health record of a person over a lifetime. With universal content definitions, the content of data transferred between two facilities is clear, even if one of the facilities uses an alias term. An alias term would translate back into the formal term and definition. For example, if the formal term is "patient identifier (number)," a facility could choose to call the patient identifier a "medical record number." "Medical record number" would then be an alias term for "patient identifier." The electronic exchange of data, or EDI, at a meaningful content level requires the use of common data definitions.

As with The Joint Commission standards, ASTM standards are voluntary. They are developed through a consensus process and improved through feedback from users. Reviews are conducted frequently to verify the validity of published standards. In 1991, the ASTM published the initial version of standard (E1384) as a guide to the content and format of an electronic health record. This standard was revised in 1998 and 2002. Readers interested in obtaining a current version of the full standard should contact ASTM at *www.ASTM.org.*

The ASTM Continuity of Care Record (CCR) was developed in response to the need to organize and make transportable a set of basic information about a patient's health care that is accessible to clinicians and patients. It is intended to foster and improve continuity of care, reduce medical errors, and ensure a minimum standard of secure health information transportability. Adoption of the CCR by the medical community and information technology vendors is a step toward achieving interoperability of medical records (one of OCHiT's [Office of National Coordination for Health Information Technology] *guiding principles*). This document specifies the data content and a method of universal data exchange *(ASTM.org or http://www. centerforhit.org/x201.xml).*

ASTM E1384 Content Guide for the Electronic Health Record

ASTM standard E1384 applies to all types of health care services, including those given in acute care hospitals, nursing homes, skilled nursing facilities, home health care, and specialty care environments as well as ambulatory care (Table 4-12).[1] The standard applies to both short-term contacts (e.g., ED services and emergency medical service units) and long-term contacts (e.g., primary care physicians and other health care providers with long-term patients).

The standard delineates the components and content of the patient record and includes definitions that conform to standard nomenclature. It is divided into segments that are grouped within or around an entity that organizes them into broad categories, such as patient, provider, problem, or observation. These broad groups are another way of depicting data in object-oriented systems design (Table 4-13).

Often the data from like or similar activities are placed together (e.g., computer screen formats, paper forms). In the paper-based health record, forms are created to allow documentation of similar activities on one form or a related series of forms. For example, inpatient nursing activities may be recorded in one section of the record on a series of related forms. As the activities of care and the methods for delivering care change, the forms are redesigned. Once recorded on paper, the data are static and cannot easily be reorganized or integrated with other data. Data entered using the computer screen format can be manipulated and reorganized.

If you conceptualize the data required to describe the activities of health care as data elements not tied to a paper form, you can begin to think of the patient data as a **database.** A database must be well organized and contain all the data elements necessary to describe the health care process. It is much more flexible in the ways data can be organized, reorganized, and retrieved to give various **views** of the data or to show trends. For example, the data, or view, needed by admitting staff is not the same view as that needed by the laboratory staff to carry out their responsibilities. A clinician may want to see the trend of blood glucose test results from the past 3 days mapped to insulin dose, meals, and activity. The data in a database can be extracted and reorganized to provide this view both as raw data and as a graph.

Major effort is being invested in developing data models for health care. The natural result of these data models is the databases needed to describe and carry out health care activities. One of the major components is the EHR. This record in its final evolution is a sophisticated database. To help arrive at the EHR, those in the field must agree on definitions of terms and content. Although it is possible to create crosswalks between systems and to use alternative or alias terms, it is still essential that there is basic agreement on content definitions. For example, if HIM professionals are exchanging authorized data for a patient and the request is for "Medical Alerts–Allergy Section," then the data to be transferred should be retrievable and translatable into a message standard format, but most important, the *content must be any known allergies to medication, food, or other substances* for this patient.

ASTM E1384 Major Segments

The major segments are presented in this chapter to help the reader begin to conceptualize the patient record as a database within which all users would agree on data definitions (see Table 4-13). Further discussion of EHRs is provided in later chapters.

SEGMENT 1: DEMOGRAPHICS
Demographics are personal data elements, sufficient to identify the patient, collected from the patient or patient representative and not related to health status or services provided. Some elements may require updating at each encounter or episode and must satisfy various national standards and regulations, such as The Joint Commission standards, *Conditions of Participation* for Medicare, UHDDS, UACDS, MDS 2.0, and OASIS. The data elements of the demographic segment characterize the patient. This segment is the root of the record; all other segments branch from it as required.

SEGMENT 2: LEGAL ELEMENTS
Legal elements indicate legally binding directions or restraints on patient care, release of information, and disposal of body or body parts, or both, after death. This segment records the legal data that characterize the patient's

Table 4-12 PURPOSES OF THE STANDARD GUIDE FOR DESCRIPTION FOR CONTENT AND STRUCTURE OF THE ELECTRONIC HEALTH RECORD (E1384)

- To identify content and logical structure of an EHR
- To define the relation of data coming from diverse source systems (e.g., clinical laboratory information management systems, order entry systems, pharmacy information management systems, dictation systems) and the data stored in the EHR. Recalling that the EHR is the primary repository for information from various sources, the structure of the EHR is receptive to the data that flow from other systems.
- To provide a common vocabulary, perspective, and references for those developing, purchasing, and implementing EHR systems
- To describe examples of a variety of views by which the logical data structure might be accessed or displayed to accomplish various functions
- To relate the logical structure of the EHR to the essential documentation currently used in the health care delivery system within the United States to promote consistency and efficient data transfer

Table 4–13   PATIENT RECORD CONTENT STRUCTURE:
DATA CATEGORIES, SEGMENTS, AND ENTITY RELATIONSHIPS

Date	Category and Segments	Entity
Administrative Data		
I	Demographics	Patient
II	Legal agreements	Patient
III	Financial information	Patient
IV	Provider/practitioner	Provider
Clinical Data: Problems/Diagnoses		
V	Problem list	Problem
Clinical Data: History		
VI	Immunization	Service instance
VII	Hazardous stressor exposure	Observation
VIII	Health history	Observation
Clinical Data: Assessments/Examinations		
IX	Assessments	Observations
	Patient-reported data	Observation
Clinical Data: Care/Treatment Plans		
X	Clinical orders	Orders
Clinical Data: Services		
XI	Diagnostic tests	Observations
XII	Medications	Service instance
XIII	Scheduled appointments/events	Encounter
Administrative Data: Encounters		
XIV	Administrative data	Patient
	Encounter disposition	Encounter
Clinical Data: Encounters		
	Chief complaint/diagnoses	Observation
	Clinical course	Observation
	Therapy procedures	Service instance

agreements to care and caveats regarding that care or the disposal of his or her effects.

SEGMENT 3: FINANCIAL ELEMENTS
Financial elements are identifying data elements on all parties responsible for payment for patient health care services. This segment contains the references to the financial bodies that will cover the cost of care. It may be referred to from within the record, as during encounters or episodes. Such reference would eliminate the need for redundantly collecting this type of data during the visit.

SEGMENT 4: PROVIDER DATA
Provider data identify the primary organization, establishment, or practitioner responsible for the availability of health care services for this specific episode or encounter. Practitioners are individuals who are licensed or certified to deliver care to patients, who had face-to-face contact with the patient, and who provided care on the basis of independent judgment. Type of health care setting or practice type, including sites of care, is included.

SEGMENT 5: PROBLEM LIST
The problem list contains a summary, an up-to-date list of clinically significant problems and diagnoses, health status events and factors (resolved and unresolved) of a patient's past and existing diagnoses, pathophysiological states, potentially significant abnormal physical signs and laboratory findings, disabilities, stressor exposure, and unusual conditions. Social problems, psychiatric problems, risk factors, allergies, reactions to drugs or foods, behavioral problems, or other medical alerts may be included. The problem list is amended as more precise definitions of the problems become available. The problem list is a master list of all of a patient's problem diagnoses or ICD-coded diagnoses. It may be referenced in presenting the diagnostic summary beginning each encounter or episode. All problems or diagnoses initially recorded in a specific encounter or episode are also entered in this master list. The segment listing of this special problem type contains all alerting conditions that may adversely affect the patient when he or she is received for care. It may be duplicated on personal cards or devices for use in

emergency situations. The medical alert section does not exist as a separate, defined segment. It is a subset of the problem list.

SEGMENT 6: IMMUNIZATION RECORD

The immunization record represents acquired (active or passive) or induced immunity or resistance to particular pathogens produced by deliberate exposure to antigens. This segment contains a chronological list of all immunizations administered to the patient and their current status. This synopsis may also be copied to an emergency record to accompany medical alert data.

SEGMENT 7: EXPOSURE TO HAZARDOUS SUBSTANCES

The what, where, when, and how data on actual or potential exposure to all biological, physical, or chemical agents that might be associated with adverse health effects are listed in this segment. This segment should provide data for epidemiological studies to determine correlations of disease with exposure to environmental stressors. Because of the potentially long latency period in exposure to stressor substances before the appearance of effects, the chronological record of exposure to hazardous chemical, physical, biological, or radiological stressors to the body, whether in the workplace or in some other environment, is contained in this segment.

SEGMENT 8: PATIENT MEDICAL OR DENTAL HISTORY—FAMILY/CUMULATIVE/MEDICAL

A synopsis of relevant natural family and patient history and signs that might aid practitioners in predicting or diagnosing illness or predicting the outcome of the patient's care, or both, can be found in this segment. The historical record of previous signs and symptoms complements the problem list in itemizing, in an integral way, the manifestations of prior disease not documented in the problem list and characterizing those already present in that list.

SEGMENT 9: PHYSICAL EXAMINATION AND ASSESSMENT

Depending on the setting, this segment may include a physical examination or assessments by nursing, dietary, patient activity, social service, and therapy specialists. The assessments may be all inclusive or may be related only to specific problems (e.g., particular body systems, dental, vision, mental health, communication). All data pertinent to prenatal and perinatal care, including monitoring during delivery, are included in a postdelivery examination and assessment. Details of the delivery are entered in the section that contains health factors of the neonate.

This segment records the observations of the practitioner during structured and systematic examinations and assessments of the patient during encounters or episodes. It includes objective observations and measurements that quantify attributes of each body system. These are the body systems

about which patient questions are asked during the history or review of systems. Such common categories allow characterization of expressed problems with observational evidence in explicit common terms and measures that, over time, allow practitioners to follow the course of illness and recovery. These observations complement the diagnostic terms described in the medication and encounter or episode segments.

SEGMENT 10: ORDERS AND TREATMENT PLANS

This segment directs a patient's treatment and includes detailed data on the orders and treatment plans and compliance with diagnostic or therapeutic orders or treatment plans. This group of data elements documents events or outcomes that are exceptions to the routine process of care. These elements flag such events or outcomes so that they can be easily recognized for review. Their review is also documented in the quality assurance process or system to ensure that significant findings are not overlooked.

A clinical order is an action-oriented message describing an intervention in the health of a specific patient that is originated by or under the supervision of a specific physician or some other duly authorized practitioner. It draws on already captured data and links the action to a therapy-specific problem or diagnosis. The clinical order acts as a communication and coordinating mechanism for all the practitioners and ancillary professionals who may participate in the explicit and implicit actions set in motion by the order. A clinical order also has legal and quality assurance implications regarding responsibilities for the ordered intervention. The clinical order structure is complex and may be thought of as a network structure because of the relationship between specific data elements within the clinical order and other data elements in the record.

SEGMENT 11: DIAGNOSTIC TESTS

Significant details of tests performed to aid in the diagnosis, management, and treatment of the patient are contained in this segment. Documentation of results from the pathology and clinical laboratory, radiology, nuclear medicine, respiratory, and any other diagnostic examinations is included.

This segment contains the chronological list of all diagnostic tests ordered and conducted on the patient. The attribute data about each such test reference the order, problem list, and appropriate physical examination, assessment, or medication segments that may be related to the monitoring of therapeutic interventions to either measure therapeutic effects or detect adverse effects.

SEGMENT 12: MEDICATION PROFILE

The medication profile is a list of all long-term medications and significant details on all medications prescribed or administered, or both. This segment contains data about the therapeutic chemical substances and treatments that have been prescribed as interventions in the disease process. All the attributes of the order described here are linked to this record by reference to the orders and treatment plans segment. Additional attributes provided by the pharmacist are also entered in the record, including adverse effects reported in the history segment or physical examination segment, or both. The problem list, which identifies the problem being treated, may also be referenced.

The segments that follow contain clinical data from multiple sources. These data may also be used to update the accumulative data segments. (See Segments 1 to 12.)

SEGMENT 13: SCHEDULED APPOINTMENTS

This segment includes a list of planned or scheduled appointments that implement the treatment plan. It includes the attributes or data that characterize the planned services and the locations and names of the practitioners who constitute the plan.

SEGMENT 14: ENCOUNTER OR EPISODE

Every encounter or episode included in the primary patient record in the course of a patient's lifetime is sequenced by means of a date and time. The subsections are organized to reflect the logical repetitions of care events that make up the continuing development of the patient record. Detail levels extend according to the specific care site. Hospitalizations and ambulatory visits are examples.

An encounter is a face-to-face session of the patient with a practitioner during which information about the patient's health status is exchanged. Under certain circumstances, telephone evaluations are also recorded. The encounter record captures the facts related to the events that took place, whether they occur in an inpatient setting or an ambulatory care environment.

A. Administrative and Diagnostic Summary Data elements clarifying time and date, location, type, and source of an encounter or episode as they differ from the information contained in previous segments appear here. They should include the problem list, narrative, and coded descriptions of admitting and principal diagnoses as well as all other diagnoses that are a factor in the patient's care during the specific episode or encounter.

This subsegment contains all the data that characterize the origin of the episode and the manner of arrival at the provider's facility, including the condition of the patient. It also summarizes the administrative and diagnostic conditions concerning the termination of treatment, except for the disposition, which is contained in a later subsegment.

B. History of Current Illness This subsegment describes the medical or dental history of the patient, including chief complaint or reason the patient is seeking care. It includes a review of systems as appropriate to the individual case. It is a summary of the systematic review of the status and functioning of the body's systems and regions.

C. Progress Notes and Clinical Course Components that form a continuing chronological picture and analysis of the clinical course of the patient during an encounter or episode are included here. This segment is applicable for any health care setting. These elements serve as a means of communication and interaction between members of a health care team. They may also occur as narratives or flow sheets.

D. Therapies This subsegment provides significant details of all preventive or therapeutic services performed at the time of the encounter or episode or scheduled to be performed before the next encounter or episode. It does not include any surgery performed in an operating room or that might be documented under later subsegments. Transfusions and physical, occupational, respiratory, rehabilitative, or mental health therapies are included. These elements are recorded to characterize all the conditions of non-pharmacological therapy and represent interdisciplinary therapy programs and results.

E. Procedures Significant data elements on all procedures performed in an operating room for diagnostic, exploratory, or definitive treatment purposes are included here. This subsegment contains data that characterize the procedural events that accompany treatment of the patient, exclusive of laboratory phases of diagnostic procedures (recorded in segment 11).

F. Disposition This subsegment identifies the circumstances under which the patient terminated the encounter or episode and includes data about the length of stay, condition of patient on discharge, recommended treatment, and other information necessary for follow-up care. It contains data that characterize the conditions under which the encounter or episode was completed and the arrangements for appropriate follow-up by either the current provider or other providers. It also contains information needed to maintain continuity of care over multiple encounters or several episodes.

G. Charges Charges represent billing for procedures and services rendered by the provider or practitioner and associates during the encounter or episode. All charges for procedures and services rendered by the provider or his or her associates during or in conjunction with the episode are shown here. It includes procedures that occurred after the episode but were ordered during the episode and the facility fee if billed separately from the professional fee.

SUMMARY AND MANAGEMENT ISSUES

Health care decisions may make the difference between life and death for patients and between success and bankruptcy for providers. There is little room for error. Timely and accurate information is needed to make these decisions with the highest possible degree of confidence. A prerequisite to such quality information and decision making is quality data. Data items that are well defined, selected, and collected make efficient use of human and computer processing resources and produce valuable information. Awareness of the needs of users, the flow of data throughout the facility, and the health care delivery system, as well as standards and content directives, positions the HIM manager at the hub of the health care decision-making process. (See the activity on the role of the health information manager.)

Key Concepts

- Sound decision making depends on having good data.
- The health record has five unique roles: a patient's health history; a method of clinical communication and care planning; a legal document describing health care services; a source of data for clinical, health services, and outcomes research; and a major resource for health care practitioner education.
- The health care delivery system includes ambulatory care, acute care, long-term care and rehabilitation, home care and hospice, and behavioral health care. All records share basic content and documentation characteristics. It is also important to be aware of variations for particular care settings.
- Users include the patient and practitioners, providers, third-party payers, agencies, and researchers.
- Cost-effectiveness includes resisting the more-is-better philosophy.
- The reason to collect data is that there is an identified purpose for their retention, retrieval, and use.
- The purpose of MDSs is to improve uniformity and comparability of data. They exist in ambulatory care, acute care, long-term care, and home care.
- Information and data sets, the *Conditions of Participation* for Medicare, and the accreditation standards of The Joint Commission and others have a profound impact on defining data items to be collected.
- Once the essential data items are identified, it is generally agreed that data should be captured only once and be accessible to all portions of the system that use that particular data item.
- Unique personal identifiers (UPINs) are used to identify the patient, practitioner, and provider.
- Confidentiality for the patient related to the inclusion of the social security number as a means of identification is a substantial concern regarding the EHR; encryption is considered essential.
- Paper-based health records may be arranged in one of three formats: source oriented, problem oriented, or integrated.

- The POMR includes a database, problem list, initial plans, and progress notes in the SOAP (subjective, objective, assessment, plan) format.
- ASTM E1384 is designed to define the data items in a comprehensive EHR.

REFERENCES

1. American Society for Testing and Materials: E1384-02a: *Standard guide for description for content and structure of an automated primary record of care,* Philadelphia, 2002, American Society for Testing and Materials.
2. Department of Health and Human Services: *Core Health Data Elements. Report of the National Committee on Vital and Health Statistics,* 1996, Department of Health and Human Services. http://aspe.hhs.gov/datacncl/ncvhsr1.htm. Accessed August 21, 2006.
3. Joint Commission on Accreditation of Healthcare Organizations: *Comprehensive accreditation manual for hospitals,* Chicago, 2006, Joint Commission on Accreditation of Healthcare Organizations.
4. Feste LK: *Ambulatory care documentation,* Chicago, 1989, American Medical Record Association.
5. Lewis KS: Medical record review for clinical pertinence, *Top Health Rec Manage* 12:52-59, 1991.
6. Department of Health, Education, and Welfare: *The uniform hospital discharge data set,* Washington, DC, 1974, Department of Health, Education, and Welfare.
7. Department of Health and Human Services: *The uniform ambulatory care data set. Report of the National Committee on Vital and Health Statistics and Its Interagency Task Force in the Uniform Ambulatory Care Data Set,* Washington, DC, 1989, Department of Health and Human Services.
8. Department of Health and Human Services: *Long term health care: minimum data set: Report of the National Committee on Vital and Health Statistics,* Washington, DC, 1998, Department of Health and Human Services.
9. Department of Health and Human Services: *Outcome and assessment information set (OASIS),* Washington, DC, 1999, Department of Health and Human Services.
10. Abraham PR: *Documentation and reimbursement for home care and hospice programs,* Chicago, 2001, American Health Information Management Association.
11. www.healthypeople.gov/Document/pdf/vol2/18mental.pdf. Accessed August 21, 2006.
12. American Health Information Management Association: Issue: Data quality management model [practice brief], *J Am Health Inform Manage Assoc* 69(6):suppl 7 p. following 72; quiz 73-74, 1998.

ADDITIONAL RESOURCES

Amatayakul M: *Electronic health records: A practical guide for professionals and organizations,* ed 3, Chicago, 2007, American Health Information Management Association.
American Health Information Management Association: *Ambulatory care section: Ambulatory care documentation,* rev ed, Chicago, 2001, American Health Information Management Association.
American Health Information Management Association: *Documentation and reimbursement for behavioral healthcare services,* Chicago, 2005, American Health Information Management Association.
American Health Information Management Association: *Position statement: Issue: Documentation timeliness,* Chicago, 1994, American Health Information Management Association.
Aspend P, Corrigan JM, Wolcott J et al., editors, for Institute of Medicine, Committee on Data Standards for Patient Safety: *Patient safety: Achieving a new standard for care,* Washington, DC, 2004, National Academies Press.

Ball MJ, Collen MF: *Aspects of the computer-based patient record,* New York, 1992, Springer-Verlag.

Centers for Disease Control and Prevention, National Center for Injury Prevention and Control: *DEEDS: Data Elements for Emergency Department Systems,* Atlanta, 1997, Centers for Disease Control and Prevention.

Clark JS: *Documentation for acute care,* rev ed, Chicago, 2004, American Health Information Management Association.

Cofer J: JCAHO focus on record content, *Med Rec Briefing* 8:3-4, 1993.

Commission on Accreditation of Rehabilitation Facilities: *Medical rehabilitation standards manual,* Tucson, AZ, 2006, Commission on Accreditation of Rehabilitation Facilities.

Department of Health and Human Services: *Charter of the National Committee on Vital and Health Statistics,* Washington, DC, 1998, Department of Health and Human Services.

Department of Health and Human Services: *Conditions of participation—comprehensive outpatient rehabilitation facilities, Code of Federal Regulations, Title 42,* Washington, DC, 1987, Department of Health and Human Services.

Department of Health and Human Services: *Conditions of participation—hospice care, Code of Federal Regulations, Title 42,* Washington, DC, 2005, Department of Health and Human Services.

Department of Health and Human Services: *Conditions of participation—hospitals, Code of Federal Regulations, Title 42,* Washington, DC, 1992, Department of Health and Human Services.

Department of Health and Human Services: *Conditions of participation—skilled nursing facilities, Code of Federal Regulations, Title 42,* Washington, DC, 2003, Department of Health and Human Services.

Dick RS, Steen EB, editors: *The computer-based patient record,* Washington, DC, 1991, National Academy Press.

Fox LA, Anderson RJ, Joseph ML: *Data dynamics: meeting the challenge of the information age,* Chicago, 1988, American Medical Record Association.

Fuller S, O'Gara SA: Techniques for dataset design: a utilization management system model, *Top Health Rec Manage* 12:8-16, 1992.

Green MA, Bowie MJ: *Essentials of health information management: principles and practices,* Albany, NY, 2005, Thompson Delmar Learning.

Grzybowski DM: The transition from signature to authorship, *J Am Health Inform Manage Assoc* 64:90, 1993.

Hanken MA, Waters KA: *Glossary of healthcare terms,* rev ed, Chicago, 1994, American Health Information Management Association.

Huffman EK: *Health information management,* ed 10, Berwyn, IL, 1993, Physician's Record Company.

James E: *Documentation and reimbursement for long term care,* Chicago, 2004, American Health Information Management Association.

Johns ML, editor: *Health information management technology: an applied approach,* ed 2, Chicago, 2006, American Health Information Management Association.

Johns ML: Information management: a shifting paradigm for medical record professionals? *J Am Health Inform Manage Assoc* 62:55-63, 1991.

Johns ML: *Information management for health professions,* Albany, 1997, Delmar Publishers.

Joint Commission on Accreditation of Healthcare Organizations: *Comprehensive accreditation manual for ambulatory care (CAMAC),* Chicago, 2006, Joint Commission on Accreditation of Healthcare Organizations.

Joint Commission on Accreditation of Healthcare Organizations: *Comprehensive accreditation manual for behavioral health care (CAMBHC),* Chicago, 2006, Joint Commission on Accreditation of Healthcare Organizations.

Joint Commission on Accreditation of Healthcare Organizations: *Comprehensive accreditation manual for home care (CAMHC),* Chicago, 2006, Joint Commission on Accreditation of Healthcare Organizations.

Joint Commission on Accreditation of Healthcare Organizations: *Comprehensive accreditation manual for hospitals (CAMH),* Chicago, 2006, Joint Commission on Accreditation of Healthcare Organizations.

Joint Commission on Accreditation of Healthcare Organizations: *Comprehensive accreditation manual for long term care (CAMLTC),* Chicago, 2006, Joint Commission on Accreditation of Healthcare Organizations.

Kohn B, Corrigan JM, Donaldson MS, editors: *To err is human: building a safer health system, Committee on Quality Health Care in America,* Washington, DC, 2000, Institute of Medicine.

Kost B, Muller PE, Smith AM: Coding and abstracting. In Mangano JJ, editor: *Health information management,* Los Angeles, 1993, Practice Management Information.

LaTour KM, Eichenwald S: *Health information management: concepts, principles and practice,* ed 2, Chicago, 2006, American Health Information Management Association.

Lee FW: Using database software for quantitative review and active caseload lists in a community health setting, *Top Health Rec Manage* 13:35-44, 1992.

Murphy GF, Hanken MA, Waters KA: *Electronic health records: changing the vision,* Philadelphia, 1999, WB Saunders.

Schechter KS: Conversion issues and data integrity: a consultant's perspective, *Top Health Rec Manage* 9:62-69, 1988.

Skurka M: *Introduction: Health information management: principles and organization for Health Information Services,* Chicago, 2003, American Hospital Association.

Stewart M: Notes from the ambulatory care section, *J Am Health Inform Manage Assoc* 64:22, 1993.

chapter 5

Electronic Health Record Systems

Gretchen F. Murphy
Susan Helbig

 Additional content,
http://evolve.elsevier.com/Abdelhak/

Review exercises can be found
in the Study Guide

Chapter Contents

Electronic Health Records: The Case for Quality and Change
The Patient Record

What Are Electronic Health Records and Electronic Health Record Systems and Their Functions?
Electronic Health Records
Electronic Health Record Systems and Their Functions
Standards Development and the Electronic Health Record
Legal Health Record
    The Personal Health Record
Designated Record Set
Electronic Health Record System Functions and Patient Record Development
    Patient Registration, Identity Management, and Admission
    Ordering and Documentation at Admission to Hospitals/Residential Settings
    Results Management—Laboratory and Transcribed Documents—Radiology, Operative Reports
    Communication Links
    On-Line Documentation
    Decision Support Systems
    Administrative Uses
    System Capabilities

Why Do Current Industry Forces Advance the Case for Electronic Health Record Systems Successfully Today?
Industry Forces That Advance Electronic Health Record Adoption
Patient Safety and Data
National Focus on Improving Health Information and Technology
Paper Record Drawbacks
Cost Containment and Return on Investment

How Do Technical Infrastructure, Data Requirements, and Operations Workflow Fit in Electronic Health Record Systems?
Technical Infrastructure and Data Requirements
Data Requirements for the Electronic Health Record

Key Words

Authentication
Bedside documentation systems
Biomedical device
Clinical data repository
Clinical guidelines
Classification system
Computer-based patient record
Confidentiality
Data
Data dictionary
Data-driven rules
Data interface standards
Data security
Data warehouses

Document
Electronic health care record
Electronic health record
Event engine
Health care information
Health informatics
Information
Information warehouses
Infrastructure
Internet
Knowledge
Multimedia
Natural language processing
Nonrepudiation

Niche vendors
Patient record
Patient record system
Primary patient record
Privacy
Registration—admission, discharge, and transfer
Script-based systems
Secondary patient record
Template
Text processing
Vocabularies

Clinical Data Repositories

Vocabularies and the Electronic Health Record

How Do Issues and Barriers Affect Electronic Health Record Planning and Implementation?

Selected Issues and Barriers

Cost Issues

Infrastructure Requirements

Laws and Progress

Confidentiality and Security

Health Care Information Standards and Interoperability

When Are Electronic Health Record Systems Part of Migration Paths in Health Care Organizations?

Organizational Migration Benchmarks

Who Offers Relevant Benchmark Data About the Electronic Health Record Experience?

Brigham and Women's Hospital and Partners Healthcare System

How Do Health Information Management Business Processes Change in the Electronic Health Record Environment?

Changing the Business Process of Health Information Management

What Management Questions/Topics Need to Be Discussed as We Move to the Virtual Health Information Department?

Introduction

Documentation Principles

The Physical Past

The Emerging Present

Patient Identity Management

Copying and Pasting

Storage and Retention

Thinning Records

Coding

Health Record Review

Release of Information

The Future Now

How are Organization Policies and Business Rules Changing to Guide Electronic Health Record Users and Systems?

Policies

Business Rules

Versioning

Templates

Titles

Electronic Record Maintenance

Completion and Authentication

Printing

Virtual Health Information Management Department

Challenge to Health Information Professionals

Summary

Objectives

After reading this chapter, the reader will be able to do the following:

- Define key words.
- Describe electronic health records in various care settings.
- Build a case for electronic health records as central components in integrated and networked systems.
- Explain functional requirements and expectations for electronic health records.
- Describe the obstacles encountered in progressing toward electronic health records.
- Discuss clinician and other user needs in an electronic health record environment.
- Discuss document, data, and information concepts for health information systems and electronic health records.
- Review the progress in electronic health record development.
- Describe technical building blocks and illustrate information system components.
- Develop an understanding of transition management in planning and implementing new technology required.
- Identify common health information management operational issues in a hybrid and electronic health record environment.
- Identify resources and strategies needed by health information management professionals to lead and participate in electronic health record projects.

Abbreviations

ADT—Admission, discharge, transfer

AHIMA—American Health Information Association

ANSI—American National Standards Institute

ASTM—American Society for Testing and Materials

BICS—Brigham Integrated Computing System

CPOE—Computerized physician order entry

CPR—Computer-based patient record

CPRI—Computer-based patient record institute

CPT—Current Procedural Terminology

DICOM—Digital Imaging and Communications in Medicine

DSTU—Draft Standard for Trial Use

ECG—Electrocardiogram

EHR—Electronic health record

ESC—Evidence of Standards Compliance

GUI—Graphical user interface

HGML—Hypertext markup language

HIM—Health information management

HIMSS—Health Information Management Systems Society

HIPAA—Healthcare Insurance Portability and Accountability Act

HISB—Health Care Informatics Standards Board

HL7—Health Level 7

Continued

HMO—Health maintenance organization

ICD—*International Classification of Diseases*

IEC—International Electrotechnical Commission

IEEE—Institute of Electrical and Electronics Engineers

ONCHIT—Office of the National Coordinator of Health Information Technology

IOM—Institute of Medicine

ISO—International Standards Organization

IT—Information technology

JCAHO—Joint Commission on Accreditation of Healthcare Organizations (now The Joint Commission)

LHR—Legal health record

MPI—Master patient index

NCPDP—National Council on Prescription Drug Programs

PACS—Picture archiving and communication system

PHR—Personal health record

REG-ADT—Registration—Admission, Discharge, Transfer

RHIO—Regional health information organization

RIO—Release of information

SGML—Standard generalized markup language

SNOMED—*Systematized Nomenclature of Human and Veterinary Medicine*

SSN—Social Security number

XML—Extensible markup language

ELECTRONIC HEALTH RECORDS: THE CASE FOR QUALITY AND CHANGE

The desire to leverage technology to improve patient safety, reduce costs, and improve care—long endorsed by healthcare providers, and more recently championed by government and standards organizations is creating enormous momentum for the EHR.[1]

The pace of commitment to adoption of the electronic health record (EHR) is accelerating. Yet the challenges are significant and we are still a long way from EHR products that are easy to install, fully functional, and interoperable that can truly take the place of the paper record systems that litter health care institutions around the country. Health information management (HIM) now and in the future requires knowledge of EHR systems, organizational leadership, and change management skills to advance the implementation of quality EHR systems.

The previous chapter features patient records in primarily paper record systems; this chapter focuses on the current status and development of the EHR and EHR systems and their impact on the care delivery process and on HIM. Even before EHR systems are acquired, incremental changes occur as patient record components are maintained electronically. Disparate systems and products are linked to form part of an EHR system. Many organizations are in transition with one or more pieces of an EHR in place. As organizations experience the benefits of an EHR system they are often more willing to invest in an integrated system with capabilities far beyond those found in paper record systems. HIM professionals are being better prepared to manage systems in transition and understand how new technology fundamentally changes what happens on a daily basis and in the longer term. HIM professional responsibilities change in the EHR environment. HIM professionals are now managing systems' initiatives and relevant life cycle activities, brokering health record data, and helping patients participate in their

own health management processes through an EHR. Overarching questions provide a framework to describe EHRs, explain their components, and examine how they operate within the health care system. The following are some of the key questions that frame the discussion of EHRs and EHR systems from the what, why, how, and where perspective:

- What are EHRs and EHR systems and what are their functions? How do standards support the advancement of systems, especially standards related to exchange of data, interoperability, and data content?
- Why do current industry forces advance the case for EHR systems successfully today? How do the expectations for improving patient safety and outcomes of care support use of an EHR?
- How do technical infrastructure, data requirements, and operations workflow fit in EHR systems? How are legacy systems addressed in the process of migration to an EHR? Is the EHR experience different in large organizations versus the smaller clinic or individual physician's office practice?
- How do issues and barriers affect EHR planning and implementation?
- When are EHR systems parts of information technology (IT) migration paths in health care organizations? Who offers relevant benchmark data about the EHR experience?
- How do HIM business processes change in the EHR environment?
- How are organizational policies, procedures, and business processes changing to guide EHR users and systems?
- How is the health information professional involved in the EHR transition process?

The Patient Record

As described in the previous chapter, the patient record is the principal repository for information concerning a patient's health care, uniquely representing patients and serving as a dynamic resource for the health care industry. Over time, it paints a longitudinal picture of health problems and services. Until recently, despite significant advances in technology, it had changed little over the past 50 years. Although still primarily paper based, it is changing and, in many settings, has migrated to an electronic format. Chapter 4 outlined a substantial list of uses and users of the patient record. As the migration to electronic records proceeds, these users need to be able to rely on the transition record system to meet their needs while working toward a fully electronic system that can provide additional data and capabilities.

WHAT ARE ELECTRONIC HEALTH RECORDS AND ELECTRONIC HEALTH RECORD SYSTEMS AND WHAT ARE THEIR FUNCTIONS?

Electronic Health Records

EHRs were initially defined from a national perspective by an Institute of Medicine (IOM) committee in 1991. Originally named the "Committee on Improving the Medical Record in Response to Increasing Functional Requirements and Technological Advances," the committee's charge was as follows:

- Examine the current state of medical record systems, including their availability, use, strengths, and weaknesses
- Identify impediments to the development and use of improved record systems
- Identify ways, including developments now in progress, to overcome impediments and improve medical record systems
- Develop a research agenda to advance medical record systems
- Develop a plan, design, or other provisions for improved medical record systems, including a means for updating these systems and the research agenda as appropriate
- Recommend policies and other strategies to achieve these improvements

The committee noted that patient record systems could be part of hospital information systems, medical information systems, or a type of clinical information system. They proposed the term "computer-based patient record" (CPR) as "a longitudinal record of events that may have influenced a person's health and resides in a system specifically designed to support users by providing accessibility to complete and accurate data, alerts, reminders, clinical decision support systems, links to medical knowledge and other aids."[2]

This IOM report focused attention on the potential value of computerized patient records—containing compre-

hensive data content and "intelligence" to actively use alerts, reminders, and expert systems directly in the care process. Over the next 15 years, many additional definitions were published.

The use of the term CPR has faded. It was an abbreviation that was already in use in health care for cardiopulmonary resuscitation. More recently, the term "electronic medical record" or "electronic health record" has emerged as the term of choice. The term "electronic health record" has the broadest interpretation as a record of all types of care to prevent and treat illness. Ideally, the record is maintained over a long time period in a manner that is accessible to caregivers, the patient, and others who need access to specific information or to aggregate information to prevent illness and improve future treatment.

Another HIM working definition, the "Murphy definition," defines the EHR as "any information relating to the past, present or future physical/mental health, or condition of an individual which resides in electronic system(s) used to capture, transmit, receive, store, retrieve, link and manipulate multimedia data for the primary purpose of providing health care and health-related services."[3] This definition is written to include concepts related to individual health status and conditions to encompass preventive medicine, illness, and patient-contributed data and to reflect system functions that address the broadest capability for using and delivering data, and to denote multimedia to identify the scope of all possible electronic tools

In 2003, the Health Information Management Systems Society (HIMSS) defined the EHR as a "secure, real-time, point-of-care, patient-centric information resource for clinicians. The EHR aids clinicians decision-making by providing access to patient health record information where and when they need it and by incorporating evidence-based decision support."[4]

Today's EHRs are being designed for large hospitals, group and single practices in ambulatory care, long-term care, behavioral health, home health, and hospice settings. Increasingly, EHRs are implemented in integrated delivery systems that contain multiple levels of care delivery. In all these settings, the basic content of patient records is becoming part of one or more databases.

An EHR works best if the user's workstation has a large, easy-to-read screen and sophisticated navigational tools. Clinicians must be able to access, retrieve, and capture data from a variety of sources and point-of-care settings and make use of available clinical and technological tools. The goal is to make information readily available and to improve health services workflow. Clinician access to practice management modules that support a specific health care documentation function for individual disciplines or departments, such as surgery, radiology, or laboratory, and access to decision support and expert system tools are components that the clinician must be able to easily retrieve and view from their workstations. EHR systems are complex in complex work environments and straightforward in single user environments. The breadth of information brought together on behalf of patients and the technology required to access and use it within EHR systems is clearly beyond the historical view of patient records as a set of data to be collected during the care process.

Electronic Health Record Systems and Their Functions

EHR systems can be one system that contains all the elements required or a suite of systems that are linked together to provide all the functions needed. Consistent descriptions of key functions help build collective expectations of what such systems need to do. In 2003, the IOM issued a letter report, "Key Capabilities of an EHR System," calling for basic functions or applications to be included in EHR systems; this report reinforced the view that EHR systems were a series of linked applications or functions. These applications are as follow:

- Health information and data
- Results management
- Order entry/management
- Decision support
- Electronic communication and connectivity
- Patient support
- Administrative processes
- Reporting and population health management[5]

This list of functions or applications builds on the initial concepts of an EHR system and includes the scope of capabilities ranging from health data to connectivity and resource availability, regardless of where or how these components originate. Multiple functions happen through multiple, linked applications. Amatayakul[6] features more specific capabilities of EHR systems as an expansion of the IOM list. All EHR system products may not include the entire suite of EHR system functions described by Amatayakul, but the following list presents a broad array of functions that benchmark experience has shown to be EHR system components. EHR systems today may include the following:

- Data repositories that collect and store data from feeder systems and deliver patient record information to users through workstations
- Document scanning/imaging systems that capture paper documents and capture and store of diagnostic images
- Order communications/results retrieval systems that allow staff to enter orders from paper records and view the status of the orders and the ancillary diagnostic results
- Computerized physician order entry (CPOE) systems designed for providers to enter orders on-line with capability to link to advice that can be used in the care process
- Clinical messaging systems that streamline communication between providers, providers and systems, and

patients and providers often through Web browser style user workstations
- Provider-patient portals that use the Internet to enable patients to access their health information, communicate with their providers, and arrange for health services such as appointments and prescription renewals
- Patient care charting to capture continuing documentation that replaces traditional paper-based progress notes and, depending on the scope of the documentation capture, transcribed documents
- Clinical decision support systems that link patient data to medical knowledge resources and offer feedback directly to clinicians responsible for patient care
- Personal health records (PHRs) that are maintained by the patients in electronic form that can be authorized for access by the patient's provider
- Population health reporting that serves epidemiology and research[6]
- Electronic Medication Administration Record automates processes of hospital medication administration

Figure 5-1 illustrates how the components of an EHR system link together and are accessed through a user workstation. Notice the breadth of systems that are contributing to the working EHR. Not only are traditional administrative systems such as the Master Patient Index and the Registration—Admission, Discharge, Transfer (Reg-ADT) administrative applications providing data, the diagnostic testing data resources are extensive. Laboratory results, pathology reports, picture archiving and communication systems, (PACS), electrocardiograms (ECG), and echocardiograms are on-line. Biomedical devices are coming on line as well. And historical and persistently paper documents, such as patient consents and advance directives, are captured in document imaging systems that can be viewed through EHR workstations.

Standards Development and the Electronic Health Record

There are many health care standards published and under development that play a role in the progress toward EHR systems. The Health Level 7 (HL7) Standards Development Organization is working closely with the American Health Information Management Association (AHIMA) and other organizations on the functional capabilities of the EHR. In 2004, HL7 published a draft standard for trial use (DSTU) for EHR systems to guide the work in designing and developing EHR systems and to offer a resource to the health care industry.[7] This standard proposes more than 125 functions. It organizes the functions into three main components: direct care, supportive, and information infrastructure. Figure 5-2 illustrates how these functions are connected; note the scope of content and the traditional patient record forms titles. The direct care section addresses

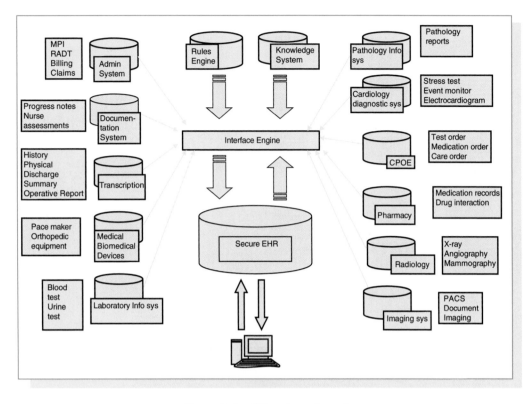

Figure 5-1 EHR system schematic.

care delivery functions. The supportive section addresses functionality for administrative and financial requirements related to care delivery. The information infrastructure section addresses the information infrastructure and technical capabilities needed to support the care process.

The HL7 standard identifies health record information and management in the purpose statement: "Manage EHR information across EHR-S applications by ensuring that clinical information entered by providers is a valid representation of clinical notes; and is accurate and complete according to clinical rules and tracking amendments to clinical documents. Ensure that information entered by or on behalf of the patient is accurately represented."[8] This standard is suitable for multiple care settings and reinforces the overriding objective for validity, accuracy, and completion of the clinical content within an appropriate legal context.

The direct care management functions of the HL7 standard include provision for health information capture, management, and review that addresses health record content. Care plans; guidelines, protocols, and patient education; medication ordering and management; orders, referrals, and results management; consents and directives; and decision support are addressed in this standard. This is a standard that will be revised with use. The standard offers specific details and describes products that should be available through EHR systems. For example, the standard describes a series of lists (problem list and others) that should be routine output of the system. It provides enough explanation of technical capabilities that system developers

can be guided on specific features. Figure 5-3 illustrates a "drill down" example. The American Society for Testing and Materials (ASTM), another accredited standards development organization, has a number of standards related to the development and use of EHRs. The ASTM Standard on Electronic Health Record Content and Structure (E1384) focuses on the data contained in the patient record whereas the HL7 standard adds technical system "how to" to the picture. These resources are valuable to vendors, health care organizations, and HIM professionals as they develop the functional requirements for their organization in preparation for acquiring an EHR system and evaluating the capabilities of EHR systems on the market.

Legal Health Record

As more and more data historically contained in paper patient records are stored in databases and as data are available in multimedia formats, the boundaries between patient record data and other patient data are changing. It is necessary to address what constitutes the health record. Does it include the same content or is it just in a new format? Are there new data that will simply reside in electronic systems but never become part of the "official" patient record? For example, a pharmacy record of patient prescriptions including who processed the prescription may reside in the pharmacy system and be available for viewing on-line through the pharmacy system, but that information is not included in the paper record. AHIMA, with the urging of its

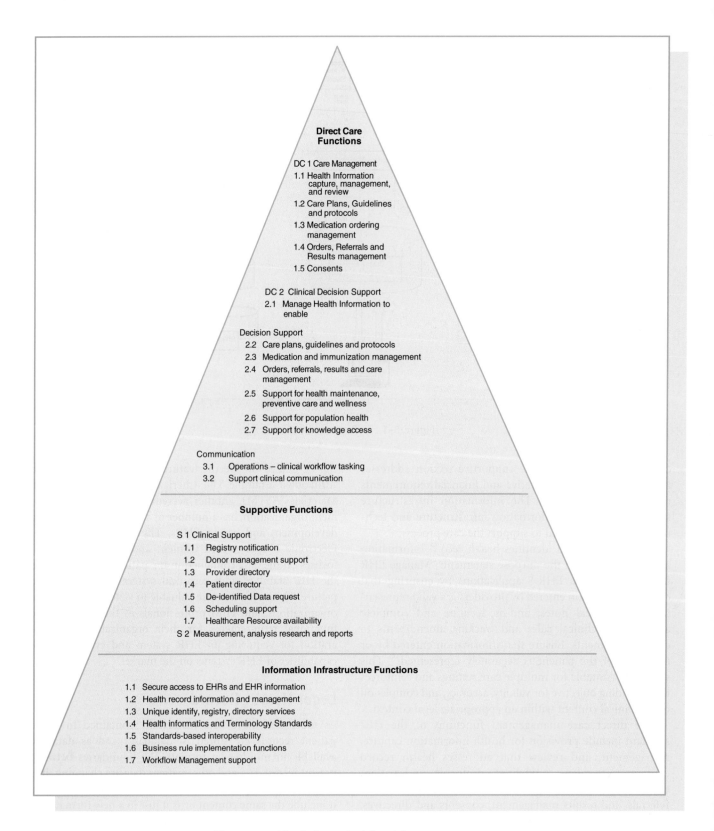

Direct Care Functions

DC 1 Care Management
1.1 Health Information capture, management, and review
1.2 Care Plans, Guidelines and protocols
1.3 Medication ordering management
1.4 Orders, Referrals and Results management
1.5 Consents

DC 2 Clinical Decision Support
2.1 Manage Health Information to enable

Decision Support
2.2 Care plans, guidelines and protocols
2.3 Medication and immunization management
2.4 Orders, referrals, results and care management
2.5 Support for health maintenance, preventive care and wellness
2.6 Support for population health
2.7 Support for knowledge access

Communication
3.1 Operations – clinical workflow tasking
3.2 Support clinical communication

Supportive Functions

S 1 Clinical Support
1.1 Registry notification
1.2 Donor management support
1.3 Provider directory
1.4 Patient director
1.5 De-identified Data request
1.6 Scheduling support
1.7 Healthcare Resource availability
S 2 Measurement, analysis research and reports

Information Infrastructure Functions

1.1 Secure access to EHRs and EHR information
1.2 Health record information and management
1.3 Unique identify, registry, directory services
1.4 Health informatics and Terminology Standards
1.5 Standards-based interoperability
1.6 Business rule implementation functions
1.7 Workflow Management support

Figure 5–2 HL7 draft standard for trial use components.

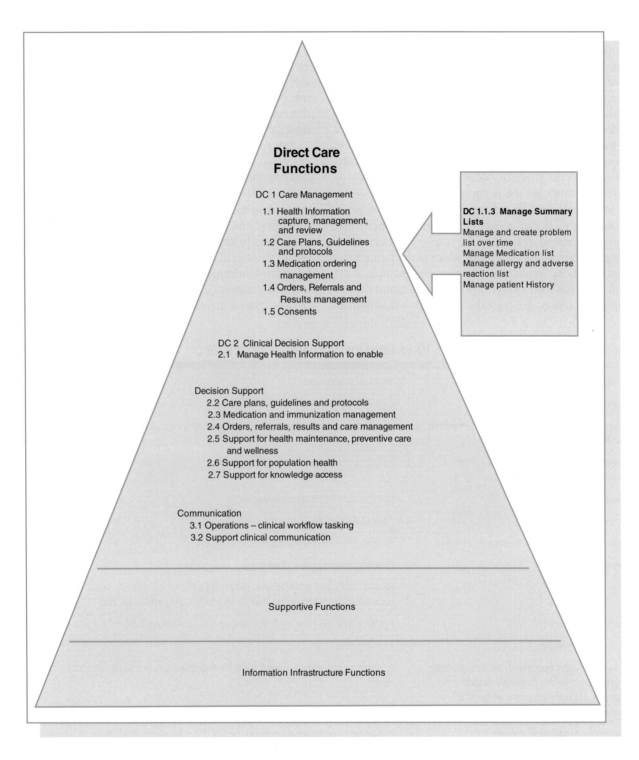

Figure 5-3 HL7 draft standard for trial use detail.

members, appointed a task force to study the issues about the legal health record (LHR). The results of this work are published in an AHIMA practice brief. The "legal record" for this purpose identifies what would be released or disclosed if an organization received a request for a copy of a patient record. Each organization needs to identify what is included in its "legal medical record." The AHIMA task force report guides the decision process for an organization. More discussion of the release or disclosure of information is found

in Chapter 15. Typically, each organization is evaluating the legitimacy of the request, what data are actually needed, whether the patient has authorized release, and other factors when responding to a request for a copy of a patient record.

AHIMA's working definition of an LHR is "the documentation of the healthcare services provided to an individual during any aspect of healthcare delivery in any type of healthcare provider organization. It is consumer or patient centric. The LHR contains individually identifiable data, stored on any medium, and collected and directly used in documenting healthcare or health status."[9] The LHR meets acceptable laws and standards, records care in any health-related setting, may physically exist in multiple mediums, and is the legal business record generated by the health care organization at the time of service to a patient. In issuing this practice brief, AHIMA affirms previous concepts of the record as a business record, accommodates hybrid record models, acknowledges the breadth of data involved in providing care, and recognizes the increasing scope of media for storage.

Hybrid records are the norm in the majority of health care settings. Hybrid records are a combination of paper records and data stored in electronic systems. If a particular document is stored in both media (paper and electronic), the organization should determine which of the formats it is recognizing as its "legal documentation." For example, if the organization has both a paper copy and an electronic copy of an operative report, the copy that is signed is traditionally considered the legal copy. There is no reason to sign both paper and electronic reports of the same document. Electronic signatures and handwritten signatures are acceptable for the legal record. Policies and procedures establish the organizational decisions in hybrid record systems to determine which documents, in which format, constitute the legal patient record for an individual organization.

Laws, regulations, and practice principles must be examined and perhaps changed in some states to better describe the legal medical record in an electronic environment. Table 5-1 shows the AHIMA Legal Health Record description by type of content.[9] The AHIMA practice brief identifies how an organization can use policies and procedures to identify the source systems where some of the record is stored electronically. Source systems might be laboratory information systems, pharmacy systems, and imaging systems. Table 5-2 illustrates how hybrid health records systems identify the content of the record using the

Table 5-1   DATA AND DOCUMENTS TO BE CONSIDERED PART OF THE RECORD

Advance directives	Nursing assessments
Allergy records	Operative and procedure reports
Alerts and reminders (see "Alerts, Reminders, and Pop-Ups," above)	Orders for treatment including diagnostic tests for laboratory and radiology
Analog and digital patient photographs for identification purposes only	Pathology reports
Anesthesia records	Patient-submitted documentation
Care plans	Patient education or teaching documents
Consent forms for care, treatment, research	Patient identifiers (medical record number)
Consultation reports	Photographs (digital and analog)
Diagnostic images	Post-it notes and annotations containing patient-provider or provider-provider communications regarding care or treatment of specific patients
Discharge instructions	Practice guidelines or protocols and clinical pathways that embed patient data
Discharge summaries	Problem lists
E-mail messages containing patient-provider or provider-provider communications regarding care or treatment of specific patients[5]	Progress notes and documentation (multidisciplinary, excluding psychotherapy notes)
Emergency department records	Psychology and psychiatric assessments and summaries (excluding psychotherapy notes)
Fetal monitoring strips from which interpretations are derived	Records received from another health care provider who was relied on to provide health care to the patient (see "Continuing Care Records," above)
Functional status assessments	Research records of tests and treatments[7]
Graphic records	Respiratory therapy, physical therapy, speech therapy, and occupational therapy records
History and physical examination records	Results of tests and studies from laboratory and radiology
Immunization records	Standing orders

Table 5-1 DATA AND DOCUMENTS TO BE CONSIDERED PART OF THE RECORD—cont'd

Instant messages containing patient-provider or provider-provider communications[6]	Telephone messages containing patient-provider or provider-provider communications regarding care or treatment of specific patients
Intake and output records	Telephone orders
Medication administration records	Trauma tapes
Medication orders	Verbal orders
Medication profiles	Waveforms such as ECGs and electromyograms from which interpretations are derived
Minimum data sets (MDS, OASIS, IRF, PAI)	Any other information required by the Medicare Conditions of Participation, state provider licensure statutes or rules, or by any third-party payer as a condition of reimbursement

Source: American Health Information Management Association, update: *Guidelines for defining the legal health record for disclosure purposes* (website): http://library.ahima.org/xpedio/public/documents/pub_bok1_027921.html.
ECG, Electrocardiogram; *IRF*, inpatient rehabilitative facility; *MDS*, minimum data set; *OASIS*, outcomes and assessment information set; *PAI*, patient assessment instrument.

Table 5-2 DEFINING HYBRID RECORDS—PAPER TO SOURCE SYSTEMS ILLUSTRATED

Patient Record Report	Media	Source Systems
Admission history and physical examination	Paper	Transcription
Physician orders	Paper	Paper record
Clinical laboratory results	Electronic	Laboratory information system
Radiology reports	Electronic	Radiology information system
Medication records	Electronic	Bedside documentation system
Preoperative progress notes	Paper	Paper record
Progress notes	Paper	Paper record
Consents	Electronic	Optical scanning system

source systems such as transcription, laboratory, radiology, pharmacy, and more. No matter what EHR transition status an organization is in at any particular moment, health information management staff must ensure that the organization has a complete medical record. This means changing business processes to accommodate electronic source systems that maintain original care documentation to ensure that the "legal health record" can be provided as needed.

The Personal Health Record

The IOM found that "When patients see multiple providers in different settings, none of whom have access to complete (health) information, it becomes easier for things to go wrong."[10] Each health care provider maintains his or her own separate patient records for patients treated. This means that health information is fragmented among the many individual and organizational providers where the patient has received care, which can lead to an incomplete story about a patient's health. What is needed is a way to coordinate the documentation among all the clinical stake-

holders in a patient's care. One obvious coordinator is the patient! The tool a patient needs to do this is called the PHR.

In 2004, AHIMA established an e-HIM work group that developed a definition and model of an electronic PHR. The definition states, "The personal health record is an electronic, lifelong resource of health information needed by individuals to make health decisions. Individuals own and manage the information in the PHR, which comes from healthcare providers and the individual. The PHR is maintained in a secure and private environment, with the individual determining rights of access. The PHR does not replace the legal record of any provider."[11]

Key considerations for the health information manager is the PHR's format and content, privacy, access and control, maintenance and security, and interoperability. Ideally, a PHR does the following:

- Eases the transition from paper to electronic record keeping
- Allows the patient to refill prescriptions electronically

- Addresses health literacy skills (reading and writing) in the context of language and culture
- Is designed so that interfaces are patient friendly
- Can custom tailor views
- Enables information sharing among patient and providers
- Is portable *and* remains with the patient
- Helps organize personal health information
- Assists patients with decision making, wellness, self-care plans, and patient safety alerts

In fact, PHR proponents believe that patients who keep their own complete, updated, and easily accessible health records are taking a more active role in their own health care. The growth of the World Wide Web combined with easy access to huge amounts of health information has led to the concept of consumer health informatics: "the branch of medical informatics that analyzes consumers' needs for information; studies and implements methods for making information accessible to consumers; and models and integrates consumers' preferences into medical information systems."[12] A patient could decide to use a portion of the PHR to organize health information gleaned from the Internet.

PHRs can be stored on paper or electronically. If patients, including ourselves, keep medical records at all, they are most likely paper based—copies of various reports from family practitioners, obstetrician-gynecologists, and so forth. In 2006, most primary health providers still maintain their records on paper. Or, PHRs can be maintained in a PC by the patient typing in specific health information or scanning copies of medical record reports. Other technology is used for PHRs: There are Web-based PHR products where the patient's information is securely stored on a Web server and is accessible through an Internet connection. Various portable devices (USB, PDAs, smartcards, etc.) can be used in connection with other PHR solutions.

Data elements are similar to those you have already learned about, with one exception: the PHR can contain patient-entered data. For example, if the patient is a diabetic, he or she may enter daily blood glucose levels so that the provider can track the patient's progress. A mother might choose to enter the names and dates of her children's immunizations. Table 5-3 shows how this might look.

Table 5-3 COMMON DATA ELEMENTS IN PERSONAL HEALTH RECORDS

Personal information	Surgeries
Emergency contacts	Medications
Health care providers	Physician visits
Insurance providers	Hospitalizations
Legal documents	Clinical test results
General medical information	Insurance types
Drugs/allergies	General conditions
Conditions	Patient-entered data

To promulgate adoption of PHRs, AHIMA developed a community-based public education campaign with several objectives:

- To increase public awareness and understanding of the issues surrounding personal health information and health records.
- to provide individuals with the information they need to better manage their personal health information and to encourage them to maintain a PHR to improve the quality of care they receive.
- To create greater public awareness of the HIM professional and the important role HIM professionals play in effective management of personal health information needed to deliver quality health care to the public.[12a]

AHIMA provides free community-based public education seminars and a public education site, *www.myphr.com.* The site contains information about health information rights, a step-by-step guide for creating a PHR, a guided tour to help the public learn more about how health information is collected, where it goes and how it is used, and an on-line form to request a local HIM professional to deliver a free public education seminar to groups and organizations. *Note:* AHIMA does not make, sell, or endorse any PHR products.

Designated Record Set

The Healthcare Insurance Portability and Accountability Act (HIPAA) is an important federal law that reinforces the privacy protection given to individually identifiable health data created and held by health care organizations and other groups designated in the law. The administrative simplification portion of the HIPAA legislation uses the term "designated record set." Designated record sets are defined in a manner that covers all types of organizations that maintain health information. For health organizations that provide health services, the patient and billing records are the typical records addressed by HIPAA. Third-party payers and other organizations also maintain records about individual's enrollment, payment, claims adjudication, or case management records that are used in whole or part to make decisions about the patient.[13] Again the "designated record set" is the record that would be released on the basis of a request for a record. This record set will vary on the basis of the requestor and the requestor's rights and needs because another component of HIPAA provides that the minimum necessary—meaning the minimum amount of data necessary to accomplish a request for information—should be released. The law specifies much more detail about its application. The primary purpose of HIPAA privacy regulations is to protect the privacy of individually identifiable information. Because organizations determine their designated record set, they also address the hybrid record status in their institutions and determine the best sources for assembling specific data into the record set.

Electronic Health Record System Functions and Patient Record Development

In Figure 4-6 in Chapter 4, the process of assembling the patient record, gathering the physical components of the record, is linked to the patient care process. In an EHR environment, the patient record supports the same care process but may look different. For example, when a patient arrives for health services in an organization where an EHR has been in place for a period of time, the patient's historical health record data are maintained in an electronic form that can be accessed and searched for prior information. With historical data available electronically, only updated and new information is needed to begin the care process.

Patient Registration, Identity Management, and Admission

Patients who are admitted for care in a hospital or in an outpatient setting begin with the fundamental registration function, which is directly linked to the institutional master patient index. This administrative application combines demographic data captured in the registration (master patient index) application with administrative census (admission, discharge, and transfer [ADT]) applications in hospitals. The registration/ADT application is used to initiate or update basic demographic data, establishes and tracks the location or service of the patient, and feeds data to other systems such as billing or the laboratory. In ambulatory care settings, the demographic data collected by the registration application is also shared with appointment scheduling applications to arrange patient appointments.

Ordering and Documentation at Admission to Hospitals/Residential Settings

Once admitted to a hospital or other type of residential or structured care program, patient care begins through an order entry or CPOE application. The order entry/ management capability streamlines the fundamental workflow of the care process, allows orders to be monitored electronically, and links them to the ordered test results for on-line viewing. Think of this capability as the initial foundation of on-line orders and results. The more advanced version of order entry, CPOE, is more powerful and includes linking patient data to intelligence options. CPOE enables physicians and other independent practitioners to enter their own orders on-line with links to decision support so that feedback on the order can be provided and any appropriate changes made at that point. The objective is to improve the quality of care and to make health care safer. An example of decision support is linking an order for medication to an individual patient's health

data and a pharmacy system's resources on drug allergies or drug contraindications. An immediate feedback alert to the ordering physician allows the order to be modified and an alternative medication selected.

History and physical examinations and nursing assessments are performed at admission. The documentation of these services may use a combination of dictation or voice activation applications and direct data capture so that information is organized and available for on-line viewing.

Results Management—Laboratory and Transcribed Documents—Radiology, Operative Reports

Providing on-line "results" to the care team is one of the major components in developing EHR capability. This function is often an early step in an EHR migration process and provides immediate benefits to busy practitioners. Amatayakul[6] presents the "results" functions in two levels. Results review allows the care team to view ancillary test results and other information items such as transcribed documents that are in electronic form. Test results in this review function are presented in a "look up" fashion with the information shown in a mode similar to how test results are presented in paper mode. In many cases, information may be looked up through secure Web access from outside the hospital. The advent of handheld devices holds promise for even more flexible access.

In more sophisticated results management applications, additional functionality allows the care team to access a specific patient's test results, radiology images, transcribed reports, and other information and view them on-line with additional features. There may be the capability to flag the most recent findings, highlight out-of-range or contrast alternative test results, or view data in historical patterns or other formats. In these cases, depending on the state of adoption of the electronically stored patient data, test results may be printed out and added to paper records or stored electronically.[6]

Communication Links

Electronic communication and connectivity by networks is used to link applications together for data access and exchange purposes. Providers and administrative staff use electronic communication for clinical and administrative purposes to support the care team and expedite messages needed to clarify orders or discuss results. Few organizations can imagine functioning efficiently today without the benefit of electronic mail and other communication mechanisms. The same is true for the health care environment.

On-Line Documentation

As a hospitalization or an encounter progresses, clinicians use workstations with EHR software navigational tools to document care and services on-line. Vital signs, medication administration, care plan notes, and progress notes replace handwritten notes.

Clinicians may use free text or "unstructured" data to enter information directly on-line or may continue to dictate their notes directly or with voice-activated dictation. They may use structured data entry in which they draw from standard phrases or pick lists and pull-down menus to help guide the entry and ensure that complete information is included. These data "tools" make use of predefined text scripts, lists, and terminology. Specialized templates also help to organize the data for both the author and eventual readers. The template is structured to improve ease of access or capture. It can provide a means of breaking narrative into several smaller recognized segments. It may also draw from data already collected and allow the clinician to modify and complete information. Significant work is under way to develop standards for templates so that consistency in content can be achieved. Workstation design also can help support accuracy, completeness, and access of data. Especially when the clinician is collecting and entering the data in the presence of the patient, ergonomic design is important to support the clinician-patient interaction.

Evidence from EHR systems that have been implemented in hospital and ambulatory care settings provide helpful suggestions for future planning. The EHR team at the Geisinger Clinic (50 locations) stresses the value of simplicity as the "heart of clarity and the single most important usability guideline" for workstation design. Noting that the design must help the clinician to focus rapidly on the most relevant information and be mindful of how clinicians use patient information, the team emphasized that this is key to realizing workflow benefits.[14]

Over the course of a hospitalization, administrative data, orders, test results, transcribed reports, and patient care documentation applications are used to assemble the information so that clinicians may access and manage data through electronic means. Patient care coordination and the care team's workflow both benefit from readily available data that provides up-to-the-minute information to the clinicians at the bedside and through workstations at their offices and through hand-held devices. These tools strengthen more consistent information use and improve efficiency in the care process.

Some EHR products provide a visit summary designed to summarize the visit and instructions to the patient provided at the end of each visit. More and more institutions are encouraging patients to access their health information on-line and, in some chronic disease situations, the on-line record system assists the clinician and the patient in monitoring key indicators that the patient reports by electronic mail. In fact, 74% of Americans report they want to go beyond self-care and e-mail their physicians.[15] Patients want to access test results, the ability to refill/renew prescriptions, check on referrals, report monitoring of chronic disease tracking measures, and learn how to help manage their own health.

Decision Support Systems

Decision support systems are integral components of EHR systems. Decision support applications use rules engines to program the logic that links patient data with clinical guidelines, disease-specific protocols, and expert systems to provide alerts and reminders directly to clinicians through the EHR workstation. The alerts and reminders may be electronic mail messages with a high-priority indicator or a clinical messaging application designed to send information to a physician's electronic inbox or a pop-up reminder that is generated when a physician signs on to the system. Hand-held devices also serve as a conduit for sending messages to the clinician about significant alerts about patients. Patient safety improvements are well documented when the care process has the benefit of these resources.[16] Figure 5-4 illustrates how decision support operates.

Administrative Uses

The EHR enhances the capacity to use and work with data. Along with clinical activities, administrative processes such as patient registration, master patient index maintenance, scheduling, referral management, record/document completion, disease and procedure coding, revenue cycle management, data analysis, abstracting, billing, financial processing, auditing access to the record, handling requests for data from patient records, quality improvement studies, and providing internal and external reports are supported by an EHR system. The data in the record serve many internal and external needs. One of the uses that is easier with an EHRS is monitoring chronic diseases. The process of required reporting such as that required for vital statistics, infectious disease reporting, and cancer reporting can be done electronically. The Public Health Informatics Standards Consortium identified extensive additional data uses to improve the health of citizens with the implementation of EHR systems. The benefits to individual patients and to society as a whole through improved process and better public health surveillance are well documented.[17]

System Capabilities

The range of EHR systems from single-practice ambulatory vendor products to large, complex institutional systems in health maintenance organizations (HMOs), hospitals, and integrated delivery system settings reflects a common core of functions, but there is often a wide variation in the functions offered by different vendors.

In cases where EHR system vendors market products that include only selected modules, they partner with the customer to link those modules with existing legacy systems. To illustrate, a product collects data from existing legacy administrative applications such as hospital ADT systems and ancillary systems and then combines and maintains it with historical patient health data within a clinical data repository for rapid retrieval through a workstation. As noted in Figure 5-1, the workstation serves as a window to all the contributing applications that send data to the repository. The EHR system products designed for large hospital and integrated delivery settings have been in place for some time and their core functions are reasonably stable and their system support is reliable. There are a limited number of long-term

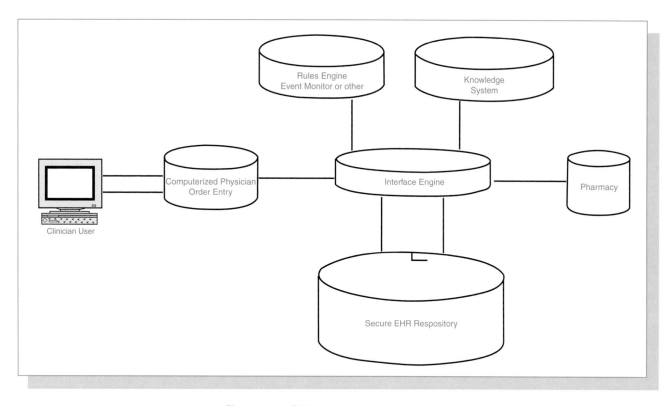

Figure 5-4 Clinical decision support process.

EHR system vendors serving the market for hospitals and larger HMOs and ambulatory centers. These vendors often look to user groups to provide feedback and to influence product upgrades. This is less the case in other environments. Many smaller vendors still come and go in the marketplace, a fact that does not encourage provider's investments in EHR systems.[18]

So, once components are in place and an EHR system is acquired or under development, how do individuals use it? What does such an EHR system actually do? Regardless of the care setting and the EHR system, users must be able to perform basic processes on data. EHR systems must allow users to do the following:

- Access health record data and documents through a variety of patient and health information systems in the organization
- Retrieve and capture data through well-designed workstations with PC, tablet, and wireless tools
- Use communication and network technology to access applications and communicate with peers and patients
- Apply readily available clinical decision support tools and references while engaging in the care process
- Use appropriate security mechanisms

and still support fundamental administrative and clinical processes.

With industry benchmarks, consolidation of a more consistent definition of the components of EHR systems, and evidence of the value of advancing IT in health care,

progress is visible. Since 2003 there is more energy and momentum to develop and implement EHR systems.

WHY DO CURRENT INDUSTRY FORCES ADVANCE THE CASE FOR ELECTRONIC HEALTH RECORD SYSTEMS SUCCESSFULLY TODAY?

Industry Forces That Advance Electronic Health Record Adoption

Patient safety concerns, health services quality, paper record shortcomings, and cost containment demands have strengthened the historical drivers to EHR adoption. National debates and reports are shining a spotlight on health care facts that call for correction and for using technology more effectively. Among six trends identified by the Gartner Research Group on Information Technology, "A 50% growth in healthcare software investment could enable clinicians to cut the level of preventable deaths by half in 2013."[19] This prediction reflects the gathering energy for applying technology to the health care process.

Patient Safety and Data

The IOM issued a series of critical reports on the nation's health care on the basis of a concerted, continuing effort focused on a 1996 initiative to assess and improve the nation's quality of care. In a key report "To Err Is Human: Building a Safer Health System," the authors cite that between 44,000 and 98,000 U.S. deaths per year were caused by medical errors.[10] In the follow-up report, *Crossing the Quality Chasm: A New Health System for the 21st Century,* the authors call for better systems and better data.[20] During the next 5 years, endorsements for industry investment in EHRs and better information sharing grew substantially. Industry leaders, professional organizations, and payers added their perspectives. Notable work by the Markel Foundation's public-private collaborative, Connecting for Health,[21] and the Leapfrog Group invested in partnerships with government, industry, health care, and consumers expanded the discussion and strengthened the drive to focus on patient safety through improving the health information needs for the country.[22] In fact, an overwhelming 94% of the health care leaders responding to a survey for Futurescan predicted that hospital EHRs would be in widespread use by 2010. Another 76% predicted that complete EHR systems, including inpatient, outpatient, and physician components would be in use by 2010.[23]

Substantial progress in hospital EHR systems in the Veteran's Administration offers significant evidence that care can be improved and become more efficient when these systems are used.[24] Payers got into the act as well. A Governance Institute White Paper issued in the fall of 2004 cited that the Boeing Company, which had invested heavily in using payment incentives to encourage hospitals to adopt safety initiatives, announced that it will continue to pay 100% of employee hospital bills where hospitals meet Leapfrog's safety goals.[25]

National Focus on Improving Health Information and Technology

In April 2004, President Bush called for "the majority of Americans to have interoperable electronic health records within 10 years" and issued an executive order naming Dr. David Brailer as National Coordinator for Health Information Technology.[26] Dr. Brailer, through the Office of the National Coordinator for Health Information Technology (ONCHIT), delivered a critical new strategic framework and a set of four goals:

- Inform clinical practice by providing incentives for EHR adoption, reducing risk, and promoting diffusion in underserved areas
- Interconnect clinicians through regional collaborations and networks and coordinating federal health information systems
- Personalize care by encouraging PHRs, enhancing informed consumer choice for clinicians and services, and promoting telehealth systems
- Improve population health by unifying public health surveillance architectures for interoperability, streamlining quality and health status monitoring, and accelerating research

Creation and diffusion of EHRs, interconnecting physicians and care sites for sharing patient information, using technology tools to support and remind clinicians about care and safety matters, and charging the American consumer with adopting PHRs are key elements for advancing IT in health care. With more comprehensive technology support, improved health surveillance, health status monitoring and research can advance rapidly.[26] In June 2005, ONCHIT formed the national collaboration, the American Health Information Community, to help with nationwide transition to EHRs—including common standards and interoperability. Federal dollars and funded research are beginning to help move the work forward.[27] See Chapter 3 for more information on the national efforts to increase the application of IT to health care information.

Today, examples of transition to EHRs are a reality in all types of health care settings. Increasing adoption requires the capacity to initiate change effectively, moving from paper-based and scattered information systems environments to fully integrated interconnectivity and functioning institutional EHRs. Ideally, as organizations recognize the value of EHR systems, they will also recognize the value of standards applied to both data content and data exchange.

The HIM profession plays a pivotal role in advancing the transition to EHRs. HIM professionals are challenged to understand, lead, and manage a transition between paper and electronic media and ensure the quality and availability of patient data in a changing environment. The goals set for health care in the new millennium are ambitious. HIM professionals work side by side with medical and clinical informatics colleagues as electronic health information management, also referred to as applied health informatics, brings us to the objective of improved patient care and improved health information systems.

For **health informatics,** which is the "science that deals with health information, its structure acquisition, and uses," the foundation role of EHRs has been a clearly stated goal.[28] The infrastructure, hardware, software, communications, and building block systems required to implement EHR systems are better understood today, although the vision of the potential of electronic health information systems continues to evolve. Today's view draws on a synergistic reality. Current systems tend to pull data from multiple applications, organize it, store it in a database and then link applications with data integration, communications, decision support capability, and workstation navigational tools to establish a functional EHR system. This suite of applications and tools may be unique to health care organizations. It is the data, the connectivity, and the user interface that brings it all together. Monda and Nunn[29] illustrated this complex concept, termed the CPR, "a corporate information factory," as shown in Figure 5-5.

The health care environment is currently exploring how to move to an integrated delivery and information system that respects individual privacy rights. More than ever, we understand the need for longitudinal information to support patient treatments to achieve better outcomes. Health IT initiatives

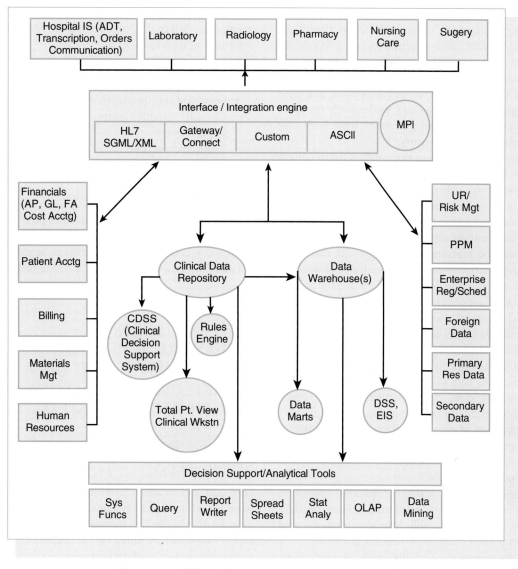

Figure 5-5 EHR: health care's corporate information factory.

are influenced by government and payers. The HIPAA legislation that mandated electronic claims processing through standard transactions and code sets is an excellent example of a government initiative. As organizations acquire and refine administrative and clinical systems, the pressure is on for health care organizations to use their information systems to do the following

- Deliver data for the more efficient operation of daily business activities
- Demonstrate cost-effectiveness
- Provide extensive patient data to a growing number of authorized users within and beyond the organization
- Contain easy tools for management analysis
- Offer streamlined data capture, particularly for use by direct care providers
- Make summary and aggregate data readily available for administrative and clinical decision support
- Standardize communications

- Define and deliver data as an organizational resource through **clinical data repositories** and **data warehouses**
- Establish a network infrastructure to enable linkages within and beyond organizations to community, regional, and national data systems
- Maintain effective data security measures[30]
- Be capable of efficient connectivity so that the assembly and use of the data by repositories and warehouses yield timely, accurate, and increasingly comprehensive views of an individual's EHR

More detailed discussion of the technical architecture and applications that serve as a foundation for EHR systems can be found in Chapter 8.

Paper Records Drawbacks

The limitations of paper records continue to present problems. As a physical entity, the record is in a single location for a single use and is restricted to one user at a time. By its very nature, the paper record cannot meet the needs of complex care environments; its use is becoming unrealistic in the presence of pressures to control operational costs and deliver information effectively. The complexity of the health care delivery process in managed care and integrated delivery systems underscores the need for effective health information systems to meet both care and care coordination requirements.

The style and completeness of documentation in patient records varies from one setting to another. Many of the traditional paper record entries rely on open-ended narrative. It is difficult in many paper systems to easily identify what facts are missing. There is no easy way to check for data and information inconsistencies in paper records. The data cannot be rearranged for display in alternative formats that might help view data relationships in new ways. The record is limited to the fundamental chronological flow of information. Caregivers and researchers must page through thick documents to connect related information from many and often diverse locations. The paper record's weaknesses in understandability, legibility, chronology, and data organization are difficult if not impossible to overcome.

Health care needs data in aggregate form to understand the effectiveness of care. Health services research needs aggregate data for evaluation of cost and quality. Although a considerable amount of data is available through national and regional public databases, these data have limitations. EHR systems will offer new resources to both internal and external studies of patient care.

Patients and providers want the patient record to function beyond a basic data repository. Adding decision support tools, for example, will help organizations and clinicians meet patient safety improvement goals.

Although the technical capability exists to send documents and images produced by external resources such as radiologists, other care settings, special study programs, and education, the business framework and policies lag behind. One reason for this is that unlimited information in such varied formats is difficult to manage in a system where the users expect almost immediate response time. As technology offers more **multimedia** capacity for voice, data, image, and video and faster electronic transmission of data, this is changing. Multimedia capacity will allow incorporation of additional information on patients from internal and external sources.

Cost Containment and Return on Investment

Implementing EHR systems will save some costs and add efficiency to organizational patient services. In addition to the obvious, such as eliminating paper supplies and the clerical staff needed to process paper records, reducing transcription costs, and eliminating copy service, a business case for adopting EHRs can be made from a broader perspective. Ball et al[31] point out major metrics to be used in determining the business case:

- Cost savings
- Cost avoidance
- Improved staff productivity
- Clinical quality improvement/medical outcome improvement
- Reduced cycle time
- Improved process accuracy
- Improved customer (physician/patient) satisfaction
- Improved employee satisfaction

In addition, data availability, provider productivity, service efficiency, and operational savings can be measured. Evidence mounts that benefits of EHR systems can be realized, although not all of the known benefits can be tied to metrics.

HOW DO TECHNICAL INFRASTRUCTURE, DATA REQUIREMENTS, AND OPERATIONS WORKFLOW FIT IN ELECTRONIC HEALTH RECORD SYSTEMS?

Technical Infrastructure and Data Requirements

Technical infrastructure refers to the technology architecture required to maintain systems. Technology infrastructure includes the hardware, software, network, and communication resources required as underpinning to an EHR system. Of course, workstations must be deployed across the organizations so that user access is facilitated. Analogous to a transportation infrastructure, voice, data, image, and video need adequate size transport (networks) to get the job done. Chapter 8 details how infrastructure fits together to support health information systems, their functions, and interoperability. What is important to note is that infrastructure provides the foundation to link legacy systems with new applications and must be robust enough to handle "industrial strength" secure data processing, storage, and widespread access and retrieval.

Data Requirements for the Electronic Health Record

Along with the technology infrastructure, data requirements must be addressed in migrating to an EHR environment. **Data** elements themselves can be viewed as the raw material of information systems. Users require data that are transformed into information and then into knowledge. Van Bemmel and Musen[32] noted that a patient or a biologic process generates data, which are observed by the clinician with subsequent information derived from interpretation. Uninterpreted data elements are given to the problem solver. This includes data as elementary as age, pulse rate, test result, diagnostic code, height, and weight.

On the other hand, **information** refers to a collection of data that contains meaning when data are processed, resulting in a display or report containing information. In this context, data and information can be stored in a permanent, accessible database. The EHR, stored or accessible on-line, would include data and information resulting from the analysis and processing of other data. For example, results reported from laboratory tests and presented through a computer workstation flow sheet provide time-oriented information to the provider of care.

Knowledge is defined as the "formalization of the relationships among elements of information and data" (p. 60).[33] That is, new data or information can be inferred from the data and information already present. For example, test results (data) can be organized into a diabetic care management flow sheet (information) and a clinician can assess that a patient's condition has undergone a change (knowledge). Perhaps the most easily understood description of knowledge in this context is the use of rules that are applied to the data and information that enable providers to apply medical judgment to the care processes.

Covey[33] noted that the "contents" of EHRs and health information systems can be expressed as data types or as data elements. Table 5-4 lists the variety of data types required in patient record systems. Data types should be presented in ways that provide information when comparisons, trends, and confirmation of differential diagnostic investigations are sought by clinical providers. If we understand the role of data types more clearly, we can better comprehend the complexity of moving from data to information to knowledge. Significant thought must be given to transforming data into information for the pur-

poses of medical knowledge. The ability to collect, organize, analyze, and retrieve data by computers in a meaningful way extends and expands the discriminating capacity and problem-solving abilities of providers and the value of EHRs.

Data interface standards such as those developed by X12 and HL7 standards development organizations, vocabulary dictionaries, and interface engines are used to transfer data. Sometimes data are translated or reformatted as required. HIPAA legislation imposed standards on the data exchange of billing data. Certain coding systems and an X12 schema for data transfer are required. The intent of this change is to reduce the administrative costs associated with the billing process. In many cases, data are transferred to institutional or community repositories for future use. The data definitions and codes need to be standardized to provide useful data.

Clinical Data Repositories

Depending on the institution and its information systems plan, the clinical data repository may be one of the components of an institutional data warehouse that is designed to collect, organize, and analyze all institutional business and clinical data that have been summarized and aggregated for that purpose. They are designed to deliver the individual patient's information to the care team through the clinical workstation. It is here that the content and presentation capability takes over.[3]

Data can be presented in a series of clinical views or profiles designed to deliver the EHR content to users. Golob[34] characterized the purposes of a clinical data repository as follows:

- Provides easy access to patient information for providers and demonstrates time saved over paper record use
- Expedites results reporting through customizable displays
- Provides quick and easy access to longitudinal patient data
- Supports a common user interface for accessing patient information, usually through a workstation
- Provides information in a comprehensive, integrated manner rather than by departmental orientation
- Provides an easy vehicle for applying population management for the prospective clinical planning needed today
- Supports monitoring and analysis of patient care outcomes

Many health care organizations also establish information (or data) warehouses that receive clinical data from a transactions system such as a pharmacy system or a radiology system and combine them with other organizational data from administrative and financial systems. State and other data systems that require data from hospitals or participating organizations are examples of data repositories. In

Table 5-4   DATA TYPES REQUIRED FOR ELECTRONIC HEALTH RECORDS

Data Type	Examples
Text	Hospital discharge, summary, history and physical examination, narrative operative reports
Numbers	ICD-9-CM codes CPT codes Blood pressure value recording
Voice	Stored dictation accessed by phone or personal computer. voice recognition or radiology dictation films
Image	Radiology film, document image
Video	Echocardiogram
Drawings	Drawing of burn distribution on body surface
Signal	Electroencephalogram or ECG tracings

fact, the advances made in community-based health information systems have relied on the principles and benefits of the repository approach. Its ability to provide data and information across institutional settings makes the repository valuable to participating providers. Even organizations taking a slower approach to acquiring an EHR in their institutional settings may already be involved in community-based health information through their participation in state data systems or, more recently, regional health information organizations (RHIOs).

Vocabularies and the Electronic Health Record

To establish EHR systems with predictable data requires standardized vocabularies that are used to represent concepts and to communicate them, including symptoms, diagnoses, procedures, and health status. A controlled vocabulary refers to a code or **classification system** that requires information to be represented in a pre-established recognized system such as the *International Classification of Diseases,* Ninth Edition, *Clinical Modification* (ICD-9-CM), or *Systematized Nomenclature of Human and Veterinary Medicine* (SNOMED). Some coding systems are classification systems and some are nomenclatures. For a more extensive discussion of this topic, see Chapter 6. Over the years, summarized data from patient records were typically represented by codes. Today, a variety of ways are being explored to represent data in patient records.

Coded data are exemplified by the use of standard coding systems such as the ICD-9-CM, SNOMED, and *Current Procedural Terminology* (CPT) systems or by special vocabularies such as those developed to represent nursing concepts. A health care organization is likely using multiple coding systems in its efforts to organize and communicate its computerized data. Coded data have the advantage of consistency of expression for diagnoses, procedures, laboratory tests, drugs, and so on. Yet, because of the strengths and weaknesses in these systems, none completely addresses the clarity and precision required to capture and represent all clinical facts contained in patient records. The National Library of Medicine project to establish the Unified Medical Language System is an ambitious attempt to bring together diverse coding schemes with general medical terms to create a vast thesaurus linking related clinical terms for the benefit of diverse users.

Many health information system developers spend significant energy improving coding systems used for claims processing, billing, and epidemiologic and outcomes research efforts. These efforts are focused on using ICD-9-CM and the *International Classification of Diseases,* 10th edition (ICD-10). SNOMED-CT, a nomenclature, is identified as having the most potential to handle the complex data representation required in EHRs.

Advocates believe that strong coding schemes are essential components of health information systems and that the fastest way to establish and secure consistent data from health care organizations is through standard coding systems. There continues to be national and international interest in identifying an "ideal" coding system to secure accurate, efficient data capture from the care delivery experience that accurately represents the clinical concepts. Coding systems are critical to capturing and processing clinical data consistently. Codes are used to represent information in a predictable, consistent, and reproducible manner.[3] ICD and SNOMED tools address part of the problem but do not fully support current models of thinking used by physicians and other health care team members in the care delivery process.

Vocabularies are used to represent concepts and to communicate these concepts. A major component of the patient record in most organizations is unstructured text. This is the most natural medium of expression and, to date, best represents the thinking and conclusions of those planning and delivering care. In fact, the majority of the content of paper records is narrative text. Because of this, the value of technology for natural language processing is well recognized. "Medicine needs a system based on an architecture that can capture medical data in natural language form, structure it in alternative ways and retrieve it through queries that allow users to retrieve and display information in multiple forms including conversion into standard codes as well as natural language expressions. **Text processing** may be defined as the computerized processing of natural language."[3] This is a far more sophisticated endeavor than searching text by key words, a process well known in library research today. Text processing requires comprehensiveness and completeness of content such that a given domain of medicine is adequately represented. **Natural language processing** for cardiology, for instance, would need to include all the terms and expressions used by cardiologists in their models of thinking. Symptoms, related medical terms, and specific cardiology expressions (including semantic linkages and relationships) would all be required elements

Script-based systems, an alternative form of structured text, combine key words and scripts. A script may be a predesigned expression that represents information about consequences of care processes. Scanning for key words invokes a particular script. The script itself then serves as a building block for the remainder of the text-processing event. It may act as a template that specifies necessary components and the properties required. Medical transcriptionists apply a similar concept when they develop and maintain stored phrases that can be invoked to assemble reports such as history and physical examinations quickly. This allows single key words to be indexed to longer medical expressions. Physician dictation, for instance, is significantly streamlined when such tools are used.

Newer approaches to handling narrative text organize the text in a consistent manner and establish standard tags to label the text. Standard generalized markup language (SGML), hypertext markup language (HTML), and extensible markup language (XML) are used to organize the data within documents by displaying information in standard ways to allow users to launch from key words in one document to other documents. Transcribed reports are then organized according to predetermined formats that can be labeled and retrieved for manipulation. Chapter 8 offers additional detail on these topics.

HOW DO ISSUES AND BARRIERS AFFECT ELECTRONIC HEALTH RECORD PLANNING AND IMPLEMENTATION?

Selected Issues and Barriers

To achieve the benefits sought in the health information systems and associated EHRs discussed in this chapter, the health care industry must address a number of issues and barriers. Issues to be addressed to successfully acquire EHR systems include the following:

- Cost requirements to get EHR system projects under way
- Technology infrastructure and customer expectations
- Legislation that lags behind the uses of technology
- Confidentiality and security concerns
- Inadequate health informatics standards

Cost Issues

Costs associated with EHRS are a major concern. Because EHRs are still relatively new, few definitive studies exist that provide useful information on economic benefits. In fact, it has been pointed out that evaluating components of EHRs will produce conflicting results.[3] It is difficult to measure individual areas of decision support and more effective information management. Examples of cost items beyond the products are project development and management, vendor selection, consultants, system implementation, interfaces and networks, and training. Once the system is in place, many values have been identified. Value opportunities of the EHR stem from several attributes including the following:

- Enhanced knowledge asset for clinical and administrative purposes
- Standard data set
- Standard descriptive nomenclature
- Utilization review– and quality assurance–driven rules
- Storage of discrete clinical data with expanded opportunities for users
- Improved care process driven by information availability
- Interdisciplinary, fully integrated critical paths
- Integrated medication cycle with potential for improving patient safety

- Alerts and reminders for the care process and health services
- Protocols (care algorithms)
- Improved documentation
- Improved operational processes from the care cycle to information management
- Instant records access for clinical and administrative purposes
- Faster claims processing
- Coding efficiencies
- Revenue cycle enhancements
- Enhanced medical management
- Support for strategy
- Master patient index
- Customer satisfaction—patients, clinicians and administrative staff
- Decision support
- Patient safety
- Support for strategic initiatives[3]

This list exemplifies the range of potential cost impact. It includes some basics that aid HIM managers and others to advance the case for EHRs for their organizations within an issues document or a white paper that presents current costs in HIM business processes. Facts about operational workflow from existing and anticipated viewpoints can incorporate benchmark data for decision making and contribute to the strategic planning process when organizations mount institutional initiatives for acquiring EHR systems.

Infrastructure Requirements

As already discussed in this chapter, fundamental infrastructure is essential to EHR developments. The computing power must be established with appropriate networks and adequate workstations. The enterprise information technology strategy dictates the potential for all systems. Customers expect access to and easy navigation in crucial health information. The care team relies on sufficient deployment of workstations to aid daily care activities. Even in the initial development of EHR capability, the basic retrieval of clinical data such as test results, images, and transcribed reports is a common expectation.

As efforts advance to strengthen data capture at the point of care, workstations (stationary or mobile) need to be near the delivery of care. EHRs must be accessible by those who direct care from mobile, external, and internal sites. As data repositories grow and access to expert systems and research expands, the customer expects that the necessary infrastructure will move and deliver data and images—not to mention video—at a credible speed. Continuous assessment and expansion of the technology infrastructure go hand in hand with EHR developments. The infrastructure required to for EHR systems depends on investment in infrastructure, continuing support, and a tolerance for adding emerging technological tools.

Laws and Progress

There are state-by-state variations in laws related to EHR systems—electronic signature, format and retention, but in most states general business laws recognize the use of computerized records and digital signatures. However, because of some state laws and the concern about the long-term accessibility of digital data, many organizations feel compelled to retain paper record printouts of EHRs. The focus on developing the EHR system has been primarily from a clinical and billing perspective of getting the data into the system and meeting short-term use requirements. Easy access to data over long periods of time requires much more planning and maintenance. Costs associated with keeping dual systems, paper and electronic, reduce value and benefits of the EHR.

Confidentiality and Security

Confidentiality and security are continuing topics of discussion and the subjects of state and national legislation. If the goal is to implement EHRs within the next 10 years, EHR systems need to protect the confidentiality of patient data, provide appropriate access, and use recognized data security measures.[35] "This is not entirely a "systems" issue. Providing a secure and confidential system involves people. Many of the measures that will provide confidentiality and security are embedded in commitments from the people who handle health information. These individuals must be trained, know the constraints on the use of health information, and be subject to penalty for misuse of the information. HIM professionals have always been part of the system's effort to protect the confidentiality and security of health information. In today's environment, HIM professionals often have more comprehensive roles in enterprise privacy and security oversight. The privacy and security standards in the HIPPA of 1996 reinforced this activity.

Privacy is the right of individuals to control disclosure of their personal information. **Confidentiality** is an ethical and a legal concept endorsed by health professionals to meet the expectation of patients that their information, when provided to an authorized user, will not be redisclosed or misused. **Data security** refers to the technical and procedural methods by which access to confidential information is controlled and managed. Laws frequently guide how confidentiality and privacy concepts are applied. Incorporating these concepts into policies for health information systems and the EHR brings new challenges. Access to health information within and organizational context is based on users' legitimate need to know to perform their jobs. Providers restrict access to specific applications or elements of patient health information according to the requesting individuals' role in the organization and audit or verify that individuals stay within the boundaries of appropriate use.

Within organizations, on the operations side, health information professionals are typically responsible for over-seeing confidentiality matters and updating organizational policies and procedures. Many of these policies and procedures have their roots in paper-based systems and need to be updated. The privacy polices need to be supported by the technical systems design. Comprehensive system and physical security tools are in place in most organizations. (See Chapter 8 for additional discussion of security measures.) The goal is have sufficient protection from unauthorized or inadvertent access, disclosure, modification, or destruction. As more data become available in electronic format, more users will want access from a wider variety of locations with relative ease. The access and use will need to protect an individual's privacy by use of approaches that apply people and system security measures. To manage the confidentiality and data security needs in health information systems effectively, we need to establish the following:

- Institutional oversight groups to recommend policies, approve procedures, and recommend appropriate access and management strategies
- Operational policies and procedures including confidentiality statements signed by all staff
- Thorough education programs for all health facility staff on confidentiality and data security responsibility and accountability
- Individual user identification for all staff keyed to their "need to know" to perform their job functions
- Individual passwords, key cards, and biometric or other means for precise registering of system access
- Monitoring and audit capability for access tracking and follow-up
- Management reports on access and potential confidentiality breaches for line managers to use in supervising staff
- Human resources policies to manage the consequences when staff breach confidentiality

Health Care Information Standards and Interoperability

The role of standards in the health information system environment is paramount. Standards are agreed-on conventions for using terms, code schemes, and processes. They are used to establish information system requirements and processes and designate technical specifications. In health care, we have worked with standards for patient record content and organization, beginning in 1918 with the American College of Surgeons and continuing over the years with the Joint Commission on Accreditation of Healthcare Organization, the federal government, ASTM, HL7, Digital Imaging and Communications in Medicine (DICOM), Institute of Electrical and Electronics Engineers (IEEE), and other standards development groups. Coding systems are standards. Computer systems that use common data definitions recognized throughout a particular industry are using standards. The AHIMA *Glossary of Health Care Statistical Terms* established standards for statistical data.

To meet the goals of consistent and reliable access to longitudinal health care information on patients, we must address standards development in crucial areas. We must agree on the following:

- A vocabulary so that the meaning of terms can be trusted and that information can be compared among institutions
- Conventions to be used to transmit data from one computer system to another to meet interoperability requirements
- Communications protocols if an electronic super-highway is to be achieved for the health care industry
- Technical security standards to be used within the information infrastructure if the American public is to accept the technology benefits inherent in patient data automation

Work on developing standards for these areas has been under way for more than 30 years in voluntary standard setting groups and the federal government. Thoughtful planners, clinicians, and systems developers have recognized that agreements on standards would be essential to successful advancement of interconnected systems. Although individual system developers build and market individual systems that meet the needs of one or more organizations, it is clear that compelling forces such as health care reform, market advantage, cost containment, and the changing nature of health care delivery itself demand that standards development be pursued cooperatively rather than competitively. The need for standards is clear. Both the federal government and private sector recognize the value of standards. Standards are sometimes very specific, such as a decision that only ICD-9-CM codes will be accepted by payers to described diagnoses. Standards are sometimes a guide to action. Standards are not cast in concrete; they need to be changed and updated. Standards require both political will and financial commitment.

The standards initiatives have been reinforced through HIPAA. This legislation called for standards methods to transmit codes for billing and claims. The Medicare drug legislation requires standards for transmitting prescription data electronically with use of National Council on Prescription Drug Programs (NCPDP) standards. Table 5-5 features key standards associated with EHR systems, their source development organization, and their general purpose.[36] Figure 5-6 illustrates the relationship between exchange standards and the EHR.

The significance of continuing standards development and refinement cannot be overstated. The core problems of common data terminology and data exchange methods require standards to support significant progress toward the national goals for health information systems.

WHEN ARE ELECTRONIC HEALTH RECORD SYSTEMS PART OF MIGRATION PATHS IN HEALTH CARE ORGANIZATIONS?

Organizational Migration Benchmarks

Some organizations have selected one vendor's integrated product; some have elected to combine multiple vendors. Other organizations have adopted preliminary strategies for increasing automation in a stepwise manner, moving toward integration at some point in the future. In these cases, it is thought that there is time to take some key steps and wait to

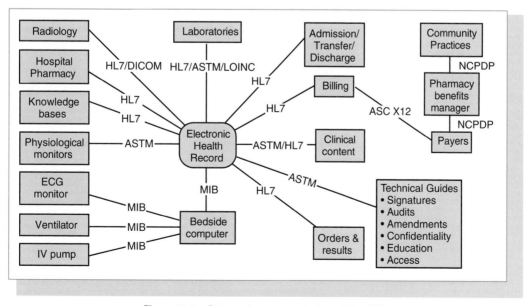

Figure 5-6 Data exchange standards and the EHR.

Table 5-5 HEALTH CARE INFORMATICS STANDARDS AND ELECTRONIC HEALTH RECORDS

Standard	Standards Organization	Purpose	How Standard Contributes to EHR Systems
Data Exchange/Messaging			
Messaging Standards Version 2 and 3 (HL7 V2.X3 and V3)	Health Level Seven www.hl7.org	Electronic message formats for clinical, financial, and administrative data. V2 is common in commercially available software. V3 was launched in January 2005.	Establishes standard message format and "envelope" through which data can be exchanged from one computer system to another. Can be used to support interoperability among applications that may send data to an EHR system
DICOM	National Electronics Manufacturers Association www.nema.org	Format for communicating radiology images and data	Allows information from imaging devices to be accessed and viewed through EHR system
National Council for Prescription Drug Programs (DCISC)	National Council for Prescription Drug Programs www.ncpdp.org	Structure for transmitting prescription requests and fulfillment	Provides standard protocol for sending prescription information between provider EHR applications to pharmacies for billing and claims
Accredited Standards Committee X12 (ANSI ASC X12)	American National Standards Institute (ANSI), Accredited Standards Committee www.x12.org/x12org/index.cfm	Electronic messages for claims, eligibility, and payments	Allows EHR system clinical and administrative data (e.g. diagnostic codes) to be organized for standardized eligibility, claims, and payment purposes.
IEEE 1073	Institute of Electrical and Electronics Engineers Standards Association standards.ieee.org/sa/sa-view.html	Messages for medical device communications	Connects patient data from medical devices such as patient monitors and ventilators, offers practitioners to view those data on applications linked to or part of EHR systems
Terminology			
ICD-9	World Health Organization www.who.int/en	Diagnosis and disease codes commonly used in billing and claims. Version 9 is often used in United States for billing and reimbursement	ICD9-CM codes are assigned on the basis of clinical content and health services documented in her systems to meet research and financial needs.
Logical Observation Identifiers names and Codes (LOINC)	Regenstrief Institute for Health Care www.loinc.org	Concept-based terminology for laboratory orders and results	Provides standard terminology for laboratory test names and results that can be used in EHR systems
SNOMED-CT	College of American Pathologists www.cap.org	Mapping clinical concepts with standard descriptive terms	Provides electronically supported nomenclature representation of patient clinical data in EHR systems. Codes offer the most granular representation of concepts.
Unified Medical Language System (UMLS)	National Library of Medicine www.nim.org	Database of 100 medical terminologies with concept mapping tools	Allows EHR system (program) to understand meaning of the language of biomedicine and health

Table 5-5   HEALTH CARE INFORMATICS STANDARDS AND ELECTRONIC HEALTH RECORDS—cont'd

Standard	Standards Organization	Purpose	How Standard Contributes to EHR Systems
Document Continuity of Care Record (CCR)	ASTM International, E31 Committee on Health Informatics *www.astm.org*	Document format that gives snapshot of patient's core data and recent encounter (allergies, medications, treatment, care plan) and makes it available to next caregiver	Defines core set of clinical data for continuity of care purposes and sets XML standards for data organization of clinical content for electronic data exchange
Clinical Document Architecture (CDA)	Health Level Seven *www.hl7.org*	Standard exchange model for clinical documents such as discharge summaries and progress notes. Formally known as Patient Record Architecture	Provides model to use for document formats for specific clinical documents to be maintained in EHR systems and used when sending and receiving clinical documents
Clinical Document Type Definitions (ASTM 2183-02) (ASTM 2182-02)	ASTM International, E31 Committee on Health Informatics *www.astm.org*	Provides standard specification for XML document type definitions that match electronic document requirements in health care industry (e.g., patient history, discharge summary)	Provides tools to represent clinical data using XML to organize document content and enable Web browser to access information. Provides specifications to organize and apply tags to content (DTD) in healthcare documents to represent content for data exchange purposes.
Content and Structure of Electronic Health Records (ASTM E1384, ASTM E1633)	ASTM International, Committee on Health Informatics *www.astm.org*	Describes content to be included in EHR. Content descriptions range from data elements (defined) to documents	Provides comprehensive data content model to serve as a resource for EHR systems including data element dictionaries and coded data guidelines and definition of longitudinal content with minimum data set specified.
EHR Systems: Draft Standards for Trial Use (HL7: DSTU)	Health Level Seven *www.hl7.org*	Proposed comprehensive functionality for EHR systems; includes health data	Offers draft model of EHR system functions that can assist organizations planning for EHR in determining basic requirements to be considered.
Infrastructure/Policy Information Access Privilege (ASTM E1986-98)	ASTM International, Committee on Health Informatics *www.astm.org*	Standard guide for access privilege for EHR, including emergency setting	Provides comprehensive model to use for information access privilege by health workers
Authentication and Electronic Signature (ASTM E 1762-03) (ASTM E 1985-00) (ASTM E 2084-00)	ASTM International, Committee on Health Informatics *www.astm.org*	Standards guides for establishing and managing authentication and electronic signature	Provide guidelines for policy and procedures and business rules for user requirements for designing/selecting electronic mechanisms to enable authentication and electronic signatures for EHR systems.
Audit and Disclosure Logs (ASTM E 2147-01)	ASTM International, Committee on Health Informatics *www.astm.org*	Describes specifications for audit trials in manual and EHR environment	Provides structures of information disclosure logs/audit trails
Amendments to Electronic Health Information (ASTM E 2017-99)	ASTM International, Committee on Health Informatics *www.astm.org*	Addresses criteria for amending individually identifiable health information	Serves as a basis for policy development and user requirements for processing amendments in EHR systems

adopt a single-focus direction. The benefits of working with one vendor are speed of implementation and tight integration of applications. A number of vendors offer EHR software and include multimedia functionality in their products. For many hospitals and other health care organizations, this is the best approach. Organizations often rely on a vendor's history, experience, and support of the necessary interfaces to existing applications in their organizations in making purchase decisions.

Many of these vendors have experienced health information professionals in positions ranging from design consultants to vice presidents. This strengthens their products from the patient record management perspective. Health information professionals have made significant gains in leading efforts to transform the paper record into electronic formats. One early strategy was to begin with on-line storage of transcribed significant reports such as discharge summaries and operative and radiology reports. On-line storage, access to transcribed reports, and links to other legacy systems such as the laboratory and the pharmacy offered a rudimentary beginning to an EHR system. The increased availability of personal computer workstations also enhanced the interest in EHRs.

There are, of course, management issues concerning the volume and organization of data in major organizational efforts to implement an EHR system. As yet, no vendor can deliver all the components of an EHR system with the consistent strength to produce the EHR as it is envisioned today. Most organizations and vendors acknowledge the value of an integrated system, but producing an integrated system that does everything well is difficult. One approach of vendors is to combine the data from legacy systems and new applications within a single organization—data transferred from diverse applications (perhaps running on different computer platforms)—and reorganize the data into a clinical data repository. Developing a data repository offers organizations the ability to establish the database and provide access to patient data normally contained in patient records. This repository is designed to deliver the longitudinal collection of data about individuals to providers, have the capability of a database for reporting, and have some patient record functionality.

Who Offers Relevant Benchmark Data About the Electronic Health Record Experience?

Brigham and Women's Hospital and Partners Healthcare System

The Brigham and Women's Hospital and Partners Healthcare System has extensive experience in "growing" enterprise-based EHR systems. The Brigham and Women's Hospital and Partners Healthcare System includes seven hospitals and more than 250 practice sites, including large suburban practices and single-provider rural practices. The developers of this EHR application focused on workflow analysis, believing that the solutions must improve current practices and designing the application components to do just that. For example, the outpatient notes are computerized but the inpatient notes are not.[3]

The developers built the EHR on a foundation of major clinical applications. They applied the philosophy that each new feature would add value and make sense for the users. Strong support in implementation was a behavioral tenet, and e-mail feedback was a particularly helpful tool for the implementation process. In addition, an emphasis on clinical decision support provides the most visible impact of the system. Order entry is used to write all orders for adult inpatient services. About 14,000 orders are entered daily by resident and attending physicians, nurses, nurse-midwives, physician assistants, and students. Order templates have been developed to facilitate order types and special-purpose cases. The order entry application uses cost and quality monitoring criteria. Teich noted that "order entry has been the single most effective tool in improving the quality of care via the computer."[3] Along with the order entry capacity to alert providers, an **event engine** tracks unexpected data. For example, this tool uses a logical inference engine that notes laboratory result "triggers" and notifies the providers by e-mail and beepers that something unusual has occurred.

The Brigham Integrated Computing System (BICS) ambulatory record is a paperless record that includes full notes, problem lists, medications, allergies, vital signs, advance directives, health maintenance information, flow sheets for specific problems, and other aids and supports. In addition, laboratory results, discharge summaries, and all other on-line clinical information are viewed from workstations located in offices, examination rooms, and patient intake areas. An interesting feature is "patient at a glance," which summarizes key data on one screen. Problems, medications, allergies, and recent visit data are immediately available. This record is available at any time, at any location. It maintains consistency in data presentation so that the user can count on the same data availability in the same format at each access. Among the unique features is a health maintenance section that is designed to maintain monitoring data such as Papanicolaou smear results and cholesterol level test results. Reminders are issued when specific monitoring tests are due.[3]

This illustration is not unique in the development of EHR systems. Health care enterprise organizations such as Columbia-Presbyterian Medical Center, the Veterans Administration Computerized Patient Record system, and many others enjoy significant progress in EHR developments. These organizations are notable for their inclusion of key elements of the computer-based patient record goal articulated in the previous decade. These organizations represent evidence of real progress toward the goal of a fully electronic health record system.

How Do Health Information Management Business Processes Change in the Electronic Health Record Environment?

Changing the Business Processes of Health Information Management

The technology influence on the record in hybrid and electronic settings changes the way business is done. By use of the general chronology of HIM business processes, the following section reviews major HIM business processes in health care organizations and how these activities are changing from the transition environment of hybrid records to the environment of fully electronic health records. Understanding the processes and HIM roles and how they change with EHR systems is important in preparing for current and future professional practice.

WHAT MANAGEMENT QUESTIONS/TOPICS NEED TO BE DISCUSSED AS WE MOVE TO THE VIRTUAL HEALTH INFORMATION DEPARTMENT?

Introduction

The patient and his or her information are the center of the health care delivery system. Without patients, the health care system would not exist; without a health care system of some type, patients would not come to be listened to, examined, tested, diagnosed, and treated. Whenever a patient and provider interact within the health care delivery system, whether the communication is clinical or administrative in nature, face to face, on the telephone, or conducted by use of a new technology, information is set down in a record to preserve knowledge of what happened. The documentation in the record is the patient's health information, which means different things to different people depending on the context in which it is being used or discussed. Original health information, created during an interaction between a patient and a health care professional, has a life cycle of its own and often goes through many permutations before it is filed and complete. During the course of a lifetime, a person's health records are created and maintained in many different settings, for example, the hospital where they were born, the clinics and physician offices where they were treated, schools, the military, and so forth. Technological innovations are radically altering the processes that are used to collect, process, and store and retrieve health information. The health record itself, at one time simply a collection of various documents stored in a manila folder, is also in the midst of a major transformation.

Because health information and health record processes and technologies are changing, traditional HIM professional management of both an individual patient's health record and multiple health records is shifting as well. Standards, laws, and regulations are being modified to reflect changes in technology and processes. What is not changing are the basic reasons that health information is recorded and the core documentation principles.

To understand the evolving health record, one must understand the types of health information content that make up a health record, the modalities used to capture the content, and the processes used to manage each. All these elements are undergoing a major change and will continue to do so. As the elements change and evolve, so will the HIM roles. It is incumbent on current and emerging HIM leaders to envision the new EHR reality and make a conscious choice to assist in the transition from manual, paper-bound departments to a mature organization-wide EHR.

Documentation Principles

Recall that the basic purpose of recording health information is simply to preserve what went on between the patient and the provider. How and what clinicians document in the health record is based on their original training, their experiences as residents/trainees working under attending physicians or preceptor guidance, reimbursement requirements, and the type of training they have received from HIM documentation specialists. In addition, documentation principles are derived from accreditation standards, clinical specialty societies, and state licensing bodies. Federal laws, reimbursement guidelines, and clinical coding organizations advise or mandate certain aspects of clinical documentation. It is critical to understand that the standards remain the same for both manual and electronic health records; it does not matter how the information is captured or how it is reported.

Unique patient identification. The documentation and data must always be linked to the correct patient's identification (usually at least the patient's name and unique identification number) at the time of capturing information, generating reports, and accessing the information. The system should provide linkage between the different identities of the same patient, identification of potential duplicate numbers of the same patient, and a method to merge/correct them and distinguish between patients with similar names.

Legibility. Documentation, including signatures, must be legible (i.e., it must be easily readable). If not legible, documentation becomes a major patient safety issue. Orders can be misunderstood, medications or dosages may be misread, and patient care can be compromised. An EHR where all documentation is entered directly through keyboarding or is transcribed and uploaded to the system is, of course, legible. A scanned handwritten document, however, is really only as legible as the original handwriting. Yes, in many systems, one can magnify portions of the scanned document, but this is an extra step that takes time and should not be considered a normal practice.

Accuracy. Information throughout a report and the record itself needs to be accurate and consistent and not contradict itself.

Completeness. The document and record must be complete according to standards adhered to by the organization. What content is required for a particular health care intervention (e.g., what are the required elements of a history and physical? an operative report? an informed consent? an authorization for disclosure? an initial assessment outpatient note? a transfer summary? a discharge summary? etc.)? If there is an addendum to the document, can it be retrieved with the original document? Is an addendum clearly marked for the reader? Accrediting bodies, regulatory bodies, clinician specialty, organizational policies. and reimbursement rules drive the content considered necessary.

Timeliness. Timeliness of documentation is linked to accurate documentation. Individual documents in the record must be created in a timely manner, again according to standards used by the organization. If documentation is created too distant from the patient care encounter, the accuracy of the documentation can be questioned. Because a clinician is treating many patients every day, it is difficult to believe he or she can remember enough detail to fully record the encounter if it is not done soon after the encounter. Timely documentation is key for the continuum of care when another provider who needs information from previous encounters sees the patient. In an EHR, timeliness tracking is an inherent process of the computer where the documentation is taking place. In the paper world, time is often left out when handwriting a note.

Integrity. Integrity in a health record means that data or the content in an order or a text document such as a history and physical examination, operative report, progress note, discharge summary, laboratory result, and so forth has not been altered or destroyed in an unauthorized manner.[37] In the paper world, any changes in an original document or report were accomplished by drawing a line through the erroneous entry, handwriting the changes, and then dating and initialing the entries. When one enters a hybrid entry in an electronic environment, health record integrity becomes a significantly larger issue, one in which the HIM professional is uniquely qualified to set policy and business processes that ensure the organization's EHR integrity. Content integrity is coupled with both document authentication and security. (See Chapter 8 for a discussion on security.) Health record integrity management requires an exquisite understanding of the various, authorized ways in which document content may be changed.

Authentication. Each entry in the health record must identify who (or what in the case of machines) created the entry or document and who is responsible for its accuracy, timeliness, and completion. Its author must authenticate each entry or document. Authentication is the process of identifying the source of health record entries by attaching a handwritten signature, the author's initials, or an electronic signature. In a paper system, authentication means a legible, handwritten signature.

In an electronic system, the electronic signature must ensure that the signed document was not modified after the signature was affixed. Additionally, the electronic signature must ensure that only the signer could have created a signature. This requirement is called nonrepudiation. After the signature has been affixed, any change in the document's information must cause the signature verification process to detect that the information has been changed. This ensures the integrity of the author's content and prevents others from altering the information. Some systems guarantee document integrity by "locking" the document after the electronic signature has been affixed. To display a change, therefore, the same or different author must write an addendum to the original document that requires an electronic signature as well with the same functionalities.

Privacy, Confidentiality, and Security. Health information must adhere to federal and state laws to protect both the patient and the organization. This is discussed in more detail in Chapters 8 and 15.

Although core documentation principles remain basically the same in both paper and electronic formats, how they are defined or implemented within a specific organization may vary, depending on the organization's process in implementing an EHR system. For example, authentication on a paper document could mean a physical signature by a physician, appended by his professional degree, MD, and his specialty, cardiology. In an electronic document, a standard (or organizational policy) might also require his PIN (provider identification number) as well. Each of these elements can be defined somewhat differently depending on a standard, law, reimbursement requirement, and so forth, as well as the organization in which the clinician is practicing. The Joint Commission has core documentation standards, many of which are found in the *Management of Information* chapter in their various manuals. Certain other documentation standards are found in the *Provision of Care, Treatment and Services* chapter.[37] These standards are often revised; it is important, therefore, to stay abreast of changes by visiting The Joint Commission Web site on a regular basis.

The Physical Past

Most health care organizations are just beginning to emerge from a manual, paper health record system. In this type of manual, paper-based system, health information is stored as various types of paper documents in manila folders, the health record, each of which identifies the patient, usually with a unique patient medical record number. The documents may include computer-generated registration information, handwritten or transcribed clinical documents, various kinds of laboratory results and reports, and administrative and medical correspondence from other health care providers.

The systems are physical; the health records (the "charts") are stored on shelves in various types of file rooms or on racks on inpatient wards. Managing physical chart movement is a major HIM function in a traditional paper-based health record system. The charts must be physically moved from place to place and each movement tracked with some sort of manual or computerized tracking system. Knowing where each chart is at all times is critical because various authorized users of the chart may need it at the same time. Only one person can use/view the chart at one time. For example, a clinician wants the chart to finish dictating his discharge summary. An HIM coder needs the chart to code the chart to meet the billing deadline. An HIM release of information (ROI) technician needs the chart to release information to another outside provider. And, of course, if the patient is presenting for care, the chart must be provided to the clinician, preferably in advance of the encounter.

Individual documents, loose reports, must be manually filed one by one in the correct patient record. If the record is not in the file room, then the file clerk must drop file reports in an outguide that is placed in the location where the health record will be returned.

In a traditional, manual environment, most HIM functions and provider/patient interactions are totally dependent on having the hard copy health record to perform their tasks. For that matter, the organization is also dependent on a well-managed paper health record system that requires the health record to be physically present for the reader to access and use the information contained in it. And, the documents must be filed accurately and include all up-to-date information. HIM managers of paper health record systems are under tremendous pressures to ensure record availability and completeness, especially in large organizations that have active, ambulatory care with more than 2500 scheduled and unscheduled visits each day. How well a traditional HIM department functions is predicated, to a large part, on the efficient and effective management of the file unit.

The Emerging Present

As organizations leave a mostly manual, paper-based environment, they are entering a hybrid health information world where some parts of the health record itself and some of its processes may be manual or electronic. The HIM professional must view himself or herself as a change master and develop the skill to conceive, construct, and convert current behavior into a new, living organizational reality.[38] This means clearly understanding current HIM practices from clinical documentation to management of HIM functions at all levels. Almost all medium and large health care organizations generate or store some part of health information in an electronic format. (See Chapter 8 for a discussion of health information systems.) Many of the business processes that are managed by HIM are actually systems themselves. As Scholtes[39] describes, system refers to interactions and interdependencies on a large scale;

processes refer to components of the system. Processes have purposes and functions of their own, but by themselves processes cannot accomplish the purpose of a system. When viewing an HIM department in an organization, we are looking at a complex social system and a technical system consisting of several subsystems and processes. The health record system is but one interacting, interdependent part of the larger system. When an organization or a section of an organization begins to move from a paper to a hybrid environment, the changes may be uncomfortable for all levels of staff. This is a normal reaction to change and it is important for the HIM professional to understand this about one's self as well as for clerks, coders, transcriptionists, administrators, nurses, physicians, and so forth. Planning in as much detail as possible is critical. In fact, it is important to visualize the eventual positive outcomes and then work backward to identify the necessary tasks. Project management is a necessary skill for anyone who is working in a hybrid system going to a total electronic health record system.

Although the business processes that a HIM department manages may differ in sequencing in various organizations, the flow described in Figure 5-5 is typical. Using somewhat different terminology, following are some common information processes that support clinical activities that need to be evaluated as an organization moves into a hybrid environment.

Patient Identity Management

Although the operational unit that handles patient registration and admissions ordinarily performs the daily operational tasks of registering and admitting a patient, it is the HIM department that carries out quality control reconciliation processes when duplicate names or numbers appear. This may mean correcting the master patient index (MPI) entries of one or more patients or tracking down document and data in both paper and electronic systems to ensure that the patient's information is flowing correctly from one system to the other. In a paper health record system, HIM staff members often physically correct patient identity information by hand on every single page of the record. In an EHR, however, corrections may be done by keyboarding changes without necessarily accessing a paper document. There are three linking methods that may used to determine the correct patient:

One method compares records on selected data elements, usually name, birth date, social security number (SSN), or sex. Exact match and deterministic linking are examples. In an exact match, all specified data elements must be identical. With a deterministic method, specified data elements must be an exact match or a partial match. Partial matches can include substring matches (e.g., first three letters of the last name or last four numbers of the SSN) or phonetic matches (e.g., Soundex).

An intermediate method enhances exact match and deterministic tools with additional logic and arbitrary or subjective scoring systems including subjective weighting, ad hoc weighting, fuzzy logic, and rules-based algorithms. With this type of method, the health care organization assigns a value to key patient identifying attributes such as the last name, first name, date of birth, and so forth.

The most advanced set of identity management tools for matching records relies on mathematical theory. Mathematical algorithms are used to supplement or enhance the tools available in the basic and intermediate methods. Probabilistic, bipartite graph theory/mathematical modeling, machine learning, and neural networks are examples of advanced matching tools.[40]

Only when the MPI is in an electronic form can these more sophisticated matching techniques be used.

Providing Prior Information. Once a patient arrives for care, either as a scheduled or unscheduled admission or visit, or after registration and admitting staff has verified the patient's identity, HIM is responsible for providing previous health records to the caregivers. In a totally manual environment, this means pulling the record from the file unit and most likely delivering it to the inpatient unit or outpatient location where the patient will be seen. The organization may have some of the patient's previous administrative and clinical information stored electronically. Or, the organization may store the information both in the hard copy health record and in a computerized repository. The information may include the patient's demographics, transcribed reports such as previous history and physical examinations, radiology reports, "final" laboratory reports, allergies, discharge summaries, and a problem list. Depending on the organization's practices and EHR implementation strategy, these reports may be available for viewing at workstations and for reading as printed, paper documents that are filed in the hard copy health record. In most cases, HIM is responsible for physically moving the health record to the needed location. In some cases, HIM is also responsible along with the IT department to ensure that all of the documents that are stored electronically are indeed complete and viewable.

Who Is Authorized to Make Entries in the Health Record?
Who can actually write in the health record must be clearly defined in the organization's policy. The Joint Commission's element of performance states, "Only authorized individuals make entries in the medical record."[41] In a paper world, this was not too difficult a task. A list of the type of staff allowed to document was often enough. In a more electronic environment, however, one cannot simply go to a computer and document care. One needs specific privileges, menus, or functions to access the computer system and document and electronically sign the entry. One needs to think out very clearly who and why certain types of staff are "authorized" (to use The Joint Commission terminology) to document in the record. This policy is one that needs to be fully discussed

and approved by the organization's medical record committee. Depending on the type of entry (notes, orders, administrative information, etc.), different policies will need to be developed.

Documenting Care. Clinicians document care by several different methods:

- Handwriting
- Speech
- Direct input
- Document imaging
- Device capture
- Clinical imaging

Handwriting. In a paper-based system or a document imaging system that digitizes (scans) documents, the most common way to document care is to handwrite it on medical record forms that have been approved by the organization's medical record forms (sub)committee. The HIM director or designee often chairs the forms committee to ensure that forms design meets clinical documentation needs and content criteria. Handwriting is known by all clinicians, is an easy way to document, and can be signed by the author at the time of recording. It has its pitfalls in that it may not be readable, and other than digitizing the document, it cannot be integrated into an EHR system by reusing all or some of its information in other notes. A controlled vocabulary is not really possible because the author uses terminology that he or she is most familiar with. To determine whether handwritten documentation meets accreditation or a legal, billing and organizational requirement obliges HIM and an interdisciplinary team to manually audit documentation note by note. In an inpatient setting, clinicians may handwrite history and physical examinations, progress notes, and orders. A paper-based system requires the HIM department to actively manage the folders and forms that make up the manual health record.

Speech. Speech is the second most common way to document care. It is known as dictation and transcription. Dictation/transcription is a dual process that combines both information capture and report generation. Physicians dictate clinical information, and medical transcriptionists convert this verbal information into written information. The transcribed products are formatted into reports such as history and physical examinations, operative reports, consultation reports, radiology reports, emergency department reports, discharge summaries, and so forth. As the document is being generated, medical transcriptionists transcribe, edit, and format it so that it is ready for review and authentication by the author. Macros or templates may be used during the process.

Speech is also captured for automatic transcription by speech recognition software. After the recognition process is completed, either the author or a medical transcriptionist edits it.

The output can be printed and authenticated with a "wet" signature (handwritten) on a paper document or it can retained in electronic form and authenticated with an electronic signature. HIM must establish business processes that track incomplete documents (i.e., those documents lacking the author's signature). Transcription is a costly process in terms of needed hardware and software and because there are not enough trained, expert medical transcriptionists available. In the traditional dictation/transcription process, there is lag time between dictation and the time when the report becomes available for viewing in either paper or electronic form. HIM business processes require monitoring of the status of dictated and transcribed reports to meet certain organizational standards.

HIM business processes that manage transcribed output change when the output is no longer printed and physically sent to another location (e.g., an operative report sent to an inpatient unit) or physically filed in the hard copy health record. With paper-based output, processes are designed to send and track the "original" document to the physician for wet/handwritten signing. Copies of authenticated or unauthenticated documents, depending on the organization's policies and procedures, may also be sent to the billing office, to referring providers, to other designated clinicians within the organization, and so forth. Paper output processes often require printing an envelope, stuffing it with the report and mailing it. Managing printed, transcribed reports is a labor-intensive process.

The organization may decide to no longer print reports for internal needs and store them instead in a document repository that may or may not be part of an EHR system. No longer printing documents is a major decision that will affect all users of the health record. When this decision is made, policies and processes need to be created that support this change. For example, will the organization allow on-line viewing of unauthenticated reports? If so, how will the organization ensure that no changes are made to the report before the electronic signature? Will an electronic signature lock the report's content? What process will alert a clinician that he or she needs to electronically sign reports? How, for that matter, will HIM track electronic incomplete documents? How will the billing office know when a report is available for their use? How will the organization control printing reports outside the HIM department? Or, does the organization control where reports are printed? How will the organization protect the confidentiality of the information if reports are printed in various locations? When printing is allowed, who is responsible for printing and ensuring that printed documents with identifying health information are secured? For example, are printed documents shredded at the point of printing when no longer needed? Or are they placed in a specialized, secure container for confidential documents?

These are examples of the kind of technical questions HIM professionals must ask themselves as they migrate from manual to hybrid electronic systems. It is a challenge to identify and understand, as much as possible, the interests and purposes of the interacting, interdependent components of the organization's systems.

The human aspect of such a major change as ceasing to print documents to hard copy cannot be ignored. It is no small thing to require users to view the health record online rather than read and turn pages in a hard copy record. In the beginning, until they become comfortable with viewing on-line, it will take longer for users to find and use what they need in the record

Direct input. Direct input means care documentation is accomplished by clinician keyboarding, clicking a mouse, or touching a screen. The information can be entered as free text as in handwritten notes or it can be entered using templates. *Note:* Templates are discussed in greater detail in a later section in this chapter. Just as with handwritten notes, authentication can be accomplished immediately after completing the documentation. This means there is no lag time to wait for authentication. When clinicians directly enter their documentation into the computer, the HIM role changes to one of assisting the clinician at the point of documentation. It is important to realize that in the early 2000 decade, there are four generations of workers in the health care field. Those in older generations do not always easily use a computer keyboard nor find their way intuitively around computer functionality. One of the HIM roles and therefore necessary processes is the ability to provide adult education classes and one-on-one tutorials for clinicians using direct input. Direct input of notes and orders plunges the organization onto the path of a fully functioning EHR system. It is necessary for HIM staff specialists to fully understand the clinical processes that clinicians go through and how care documentation can be integrated into care processes. Teaching clinicians the intricacies of documenting in an EHR means the HIM specialist needs to pay compassionate attention to the learning needs and constraints of each trainee.

Document imaging. Document imaging (or document digitizing) involves prepping, scanning, indexing, and performing quality control on paper documents that are being entered into a computer system. Paper documents, created through handwriting or transcription, can be transferred into digital form with image scanning, optical recognition, or a combination of the two. The ability to easily identify and retrieve individual documents depends on indexing that must be precise, unalterable, and correct. Document imaging requires HIM to develop processes and for each of it steps. Document imaging is discussed in more detail in Chapter 7.

Device capture. Device capture is a process by which a system captures health information directly from a medical device such as an electrocardiogram, thermometer, or ventilator. The machine-generated information must be read and interpreted by a clinician and validated. In the paper world, the output from a medical device may or may not have been filed in the paper chart. Fetal monitoring strips are an example of output that is normally filed in the hard copy chart. With an EHR and an appropriate interface, these types of output can be stored and viewed electronically.

Clinical imaging. Clinical imaging involves data capture using photography or various imaging devices used in conjunction with diagnostic testing such as radiology, magnetic resonance imaging, and so forth. If the organization defines photographs as being part of the (legal) health record, then the HIM department must develop processes to ensure that the photographs are filed in the hard copy record. As the EHR develops and it becomes possible to attach digital photographs to electronic notes, then HIM must work with the medical photography unit and units who routinely take photographs (e.g., dermatology) to develop consistent processes to ensure uploading to the EHR. The ability of clinicians besides radiologists to view radiographic images on screen affects the radiology file unit in much the same way it does in the medical record file unit. Clerks are no longer needed to file films in folders and pull them when needed by radiologists. There is no more film, only digitized images that can be viewed from local and remote workstations.

It is important to realize that an EHR may consist of discrete data fields, images, and text documents.

Copying and Pasting

The electronic function of copying and pasting is a powerful tool that can, when used appropriately, increase a clinician's documentation efficiency. Copy and paste refers to duplicating selected text or graphics and inserting it in another location, leaving the original unchanged. Copying and pasting from other areas of the EHR must, however, be done with caution. Clinical, financial, and legal problems may result when text is copied in a manner that implies the author or someone else obtained historical information, performed an examination, or documented a plan of care when the author or someone else did not personally do it. When organizations begin implementing an EHR, they do not always understand the ramifications of inappropriate copying and pasting. Copying information does not always assist the reader and often makes the documents longer, making the chart more difficult and time consuming to read. It behooves the organization to set clear policy guidelines as to what is and is not appropriate copying and pasting practices.[42] For example, the organization might provide guidelines similar to those in Box 5-1. The organization's medical record committee should include a way to monitor this type of policy. Be warned that monitoring is difficult unless the EHR system itself was designed to track the use of copying and pasting.

Storage and Retention

Storage and retention of health records and health information is a major management challenge for the HIM

Box 5-1 SAMPLE COPY AND PASTE GUIDELINES
• Plagiarized data in the health record is prohibited. Make sure to attribute the content you are copying to whoever originally wrote it. Using quotation marks around the copied data is acceptable.
• Never copy the electronic signature block from one note into another note (e.g., a nurse must never copy the content or information that a physician has written).
• Never copy data or information that identifies a health care provider as involved in care that the health care provider is not involved in (e.g., the results of a physical examination done by someone else).
• Do not copy entire laboratory findings, radiology reports, and other information verbatim into a note. Data copied into a note needs to be specific and pertinent to the care provided during that specific encounter.
• Do not re-enter previously recorded data.
• Authors are responsible and liable for the content of copied items within the notes they authenticate.

---

department whether the records are physical, electronic, or a combination. Traditionally, HIM professionals were and are responsible for the department's filing systems, policies, and procedures, that they comply with federal and state regulations and accepted standards of practice and meet the clinical and administrative needs of the organization. Filing, storage, retention, and destruction of health records and health information all require policies and procedures. Unless a new health care facility opens "paperless," using an EHR, where there is no need for physical storage of hard copy health records, the HIM professional must manage the physical storage of hard copy health records. The first consideration is to ensure that hard copy records can be retrieved and delivered in a timely manner for patient care or other authorized purposes. AHIMA's *Practice Brief: Retention of Health Information* recommends excellent guidelines for establishing retention schedules for all media including paper, images, optical disk, microfilm, and CD-ROM.[43] Although operational responsibility may be redelegated to the IT department when the records are stored electronically, it is still HIM's role to ensure that the organization's retention and destruction policies follow state and federal laws and accreditation requirements.

Because health records and health information are increasingly stored in various types of media, it is also crucial that HIM be a strong advocate for ensuring that patient information is retrievable in a reasonable amount of time. For example, if older health information is only available on imaging platters, will the organization be able to retrieve the information when that technology is no longer current? If health information is written to tape, how fast can IT find the specific information that is being requested? HIM professionals must stay current on evolving storage technologies and must be ever vigilant to ensure that historical health information is retrievable as needed.

Thinning Records

When a patient has a long inpatient stay and remains an inpatient, nursing services may ask HIM staff to thin paper records because nursing has run out of physical space on the inpatient units to store all of the data and documents that have been generated during a specific patient's stay. Once again, this is a manual process that HIM performs using guidelines developed by the HIM department in conjunction with nursing services. The thinned portions of the records are returned to the main file room and are filed in the appropriate location. In an EHR, the process of thinning records on an inpatient unit does not exist. If the organization is still in an early transition to a hybrid environment, the nursing unit may still be printing orders, progress notes, and other results and may need to shred them after they are no longer needed. All the information would still reside in the EHR's clinical repository.

Coding

After a patient is discharged (or sometimes during the hospitalization itself), the HIM department codes the inpatient stay, which may include both facility and professional coding, involving at least two different coding systems. Even in organizations with a paper-based health record, most use an encoding software system to assist professional coders with their tasks of coding and grouping diagnoses and procedures. In a paper-based system, however, it is incumbent for HIM to have streamlined processes in place to acquire the hard copy record as soon as possible after discharge so that coding and therefore billing can take place. There is tremendous pressure on HIM directors to quickly and accurately complete coding so that billing can occur and the organization can receive its payment. In a paper-based system, this is no easy thing to accomplish because the chart may not be complete when it is received in the department and "loose paper" can continue to trickle into the department for some time. When the organization implements an EHR for inpatients, coders can perform their tasks without reading the hard copy chart. This is a major change for the coders because they will not be using the physical chart to read the documentation. They will read and code on-line. Processes will need to change. No longer will a supervisor be able to simply look at the number of charts needing coding by date of discharge; there can be a computer work queue that coders access to find the next case to code. When the entire inpatient episode is on-line either through an EHR or because everything is part of a document imaging system, it is possible to move the coders offsite either to a different location, to their homes, or to an outsourcing vendor who may have coders in many geographic locations. To do this requires clear policies and procedures as to how the work is accomplished, what kind of workstations are needed, how they will be maintained and updated, and security procedures to protect the confidentiality of the information, and so forth.

Health Record Review

Health care organizations should design and implement a health record review program as part of their site's overall information management, performance measurement, and quality management systems. The health care record review program will need to continually change and improve as regulations and accreditation standards evolve to meet increasing demands for accountability. Health record reviews meet many requirements, including mandatory reporting for regulatory and accreditation and for performance monitoring, record completion, and quality improvement. The HIM role in the design and deployment of a health record review program is a vital part of the umbrella of information management.[44-46]

In setting up or modifying an already existing health record review function, an important guiding principle is to incorporate all health record review activities into one encompassing, integrated health record review program, even if the program crosses organizational boundaries. All staff involved in any aspect of the health record review program need to understand the scope of review activities to minimize redundant reviews and conflicting data definitions.

At the heart of this review is documentation analysis of various aspects of the health record. Sometimes organizations use the term "abstracting" to refer to the actual collection of data from the health record. Traditionally, HIM staff and others in the organization such as quality managers, utilization review coordinators, cancer registry staff, and so forth, reviewed individual records against certain criteria. It was and still is, for the most part, a manual process. The Joint Commission has always included standards that incorporate some type of continuing health record review. Since January 1, 2004, however, The Joint Commission is no longer prescriptive. Instead, the patient-specific information standards (IM.6.10 through IM.6.60 for the 2006 hospital standards) require an organization to demonstrate and report Evidence of Standards Compliance (ESC).[38] To know how well the organization is doing on information management and other standards, the organization needs to collect and analyze data. Consider the following:

What Health Record Content and Standards Need Monitoring?
- What are current organizational priorities, accrediting or regulatory agencies?
- Of these priorities, what areas lend themselves to health record review? What performance measures would provide information to make a difference in how the organization is doing, if it is meeting its goals, if its customers are satisfied, if processes are in control, or if and where improvements are needed?
- What aspects of care and documentation need or require 100% monitoring or review?
- What aspects require periodic monitoring, how often, and what sampling methods may be used? What is an

appropriate sampling size? Note: The most recent Joint Commission accreditation manual presents required sampling sizes for demonstrating compliance.[38]

- How frequently should each review be conducted or reported?
- Where can data collection, analysis, and display make a difference? How much realistically can be done?
- What "canned" reports or automated data are available?

Who are Collaborative Stakeholders?

- Who are the organization's executives who are responsible to ensure that a review process is in place?
- Which clinical staff members are willing to champion the review process?
- Who already conducts or could participate in health record reviews? Usually one thinks of HIM and quality management data analysts. There are others who could also perform this type of review: department managers, administrative officers, business managers, clinicians, etc.
- What would motivate stakeholders to participate in such a program?
- Who decides when and what to collect?
- Who creates and maintains the data dictionaries? (Yes, these are indeed needed!)

Reporting Structure. What reporting structure makes sense in the organization? Remember, it is important to provide the entire organization with a "picture" of how well the organization is performing and the areas needing improvement. It is also important to report results to leaders who will be able to understand the importance of the data and who will plan appropriate action.

Data Presentation. Data should be presented in such a way that information and trends can be readily understood. Graphical displays should always include a narrative description of what is being measured, including the standards; what the data mean; where, when, and how they were collected; a summary of findings; recommendations for improvement; and when and how the changes are being followed up, including a date for rereview.

Types of Review. As mentioned above, health record review topics are left up to the discretion of the individual health care organization. The Joint Commission does, however, require that health records are reviewed "on an ongoing basis at the point of care." They further state that the review is based on "hospital-defined indicators that address the presence, timeliness, readability (whether handwritten or printed), quality, consistency, clarity, accuracy, completeness, and authentication of data and information contained within the record."[38]

Focused reviews, special projects, and documentation improvement activities may all give rise to health record criteria or health record reviews. HIM may be charged with coordinating or performing these reviews. Again, it is important to use consistent data definitions and prevent wasted time through redundant reviews. It may be that data previously collected can be analyzed from a different viewpoint to meet a new need. For example, data collected to track health record delinquency can also be used to pinpoint the timeliness of documentation.

Record Completion Process. In this process, tracking is done primarily for the presence, timeliness, and authentication of health record documentation.

Performance Improvement Plans. Whatever group is receiving a health record review report should be responsible for planning or delegating actions for implementation, when required.

Reports. As mentioned above, the data collection process is still manual except in those organizations that have a health data repository. If some or all health record data are collected electronically as discrete fields during the documentation process, then it may be possible to use data mining tools to identify patterns or exceptions. If text documents such as the history and physical examinations, progress notes, and so forth are not in discrete fields, most likely a health record analyst will need to read the health record and abstract necessary information. There are electronic data collection tools designed specifically to collect and report on this type of data. Or, an organization can decide to build its own tool. Following are examples that used an electronic data collection tool built and maintained by an HIM specialist. Microsoft Access was used to take advantage of its automated data tabulation and extraction functionality. Forms used to collect data are created and completed in an Access database (Figures 5-7 to 5-9).

Release of Information

Once the health record is stored in an electronic format, the release-of-information function processes change dramatically over time. The electronically stored record can be either a true EHR or it can simply be a scanned health record. The term "over time" is important to understand. When requests for information come to HIM, they often include requests for older documents. Those documents may be contained in historical paper health records or a previously used imaging system. The HIM processes will need to address both paper and electronic retrieval and tracking while in a hybrid state. As more and more health information is stored in the EHR system, the processes will need to be redesigned to fit the media in which the health information is stored and retrieved. When all the information retrieved is electronic, it is also possible to provide the information to the requestor in an electronic format such as a CD, DVD, or electronic transfer. This is practice in some organizations as of 2006.

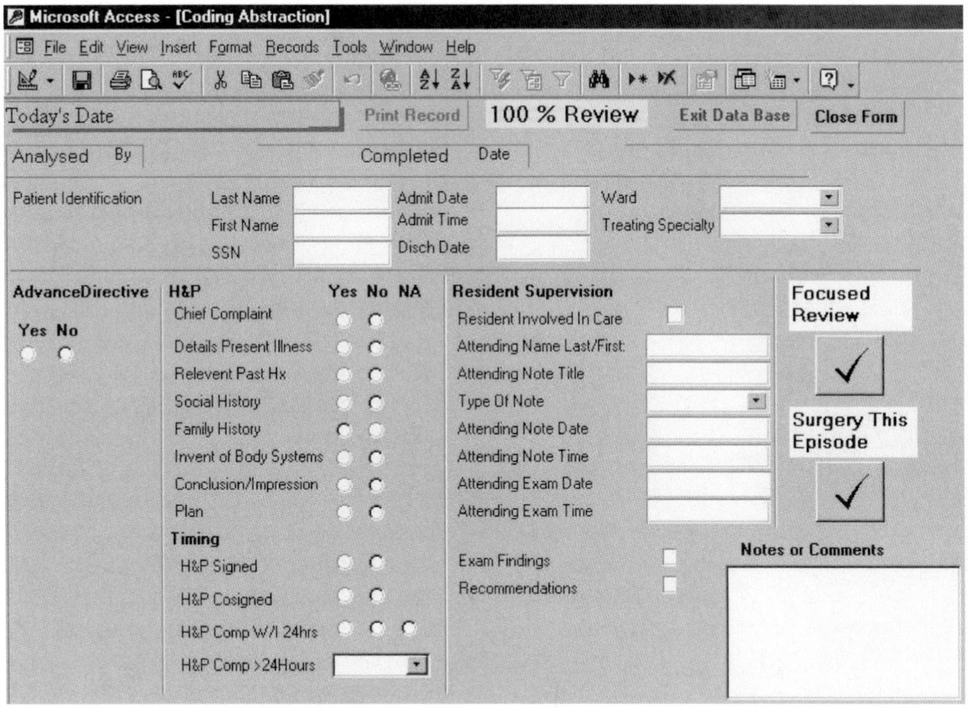

Figure 5-7 Admission event review.

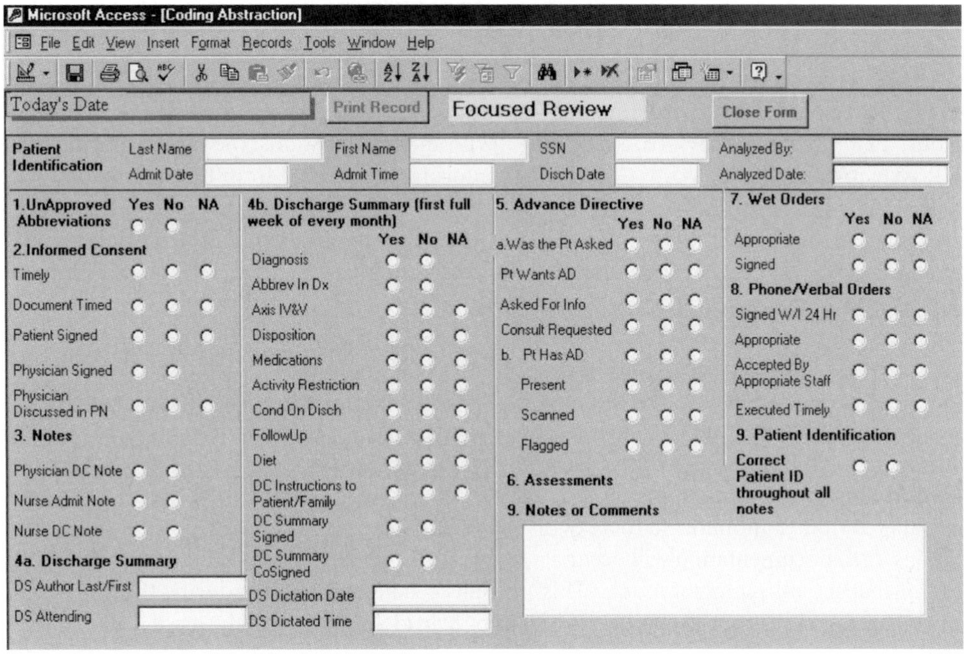

Figure 5-8 Focused review form.

THE FUTURE NOW

Management of EHRs is already changing the HIM professional's role in how an individual record is created, maintained, and retrieved. Recall that the purposes and principles for generating and maintaining a health record remain the same, no matter in what media it resides. No matter where an organization is in relation to transitioning to an EHR, the HIM professional needs to clearly identify what part of the record is paper and what part is electronic. At the same time, the HIM professional needs to envision

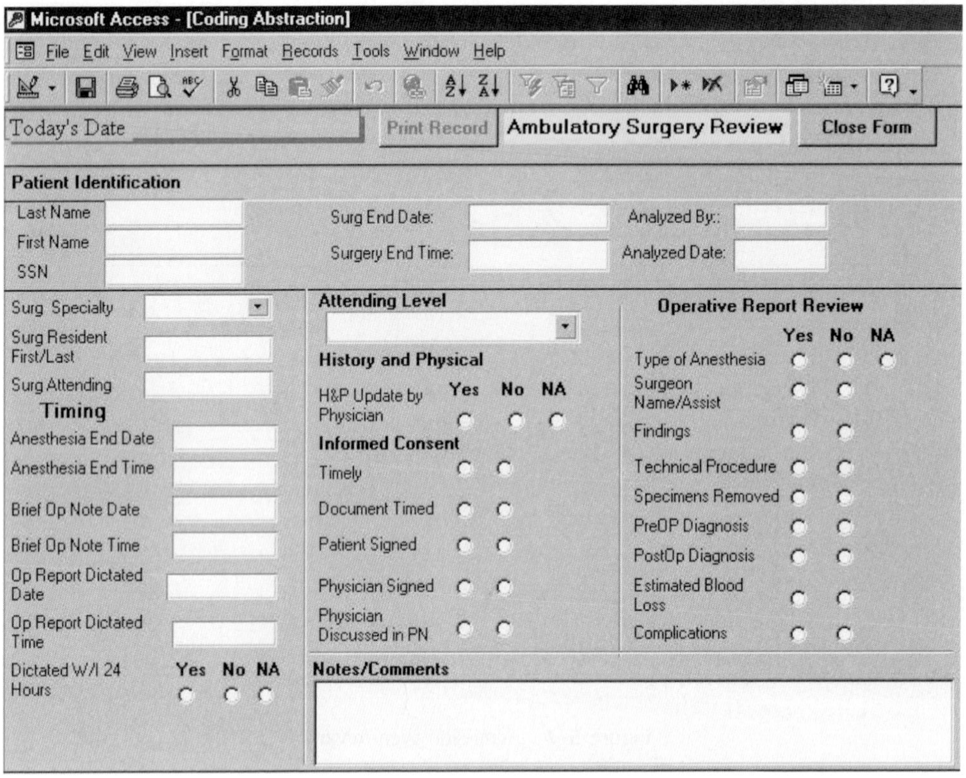

Microsoft Access - [Coding Abstraction]

File   Edit   View   Insert   Format   Records   Tools   Window   Help

Today's Date   Print Record   **Ambulatory Surgery Review**   Close Form

Patient Identification

Last Name   Surg End Date: Analyzed By::
First Name   Surgery End Time: Analyzed Date:
SSN

Surg. Specialty   **Attending Level**   **Operative Report Review**
                                                                      Yes   No   NA
Surg Resident   Type of Anesthesia
First/Last   **History and Physical**   Surgeon
Surg Attending   Name/Assist
Timing   H&P Update by   Yes No NA   Findings
                           Physician
Anesthesia End Date   **Informed Consent**   Technical Procedure
Anesthesia End Time   Timely   Specimens Removed
                                                           PreOP Diagnosis
Brief Op Note Date   Document Timed   PostOp Diagnosis
Brief Op Note Time   Patient Signed   Estimated Blood
Op Report Dictated   Loss
Date   Physician Signed   Complications
Op Report Dictated   Physician
Time   Discussed in PN
Dictated W/I 24   Yes No NA   **Notes/Comments**
Hours

Figure 5-9 Outpatient surgical review.

new action possibilities—new policies, new behaviors, new patterns, new methods, new HIM services—based on a reconceptualized EHR system.

Technology is also changing where and how care is being provided, which often affects documentation practices. For example, technology allows certain types of patient care to be set up when the patient is in one location and the physician is in another. Often, the physician is located at one organization and the patient is located at another organization. The physician can interview the patient through live computer video; there may be another clinician, such as a registered nurse, who may take the patient's vital signs or perform certain procedures under the direct supervision of the physician through the computer monitor. If there is a provider at both locations, then documentation will occur at both locations, either on paper or by the computer. This technology and care is called telehealth. Such a scenario presents a creative challenge for health information staff to develop processes to ensure that documentation and coding standards are met as well as privacy, confidentiality, and security requirements. A similar scenario called tele-monitoring occurs when the patient has monitoring equipment installed in his or her home and communicates with the health care provider by telephone or computer on scheduled and as-needed times. The documentation may be "fed" to the organization's EHR system and a health care professional such as a nurse may monitor it at scheduled times. Or, if the home monitoring system is not interfaced with the organizations, the nurse[3] may document pertinent information gleaned from the stand-alone system on either paper forms or in the organization's computer system. As in the first scenario, there will need to be policies and documentation processes that are agreed on and followed.

How Are Organization Policies and Business Rules Changing to Guide Electronic Health Record Users and Systems?

Policies

It is critical that an organization's policies be rewritten to reflect changes occurring during the transition from manual to hybrid and, ultimately, to a total EHR system. ABC Hospital's overarching policy description (Box 5-2) of its health record makes this point very clearly. Notice the goal is to "standardize the record..." Standardization, an oft-stated aim of EHRs, is an ambitious goal. To accomplish this requires looking at how to normalize documentation for many types of clinicians who learned observation and documentation techniques at different colleges, universities, and training grounds and who have differing subject matter expertise. Even in the paper world, organizations attempted standardization through the forms committee that had

Box 5-2 SAMPLE HEALTH RECORD POLICY

ABC Hospital

Health Record Policy
ABC's health record consists of the EHR, scanned documents and the paper record, combined. Existing policies and procedures pertaining to paper health records apply to computer-generated medical records, including but not limited to, health record delinquencies and deficiencies, responsibility for the accuracy, and authority to make entries and changes in the medical record.

The goal is to standardize the record in relation to its content, creation, maintenance, management, and processing, including quality measures. Electronically stored or printed health information is subject to the same medical and legal requirements as handwritten information in the health record.

Box 5-3 EXAMPLE OF A HEALTH RECORD STEERING COMMITTEE POLICY

ABC Hospital

Health Record Steering Committee
The Health Record Steering Committee is responsible for overseeing the contents and quality of the health record. Membership includes the Associate Chief of Staff for Clinical Information Management, the Director of Health Information Management, Clinical Application Coordinators or Health Information Specialists, clinical staff, and other representatives as appointed by the Chief of Staff. The HRSC is cochaired by the Associate Chief of Staff for Clinical Information Management and the Director of Health Information Management. Subcommittees may be created to address specific issues or needs.

authority to approve or disapprove medical record forms. The forms committee is often a subcommittee of the organization's medical record committee. In the hybrid and electronic worlds, this function becomes critical if the organization decides to use templates to guide documentation of text documents such as an history and physical examination, various types of progress notes, operative reports, discharge summaries, and so forth. Again, it is important to state who has the authority over template design and construction (Box 5-3).

Business Rules

Besides policies, organizations must create business rules. In a paper world, procedures implemented policies (Box 5-4). In a hybrid and electronic world, both procedures and business rules implement policies. Policies, procedures, and computer business rules must be in concert with the

Box 5-4 EXAMPLE OF FORMS POLICY

ABC Hospital

Health Records Forms
All health record forms (paper and electronic templates), overprinting, assembly, and use thereof are under the surveillance and control of the Medical Record Committee. All requests for new health record documents, including templates, must be reviewed by the Health Information Management Director/designee to ensure compliance with policy before submission to the committee for approval. Repetitive fill-in data are the only data authorized to be overprinted on forms approved for use.

organization's medical staff bylaws and rules and regulations if the organization has an organized medical staff. Business rules are:

- Prescribed statements
- Usually written as computer procedures, sets of conditions, or formulas and
- Useful to define what roles certain or individuals are allowed to fill.

For example, documentation business rules might address the following:

- Who can read entries in the EHR
- Who can write only a specific or all clinical documents
- Who can dictate documents
- Who can sign documents
- When a cosignature is required
- Who can edit a document and when
- Who can change (amend) a medical record entry
- When a document can be viewed
- Who can retract documents
- Who can scan documents

It is important that the HIM professional be closely involved in writing or reviewing all business rules that affect health record documentation to be sure they accurately reflect the organization's policies. For example, well-written policies, procedures, and computer business rules ensure that only authorized individuals can document in the health record.

Versioning

EHR systems save different iterations of the same document. It is important to save different versions because care decisions can be made at any point when the document is viewable. When are documents viewable? Depending on a specific EHR system, there may or may not be multiple version functionality. What this means is that once a document is edited, previous versions may or may not be available. It is *critical* for the HIM professional to understand whether versioning capability exists, at what point change

---

Box 5-5   CASE STUDY FOR DISCUSSION

- Resident signed a dictated discharge summary that included a diagnosis of CA Chest (which is what the transcriptionist heard).
- The discharge summary document was viewable by others at this time.
- The attending physician edited and cosigned the summary with a corrected diagnosis of CHF.
- Which version of the discharge summary was used for what decisions?
- *It is critical to address when a document is viewable on the basis of the EHR system's capability.*

---

versions are saved, and who can view previous versions. See Box 5-5 for a case study.

Templates

Template design and management is an emerging need in any kind of EHR and requires exquisite attention to detail and a thorough understanding of health record content requirements. It is critical, therefore, for health information specialists to step forward and acquire this skill for whatever EHR system is being implemented in the organization in which he or she is working. Template formats are driven by both computer and aesthetic considerations, dependent, again, on the system being implemented. A template is a pattern used in computer-based patient records to capture data in a structured manner; it may contain both text and data objects.[47] Templates can be used for progress notes, consultation requests and reports, history and physical examinations, operative reports, and discharges summaries—any document that requires textual health information. There may be different types of templates used by the EHR system from simple plain text templates tool to dialogue and reminder templates. For example, reminder template content may satisfy a clinical reminder such as a diabetic foot examination or a flu shot. It is important for a health information specialist to learn the terminology and requirements of whatever system they are working in. Before requesting a new or edited template, there are certain considerations:

- Does similar content already exist in another template? If yes, can the other template be deactivated?
- Is there some type of mandate for this template?
- Does the proposed content meet required standards (e.g., The Joint Commission, Commission on Accreditation of Rehabilitation Facilities [CARF], organizational policies)?

Templates have format requirements that are driven by whatever template software is being used. Template guidelines should require basic grammar requirements that help ensure that a reader understands the content in the template-generated document:

- Is consistent tense used throughout the template?
- Are pronouns consistent?

- Are abbreviations spelled out the first time used?
- Are periods used only after a full sentence and not after a term or phrase?
- Has everything been spell checked?

Because the ultimate purpose of any documentation is to inform the reader about the care encounter, template builders need to remember that many different types of people, users, may read the note. Users become accustomed to their own view of the health record. A view is simply how the reader sees the information on the workstation screen. It is important, therefore, to assist readers in finding information quickly. Proper template design can aid the reader by considering the following:

- Group information into small, manageable units. A manageable unit is one consisting or 7 ± 2 pieces of information.
- Group similar information together.
- After information is organized, provide a label or header for each unit of information.
- For similar subject matter, use similar words, formats, organizations, and sequences.
- Put *what* the reader needs where the reader needs it.

Titles

Closely aligned with templates are document titles. Before the introduction of word processing to health care organizations in the 1980s, most forms were pre-printed and there was very little modification of a form's title. A progress note was a progress note, no matter who wrote on it. An orders form was an orders form. Often, these forms were color coded to make it easy for a reader to find the type of information he or she needed to read or to document. With the introduction of word processing, however, this changed. It was possible to easily create new forms and new titles. Forms "control" began to slip away from the forms committee as various clinical entities in the health care organization decided on new forms that would make their documenting responsibilities easier. They did not always think about the reader who needed to find this information. With word processing, printing is typically on white paper without colored borders. It was not uncommon for a teaching hospital to have more than 1800 different document titles! In the electronic world, it is just as important to consider how a reader of the health record finds needed information. If there are too many titles, the same problem exists. Titles must also come under the oversight of the medical record committee or its forms and template subcommittee.

Electronic Record Maintenance

Besides template design and management, there are other individual record management functions that are different in the electronic world. One of the key functions requiring HIM expertise is managing and performing correction of erroneous documents. The EHR demands a precision that is

Box 5-6 SAMPLE FROM AN ELECTRONIC HEALTH RECORD DOCUMENT

... from an ABC Hospital policy document—document correction:

To protect patients while preserving a complete record of their care, this section establishes procedures to identify when it is appropriate to (1) write an addendum, rescind, reassign, retract, or delete erroneously entered electronic text documents, including progress notes, discharge summaries, surgery reports, addenda, images, and so forth, and to identify when it is appropriate to (2) rescind documents from active use that are no longer applicable, including advance care directives, alerts regarding allergies, adverse reactions, warnings, and agreements to participate in research, and so forth.[48]

more detailed than in a manual health record. The stated purposes, therefore, must be elucidated in a policy document. (See Box 5-6 for an example.)

The HIM director and the health record committee need to clearly define all of the terms contained in this type of policy. Depending on the system and policies, following are examples of terms needing definition[48]:

- An *addendum* for a *correction* must be written by the document's author and includes additional information for the source document. Addendum is not to be confused with an *amendment* which, by definition, is something that the patient requests.
- To *reassign* a document means to change the encounter or patient to which the document is attached.
- To *remove* means to erase the document or a data field within a document as if it never existed. Depending on the system, this action may require a programmer.
- To *retract* an erroneous document means the content is shielded from general view. Viewing is limited to only certain users (e.g., the HIM director).
- To *delete* a document can occur only for unsigned documents that have never been viewed except by the author. The date, time, title of documents, author, and content are completely erased from the system. Notice the difference in definitions between removal and deletion.

ABC's policy document might state the following:

From a policy document...
To preserve health record integrity, erroneously entered notes will not be deleted from the database. Depending on the individual case, erroneous notes may be corrected by adding an addendum or by retracting or rescinding the information.

Errors occur in the electronic record for a variety of reasons, some of which are listed below:

- Document is created on wrong patient (e.g., the clinician mistyped the medical record number by one digit).

- Signed document is linked to the wrong clinic visit (e.g., a transcribed document is being signed by the clinician who dictated it and chooses an earlier visit to link the transcribed document to).
- Document has an incorrect designated cosigner (when resident documentation requires an attending physician's signature) (e.g., the resident added the current month's attending physician rather than last month's attending physician when the document was originally written or Dr. Jones was scheduled to be the attending surgeon but was sick the day of surgery and now Dr. Smith is the correct attending surgeon).
- Wrong title used and the document's author wishes to change the title (e.g., a note by the emergency department staff was titled "Urgent Care Note" but should have been titled "Employee Health Note." Employee Health Notes raise other issues about privacy and the correct location of the data.).
- Signed consultation report is linked to the wrong consultation request or not attached to a consultation request at all. In an EHR the consultation report should be linked to the request that generated the encounter (e.g., an outpatient, nonurgent consultation was requested of a cardiologist. The patient was subsequently admitted and an urgent cardiac consultation is requested and completed. However, the inpatient report gets attached to the outpatient request, meaning the hospital team may not be notified of the results and the results would show up as part of the outpatient record instead of the inpatient record. Of course, if the result was abnormal or critical result, most often a phone call would be made to the attending physician.).
- Signed document is for the correct patient but the text is so egregiously in error that an addendum to the document will not be clear to a reader (e.g., in an operative report, the surgeon dictates left knee when in fact it is the right knee on which the surgery was performed. Or, in an emergency department note, "patient reports taking codeine for pain" as opposed to "patient reports using cocaine for pain").

In addition to policy statements, procedures need to be identified for each of the policies, including who is responsible for carrying out the procedures.

Completion and Authentication

The traditional HIM role of monitoring the completion and authentication of key documents in the medical record does not go away in the electronic environment. Depending on the EHR system installed, there may be electronic tools to identify, sort, and alert clinicians who need to complete their documentation. In the paper world with stand-alone departmental systems, the HIM staff would physically identify what signatures and documents were missing from the discharged patient's record. Staff would generate letters on a monthly basis and send them to physicians. With an organization-wide health information system, it is possible to alert the affected clinicians within a secure electronic e-mail system or when they sign onto the EHR system. Reports may still need to manually be rolled up from spreadsheets or databases. In an even more sophisticated environment with standardized document titles, it may be possible for the EHR system to perform almost real time monitoring and alerts for documentation needs. For example, if a patient is admitted and there is no history and physical examination in the record within 8 hours of admission, the system could automatically page the identified HIM staff to contact the responsible clinician's office or the system could directly page the admitting clinician. It is possible to design reports and graphs that are automatically generated by clinical services and individual clinicians. As mentioned previously, this function may be subsumed in an organizational health record review program.

Printing

The HIM professional must seriously consider the printing issues in an EHR environment. Does the EHR system support printing functionality? Most of these systems are not designed to produce paper. When printing from an EHR, the volume of paper increases by at least 25% and even much more if only one side of the paper is printed. When a document is printed, it must be in a format that is understandable by the reader. Often, because the systems were not designed for printing, printed output is not useful for the reader. For example, when printing progress notes, the program may simply run them together, making it difficult for the eye to find the particular needed notes. HIM professionals who have implemented EHR systems strongly discourage printing electronic data and documents and recommend from the very beginning of any EHR implementation project that the concept of "no printing" be discussed and a transition date be set to go "no printing." In the meantime, decide whether the print functionality can be restricted by role description. If "print screen" is an option in the system, can it be controlled? Decide who can print, why printing a document is necessary, what and when a user can print. Decide who is authorized to print the entire medical record and if there will be designated areas for printing. For example, HIM could be authorized to print documentation for release of information, transfer of records, and archiving records. Be sure to consider privacy issues of printed documents whether printing in one's own organization or printing remotely.

There needs to be accountability for printing. If possible, the user name and ID should be printed on each document. Use caution, however, with printing the user's name. The organization's name and location should also be on each page of the printed document. There should be a statement in the document footer or header that reads, "If document received in error, please contact the corporate privacy officer at XXX-XXXX."

Decide on a strategy on how to stop routine printing. For example,

- Make sure there are enough workstations for viewing
- Mandate computer entry for all staff through official committees
- Phase printing out and electronic entry in. Remember, however, they are asynchronous because they are phased in and out at different rates.
- Identify when there are enough documents in the system to stop printing
- Make sure users know where to find the information in the EHR
- Publicize what you are doing broadly. Make sure both staff and patients are aware as changes are being planned.
- Decide when you can routinely stop delivery of the hard copy chart. This can be phased in by location depending on receptivity of the staff.
- Continue to educate
- Publicize and celebrate milestones

Recognize that a print function will be required and that there should be some planning related to printing documents in readable formats.

Box 5-7 shows a snapshot of how one health care organization migrated to the EHR.

VIRTUAL HEALTH INFORMATION MANAGEMENT DEPARTMENT

The "future now" means living and working as if the future EHR is already here. What might this mean to a traditional HIM department that is bound by physical constraints because the business processes must take place near where the physical, paper record is located? If the organization is transitioning to a hybrid or EHR status and business processes will no longer be tied to the paper, physical record, the HIM department must consider the possibility of a virtual health information management department—one where many HIM business processes are conducted outside the physical organization. If the file room will soon only reside in computer servers, if coding and transcription are done from home, if one can have meetings by phone or Internet, what are the challenges HIM professionals must address as we migrate to different and more sophisticated technologies for supporting patient care documentation?

Challenge to Health Information Professionals

Sustaining quality through transition to a true EHR is the continuing challenge. Mastering the future requires a solid "feet on the ground" understanding of how the basic information processing activities function in health delivery

Box 5-7 BENCHMARK DATA—VETERANS ADMINISTRATION PUGET SOUND HEALTH CARE SYSTEM'S TRANSITION TO THE ELECTRONIC HEALTH RECORD

The way we were

Up until the late 1990s, this hospital had a limited hybrid environment. Basically, laboratory and radiology reports were electronic but still filed in the hard copy chart. All other documentation was either handwritten or transcribed, "wet signed"/handwritten and filed in the hard copy chart. In the 1990s, the paper record included the following:

- Progress notes
- Physician orders
- Consultations
- Medication flow sheets
- Discharge summaries
- Other flow sheets
- Printed laboratory reports
- Consents
- Printed x-ray reports
- Printed ECGs
- Printed pathology reports
- Diagnostic studies
- Procedure reports

As in any hybrid system, the paper chart was pulled for scheduled and unscheduled appointments and admissions, for coding, for quality review, for utilization review, and so forth. Some processes had to wait until the record could be "corralled" long enough to complete the work. Even with an excellent chart tracking system, charts were available to clinic appointments only 95% of the time, and when other processes needed the chart, such as coding, the chart may have been taken before the record was coded, necessitating another retrieval and use of staff time. Filing documents into the paper record was difficult because the records were constantly moving into and out of the medical record file unit. If a clinician wanted the most up-to-date information and requested the hard copy chart, it was often not available because the filing was waiting for the chart to remain long enough in the unit for filing to occur.

What we decided

In the mid 1990s, much discussion focused on what the organization needed from a health record system. Availability was one of the key identified needs. Other major needs included saving space (decreasing the amount of paper in the chart and the physical size of the file area), ease of clinician documentation and timeliness of document completion, readability (making documents more consistent in their formats), and legibility. Clinicians clearly stated a preference to only refer to *one source* for each type of information, meaning they did not want to look in the computer and in the paper chart for laboratory results or progress notes and so forth. The organization decided that an EHR implementation was required to meet the identified major needs. It was recognized that this required a substantial

investment of resources, in technology, hardware, software, hiring specialized staff, and an enormous educational effort for every level of clinical and administrative staff.

What we did

Starting about 1995, clinician order entry was mandated for all inpatient orders and was allowed for any outpatient order. To require clinician direct order entry at the beginning of an EHR implementation is unusual for most EHR implementations. The decision was largely driven by patient safety and the need to get the clinicians on board. Pharmacy was another advocate for direct order entry for prescriptions. With direct order entry, prescriptions could be filled faster because pharmacists would no longer need to contact clinicians because of legibility issues for both the actual prescription and the prescriber. Physician order entry resulted in fewer erroneous or duplicate tests and allowed near real time electronic results reporting back to the ordering physician who knew the results were ready because he or she received an electronic alert. Despite some resistance, the transition went quickly and fairly smoothly and resulted in a clinician base that was beginning to be comfortable using a computer to input and receive clinical information about their patient. By mid 1997, radiology and laboratory results, orders, and order results were available on-line.

In 1997, we decided to expand the use of the EHR and established a rough time frame to phase in various components. Beginning almost immediately, all discharge summaries for inpatient stays more than 48 hours were required to be either direct entered or dictated, transcribed, and uploaded to the EHR. Stays less than 48 hours could still be handwritten on a special form. The mandated use of electronic progress notes was phased in by one clinical service at a time and by one inpatient ward at a time. At this point, outpatient use was voluntary and some clinicians chose to directly enter their progress notes in the clinics.

In 1998, the decision was made to stop printing radiology and laboratory results because clinicians were used to viewing the results on the computer screen. That meant the file unit no longer had to file these voluminous reports. HIM, however, was still delivering hard copy charts to both inpatient units and clinics. As stated earlier, clinicians had always wanted "one stop shopping" for reviewing patient history. At this point, HIM was still printing every progress note and filing it in the paper chart. In fact, we continued printing and filing until 1999.

By January 1999, all levels and types of clinicians on all inpatient units were using electronic progress notes and orders. This meant they both entered data through the EHR and viewed the information on computer screens. At this point, inpatient orders and inpatient progress notes ceased being printed daily but were still being printed at discharge and filed in the paper chart because there was a clinical concern that there be hard copy documentation if the computer system went down.

Continued

Box 5-7 BENCHMARK DATA—VETERANS ADMINISTRATION PUGET SOUND HEALTH CARE SYSTEM'S TRANSITION TO THE ELECTRONIC HEALTH RECORD—cont'd

To address the very real patient safety issue of what to do when there was computer down time, scheduled or unscheduled, the organization came up with a very creative idea. Each inpatient unit, the emergency department, and several outpatient areas were issued special "downtime computers." These devices had dedicated power supply and memory robust enough to accept regular downloads several times an hour for all current inpatients (on inpatient units) and all *scheduled* outpatients for the previous day, the current day, and the next day (in the emergency department and outpatient areas). A summary document is created for each patient and includes a variety of components: the last three discharge summaries, the last 7 days' progress notes for inpatients, the last year of outpatient progress notes for outpatients, current medication lists, problem list, laboratory and radiology results, and so forth. The system rolls up the components, creates the summary document, and pushes all of the summaries to each downtime computer.

Meanwhile, in the outpatient arena, a similar phased approach was being implemented beginning in mid 1998. Primary care volunteered to be the pilot. By June 2000, all outpatient clinics were required to enter progress notes directly into the computer. Initial assessments were allowed to be dictated, transcribed, and uploaded; all other notes were required to be directly entered.

By June 2000, it was recognized that no one was referring to the hard copy chart for inpatient orders or notes. Therefore, all printing ceased for inpatient cases. In the outpatient setting, many clinicians felt they needed a 2-year history before they could give up the hard copy chart. HIM negotiated halting printing on a specialty-by-specialty basis and stopped printing outpatient progress notes in July 2000 and began phasing out chart deliveries 6 months later, again, specialty by specialty. By 2004, only the eye clinic still required paper charts because of the eye drawings and noncomputerized testing equipment where handwritten results were used. The eye testing equipment could not be interfaced into the EHR. In 2005, however, new eye testing equipment was purchased that will allow direct entry into the EHR of these important tests.

During 2003, the organization began scanning selected documents, including advance directives, power of attorney for general and health care, and certain financial records. Because of the phased in use of electronic notes, it was decided *not* to backscan previous health record documentation. Any scanned documentation was viewable on the same clinical workstations.

By June 2000, a mandate stated that any clinical documentation that could be entered into the EHR had to be done electronically. By June 2001, anything that was in the EHR was no longer printed

for inclusion in the paper record. There were, however, certain exemptions granted by the Medical Record Steering Committee that allowed handwritten documentation, either because of software limitations or staffing issues. Also, because of software limitations, medication and intensive care unit flow sheets remained handwritten.

What goes in the paper chart now

In 2006, the organization continues to mandate the use of the EHR exclusively where that is possible. HIM receives some loose filing for inclusion in the paper chart. HIM still files the following:

- Intensive care unit and certain other flow sheets
- Hand drawings
- Outside documents (We scan certain outside documents such as discharge summaries, consultation reports, and operative reports and other documents as specifically requested by clinicians)
- "Downtime" documents. (Any handwritten documents created during a downtime.)
- Consents. (We are in the process of phasing in an on-line patient consent program where the patient will sign on-line, as will the clinician and witness.)

Lessons learned

- HIM should be involved in the early discussions and planning for an EHR implementation to ensure that information and documentation principles are considered in the design. It is far more difficult to make a change in an implemented system than to design it in the first place.
- Regular, scheduled downtime (for system maintenance, updates, patching, etc.) decreases the amount of unscheduled downtime and allows staff to plan and become familiar with downtime contingency processes.
- Although not discussed in the case, a strong clinical champion is absolutely the most important element in a successful implementation.
- A strong, collegial HIM director who can work with the clinical champion, executive leadership, and clinical and administrative staff is also key to a successful implementation.
- Celebrate successes often; publicize them. Clearly define milestones when objectives will be met.
- Be open to change and protect the integrity of the health record in whatever form(s) it happens to be at any specific moment.
- Remember, plans change as implementation progresses; be flexible and adapt to what the organization needs.[51]

settings in both paper and hybrid environments and the capacity to track, anticipate, and plan for the future reality. What actions need to be taken to both advance the EHR initiatives in individual organizations and maintain fundamental quality in patient data and data systems fundamental to day-to-day operations? As a future HIM professional, consider what strategies you will choose and commit to as you embark on various transition projects on the way to an EHR.

1. *Educate health care organizations, practitioners, and consumers to prepare for change.* Health care is increasing the use of technology in everyday operations and adapting innovative ways for those in health care organizations to communicate with their peers, their practitioners, and their patients. Organizations and institutions are educating users to rely on computers as tools to supply their data needs. To educate effectively, we need to proactively track the progress of EHR developments through the hybrid iterations. As organizations migrate from paper record systems, teaching others about the incremental benefits and challenges underscores the progress and uncovers work issues along the way. We already know how EHR advances affect documentation and patient data availability for the care process. For instance, record availability issues decrease when information can be retrieved through workstations within and beyond the physical care site. The consumer needs education as we become more efficient in delivering and coordinating consumers' care information through computers, already happening through secure portals where they can access their own medical records. Because providers can rely on up-to-the-minute data and research to communicate with patients, we will foster a different kind of patient—one who can function as a stronger member of the health care team.

2. *Recognize that technology infrastructure must be in place to support EHR functions.* Electronic data systems and the networks required to link them within organizations continue to be dependent on fundamental and affordable technology. Foundation systems are needed to provide daily transaction processing for all health services, and enough workstations, including tablet and hand-held devices where adopted, must be deployed to afford clinicians ready and near-to-care access. Until the infrastructure is in place, the shift to replacing the dependence on paper and increasing direct use of computer systems by providers will not occur. For many organizations, however, progress is well on the way. The HIMSS 2006 survey reports that 81% of surveyed hospitals have an EHR or plan to purchase one.[49] On the business operations side, managers are already expected to use computers in their own daily activities, including budgeting, data analysis, and writing and communication. Active participation in planning, advocating, and implementing appropriate technology within organizations will strengthen managers' skills and better prepare them to understand technologic needs.

3. *Address the crucial acceptance factors.* Still a major component, success relies on how effectively organizations work to secure sponsor endorsement, engage clinical "champions" to assist in marketing to their peers, adopt demonstration pilots to move ahead in incremental steps, and analyze the lessons learned from others to enrich the analysis and planning for the organization. For instance, a key acceptance factor, the dashboard design of the clinical user interface, often Windows-style navigation, is a crucial acceptance factor for workstations. Another acceptance issue is the necessary preparation to manage confidentiality adequately by determining how the confidentiality and security policies and procedures will be operational in an EHR setting. Patients and those associated with the user communities are concerned about privacy and worry about who has access to their data. Patient forums such as focus groups and information sessions are valuable options for exploring patient concerns.

4. *Model quality and cost incentives to encourage individual organizations to adopt aggressive programs.* A sound business cost-benefit rationale is required. Closer scrutiny is directed to systems development projects to be sure that clear cost containment targets are included in the planning. The opportunity for "nice-to-have computer systems" is giving way to "cost-justified computer systems." Managers apply cost-benefit tools in their forecasting with greater discipline than ever before. A realistic analysis is essential. Strategic steps, such as bringing transcription reports or consultation referral letters on-line along with diagnostic test results, are well received components that bring immediate benefits and fit nicely into an overall migration plan to build toward enterprise EHR systems. As an HIM manager, be sure you fully understand the business process and current costs of transcription. Gather the facts about on-line transcription from experienced peer organizations, including production increases or decreases, to demonstrate full understanding of cost. Then make the case using white papers and other strategic planning devices.

5. *Upgrade organizational policies and procedures to redefine the patient record and move from a paper record to a combined paper and clinical information data systems record.* This work is modeled at national and state association levels as well as within individual institutions. Hybrid "how to's" offer road maps and recommend concrete measures to support the hybrid to electronic developments. Plan for multimedia patient health information to grow in a clinically designated "virtual" record. This helps formalize the data system's content as part of the patient record.

6. *Coordinate programs that stage EHR-related development within information systems master plans.* This endorses the concept of a unifying principle. Research and conceptualize how EHR systems come on-line and identify how a migration master plan could work. Benchmarks are available to help identify examples. Apply them. Some of these go hand in hand to cover the most return on investment and, at the same time, extend value added to multiple customers. Systems must become more affordable, dependable, and useful to more customers. A new clinical laboratory system, added to a large organization's integrated clinical systems development plan, can drive the results reporting for clinicians and send data to a clinical repository in which a growing EHR is maintained. It may also offer a new service. Previously mailed test result reports to patients may now be made accessible through on-line patient portals. If your organization is in the process of providing increasing patient data from laboratory and pharmacy to radiology images, electrocardiograms, and more to a clinical data repository or data warehouse, be aware of the value of contributing to your master IT plan to monitor and support the evolving activities as progress is accomplished.

7. Actively support revised legal frameworks so that federal and state legislation allows the transition from paper to electronic media to occur. State laws are in the process of being realigned with federal requirements in these areas. New definitions of the patient record, accepted changes in storage requirements, and automated authentication techniques are all needed to advance the work. Legislation on digital signatures[50] paved the way to electronic authentication at a new level.

8. Find ways to deliver better clinical information from the current information systems now. Propose that EHR components be introduced, evaluated, and rapidly deployed. A good illustration of this strategy is the production of minisummaries that show the "patient at a glance," for example, problem list, medications, and laboratory test results or a specific patient care plan, perhaps designed to manage a chronic disease. This strategy focuses on the experience that bringing technology to the eager customers first—particularly clinicians—accelerates technology diffusion. Happy customers market the technology most effectively. At this point in health information systems development, there are many demonstrations that illustrate this experience. If we provide new data such as chronic disease monitoring information or data in new and more effective formats such as on-line transcription, clinical customers will be more willing to modify their data collection behaviors and accept on-line data capture when these component applications are adopted.

9. Monitor continuing work on clinical guidelines and protocols and find ways to introduce them into the organization. Not only are they needed for reasonable support to medical providers, but they are clearly a resource for inclusion in EHR systems. In the simplest form, guidelines can be stored electronically and look-up features can be provided. Commercial products are already in use with hand-held devices. In sophisticated approaches such as computerized provider order entry, organizations tailor guidelines for internal use and incorporate advice and reminder protocols. Connecting individual patient data to expert knowledge through event monitoring with alerts and reminders to offer feedback before, during, and after the care delivery process characterize current model EHR systems.

10. Study the known barriers already published to develop action plans to overcome them—learn from others' mistakes. Success benchmarks are notable and HIM roles are represented in professional practice briefs and national education opportunities from AHIMA and the American Health Informatics Association, Health Information Systems Society, and others. Sharing experiences with other organizations helps develop a collective wisdom as we move to such a new environment. To illustrate a simple case, many health professionals have not learned to type. This means that introducing computer systems—even point-of-care systems—to personnel who do not possess simple keyboarding skills will require expensive pretraining in the technology itself before a specific application can be taught. Time is also needed to adjust from character-based terminal screens to the newer graphical user interfaces (GUIs). It must be clear that newer user interface styles are going to be more effective. In some cases, such as a high-volume prescription data entry function, icons and a Windows user interface style may not be the most efficient for the organization, but evidence to date indicates that the GUI benefits have led to easier and more intuitive learning for information system users.

11. Lead and participate in re-engineering current user processes. We need to prepare the operational environment for change. One of the driving forces of this decade is re-engineering. We have learned that simply installing computer systems for existing business processes fails to realize the benefits. Business processes, the way we move patients through appointment, check-in, care, and follow-up, must be re-examined. Along with other business processes, track the data flows in detail. These workflows require careful review to see whether there are more efficient ways to accomplish them. This applies to the way we organize and use the patient record content and formats. The notion of continuously improving our business processes to be sure that the best methods are in place fits in with the total quality management philosophy and practices that have been used with positive results since the late 1980s. We can expect to re-engineer patient-related care processes, update the processes used to capture, document and transfer the resulting health information, and design better ways to use this information. Re-engineering means fundamental rethinking and transforming business processes to achieve dramatic performance improvements with radical redesign. Cost, quality, service, and speed of operations can be improved. Considering that providers are expected to incorporate new technology in direct care practices, examining how data capture and retrieval can occur most efficiently, particularly across functional processes and departments, can lead to better alternatives.

12. Once an EHR project is under way, incorporate a thorough knowledge of the impact of change on the workforce into strong project leadership from a top-down approach. We know that technology affects organizational culture, including structure and design. It changes work flows and brings in new job designs and responsibilities. Staff requires new skills and knowledge to perform their work. Worker motivation and incentives call for new communications and operations policies and procedures to build the kind of strong teamwork required to absorb change. Human resources personnel are strategic partners for all managers in the long-term change agent tasks, and new skills are required for managers as well as workers.[3] Assembling and participating in strong teams are essential. HIM professionals are already assuming leadership roles with project management requirements. An EHR project is mapped out in Figure 5-6.

SUMMARY

Transition marks the current state of patient record systems and requires HIM professionals to apply theories and practices to parallel realities. Determining the future reality and recognizing the pathway to reach it is a fascinating and challenging task. The fundamental change involved in moving from paper record systems under one operational unit to EHR systems that expand operational boundaries and enable enterprise-wide patient information to be used, processed, protected, and resourced opens the door to expanded professional influence and responsibilities. To understand what the future looks like and how it may function—along with issues and barriers that must be considered—is essential. This chapter addressed the what, why, where, when, and how aspects of the future and proposed concrete steps to manage the transition from paper to electronic records. Given the changing boundaries and professional challenges required today, more complex roles have been described to prepare for leadership and teamwork in EHR projects of all kinds. When "at the table" as EHR systems projects are planned and implemented, the required set of working tools include knowledge of EHR systems and their functions, assessment, and syntheses of benchmark experiences; alternative "maps" of successful migration paths for EHR systems; change management principles and skills understanding; and facts about costs and clear details of how the EHR system components meet the patient care and patient record business processes from hybrid to electronic cases. The virtual HIM department has been characterized examples of emerging business processes. The gathering energy to improve health information from individual practices from practitioners to comprehensive health care settings within an expanding national health information infrastructure is well underway. Health information demands from those who provide health care and those who receive it will be met. Your challenge as an HIM professional is to seize the transition opportunity to help build and improve our nation's EHR systems.

REFERENCES

1. Miller J: *PHIMSS: Implementing the electronic health record,* Chicago, 2005, HIMSS.
2. Dick RS, Steen EB, editors: *The computer-based patient record: an essential technology for health care,* Washington, DC, 1991, National Academy Press.
3. Murphy GF, Hanken MA, Waters K: *Electronic health records: changing the vision,* Philadelphia, 1999, WB Saunders.
4. Handler GT, Holtmeier R, Metzger J et al: *HIMSS electronic health record definitional model, version 1.0, EHR definition, attributes and essential requirements, version 1.0,* Chicago, 2003, Health Information Management Systems Society.
5. Tang P, Coye M, B E et al: *Letter report: key capabilities of an electronic health record system,* 2003, Committee on Data Standards for Patient Safety, Institute of Medicine. www.iom.edu/ CMS/3809/4629/ 14391. aspx. Accessed December 6, 2006.
6. Amatayakul MK: *Electronic health records, a practical guide for professionals and organizations,* Chicago, 2004, American Health Information Management Association.
7. Dickinson G, Fischetti L, Heard S, editors: *HL7 EHR system functional model draft standards for trial use,* Ann Arbor, MI, 2004, HL7 Inc.
8. Dougherty M: Understanding the EHR system draft standard for trial use (AHIMA practice brief), *J AHIMA* 76(no. 2):64A-D, 2005.
9. Addison K, Braden J, Cupp J et al: Update: guidelines for defining the legal health record for-disclosure purposes, *J AHIMA* 76:64A-64G, 2005.
10. Kohn LT, Corrigan JM, Donaldson MS editors: *To err is human—building a safer health system,* Washington, DC, 1999, Committee on Quality of Health Care in America, Institute of Medicine, National Academy Press: http://www.nap.edu/catalog/9728.html. Accessed August 16, 2006.
11. AHIMA e-HIM Personal Health Record Work Group: The role of the personal health record in the EHR, *J AHIMA* 76:64A-64D, 2005.
12. Eysenbach G: Consumer health informatics, *BMJ* 320: 1713-1716, 2000.
12a. *Your personal health information: how to access, manage, and protect it.* A community-based public education campaign. Educational handout used at the AHIMA Community Education Coordinator training session, Chicago, June 2005.
13. Health Insurance Portability and Accountability Act of Administrative Simplification, 1996. www.CMS.hhs.gov/HIPAAGenInfo. Accessed August 21, 2006.
14. Walker JM, Beiber EJ, Richards F, editors: *Implementing an electronic health record system,* London, 2005, Springer, 2005.
15. Cummings J: Few patients use or have access to online services for communicating with their doctors, but most would like to, *Harris Interactive Health Care Poll, September 22, 2006:* www.Harrisinteractive. com. Accessed December 2006.
16. Krall M: Patient safety and the EHR. Presented at the Second Annual Northwest Conference on Patient Safety, May 17, 2005, SeaTac, WA.
17. Caeser C, Claudio Y, Carmor K et al, Ad Hoc Task Force on Electronic Health Record-Public Health (EHR-PH): Report to the HL7's electronic health record special interest group [white paper], Public Health Informatics Data Standards Consortium, Baltimore, 2004.
18. Middleton, B, Hammond W, Brennan PF, Cooper G: Accelerating U.S. EHR adoption: how to get there from here, Recommendations based on the 2004 ACMI retreat, *J AHIMA* 12:13-19, 2005.
19. Plummer DC: Gartner predicts 2006 and beyond: http://www.gartner.com. Accessed November 28, 2005.
20. Briere R, editor: *Crossing the quality chasm: a new health system for the 21st century,* Washington, DC, 2001, Committee on Quality of Health Care in America, Institute of Medicine, National Academy Press.
21. Attitudes of Americans regarding personal health records and nationwide electronic health information exchange, survey, Markel Foundation—connecting for health: http://www.connectingforhealth. org. Accessed October 2005.

22. Brown EG: The next generation of wired physicians, *Forrester Res:* www. forrester.com. Accessed August 24, 2004.

23. Seymour D, editor: *Futurescan: healthcare trends and implications 2005-2010,* Chicago, 2005, Society for Healthcare Strategy and Market Development, Health Administration Press.

24. Longman P: The best care anywhere, *Washington Monthly* 1-5, November 2005.

25. Garets D, Davis MW: *The U.S. hospital clinical system environment: market dynamics drive adoption models* [white paper], Chicago, 2004, Governance Institute, HIMSSanalytics.

26. Brailer DJ: The decade of health information technology, delivering consumer-centric and information-rich health care: framework for strategic action. Letter accompanying the report to Secretary T. G. Thompson, July 21, 2004.

27. Office of the National Coordinator for Health Information Technology: http://www.hhs.gov/healthit/ahic/html. Accessed August 16, 2006.

28. Stead WW: The challenge to health informatics for 1999-2000, *J Am Med Informatics Assoc* 6:88-89, 1999.

29. Monda DT, Nunn S: Understanding CPR architecture: a HIM professional's guide, *J AHIMA* 2:30-37, 1999.

30. Ball MJ, Douglas JV, O'Desky R et al, editors: *Healthcare information management systems,* New York, 1991, Springer-Verlag.

31. Ball MF, Weaver CA, Keil JM, editors: *Healthcare, information management systems,* ed 3, New York, 2004, Springer.

32. van Bemmel JH, Musen MA, editors: *Handbook of medical informatics,* Houghten, The Netherlands, 1997, Springer.

33. Covey HD: The digital hostage takers syndrome: reflections on the computer-based patient record, *Managed Care Q* 1:60, 1993.

34. Golob R: Securing a bridge to the CPR: Clinical data repositories, *Health Information* 11:50, 1994.

35. American Society for Testing and Materials: ASTM E1869 standard guide for confidentiality, privacy, access and data security principles for health information including computer-based patient records, 14:832, 1998.

36. Kim K: *Clinical data standards in health care: five case studies, health reports,* 2005, Report of California HealthCare Foundation, Oakland, CA.

37. ASTM E 2084-00 standard specification for authentication of healthcare information using digital signature, ASTM International Committee on Health Informatics (2000): www.astm.org. Accessed August 15, 2006.

38. Kanter RM: *The change masters,* New York, 1983, Simon & Shuster.

39. Scholtes PR: *The leader's handbook,* New York, 1998, McGraw-Hill.

40. Fernandes L, O'Connor M: The future of patient identification, *J AHIMA* 77:36-40, 2006.

41. Joint Commission on Accreditation of Healthcare Organizations: *2006 Comprehensive accreditation manual for hospitals: the official handbook,* Chicago, 2006, Joint Commission on Accreditation of Health Care Organizations.

42. Hammond KW, Helbig ST et al: Are electronic medical records trustworthy? Observations on copying, pasting and duplication. In Proceedings of American Medical Informatics Association Symposium, pp. 269-273, Bethesda, MD, 2003 American Medical Informatics Association.

43. American Health Information Management Association: Practice brief: Retention of health information, Chicago, 2002, American Health Information Management Association.

44. Clark JS: *Information management, the compliance guide to the JCAHO standards,* ed 4, Marblehead, MA, 2004, HCPro.

45. Pinder RS, Osborne FH: *Automate ongoing records review,* Oakbrook, IL, 2002, Opus Communications/HCPro.

46. Spath PL: *Fundamentals of health care quality management,* Forrest Grove, OR, 2000, Brown- Spath & Associates.

47. Heller T, Aanes D: Unleashing the power of personal templates, class 240, VHA eHealth University (2005): www.vehu.med.va.gov. Accessed August 21, 2006.

48. American Society for Testing and Materials: *ASTM 2017-99 standard guide for amendments to health information,* West Conshohocken, PA, 1999, American Society for Testing and Materials.

49. Health Information Management Systems Society: *2006 Survey of health professionals,* Chicago, 2006, Health Information Management Systems Society.

50. Washington State Electronic Authentication Act RCW 19.34 (1999).

51. Veterans Administration, Puget Sound, WA.

ADDITIONAL READINGS

American Health Information Management Association: Defining the personal health records: http://library.ahima.org/.

American Society for Testing and Materials: *E 1762-95 Standard guide for electronic authentication of health care information*, West Conshohocken, PA, 2004, American Society for Testing and Materials.

Beinborn J, Herbst M et al: EHR fundamentals, audio seminar, AHIMA Continuing Education, Chicago, 2006.

Department of Veterans Affairs, Health Information Management and Health Records: *VHA handbook, 1907.1*, Washington, DC, 2004, Veterans Health Administration.

Harmon L: *Ethical challenges in the management of health information*, ed 2, Boston, 2001, Jones and Bartlett.

HIMS Management Team, Medical Record Review Program: *Access data base and data dictionary*, Seattle, WA, 2005, Veterans Administration Puget Sound HIMS.

Horn RE: *Developing procedures, policies and documentation*, Waltham, MA, 1989, Information Mapping.

Veterans Administration Puget Sound Health Care System, Medical Record Management: *management of information memorandum IM-03*, Seattle, 2003, Veterans Administration Puget Sound Health Care System.

Waegemann CP, Tessier C, Barbask A et al: *Healthcare documentation: a report*, Newton, MA, 2001, Medical Records Institute.

Classification Systems, Clinical Vocabularies, and Terminology

Gail Graham
Kathleen Strouse
Marlene Haddad

Additional content,
http://evolve.elsevier.com/Abdelhak/

Review exercises can be found
in the Study Guide

Chapter Contents

Terms About Terms
Administrative Terminologies
  International Classification of Diseases
    International Classification of Diseases, Ninth Revision
    International Classification of Diseases, Tenth Revision
    International Classification of Diseases, Tenth Revision,
      Procedural Coding System
  Derivations of the International Classification of Diseases
  Current Procedural Terminology
  Healthcare Common Procedure Coding System
  Diagnosis Related Groups
  Adaptation of Administrative Terminologies
Clinical Terminologies
  Systematized Nomenclature of Medicine
  Logical Observation Identifiers Names and Codes
  Drug Terminologies
  Nursing Terminologies
  The Role of the Unified Medical Language System
Terminology Characteristics
Health Data Standards
  Consolidated Health Informatics
  National Committee on Vital and Health Statistics
  Interoperability: The Lingua Franca of the Electronic
    Health Record World
  Development and Selection of Health Data Standards
  Electronic Health Record Functional Model
  A National Network for Health Information Exchange
  Benefits of a National Network

Abbreviations

AAFP—American Academy of Family Physicians
AAP—American Academy of Pediatrics
ACP—American College of Physicians
AHCPR—Agency for Health Care Policy and Research

Key Words

Basic interoperability	Data standards	Nomenclature
Classification	Encoding	Nonsemantic concept identifier
Clinical reference terminology	Formal definitions	"Not elsewhere classified"
Clinical terminology	Functional interoperability	Nursing classification schemes
Code	Functional model	Polyhierarchy
Coding	Granularity	Recognized redundancy
Coding system	Interoperability	Semantic content
Code set	Mapping	Semantic interoperability
Concept permanence	Messaging standard	Terminology
Context representation	Multiple consistent views	Vocabulary
Content	Multiple granularities	

AHIC—American Health Information Community

AHIMA—American Health Information Management Association

AHRQ—Agency for Healthcare Research and Quality

AMA—American Medical Association

ANA—American Nurses Association

ANSI—American National Standards Institute

AP-DRG—All Patient Diagnosis-Related Groups

AMA—American Medical Association

APR-DRG—All Patient Refined Diagnosis Related Groups

ASTM—American Society for Testing and Materials

CAP—College of American Pathologists

CCHIT—Certification Commission for Healthcare Information Technology

CDC—Centers for Disease Control and Prevention

CHCF—California Health Care Foundation

CHI—Consolidated Health Informatics

CINAHL—Cumulative Index of Nursing and Allied Health Literature

CIS—commercial information system

CMS—Centers for Medicare and Medicaid Services

CPRS—Computerized Patient Record System

CPT—Common Procedural Terminology

CT—computed tomography

DICOM—Digital Imaging and Communications in Medicine

DOD—Department of Defense

DRG—Diagnosis Related Groups

DSM—Diagnostic and Statistical Manual of Mental Disorders

EHR—electronic health record

EO—Executive Order

FDA—Food and Drug Administration

HCPCS—Healthcare Common Procedure Coding System

HHS—Department of Health and Human Services

HIM—health information management

HIMSS—Health Information Management Systems Society

HIPAA—Health Insurance Portability and Accountability Act

HITPA—Health Information Technology Promotion Act

HITSP—Health Information Technology Standards Panel

HL7—Health Level 7

ICD-9—International Classification of Diseases, Ninth Revision

ICD-9-CM—International Classification of Diseases, Ninth Revision, Clinical Modification

ICD-10—International Classification of Diseases, Tenth Revision

ICD-10-PCS—International Classification of Diseases, 10th Revision, Procedural Coding System

ICD-O—International Classification of Diseases for Oncology

ICU—intensive care unit

IEEE—Institute of Electrical and Electronics Engineers

IOM—Institute of Medicine

ISO—International Organization for Standardization

JCAHO—Joint Commission on Accreditation of Healthcare Organizations (now The Joint Commission)

LOINC—Logical Observation Identifiers Names and Codes

MESH—Medical Subject Headings

NANDA—North American Nursing Diagnosis Association

NAHIT—National Alliance for Health Information Technology

NCHS—National Center for Health Statistics

NCPDP—National Council of Prescription Drug Programs

NCVHS—National Committee on Vital and Health Statistics

NDC—National Drug Codes

NDF-RT—National Drug File Reference Terminology

NEC—Not Elsewhere Classified

NIC—Nursing Interventions Classification

NLM—National Library of Medicine

NOC—Nursing Outcomes Classification

ONCHIT—Office of the National Coordinator of Health Information Technology

PCS—procedural coding system

PBM—pharmacy benefits management

PMRI—patient medical record information

PNDS—Perioperative Nursing Data Set

RELMA—Regenstrief LOINC Mapping Assistant

SCD—Steering Committee of Databases to Support Clinical Nursing Practice

SDO—standards developing organization

SNODENT—Systematized Nomenclature of Dentistry

SNOMED CT—Systematized Nomenclature of Medicine, Clinical Terms

SNOMED RT—Systematized Nomenclature of Medicine, Reference Terminology

SNOP—Systematized Nomenclature of Pathology

UMLS—Unified Medical Language System

VA—Department of Veterans Administration

VAMC—Department of Veterans Affairs Medical Center

WHO—World Health Organization

Objectives

- Explain the difference between a classification, a nomenclature, and a vocabulary
- Outline the primary uses of coded data
- Describe the value of clinical terminologies in relationship to the electronic health record
- Trace the evolution of International Classification of Diseases-related systems
- List the primary purposes of the International Classification of Diseases (ICD), Current Procedural Terminology (CPT), and Healthcare Common Procedure Coding System (HCPCS)
- Differentiate between Systematized Nomenclature of Medicine and International Classification of Diseases capabilities
- Describe the purpose and applicability of the Logical Observation Identifiers Names and Codes (LOINC) system

Continued

- Describe the purpose and applicability of key nursing terminologies
- Explain how the Unified Medical Language System (UMLS) supports clinical terminologies
- Identify the key characteristics of a clinical terminology
- Explain the value of data standards in health care
- Identify the primary activities and the key organizations developing and using standards

The health care environment has always been characterized by the need for timely, reliable, and easily accessible health care information to support patient care. As more providers adopt electronic health record (EHR) systems, the demand for such information has grown. Today's EHRs are not simply paper records that have been stored electronically. Clinical decision support tools that generate alerts, reminders, or practice guidelines based on the information in the patient's record can maximize the value of that information and help clinicians provide more personalized care to each patient.[1,2] Standardized clinical terminologies are essential for capturing clinical information in a form that is usable by both computers and people, and are the foundation for the meaningful sharing of health data between clinicians, among health care organizations, and between patients and their health care providers. The use of EHRs supported by clinical terminologies has implications for virtually all aspects of health care, from direct patient care to public health reporting.[3]

> Consider the case of Elton Ramsay, a 64-year-old man vacationing with his family in Arizona. While visiting his son, Mr. Ramsay experiences mild weakness in his left arm and asks to be taken to the Department of Veterans Affairs (VA) medical center a few minutes away. On arriving at the emergency department, Mr. Ramsay experiences a generalized left-sided hemiparesis and shortly thereafter loses consciousness. A computerized tomography (CT) scan reveals a large hemorrhagic infarct involving the right hemisphere. It becomes obvious that Mr. Ramsay needs surgical intervention; however, his family does not know what medications Mr. Ramsay is taking—only that his considerable health history includes diabetes, hypertension, and "something with his legs or feet." Fortunately, Mr. Ramsay routinely receives care at the VA medical center in St. Louis and his medical record is accessible across all VA sites. The emergency department physician in Arizona checks Mr. Ramsay's EHR to review his medications, allergies, medical history, laboratory results, radiology examinations, and cardiology reports and finds that Mr. Ramsay is taking captopril, insulin, and clopidogrel bisulfate (Plavix) for his hypertension, diabetes, and peripheral vascular disease. With access to this information, VA surgeons in Arizona know that the patient is taking an antiplatelet agent that could contribute to hemorrhage. Without this information, they might have assumed that a normal platelet level was adequate for this patient before surgical intervention—with serious consequences for Mr. Ramsay.

This fictional scenario illustrates the power of health information technology to affect health care for both patients and clinicians. A key to the successful use of health information technology is the ability to capture, interpret, and transmit relevant health data for a host of clinical, financial, and administrative purposes. Clinical terminologies are needed to support the different uses—and different users—of health data.

Health information management (HIM) professionals play an important role in helping health care organizations achieve the benefits of health information technology. David Brailer, MD, PhD, the first national coordinator for health information technology, noted that, "HIM professionals know what to do with records, how they flow through the systems, who uses them, who has access to them, and how to release information appropriately." With expertise in health information, data standards, EHR functionality, and supporting business processes in a variety of health care settings, health information managers can serve as advocates and subject matter experts, helping to resolve a range of health information technology issues from data standardization to privacy. To be effective in this evolving role, HIM professionals must understand the uses and limitations of different health care terminologies and be able to assist in the selection of appropriate terminologies for use with EHR systems.

TERMS ABOUT TERMS

The development and use of EHRs have brought together many different users of health data—including clinicians, HIM professionals, billing and reimbursement staff, medical informaticists, health economists, medical researchers, and data modelers. Although these users often rely on the same data to do their jobs, they do not always interpret that data the same way or even use the same words to talk about health data and information technology characteristics.

For example, the words *classification*, *code*, *vocabulary*, *nomenclature*, and *terminology* are used throughout health care to describe different forms and formats of data. Yet there is a great deal of variation in how these words are defined, and people often use them interchangeably when it is not appropriate to do so.

The word **classification** is typically used to describe a scheme for grouping similar things in a logical way on the basis of common characteristics. A given classification might organize related items alphabetically, chronologically, or by major category. Classification systems vary in their level of detail; some offer very general groupings, whereas others allow more detailed groupings and subgroupings, enabling the user to capture a greater degree of specificity, or granularity, of data.[4] One of the most commonly used classifications in health care is the *International Classification of Diseases* (ICD), maintained by the World Health Organization (WHO).

A set of terms and their corresponding definitions is known as a **vocabulary**. A **nomenclature** is a system of names that have been assigned according to pre-established rules. There is often overlap between these two terms. For example, the Systematized Nomenclature of Medicine, Clinical Terms, known as SNOMED CT, is both a vocabulary and a nomenclature.[5]

A **code** is a unique identifier assigned to a specific term, description, or concept. A list of codes and the terms or descriptions with which they are associated is known as a **code set**. In some code sets, the codes serve as a kind of shorthand—a way of conveying meaning with a minimum of complexity. For example, in the fourth edition of the *Current Procedural Terminology* (CPT), developed by the American Medical Association (AMA), codes between 80048 and 89356 are all related to pathology and laboratory.

Classifications, code sets, vocabularies, and nomenclatures all come under the umbrella of **terminology**.[6a] Terminologies have been developed to represent diseases, procedures, interventions, medications, devices, anatomy, functional status, demographics, and other types of information. Clinical terminologies are used for many different tasks, from simple archiving and retrieval of medical information to complex clinical decision support and data sharing between systems.

In the field of HIM, coding commonly refers to the selection of alphanumeric codes to represent diseases, procedures, and supplies used in the delivery of health care. Administrative coding may be done manually by using code books and other reference sources or with the assistance of electronic tools.[7]

However, when used in the broader context of EHRs, coding (or encoding) refers to the assignment of unique identifiers to the terms within a particular clinical terminology. Rather than being assigned manually, codes are assigned according to some predetermined algorithm, usually without any manual intervention. In a well-designed terminology, no meaning can be discerned from a code itself; it is simply a unique identifier that represents a more detailed description, concept, or term. The codes themselves remain unknown to most users; when a user selects a term to use, the associated code is stored electronically. These codes are used to transmit health data from one electronic system to another, for analysis, aggregation, or use at the point of care.[8]

Codes provide a more concise and efficient means of storing and transmitting detailed information than free text does. Reliance on free text information limits our ability to aggregate and compare information from different sources and presents challenges to the designers of advanced EHR tools. With encoded data, information can be displayed in a form that human beings can read and understand and stored in a form that computers can exchange and manipulate.[6] Clinical terminologies that use codes to represent detailed concepts provide a way to combine the expressiveness and flexibility of free text information with the clarity and computability of encoded information.[9]

ADMINISTRATIVE TERMINOLOGIES

Classification and coding systems commonly associated with health care, such as ICD-9, CPT, and the Healthcare Common Procedure Coding System (HCPCS), are primarily designed to support the administrative, financial, and regulatory functions associated with care. These terminologies serve as the primary communication tool between those providing services (e.g., physicians and hospitals) and those paying for services (e.g., insurance companies). They are also used by providers, payers, researchers, government agencies, and others for the following:

- Measuring the quality, safety, and efficacy of care
- Managing care and disease processes
- Tracking public health and risks
- Providing data to consumers regarding costs and outcomes of treatment options
- Payment system design and processing of claims for reimbursement
- Research, epidemiological studies, and clinical trials
- Designing health care delivery systems and monitoring resource utilization
- Identifying fraudulent practices
- Setting health policy[6,10]

Some common administrative terminologies used in the United States are described below.

International Classification of Diseases

ICD is a system used to classify inpatient and outpatient diagnoses and inpatient procedures. The foundation for ICD was established in 1893, with the development of the *Bertillion Classification of Causes of Death*. Although the system was initially used to classify mortality data from death certificates, it was expanded and adapted for other uses throughout the next century.

International Classification of Diseases, Ninth Revision

In 1977, WHO published the *International Classification of Diseases, Ninth Revision* (ICD-9).

In response to concerns that ICD-9 did not provide sufficient coverage for general coding and specific specialties, the National Center for Health Statistics (NCHS) initiated work to adapt ICD-9 for use in the United States. NCHS subsequently published a set of "clinical modifications" to ICD-9, which reflected the broader use of ICD-9 in the areas of reimbursement, epidemiology, and health sciences research. ICD-9 uses a core classification of three-digit codes, supplemented by a fourth digit (in the first decimal place) that provides additional detail and specificity.[11]

The version of ICD currently in use in the United States is the Ninth Revision with Clinical Modification, known as ICD-9-CM. ICD-9-CM includes a fifth digit to allow for another level of detail. In ICD-9-CM, terms are arranged in a strict hierarchy, which is reflected in the codes themselves: three-digit codes are at the highest level of the hierarchy, with four-digit codes at the second level, and five-digit codes at the third level.[11,12]

International Classification of Diseases, Tenth Revision

In 1992, WHO published ICD-10, the tenth revision of the ICD system. (WHO no longer supports ICD-9.) The United States began to use ICD-10 to report mortality statistics to WHO in 1999. As with ICD-9, NCHS developed a clinical modification for ICD-10 for use in the United States. ICD-10-CM contains significantly more codes and covers more content than ICD-9-CM, including additional information related to ambulatory and managed care encounters, expanded injury codes, combination diagnosis/symptom codes for more concise coding, and laterality codes. Codes in ICD-10-CM are alphanumeric and can contain up to seven digits.

With use of ICD-10, Mr. Ramsay's hemiparesis can be further defined by its underlying etiology of intracranial hemorrhage, as shown in the comparison below.

HEMIPARESIS

ICD-9-CM	ICD-10-CM
438.2 hemiplegia/ hemiparesis	**I69.25** hemiplegia and hemiparesis after other nontraumatic intracranial hemorrhage
438.20 unspecified side	I69.251 affecting right dominant side
438.21 affecting dominant side	I69.252 affecting left dominant side
438.22 affecting nondominant side	I69.253 affecting right nondominant side
	I69.254 affecting left nondominant side
	I69.259 affecting unspecified side

International Classification of Diseases, Tenth Revision, Procedural Coding System

Under a contract with the Centers for Medicare and Medicaid Services (CMS), 3M Health Information Systems developed the Procedural Coding System (PCS) to replace the list of procedure codes included in ICD-9-CM. ICD-10-PCS offers a much broader range of codes than ICD-9-CM, with room for expandability and greater specificity. ICD-9-CM is outdated and cannot adequately represent current medical practice and available medical technology; as a data capture tool, CPT does not adequately represent services provided in an inpatient hospital setting. Thus, neither terminology allows hospitals to provide complete, accurate, and precise reporting of clinical care. ICD-10-PCS would provide nearly 198,000 procedure codes, enabling hospitals to collect more specific information for use in patient care, benchmarking, quality assessment, research, public health reporting, strategic planning, and reimbursement.[13]

Although ICD-10-CM was originally targeted for release in 2001, neither the federal government nor the private sector had begun to implement ICD-10-CM or ICD-10-PCS as of 2006. The delay in implementing ICD-10 could have serious consequences for the nation, affecting the quality of data used for quality measurement, public health reporting, medical error reduction, service reimbursement, and bioterrorism response, as well as the nation's ability to support interoperable health data exchange. The National Committee for Vital and Health Statistics (NCVHS), which serves as an advisory committee to the Secretary of Health and Human Services, has recommended that the federal government make the necessary regulatory changes to require use of ICD-10-CM and ICD-10-PCS codes in the United States.[14] The American Health Information Management Association (AHIMA) has endorsed the adoption and implementation of ICD-10-CM and ICD-10-PCS and has called for the Department of Health and Human Services (HHS) to initiate the regulatory processes necessary to do so. The Health Information Technology Promotion Act of 2005 (HITPA) bill, which was introduced in the US House of Representatives on October 27, 2005, calls for the adoption of ICD-10-CM and ICD-10-PCS by October 1, 2009.

Derivations of the International Classification of Diseases

The Diagnostic and Statistical Manual of Mental Disorders (DSM), developed by the American Psychiatric Association, is a derivation of ICD that is used in behavioral health settings. It includes definitions and diagnostic criteria for mental disorders, with code numbers for each diagnosis.[15] All diagnostic codes in DSM-IV, the current version of DSM, are valid ICD-9-CM codes. DSM-IV systemizes psychiatric diagnosis using five axes:

Axis I	Major mental disorders, developmental disorders, and learning disabilities
Axis II	Underlying pervasive or personality conditions and mental retardation
Axis III	Any nonpsychiatric medical condition ("somatic")
Axis IV	Social functioning and impact of symptoms
Axis V	Global Assessment of Functioning (GAF) (on a scale from 100 to 0)

Not all axes must be used. An example of a multiaxial evaluation using DSM is shown on the following page.

Axis I   296.23 Major Depressive Disorder, Single
          Episode, Severe without Psychotic Features
          305.00 Alcohol Abuse
Axis II   301.6 Dependent Personality Disorder
          Frequent use of denial
Axis III None
Axis IV   Threat of job loss
Axis V   Global Assessment of Functioning (GAF)
          = 53 (current)

The International Classification of Diseases for Oncology (ICD-O) is another system derived from ICD. It is used to classify neoplasms according to their site, behavior, and morphological characteristics. Site codes are based on the malignant neoplasm codes in ICD-10. Like ICD, ICD-O is maintained by WHO.[16]

Current Procedural Terminology

CPT was developed by AMA nearly 40 years ago to provide a uniform language for effective communication among physicians, other health care providers, patients, and third parties.[17] When it was published in 1966, CPT helped encourage the use of standard descriptors to document procedures in the medical record. CPT includes descriptive terms and the identifying codes associated with them. The first edition of CPT contained primarily surgical procedures; subsequent editions provided an expanded set of terms and codes to represent diagnostic and therapeutic procedures in surgery, medicine, and the specialties. The 2005 CPT update contains 8568 descriptors and codes.

Today, CPT is used extensively throughout the United States as the preferred system of coding medical, surgical, and diagnostic services. It is widely used in administrative applications, particularly for billing and reimbursement purposes. However, given the availability of CPT data, it is often used for purposes for which it was not designed—for example, as a basis for performance monitoring and measurement, for research related to professional services, and even to evaluate physician efficiency.

CPT is continually reviewed, revised, and updated to reflect changes in medical technology and clinical practice and to accommodate new uses and users of CPT data. The current edition is CPT-4; updates to CPT-4 are published in the fall and take effect the following January 1. To extend the applicability of CPT, AMA is overseeing the development of CPT-5. This new version will include three categories of codes: one for procedures and services, a second to support performance measurement, and a third to facilitate assessment of new services and procedures and other emerging technologies.[17]

Healthcare Common Procedure Coding System

CPT serves as Level I of the Healthcare Common Procedure Coding System (HCPCS), which is used to report physician services and other health care services and medical supplies, orthotic and prosthetic devices, and durable medical equipment. HCPCS Level II, also called alphanumeric HCPCS, consists of national codes for durable medical equipment, drugs, supplies, and services not included in Level I. Level II codes are maintained by CMS. Before 2003, HCPCS included Level III codes, which were used by Medicare carriers, fiscal intermediaries, health plans, and insurers for specific local needs. Although HCPCS Level III was virtually eliminated under the Health Insurance Portability and Accountability Act (HIPAA), many users still had a need for the information formerly captured through the use of Level III codes. Additional Level II codes are used to compensate for the loss of the Level III codes.[15]

Diagnosis Related Groups

Diagnosis Related Groups, or DRGs, are used to categorize patients on the basis of principal and secondary diagnoses, principal and secondary procedures, age, sex, complications, discharge status, and comorbidities.[18] DRGs were designed as a way to group services and estimate costs to support prospective payment under Medicare. The basic DRG method is used by CMS for hospital payment for Medicare beneficiaries. DRGs have has been widely adopted in the United States by Medicaid programs and by other third-party payers. For some populations, such as pediatric, rehabilitation, or psychiatric patients, it is difficult to establish utilization norms based on diagnosis and major procedures because there are wide variations in the resources consumed for a particular diagnosis. Two other versions of the DRG method, All Patient DRGs and All Patient Refined DRGs, are designed to address these limitations.[19] All Patient DRGs (AP-DRGs) provide an expanded version of the DRG model that is more representative of non-Medicare populations. All Patient Refined DRGs (APR-DRGs) further refine AP-DRGs by taking into account severity of illness.[19] More information about DRGs and financial management issues can be found in Chapter 18.

Adaptation of Administrative Terminologies

Terminologies developed for one purpose are often adapted or expanded to support others. For example, ICD—a system originally developed for collecting morbidity and mortality statistics—evolved into a system to support billing and reimbursement and is used for clinical research, quality improvement, and other purposes. However, not every terminology is appropriate for every task, and terminologies designed for one purpose may not work well for others.

Simple decision-support features, such as clinical reminders to perform interventions for chronic disease, are often based on CPT and ICD-9-CM codes. CPT codes are used by VA for workload capture, clinical reminders, and decision support. The presence of the ICD-9-CM code for diabetes mellitus can be used to prompt an annual preventive interventions such as foot examinations, eye examinations, and tests for hemoglobin A1c.[20,21]

Administrative data can also be used to refine decision support features so that clinicians are not overloaded with reminders and alerts. For example, an EHR system could remind a clinician to perform an annual prostate examination for male patients over 40 years of age, unless the patient's record indicated that he was post prostatectomy, in which case the alert would be deactivated.

Although administrative terminologies can be used to support clinical applications, they were not designed for the primary documentation of clinical care and thus are not the most clinically relevant data sets on which to base clinical decision support.[22] Terminologies designed primarily for administrative purposes do not have the granularity of a comprehensive clinical terminology and cannot adequately capture the complexity required for advanced decision support.

Administrative data collection is often limited to billable diagnosis and procedure codes, and miscoding can compromise the validity of ICD and CPT data for clinical uses. Even variations between inpatient and outpatient coding rules can affect the usefulness of administrative data for decision support. For example, current ICD-9 coding conventions require that an inpatient admission for unconfirmed diabetes mellitus be coded. These data remain a part of a patient's EHR as an ICD-9 code even in the event that the diagnosis is later eliminated. In the VA, a diabetes diagnosis will trigger a set of preventive reminders to assist clinicians in managing and improving quality of care. Populations are also tracked for quality-of-care issues, recidivism, and disease management. Reminders will continue to erroneously display as part of this patient's medical profile until they are manually deactivated.

One of the challenges facing health care is how to represent clinically specific data in a form that is usable for clinical decision support and data analysis.[23] Rather than attempting to stretch the use of administrative terminologies to accommodate clinical requirements, providers are now seeking terminologies specifically designed with clinical applications in mind.

CLINICAL TERMINOLOGIES

At the most basic level, a clinical terminology is used to represent the information in a medical record, whether that record is in paper form or electronic form. To understand the need for clinical terminologies, it is helpful to think about the evolution from paper-based records to EHRs. In early EHR systems, much of the information was entered in the medical record as free text—just as it had been entered in a paper record. For example, to enter a progress note in the EHR, a clinician typed a few sentences on a computer rather than writing them on paper. Although another clinician

could understand these sentences regardless of whether they were on paper or on a computer screen, another computer could not.

Human readers can easily interpret narrative information and automatically add context that helps them interpret that information. In reviewing another clinician's progress note about a patient, for example, a physician might recall a previous conversation that was not documented in the record, think about practices at the other hospital where the patient had been treated, or even consider who wrote the note to capture subtleties that a computer might miss.

In contrast, computers are quite literal in their interpretation of data. A classic example of this is illustrated by the sentence, "Baby swallows fly." This sentence could be interpreted in different ways, depending on whether the verb in the sentence is "swallows" or "fly" and on whether "baby" is a noun or an adjective.[4]

Health data can also be ambiguous. The word "cold," for example, can refer to many different things, including temperature, mood, illness, and influenza. For example, a patient might report to her physician that she has a cold or that she feels cold all the time. If the letters "cold" were transmitted from one provider to another as part of the patient's medical record, the recipient might wonder whether the patient had chronic obstructive lung disease unless additional information were provided to clarify the use of the term. When clinical terminologies are used, much of the ambiguity inherent in natural language can be eliminated.[24,25]

Systematized Nomenclature of Medicine

SNOMED CT is a comprehensive clinical reference terminology developed and maintained by the College of American Pathologists (CAP). SNOMED stands for Systematized Nomenclature of Medicine.[26] The terminology evolved from SNOP, the Systematized Nomenclature of Pathology, a four-axis system of terms and codes designed specifically for pathologists. In 1974, CAP released the first version of SNOMED, which extended the terminology to other specialties with the inclusion of a broad array of clinical terms.

The second edition of SNOMED, released in 1979, included 44,587 terms and was endorsed in this country and the United Kingdom as the preferred terminology for clinical and anatomic pathology. The third edition of SNOMED, released in 1993, is recognized as a work of enormous significance. With 130,580 terms and codes organized in 11 modules, SNOMED III provided a multidimensional, structured nomenclature for indexing medical diagnoses and treatments. It was translated into several foreign languages, gaining wide acceptance throughout the international health care community.[27]

In 1995, CAP began a collaboration with Kaiser Permanente, revising the structure of SNOMED to reflect advances in medical informatics and computer science. The SNOMED Reference Terminology (SNOMED RT), launched in May

2000, was designed as a unified clinical terminology for health states, disease states, pathophysiology, treatments, and outcomes.

SNOMED has been refined and expanded for more than four decades, and it is now considered the most comprehensive international and multilingual clinical reference terminology in the world. The SNOMED CT core terminology offers a consistent language for capturing, sharing, and aggregating health data across specialties and sites of care.

SNOMED is based on concepts. Each concept represents a unit of thought or meaning and is labeled with a computer-readable unique identifier. The phrases in human language used to describe the concept are called "descriptions" or "synonyms." Each concept has one or more descriptions linked to it. SNOMED provides a rich set of logical interrelationships between concepts. Through the use of these relationships, computer-readable definitions of medical concepts can be provided. These definitions greatly enhance the value of the data collected, allowing it to be searched, retrieved, reused, or analyzed in a variety of ways.

Hierarchical relationships define specific concepts as children of more general concepts. For example, "appendicitis" is defined as a kind of "inflammatory disorder of the intestine." In this way, hierarchical relationships provide links to related information about the concept. This example shows that appendicitis also represents a part of the body and has a morphology of inflammation (Figure 6-1).

In medicine, there are many ways to state the same concept. By linking synonyms to a single concept, SNOMED CT allows computer systems to recognize the common meaning of synonymous terms. Description logic assists in providing a complete and fully defined definition. There are several types of relationships. Figure 6-2 illustrates a more detailed representation of the "is-a" relationships by use of the diagnosis of coronary atherosclerosis.

One of the greatest strengths of SNOMED is that it was designed with electronic systems in mind. In addition to EHR applications, SNOMED CT is being used for intensive care unit (ICU) monitoring, medical research studies, clinical trials, disease surveillance, image indexing, and consumer health information services. As of July 2005, the core terminology contained more than 366,170 health care concepts, 993,420 descriptions, and approximately 1.46 million semantic relationships. SNOMED has also integrated various domain-specific vocabularies into its terminology such as the nursing vocabularies, laboratory Logical Observation Identifiers Names and Codes (LOINC), and Systematized Nomenclature of Dentistry (SNODENT).[28] SNOMED has been mapped to other clinical terminologies, including LOINC, ICD-9, and ICD-10, streamlining data capture and facilitating billing, health reporting, and statistical analysis. The mapping resources include simple many-to-one tables such as SNOMED to ICD-O topography, more complicated lists of alternatives (to ICD-9 or ICD-10), and nursing classifications systems (Perioperative Nursing Data Set [PNDS], Nursing Interventions Classification [NIC], Nursing Outcomes Classification [NOC], and North American Nursing Diagnosis Association [NANDA]).[27,29]

Logical Observation Identifiers Names and Codes

LOINC is another example of a terminology designed for use in EHR systems.[30] LOINC stands for Logical Observation Identifiers Names and Codes. It is a system of 36,000 concepts used to represent laboratory and clinical measurements, survey questions, clinical documents, and diagnostic reports. The concepts include names, codes, and synonyms.

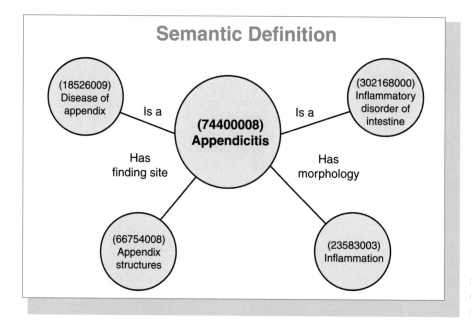

Figure 6-1 SNOMED CT® appendicitis. (From the College of American Pathologists.)

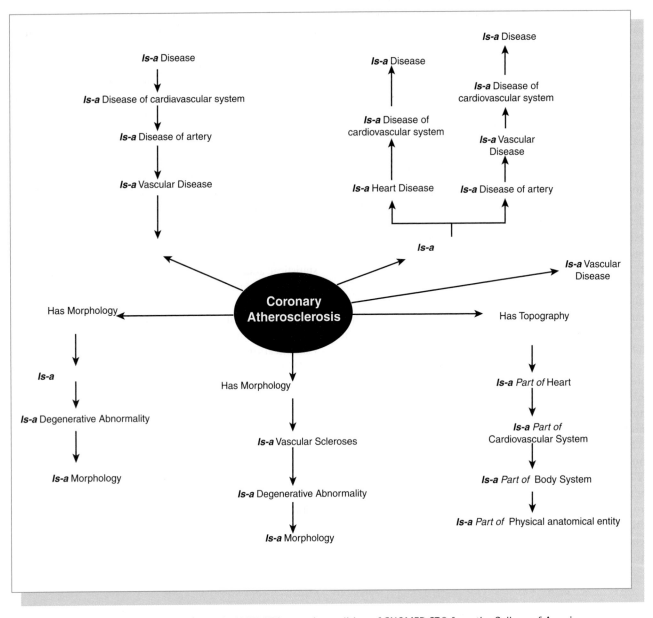

Figure 6-2 SNOMED atherosclerosis. (From SNOMED RT,® a previous edition of SNOMED CT,® from the College of American Pathologists.)

LOINC was designed to facilitate the exchange and aggregation of results—such as blood hemoglobin, serum potassium, and vital signs—for clinical care, outcomes management, and research.

The LOINC database and supporting documentation are maintained by the Regenstrief Institute,[31] with funding by the National Library of Medicine, John A. Hartford Foundation of New York, and the Agency for Health Care Policy and Research (AHCPR) and through a grant/cooperative agreement from the Centers for Disease Control and Prevention (CDC).

Regenstrief LOINC Mapping Assistant (RELMA) is the tool that is used to view and search the LOINC database. The power of LOINC is in the ability to facilitate the exchange of information between health care entities. It is used

in the Regenstrief information exchange project that began in Indianapolis, which has expanded to be the Indiana Health Information Exchange Project. LOINC has expanded beyond the laboratory realm to include clinical measurements, assessments, and clinical document references.[11] Dr. Stan Huff and his colleagues at Intermountain Health Care in Salt Lake City used LOINC to establish an information model to capture the data needed to effectively treat patients undergoing organ transplantation. The model enables them the ability to record not only information about the patient but information about the donor as well. It is a reusable model for circumstances when it is necessary to refer to one patient's data from another patient's EHR, as is needed in situations such as transplants and mother-child relationships.[32]

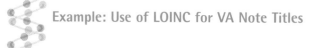

Example: Use of LOINC for VA Note Titles

Virtually all clinical documents created by VA providers are stored in VistA; as a result, patient records containing hundreds or thousands of notes are becoming common. As of December 2005, VistA systems contained nearly 779 million progress notes, discharge summaries, and reports; 1.54 billion orders; and almost 425 million images. More than 577,000 new clinical documents, 906,000 orders, and 608,000 images are added each work day—a wealth of information for the clinician. As the volume of on-line information increases, the task of finding a specific note or report can be difficult, particularly when different clinicians and sites assign different names to similar documents.

In using the Computerized Patient Record System (CPRS), a graphical interface to the information in VistA, clinicians use an on-screen menu to select a document based on its title. However, the readability of document titles varied widely from site to site and from author to author. Titles such as *UR 67CD (T) (K), CIH/STAR II CONSUL, or PATIENT HEALTH EDU POINT AND CLICK,* for example, might be clear to the author but are difficult for other users to decipher. Users were often frustrated with the time required to find relevant notes among hundreds of irregularly structured titles.

To speed the retrieval of clinical information, a team of VA clinicians, developers, terminologists, and HIM professionals collaborated to establish standard conventions for naming and transmitting clinical documents created in VistA. After researching existing LOINC and Health Level 7 (HL7) standards, the team extracted 156,000 document titles from 128 site-based databases, analyzed every term within the extracted titles, and categorized them in accordance with LOINC naming standards and HL7 messaging standards.

The LOINC document naming nomenclature contains five axes: subject matter domain, role, setting, service, and document type. A standard title is created by combining a term from each axis into a composite title. Not all axes are required to create a valid document title; some may be left blank as long as the correct order is maintained.

The use of standardized note titles will make it easier for users to find relevant clinical documents and to transfer and incorporate documents created at other VA and non-VA sites. To minimize disruption at the local level, VA facilities were not required to rename clinical documents already stored in VistA. Instead, the titles of existing documents are mapped to the new standard title format before the documents are transmitted to a national clinical repository; where they are accessible to providers throughout VA.[24,33]

Drug Terminologies

National Drug Codes (NDCs) were developed by the Food and Drug Administration (FDA) for labeling drug packages.

Drugs administered in health care settings are reported under HIPAA billing transactions; either HCPCS Level II or NDC may be used for this purpose. The National Library of Medicine and the VA are working on new drug terminologies that will be more appropriate for use in clinical care and will support institutional and provider reporting. The VA developed the National Drug File Reference Terminology (NDF-RT), a nonproprietary terminology used to classify drugs by mechanism of action and physiological effect.

Nursing Terminologies

The American Nurses Association (ANA) developed nursing classification themes to describe the nursing process, document nursing care, and facilitate aggregation of data for comparisons at the local, regional, national, and international levels. The ANA established the Steering Committee of Databases to Support Clinical Nursing Practice (SCD) to monitor and support the development and evolution of the use of multiple vocabularies and classification schemes.[13]

NIC and NOC are comprehensive, research-based, standardized systems used to classify the interventions that nurses perform and outcome evaluations based on those interventions.[34,35] NIC and NOC are useful for clinical documentation, communication of care across settings, integration of data across systems and settings, effectiveness research, productivity measurement, competency evaluation, reimbursement, and curriculum design. NIC and NOC can be used in all settings (from acute care intensive care units, to home care, to hospice, to primary care) and all specialties (from critical care to ambulatory and long-term care).

NIC interventions include both the physiological (e.g., Acid-Base Management) and the psychosocial (e.g., Anxiety Reduction). Interventions are included for direct care, as in illness treatment (e.g., Hyperglycemia Management), illness prevention (e.g., Fall Prevention), and health promotion (e.g., Exercise Promotion). Although most of the interventions are for use with individuals, many are for use with families on behalf of patients (e.g., Family Integrity Promotion), and some are for use with entire communities (e.g., Environmental Management: Community). Indirect care interventions (e.g., Supply Management) are also included. Each intervention as it appears in the classification is listed with a label name, a definition, a set of activities to carry out the intervention, and background readings. NIC can be used by other nonphysician providers to describe their treatments. NIC is recognized by The Joint Commission as one nursing classification system that can be used to meet the standard on uniform data. Both NIC and NOC are registered in HL7 and have been mapped to SNOMED.[44]

NOC is a three-level classification system currently composed of seven domains, 29 outcome classes, and 260 outcomes. An outcome is a measurable individual, family, or community state, behavior, or perception that is measured along a continuum and is responsive to nursing interventions. Although the entire classification describes the domain of nursing, some of the interventions in the classification are also performed by other providers. Each outcome is associated with varying quantities of indicators. Each indicator is given a score on one of 17, five-point Likert-type scales. This structure allows for measurement and comparison at any point along a continuum. Examples of outcomes influenced by nursing interventions include: Ambulation, Caregiver Emotional Health, Mobility Level, Nutritional Status, and Cognitive Orientation.[36]

The Omaha System was one of the first taxonomies or terminologies recognized by ANA. It is a research-based, comprehensive, and standardized taxonomy designed to enhance practice, documentation, and information management. It consists of three relational, reliable, and valid components: the Problem Classification Scheme, the Intervention Scheme, and the Problem Rating Scale for Outcomes. Initial adopters included home care, public health, and school health practice settings and some educators in the United States. Omaha System terms and definitions are not held under copyright so are available for use without permission. However, the source of the terms, definitions, and codes must accompany their use. Other sections of the new book are held under copyright.

The Problem Classification Scheme (nursing diagnosis) is organized into four levels:

Level 1: Domain	There are four general domain areas: Environmental, Psychosocial, Physiological, Health-Related Behaviors
Level 2: Problems	There are 42 specific health-related concerns
Level 3: Modifiers	Type of problem: Actual, Potential, Health Promotion
	Client Type: Individual, Family, Community
Level 4: Signs and Symptoms	Evidence of a patient problem

Example of Omaha System within Domains and Sample Problems

Level 1	Level 2
Environment	Income, Sanitation
Psychosocial	Mental Health, Grieving, Abuse
Physiological	Hearing, Vision, Speech, Circulation
Health Behavior	Nutrition, Medication Regimen

Table 6-1 contains the thirteen data element sets and terminologies that the ANA recognizes as supporting nursing practice.

The Role of the Unified Medical Language System

No single terminology is appropriate for all uses or meets the needs of all users, and a great deal of work is being done to define appropriate uses of available health care terminologies and the relationships between them. The National Library of Medicine's (NLM) Unified Medical Language System (UMLS) is a valuable resource for interrelating terminologies by supporting mappings and cross-references among them. UMLS is a relational database that connects scores of vocabularies, classifications, and other sources by concept, allowing users to map data from one terminology to another. **Mapping** is valuable for retaining the value of historical data when migrating to newer database formats and terminology versions (e.g., migration from ICD-8 to ICD-9). Mapping also enables users to use data for multiple purposes without having to capture the data in multiple formats. The UMLS, begun in 1986, uses one identification code to represent the same concept from different vocabulary sources, such as NLM's Medical Subject Headings (MeSH) and ICD-9. An EHR could use this link to generate an automated literature search based on a patient's ICD-9 diagnosis code, enabling the treating physician to retrieve relevant literature through a MeSH-based query to NLM's PubMed system.

NIC, NOC, and the Omaha System have been mapped to SNOMED CT and integrated in LOINC and are included in the NLM Metathesaurus for a Unified Medical Language and the Cumulative Index of Nursing and Allied Health Literature (CINAHL).

In 2003, HHS, in conjunction with VA and the Department of Defense (DoD), entered into an agreement with CAP to license SNOMED CT for use in the United States. The agreement includes English and Spanish editions of SNOMED CT and cross-maps between SNOMED CT and ICD-9-CM, ICD-03, LOINC, NIC, NOC, NANDA, and PNDS.

TERMINOLOGY CHARACTERISTICS

As EHRs have become more sophisticated, so has our understanding of the uses and limitations of health data and the systems we use to organize and exchange health data. To interpret and use a terminology correctly, it is important to understand its structure, design, and intended purpose and the process by which codes are assigned to individual terms.

In 1998, a medical informaticist named James Cimino, MD, identified 12 *desiderata*, or desirable characteristics, that would make clinical terminologies more useful.[37] These desiderata have since gained broad acceptance and are now considered the fundamental principles for the development and integration of clinical terminologies. The twelve characteristics are as follows:

1. Content
The usefulness of a given terminology is largely determined by its *content.* Terminologies that have a very narrow

Table 6-1   AMERICAN NURSES ASSOCIATION–RECOGNIZED TERMINOLOGIES AND DATA ELEMENT SETS[35]

Data Element Sets	Setting Where Developed	Content
1. NMDS Nursing Minimum Data Set currently recognized	All nursing	Clinical data elements
2. NMMDS Nursing Management Minimum Data Set currently recognized	All settings	Nursing administration data elements
Interface Terminologies **3. CCC** Clinical Care Classification currently recognized	Home care	Diagnoses, interventions, and outcomes
4. ICNP International Classification of Nursing Practice currently recognized	All nursing	Diagnoses, interventions, and outcomes
5. NANDA North American Nursing Diagnosis Association International currently recognized	All nursing	Diagnoses
6. NIC Nursing Intervention Classification currently recognized	All nursing	Interventions
7. NOC Nursing Outcome Classification currently recognized	All nursing	Outcomes
8. OMAHA SYSTEM Omaha System currently recognized	Home care, public health, and community health	Diagnoses, interventions, and outcomes
9. PCDS Patient Care Data Set retired	Acute care	Diagnoses, interventions, and outcomes
10. PNDS Perioperative Nursing Data Set Currently recognized	Perioperative	Diagnoses, interventions, and outcomes
Multidisciplinary Terminologies **11. ABC** Alternative Billing Codes currently recognized	Nursing and other	Interventions
12. LOINC Logical Observation Identifiers Names and Codes currently recognized	Nursing and other	Outcomes and assessments
13. SNOMED CT Systematic Nomenclature of Medicine Clinical Terms currently recognized	Nursing and other	Diagnoses, interventions, and outcomes

Source: American Nurses Association. http://www.nursingworld.org/npii/terminologies.htm. Accessed March 2006.

focus may be quite useful for a specific purpose but have limited value for other purposes. Yet terminologies that cover a broader range of concepts are not necessarily better if they are poorly designed or maintained. There must be a formal method for adding content when gaps in content coverage are discovered. AMA has clearly stated the context in which CPT should be used and as such it is now widely used for billing and reimbursement of professional services. CPT-4 is maintained by a CPT editorial panel that revises, updates, and modifies CPT codes. Modifiers are used extensively to add or refine information about the provided service. It is not a comprehensive coding system and is not marketed as such.

2. Concept Orientation

Each terminology should have a *concept orientation*— that is, each term should correspond to a single concept and that concept should have a single, coherent meaning. A given concept may be interpreted differently when used in different contexts; for example, a condition recorded under the personal history of a patient may have different implications than the same condition recorded under family history. SNOMED is a concept-based terminology, with each concept representing a unit of meaning. Consider the example of a patient who has undergone a total abdominal hysterectomy. CPT would assign a code of 58150; however, this code would not indicate whether the patient had a removal of tubes, a removal of an ovary, or a combination of the two. SNOMED does not exhibit such ambiguity and allows for the necessary degree of specification.

3. Concept Permanence

Concept permanence means that once a concept has been created within a terminology, its meaning cannot change and it cannot be deleted. The preferred name of the concept can change, or the concept may be deemed inactive, but its meaning must remain fixed as long as the terminology is in use. The name for the concept "non-A-non-B hepatitis," for example, cannot be changed to "hepatitis C" because the two concepts are not synonymous. Concept permanence helps prevent the users from misinterpreting historical data. ICD-9-CM is a stable classification system that allows for long spans of review. However, this stability has come at the expense of responsiveness to change. Although no system is perfect in this regard, changes can be tracked. SNOMED CT is an example of a clinical reference terminology that allows for concept permanence.

4. Nonsemantic Concept Identifier

There must be a *nonsemantic concept identifier* associated with each term. This means that an identifier does not carry any meaning in itself and does not indicate the hierarchical position of the term it represents. This characteristic is important so that classification systems can expand and can be reclassified or categorized in more that one area if needed. However, neither CPT nor ICD-9-CM exhibits this characteristic. In ICD-9-CM, for example, meaning can be inferred by the numerical placement of the concept. The use of a hierarchical numbering convention limits the number of concepts that can be represented by the terminology; in ICD-9-CM, very few unassigned codes are available to accommodate new diagnoses and procedures.

5. Polyhierarchy

Many terminologies are arranged hierarchically. A hierarchical structure can help users locate concepts, group related concepts, and add context. It is not necessary to have a single hierarchy—in fact, *polyhierarchy* is necessary to support different users and uses of the same terminology.

Let's examine the diagnosis of Pneumonia. ICD-9-CM lists Salmonella Pneumonia (003.22) as a descendent in the 003 section (other Salmonella Infections) and not under either 482 (Other Bacterial Pneumonia) or 484 (Pneumonia in Infectious Disease Classified Elsewhere). The strict hierarchical structure of ICD-9-CM precludes its ability to classify terms in more that one way. SNOMED accomplishes polyhierarchy through the use of "is-a" relationships.

6. Formal Definitions

Formal definitions are those that follow a formal structure, that is, definitions that are represented in a form that can by manipulated by a computer, as opposed to narrative text definitions intended for human readers. These definitions can be expressed through the use of "is-a" relationships connecting concepts in a vocabulary. Using our previous SNOMED example, the concept "Coronary Atherosclerosis" can be defined with an "is-a" link to the concept "Arteriosclerotic Vascular Disease" and a "site" relationship to "coronary artery." There are a number of ways this information can be expressed; the important point is that the information can be manipulated through the use of a computer, as opposed to the variety of ways this information can be displayed by health care professionals using narrative text.

7. Reject "Not Elsewhere Classified"

Not Elsewhere Classified (NEC) terms are used to collect concepts that are not covered elsewhere in a terminology. Although NEC terms can be convenient to those developing a terminology, they can cause problems for the user. Because NEC terms are defined by exclusion, their meaning can change every time a new concept is added to the terminology. The *Reject "Not Elsewhere Classified"* characteristic requires that a terminology does not include NEC terms. The use of NEC in ICD-9-CM is one of the principal limitations of the terminology for storage and retrieval of clinical data.

8. Multiple Granularities

Granularity refers to the degree of specificity and refinement of a term. Different users are likely to require different levels of granularity. Terminologies that include *multiple granularities* of the same content can support many more users that those with a single level of granularity. Classifications are intended to aggregate information by skipping nonessential characteristics so that similar items can be grouped together. For EHR use, clinical terminologies must allow users to distinguish between similar items by highlighting the different between them. For example, the concept "diabetes" is too general to be very useful, whereas "insulin-dependent type II diabetes" has greater granularity depending on the purpose of the information or the knowledge known at the time. CPT and ICD-9-CM have the capability to provide some level of granularity but not to the level of SNOMED.

9. Multiple Consistent Views

Multiple consistent views are required to support the different views of the vocabulary depending on the utility. Cimino[37] states that polyhierarchical terminologies with multiple levels of granularity must not permit inconsistent views of a single concept.

10. Context Representation

A well-designed terminology must allow for *context representation.* It should include formal, explicit information about how concepts are to be used.[37] This means that there is a "grammar" that can be used to manipulate data and that there is also context-specific information about what is "sensible to say." For example, it would be sensible to see the word "rupture" used in relation to "appendicitis" but not to the term "eyebrow." The ability to represent context is essential to avoid the misinterpretation of health data.[13]

11. Graceful Evolution

The structure and content of a terminology must change over time to reflect scientific advances, administrative changes, and other relevant factors. A terminology created in

1970, for example, might include the concept "non-A-non-B hepatitis." Without the subsequent addition of "hepatitis C," however, the terminology would not have sufficient content to describe current medical practice. There must be a formal method for adding content to the terminology so that does not become obsolete as the field of medicine evolves, and all changes should be described and documented in detail. As noted under Concept Permanence, not all types of changes are desirable. For example, the reassignment of codes or redefinition of a concept can render a terminology unusable.

12. Recognized Redundancy

Redundancy is a characteristic of language. Redundancy occurs within a terminology when there is more than one term with the same meaning. This is desirable as long as the redundancy is recognized. *Recognized redundancy* means that terms with the same meaning are treated as synonyms and are represented by the same identifying code. Ideally, these redundant entries map to the same concept; for example, Myocardial Infarction and Heart Attack are synonyms and should be treated as though they represent the same concept. If synonymous terms are not recognized within the terminology, data aggregation becomes incomplete and inconsistent. The evolution of medical knowledge ensures that controlled vocabularies need to change over time.

On the basis of experience in implementing a clinical terminology for Kaiser Permanente, Campbell identified six additional desirable characteristics[28]:

1. Copyrighted and licensed

The terminology should be licensed, copyrighted, and maintained by a single organization to prevent local modifications that might make the data incomparable across different sites, systems, or organizations.

2. Commercial information system (CIS) vendor-neutral

The design of the terminology should not give any advantage to a particular CIS vendor. This will ensure that the terminology is available nationally (or internationally), prevent limits on its use for profit reasons, and protect the terminology from events that adversely affect a vendor. ICD-9, CPT, and SNOMED are all vendor-neutral.

3. Scientifically valid

The terminology should be understandable, reproducible, useful, and reflective of the current understanding of science.

4. Well-maintained

There must be a central authority responsible for keeping the terminology current and for providing rapid response to new terms. Both ICD and CPT are updated on a regular basis. The ICD-9-CM Coordination and Maintenance Committee reviews proposals to update ICD-9-CM; changes are effective October 1 each year. Proposed changes to CPT are reviewed by the CPT Editorial Panel and experts from affected medical subspecialties, and they are effective January 1 each year.

5. Self-sustaining

The terminology should be supported by public or endowment funding or by license fees to cover development and support costs. CPT is licensed by the AMA; ICD by the AHA. With the $32 million federal investment in SNOMED CT, users throughout the United States will be able to use the terminology maintained by CAP without incurring licensing costs.

6. Scalable infrastructure and process control

Tools and processes used to maintain the terminology should be scalable to the number of users so that timely maintenance is not jeopardized.

HEALTH DATA STANDARDS

Although the need for common clinical terminologies has been recognized for decades, such terminologies are not in general use. The lack of agreed-on clinical terminologies for the capture and exchange of health information presents a significant impediment to the expanded use of EHR systems. Providers can certainly exchange health information without using clinical terminologies (as they do now when they copy and send paper records); yet the reliance on nonstandardized data or narrative information can limit the benefit of EHRs and other health information technology tools.

Widespread adoption of standard clinical terminologies will enable health care providers and systems to exchange clinically specific data without human intervention. The use standard terminologies, coupled with the broader adoption of EHR technology, will support the following:

- Higher quality health care for patients
- The development of more sophisticated tools for clinical and administrative staff
- Greater interaction among providers, public health organizations, and other health care partners and, as result,
- More cost-effective use of health care resources

The development and adoption of health data standards is key. Data standards are documented agreements on representations, formats, and definitions of common data. The International Organization for Standardization (ISO) defines a standard as "a documented agreement containing technical specifications or other precise criteria to be used consistently as rules, guidelines, or definitions of characteristics to ensure that materials, products, processes and services are fit for their purpose."[38] Standards affect nearly every facet of our lives and can have a profound influence on the safety, reliability, effectiveness, and durability of products we use every day, from milk cartons to telephones.

Standardized data are easier to store, exchange, and interpret than are nonstandardized data and, as a result, are more powerful for the user. There are many different types of health data standards. A standard may dictate which terminology is used, what format is used to transmit it from one party to another, or how each term is defined. A health care organization may elect to store data, display, and transmit to a partner organization in a third format for compliance.

The need for data standards is not limited to complex clinical concepts and applications. Consider two simple terms: yes and no. In many computer systems, the numeral "1" is used to indicate "yes," and the numeral "2" is used to indicate "no." In some systems it is reversed: "1" means "no" and "2" means "yes." Some systems use "0" and "1" instead of "1" and "2." In still other systems, "Y" is used to indicate "yes" and "N" is used to indicate "no." Sometimes lower case "y" and "n" are used. Sometimes "yes" is actually stored as "y-e-s" and "no" as "n-o."

VA's EHR contains more than 100 separate applications. When VA established a formal data standardization program in 2003, VA analysts found 30 different combinations of codes for "yes" and "no" stored in nearly 4000 different data fields in the VA's EHR.

The problems created by a lack of standardized data are magnified when data are exchanged with other organizations. Even seemingly straightforward data can be misconstrued when interpreted by different organizations, systems, or users. VA, for example, can standardize its representation of "yes" and "no" and other data values within VA computer systems, but unless its health care partners use the same standards to exchange data with VA, inconsistencies and misinterpretations are very likely to occur.

 ### Example: Standardizing VA Allergy Data

The VA was an early leader in the development of EHR systems. VA's VistA system is recognized as one of the most comprehensive EHRs in use today. When VA developed its first EHR, the technological environment in VA hospitals—as in other hospitals at the time—was very different from the environment today. There was not a computer on every desk. There were no graphical user interfaces or pull-down menus, only text-based displays on "dumb terminals." When users wanted to enter data in the EHR, they did not point and click; they typed.

For example, when a clinician wanted to document a patient's allergy to penicillin, he typed the word "penicillin" in the allergy section of the patient's EHR. To save time, many clinicians entered "PCN," a common abbreviation for penicillin.

When VA analysts reviewed the allergy data that had been collected over the years, they found that "penicillin" and "PCN" had been typed in thousands of times—and in thousands of cases, these entries had been misspelled. VA recognized that the reliance on free-text data entry for allergy information was time consuming for the clinician and, more important, introduced a potential patient safety issue.

Suppose a veteran comes in for a checkup and tells the physician that he is allergic to sulfa drugs. The physician enters this information in the patient's record under allergies, but because she is typing quickly, she inadvertently misspells the word "sulfa." Suppose that on a subsequent visit, another clinician orders sulfamethoprim, which is a type of sulfa drug. Whenever a clinician orders a medication, the EHR checks the patient's record to see if the patient is allergic to the medication. Although the system checks for common misspellings, it cannot predict every possible misspelling of every medication. In this case, the EHR might not alert the second physician that he had ordered a drug the patient was allergic to, simply because the word "sulfa" was misspelled when it was entered by the first physician.

To eliminate misspellings and other data entry errors, VA encoded commonly used allergy information and made standard selections available to clinicians in a pull-down menu. Now, rather than typing "penicillin," a VA clinician can simply select it from a list by pointing and clicking. Although the word "penicillin" appears on the screen, the information is stored in its encoded form. The use of encoded data supports patient safety and the clinical decision-making features of VistA with greater reliability than free-text data do. The use of a standard set of allergens across VA sites ensures that medication order–checks work as intended and that information can be exchanged reliably between sites.

For nearly every kind of clinical data—from diseases, procedures, and immunizations, to drugs, laboratory results, and digital images—there are multiple sets of standards from which to choose. For example, there are at least 12 separate systems for naming medications and the ingredients, dosages, and routes of administration associated with them. It is often necessary to use a combination of data standards to transmit a single message from one system to another. As a result, even health care organizations committed to using standards have a difficult time figuring out which standards to use.

Consolidated Health Informatics

Consolidated Health Informatics (CHI) is an eGov initiative involving federal agencies with responsibility for health-related activities and information.[39] CHI participants evaluate and choose health data and communication standards to be incorporated into their information technology systems, which maintain, process, or transmit health-related information. VA was instrumental in the formation of CHI and works closely with DoD, HHS, and other CHI partners to help foster the federal adoption of the endorsed standards as part of a joint strategy for developing federal interoperability and sharing of electronic health information. The CHI portfolio now encompasses 27 health data domains. To date, CHI has endorsed 20 communications and data standards in areas such as laboratory, radiology, pharmacy, encounters, diagnoses, and nursing information, as well as drug information standards developed collaboratively by VA and HHS.[39] These standards will be used by all federal health agencies in implementing new health information technology systems and, in some cases, modifying existing systems and related business processes.

CHI standards (Table 6-2) will work in conjunction with HIPAA transaction records and code sets and HIPAA security and privacy provisions. CHI is now focusing on the implementation, maintenance, and identification of new and adopted standards. As of this writing, CHI work products are being incorporated into the standards harmonization effort of the Health Information Technology Standards Panel (HITSP) under contract to the ONCHIT.

National Committee on Vital and Health Statistics

Under HIPAA, the National Committee on Vital Statistics (NCVHS) was charged with assessing existing terminologies to define the scope of patient medical record information (PMRI) and determine selection criteria for terminologies that could capture this information. In August 2000, the committee published a framework and a set of guiding principles for the selection of uniform data standards for PMRI.[29] The first set of specific PMRI standards recommended by NCVHS was for PMRI message formats; these standards were adopted by HHS in March 2003 as part of the CHI initiative. In August 2002, NCVHS began soliciting input from medical terminology experts and evaluated 46 candidate health care terminologies. NCVHS concluded that no single terminology would provide adequate domain coverage for PMRI and in November 2003 recommended that a "core set" of terminologies be adopted as a national standard. The core set includes the minimum set of terminologies that (1) are adequate to cover the scope of patient medical record information and (2) meet essential technical criteria to serve as reference terminologies for PMRI.

The core set of PMRI terminologies recommended by NCVHS includes the following:

- SNOMED CT
- LOINC
- Federal drug terminologies
  - RXNorm
  - The representations of the mechanism of action and physiologic effect of drugs from NDF-RT
  - Ingredient name, manufactured dosage form, and package type from the FDA NDCs[40]

Interoperability: The Lingua Franca of the Electronic Health Record World

In the EHR world, interoperability and data standardization go hand in hand. In fact, NCVHS defines data standards as "methods, protocols, and terminology agreed on by the industry to allow disparate information systems to operate successfully with one another"—a definition that focuses on

Table 6-2 SUMMARY OF CONSOLIDATED HEALTH INFORMATICS ADOPTED STANDARDS

Domain	Standard Adoption Recommendation
Anatomy and Physiology	SNOMED CT National Cancer Institute (NCI) Thesaurus
Billing/Financial	Transaction Code Sets
Chemicals	Conditional: Substance Registry System (SRS)
Demographics	HL7 Version 2.4+
Disability	No standard is recommended for adoption at this time for disability content needed by the federal government. However, recommendations are offered to guide research that will facilitate the development of (1) needed disability and functional content into existing terminologies and classification systems and (2) algorithms that can be used to equate the alternative scaling concepts used across federal classification systems. This research should be a collaborative effort between the disability community and terminology
Diagnosis and problem lists	SNOMED CT
Clinical encounters	HL7 Version 2.4+
Genes and proteins	Human Gene Nomenclature (HUGN) for genes. None for proteins
History and physical examination	None: work deferred to CHI Phase II
Nonlaboratory interventions and procedures	SNOMED CT
Immunizations	HL7 Version 2.3.1+ labeling sections

Continued

Table 6-2 SUMMARY OF CONSOLIDATED HEALTH INFORMATICS ADOPTED STANDARDS—cont'd

Domain	Standard Adoption Recommendation
Laboratory result contents	SNOMED CT
Units	HL7 Version 2.X +
Interventions and procedures: laboratory test order names	LOINC
Medications subdomain: clinical drugs	SCD of RxNorm
Medications subdomain: special populations	HL7 Version 2.X +
Medications subdomain: drug classifications	NDF-RT
Medications subdomain: manufactured dosage form	FDA/CDER Data Standards Manual
Medications subdomain: active ingredients	FDA Established Name for active ingredient & FDA Unique Ingredient Identifier (UNII) codes
Medications subdomain: package	FDA/CDER Data Standards Manual
Medications subdomain: drug product	NDC
Medications subdomain: structured product labeling sections	LOINC
Multimedia	None: Work deferred to CHI Phase II
Nursing	SNOMED CT
Population health	None
Medical devices and supplies	None: Monitor industry work
Text-based reports	HL7 CDA Release 1.0-2000

interoperability between different computer systems or organizations. In preparing its recommendations for a core set of terminologies, NCVHS assessed the extent to which different terminologies enabled interoperability between information systems.

Perhaps it is no surprise that health care, which lacks agreement on any number of standards related to interoperability, lacks a standard definition of interoperability itself. The member organizations of the National Alliance for Health Information Technology (NAHIT) have produced a useful one, intended as a guiding principle rather than a technical specification. In health care, writes the alliance, "**interoperability** is the ability of different information technology systems and software applications to communicate, to exchange data accurately, effectively, and consistently, and to use the information that has been exchanged."

There are different levels of interoperability. **Basic interoperability** means that one computer system can send data to another but does not necessarily mean that the receiving system can interpret that data. **Functional interoperability** (or syntactic interoperability) specifies the syntax or format of the transmitted message so that it can be parsed and stored by the receiving system. **Semantic interoperability** is the most sophisticated level of interoperability, incorporating the **semantic content** (i.e., the

meaning) of the message. At this level, data received from another system can displayed, interpreted, and manipulated as if generated locally.[41]

Interoperable EHRs with embedded standardized clinical terminologies offer significant benefits, including the following:

- Clinician access to critical health information at the point of care
- Improvements in patient safety through decision support and enhanced communication
- Decreased health care costs attributed to unavailability of information
- Improved biosurveillance capabilities
- Increased sophistication in the area of clinical decision support

Development and Selection of Health Data Standards

Chapter 4 introduces some standards developing organizations (SDOs), the processes they use to develop and maintain standards, and standards related to the content of clinical record. Chapter 5 discusses a number of standards that are relevant to the EHR and its use. In the United States, standards are created in three different ways: by the public sector, by the private sector, or through common use. Microsoft operating systems and applications are example of products that are so commonly used that they are considered "standard." The government rarely endorses such standards, however, because they can be viewed as stifling competition.

Although standards are sometimes created by government entities, the government generally prefers to adopt standards created by the private sector. Ideally, standards are developed through the collaborative efforts of SDOs that adhere to a strict and well-defined set of operating procedures that ensure consensus, openness, and balance of interest among volunteer participants as the standards are developed and balloted.

The American National Standards Institute (ANSI) is the body that oversees and accredits private SDOs in the United States and coordinates with international bodies. The primary ANSI-accredited SDOs in health care focus on specific domains of health care, such as HL7 for management and delivery of health care services, the National Council of Prescription Drug Programs (NCPDP) for pharmacy information, the Institute of Electrical and Electronics Engineers (IEEE) for medical devices, Digital Imaging and Communications in Medicine (DICOM) for imaging, X12 Insurance Subcommittee for financial transactions, and ASTM International E31—Healthcare Informatics Committee for the policies, content, and technical issues related to EHRs, privacy, security and other health care informatics topics.[42]

HL7's mission is to create standards for the exchange, management, and integration of electronic health information that support clinical patient care and the management and delivery of health care services by defining the protocol for exchanging clinical data between diverse health care information systems. This encompasses the complete life cycle of a standards specification: development, adoption, market recognition, utilization, and adherence.[43]

"HL7" is also used to refer to messaging standard developed by the HL7 SDO. HL7 messaging standards have been widely adopted throughout health care for administrative and clinical purposes.

Electronic Health Record Functional Model

Despite the appeal of EHRs and the visibility of federal health information technology efforts, some practices—particularly small providers—have been slow to adopt EHRs. One reason is that it is difficult for potential users to compare available EHR systems and to determine which capabilities are necessary for a given specialty or setting and which capabilities are not essential.

At the request of CMS, VA, the Agency for Healthcare Research and Quality (AHRQ), and other federal health organizations, the Institute of Medicine (IOM) identified

core capabilities of the EHR.[21] Using IOM's findings as a base, HL7 developed a draft "functional model" for EHRs. The HL7 EHR System Functional Model is intended to describe EHR system (EHR-S) capabilities from a user's perspective, so that users can compare different systems to determine which one is appropriate for them.

The EHR-S Functional Model is composed of a functional outline, functional profiles, and the priority associated with each function in a given profile (e.g., essential, desirable, optional). The EHR functional outline includes more than 100 individual functions, each with a Function Name, Function Statement, and Conformance Criteria, as well as associated reference information (such as a description of the function). The outline is organized into three sections: Direct Care functions, Supportive functions, and Information Infrastructure functions; these three main sections are divided further into 13 subsections. A hierarchical numbering scheme is used to indicate parent-child relationships between the functions. For example, function *DC.1.1 Health information capture, management, and review* is a parent function that includes the child function *DC.1.1.1 Identify and maintain a patient record.*

The HL7 Functional Model is the result of a broad public-private partnership and reflects input from hundreds of individuals around the world. Some functions are setting specific, whereas others apply across health care settings. Although the HL7 model is intended to include all reasonably anticipated EHR-S functions, most users will only require a subset of the functions included in the HL7 functional outline. Similarly, many EHR systems will support only a subset of the functions in the outline. By specifying and prioritizing EHR features by health care setting, the HL7 Functional Model will help potential users find EHR systems that meet their needs, thus supporting federal efforts to accelerate the implementation of EHR nationwide.

A National Network for Health Information Exchange

Over the past few years, the collaborative efforts of public and private sector health organizations have received more visibility as the federal government has sought to encourage the promotion of health information technology to meet a variety of needs.

In April 2004, the President signed Executive Order 13335 (EO) announcing his commitment to the promotion of health information technology to lower costs, reduce medical errors, improve quality of care, and provide better information for patients and physicians. In particular, the President called for the widespread adoption of EHRs so that health information could follow patients through their care in a seamless and secure manner. ONCHIT was established by the Secretary of HHS as directed by the EO. Recognizing the need for public- and private-sector collaboration to achieve the outlined goals, the EO charged the national coordinator with facilitating outreach and consultation with public and private parties of interest, including consumers, providers, payers, and administrators. As a result of the collaboration, the American Health Information Community (AHIC) was created to advise the secretary and recommend specific actions regarding the achievement of a common framework for interoperable health information technology to the secretary of HHS.

Broad goals for improving health care were set forth in an early ONCHIT report. One of the key actions listed to support those goals was *the private-sector certification of health information technology products.* Financial incentives were offered from a broad range of health care payers in both the private and public sectors, but only if they could ensure that the EHR products delivered would be robust enough to deliver benefits. Physicians, particularly those in small practices, were hesitant to buy a product that might not be suitable, interoperable, or portable, or that might not deliver the needed level of quality. In response to this challenge, three leading health information technology industry associations—AHIMA, Health Information and Management Systems Society (HIMSS), and the NAHIT—joined forces in July 2004 to launch the Certification Commission for Healthcare Information Technology (CCHIT) as a voluntary, private sector initiative to certify health information technology products. The three associations committed resources to support the commission during its organizational phase. Additional funding support came in 2005 from the American Academy of Family Physicians (AAFP), the American Academy of Pediatrics (AAP), the American College of Physicians (ACP), the California HealthCare Foundation (CHCF), Hospital Corporation of America, McKesson, Sutter Health, United Health Foundation, and WellPoint Health Networks, Inc.

In September 2005, HHS awarded CCHIT a 3-year contract to develop and evaluate certification criteria and an inspection process for EHRs in three areas: ambulatory EHRs, inpatient EHRs, and the infrastructure components through which they interoperate.

Benefits of a National Network

As VA experience has shown, the use of EHRs and other information technology tools in a single medical office or health system can improve health care quality, reduce medical errors, improve efficiency, and reduce costs. However, the full benefits of health information technology will be realized when there is a coordinated, national network in place to allow the secure exchange of clinical data to support patient care, regardless of where the patient is treated.

In the future, patients such as Elton Ramsay, whose VA primary care provider already uses EHR technology, will see a greater coordination of care among different providers. What would this look like? Suppose Mr. Ramsay has severe diarrhea, nausea, and vomiting while at a meeting in Virginia and presents to a regional health care facility there. Mr.

Ramsay's glucose levels are very low and he has an electrolyte imbalance. During Mr. Ramsay's medical examination he is asked if he's traveled outside the country, been camping recently, or changed his medications. Mr. Ramsay states that he has not been out of the country but just returned from helping hurricane Katrina victims in the Gulf Coast, that his physician has recently changed him from an oral hypoglycemic to insulin, and that he can't remember all the names of his other medications. With the National Health Information Network in place, the facility queries the Record Locater Service to determine where Mr. Ramsay has previously received medical services. Given that a treating relationship has been established with Mr. Ramsay, the facility is authorized to access medical data identified through the query. The clinician promptly receives electronic copies of progress notes, medication lists, procedure reports, and other medical information from the VA, Mr. Ramsay's local physician, radiology and laboratory service providers, and his pharmacy benefits management provider. As the diagnosis information is entered into the EHR, an alert appears that a cryptosporidiosis outbreak has occurred in Louisiana. Special laboratory tests are ordered and a diagnosis of cryptosporidiosis is confirmed. Mr. Ramsay is hydrated, started on a course of nitazoxanide, and given instructions regarding his insulin dose.

With this information in hand with EHR tools, the clinician is able to quickly assess the problem and provide prompt, appropriate treatment without ordering unnecessary tests or prescribing conflicting medications. The regional medical health care provider is able to ensure that all the treating providers are aware of Mr. Ramsay's episode of care. This continuity saves time and money. More importantly, Mr. Ramsay receives the right care when he needs it.

REFERENCES

1. *Comprehensive guide to electronic health records: the definitive resource for strategic planning, technology, standards, security, legislation and regulation,* New York, 2000, Faulkner and Gray.
2. Lobach DF: Computerized decision support based on a clinical practice guideline improves compliance with care standards, *Am J Med* 102:89-98, 1997.
3. Institute of Medicine. 2003. Key capabilities of an electronic health record. Letter report. Washington, DC: The National Academies Press.
4. Amatayakul M, Cohen M: *Electronic health records: strategies for implementation,* Marblehead, MA, 2004, HCPro.
5. http://www.snomed.org. Accessed December 21, 2006.
6. National Committee on Vital Health Statistics, Department of Health and Human Services: Report on uniform data standard for patient medical information: http://www.ncvhs.hhs.gov/reptrecs.htm. Accessed December 21, 2006.
6a. National Committee on Vital Health Statistics Report to the Secretary of US Department of Health and Human Services on Unified Standards for Patient Medical Record Information, July 2000, p. 33.
7. AHIMA e-HIM Work Group on Computer-Assisted Coding: Delving into computer-assisted coding [practice brief], *J AHIMA* 75 10):48A-48H, Nov-Dec 2004.
8. Case JT: Are we really communicating? Standard terminology standards in veterinary clinical pathology, *Vet Clin Pathol* 34:5-6, 2005.

9. Vardy G: Israeli coding medical information: classification versus nomenclature and implications to the Israeli medical system, *J Med Syst* 22: 203-210, 1998.

10. McDonald CJ, Huff SM, Suico JC et al; LOINC, a universal standard for identifying laboratory observations: a five year update, *Clin Chem* 49:624-633, 2003.

11. National Center for Health Statistics Classification of Diseases and Functioning and Disability: http://www.cdc.gov/nchs/about/otheract/icd9/abticd10.htm. Accessed December 21, 2006.

12. Fenton S: *Clinical classifications and terminologies,* Chicago, 2002, American Health Information Management Association.

13. Demetriades J, Kolodner R, Christopherson G: *Person-centered health records: toward healthy people,* New York, 2005, Springer Science + Business Media.

14. Letter to the Secretary of the Department of Health and Human Services from Chair of the National Committee on Vital Health Statistics, February 27, 2002.

15. Abdelhak M, Grostick S, Hanken MA et al, editors: *Health information: management of a strategic resource,* ed 2, 2001, Philadelphia, WB Saunders.

16. Alexander S, Conner T, Slaughter T: Overview of inpatient coding, *Am J Health Syst Pharm* 60(6 suppl):S11-S14, 2003.

17. American Medical Association: http://ama-assn.org. Accessed December 21, 2006.

18. Ingenix: *DRG desk reference: the ultimate resource for improving DRG assignment,* 2007.

19. Averill R, Goldfield N, Steinbeck B et al: *All patient refined diagnosis related groups (AR-DRGs), version 2.0, methodology overview,* 2003, 3M Health Information Systems.

20. Institute of Medicine: *Report: who will keep the public healthy: educating public health professionals for the 21st century.* Washington, DC, 2002, Committee on Educating Public Health Professionals for the 21st Century.

21. Institute of Medicine: *Letter report: key capabilities of an electronic health record system,* Washington, DC, Committee on Data Standards for Patient Safety.

22. Institute of Medicine, Committee on Enhancing Federal Healthcare Quality Programs: *Leadership by example: coordinating government roles in improving healthcare quality,* Washington, DC, 2003, National Academy Press.

23. Chute CG, Cohn SP, Campbell KE et al: The content coverage of clinical classifications, *J Am Med Inform Assoc* 3:224-233, 1996.

24. Graham G, Nugent L, Strouse K: Information everywhere: how the EHR transformed care at VHA. *J AHIMA* 74:20-24, 2003.

25. American Health Information Association: http://library.ahima.org/xpedio/groups/public/documents/ahima/bok1_02982_hcsp. Accessed December 21, 2006.

26. Wasserman H, Wang J: An applied evaluation of SNOMED CT as a clinical vocabulary for the computerized diagnosis and problem list, pp. 699-703, *AMIA 2003 Symposium Proceedings,* Washington, DC, 2003.

27. SNOMED: http//www.snomed.org. Accessed December 21, 2006.

28. Goldberg LJ, Werner C, Eisner J et al: The significance of SNODENT, Medical Informatics Europe (MIE 2005), Geneva, *Stud Health Technol Inform* 116:737-742, 2005.

29. Bakken S, Cimini JJ, Hripsak G: Promoting patient safety and enabling evidence-based practice through informatics, *Med Care* 42(2 suppl):II49-56, 2004.

30. Huff SM, Rocha RA, McDonald CJ et al: Development of the logical observation identifier names and codes (LOINC) vocabulary, *J Am Med Inform Assoc* 5:276-292, 1998.

31. Regenstrief Institute, Inc: http://www.regenstrief.org/loinc/. Accessed December 21, 2006.

32. Institute of Medicine: *Leadership by example: coordinating government roles in improving healthcare quality,* Washington, DC, 2002, National Academy Press.

33. Brown SH: Derivation and evaluation of a document-naming nomenclature, *J Am Med Health Informatics Assoc* 8:379-381, 2001.

34. Henry SB, Mead CN: Nursing classification systems: necessary but not sufficient for representing what nurses do, *J Am Med Informatics Assoc* 4:222-232, 1997.

35. American Nurses Association: http://www.nursingworld.org/npii/terminologies.htm. Accessed March 2006.

36. *HIMSS Standards Insight: an analysis of health information standards development initiatives:* http://www.himss.org/content/files/StandardsInsight/2003/07-2003.pdf. Accessed January 2006.

37. Cimino J: Desiderata for controlled medical vocabularies in the twenty-first century, *Methods Inf Med* 37:394-403, 1998.

38. International Organization for Standardization: http://www.iso.org/iso/en/faqs/faq-standards.html. Access December 21, 2006.

39. United States Department of Health and Human Services: http://www.hhs.gov/healthit/chiinitiative.html. Accessed December 21, 2006.

40. Sujansky W, Subcommittee on Standards and Security of National Committee on Vital Health Statistics: *Scope and criteria for selection of PMRI terminologies: a report to the National Committee on Vital and Health Statistics Subcommittee on Standards and Security, version 3, December 23, 2003,* 2003, The Committee: ncvhs.hhs.gov/031105rpt.pdf. Accessed December 21, 2006.

41. Heubusch K: Interoperability: what it means, why it matters, *J AHIMA* 77:26-30; quiz 33-34.

42. ASTM International: http://astm.org. Accessed September 15, 2006.

43. HL7 Health Level 7: http://hl7.org. Accessed September 15, 2006.

ADDITIONAL RESOURCES

Consolidated Health Informatics: http://www.hhs.gov/healthit/chiinitiative.html.

Health Level 7 functional model: www.HL7.org.

LOINC® (free download): www.loinc.org.

chapter 7

Data Access and Retention

Stanley P. Greenberg
Darice M. Grzybowski

Additional content,
http://evolve.elsevier.com/Abdelhak/

Review exercises can be found
in the Study Guide

Chapter Contents

Access and Retention of Paper-Based Records
Record Identification
Alphabetical Identification
Numerical Identification
Filing Equipment
Filing Cabinets
Open-Shelf Files
Motorized Revolving Units
Compressible Units
Space Management
Centralized and Decentralized Files
Filing Methods
Alphabetical Filing
Straight Numerical Filing
Terminal Digit Filing
Master Patient Index
Content
Creation of the Index
Records Management Issues
File Folders
Color Coding
Record Security
Storage of Inactive Records
System File Conversion
Record Tracking
Manual Record-Tracking Systems
Automated Record-Tracking Systems
Application in Use: University of Texas-James W. Aston
Ambulatory Care Center

Key Words

Access time	Local area network	Purge
Active record	Magnification ratio	Record tracking
Alphabetical identification	Mainframe	Reduction ratio
Bar code device	Master patient index	Redundant array of independent disks
Cache memory	Microcomputers	Requisition
Centralized filing	Microfiche	Retention period
Client-server technology	Microfilm jacket	Roll microfilm
Color coding	Microfilm reader	Scanner
Computer output microfiche	Microform	Serial numbering
Computer output to laser disk	Minicomputers	Serial-unit numbering
Cooperative processing	Mirroring	Statute of limitations
Cross-reference	Multifunctional device	Symbology
Decentralized filing	Multimedia	Terminal
Destruction letter	Numerical identification	Terminal digit filing
Disaster recovery	Open architecture	Thin
Electronic data interchange	Open system	Transfer notice
Encounter	Optical character recognition	Uninterruptible power supply
Exchange time	Outcard	Unit numbering system
File guide	Outguide	Unit record
File server	Payback period	Voice recognition
Graphical user interface	Pen-based device	Wide area network
Hardware	Personal data assistant	Workstation
Inactive record	Picture archiving and communication	Write once read many
Internet	system	
Jukebox	Proprietary system	

Application in Use: University of Iowa Hospitals and Clinics

Record Retention
Federal Statutes and Regulations
State Statutes and Regulations
Organizational Needs
Retention Schedule
Facility Closure

The Legal Record Definition

Disaster Recovery for Paper-Based and Electronic Records

Computer Technology in Automated Data Access and Retention

Hardware

Input, Output, and Storage Devices

Terminals and Workstations

Pen-Based Devices

Radiofrequency Identification

Document Imaging Devices

Voice Recognition

Computer-Assisted Coding Tools

Communications
Local Area Networks
Wide Area Networks

Client Server Technology

Access and Retention of Image-Based Records

Micrographics
Microforms
Equipment
Legal Considerations
Cost Analysis
Application in Use: Kurten Medical Group in Racine, Wisconsin
Application in Use: New York Hospital–Cornell Medical Center in New York City

Electronic Document Management
Electronic Health Record and Electronic Document Management
System Components
System Benefits and Advantages
Evaluating System Requirements
Implementation Strategies
Legal Considerations
Application in Use: Memorial Hospital and North Park Hospital, Chattanooga, Tennessee

Abbreviations

CAR—Computer-assisted retrieval
CDR—Clinical data repository
COLD—Computer output to laser disk
COM—Computer output microfiche
EHR—Electronic Health Record
EDI—Electronic data interchange
EDM—Electronic document management
GUI—Graphical user interface
HL7—Health Level Seven interface language
LAN—Local area network

MFD—Multifunctional device
MPI—Master patient index
OCR—Optical character recognition
PACS—Picture archiving and communication system
PC—Personal computer (microsystem or minicomputer)
PDA—Personal data assistant
PPI—Pixels per inch
RAID—Redundant array of independent disks
SAN—Storage area network
UPS—Uninterruptible power supply
WAN—Wide area network
WORM—Write once read many

Objectives

After reading this chapter, the reader will be able to do the following:

- Define key words.
- Discuss the various numbering systems for health information.
- Compare and contrast the filing options for the paper record.
- Compare and contrast microfilming of records versus commercial storage and identify when each method is desirable.
- Identify key milestones in a file conversion.
- Identify considerations important to the selection of file folders.
- Describe the benefits of color coding to any of the filing methods.
- Describe how an automated record-tracking system can be developed and implemented.
- Identify how bar code technology interacts with an automated record-tracking system.
- Explain how the statute of limitations pertains to record retention.
- Describe the different hardware options available when designing an automated data access and retention program.
- Identify the different microform options available when designing a micrographics storage and retrieval system.
- List the necessary components of an optical imaging system and the various cost factors involved in implementing an optical imaging system.
- Identify possible steps in the implementation of an optical imaging system.
- Describe why electronic storage of data is a prerequisite to the successful implementation of the electronic health record.
- Examine a current storage and retrieval system and determine alternative solutions to solve identified problems.
- Prepare strategies for planning and implementing solutions to information system problems.

Health care is information dependent and cannot be provided efficiently without facts regarding the patient's past and current conditions. Various systems are necessary to ensure that the information is available where and when it is needed for patient care at a reasonable cost.

The patient record provides the data to establish the who, what, when, where, and how of patient care. It is the documentation of everything that takes place during the provision of health care. These data are maintained to provide better quality health care, to support billing accuracy, to minimize litigation losses, to comply with applicable laws and regulations, and to aid in medical research efforts. Retaining the data so that they are available for use in the future is a major concern of all health information professionals.

This chapter describes various ways in which patients' health information can be accessed and retained. The discussion begins with the paper record and progresses with computer technology to microforms, optical imaging to electronic document management (EDM) to the electronic health record (EHR).

The role of the health information professional is to evaluate past and current methods and current and future needs and to select the best system to meet those needs. This may involve converting to new filing methods or filing media, maintaining current systems more efficiently, or making decisions regarding the destruction of nonuseful material. In addition, health information professionals must keep their knowledge of technologies current so that plans can be made to keep the data retention program current with the technology. Just as an IBM 286 personal computer (PC) with a $5\frac{1}{4}$-inch disk drive is not current technology today, the state of the art today may no longer be usable or accessible for data retrieval in the next 5 to 10 years. Data access and retention mean ensuring that no data are lost to technology obsolescence. Every effort must be made to ensure that, as technology advances, either the old technology is maintained to ensure access or the new technology can access the old data.

The health information professional's knowledge of information management consists of more than information systems concerning the formal patient record. Information management knowledge can easily be applied to other areas as well, such as radiology film storage, human resource management, and administrative records. No other field of study within the health care arena provides information management background, although each discipline maintains patient health care records. Wise facility managers use the health information professional as an in-house consultant to these other areas to improve overall facility efficiency. Therefore, the concepts covered in this chapter present ways of accessing and retaining information, regardless of the scope, size, or shape of the information or storage media involved.

ACCESS AND RETENTION OF PAPER–BASED RECORDS

Although there is an active transition occurring in our profession to the paperless record, health care facilities maintain a substantial portion of their patient records in a paper-based format. The first portion of this chapter discusses maintenance of the paper-based format of the patient record and methods of identifying the record.

Record Identification

Alphabetical Identification

Identifying the record by patient name, called **alphabetical identification,** is the most basic identification system used in health care. Although it sounds simple, the system can be more difficult to maintain than it appears.

In maintaining an alphabetical identification system, the correct patient name is the vital piece of information. All patient names, both first and last, must be spelled accurately to be sure that the record can be located in the future. All name changes must be indicated on the patient record folder, creating a **cross-reference** for the previous location in the file. Alphabetical identification systems can be maintained without a separate **master patient index** (MPI) because the records themselves form a large patient index. If a separate index is used, cross-referencing of name changes must also be completed in the index; this requires extra work.

An advantage of the alphabetical identification system is that the record can be located using information obtained directly from the patient. The disadvantage of the system is the complex spelling of many names. In addition, not everyone knows instinctively how to file names alphabetically. To achieve the consistency needed for successful future retrieval, the record maintenance staff must be taught the filing rules adopted by the facility and reference them while completing their work.

Numerical Identification

An alternative method of identification is to use a number to identify the patient record; this is called **numerical identification.** Assigning a number to a patient record requires the use of the MPI, which contains a minimum of the patient name and the patient identification number. Additional data elements to be included in this index are covered later. In the manual version of this identification system, the MPI cards are filed alphabetically and referenced to find the patient identification number. In an automated format, a computerized database serves as the MPI. The computer file is searched for the required name or a similar combination of letters. The correct name is determined, and the associated identification number is displayed on the computer screen.

The manual version of this method has some of the same problems as the alphabetical filing of patient records. The computerized version provides the added advantages of allowing access to the identification number by multiple users at one time and consistently sorting the database in the same way for each user. The computer also provides the flexibility of producing reports in both alphabetical and numerical order for reference.

Methods of Numbering. A number identification system can be designed in several ways. Serial, unit, and hybrid serial-unit numbering are discussed here.

Serial Numbering. **Serial numbering** is a system of number assignment in which a patient receives a number for each encounter at the facility. The patient could have multiple numbers, all of which require entry onto the manual index card or maintenance in the computerized database. This method is time consuming and makes computer database space difficult to allocate, especially in a facility with a high volume of encounters. This method also has a higher supply cost because each encounter at the facility requires the use of a new file folder. Each new folder is filed in a different location, requiring the searching of multiple locations to retrieve one patient's entire record, a time-consuming process. Serial numbering can be used effectively when the patient return rate is low or the population served is transient.

Unit Numbering. To avoid the extra effort of assigning a new number for each encounter and the searching of multiple locations for record folders, the unit numbering system was developed. In the **unit numbering system,** each patient receives an identification number at the first encounter and retains that number throughout all contacts with the facility. With this numbering system, a facility can easily create a **unit record** for the patient, filed in one location in the file.[1] Labor costs are reduced because the number is entered into the MPI only once, and supply costs are lower because the same folder is used for all encounters except where the number of encounters exceeds the storage capability of the folder, thus resulting in additional folder(s).

Technically, any number could be chosen as the unit number identifier, but most facilities prefer to assign numbers sequentially, starting with the number 1. Some facilities, such as those that are government sponsored, have chosen to use the Social Security number as the unique patient identifier and they ask the patient to provide it. In this system, any patient without a Social Security number receives a pseudo-number, or fake number, as the identifier until a number is permanently assigned.

In a variation of the unit numbering system, a number is assigned to a family rather than to an individual. This numbering system is common in community health centers that treat a family as a unit. This approach allows common identification of a family unit, even if the family members have different last names. If this method is chosen, consideration must be given to assigning each family member his or her own identifier as an additional number and giving the person his or her own folder.

Serial-Unit Numbering. In an attempt to combine the ease of number assignment from serial numbering and the unit record concept from unit numbering, the **serial-unit numbering** method was developed. Numbers are assigned serially, but as each new encounter takes place, all the former records are brought forward to the most recently assigned record number and filed as a unit.

Table 7-1 shows a comparison of these three numbering systems. In the future, the concept of a unique (unit) identifier for each patient will become more attractive. Some form of unique identifier can provide the common link for all the information contained in the multiple computerized databases of information maintained on individual patients.

Filing Equipment

Making a decision about how to store patient records and other record-related material is a situation that all health information professionals face at some point in their careers. Although sales personnel are trained to assist in the decision-making process, it is helpful to know the advantages and disadvantages of the different types of storage equipment before the process begins. Table 7-2 compares the available types of storage equipment according to physical description, strengths, weaknesses, and facility types where they are best suited. Figure 7-1 shows an aerial view of open shelves and compressible units.

The Occupational Health and Safety Administration (OSHA) requires that certain minimum allowances be made for aisles and spaces between equipment. OSHA requires

Table 7-1 NUMBERING SYSTEMS

System	Number Assignment	Filing Concepts
Serial numbering	A new number is assigned for each encounter.	Each record is filed separately using the number that has been assigned for that visit.
Unit numbering	One number is assigned at the first encounter and used for all future encounters.	The record is filed using the unit number.
Serial-unit numbering	A new number is assigned for each encounter.	The record containing each number is brought forward and filed using the newest number assigned.

Table 7-2 COMPARISON OF DIFFERENT TYPES OF STORAGE EQUIPMENT

Equipment	Physical Description	Strengths	Weaknesses	Best Suited For
Filing cabinets	Three to five drawers, vertical or lateral arrangement	Can be purchased as a fireproof cabinet Can be purchased with locks Protects records from the environment	Requires dedicated aisle space Difficult and time consuming to open each drawer Can open only one drawer at a time	Small facilities Dirty environments High fire dangers Low file activity requiring high security
Open-shelf files	Five to eight shelves with full access to the front (similar to bookshelves)	Easy access to any part of the shelves and multiple shelves at a time Can accommodate multiple workers at one time	Requires a 36-inch dedicated aisle between shelving units Records open to the environment	High-volume files with multiple file maintenance workers Relatively clean environments with sufficient space for aisles Works well in a clinic facility for active records and in hospitals for outpatient records
Motorized revolving units	Shelves move around central spine like a Ferris wheel with records carried on bucket shelves; run by a motor	Little aisle space needed All work is at one height level Records can be covered and locked	Must be carefully loaded and unloaded in a balanced manner or it will not run Motor or power failure causes record unavailability High initial cost, maintenance contract costs	Limited space with low file activity and one primary file maintenance worker Dirty environments
Compressible units	Open-shelf files that move in parallel lines to form an aisle opening Motor-assisted movement or hand cranked	Saves space of unused aisles Easy access to shelf currently opened to the aisle One dedicated aisle required	Time needed to locate where the access aisle is needed and to open the mechanism to the aisle Limited number of aisles Mechanical failure causes record unavailability Maintenance contract costs	Limited space with low to medium file activity and two to three file maintenance workers Works well in a hospital facility for inpatient records or inactive records

that main aisles leading out of a room or to a fire exit be a minimum of 5 feet wide and that secondary aisles, such as between shelving units, be a minimum of 3 feet wide. These minimums are set to provide adequate work space for all workers as well as access to exits.

Filing Cabinets

Vertical filing cabinets are the traditional type of drawer files seen in many offices. They vary in height, width, depth, and number of drawers. These cabinets are specifically constructed to hold cards, letter files, and legal files, or they can be constructed as a combination of card file drawers and larger drawers.

Lateral filing cabinets are also available. The file drawers in a lateral filing cabinet open from the long side, and the entire cabinet resembles a chest of drawers. Because these cabinets have drawers that are not deep, they are well suited to narrow spaces, such as along walls. or as room dividers.

Both vertical and lateral filing cabinets are available with two to five drawers and can be purchased with special fireproof wall and drawer construction or with locks. Although they protect records from the environment, considerable effort is required to open each drawer when filing or retrieving a record. These files are best suited to small settings such as physician practices or nursing homes in which record retrieval is limited and performed by one or two people.

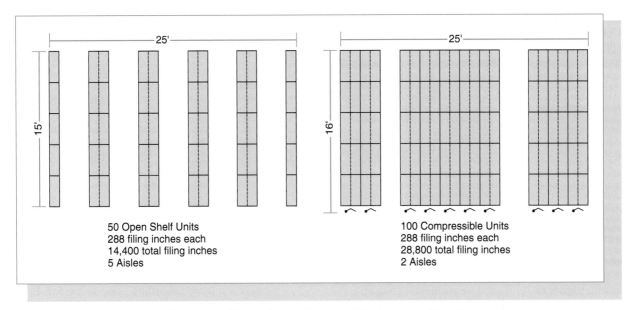

Figure 7-1 Overhead view of open-shelf and compressible units.

Open-Shelf Files

Open-shelf files resemble bookshelves and provide ready access to records without having to open any drawers. They are available with five to eight shelves per section and they are usually adjustable to accommodate different heights of folders. Adjustable shelf dividers help support the file folders on the shelves. The files, which require a dedicated 36-inch aisle, leave records open to the environment. Open-shelf files are the storage equipment of choice for high-volume file rooms in which many people require simultaneous access to the shelves, such as in clinics.

Motorized Revolving Units

The motorized revolving file contains 16 shelves that rotate around a central spine like a Ferris wheel. The records are placed on a shelf similar to an open shelf or on a bucket shelf in a lateral file. Files must be loaded or unloaded from the machine in a balanced manner, just as passengers are alternately loaded onto and off a Ferris wheel. If the load is unbalanced, the machine stops to avoid damaging the internal mechanism. These files are best suited to small facilities in which record retrieval is limited and performed by one person, such as solo physician or dental practices.

Compressible Units

These movable-aisle systems, or compressible units, are similar to open-shelf files but are mounted on tracks secured to the floor. The shelf units move on the tracks, and the operator opens the file at the appropriate place to create the aisle where needed. They are available in both manual and motor-assisted models. Although this type of file saves considerable floor space, access to files is limited because only one or two aisles can be created at a time. Compressible units are best suited to files with low to medium file activity

with only a few people working in the files at one time. In the electronic style (motorized) models, electrical wiring is necessary. Electrical models are priced more intensively but may save greater time and labor, thus increasing staff productivity overall. The pros and cons of each option on the basis of the staffing levels and physician constraints must be considered before shelving decisions can be made. They may solve some space issues for health information departments.

Space Management

Centralized and Decentralized Files

Facilities can use a centralized or a **decentralized filing** method. In centralized filing, there is a single location for all records created throughout the facility. This centralized file location is staffed by specialized personnel who provide records that have been requested by authorized users.

In the **decentralized filing** method, parts of the record are filed in different locations in the facility. Outpatient and emergency departments (EDs) frequently file their records in their own departments. In clinic facilities, decentralized records may be created when specialty departments maintain their own records. Table 7-3 shows the advantages and disadvantages of the centralized and decentralized record management alternatives.

Filing Methods

Designing a numbering and filing system within a facility is a major responsibility, and the decisions can affect other functions in the facility. Understanding each of the options is important. Although the term "filing" does not connote a high degree of professionalism, the efficient management of

Table 7-3 COMPARISON OF CENTRALIZED AND DECENTRALIZED RECORD MANAGEMENT ALTERNATIVES

Centralized Files	Decentralized Files
Overall supply costs are lower.	Supply costs for storage equipment and multiple folders are increased.
High level of security with record control is easy to maintain.	Record control is more difficult to maintain.
Standardized procedures for file maintenance can be developed.	File format can be flexible to meet the unique needs of the patient and providers.
Specialized staff can be trained to perform file maintenance as their primary duty.	File maintenance staff are harder to train consistently, and file maintenance may be a low priority for staff with other duties.
Consistent supervision is available for file maintenance staff.	Supervision is provided by department staff in the area where the records are located.

files in any format is an important asset provided by a health information professional to a facility.

Alphabetical Filing

How to Use. An alphabetical identification system and the alphabetical filing method must be used together. The alphabetical filing method starts with last names that begin with A and continues through all the names, ending with Z. For records of patients with identical last names, the first name and then the middle initial are used to determine the exact filing order. When first names are a single initial or no middle initial is given, the rule of nothing before something is used to determine filing order. Each name (last, first, middle) or the corresponding initial is treated as a group when filing. A single-initial name is the shortest name possible and would be filed first. The file would look like this:

Henri, Martha
Henry, J
Henry, J T
Henry, John T
Henry, Judy
Henry, Judy R

Box 7-1 ALPHABETICAL FILING RULES

1. Place the last name first and then the first name followed by the middle name or initial according to strict alphabetical order.
2. If there are two or more identical last name and first name combinations, use the middle initial to determine the order. If the middle initial is the same or no middle initial is given, use the birth date, filing the oldest patient first.
3. Names with prefixes (O', D', Mc, Mac, Von, etc.) are filed as if there was no apostrophe or space (O'Dell is O'-D-E-L-L). The apostrophe should be typed as one character when entering information into a database.
4. Hyphenated names are filed as if there was no hyphen (Smith-Jones is S-M-I-T-H-J-O-N-E-S). The hyphen should not be included when entering information into a database.
5. If an initial is given instead of a first or middle name, use the "nothing before something" rule to file J T Henry before John T Henry. Periods should not be entered as characters when entering information into a database.
6. Do not abbreviate names in alphabetical filing. However, if the name is abbreviated, file it as it is spelled (Wm is W-M).
7. Do not include seniority designations (Sr, Jr) or titles (MD, PhD) in alphabetical filing. If found, do not use in determining file order.

Modified from Johnson M, Kallaus W: *Records management*, Cincinnati, 1982, Southwestern Publishing.

Specific alphabetical filing rules are shown in Box 7-1.

Names that contain nonalphabetical characters, capitals, or spaces, such as O'Dell, McCallum, and Van Braun often cause variations in filing accuracy. Add to this the complexity of numerical modifiers such as Sr., Jr., and III. Each facility should maintain consistency in filing by deciding how special filing situations are to be handled, documenting the correct order, and referencing the documentation as the filing process is completed.

Space Planning. Letters of the alphabet appear in any given volume of records with an average frequency. These frequencies can be used to predict the percentage of file space that should be allowed for each letter of the alphabet (Box 7-2).

File Guides. File guides are used to aid in the filing process. These guides list the letter of the alphabet and any vowel subdivisions within the main letter category, such as Da, De, Di, Do, Du, all within the main letter category of D.

Benefits and Considerations. Alphabetical filing systems work well for facilities with fewer than 5000 records, a stable patient population, and little or no computerization. They may not work well in ethnically homogeneous areas in which last names are frequently repeated.

Straight Numerical Filing

How to Use. Facilities that have more than 5000 records, have frequently changing populations, or have become

Box 7-2 FREQUENCY DISTRIBUTION OF THE ALPHABET

A 3.00%	M 9.50%
B 9.38%	N 1.85%
C 7.18%	O 1.52%
D 4.84%	P 4.93%
E 1.87%	Q 0.17%
F 3.72%	R 5.05%
G 5.05%	S 10.20%
H 7.38%	T 3.37%
I 0.38%	U 0.24%
J 2.59%	V 1.24%
K 4.24%	W 6.31%
L 4.85%	X, Y, Z 1.14%

From Waters KR, Murphy GF: *Medical records in health information*, pp. 449-450, Germantown, MD, 1979, Aspen Systems.

computerized usually assign numbers to their patients. They may choose to file their records in straight numerical or sequential order, a basic system that starts with a record of the lowest number value and ends with a record of the highest number value. New records are always added at the end of the number series, concentrating most of the filing activity in one area of the file. Accountability for filing accuracy is harder to track when most of the record maintenance staff is focused in one area of the files.

File Guides. File guides are used in this system to help the eye determine the change in digits. If the folders are thick, file guides should be placed every 100 records. If the folders are thin, one guide for every 1000 records may be sufficient.

Space Planning. To plan space adequately for a straight numerical filing system, consideration should be given to thinking of the file room as a circle. As **inactive records** are removed from the lower-numbered areas, these areas can be consolidated forward, creating additional room for the end of the number series to grow into. This method is far easier than moving the entire contents of the file area back to the starting point whenever the end of the number series has come to the end of the filing space. Inactive records are also discussed under record management later in this chapter.

Terminal Digit Filing

How to Use. The **terminal digit filing** method is based on a patient identification number that is divided into three parts. Most facilities use a minimum of six digits (filling any unused digits on the left for numbers lower than 100,000 with zeros), and other facilities use the terminal digit method with numbers as large as the nine-digit social security number.

See the following example of a standard six-digit identification number.

Example of a Standard Six-Digit Identification Number

12	34	56
Tertiary digits	Secondary digits	Primary (or terminal) digits

The number is read from left to right for identification purposes and from right to left (from the terminal end) for terminal digit filing purposes. To understand the filing concepts, it is best to visualize the file layout in a terminal digit system. If the file room has 100 sections of filing equipment, each would contain the records labeled with one of the 100 possible primary digit combinations (from 00 to 99). Using the preceding example, the 56 section would be further visually subdivided into 100 possible locations for records. Record number 12-34-56 would be in the thirty-fourth subdivision (secondary digits of 34), or about one third of the way into primary section 56. Within the thirty-fourth subdivision, records are filed in straight numeric order by the tertiary digits. In this example, the record is number 12, following record 11 and preceding record 13. File sections 56 and 57 would look like this:

11-34-56
12-34-56
13-34-56 ... to 99-34-56, with the next folder being
00-35-56
01-35-56 ... until 99-99-56 is reached, with the next folder being
00-00-57
01-00-57 and so on.

The steps in finding record 12-34-56 are as follow:

1. Go to section 56.
2. Within section 56, go to the subdivision of 34s.
3. The record is the twelfth record in subdivision 34 if all records are present.

The same concepts used in our monetary system, 100 pennies in a $1 bill and 100 dollar bills in a $100 bill, apply here. In this system, the pennies are records.

File Guides. File guides are used to mark primary digit sections in small files. In larger files, each group of 10 secondary digits is guided, in addition to the primary digit sections. Space planning is easiest in a terminal digit system. Because new numbers assigned sequentially are evenly distributed among all 100 filing sections, the file grows evenly. Time has shown that records become inactive at a relatively even rate of distribution, allowing the file to increase or decrease evenly in size.

Space Planning. To determine the size of each primary section in a new file area, calculate the available inches of filing space by measuring the lengths of the actual shelves or drawers available. Divide the total number of inches of filing space by 100. The result is the number of inches of filing space to allow for each primary digit combination. Remember to start allocating space for number 00, not 01. This may leave considerable space between primary sections but saves the time of shifting the records later as the file grows. Theoretically a terminal digit filing system would grow equally and take up an equal amount of space per terminal digit. Realistically however, they may not grow equally. For this reason, it is important to not plan to fill up the shelving to full capacity. Filing units should be purchased in multiples of 5, such as 5 units (or cabinets), 25 units, 50 units, or 100 units, if space permits. This allows each terminal digit number to reside in an area of a filing unit. If 50 units of storage space are purchased, two terminal digit numbers are placed in that shelving unit or cabinet. Table 7-4 compares the advantages and disadvantages of straight numerical filing and terminal digit filing.

Master Patient Index

The MPI is the key to locating the patient record in any filing or computer system. It identifies all patients who have been treated by the facility and lists the number associated with the name. The index can be maintained manually or as part of a computerized system. In either case, the MPI should be maintained permanently.[1]

Content

The MPI should contain enough demographical data to readily identify the patient and his or her record. There are usually two levels to the MPI. The first is the demographic

level, which contains information about the patient that usually remains consistent from visit to visit and does not reflect episode-specific data. The second, or episode level, reflects visit or account information that varies by the date of service. The content of the MPI usually includes the following:

Demographic Level
Full name (last, first, and middle)
Patient sex
Patient date of birth
Patient identification number: Medical record/unit number. (This is a lifetime number that follows the patient throughout all visits. It usually determines the type of filing index system used to access patient records, such as serial or terminal digit reference.)
Other cross-reference numbers or names
Other demographics that represent the patient at the time of encounter: address, phone number, Social Security number, guarantor, and so on
Visit Level
Specific account or episode numbers
Encounter date(s) (i.e., admission and discharge)
Patient type or service
Admitting diagnosis
Attending physician name

In most settings the MPI is an electronic database that serves many purposes. It is the link to other databases and, if an organization has a numerically filed paper-based record system, the MPI is the key to record location. It is also used for report routing, statistics, and historical identification of activity within the facility. It is not intended to be used as a marketing or community database because it is not updated with name or address changes, expirations, or other personal addenda, unless the patient returns to the same facility. It is also not intended to be manipulated for billing, payment, or insurance purposes. Episodes of care must be unique and reflect only individual occurrences and must not be combined for the purpose of combined billing. Gaps in recurring

Table 7-4   CHARACTERISTICS OF STRAIGHT NUMERICAL FILING AND TERMINAL DIGIT FILING

Straight Numerical	Sample Order	Terminal Digit	Sample Order
Training period is short.	29160	Training period is slightly longer.	24-29-04
File grows at the end of the number series, requiring backshifting.	30158 / 101412	File grows evenly throughout 100 sections— no backshifting required.	25-29-04 / 10-14-12
Inactive records are pulled from one general area.	107412 / 107643	Inactive records are purged evenly throughout the 100 sections.	49-32-12 / 10-74-12
File staff is "bunched" in the highest numbers, causing less accountability for filing accuracy.	107644 / 123456 / 242904	Work is evenly distributed throughout the 100 sections, causing accountability for accuracy in that section.	10-76-43 / 10-76-44 / 12-34-56
Number is dealt with as a whole, causing mental fatigue, transpositions, and misfiles.	252904 / 493212	Number is dealt with in two-digit pairs, easing mental fatigue and causing fewer transpositions and misfiles.	03-01-58 / 02-91-60

care, unless identified through other means, must be separated by use of individual accounts.

Alias names are not recommended for use in an MPI because they must eventually be cross-referenced to the actual name and may draw more attention to the individual than is necessary in a health care setting. As an alternative, appropriate security controls and flags indicating not to display information where not needed by those directly involved in the care should be used. Figure 7-2 is a sample Alias Policy and Waiver form for the MPI.

Creation of the Index

If an electronic system is not available, a manual MPI can be maintained according to alphabetical filing rules (see Box 7-1),

keeping in mind the need for consistency in filing. Computerized indexes must have the same consistency and careful data entry. Database software is not intelligent. It retrieves only what it is given. Therefore, names with special characters or spaces must be entered in the same manner each time to be retrieved when needed.

Whether manual or computerized, hyphenated names present a challenge in the MPI because they are retrieved differently from the same two names combined without a hyphen. In most computerized systems, hyphens are excluded from the name. Also, prefix names entered without a space (such as McDonald) are retrieved separately from those entered with a space (Mc Donald). When numbers are assigned in a unit numbering system, these database

---

Patient Waiver for Use of an Alias

Philosophy: This facility believes mechanisms should be available to provide an extra level of online security access in extraordinary circumstances. This facility also believes that this mechanism should provide for long term integrity of the patient data and master patient index as well as continuity of care, and thus should be administered according to detailed procedures that help support confidentiality as well as validity of information.

Procedure:

General Security:

1. All patient information is protected by general release of information policies and is available only on a need to know basis within the scope of work or with appropriate patient or legal guardian authorizations.

2. All behavioral medicine patients are protected with an extra level of computer access security based on the patient type utilized within the hospital information system upon patient registration.

Extraordinary Circumstances:

1. Typically, an individual requesting use of an alias makes contact with a facility staff member.

2. Staff notifies supervisor or appropriate charge person.

3. Supervisor is to evaluate request against the following criteria for validity:

    a) Is patient a VIP requiring anonymity due to public notoriety?

    b) Is patient's safety or care endangered if identity is revealed? (i.e., criminal, victim of rape, incest, or other abuse)

    c) Has physician ordered, and patient agreed, to use of an alias?

4. If request is received outside of Patient Registration and falls into approved criteria, supervisor is to notify Patient Registration Charge Person to initiate the alias process.

5. Registration Procedure:

    a) Patient is to sign waiver for use of an alias form. Alias will not be used unless the patient signs the waiver.

    b) Patient is registered for this episode of care using legal name (may or may not already exist in the MPI) in order to originate or use correct unit number (MRN).

    c) Patient signs all consent/authorization and other legal forms throughout the episode care using their legal name.

    d) After registration is complete, registrar will change legal name within the computer system to the alias of the patient's choice as documented on the waiver form. Legal name will be retained as an alias within the system during the current episode of care.

    e) The face sheet will be sent to the unit supervisor with the original of the alias waiver form. These are to be retained as a permanent part of the medical record.

6. Discharge Procedure:

    a) On the day of discharge, immediately prior to the actual discharge, the supervisor on the discharging nursing unit will notify the Patient Registration Charge Person of the impending discharge.

    b) Patient Registration will change the alias back to the patient's legal name, now retaining the alias as a previous name in the computer system. It is important to do this prior to discharge to insure billing will occur correctly.

Figure 7-2 Patient waiver for use of an alias.

Continued

Waiver for Use of an Alias

You have requested to use an alias (pseudonym) while you are a patient. When using an alias, there are certain consequences which may occur. While an alias may superficially help protect your confidentiality to a higher level, it may also actually draw attention to your presence in the facility, due to the number of steps necessary to implement a pseudonym. Therefore, we ask that you read the following information and give your consent to the use of the alias you have chosen.

I understand:

1. My insurance company may not verify coverage using an alias. I will provide the facility with my legal name and sign all the paperwork using my legal name for billing as well as medical consent purposes. I will be liable for any bills my insurance company refuses to pay because of the use of an alias.

2. Information I provide about next of kin will not be changed to an alias.

3. Previous medical information or information provided by other health care providers may not be readily available if I choose to use an alias. I understand if I do not use the same alias each time I choose an alias, my medical records may not be recognized and retrieved in a timely manner to assist with my care.

4. My alias will be returned to my legal name within the computer system after my episode of care is completed. My alias name will be cross-referenced to my legal name at that time.

5. Portions of my medical record will contain both my legal name and alias name depending on when the results are printed.

6. The pharmacy and other ancillary areas of the facility may not be able to release prescriptions and results to me while I am using an alias, unless proper identification of my legal name is available.

Legal name is: (print) ————————————————————————

Alias name is: (print) ————————————————————————

Signature of patient/legal guardian ——————————————— Date ——————

Witness Signature ——————————————————————————————

Figure 7-2, cont'd   Patient waiver for use of an alias.

retrieval problems can cause the patient to be incorrectly assigned an additional number. New MPIs should be entered consistently, and continuing indexes should be verified for possible problems with inconsistent data entry. Figure 7-3 shows a sample basic MPI screen for a facility that uses unit numbering.

Policies and procedures must be set up to ensure MPI data validity. The MPI is generally originated on patient scheduling or registration; maintained or added to during the course of clinical care; and validated, updated, and maintained by health information professionals. Duplicate number assignment can result in the need to merge visits, which must include updating any and all corresponding

Name:	Smith, John James	MR#:	12-34-56
DOB:	03-03-1936	SS#:	294-55-3235*
Sex:	M		

Dates of Admission:	01-10-84	Discharge:	01-15-84
	06-05-91		06-07-91
	10-20-94		10-26-94

* Social Security numbers are obtained voluntarily from patients

Figure 7-3   MPI screen.

reports, records, and databases in a health care facility (paper and electronic) for consistency. Figure 7-4 shows a sample MPI Creation Policy and Procedures, and Figure 7-5 shows a sample data validity tracking form. Many facilities engage in a daily reconciliation and validity checking process for the MPI to ensure that duplications and errors are cleansed.

Master Patient Index Creation Policy and Procedure

Philosophy: A computerized Master Patient Index (MPI) legal record to be maintained permanently for all patient episodes of care. These episodes are identified by a unique unit number (also known as medical record number - MRN) and account numbers for each case or series of care. Maintenance of an accurate and timely master patient index is essential to the operations of the facility. Patient Registration areas are responsible for the accuracy of the information entered into the computer system upon registration or pre-registration. Clinical/Ancillary areas are responsible for the data integrity during patient care that is required to accurately reflect activity. Health Information Management will facilitate revisions needed after patient discharge to maintain data validity.

I. Master Patient Index Creation Guidelines
  A. Upon registration, only legal names shall be entered into the computer system unless specific policy dictates otherwise.
    1. Verify with proof of identification (preferably Driver's License) at the time of registration whenever possible.
    2. Nicknames or alias are not to be used unless there is a risk to patient safety. (See Alias Policy and Procedure.) In the rare circumstance that an alias is utilized, appropriate Alias Waiver will be utilized.
    3. Do not use punctuation, spaces, or symbols in a name. Hyphenated names are to be entered as a single continuous name without a hyphen.
    4. Enter middle name only if entire name as listed on legal ID fits in designated space. Otherwise, use middle initial only.
    5. Do not use title (religious, medical, etc.)
  B. Check for previous name or numbers (which must be done at EACH REGISTRATION).
    1. Check the Master Patient Index by entering last name and first initial.
    2. Use birth date, address, mother's maiden name and/or social security number as an additional check.
    3. Use phonetic search if no name is found.
    4. Never enter middle initial or middle name when searching the MPI for purposes of registration.
    5. Verify with the patient or family member that no other name may have been given when registering previously.
  C. Unidentified Patients:
    1. Until accurate information can be obtained:
      a. Females should be entered as Doe, Jane with a birth date of January 1 of the current year.
      b. Males should be entered as Doe, John with a birth date of January 1 of the current year.
      c. If multiple Does are entered, the middle initial should be entered in alphabetical order (i.e., Doe, John A).
      d. Trauma patients are entered as TRAUMA, ###### (# representing the number they are given in a trauma situation).
    2. Social security number should be entered as all zeros for unidentified cases.
    D. Newborn babies are to be entered upon birth as "Last name, Baby boy". (or Baby girl) (i.e., Jones, Baby boy)
II. Demographic Data Changes
  A. Incorrect patient name:
    1. If patient has been registered under a previous name which is not the legal name (but is a name the patient may have given at the time of the previous registration), correct the previous name. Only the legal name should be retained.
    2. If a patient has been registered under a previous name which was the legal name previously (i.e. the maiden name), both names are to be retained. Keeping a previous name creates an alias.
    3. If a patient has been registered under a previous name which has an incorrect spelling, correct the previous name. Do not retain the incorrectly spelled name.

Figure 7-4 MPI creation policy and procedure

Continued

4. For newborns, adjust the permanent name from the original. Newborns will
   be changed from "Last name, Baby boy" format to the "Last name, First
   name" format without retaining an alias. However, for newborns whose
   legal name is different from that given at registration and/or different from
   the mother's name, two name changes will be required. First, from baby to
   given first name, which does not require an alias, and second, from name
   upon registration (with the updated first name) to legal name appearing on
   the birth certificate, which will require an alias to be retained.
   Example A: Jones, Baby boy (name change without alias retention) to Jones,
       Michael
   Example B: Jones, Michael (name change with alias retention) to Smith, Michael

III. Duplicate Unit (Medical Record) Number
  A. If one or more duplicate unit numbers are discovered:
    1. Register the patient's new account under the earliest (oldest or lowest
       number) in the system. This is the "correct" number.
    2. Notify H.I.M. of the duplicate number by completing the duplicate unit number
       report form. A copy will also be given to the Patient Registration Manager.
       Items to be recorded include:
       a. Patient Correct/Legal Name
       b. Date of Birth (DOB)
       c. Correct (original) Unit Number
       d. Wrong Unit Number (duplicate)
       e. Last Account Number created in incorrect unit number
       f. Registrar Initials
    3. All patient records, centrally or de-centrally stored, and applicable databases
       will be reconciled by managing departments to concur with correct and
       cross-referenced unit numbers.
    4. If patient is registered under another patient's unit number, transfer account
       from one unit number to the other.
  B. If one or more duplicate unit numbers are discovered when the record is being
     processed:
    1. Complete the Patient Data Validity and Correction Form and route to the
       manager.
  C. Correcting Inpatient/Outpatient Records and Databases after the unit numbers
     have been merged:
    1. Obtain report of daily MPI merging activity.
    2. Locate the record using the invalid unit number.
    3. If the record is in the permanent file:
       a. Cross out the invalid number on the facesheet and document (in red)
          the valid number.
       b. Update the letter color labels if necessary.
       c. If the patient has had previous admissions under the valid unit number,
          file the record under that valid number.
       d. If the patient has not had previous admissions, update the folder to reflect
          the valid unit number and patient name, file in correct terminal digit
          location.
    4. If the record is anywhere outside of permanent file:
       a. Cross out the invalid unit number and patient name on the facesheet and
          document (in red) the valid number.
       b. Update the letter color labels if necessary.
       c. Return the record to the proper location.
       d. Notify the Incomplete Record Area staff of the merge so that proper
          updating in the Deficiency System is made if the record is incomplete.

Figure 7-4, cont'd MPI creation policy and procedure.

Others use specialized software that is designed to screen and identify existing or possible discrepancies at the time of creation of the MPI or afterward in a batch mode. This area of the profession has become so specialized that today companies have been established to handle MPI maintenance, elimination of duplication, and general overall validation.

Backup of the MPI is extremely important because this is a primary index for record retrieval functions in a paper-based clinical record system. Therefore, where an automated MPI exists, computer output microfiche (COM) output or paper backup files must regularly be prepared and available for staff to use in case of computer downtime.

Patient Data Validity and Correction Tracking Form

Date: _____

TO: ——— Patient Business Office/Patient Registration
——— Nursing Assistant Director: Unit/Dept:
——— Other:

FROM: Health Information Management:

This form has been designed to give you feedback regarding data discrepancies identified during record processing activities. Please take this opportunity to investigate how this problem may have occurred, share the information with appropriate staff, and initiate any educational, preventative, or corrective action to avoid this situation in future cases.

The Shaded Box Reflects Current Info Which May Be Incorrect. The Corrected Information is Shown Below The Shaded Box.

DATE DISCREPANCY IDENTIFIED: ——————— BY WHOM: ———————————

PATIENT NAME: (L) ——————— (F) ——————— (M) ———————

ADMIT DATE: ——————————— DISCHARGE DATE: ———————

ACCOUNT NUMBER: ——————— UNIT # (MRN): ———————

DISCHARGING NURSING UNIT: ——————— PT TYPE: ———————

WRONG DEMOGRAPHIC DATA: ——————— Correct Data is: ———————

DUPLICATE ACCOUNT #: ——————— Correct Account # is: ———————

WRONG PATIENT TYPE: ——————— Correct Pt Type is: ———————

WRONG ADMIT/DISCH DATE: ——————— Correct Date is: ———————

OTHER ISSUE(S)/QUESTIONS(S): ———————————————————

RESPONSE/ACTION: Please return this form to the Health Information Department with a response if action is needed. ———————————————————

Health Information Database Correction Use Only:

Computer System ——————— Initials: ——— Date: ———————————

Patient Record ——————— Initials: ——— Date: ———————————

Cancer Registry ——————— Initials: ——— Date: ———————————

Figure 7-5 Patient data validity and correction tracking form.

The use of corporate or enterprise-wide identification numbers is popular so that patients can be identified to the demographic level within a health care system. This usage also allows such entities to continue to use a separate and unique numbering system without losing the ability to identify shared patient information within the corporation (Box 7-3). Howe-ver, care must be taken when working within a corporate health system not to merge the MPI, unless there is also a way to *unmerge* the same index in case of separation of entities within a system. If multiple facilities are serviced through one index, such as in a multihospital system, the index should indicate the facility in which the admission or encounter occurred.

Box 7-3 CASE STUDY: MPI SOFTWARE CLEANS UP AND PREVENTS DUPLICATE MEDICAL RECORD NUMBERS

This case study concerns how two hospitals with a combined total of nearly 40,000 inpatient discharges and 185,000 outpatient visits a year with different information technology and different data fields came together beginning with a corporate person index (CPI). The challenge was to implement a common CPI for two hospitals while performing a data integrity improvement of each of the existing MPIs. The target date for completion was 12 months.

The medical records department was assigned responsibility for identifying "duplicate" patients in the CPI between the two facilities and updating the respective separate MPIs to reflect the most current information. The process began with a traditional deterministic search method to identify duplicates within each facility's MPI. (Figure A).

The following elements were researched in an exact deterministic match on all elements:
- Last name, first name
- Social Security number
- Date of birth

The problem with this method is that it is not possible to detect duplicates caused by errors in name spelling or number transposition. Also, there is no easy way to cross-reference merged duplicate numbers.

After a year of manual clean-up effort and more than $60,000 in manpower, time had run out. When the two hospitals' MPIs were loaded into the CPI, another 78,000 duplicates occurred within the CPI. An immediate and cost-effective solution had to be found. At that point the director of patient financial services recommended using a computerized process that searched the MPI files by using algorithms. Because time was of the essence, a product and a vendor who had an immediate solution had to be selected. Medibase, Inc. was the vendor selected to install electronic clean-up software. Medibase, Inc. accomplished the installation and had the software operating in less than 3 months.

The software was able to identify duplicates by using the following:
- Phonetic search
- Deterministic search
- Probabilistic algorithms that rank the information from 100 to 1 as a probable duplicate record number

In addition, the software used name normalization, address normalization, and a stoplight method of highlighting potential duplicate data fields, thus expediting the process of duplicate number decisions by the clerical clean-up team.

At the time the two hospitals decided to embark on this partnership, there was a multidisciplinary conversion team formed that included all ancillary departments, patient financial services, the internal audit manager, computer services, and medical records. The high volume of duplicates affected the ancillary departments. In addition, as the clean-up was occurring, the medical records department became frustrated that duplicates continued to occur as a result new duplicates being generated every day during registration.

In addition to the conversion team, a registration team was formed. This team worked with the director of HIM and the medical records support manager responsible for making recommendations about decision rules for the clean-up process. The decision rules regarding which medical record number would "survive" as the permanent number was a collaborative effort among the vendor experts, computer services, and the medical records professionals. The registration team worked on data element standardization between the two facilities so the data element sex, for example, was "F" for female in both sites and "M" for male versus using "b" for boy and "g" for girl. The MPI team started with the highest probabilistic matches because the team was simultaneously cleaning the MPI and the CPI. However, as the clean-up project continued, it was apparent that new duplicates continued to be created every day. The director of medical records felt that the project value was mitigated without "up front" (at the time of registration) prevention of new duplicate numbers. This viewpoint was strongly supported by the ancillary departments. The blood bank, for example, was very supportive of duplicate prevention software. As a result of the team support, the hospital elected to add upfront duplicate prevention software.

Unfortunately, the problem of duplicate medical record and guarantor numbers in health care provider settings is not unique. What makes this case study interesting is that the electronic solution of the 78,000 CPI duplicates was completed in less than 4 months, including 22,000 physical chart merges. Today the MPI remains very clean with a computer "refresh" run every 6 months. The computerized refresh presents only duplicate numbers that have been issued since the last refresh and does not present duplicates that have been rejected as "not a duplicate" (Figure B). The medical records department has initiated an imaging solution to having two separate medical records departments. The imaging project is moving forward smoothly largely in part as a result of a clean MPI and CPI.

Definitions
1. *Corporate person index (CPI):* A person index that contains person names and medical record numbers for multiple facilities. Person names may be the patient or guarantor of the account
2. *Cross-reference:* Archive of numbers file that when created electronically all numbers that pertain to the same patient are filed together in the cross-reference
3. *Deterministic:* Able to establish an association between two files by searching for an exact match against a set of given criteria (e.g., medical record number). (AHIMA practice brief November 1997).
4. *False positive:* If a record is reported as a duplicate but on review is determined not to be a duplicate and is rejected, careful attention has to be given as to where in the 100 to 1 probabilistic scoring the majority of these occur
5. *Merge:* Once the patient number that is to survive is selected, the computer electronically merges data from nonsurvivor (retiree) encounters together with the survivor number, therefore providing continuity of patient information

Box 7-3 CASE STUDY: MPI SOFTWARE CLEANS UP AND PREVENTS DUPLICATE MEDICAL
RECORD NUMBERS—cont'd

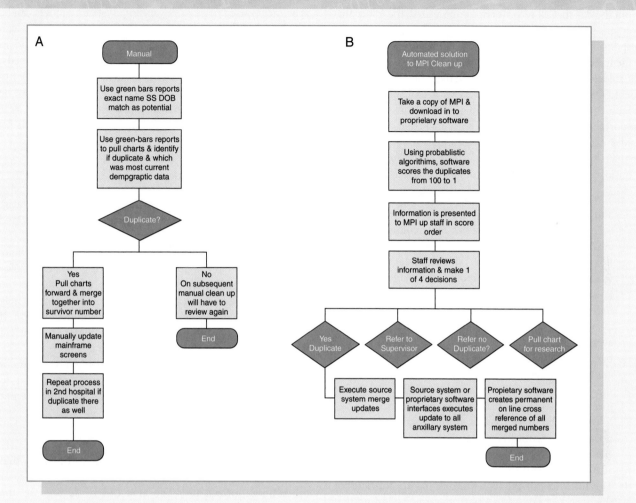

6. *Name normalization:* A process that links common names such as "William, Billy, Bill" together under one name
7. *Pairing rule:* A data element field or fields used as a key by the scoring algorithm for identifying potential duplicates
8. *Phonetic file:* A system to file and find names without regard to vowels. Used to locate names that sound alike but are not spelled the same way
9. *Probabilistic:* Capability or linking of data elements that compensate for discrepancies by using all the information recorded in two files and attach a weighted value for matching discrepancies. (AHIMA practice brief, November 1997).
10. *Refresh:* Computer capability to locate all new person/patient numbers issued since the last update excluding those designated as "not a duplicate" during the earlier number clean-up efforts. To "refresh" the file is to bring out all legitimate duplicates created since the last time the process was refreshed.

11. *Retiree:* The duplicate patient number that is determined to be sent to an archive cross-reference list and not to be used for further patient care
12. *Scoring:* Weighted or probabilistic algorithm for quantifying the relative validity of a potential duplicate
13. *Street normalization:* A table that brings "Berkshire St." and "Berkshire Street" together
14. *Survivor:* The duplicate patient number that is selected to remain in the active file and that will be used in new encounters

Suggested Reading

Pavoni MM: Technology and teamwork rescues corporate person index. Proceedings of the American Health Information Management Association National Convention and Program, October, 1999.

(Courtesy of MediBase and Mary Mike Pavoni, RHIA, FAHIMA.)

Records Management Issues

File Folders

Until the day that all records are computerized, the folder that contains patient information is important for anyone who has responsibility for the record. Many facilities may use the paper patient record as a historical document well into the future. The file folder is the most fundamental element of record management. The folder should be viewed as a tool for protecting documents and managing information. For this reason, it is important to be aware of the difference that choosing the right folder can make. All these considerations also apply to the management of other records, such as radiology films. Considerations in folder size and design are as follow:

- Standard folders for patient records are $9\frac{1}{2}$ inches high and $12\frac{1}{4}$ inches wide.
- Standard folders are manila but other color choices are available; typically up to 12 colors.
- Reinforced top and extended side panels are important when there is a high rate of record retrieval from the file.
- Folder bottoms should be scored (manufactured with indented lines that assist in creating straight folds) to allow the folder to accommodate a patient record of average size for the facility. Consider the average number of pages per discharged record, the number of annual outpatient **encounters,**[2] or both when estimating the average record size. Also consider whether the facility provides any services that are long term in nature (e.g., oncology, dialysis) or creates especially large records for documenting complex care, such as neonatal intensive care records. High-volume ambulatory practices can also produce a large amount of paper documentation.
- The thickness of the folder should be appropriate for the expected rate of use, with the understanding that heavier folders cost proportionately more. The two standard thicknesses are 11 point and 14 point, with 14 point being heavier and more durable. Manila stock is also available in 13, 14, 15, 18, and 20 points. Of these, 11, 14, and 15 point stock are the most commonly used. *Please note:* Point and *weight* are different. Point measures thickness (a point measure is equal to 1/1000 inch or 0.001"). Weight measures density (measured by weighing 1000 sheets of sized paper stock). To determine the correct weight, consider the following:
- The number of pages expected to be protected and filed in the *average* folder
- The specific retention period of the paper record
- The average number of times the folder will be removed from the shelf in its lifetime of use (the wear-and-tear factor)

If the wear-and-tear factor is low or the **retention period** for the paper folder is projected to be short (2 to 3 years), the 11-point folder is adequate. If the paper record is expected to be used for 3 or more years, the 14-point folder is a wiser investment.

There are two basic configurations of folders; end tab configuration and top tab configuration. End tab is primarily used for open shelf file systems. Top tab configuration is primarily used in pull drawer filing systems. Folders can be purchased with or without fasteners, and the fasteners can be applied in various positions within the folder to aid in organizing the data to best meet the facility's needs. Additionally, reinforced extended tabs add to the longevity of the folder. However, reinforced extended tabs may not be the best course of action when you consider adding year bands, color-coded labels, or computer generated labels on the extended tab.

Color Coding

Using **color coding** to designate certain letters or digits helps to prevent misfiles and aids in rapid storage and retrieval. Color can also provide an easy way to distribute workload and make sorting of folders much easier.

Differently colored folders can be used to designate changes in primary digits of a terminal digit system. Color bars designating letters or digits can be preprinted on the folder or added by using adhesive labels. The color bars may have both a color designation and a position designation. If either the color or the position on the folder is incorrect when it is placed in the file, it indicates a misfile.

Employees working in a color coding environment should be tested by the human resources department to ensure that candidates for working in the file room are not color blind.

Record Security

Patient records should be stored in an area or a room that can be locked to prevent inadvertent loss, tampering, or other unauthorized use. The area can be secured by the traditional lock-and-key method or with a computerized access panel that operates by activating the correct key combination. The computerized access panel has the advantage of being easily updated with a new code if a security problem is noted, rather than by attempting to physically locate all the keys. The Health Insurance Portability and Accountability Act (HIPAA) and organizational policies typically permit access on a need basis only. Security of computerized records is discussed in Chapter 8 on Technology, Applications, and Security. Additional discussions of HIPAA as it relates to the privacy of health information are found in Chapter 15 Privacy and Health Law.

Storage of Inactive Records

An organization may determine how to keep frequently needed files accessible. One perspective is to define files as active and inactive on the basis of the health care activity of the patient. Active records are stored in a location commonly referred to as the active files. Activity is determined by the frequency of encounters with the typical patient and the amount of filing space that is conveniently located. If a patient has not received treatment or had other activity associated with the record for more than 5 years, then the record could be declared inactive. Inactive records do not need to be as readily available but do need to be accessible when they are needed. For example, one hospital has limited space for its paper-based clinical records and can only maintain about 1 year's worth of records on site. Records stored off site are accessible through a contract delivery and storage service that provides twice-a-day plus on-call deliveries to the hospital. The hospital plans to transition to an electronic record system, but this interim approach meets their needs.

Alternate Location. With regard to storing inactive records that are no longer in high demand, two options are available without changing the records to another format or medium. One option is to store records in an organized filing system located in another area of the facility. Another option is to use the services of a commercial storage company.

Commercial Storage. Commercial storage companies store different types of records but may specialize in highly confidential records, such as legal or patient records. As a minimum, the commercial storage company should have the following:

- Business associate agreements compliant with HIPAA rules and regulations
- HIPAA-acceptable confidentiality policies and statements signed by their employees
- Acceptable references from health care facilities or similar business facilities
- Insurance coverage for loss, damage, personal injury, and workers' compensation
- Record return guarantee by either faxed or electronic transmission
- Reasonable retrieval fees
- No surrender fee (cost to remove all the records from storage)
- Quality control in both storage and retrieval methods

Other items to be included in contract discussions with commercial storage companies are the "hidden," or seldom thought of, questions, such as the following:

- Who pulls the files from the current storage system (who pays for it)?
- Who completes the list of what is to be stored (who pays for it)?
- Exactly when does the custody of the record change over to the storage company (whose insurance is paying for it)?
- What are the billing terms (yearly, monthly, as used)?
- What price increases to expect and frequency of these increase over the life of the contract?

Each possible storage company should be screened to evaluate its overall costs and services provided. Investigate other alternatives discussed in this chapter when developing a long-term storage and retrieval system. Calculate the costs for all options in accordance with the facility retention policy or over a minimum of 10 years to provide adequate comparison of the costs.

System File Conversion

Existing alphabetical and straight numerical filing methods often do not meet the future needs of growing facilities. Increased filing efficiency is usually sought by converting existing systems to numeric identification and the terminal digit filing method. The thought of conversion sounds intimidating, but it does not need to be if thorough planning takes place. Conversion concepts can apply to moving the contents of a department or file room to a new location (see Box 7-4). If it is decided to convert to a new filing system, consider taking a picture of the file area *before* beginning the process to be able to visually show the success afterward.

Box 7-4 CONVERSION CHECKLIST

1. _____ Take "before" pictures.
2. _____ Develop a chart of project time lines and post it.
3. _____ Purge the records if not all are to be converted.
4. _____ Assign numbers to record, if necessary, and create an index.
5. _____ Apply color coding or bar code labels, if necessary.
6. _____ Schedule an actual conversion date.
7. _____ Hold a project meeting with the staff.
8. _____ Complete test trials to determine average times.
9. _____ Complete an estimated count of the records to be converted.
10. _____ Calculate staff needs and obtain staffing commitments.
11. _____ Assign team leaders, project teams, and duties.
12. _____ Hold a project meeting with the staff.
13. _____ Train the staff in the terminal digit system; take "field trips" as necessary.
14. _____ Take "halfway" pictures (with color-coded labels out of order).
15. _____ Alert and train the medical staff about conversion.
16. _____ Hold a project meeting with the staff to establish ground rules for the conversion weekend.
17. _____ Order food for breaks and meals and tables and carts for sorting.
18. _____ Determine and label new terminal digit section placement in the file.
19. _____ Organize the chart return day for 1 day before conversion.
20. _____ Locate a secure area, with keys, for personal belongings.
21. _____ Receive delivery of tables and carts.
22 _____ Actual conversion takes place.
23. _____ Take "after" pictures (with labels in order).
24. _____ Send thank you notes.
25. _____ Hold open house party.

Planning Process. Make as many changes as possible before the actual conversion. If the files are being converted from an alphabetical arrangement to a straight numerical or terminal digit arrangement, they need to have numbers assigned to them and an index must be created. If a computer system is already in use, a patient number field must be available to store the numbers. Either assign the numbers and enter them into the computer or have the computer complete the number assignment process.

Before filing systems are converted, the following steps should be taken:

1. Be sure that all record management applications have been thoroughly explored, giving equal consideration to imaging and scanning or EDM. Software, hardware, file supplies, and employee costs are all factors in the equation. If the decision is to continue using paper-based records and to do a conversion to a new filing system, then proceed with this plan.
2. Change to new folders. In converting to an automated record-tracking systems, some manufacturers can manufacture file folders with bar codes already printed or embedded on the folder, thus saving time and money.
3. Apply color coding or other labels to ease the resorting process during the conversion.
4. Purge the files not being converted so that the fewest records possible need to be moved.

Schedule the conversion during an off-peak time for the facility, such as during the slower summer months. The move should be scheduled for a weekend from Friday at 5:00 pm to Monday at 8:00 am.[2] Trial tests should be made with a small number of records to determine the time it takes to complete each phase of the conversion work, with an average time per unit of work being multiplied by the estimated number of work units to be completed. Allow for 10% fatigue time when converting patient record folders and 15% fatigue time when converting radiology film jackets. (Radiology film jackets are much larger and far heavier than patient record folders.) Schedule enough workers to complete the conversion on the basis of the number of hours available and the average times calculated from the trial tests.

Develop a visual display of the project time lines. Post the chart in a prominent place in the department, and educate all staff members about their roles in adhering to the conversion time line. Hold as many preparatory meetings as necessary to make the staff feel comfortable with the conversion.[2] Take "before" pictures of the file room area before the conversion starts.

Train all staff to a working comfort level. Inform employees about the theory behind terminal digit filing, train them in its use, and have the employees practice the new methods.[3] Considering that most file system conversions incorporate new folders, color-coded applications, and possibly computer interface, ask your vendor(s) to assist in providing a small mock file room for practice purposes and other hardware applications necessary to train staff. Check the work of each employee to determine the employee's understanding of the new system. Also, educate the remainder of the facility staff and the medical staff about the changes that will be taking place in the department to increase their understanding.[3] Answer their questions, reassure them that service will not be interrupted during the conversion, and enlist their cooperation during the conversion time period.

Have sufficient staff and supplies available for the conversion. Use department staff and supplement them with other workers as necessary. Order folding tables for sorting and transportation carts from a rental company, or borrow them from another facility.[3]

Conversion Process. There are four project phases in the conversion, each requiring a team leader assignment:

1. Transport the records to the sort area and back to file
2. Rough-sort into 10 terminal digit sections (e.g., 00-09, 10-19)
3. Secondary-sort into 00, 01, 02, and so on
4. Fine-sort into strict terminal digit order on the file shelves

Begin the conversion by removing records from the areas prelabeled as section 00 and section 50. Remove an equal number of records from the areas that will hold each terminal digit section. This minimizes the number of records that must be off the shelves at any given time and provides a place to put records as soon as they are sorted. Team 1 transports the records to the sort area and back to the file. Team 2 rough-sorts the records onto sorting tables (or boxes on chairs), and Team 3 does an intermediate-sort into 00, 01, 02, and so on. To minimize back injury from lifting, have employees avoid placing records on the floor or lower than waist height. Use carts to transport all records.

When sufficient records are available in any given primary section where shelving is available, Team 1 transports the records back to the shelving area and places them on the appropriate shelf. Team 4 then fine-sorts the records into strict terminal digit order. Continue this process until all records have been rough-sorted and returned to the file in their primary section. At that time, Teams 2 and 3 become fine sorters with Team 4, and Team 1 assists in any shifting of files necessary within primary sections.

Teams should be scheduled in 8-hour shifts, all taking breaks and lunches together.[3] The facility food service or an outside catering service should prepare meals and break refreshments for the team staff. A secured, lockable area where personal belongings can be stored should be provided.[2] Throughout the process, expect the unexpected and adjust plans as necessary.

When the process is complete, take "after" pictures of the finished product. Tell of your success and hold an open house for the facility.[2] Today, many organizations publish an in-house newspaper for its staff and employees. This is a great vehicle to share your success and recognize those who assisted in the process. And finally, do not forget to send thank you messages to all participants.

Record Tracking

Regardless of how records are filed within the facility, one of the biggest concerns is knowing where a record is when it is needed. For a record management system to be efficient, there must be some method of tracking the current location of a patient record.

Manual Record-Tracking Systems

Manual **record-tracking** systems are the most common, with use of **outguides** and **requisitions** as their basic tools.

Outguides. An outguide is a plastic folder used in place of a record when the record has been removed from the files. It can be thought of as a placeholder. Outguides usually contain two separate see-through pockets, one to hold the requisition slip and one to hold any loose papers to be filed in the record that accumulate while the record is out of file.

Requisitions. A **requisition** is somewhat like an IOU. It is an acknowledgment that someone has taken a record and intends to return it.[4] Figure 7-6 shows a typical patient record requisition slip. Part 1 of the requisition slip is placed in the outguide as the record is removed from the file. Parts 2 and 3 travel with the record as a routing slip. Part 2 can be used by the requester as a **transfer notice** if the requester forwards the record to another location. Notification of a record transfer is important to obtain but can be especially difficult to obtain in a manual system. The notices are usually 3 × 5-inch slips that can easily be lost in transit. The transfer notices that do make their way to the file area should be given a higher priority than the retrieval of records. Filing the transfer notices first ensures that the most current location for every record is known before retrieval is attempted.

Manual record-tracking systems should also be able to determine when the record has been **purged,** or **thinned,** from the active files and either moved to an alternative storage site or converted to another medium, such as microforms or optical disks, discussed in this chapter. **Outcards** listing the new location or medium should be used for this purpose.[4] An outcard differs from an outguide in that outcards are usually cardboard to allow the patient name and record number to be written directly on them. Outcards stay in the file permanently to tell the new location of the paper record or the new medium to which it has been transferred.

Record Retrieval Steps. The steps in retrieving a record in a manual system are as follow:

1. Receive the request for a record.
2. Verify the name and number of the record.
3. Place the requisition slip in an outguide.
4. Locate the record on the shelf.
5. Put the outguide on the shelf and remove the record.
6. Forward the record to the requester.

When the record returns, refile it on the shelf and remove the outguide placing any loose filing material in the outguide in the file itself.

Color coding methods can also be applied to the use of outguides. Two common methods of color coding outguides are assigning colors for specific request reasons or assigning colors to a specific retrieval time period. Using unique colors for different request reasons alerts the staff to immediately check another location, such as the release of information area or the physicians' incomplete area.

When assigning colors to a specific retrieval time period, some departments use a differently colored outguide every week on a 4-week rotating cycle. As a new week begins, the outguides from the past 4 weeks (four different colors) are counted. All outguides older than 3 weeks are checked and updated with the new location. This provides a constant file review process for records out of file longer than 4 weeks. Other similar plans can be used to track records according to specific facility needs.

A sufficient supply of outguides is important to a record-tracking system. Past activity levels can help determine the

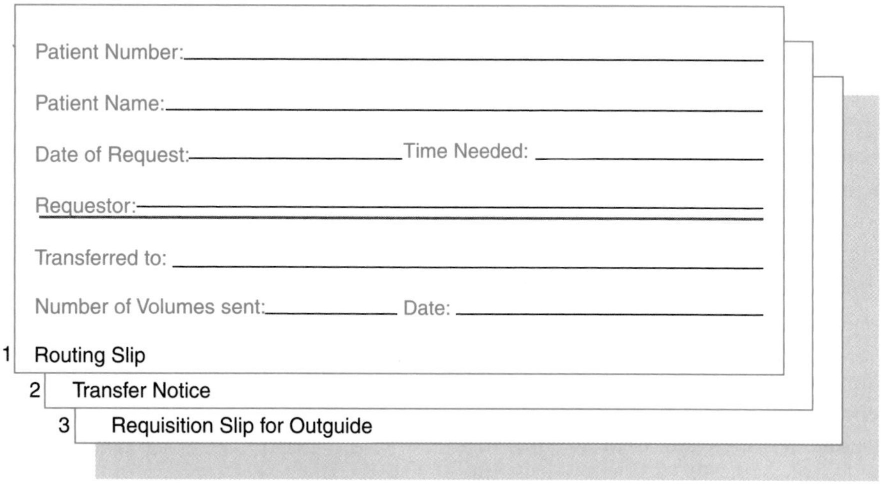

Patient Number:_____

Patient Name:_____

Date of Request:_____Time Needed: _____

Requestor:-_____

Transferred to: _____

Number of Volumes sent:_____ Date: _____

1 | Routing Slip

2 | Transfer Notice

3 | Requisition Slip for Outguide

Figure 7-6 Requisition slip.

quantity of outguides to have on hand. Be sure that the outguide pockets are large enough to accommodate both the requisition slip and any loose papers. Filing loose papers in the outguide allows the staff to forward information to a requester if the record is unavailable and allows the record to be updated immediately when it returns to the file.

Although these manual system procedures have been used for years, this tracking system is not without certain disadvantages, including the following:

- Time lags in updating record locations[5]
- Excessive time needed to file transfer notices to keep record locations current
- Illegibility of many handwritten requests[5]
- Difficulty in prioritizing workload
- High frustration levels of staff whose work is crisis oriented[5]
- Dissatisfaction of record requesters with service

Automated Record-Tracking Systems

Software Considerations. Automated record-tracking systems were developed to address the concerns just listed. An automated record-tracking system is a database that stores the current and past locations of the record. The automated system is similar to inventory control software that is used in manufacturing to track parts or similar to tracking systems used by the U.S. Postal Service, UPS, FedEx, and others. The fact that the system is automated does not mean that outguides and requisition slips are forgotten. Outguides can still aid in the refiling process and hold loose papers. However, organizations have been known to "forward" loose documents to the holder of record for filing. Requisition slips identify the name and number associated with the outguide. Once the record is retrieved, the outguide is no longer considered the source of information on the record location. The tracking system holds the information about all record requests and transfers.[6]

The tracking system is often linked to other facility systems to avoid duplication of effort. For example, linking the tracking database to the MPI eliminates the need for this second database to contain large amounts of patient demographic information. It is also efficient to link the record-tracking database to a patient scheduling system to allow automatic transfer of requests for appointment records.[7] Linking the system to a record deficiency system gives an added advantage of knowing which records need to be returned for completion.

Having an on-line request-for-records feature speeds the request process and produces legible requisitions with complete and accurate information with each printing. This feature also allows the tracking software to prioritize the requests according to date and time of need and whether the request is for direct patient care. This feature significantly decreases the need for telephone requests for records and frees the staff to spend time retrieving records rather than answering the telephone. Printers are used to printing requisitions and are placed in the file area near where the records are located (Box 7-5).

An automated record-tracking system should be able to produce both management reports and statistical reports (Box 7-6).

Data Entry Capabilities. Automated systems work extremely well when integrated with bar code technology to speed the data entry process. Bar code labels can be applied to existing folders in preparation for converting to a bar code system (Box 7-7) or as an enhancement to a current record-tracking system to increase productivity.

Bar codes have been used in medical records departments since the 1970s. The Health Industry Bar Code Council,

---

Box 7-5 FEATURES OF AN AUTOMATED RECORD-TRACKING SYSTEM

- On-line requesting of records, individually or in batch
- Prioritizing of requests done by the software
- On-line inquiry, both current and historical, from every system terminal
- Tracking of multiple volumes of the same record
- Tracking of multiple file room locations
- Updating of system done in real time
- Support of bar code technology, both hand held and portable
- Support of keyboard data entry of patient identification number or name
- Operation in a user-friendly environment
- Alerts staff when a returned record has been requested during its absence

---

Box 7-6 SOFTWARE REQUIREMENTS OF AN AUTOMATED RECORD-TRACKING SYSTEM

Dictionary Driven, User Definable
- Reasons for requests
- Out-of-file locations

Reporting Capabilities

Management Reports
- Appointment listings
- Unsatisfied requests listings
- Location listings (for use during downtime)
- Overdue listings by user-defined time frames
- Out-of-file listings by location
- Inactive record listings by alternative storage site or medium

Statistical Reports
- Total scheduled appointments and percentage satisfied
- Total walk-in appointments and percentage satisfied
- Total stat requests and percentage satisfied
- Total requests for each out-of-file location and percentage satisfied
- Grand total of all requests and percentage satisfied
- Total records refiled
- Total records retrieved from inactive storage and other media

Box 7-7 WORKSTATION OBJECTIVES

- Increase user productivity.
- Reduce data entry time and eliminate redundant data entry.
- Standardize the provider-system interface by allowing command and response specifications of an information system to be user modifiable.
- Complete the bulk of the patient care documentation during the patient encounter through on-line, point-of-service data capture—bedside and examination room.
- Improve quality of care through availability of clinical guidelines.
- Provide intervention messages for exceptional patient conditions through innovative displays.
- Facilitate the management of free text data.
- Allow for new voice input and output, handwriting recognition, and imaging technology to be incorporated in the workstation.
- Facilitate the collection of administrative, financial, and clinical data for outcomes, research, organizational assessment, and resource management studies.
- Increase accessibility of medical information through the use of clinical decisions support tools and the provision of easy-to-use links to existing medical reference databases (MEDLINE).
- Provide easy access to output processes that integrate various result data to display medical information.
- Lessen the risk of data loss and mitigate the effects of a system failure through the local collection and storage of patient data (that can be stored for transmission to the health information system after recovery).[18]

which was formed in 1984, approved a particular bar code symbology specifically for use in health care: code 39. The **symbology** of a bar code means the way the lines and spaces in the bar code are arranged. Code 39 was selected for its variable length, accuracy, and flexibility.[8] Materials management, radiology, and food service all use the same standard bar code to track supplies, radiology films, and meals, respectively. Also see Chapter 8, Technology, Applications and Security for information on bar coding.

The bar code symbology for record folders contains at least two pieces of information, the patient number and the volume number of the record. If other information is needed, it is usually retrieved by on-line access to the MPI or other database.

When a bar code is read, the software receives the characters as if they were entered by way of the keyboard and it processes the information in the same way. This is the same as the process used in a grocery store scanner that reads the universal product codes (UPC) from canned and packaged products. If the UPC is unreadable, the cashier enters the number on the keypad.

Hardware Needs. Hardware requirements for the system are laser printers, placed where new records are generated, and a variety of bar code reader devices, depending on the quantity of records to be scanned. Programmable color laser printers can be purchased that can print a strip label for the side of the folder that contains the patient's name and identification number, the bar code, and the color code bars. This method ensures that records are labeled uniformly and that the labeling process is completed with the least amount of hardware and supplies.

Bar code **scanners** are available in two types: contact and noncontact.[9] A contact scanner is sometimes referred to as a light pen or wand and must come in contact with the bar code to read its contents. Noncontact scanners can be hand held or fixed. Department store cashiers frequently use hand-held scanning "guns" to read product labels. Fixed scanners, such as grocery store scanners, read labels that are passed over or under them.

Even with all the automated assistance, the ultimate success or failure of an automated record-tracking system still depends on proper training, commitment of all staff to use it consistently, and the system's ease of use.

It is important to understand that, although health information management continues to move closer to the true EHR, record tracking will not become obsolete for many years. Entering all data contained in previous paper records would be an extremely costly project, and therefore these records need to be tracked until they are no longer useful or until the majority of historical information is entered into the EHR.

Application in Use: University of Texas–James W. Aston Ambulatory Care Center

The University of Texas Southwestern Medical Center, at its James W. Aston Ambulatory Care Center in Dallas, saw 550 patients per day during 1992. The medical record department processed 114,000 requests for records that year.[8] Because of the academic setting, the records move throughout all the facilities, and the medical record department estimated that about 50% of the medical records were out of the file at any time. The facility did not have a policy prohibiting removal of records from the facility or a policy on timely return of records.

The center has continued to grow since it was established in 1984, and it became obvious by 1992 to the administrative staff that the manual record-tracking system in place could not keep up with current volume, much less future growth. It was decided that two areas needed attention: firm policies on the return of records to file and proper tracking of files throughout the facility.

A task force of representatives from the medical record, information systems, and administrative departments met to discuss these issues and decided to purchase and implement a software package that was available from the current mainframe computer system vendor. All current mainframe users would have access to the system through their existing terminals, and regular system security would be applied as before, including user names and passwords.

The system that was chosen uses "dictionaries," or data tables, to provide consistency of data. These dictionaries were developed before implementation to standardize requester names, locations, and request reasons for reporting purposes. New requesters, locations, and reasons could be added as future needs developed.

Before implementation, two projects needed to be completed in the medical records department. The first was converting records from the old Social Security numbering system to a new six-digit terminal digit numbering system, with a number being automatically assigned by the accounts receivable system. Only records that had activity in the prior 13 months were converted. All others were converted when patients returned for appointments.

The second major project was the application of the bar code labels used with this system. These labels contained the patient's Social Security number and the new computer-assigned number; these labels were applied to all converted charts.

When the system was implemented, the facility started using the on-line requesting system for records. It also used the reports and statistics produced by the system for management of the department and monitoring of the chart return policy that was implemented. The new system was able to track record volumes and handle multiple home locations of different file rooms for the staff.

Because of the implementation of the system, the medical records job functions and job descriptions changed. Staff were added to the department and service was greatly improved. Record retrieval time averaged 15 minutes, and retrieval percentages were at 99% of all requested records after implementation of the automated record-tracking system.

Application in Use: University of Iowa Hospitals and Clinics

The University of Iowa Hospitals and Clinics is a combined health care system in Iowa City whose medical record department processed more than 600,000 patient record requests in 1989, the year they implemented an automated record-tracking system using bar code technology.[10] The previous tracking method was a standard manual system that used index cards and outguides. The manual system could not keep up with increasing volumes and demands from users. Workload volume increased by 24%, but the size and staffing of the department did not.

A facility-wide committee structure was put in place to investigate the problem, and the committee eventually decided to design its own automated record-tracking system especially for the University of Iowa. The management engineering division helped to collect data about department activities and volumes. The training division assisted in the hands-on training of 600 staff members when the system was ready to be implemented.

The medical record department staff placed bar code labels on each patient record not in storage. Each record that was out of the file had the location indicated in the computer. All records without a location in the computer were assigned to the storage location. The medical records department started using the system first, and all areas of the facility gradually began using the system over a 2-month period.

The bar code labels were printed on sheets by a laser printer and used code 39 symbology. The University of Iowa decided not to put the patient number on the bar code label but rather to preprint other numbers on the label and let the computer "associate" the two numbers in the database.

Any computer terminal in the facility can be used by authorized users to access the system, determine record locations, and update the system on record transfers. The system also displays frame and reel locations for records stored on roll microfilm. The same system security previously in use controls access to the system.

On-line requesting of records is available, with the system alerting the requester if the record is already signed out of the file, either to the requester or to another party. Requesters then notify the other party to make arrangements for retrieving the record. This on-line request system reduced telephone calls by 83% within 2 months after installation. The overall satisfaction rate for record requests went from 82% to 93% in the same 2 months.

The system also produces the basic management reports and statistics expected from an automated system. It has helped to improve significantly the quality of medical record services provided to the staff at the University of Iowa Hospitals and Clinics.

These are excellent examples of how the functions involved in access and retention of records can have a substantial impact on the efficient delivery of health care.

Record Retention

Health information professionals are frequently asked questions about how long to keep patient records. There is no universal answer to the question. Several factors need to be considered.

Federal Statutes and Regulations

The federal government has a number of laws and regulations related to record retention. Depending on the type of organization, the health care facility may be subject to one or more federal laws and regulations. For example, Department of Veterans Affairs hospitals are expected to keep their patient records 75 years from the date of last activity. Hospitals and other types of health care organizations can check federal requirements related to participation in certain programs and the length of time records should be retained to prove that services were provided in case there is a billing or payment review some years after the service is rendered.

State Statutes and Regulations

State law provides the most concrete guidance on retention. The state laws should be referenced individually to obtain the most current information related to retention requirements.

State laws may be specific to the type of organization, such as hospital, boarding home, psychiatric hospital, or behavioral health clinic. In 2002 the American Health Information Management Association (AHIMA) reviewed record retention requirements and recommended categorical time lines as guidance in the absence of a particular law. The document also reviewed federal laws and state laws on retention of records. The **statute of limitations** in each state should be considered specifically when determining a retention policy. The statute of limitations determines the period of time in which a legal action can be brought against an organization for injury, improper care, or breach of contract.[11] In most states the statute of limitations begins at the time of the event or at the age of majority if the patient was treated as a minor.

Organizational Needs

Institutional policy is another source to be considered. Because the organization maintains the record for the benefit of the patient, the physician, and the health care organization, it is the responsibility of the organization to keep the record for the use of all three parties.[12] Organizations usually require that information kept in an MPI be kept permanently. Ideally, key elements of the patient record would be maintained indefinitely. Although this is the best policy, it may not be possible from a financial or space standpoint.

An organization should also consider the rate of patient readmission and the level of commitment to research and education in the final decision on retention. An organization with a high readmission rate will find its own records extremely valuable in the future care of the patient. Longitudinal studies conducted in research facilities are difficult to complete if short retention periods are chosen for patient records.

Different types of medical organizations may have different retention requirements. In some states the record retention for long-term care facilities is 5 years. In other states free-standing ambulatory settings or physician practices may not have record retention regulations or statutes. Therefore, it is incumbent on the health information management (HIM) professional to research existing statutes, regulations, professional practices, and organizational needs to recommend an appropriate course of action.

Retention Schedule

Once a facility makes the decision about which records to keep and for how long, a record retention schedule should be developed and approved by the facility attorney, facility compliance officer, malpractice liability insurance carrier, and board of directors. The schedule should list all medical and business records and should address retention and destruction of both original records and copies of records.[11] For hospital settings, the American Hospital Association recommends retaining records for a minimum of 10 years.[12]

When destruction is determined to be appropriate and no federal or state laws preclude this guidance then, a minimum retention schedule should be as follows:

If the patient was older than the age of majority when treated, 10 years.

If the patient was a minor when treated, 10 years past the age of majority.

If federal or state laws require longer retention periods, then the federal or state laws or regulations should be followed. Records involved in an investigation or in litigation should never be destroyed, even if they are due for destruction according to the retention schedule.[11]

As an additional recommendation, the following information should be retained permanently in some format, even if the remainder of the record is destroyed:

- Dates of admission, discharge, and encounters
- Physician names
- Diagnoses and procedures
- History and physical reports
- Operative and pathology reports
- Discharge summaries[1]

Destruction of records should take place only after approval by the facility administration, facility attorney, malpractice liability insurance carrier, and board of directors. Complete details of all records destroyed must be kept indefinitely. A manifest including all patient record numbers and patient names should be created as the records are purged or removed from the files. The destruction process, either by shredding or by incineration, should take place in the presence of two witnesses who both sign a **destruction letter** that has the complete manifest as a referenced attachment.

The AHIMA issued a practice brief on the subject of health information retention in 2002. It outlines legal and regulatory requirements, accreditation requirements, recommendations, and the applicable state laws or regulations for each of the 50 states and the District of Columbia. This practice brief and others are available on line by visiting the Journal of AHIMA on the AHIMA Web site at *www.ahima.org*.

Facility Closure

Special considerations are necessary regarding record retention when a facility closes, either by sale or by dissolution of a physician practice. The two major considerations are protecting the confidentiality of patient information and ensuring that authorized parties have access to the information as provided by law.[13]

If the facility is sold to another provider of health care services, the records are usually considered an asset of the sale because they provide a considerable marketing advantage to the new owner. If the buyer is not a health care provider, records should not be considered assets of the sale and other arrangements should be made. To ensure that patients are aware of what is happening to their information, a series of notices should be published in local newspapers informing interested parties of the planned date of closure and new location of the records. The facility can then contract with another health care provider, the facility attorney, or a commercial storage company to assume responsibility for the records and provide information to authorized requesters in the future. Other considerations should be evaluated such as scanning or filming of the records. Either of these may be less expensive than a long-term storage solution. As a last option, the state department of health may assume responsibility for the records. In any case, every effort should be made to ensure that all records are complete as of the date of transfer.

AHIMA issued a practice brief on the subject of protecting patient health information after a closure in November 2003. This brief and others on this subject are available on line by visiting the AHIMA Web site at *www.ahima.org.*

The Legal Health Record Definition

Work by a task force of the AHIMA related to defining the legal health record can be found at *www.ahima.org.* A group of HIM professionals continues to discuss this topic and provide guidelines for hospitals in how to create an individualized definition of the legal health record for their facilities. With the recent proliferation of different modes of digital input and output of record text, images, and other forms of documentation, it is difficult to determine what is truly part of the 'legal' record versus which is a byproduct of the patient care process but is not considered part of that legal output. There are practical considerations with today's technology that make it unlikely that a single repository could be created to house all varieties and types of documentation able to be created, so the legal health record is must be defined in each organization.

Once a multidisciplinary team completes a full forms/computer views (paper and electronic) inventory, the subset identified as the legal health record can be confirmed. When records are stored in a paperless format, that subset defined as the legal record can be parsed out or printed on demand to created the episodic version of the health record that will be used for that facility's legal health record document of care. From a management perspective, this allows a "wrapper" to be put around the health record that is both reasonable and manageable.

Disaster Recovery

Disasters can result from fire, broken pipes, blocked drains, malfunctioning equipment, environmental storms, and floods. Water is almost always the culprit, causing paper records to become soaked and possibly contaminated with pollutants, such as sewage.

As with most things, planning ahead can make all the difference in the ability to restore wet medical records to a more usable form. Preparation for **disaster recovery** includes investigating a local or regional restoration specialist. Property insurance carriers are a good source of qualified referrals. In addition, most qualified restoration specialists are members of the Association of Specialists in Cleaning and Restoration, International (ASCR). The ASCR Web site on the Internet *(www.ascr.org)* states that when large quantities of records are water damaged, they should be frozen as soon as possible to prevent mold or mildew from forming and to prevent swelling and rippling of the paper. Smaller volumes of wet records, such as 10 average-sized records or less, can be air dried by separating the pages and exposing to the air. Restoration vendors can freeze the records while other options are being considered.

If the volume of wet records is too great to freeze immediately, changing the environment of the location will help retard mold or mildew development. The heat should be turned off and the air conditioning used to bring the temperature of the room as low as possible under 70° F and to reduce the humidity to below 60%. Fans can be used to help circulate cool, dry air and wet-dry vacuums can be used to remove water trapped in carpet or standing on floors. Wet records can be dried with a vacuum thermal drying process. A vacuum is created inside a special chamber, a source of heat is introduced, and the records are dried at temperatures above 32° F.[14] This method may cause more rippling of dried pages than other methods.

Freezing the records provides two other alternatives for restoration—freezer drying and vacuum freezer drying. In either case, restoration specialists want to know what types of paper are included within the wet records. They need to be especially careful with coated paper, such as the paper used for electrocardiograms and other medical tracings. This paper tends to stick together more than traditional bond paper. Photographs contained within the record should be dried separately by a photograph conservator.

Freezer drying of wet paper removes water by vaporizing the ice crystals without melting them and may take several weeks to several months to complete. Vacuum freeze drying involves the use of specialized equipment. A vacuum is created, a source of heat is introduced, and the records are dried at temperatures below 32° F. The process may take only a few weeks because the vacuum process speeds the overall drying time, just as pressure cooking speeds the overall cooking time for food.

Another method of preparation for a disaster is to minimize the potential for water damage from malfunctioning sprinkler systems or sprinklers that are activated during small fires. Staff should be trained to know where the sprinkler shutoff values are and to turn them off as soon as any danger has passed. An appropriate tool kit should be kept in the area of the fire extinguisher.

If records are maintained in an electronic format, a disaster plan is also necessary. Some of the same issues of protection from the elements are true with the hardware, software, and data storage components of electronic record systems. The advantage in electronic systems is that backups can always be at an off-site or remote location. If a fire or other disaster strikes one location, the other location may not be harmed. Also electronic data storage is often protected in special vaults created for this purpose. Another advantage is that moving the electronically stored data out of harm's way is typically easier because it involves moving a much smaller set of media.

In 2005, some southern states were devastated by hurricane. As a result, AHIMA suggested methods for individuals attempting to recover their health information. This and other related articles can be found on the AHIMA Web site under the category "disaster planning."

COMPUTER TECHNOLOGY IN AUTOMATED DATA ACCESS AND RETENTION

Automated data access and retention rely on information technology—hardware, software, and telecommunications—to collect, store, manage, and transmit health information. The following briefly reviews key concepts in these areas and illustrates their roles in automating the processes of data access and retention.

Hardware

Hardware is the physical equipment that makes up computers and computer systems. It includes the electric, electronic, mechanical, and other equipment. The computer requires a central processing unit with the capacity to hold data being processed and the equipment needed to carry out the data processing functions. Peripheral equipment including magnetic disks and tape drives, data input devices such as terminals, hand-held devices, and PCs, and output devices such as printers and plotters are also hardware. Computers come in mainframe, mini, and micro sizes. **Mainframe** machines are used for major applications, to maintain large databases, and for high-volume work. **Minicomputers** are often used in departmental systems such as laboratory or radiology systems. **Microcomputers** are used in individual applications such as a single-user donor registry and as workstations for larger systems. Hand-held devices or other peripheral devices interface with most hardware on the market today. Most managers use microcomputers in their daily work.

Input, Output, and Storage Devices

Data can be collected automatically from other computer systems or can be entered through a staffed data entry process. Biomedical devices such as automated electrocardiogram systems and patient monitoring systems convert data from one form to another and transmit the data to a database. Terminals, PCs, optical scanning devices, pen-based devices, and other devices are operated by users to capture and enter data into computer systems. Computers can receive input directly from remote computers through communications networks. Collen[15] noted that, with respect to medical information systems, the most important innovation in the 1980s was probably the improved connections among machines into more general, local, national, and worldwide high-speed networks. By using network technology, hospitals could unite all the different computers throughout their various departments, although the computers were located in geographically dispersed locations. This trend continues today with the intricacy of health information system networks mirroring the complex organizational structures that have developed. Table 7-5 defines and describes input and output devices.

Table 7-5 DATA INPUT AND OUTPUT OPTIONS

Keyboards and Terminals (Cathode Ray Tube or Video Display Monitor)
Link monitor screen to the computer and use for data entry and retrieval. Terminals may use a keyboard, a point-and-click device, or a touch screen on which finger touch selection guides the user through the process.

PC Workstations
PCs used for "one-stop" access and retrieval. They perform the same functions as the keyboards and terminals and contain programs that can manipulate the information locally. PC workstations often contain standard software tools such as word processing, spreadsheets, databases, and electronic mail applications.

Hand-Held Computers (Also Called Personal Data Assistants, PDAs)
Devices available for point-of-service input; travels with caregiver; can be wireless. These are also known as pocket devices.

Miniaturized Cathode Ray Tubes
Very small terminals (less than 3 inches across) that can be mounted and made available for users at eye level, freeing users from moving to check data.

Scanners and Wands
Used for quick reading of bar codes or other scannable input documents such as service billing sheet data or patient self-recorded history questionnaires. Some scanners enable the computer to read a printed or handwritten page. See optical scanning.

Continued

Table 7-5   DATA INPUT AND OUTPUT OPTIONS—cont'd

Sensors
Devices used to sense and record changes in temperature, weight, and other findings. Monitoring equipment uses sensors to collect, display, and record data.

Voice Recognition
Computer capability to understand human speech. This allows practitioners to talk directly to devices and record findings. Emergency and radiology departments have applied this technology.

Voice Response
Units that use prerecorded messages or speech synthesizers and are capable of communicating directly to users.

Printers
Used to print reports and copies of screen displays. Printers are valued according to speed, print quality, noise, reliability, and size.

Microfilm/Microfiche (Computer Output Microfilm)
Produced by computers for such uses as MPIs, these retrieve data through special readers. They are a less costly alternative to maintaining data on-line.

Disk Drive/Diskette
Part of the computer that reads software and data files into memory. As an output device, it writes information from the computer to the disk, thereby allowing backup of the complete work.

Optical Disk
A disk that is written and read by a laser beam. CDs, CD-ROMs, and video disks are recorded at the point of manufacture and cannot be rewritten. WORMs are optical disks that are recorded in user locations and cannot be rewritten.

Terminals and Workstations

Data retrieval is most commonly performed from the terminal or workstation. **Terminals** are connected to information systems and are used to enter and retrieve information. A health information system has terminals located at nursing areas for data entry such as ordering patient services and to retrieve information such as laboratory test results. Although terminals are still common in health information systems of all kinds, PCs are a more sophisticated and powerful input device. A workstation is a PC or other device that is connected to an information system. It is used to connect directly with the database in the system and to access and receive information from the system directly. When the information is passed to the workstation, it can be further processed at the workstation level. PCs and other devices house software applications as well. Electronic tools currently available such as local word processing software, spreadsheets, and database tools can be coupled with information provided through the health information system connection. The user may manipulate data on the workstation and send the data through electronic mail to another user in the system. In addition, computer users may access external resources through communications equipment such as the Internet that offer up-to-the-minute references and clinical support tools. The **Internet** is a telecommunications international computer network that serves as the gateway to a multitude of users. The workstation is planned as the ubiquitous doorway for all users (Box 7-7) and is a key concept in the computer-based patient record.[16]

Most health care practitioners today are already influenced by the power and communications options available through computer workstations. The home computer industry has done much to educate the consumer about software and the communications capabilities of computers. Managers work with electronic mail within and beyond their organizations. In small group practice settings, PCs are used to maintain patient records; retrieval is readily available for transcribed notes and for data sent through communications links from hospitals and special care centers that are linked to these settings. Indeed, the computer is becoming as common as the telephone in business environments.

Pen-Based Devices

Pen-based and hand-held computers offer a very specialized approach to the workstation. These are devices that can be carried in the pocket. They have built-in communications and organizer software. The goal is ultimately to replace beepers, mobile phones, personal organizers, facsimile (fax) machines, and laptop computers. In the health care industry, one example of **pen-based devices** is used in home health organizations, where visiting nurses use the pen-based device to record visit encounter data. In another case, a pen-based device is used to document intravenous therapy data for hospitalized patients. In both examples, the devices are used for daily tasks and are plugged into a "dock," or receiving component, that transfers the data into a larger computer system. In the past, these devices were limited in size and display capability and by lack of full recognition of handwriting. In a report published in 1993, the technology was estimated to be able to read the user's handwritten characters about 95% of the time. The capabilities of these devices have improved, and the devices promise to become an effective working tool for capturing patient information for busy practitioners.

Radiofrequency Identification

Radiofrequency identification (RFID) is a process where a tiny microchip is attached to an item (i.e., a medical record patient folder in this case) to assist in the tracking of the object. Similar to a bar code, this tag can be embedded with information that allows a user to know the location of a device. However, it is more reliable than a bar code system because it does not rely on manual intervention (scanning or checking in and out of locations) to update the location. Instead, the RFID chip acts as a sensor in which the various frequency receiving devices can "track" the location of the chart as it travels throughout a facility, providing instantaneous "update" information through a computer network. Chapter 8 on technology, applications, and security provides additional information on technology used in health care.

Document Imaging Devices

One approach to developing an EHR is to use document imaging as a way to capture and store text-based information. Some health care organizations have already initiated this process as a strategic step in moving toward a fully electronic health record. In these organizations, patient record forms are scanned by document imaging as soon as they are sent to the HIM department. When the record has been scanned, all functions needed to process it, such as quality review, coding, data abstraction, and others, can be done through a workstation that provides the capability to retrieve the scanned items. This offers fast processing and retrieval capability available through workstations around the facility, with extensive access for users.

As a data input approach, document imaging builds an effective bridge to the next generation of information processing by familiarizing providers with the general technology and the capability to retrieve needed information electronically in multiple locations. Through workstations, physicians can access records of previous visits in patient care areas. With the technology of **multimedia,** many health care organizations are combining the use of imaging storage systems with digital health information systems to offer initial multimedia features of an increasingly electronic health record. Multimedia processing incorporates data, voice, and video to communicate through a workstation.

Voice Recognition

Voice recognition is considered by many to be a key to automation of the patient record. It offers an efficient means for many practitioners to incorporate data capture into their normal routines. When the health care team works with many patients throughout the day, the methods used to capture the necessary clinical and service information must be easy to use. How do busy practitioners incorporate working with a computer workstation into daily activities in ways that conserve time? For many, the possibility of voice recognition offers the greatest promise. This technology has grown phenomenally over the past 10 years, and it continues to grow. Effective uses were noted in ED, radiology, and surgical pathology applications in the late 1980s; however, speed was generally slow and the vocabulary was limited. These systems require a voice recognition board in the computer and associated software.

Compatibility with existing software, expansion of vocabulary, techniques for establishing computer recognition of the user's voice, and cost are still issues that require work. However, voice recognition systems have improved. In one example, the use and benefits of an automated speech recognition application were explored for nursing documentation in a hospital. The system allowed nurses to create patient documentation by speaking directly to a microphone connected to a PC. There was little or no use of a keyboard. Linked directly to a hospital information system, this application provided immediate retrieval and a hard copy. This hospital acquired three voice systems that contained 10,000-word, speaker-independent vocabularies. (Speaker-independent refers to the ability of the system to recognize words regardless of who speaks.)

Nurses in two target areas, the ED and surgery, were selected as domain experts and worked with the developers to set up a nursing documentation care plan. The user spoke a few "trigger" words into the system to call up much longer phrases that were then entered into the text. For instance, a trigger word allowed the nurse to express complex observations by using several key words or phrases, thereby saving significant nursing documentation time and still capturing patient data efficiently. In this case, just 12 words triggered the system to create a 44-word passage that completely, accurately, and in accordance with standardized guidelines described the nursing assessment for a particular patient.[17] Once continuous voice recognition and extensive vocabularies become available, data capture and retrieval will grow quickly and this technology will offer rapid developments in automating data capture.

Computer-Assisted Coding Tools

Computer-assisted coding tools encompass several different types of technologies available to HIM departments to help automate the coding process in health care facilities. These tools can be as simple as an embedded link between text and codes in a table (more commonly referred to as structured text coding) or as complex as logic-based tools that interpret and translate different syntax combinations into code sets (known as natural language processing). Most commonly used today in simpler documentation settings (e.g., physician clinics, ambulatory care, radiology tests), computer-assisted coding tools have evolved from the use of a pure encoder as a logic or dictionary style assist tool to one that actually can replace portions of coding from having to be done manually (documentation to coder—translator—to coding system/generator) to one in which *electronic* documentation is reviewed solely by the software program and generates a code. This process, without human intervention, is helpful in generating a code that can be verified by a coder. Codes that are closely linked to procedures billed through a chargemaster that is carefully constructed and is kept up to date helps to generate codes for review. (Refer to Chapter 18, Revenue Cycle and Financial Management, for a discussion of the chargemaster.) Computer-assisted coding has great potential in helping to screen and process repetitive and simple documentation for coding and allowing the coding staff to focus more of its time on complex coding. Coding staff can also use preliminary output as a first phase in quality checking and editing of coding output. The use of computer-assisted coding software may help improve the consistency of coding, and the use of this type of software is expected to grow as more of the patient record components are computerized.

Communications

Communications technology has revolutionized both performance and expectations for data access, transmission, and use. As the backbone of health information systems, it was targeted in 1993 as a significant element of health care reform. Health care organizations are currently linked in alliances of all kinds. Health maintenance organizations (HMOs) and primary care networks (PCNs) are two examples. In addition, we have seen how the evolution of health care extends from ambulatory and hospital care to home health, occupational health, hospice, rehabilitation facilities, and long-term care facilities. Information systems are passing data to coordinate patient care, to process claims more efficiently, to facilitate collaborative planning and research, and to control costs. Consumers are expecting their clinical information to be transferred among providers to maintain the flow of health services. Most health information professionals are using communications technology to accomplish daily tasks, both within and beyond their immediate organizational boundaries.

Local Area Networks

Communications technology is used within individual organizations to connect the terminals, workstations, printers, and storage equipment to the computer. Information systems that operate with a mainframe computer use communications technology to form a network of the terminals located in patient care areas with ancillary areas. Communications technology has evolved from the basic terminal to computer connection to local and wide area networks and the **client server technology.**

A **local area network** (LAN) connects multiple devices together through communications and it is located within a small geographic area. An example of a LAN is a medical computing system at a primary care clinic in which seven PCs are connected to a server. The physicians and nurses all access the server for patient files as needed. The basic job of a LAN is to link together physically a few to several hundred PCs and often link them to a mainframe or minicomputer. The mainframe or minicomputer—and even some microcomputers—provides the location for all or some of the data needed by the PC users. Other data and programs needed for processing may be located on each PC locally. Communications technology consists of a variety of materials such as twisted-wire cables, fiberoptics, phone lines, and even infrared light and radio signals.

Typically, a message is sent from one PC to another. This may be a query for data, a response to a request, or an instruction to run a program that may be stored on the network. The action may require data stored locally in the PC or data maintained on the file server. A **file server** is a specialized PC, or larger host computer, that is used only to provide a common place to store all the data that the PC users may need. The configuration of the LAN enables the users to retrieve and use the data as rapidly as possible. The network must receive requests from individual PCs, handle simultaneous requests, and send messages to the appropriate requester. In effect, it must manage traffic. LAN topologies refer to the physical configurations of the networks.

Wide Area Networks

Wide area networks (WANs) are used for extensive, geographically larger environments. They are often used for computer systems connecting separate institutions. They are also used for computer systems in large single institutions. An extensive WAN was installed at the Columbia-Presbyterian Medical Center. Beginning in the late 1980s and supported by a federal grant program, this institution pioneered an extensive network that encompassed 18 buildings at seven geographically separate sites. With the goal of a workstation for "one-stop shopping," this institution combined clinical and research computing facilities with library and PC utilities such as word processing and electronic mail. Columbia-Presbyterian Medical Center has demonstrated the value of implementing this technology as an overall technical strategy in building a comprehensive information system.[18] Today, these installations are commonplace.

Client Server Technology

Client server computing involves the splitting of an application into tasks that are performed on separate computers, one of which is a programmable workstation. Put another way, client server computing is a form of **cooperative processing.** The five types of this technology are distributed presentation, remote presentation, distributed logic, remote data management, and distributed database.[19]

Cooperative processing distributes the processing tasks to different systems for optimal responsiveness. By separating shared data, for instance from the application program, it can provide more efficient computer functions. It seeks to achieve the best performance for low-volume and high-volume processing, optimal network traffic, and realistic security and control. The benefits are improved user experiences because the workstation capability improves through custom presentations and reduction of the traffic on the system network. In cooperative processing, the host computer may perform tasks associated with maintaining the application database, and the microcomputer controls the presentation of the data and the user's interaction with the data.

An example of client server technology occurs when clinical data from transaction systems, such as laboratory and pharmacy systems, are sent to a workstation. Programs housed in the workstation then direct the format of display and data. For instance, customer-designed flow sheet data display formats may differ from one medical discipline to another at the workstation level, yet the information may be retrieved from the same source (server) because the client workstation uses local application logic to retrieve that presentation.

Client server technology must combine and connect technical functions at three levels: the host server (often mainframe systems), the network functions, and the intelligent workstation capability. Simply expressed, large computer applications are in the process of using networks and their associated operating systems to distribute and extend computing operations to workstation customers who are operating diverse machines. In a large customer environment, for instance, the organization may use this approach to connect both PC and Macintosh machines. Implications for this technology are many. For those who process medical information, integrity of data is a major concern. There must be adequate data management tools to ensure the integrity of updates so that every user has reliable, timely data. Chapter 8, Technology, Applications, and Security contains additional discussions about technology and applications.

ACCESS AND RETENTION OF IMAGE-BASED RECORDS

Automated data access and retention can be divided into two main branches—image-based records and electronic records. These two subjects are covered in the remainder of this chapter.

Micrographics

The most traditional and well-known option for image-based record storage is micrographics. Micrographics is the formal name for the process of creating miniature pictures on film, commonly referred to as microfilm. Micrographics was first used commercially by the banking industry in the 1920s as a solution for the growing volume of canceled checks that banks needed to store.[4] The microfilming process has been used for years in health care for storage of patient records, and many facilities routinely microfilm their inactive records after a certain period. Microfilmed images are small negative photographs of the original documents that cannot be read with the unaided human eye. They must be magnified for viewing by specialized reading devices.

Microforms

Facilities have several micrographics options to choose from when planning a storage and retrieval program. The generic word for any micrographics format is a **microform.** Choosing the correct microform for the project requires knowledge of four key facts about the project:

1. The type and amount of information to be microfilmed, including age and current format
2. The frequency at which the material will require updating
3. The amount of access needed for patient care and other uses
4. The budget available for the microfilm conversion project

The various microforms are discussed here in relation to these four key facts.

Roll Microfilm. Roll microfilm is a continuous film strip, similar in appearance to movie film, that holds several thousand document pages, depending on the reduction ratio used when the documents were filmed.[4] The **reduction ratio** indicates the amount by which an image has been reduced in size. A standard ratio for patient records is 24×, or 24 to 1, meaning that the image is $\frac{1}{24}$ the size of the original.[4]

In a patient record environment, several patient records are normally stored on a roll of film. Patient records must be complete when filmed because roll microfilm cannot be updated. Documents must also be in a consistent order when filmed to make future retrieval possible. Roll microfilm is similar in concept to the serial numbering and filing method. Multiple records on the same patient can be found on various rolls of film if the patient returns several times over the years. Bringing these records together for current patient care purposes is difficult unless paper copies are made and used for reference. Therefore, roll microfilm is usually a choice only for extremely old records, records of deceased patients that will never need updating, or as an archival copy of records maintained in microfilm jackets. It also works well with the serial filing method.

Jacket Microfilm. Roll film can be converted to different packaging to provide the ability to update it. This can be done by cutting the film and placing it into microfilm jackets. **Microfilm jackets** are 4 × 6–inch holders that have channels, or narrow sleeves, formed by fusing together two panels of transparent material. A strip of roll microfilm can be inserted into a channel. Each jacket can hold about 70 document pages, depending on the reduction ratio used when the documents were filmed.

When microfilm jackets are used for patient record storage, each of the jackets is a patient record, maintaining the unit record concept. Records of subsequent admissions or encounters can be added to the channels as they become inactive and are filmed. The jackets are labeled, or indexed, with the patient name and identification number and normally filed by the same method used for the original paper-based records in the facility. Jackets can be purchased with differently colored strips on the top edge to provide the same color-coding scheme used in the active files.

Microfiche. Microfiche is a copy of a microfilm jacket made on a special 4 × 6–sheet of polyester film (Mylar). Copies of microfilm are useful because many facilities do not remove the microfilm jacket from the file for routine use. Instead, they make microfiche copies to circulate for patient care and provider use, protecting the original from loss or damage. These microfiche copies can be destroyed when they are no longer needed. Microfiche can also be used as the primary source document in the facility if the original microfilm jackets are stored away from the facility for safekeeping.

Microfiche copies can be added to a paper record folder in a pocket to keep the unit record intact if the patient returns to the facility. These copies can also be added to active record folders for patients whose active record is too large or cumbersome to deal with in a paper format in the active file. This means that facilities with patients who return consistently and frequently can film older portions of the record and file microfiche copies in the paper folder to use less space in the active files. This can be done without changing the retention schedule of the active file.

Microfiche can also be filmed directly from the source document. This eliminates the need to cut the roll film and insert it into jackets. Indexing of the jackets is also eliminated because the indexing is created by the camera when the images are filmed. Microfiche can be filmed at 24×, 42×, or 48×. Using a larger reduction ratio can save considerable money over the jacket method, which contains 70 images per jacket filmed at 24×.

Computer-Assisted Retrieval—Roll Microfilm. Microfilm needs to be created differently to be used in a computer-assisted retrieval (CAR) system. When the microfilm is created, the images are numbered. In the simplest form, the images are cataloged by patient name, patient identification number, roll number, and frame number. These roll and frame numbers are entered into the MPI or another database specially designed for this purpose. In a more advanced form, the database can contain more data than may be required by a particular application. In any CAR system, when a particular patient's records are requested, the roll and frame numbers are retrieved from the index and the roll is located. The roll is searched until the appropriate frames are found.[4] Some reader-printers automatically locate the frame number desired if it is entered on a keypad by counting the images that pass an internal scanner.

Computer-Assisted Retrieval—Jacket Microfilm. The same concepts can be applied to jacket film in a CAR jacket system. Sequentially numbered film frames are loaded into sequentially numbered jackets. The MPI or other database records the jacket and frame numbers of each patient's film. The needed jackets are retrieved as the patient's record is requested.

Table 7-6 shows micrographics options frequently chosen in health care. Table 7-7 shows the advantages and disadvantages of these options.

Computer Output Microfiche. Another micrographics option used in health care is **computer output microfiche**

Table 7-6 MICROGRAPHICS OPTIONS IN HEALTH CARE

Roll Microfilm	CAR–Roll Microfilm	Microfilm Jackets	CAR–Jacket Microfilm
Description: Continuous film containing about 2400 images Multiple patients can be found per roll. It can be used well with extremely old records or records of deceased patients.	*Description:* Continuous film containing prenumbered images Database references the patient by roll and frame number. Multiple patients can be found per roll. It eliminates the disadvantage of roll film's inability to be updated.	*Description:* 4 × 6-inch holders containing up to 70 images cut from continuous roll film Film is held in channels. Not all channels may be used if the record has few pages. There is a single patient per jacket. It can be used well in facilities with a high patient return rate or when a unit is vital to patient care.	*Description:* 4 × 6–inch holders containing about 70 images cut from continuous roll film Film is held in channels. All channels are completely filed with prenumbered images. Database is used to reference the patient by jacket and frame number.

Table 7-7 ADVANTAGES AND DISADVANTAGES OF MICROGRAPHICS OPTIONS

Factor	Roll Microfilm	CAR–Roll Microfilm	Microfilm Jackets	CAR–Jacket Microfilm
Cost	Least expensive method	More expensive than roll film because of database of roll and frame number	Most expensive method because of indexing and loading of jackets	May be as expensive as microfilm jackets because of jacket loading and database of jacket and frame number
Security	Images cannot be misfiled on the roll, but entire rolls may be misfiled or lost.	Image cannot be misfiled on the roll, but entire rolls may be misfiled or lost.	Jackets can be color coded and filed in a miniature version of the paper system.	Jackets can be misfiled because they are numbered sequentially and usually are not color coded.
Unit record	Difficult to create without converting to paper. Difficult to perform longitudinal studies.	Difficult to create without converting to paper; easier to create than with regular roll film.	Automatically created. Easy to perform longitudinal studies. Microfilm or a copy can be placed in a new paper folder for later use.	Difficult to create without converting to paper. Difficult to perform longitudinal studies.
Access	Film cannot be used for court or patient care without converting to paper because of multiple patients on roll.	Film cannot be used for court or patient care without converting to paper because of multiple patients on film.	Copies of film can be taken to court or given to patient care areas because there is only one patient on film.	Film cannot be used for court or patient care without converting to paper because of multiple patients on film.
Ability to update	Cannot be updated as a unit; record must be complete when filmed.	Cannot be updated as a unit but database directs the user to additional records on a different roll.	Additional records updated into space available in an open channel or additional jackets used.	Cannot be updated as a unit but database directs the user to additional records on a different jacket.
Ability to partial film	Cannot film an older portion of an active record.	Can film an older portion of an active record, but it must be converted to paper for use.	Can film an older portion of an active record and place the microfilm or a copy in the paper folder.	Can film an older portion of an active record, but it must be converted to paper for use.

(COM). COM allows large amounts of electronically stored data to be placed on microfilm quickly. In COM, the computer displays data on a special screen connected to a microfilm camera called a recorder. The recorder films the screen, reduces the image in size, and places the image directly onto a Mylar microfiche sheet. As more screens are filmed, they are added to the microfiche until it is full, usually 240 images at 48×. This process continues until the entire computer file has been copied to film.[4]

This technology is applicable to the filming of indexes, such as the MPI and the diagnostic index. Microfiche copies can then be used as a backup source for locating patient numbers or data if the computer is unavailable. This process can be accomplished 20 times faster than the creation of a computer printout and eliminates the steps of filming the printout, developing the film, and loading the microfilm jacket. Considerable savings can be realized by using this completely automated process.

Other micrographics options that are available but seldom, if ever, used in health care are aperture cards, roll cartridges, and roll cassettes. Aperture cards are used mainly to hold film copies of large documents, such as architectural drawings or radiological images. Roll cartridges and cassettes are other ways to package roll film to protect the film surface. Roll film in this format still cannot be updated. Cartridges or cassettes may be used in file systems where files are frequently referenced.

Equipment

Storage Equipment. Jackets are commonly stored in filing cabinets with shallow but sturdy drawers specifically made for microfilm. A 10-drawer microfilm cabinet is especially efficient for creating a miniature terminal digit file with microfilm. The cabinet drawers should be managed by use of the same tools discussed in connection with paper-based records, such as file guides for determining file location, outguides to mark the place of removed film, and requisition slips if original film is removed from the files.

Reproduction Equipment. Microfilm images must be read by use of a **microfilm reader.** A reader, also called a viewer, is a projection box that magnifies the image, passes light through it, and displays it on a screen. Readers can be combined with the reproduction capabilities of a copy machine to form a reader-printer combination. This allows the displayed image to be copied onto paper for use again as a paper record. It is best to have readers and reader-printers that display a full-page image, making viewing easier. Smaller viewers can be used when a large space is unavailable, but staff may find them more difficult to use.

Readers and reader-printers are constructed to accommodate one format of microform, although they can be purchased with combination adapters to allow them to view both roll and jacket film. This saves a considerable amount of space and money. The magnification ratio of the reader or reader-printer must be matched to the reduction ratio used when the film was created. The **magnification ratio** is the inverse of the reduction ratio.

Some reader and reader-printers were capable of projecting an image on a screen much like that of projection equipment. This application was useful in teaching hospitals where micro imagery systems are used.

Duplication Equipment. A duplicator for microfilm creates a copy of the film with as much clarity for use as the original film. Entire rolls can be duplicated, or jackets can be duplicated as microfiche. Duplication of film can be done for many reasons. Facilities may choose to use duplicated copies to circulate instead of the originals, or copies may be made to satisfy multiple requests received for the same record at the same time. Duplicates of microfilm jackets (Diazo) can also be sent to another facility that uses the same micrographics format when a request for the record is received.

Legal Considerations

It is important to realize that microfilm is legal in the United States. Federal legislation was passed in 1951, in the form of Public Law 129, that allows microfilm as primary evidence in court. If necessary, the facility must be able to prove that the original record was destroyed by producing the destruction letter and manifest for the court. Public Law 129 supersedes any state law to the contrary.

Cost Analysis

Storing paper records in a storage room or with a commercial storage company seems like an economical alternative to having crowded active files. The reality is, however, that converting the records to another medium may have a **payback period** (the time in which a project saves enough money to pay for itself) that is less than suspected. In the past 5 years newer technology has grown in popularity and high-volume film scanners are available for use by service organizations performing the conversion. As one might expect, this is advantageous because the facility does not have to keep reader/printer equipment for the life of the record retention policy. Furthermore, older archives can be kept electronically. The disadvantage to this is that electronic images will consume space on a server. However, as technology advances and hardware becomes cheaper, space consummation may not be an issue.

Table 7-8 shows a sample cost analysis for a paper-based system and a microfilm jacket system over the same 10-year period. After the initial investment year, the microfilm system expenses remain constant throughout the next 9 years. The paper-based system begins to have modest increases in retrieval costs and has tremendous increases in storage space and shelving costs for the 10-year period. The microfilm system actually pays for itself somewhere in the middle of the sixth year. The system pays for itself even faster if the storage space is at the facility and can be converted into revenue-producing patient care space.

When converting paper-based records to microfilm, an initial decision must be made about which portions of the record will be filmed. The easiest choice is to film the entire contents of the record. However, for purposes of economy, the record may be purged of certain items not important to continuing patient care. Examples of unnecessary items are belongings lists and detailed data that are summarized elsewhere in the record. Also, photocopies of records received from other facilities, such as documents from previous hospitalizations, need not be filmed. These records are retained by the originator of the documents.

During this initial decision-making phase, test films should be created to determine the best method for filming "difficult" documents, such as documents on colored paper and documents whose resolution is vital, such as electrocardiograms. When the extent of the project has been identified and exact methods to be used are determined, the remaining decision is how the work will be performed, either in house or by a contracted microfilm service bureau.

In-House Microfilm Processing. Even with the technology advances in imaging equipment during the last decade, it is still important to recognize that all technological options available. Microfilming records at the facility requires a large investment in equipment as well as a new body of knowledge and a new set of skills related to the use and maintenance of the equipment. A description of the equipment needed and an overview of the process are included here to provide the background information necessary in deciding whether to complete the work in house or to write an outside contract.

The pieces of equipment used in the process are a camera, a film developer, and, for a jacket system, a typewriter and a jacket loader, or inserter. An in-house microfilm program requires at least one microfilm camera of a type best suited for the records to be filmed. Microfilm cameras are large pieces of photographic equipment that can reduce the size of the photograph as the image is recorded. These cameras require periodic maintenance, usually under a maintenance contract with a qualified service vendor.

Table 7-8   SAMPLE COST ANALYSIS*

Year	Paper-Based System					Microfilm Image-Based System					
	No. of Records to Store	Retrieval Costs	Storage/Shelving Costs	Yearly Costs	Cumulative Costs	Records to Film	Film Costs	Equipment	Upkeep Costs	Yearly Cost	Cumulative Cost
1	70,000	$9,450	$11,880	$21,330	$21,330	70,000	$50,974	$7,000	$2,100	$60,074	$60,074
2	83,000	$9,750	$8,880	$18,630	$39,960	13,000	$10,241	$1,300	$2,100	$13,641	$73,715
3	96,000	$10,050	$9,800	$19,850	$59,810	13,000	$10,241	$1,000	$2,100	$13,341	$87,056
4	109,000	$10,350	$10,800	$21,150	$80,960	13,000	$10,241		$2,200	$12,441	$99,497
5	122,000	$10,650	$11,880	$22,530	$103,490	13,000	$10,241		$2,300	$12,541	$112,038
6	135,000	$10,950	$12,880	$23,830	$127,320	13,000	$10,241		$2,400	$12,641	$124,679
7	148,000	$11,250	$13,880	$25,130	$152,450	13,000	$10,241		$2,500	$12,741	$137,420
8	161,000	$11,550	$14,880	$26,430	$178,880	13,000	$10,241	$1,000	$2,600	$13,841	$151,261
9	174,000	$11,850	$15,880	$27,730	$206,610	13,000	$10,241		$2,700	$12,941	$164,202
10	187,000	$12,150	$16,880	$29,030	$235,640	13,000	$10,241		$2,800	$13,041	$177,243
Total					$235,640						$177,243

*Assumes no inflation.

The three types of cameras are rotary, planetary, and step-and-repeat. The rotary camera is the least expensive to use to produce microfilm images. It produces a lower-quality image because the paper source document moves rapidly past the camera lens as the photograph is being taken. This camera is appropriate for standard-sized documents and can also be used for continuous documents, such as monitor strips and electrocardiograms. It is not appropriate for irregular-sized documents or shingled copies, in which one sheet has multiple other sheets taped or stapled to it.

The planetary camera is more expensive to use in creating microfilm images because each paper document must be individually placed on the glass plate for the photography process. This camera is used when high-quality images are required, when fragile documents are being filmed, or when documents require special positioning for filming. Either camera can be equipped with an automatic eye to sense color and density changes on the paper source document.

A step-and-repeat camera is used only for creating microfiche. It films directly onto 4 × 6–inch Mylar sheets of film.

No matter which camera is used for the process, documents must be prepared ahead of time to speed the filming process. The steps included in the preparatory process are as follow:

1. Create an eye-readable target sheet, printed in large print, for the record. It contains the patient's name and identification number and is used as the first image to identify the record that is to follow. Additional targets can be made to identify individual admissions or encounters.
2. Remove staples and fasteners from all sheets of the record.
3. Verify all sheets for correct name, correct location in the record, and eligibility for filming within the retention schedule.
4. Repair any damaged sheets.
5. Unmount any sheets mounted with tape to another sheet.
6. Make an entry for the record on a microfilm control log. The control log follows the record through the filming process and eventually becomes the manifest attached to the destruction letter to verify that the record was filmed and then destroyed.

Once the pictures have been captured on the film, the film must be developed. Some in-house operations choose to send the film elsewhere for developing rather than buy a developing machine and the chemicals required for the process. The roll film is usually checked for image clarity by the developer.

Developed film can remain as a roll if the micrographics program uses that format. If jackets have been chosen, a supply of jackets, a typewriter, and a jacket loader (or inserter) are required. Jackets are indexed on the top strip with the identifying information, including a volume number, by use of the typewriter. Rather than indicating volume 1 of 3, jackets 1 and 2 would be coded with 1+ and 2+, respectively. Jacket 3 would be coded with only a 3, indicating that it is the last jacket in the series. If other images are added later and jacket 4 is required, a plus sign (+) would be added to jacket 3's code.

Jackets are loaded by using an inserter to cut the roll film to the appropriate length and feed it into the jacket channels. Loaded jackets should be checked to ensure that images are clear, straight, and loaded correctly, with the contents matching the indexing.

Contracted Microfilm Service Bureaus. Because most facilities do not have the volume necessary to support the purchase of a camera, a developer, and a jacket loader, they engage the services of a microfilm vendor, or service bureau. The service bureau performs microfilm conversions for multiple customers in large volume and can justify the cost of the many pieces of equipment needed for the process.

Microfilm service bureaus price their services by the cost per 1000 images, based on the specific service requirements that the customer outlines. Requesting certain procedures or methods may increase the price. It is wise to ask the vendor what the least expensive method would be in comparison with the method designed by the facility. Most vendors who routinely convert patient records to microfilm have a "standard" method that they are equipped to offer at an economical price. Choosing the standard plan may reduce the cost significantly.

Table 7-9 shows a sample evaluation matrix used to determine the best vendor for a conversion to a jacket microfilm system for 70,000 records with 1,200,000 images. An estimated 15% of the 70,000 patients would have records that have more than 70 images, requiring a second jacket. The total number of jackets projected for this system is 80,000. The prices range from $25.81 to $31.03 per 1000 images of completed microfilm, excluding the jacket cost. As Table 7-9 shows, price was not the only factor considered in determining the vendor. The evaluation matrix was used to rate all the important factors.

This evaluation matrix can be applied to any situation in which a decision needs to be made between two or more alternative systems, vendors, or methods as candidates. The steps in building an evaluation matrix are as follows:

1. Determine the items most important to the success of the project. Use these items as evaluation criteria.
2. Weigh each criterion on a scale of 1 to 5 regarding how crucial it is to the overall success of the project.
3. Place the name of each candidate at the top of a column. Assign a rating to each candidate for each criterion, using a scale of 1 to 5, with excellent being rated 5 and poor being rated 1.
4. Multiply the weight by the rating score to determine the results.
5. Total the scores for each candidate to select the best possible choice.

A matrix similar to the one in Table 7-9 helps to show how the decision was made. It also provides a large amount of information for makers of a final decision regarding which items were evaluated and the results of the evaluation.

Table 7-9 SAMPLE EVALUATION MATRIX-CONTRACT MICROFILM SERVICES

Criteria and Weight		Vendor # 1			Vendor #2			Vendor #3		
		Rating	Results		Rating	Results		Rating	Results	
Cost/1000 images	5	Excellent ($25.81) ($30,974)	5	25	Very good ($29.75) ($35,700)	4	20	Good ($31.03) ($37,236)	3	15
Cost/4 × 6-inch jacket	5	Excellent ($0.25) ($20,000)	5	25	Excellent ($0.25) ($20,000)	5	25	Excellent ($0.25) ($20,000)	5	25
Control sheet production	4	Excellent (done by vendor at no charge)	5	20	Good (facility not required to do but not done by vendor)	3	12	Fair (facility required to do)	2	8
Record pull	4	Excellent (done by vendor at no charge)	5	20	Excellent (done by vendor at no charge)	5	20	Fair (facility must do)	2	8
Jacket color selection	3	Excellent (all colors matched)	5	15	Fair (off by two colors)	2	6	Excellent (all colors matched)	5	15
Storage after filming	2	Excellent (6 months)	5	10	Excellent (6 months)	5	10	Good (2 months)	3	6
Emergency returns	2	Excellent (1 hour at no charge)	5	10	Very good (fax at no charge)	4	8	Very good (2 hours at no charge)	4	8
Payment schedule control	2	Excellent (requests honored)	5	10	Good (100 working days	3	6	Good (vendor preference)	3	6
Total				135			107			91

5, excellent; 4, very good; 3, good; 2, fair; 1, poor.

With the top candidate identified, the contracting process can proceed. Each evaluation criterion should be detailed in the contract to ensure that the expected results are agreed on. Other items to include in the contract are confidentiality provisions; quality expectations, including retakes at no charge; and the details of the destruction schedule and process.

Many vendors include an addendum to the contract that details how roll film will be labeled or how jackets will be indexed, as well as any special image requirements determined during the test phase. All aspects of the conversion should be detailed in the contract to avoid future disagreements between the facility and the vendor.

Although microfilm may seem to be an older technology, it is still frequently used to solve many storage and retrieval problems that do not require more advanced technology as a solution. Facilities that have an active and stable population, such as HMOs, may not have large volumes of inactive records. They do have large active files that cause active storage requirements to grow continually. Microfilm

provides a solution to the active storage space problem through the use of microfilm jackets. Older portions of active records are filmed by a contracted microfilm service bureau and placed in jackets. These jackets are labeled with the patient names and identification numbers and can be color coded with the same method used for the paper record. The jacket or jackets are placed inside the paper folder and are available for use by the patient care staff if they are needed.

Using microfilm in this manner does not require the purchase of storage cabinets or a microfilm duplicator. It requires the purchase of readers to be conveniently located in the patient care areas and at least one reader-printer for creating paper copies. This method converts inactive paper stored on the active shelf into microfilm, creating new and available space while maintaining a unit record system usable for patient care. It also provides a method for the facility to try a micrographics program on a limited scale without a major purchase of equipment.

A newer technology that is growing in popularity is high-volume film scanners. This allows the vendor to convert large groups of rolls or jackets to electronic images. This is advantageous because it is not necessary to keep reader/printer equipment for the life of the retention policy. As previously mentioned, the disadvantage to this application is the amount of server space needed to store these images. However, as server space continues to become cheaper, the long-term advantages could outweigh this.

Application in Use: Kurten Medical Group in Racine, Wisconsin

When the newly hired Director of Information Services and the Health Information Supervisor at Kurten Medical Group, both health information professionals, surveyed the active and inactive files, they found some disturbing situations. The facility had no overall storage and retrieval plan in place for the future and had not documented past practices.

The 114,000 active records were stored in 11 motorized revolving file units that were more than 10 years old. They required frequent servicing, sometimes weekly, from a company 30 miles away. The maintenance agreements on some of these units were not being offered for renewal in the coming year. The 19,000 filing inches in these motorized units were overcrowded and difficult for the growing staff (then 14) to access. These active records were in color-coded folders, with a 10-color system, and filed according to the terminal digit method. The only problem with the folder was a typed label that was hard to read. Because of inadequate file space, the records were purged to inactive storage after 13 months of inactivity.

There were 81,000 inactive records from 1979 to 1988, which were kept in a large storage room about 100 feet from the main health information department. These records had numbers, but many had been indexed manually and the manual index was no longer available. The records had not been entered into the facility's first computer in 1982. Therefore, all inactive records had been filed alphabetically since the late 1970s. An additional 5000 records from the early 1970s had been microfilmed and placed in microfilm jackets, all with a red stripe. These jackets were also filed alphabetically for the same reason. A group of inactive records from 1975 to 1978 were destroyed. Later requests for information from these records prompted multiple patient complaints.

All inactive records, both paper and microfilm, were labeled with the patient's name, date of birth, and record number. No numbers had ever been duplicated, and new patients were still receiving unit numbers from the same continuous number series, approaching 25-00-00 at that time.

Kurten Medical Group had recently purchased a new mainframe computer and software for on-line requesting of records, automated record tracking, and bar code label production. This health information software module was ready for installation when the department could accommodate it. The facility had been using the manual outguide and requisition method up to that time. All the past practice information was obtained by interviewing long-term employees, by investigation, and from calculations done by the director and supervisor because no storage and retrieval plan could be found.

The health information professionals began working on a storage and retrieval plan to improve the information system and allow implementation of the automated record-tracking system that was available. Their plan involved replacing the motorized units with open-shelf files, microfilming the inactive records into a jacket format, and applying the bar code labels to all active records.

Later the same year, administrative approval was obtained and a microfilm service bureau with sufficient storage space to accommodate 81,000 records was located. The service contract was written for a color-coded jacket system. Jackets were chosen because of the previous 5000 records filmed by the jacket method and the need to place the jacket microfilm in a new paper folder if the patient returned to the clinic. In addition, the jacket method allowed filming of older portions of large active records and therefore allowed control of the space used in the active files. The records in the storage room were emptied into boxes and picked up by the service bureau, and the microfilm conversion process started immediately.

The next weekend, as many of 114,000 active records as possible were moved from the motorized files into the temporary health information department setup in the storage room down the hall. This storage room was the department's home for the next 2 weeks. The remainder of the records were stored in the employee lounge and other areas not involved in patient care on large, rented, four-tier carts. A moving company was secured to disassemble the motorized revolving files and remove the used parts. The motorized units were not replaced because of the increased size of the active files and the number of file workers who needed access to the records simultaneously. In addition, no funds were available to replace all 11 units. Instead, additional filing inches were gained by reconfiguring the same space by using open-shelf filing at far less cost. The overall filing space was increased to 21,024 inches.

The removal of the motorized units, replacement of worn flooring, upgrading of the lighting, and painting of the walls took 7 week days. The new open-shelf filing units were installed on the eighth and ninth week days. On the weekend, the records were returned to their new file shelves, leaving the storage room available for other use. The 30-physician clinic continued to operate at full capacity during the conversion, and patient care was not compromised.

Next, the 10-drawer microfilm cabinet arrived for the miniature, color-coded terminal digit system, along with the reader-printer and the readers. Microfilm started arriving shortly after that. During available time periods, the reception staff checked returning film and old film for the presence of a computer record on the patient. If none was found, the patient's name, date of birth, and record number were entered as a minimal database entry, along with a record-tracking location of "microfilm" in the new automated record-tracking software. If the jacket color was wrong (all old jackets were red), new jackets were retyped and reloaded into the correct color drawer. Finally, the film was all filed in terminal digit order in the microfilm cabinet.

During the same time, the health information professional team was building requester location and reason files in the record-tracking software and were training all facility staff in the use of the automated record-tracking system. The health information department staff was applying bar code labels, which contained the patient's name, date of birth, and record number in large print, to the front of all active records. When the label application was complete, all records out of file were recorded to their requester location and all others kept the default location of "In File."

Less than 6 months from the implementation of the plan, Kurten Medical Group's health information department was using its new storage and retrieval system, with decreased costs, adequate space, and increased morale.

Application in Use: New York Hospital–Cornell Medical Center in New York City

Fetal heart monitor strips are an unusual size and pose a unique storage problem. New York Hospital–Cornell Medical Center used microfilm jackets to store their fetal heart monitor strips as part of the patient record in a smaller, more convenient form. Each microfilm jacket holds 7.64 hours of fetal monitoring records filmed with a 20× reduction ratio.[20]

The monitor strips are filmed on a special continuous-feed camera, similar to a rotary camera. The film is then cut and loaded into microfilm jackets. These jackets can be stored with the paper record throughout its active shelf life and then form the first microfilm jacket if the record is converted to jacket film later.

This facility also used microfilm for storing prescription records, requiring permanent storage. This technology is also applicable to continuous electrocardiographic tracings from stress test machines, electroencephalogram tracings, and polysomnography tracings.

Electronic Document Management

Paper volumes have continued to increase with the use of computerized point-of-care documentation software, automated laboratory, and other ancillary documentation systems. In addition, managed care, the shift to outpatient encounters, and the lowered length of stay have generated a need for portability of health care records and immediate access to information. Therefore, one of the fastest-growing areas of technology in the market of health information is EDM. This is the method of digitizing paper-based and electronic documentation onto secure electronic (typically magnetic) storage. To describe the technology, the definition of an EDM system, components of an EDM system, methods of data entry and conversions, and implementation strategies are discussed in this section.

Electronic Health Records and Electronic Document Management

As the concepts surrounding EHRs are being defined, EHRs and EDM systems are often confused because many facilities attempt to automate patient records by digitizing components of the record into electronic data before they actually capture the images of the patient record electronically. In actuality, an EDM system is one type of electronic health record; it provides a method for capturing document images in an archival manner and provides for enhancements to workflow processing and record access. In the EHR model, data become part of an electronic repository of data, which assists practitioners in determining trends in information such as laboratory results and in manipulating the data into various formats. However, an EHR repository alone does not have the ability to capture handwritten or externally received documents. Most facilities have 40% to 70% of records captured electronically, with the remainder handwritten (e.g, consent forms). Although these numbers are changing as providers of care become more automated with computerized physician order entry (CPOE) and other EHR tools, paper is still used for a number of the handwritten forms included in a patient record. Therefore many EHR systems combine electronic data and images. EHR systems and their components, development, and selection are also discussed in Chapter 5 and Chapter 9.

System Components

Scanner. A scanner converts the images on paper into digital images. Dot patterns, called bitmaps, are created in the same pattern as the dots in the paper image, much as in today's fax technology. The scanner itself looks like a copier, with an automatic document feeder, a flatbed, or both. Scanner quality is rated in pixels per inch (PPI): the higher the PPI, the higher the resolution and the clearer the document. Most scanners read in only paper-based images, but some special scanners can read in microfilm images.[21]

Certain **multifunctional devices** (MFDs) are able to serve as any combination of scanner, photocopier, fax, or printer output device. A **picture archiving and communication system** (PACS) provides rapid access to digitized film images such as for radiology applications and it can help eliminate the cost of film processing and storage. Currently, because of the pixel quality required and storage size limitation, few systems archive film, voice, or video images with other paper documents. Many scanners can accommodate double-sided scanning and can adjust to colored and variously sized source documents. Some have the ability to scan color images and photographs from the document to the screen. The PC attached to the scanner is used not only for indexing but also for quality review of the image database.

The health information professional should be aware of the speed at which a scanner can scan documents into the system. Scanner speed is rated in pages per minute (PPM), with 90 to 140 PPM signifying a faster rating. When considering a scanner purchase, actual speed should be determined by using sample forms from the current files. The speed of the scanner determines, in large part, the labor involved in placing documents in the system because work can proceed only as fast as the scanner can go. In some cases, scanning may be done concurrently at the time and site where the document is being produced (e.g., a nursing unit). At other times, it may make more sense to scan the document at the end of care in a centralized location. The scanner should be equipped with an image enhancement feature that adjusts the density and contrast of an image automatically. This eliminates the need to stop the scanner to adjust these settings manually. The scanner is usually attached to a PC, where the images can be viewed as they are being scanned.

In the scanning process, the person who operates the scanner is also responsible for indexing the images. The index is in a database format and allows the documents in the imaging system to be retrieved easily. The information can be indexed by patient name, medical record number, or other identifying information. With multiple cross-indexes, the chance of a document being lost in the computer system is rare. Determining which fields to index the individual records by is the most important part of planning an optical imaging installation. For example, portions of the record may be indexed separately, such as the discharge summary and operative report. Some facilities regularly index the physician number, diagnosis codes, and procedure codes associated with the encounter. This indexing step can be valuable if there is a need to locate a particular report quickly without having to search through the entire record database. The disadvantage of complex indexing is the time consumed in completing the process. Some companies provide Web-based services that place scanned documents directly into an active archive system, which is then managed remotely.

Optical Character Recognition. Optical character recognition (OCR) is an automated option that helps decrease the cost of indexing by speeding up the entry process. This indexing method recognizes alphabetical or numerical characters and their position and creates the index from these codes. Documents must be redesigned into standard formats that are readable by the equipment if this indexing method is to be effective. Accuracy rates can vary, especially if characters are hand entered (as in scores on a patient questionnaire), and more intensive quality checks after scanning may be necessary.

Bar Code Readers. Bar codes can be used in a variety of ways in imaging systems to automate indexing of documents and files. Patient demographics (e.g., name, account number, date of birth) can be placed on a label or laser-printed form or folder to identify the case. Individual pages of the record may have a bar code imprint that identifies the form type or number. This number can be programmed to correlate with a specific section of the imaged file so that presorting or manual indexing is not necessary. Each page may be date stamped or have the imprint of patient identification on it so that individual loose or late reports may be easily entered into the system after scanning. An example of this would be physician orders.

Bar code devices, such as wands attached to PCs by a wedge reader, and gun-style scanners serve the same purpose. Wands are generally less expensive and take up less space but tend to read the bar code unidirectionally and with less accuracy than a gun-style scanner. Wands also require human intervention (holding the pen), whereas the gun-style scanner can be used as a stand-alone platform.

Keyboard. With each PC used for scanning or review, a mouse and keyboard mode of entry for basic index or inquiry information is useful. Menu-driven table and field entry on the computer screens is available with purchased optical imaging software, with differences in the application usually vendor specific. Flexible flows, expandable fields, and unlimited index choices are marks of excellence in application for an imaging solution.

File Server. The file server takes requests for images stored in the system, prioritizes them, and, subsequently, sends the images to the requester. A minicomputer or a mainframe computer may be used as the file server. The file server acts as the data storage component of the system and literally "serves" the other components of the system, providing them with the data that are needed when requested. An important consideration in selecting a powerful enough file server is what other applications may need to reside on the file server. In some situations, for maximum efficiency, dedicated image servers may be recommended.

Magnetic Disk. Information may be stored on a magnetic disk until it is copied onto a permanent EDM. This allows rescanning of images that are of poor quality or otherwise incorrect before the images become permanent. The magnetic disk can also accept data from other facility systems by **electronic data interchange** (EDI). EDI is a computer-to-computer exchange of information based on communication standards approved by the American National Standards Institute (ANSI). These standards allow information to be exchanged between electronic media such as magnetic disks, tapes, and computer networks. The goal of EDI is paperless trading of information in a readily understandable format. The receiving system does not have to translate any information if it has been transmitted using an ANSI standard format. HL7 (Health Level Seven) messaging standards are recommended as a nonproprietary solution for any data interface or integration of the imaging system into other health care computer systems.

EDI enables other industries to become automated, as in the banking industry's widespread use of automated teller machines. EDI makes these transactions possible. The same process allows transcribed documents from a word processing system or results from laboratory equipment to be automatically entered into the imaging system, either in place of a paper copy or in addition to it. The automatic transfer of data to EDM is similar in theory to COM, in which computerized data are transformed into image-based data for use or storage. This technology, called **computer output to laser disk** (COLD), is an important part of automating document images and index functions without the degree of manual labor required in scanning.

Optical Disk Platters. An optical disk resembles a compact disk used for computer programs or music. The image can be burned into the disk's surface with a laser beam and is read with use of a laser. The surface of the optical disk can store a large amount of information. The laser technology uses light to record data in a more tightly packed form than that used by the magnetic read/write heads of a conventional drive.

One type of laser technology is called **write once read many** (WORM) because it stores the data in a permanent capacity and does not allow the user to alter the document. The document is written once and can be read as many times as necessary from the disk. WORM technology is preferred for health information storage because data cannot be misfiled, accidentally erased, or altered.

The disks are available in different sizes and are capable of holding varying amounts of data. These disks hold thousands of record images at one time, and technology provides increasing amounts of storage with each new generation of disks.

Another type of laser technology is rewritable magneto-optical platters. Although this rewritable technology does not provide unalterable images with guaranteed permanence, it does provide the ability to use optical technology for working documents. For example, a nursing graphic record of a hospitalization may need updating multiple times during a patient's stay. Rewritable technology would allow the document to be changed until the patient was discharged. The document could then be written to WORM technology for permanent storage.

Optical disks are written with a disk drive that resembles a magnetic disk drive. If the facility determines that both WORM and rewritable technology are required, multi-functional drives that accommodate both technologies are available.

Jukebox. The **jukebox** holds and retrieves individual disks as they are requested, much as a music jukebox does. With the music jukebox, the listener selects a record and the internal mechanism of the jukebox retrieves the record and plays it. The optical disk system jukebox works the same way. Each box or cabinet holds multiple disks and is capable of high-speed retrieval. In some configurations, jukeboxes are linked together, which allows even greater storage capacity. Off-site, off-line storage may increase the amount of manual labor to change disks if adequate jukebox space is not allotted.

The time it takes the jukebox to locate the disk and retrieve it is called the **exchange time.** The exchange time is the number of seconds it takes to complete the process. Users may consider 10 seconds the longest acceptable exchange time, with less than 10 seconds being optimal. Once the disk is placed in the disk drive, the appropriate image must be located for display on the terminal screen. The time it takes for this process to be completed is called **access time.** Access time is rated in milliseconds because access is an electronic process, in comparison with exchange, which is a mechanical process.

Fragmented WORM platters, or disks on which multiple images from the same record have been written to different areas of the platter or even different optical platters, can increase the access time of the system. Fragmentation can be corrected by rewriting all the images on the platter into the correct sequence on a different platter. This process is similar to defragmenting a magnetic hard drive if it was rewritten to a new hard drive. Although defragmenting platters speeds access, it makes the old platters unusable and can be an expensive process.

Secure Magnetic Storage. Secure magnetic storage, such as storage area networks (SANs), allows many applications to store data together on redundant magnetic disks. This type of storage evolved from optical disk storage. **Redundant array of independent disks** (RAID) is the typical storage device inside SAN. It provides a cheap alternative to storage compared with magnetic storage, and there are supposedly no legal issues with its use.

Retrieval Workstation. When the system is operational, users must have a retrieval workstation to access records that are stored within the system. The equipment most commonly used for this workstation is the PC. Many of the computers in use today in health care facilities can easily be converted to retrieval stations. The size of the monitor and the resolution of the images vary, depending on the user's needs. Image resolution requirements are determined by the users' needs, with radiographic film images requiring the highest resolution available. A 17- to 20-inch color monitor is recommended as a standard configuration for imaged medical records.

Cache Memory. An extremely important capability of the system is the caching of images.[21] **Cache** (pronounced "cash") **memory** is memory within the magnetic disk on the workstation. When a request is received by the file server, as many images as possible are copied onto the local magnetic disk. Future requests for images are handled rapidly because the images are in temporary local storage on the workstation magnetic disk. Some cache systems attempt to anticipate future data requirements by transferring the data from the optical disk into the cache even if it has not been formally requested.

Caching is done in optical disk systems for two reasons. The first is to reduce the time it takes to page through the record because the record, in total, is stored on the disk. Therefore, the user does not have to request each page of a record from the file server individually. This capability leads to the second reason: fewer requests are sent to the file server, which decreases access time for all users on the system. Optical systems with caching are, therefore, faster and more efficient. The number of cache drives needed increases with the amount of record access or hits to the system. Generally, 80% of all requests can be cached; the remaining 20% are emergency or unexpected requests.

Digital Document Imaging. Imaging capability and technology has changed significantly since its introduction. It will continue to change and offer more options. A significant change was the ability to scan documents into multiple formats, store these documents in digital format, and easily retrieve the documents or words stored in the documents. In addition, the use of this technology has become more affordable. Organizations now have the option of setting up full imaging management resources internally or contracting with companies that use a secure Web site to process images and then provide access to scanned documents.

Database Software. One of the most important components of any system is the imaging system software. This part of the system determines the practicality and appropriateness of the system for the environment. As with other software, there are proprietary systems and open, or public domain, systems. A **proprietary system** is owned or copyrighted by an individual or a business and is available for use only through purchase or by permission of the owner. These systems allow no modification by the user and are specifically written for a particular hardware configuration. In **open systems,** the specifications are made public to encourage third-party vendors to develop add-on products for them. These systems are designed to incorporate all kinds of devices, regardless of the manufacturer or model, that can use the same communications facilities and protocols. The **graphical user interface** (GUI) or user-friendly screen application is important for efficiency and user satisfaction for both the individuals involved with scanning and the clinicians.

Printers. All EDMs must have at least one output device. High-quality laser printers are used to reproduce images that have previously been stored or scanned onto the system. If the file server resides on a network, any connected printer device will be able to reproduce the images. As an optional component, an EDM can be combined with a fax unit, an additional output device that allows images to be sent to another location over telephone lines. The fax sends images directly from the server rather than routing them to the workstation for printing and then conventional faxing. A separate print or fax server may be needed, depending on the volume and speed desired.

Uninterruptible Power Supply. Another necessary item is an **uninterruptible power supply** (UPS) or battery to keep the system running during a power failure and to protect it from the power surges associated with power outages. All major pieces of equipment in the optical system should be connected to the UPS, including at least one printer, to ensure that vital patient records are continuously available. A redundant **mirroring** backup server is required

to ensure data validity, and full RAID technology is recommended for integrity.

System Benefits and Advantages

Space Savings. The simplest and easiest to implement use of an EDM system is as a storage and archival system to replace inactive paper-based records. Although this provides a great space savings, similar to the space saving by use of micrographics, it does not use the technology of EDM to the fullest extent or provide the dollar savings of a true imaging solution that uses workflow applications (see the following).

Work Flow Applications. Many work flow applications built into imaging software can foster improved processes to reduce labor costs in a health information or other department and provide better access to records.[22] Some examples and case studies follow:

1. *Incomplete processing.* Records need to be minimally assembled, and only portions requiring manual scanning and indexing need to be placed in sequential order. Charts can be separated into COLD versus scannable documents for temporary storage. Analysis deficiencies may be assigned automatically from an order-entry system or during the scanning portion. Application software may be able to provide "color-coded" flagging of items needing authentication, and with the availability of on-line incomplete lists within the network, the need for an incomplete staging area is eliminated.
2. *Correspondence and release of information.* Records may be requested on-line, cached, and sent automatically to requesters by printed, faxed, or electronic (on-screen) output. This application is excellent to speed internal reviews, and some external customers such as insurance companies and other providers of health care may be able to accept electronic documents rather than photocopies or faxes.
3. *Coding and abstracting.* On-line access can make coding a function that can be decentralized by including home-based staffing. A patient can be seen in one facility, records created, and then the records coded or quality audited at another physically distant facility. Access to the previous record assists in coding validity, and diagnosis-related group (DRG) optimization and reduced accounts receivable days become a byproduct of better access. Cancer registry follow-up becomes easier, and records that need to be completed by physicians are simultaneously available and are not delayed by the coding process.
4. *File and retrieval.* Permanent file and study retrieval or refile are virtually eliminated when all records are part of the optical system. During temporary holding of records, which takes place magnetically for a certain period of time, paper records can be maintained as a back up. Loose report scanning is reduced and simplified and misfiles are eliminated by use of COLD.

Back scanning is usually not done except for the case of readmissions, but staff must be allocated for previous record retrieval if any paper or microfilm records exist. Table 7-10 and Table 7-11 show sample workflow changes for the physician record completion and patient readmission processes.

Productivity Gains. An EDM system can dramatically decrease the amount of time spent moving records from one location to another. The tasks of retrieving, assembling,

transporting, and filing paper-based records are eliminated. Telephone calls to initiate record searches and requests to copy records on the photocopy machine are also eliminated. By deleting these paper-based steps from the record management process and replacing them with an automated retrieval system such as imaging, the facility realizes several important advantages.

One advantage is 24-hour access to records by authorized users, without clerical staff assistance and with a considerable reduction in retrieval time. There are also no lost or misplaced documents to be searched for, and the documents maintain their long-term quality for future use. An additional advantage is the opportunity to use available work hours to complete other tasks, such as monitoring documentation patterns and performing quality studies.

Increased Use of Computer Technology. The use of imaging and more advanced technology as it evolves encourages the use of computer technology. To retrieve an image, the user must use a workstation, and the workstation displays a familiar-looking document, much like the paper document that has always been used. This familiarity enhances user acceptance of optical images or other technological advances that are computer generated, such as laboratory values and transcription output. These systems help prepare the user for future information technologies that are completely computer based.

Multiuser Simultaneous Access. One of the greatest benefits of an EDM is that it offers multiuser access to the same information at the same time—something that neither paper-based nor microfilmed records can provide. With an EDM system, many people can view the same information at the same time because each is viewing a copy of the image. Coders, physicians, social workers, nurses, and correspondence clerks can all view the record at the same time, providing greater efficiency by eliminating the waiting time for the record before they can perform their functions. A physician treating a patient in the ED can view a record from the patient's recent visit to the hospital at the same time that administrative users are viewing it. This has a positive impact on the quality of care that can be provided and is extremely valuable when facilities provide care across a variety of settings and sites or have a large number of outpatient encounters.

On-Line Availability of Information. An EDM can create an on-line record for patients as they are admitted. The system can incorporate data from different sources as the information is created electronically at multiple points in the hospital (e.g., registration, laboratory, pharmacy, rehabilitation, radiology). The data are compiled into one record, maintained digitally during hospitalization, and viewed by many users while the patient is being treated. The images remain on magnetic or other media throughout the completion process and are then moved to SAN when the record is complete. The images are stored as a group, speeding future retrieval time.

System Security and Confidentiality. System security is maintained because images stored in the system can be

Table 7-10   SAMPLE WORKFLOW CHANGES: PHYSICIAN RECORD COMPLETION

Current (Paper) System	Proposed (Imaging) System
Physician deficiency identified	Physician deficiency identified (potentially automated with link to order entry system)
Record flows through processing (up to 1 week delay)	Records immediately available for on-line completion
Physician calls for records Records retrieved (30% refile rate)	Automated audit trails
Work completed	
Deficiencies updated	
Record refiled	
(This process is repeated an average of three times per record)	

Table 7-11   SAMPLE WORKFLOW CHANGES: PATIENT READMISSION

Current (Paper) System	Proposed (Imaging) System
Provider request	Provider request
Health information staff retrieves*	Record reviewed on line
Record outguided	Automated audit trails
Unit called to pick up or health information taff delivers	
Paper record received on unit	
Record picked up after discharge	
Record refiled and outguides reconciled	
Chart tracking system updated	

*Separate subprocess of search and retrieval if out of file.

viewed only by use of access codes with passwords. Access to viewing stations can be controlled by the same system security measures that are now used on large computer systems. This use of access control makes the EDM more secure than any paper-based or microfilm system could ever be.

User-specific retrieval of information can be implemented to increase security. Clerks can receive only the portions of the record that are required for their assigned duties. Physicians can view only cases that their facility numbers have been associated with (physician of record). A physician's billing staff can view only demographics and insurance data and only for patients whose records carry the physician's facility number. Other user-specific retrieval specifications can be developed to increase security, such as audit trails to review emergency access to cases that were outside the scope of the previous clinician of record.

Database Retrieval. The EDM software can perform database searches for specific information that has been indexed. If the diagnosis and procedure codes were indexed, the imaging software can form the MPI, disease index, operative index, and physician index that were traditionally done manually or in an abstracting system. After a database search for a specific diagnosis is performed, the software displays the list of patients with that diagnosis and can cache their records for review or retrieval.

Evaluating System Requirements

When the need for an alternative solution to a storage, retrieval, and workflow application system has been recognized, the health information professional must obtain approval from the appropriate level of authority in the facility to evaluate possible alternatives. Without this prior approval and clinical buy-in, considerable time and effort may be expended needlessly. Full commitment later usually depends on prior approval to begin the investigation process.

Analyze Problems and Conceptualize Solutions. As system requirements are being determined, the current problems must be analyzed and appropriate solutions conceptualized. All proposed automated systems must solve the major problems identified in the current system, not merely add costs.[23] If the proposed system can solve problems without creating long-term additional ones, the system should be developed in detail, including the following:

- Identifying new or different tasks that affect work flow for the new system
- Determining the current volume of work and the projected volume of each task to be completed in the new system
- Determining whether the skill levels of the staff need to be adjusted to a higher or lower level in the new system
- Developing productivity targets
- Identifying tasks that could be completed during off hours or off site

- Interviewing potential system users in the facility to obtain their view of the current system, its problems, and their future needs
- Designing a diagram of the processes in the new system for explanation and training purposes
- Determining equipment needs and specifications

Identify Potential Vendors. When the system concept has been developed and equipment needs are known, locate several vendors who are capable of providing the equipment required, the software applications needed, the system integration, and the long-term service needed. System integration is the process of combining all the necessary hardware and software into a system that functions according to the system design. The successful vendor should be able to provide a system with sufficient size and capacity, including expansion capability. The vendor must also provide training and system support, have an exceptional service record, and offer a competitive price on all equipment and services.

Open architecture is the best choice in most cases to ensure that the system can be integrated from the best possible products that provide the best speed and processing capabilities. The opposite of open architecture is a proprietary system that uses only equipment designed and manufactured by a certain vendor. Open architecture protects the facility's investment against possible vendor bankruptcy or complete closure. It also allows individual pieces of equipment to be exchanged as rapidly as technology advances, not only as rapidly as one vendor makes upgrades. It does carry the risk that one weak piece of equipment could adversely affect the entire system design.[24] This risk can be minimized by thorough investigation of all equipment choices. The system must be updated regularly to keep records available for patient care and other users as required by state and federals laws.[26]

Optimal specifications should be set for all equipment required for the system, with speed and processing capabilities used as the identifiers. Any equipment that does not meet the optimal specifications should not be considered. If the optimal specifications cannot be met or are met only to a minimum as the equipment is being evaluated, the equipment will probably be obsolete before the installation takes place.

Interview those given as references and visit other health care installations completed by the vendors being considered. Ask the users and the selection committee at the reference facility if they would use the same vendor again and how they could have proceeded differently.

Cost/Benefit Estimates. The purchase price of an EDM system or an EHR system can be difficult to justify for many facilities. Although the price of technology has been decreasing over the years, the prices can still seem exorbitant to budgetary decision makers. Those who are not familiar with long-term technology solutions in health information management may have difficulty understanding the investment required to automate a paper document system. Cost justification of a system must begin by determining the costs associated with the old and new systems and opportunities for saving and revenue enhancement with a new system. Both paper-based record costs and micrographics costs should be included if both are being replaced.

Use the approach shown in Table 7-8 for the comparison of paper-based records and microfilm systems. The cost justification could involve a comparison of all systems over a 10-year period, assuming no inflation. Rather than listing the savings of the systems involved, list the costs associated with the process in the system that uses it. For example, if 50,000 fewer photocopies will be made monthly with an optical system or an EHR system, list the cost of 50,000 copies under the paper-based system. Also include the cost of replacing the photocopier as it becomes no longer usable. If the same 50,000 copies are replaced by 35,000 retrievals on a retrieval workstation and 15,000 prints on the EDM system printer, list the cost of 15,000 prints. The number of retrieval workstations needed for the imaging system or the EHR system should be calculated but accounted for in the system configuration and overall purchase price of the system. Continuing costs and one-time costs should be included. This cost-based method allows direct comparison of costs for each system.

Direct Costs. Direct costs to include in the analysis are as follows:

Photocopy supply costs. Include the cost per copy times the number of copies made per month in each system.
Storage and supply costs. Include file folders, fasteners, dividers, boxes, warehouse or facility space, and shelving costs.
Microfilm and supply costs. Include service bureau charges, film, jackets, equipment, purging, filing, software, and supply costs.
Labor costs. The labor costs involved for all tasks associated with each system can be determined by multiplying the volume of each task by the time it takes to complete the task times the average hourly wage of the staff, including benefits. Departments outside the health information department may also have a saving in staffing and supply costs, particularly departments that keep decentralized records or record copies or that handle a great many record requests and reviews.
Outside service costs. Include courier services between facility locations or physicians' offices and remote storage.

Indirect Costs. Indirect costs, such as the loss of interest income when bills are delayed in a paper-based system, should be quantified. The faster the bill is delivered to the payer, by use of efficient methods, the faster the facility is paid and has use of the money to meet commitments and earn interest. The fax feature also speeds answering requests for information from third-party payers and outside review agencies. The facility's financial department can provide estimates in this area.

Offsetting Revenue. The financial department may also be able to provide estimates of revenue that can be produced as a result of installing an EDM or an EHR system. Revenue produced by the sale of equipment or the conversion of space should be included. The revenue produced from the eventual sale of unneeded shelving and microfilm readers, reader/scanners (reader-printers), and cabinets should be applied to help offset the cost of the system. Remember that some equipment may still be needed to maintain the old system as long as the old system is still functional. A reduction in accounts receivable days and an increase in revenue from correspondence may be a consideration and should be included if applicable.

Other revenue can be produced when vacated storage space is converted to space for revenue-producing patient care activities. For example, if a facility is interested in establishing a cardiac catheterization unit but cannot find the needed space, transferring paper-based records to an EDM or EHR system may provide the needed space. If the only factor stopping the development of a profitable catheterization unit is space, the conversion of paper-based records to an EDM or an EHR system will produce savings that can be used to compensate for the purchase price of the new system.

Unquantifiable Benefits. There are benefits associated with any system that are unquantifiable. They should be listed along with the actual cost figures for each system. The benefits and advantages of the EDM or EHR system that are listed in this chapter should be included, as well as improved patient and staff satisfaction that can be obtained by installing an efficient system.

Obtaining Commitment and Purchase Agreement. Prepare a detailed proposal for approval by the budgetary decision makers. This normally includes the following:

System diagram. This diagram is an overview in pictures, using whatever method is normally used in the facility. There should be enough detail to make it understandable but not so much that it is overwhelming. The diagram can be tested with a knowledgeable person who has not been previously exposed to the discussion of the system to be sure that person can understand the system flow.
System summary. This is a written, descriptive overview of the system, sometimes called an executive summary, that explains the system concepts. It identifies the current system and the problems associated with it as well as the proposed system and how it addresses or eliminates those problems. It also includes a description of the hardware needs by areas of the facility.
Financial summary. This is the cost/benefit analysis and may be similar to the one presented in Table 7-8. It should list which system components are to be purchased, which are to be leased or rented, and the purchase time table. Remember to include the differences between initial capital investments that can be amortized over time and the continuing cost of

supplies and service contract. (Payback is usually within 3 years of purchase of an imaging system.)

Vendor comparison and references. This is a listing of the final vendor selection criteria; it may be similar to the one presented in Table 7-9. A written summary of the reference checks and installation visits performed should be included.

Implementation plan and schedule. This is a calendar or chart displaying the phases of the implementation, projected timelines, and implementation teams. It should be realistic from both the workflow aspect and the financial aspect.

The health information professional should be prepared to give a presentation, if it is required, to defend the analysis and ensure approval of the project. There will undoubtedly be questions that even the best documentation cannot answer. If the documentation and presentation are well prepared, the necessary commitment for purchase and installation will be given.

Implementation Strategies

Phasing in the New System. There is no perfect or universal method for phasing in a new system. Some sources suggest that the initial place to start is the outpatient area or ED of the hospital or on-line patient records at admission.

Others suggest that an imaging system could be initiated by scanning inpatient discharge charts the day after discharge. Both imaging and EHR systems need to support appropriately with hardware installation to the entire facility and to interface with current electronic systems.[25] Regardless of where the implementation starts, forms should be redesigned or evaluated for design purposes. When an imaging system is implemented, forms should include bar codes for automatic indexing as soon as possible. The process of inventorying forms and providing bar codes on the forms takes time and should be initiated well in advance of the implementation. The bar codes should be placed in exactly the same location on every form and provide sufficient information to identify the patient, the form type, and the date of the documentation contained on the page. Many EHR systems also have a scanning component to handle forms received from external sources and some handwritten forms such as consent forms.

No matter how intense the planning, implementation is never easy. Strong commitment from facility administration and pretesting of all hardware and software before live conversion go a long way toward providing smooth implementation.[26] Staff training is also essential.

All medical staff members should be trained in the use of the new system as soon as the final configured system with actual documentation is available. Their office staff should also be trained thoroughly because the medical staff look to them for support when change is happening rapidly.

Redefining Jobs and Skills. The introduction of an EDM or an EHR system results in the need for internal change in the health information department more than in any other department of the facility. The department staff needs to learn as much as possible about the new technology before it is implemented and should help in the redesign of staff job functions. Positions will probably not be eliminated with the initial implementation of the system. Employees should be reassured that staffing will be changed but not eliminated. Any eventual staffing decreases that might be realized can be handled through transfers, formal retraining, or attrition.

New position titles will evolve to replace the familiar "file clerk" and "assembler/analyst." Titles decided on at the University of Cincinnati Hospital during that facility's job redesign were image processing specialist, information processing specialist, and record processing specialist.[27] The image processing specialist handles record preparation and scanning. The information processing specialist handles record completion, release of information, and coordination of input from other sources. The record processing specialist handles hard-copy reproduction and other record management activities. Decision support analysts will also play an important role in database development and retrieval and should be included as early as the planning stages for proper indexing design.

Legal Considerations

Each state can specify whether business records reproduced by a particular medium are admissible as evidence, but not all have addressed the issue of imaging. As business practices evolve into a more electronic environment, patient records in a variety of mediums are being recognized.

When states address business records as evidence, the Federal Rules of Evidence, Rule 803(6) of the Uniform Rules of Evidence, or the Uniform Photographic Copies of Business and Public Records Act is used as their basis. The facility's legal counsel should be consulted for an opinion if state statutes are unavailable or unclear. This is an excellent reason why HIM professionals need to help the facility define the legal health record (LHR). It is for this reason that the LHR is one of the biggest drivers for using EDM or an EHR system.

Application in Use: Memorial Hospital and North Park Hospital, Chattanooga, Tennessee

Contributed by Kelly McLendon, RHIA

Memorial Hospital Enterprise System

Main Facility: Memorial Hospital
Catholic Health Initiatives
365 beds
800 medical staff members
14,000 inpatient discharges per year
26,000+ ED visits per year
Outpatient services

Information Systems: ChartMaxx by MedPlus Electronic Patient Record (EPR) Meditech HIS
Lanier Transcription Meditech Lab

Additional Sites: North Park Hospital
                           80 beds
                           Acute care general hospital
                           300 medical staff members
Information System: Meditech HIS
                           The Atrium
                           Diagnostic imaging center
                           Mountain Management
                           Physician office practice

The Challenge. In the mid 1990s Memorial Hospital determined that EPR technology had advanced to the point where cost savings could be achieved for problem areas within the medical record department. The same types of issues were present in this hospital as in most other health information management departments—lack of floor space for rapidly expanding files, difficult access to the information within the files, and difficulty in managing the logistics of a paper-based system. There was an increasing demand for charts from the outpatient areas. Release of information was a non–profit-generating, contracted service. So Memorial Hospital began its search for the best EPR system to manage crucial high-volume medical record files and provide access for all clinicians and other users of the information.

When implementation of these systems was planned, it became clear that simultaneous access of the chart information was vital to the entire health care enterprise. Memorial Hospital's integrated delivery network was beginning to grow. It was determined that the information needs of the remote facilities could not be served with a paper record. It also was obvious that management of patient accounts and other nonpatient records would need to be addressed.

A Bump in the Road. Memorial Hospital began its imaging project by scanning outpatient records. Although the system chosen for this task was not fully adequate for it, hospital personnel were well trained in not only the processes associated with electronic records but also the technologies. It was determined to discontinue the scanning within this platform and search for another, more robust EPR system.

The Solution. After a functional specification for the EPR system was developed, Memorial Hospital underwent a search process and selected another EPR. Reasons for the selection included HIM expertise by the vendor, a wide scope of applications for both medical records and patient accounts, and operational interfaces and integrations with the health information system.

An integral part of this process had been to facilitate participation of the medical staff in the proposed system. Several meetings were held with physicians to educate them and to facilitate their acceptance of the selected product. The contract for ChartMaxx was signed in late 1997.

The plan developed by Memorial Hospital and the vendor established operations within the medical record department with a complete HL7 data set, a discrete interface to Meditech ADT, a Lanier Transcription interface, and a COLD Meditech Lab interface. The EPR uses on-board STC DataGate and COLD engines to facilitate the interfaces.

Deficiency analysis, chart completion, and release of information were targeted for automation with the EPR system, as well as high-volume scanning and quality review. These functions, combined with the ability to expand into patient accounts, registration, and other nonpatient areas such as human resources, were to be delivered later in the implementation process.

The system procured was a client-server UNIX processor (Hewlett Packard) with RAID, WORM optical disk jukebox, scanners, printers, and other hardware components. The system is scalable and has a redundant server configuration. All hardware components attach to the hospital 100-MB network backbone. Access is by software clients, Web, or thin clients.

Planning. MedPlus and Memorial Hospital held a kick-off meeting and began the formal implementation sequence. It was determined that backscanning of ED and outpatient charts that had been accumulating since the other imaging system was unplugged would commence before concurrent charts were scanned. Once the interfaces were established and the backscanning was well under way, ED, same-day surgery, outpatient, and inpatient chart would be started.

After all these functions were operational and budgetary considerations addressed, the system would be expanded throughout the enterprise and into patient accounts.

Implementation. Implementation of the EPR system has progressed along the lines of the original planning. Interfaces were established and backlog scanning undertaken. This allowed the scanning and quality review operators to learn the system. Enterprise-wide bar coding was initiated.

Capture of the first-visit type of concurrent records of the ED was begun in the training database. Once the system and processes were defined within the training database, live production of the charts began in March 1998, moving quickly within approximately 30 days into outpatient charts and finally to same-day surgery charts. All these visit types had associated deficiency analysis and chart completion requirements, which were instituted along with scanning and interface reconciliation. This involved physician training and security setup. Acting as a team, the site and vendor personnel began the process with physician training. Site trainers carried on after the vendor's implementation roles were accomplished.

These visit types became paperless from a medical record department perspective at this point. Continued work on the backlog scanning and preparation for the inpatient discharges were the next steps. Having a large (800-member) medical staff, Memorial Hospital determined that it would take several months to be ready to present the system to the entire group. In November 1998, live production of inpatient discharges was undertaken. Along with this process, Memorial Hospital brought the contracted release of information function back into the medical record department.

Benefits. Any project of this magnitude has its share of issues to be solved. But the working relationship between the vendor's sales, implementation, support, and development teams and the Memorial Hospital medical record and information systems teams has been productive and has allowed the issues to be resolved in a timely manner.

Early in 1999 the system was expanded to encompass all medical record staff members and many other workstations within the main building. All physicians complete their records within the system; deficiency analysis and chart completion functions are also entirely handled within the system. Chart e-mail and release of information is also accomplished with system applications.

Within the medical record department, tangible savings have been realized with reductions in staff requirements for release of information functions and file clerks. Duties have been shifted for the staff involved with these functions to the backlog-scanning project and to intense 100% image review. This highly detailed image review is being undertaken as a part of the planned sequence for system acceptance. On satisfaction of the requirements in this quality management plan, image review will be scaled back and tangible staffing benefits obtained. To date, in excess of five full-time equivalents (FTEs) have had duties shifted into these areas. Also, all revenues from release of information have been brought back in house.

Benefits achieved to date from the EPR system include the following:

- High physician satisfaction with the system; enthusiasm has increased as the project has commenced.
- Physician completion of chart deficiencies from any workstation without need to go to the medical records department.
- Physician access to the chart information from patient care areas. ED physicians are especially excited about the timely access to all chart information, including electrocardiograms.
- Elimination of permanent chart floor space requirements (except shelved backlog).
- Improved workflow of deficiency analysis and chart completion processes. No rechecking of charts is necessary after deficiencies are addressed by users.
- In-house release of information functions with reduced staff. Revenue brought back in house.
- Pulling and delivery of charts for same-day surgery, outpatient, surgery, ED, and the floors has been discontinued for records already in the system. In time, the delivery to these sites of any paper-based information will diminish; eventually it is projected to fall to below 5% of the original level. Retrieval for study and committee use is also possible.

Moving Ahead. Memorial is working to begin implementation of record management at the North Park, Atrium, and Mountain View facilities. With patient care information required simultaneously from all these sites, ChartMaxx will be expanded to encompass them. Patient accounts is also being positioned for inclusion in the project, as well as registration areas. The inclusion of patient accounts will necessitate a financial interface with UB-92, bills, and HCFA 1500 capture.

The number of users in the system is to be expanded. The next system expansion is envisioned to encompass all the remaining sites and applications. The most exciting developments have been the anticipation of the Web access application. By using a Web browser, a physician (or other user) can connect to the secure *Intranet* server through the hospital firewall and both access and complete chart information. This exciting application, which has caught the attention of the medical staff, has been in operation on a limited basis. Physician eagerness for the capability to view and complete charts from anywhere, including home or office, is driving this process quickly along.

Key Concepts

- Paper-based records are still common in health care today, although it is widely recognized that paper is not the best medium for all situations. Image-based records and electronically stored information are two alternatives.
- Records are identified by two methods—alphabetical identification and numerical identification. Alphabetical identification uses the patient's name as the identifier for the record, and numerical identification uses a number, either supplied by the patient or assigned by the facility.[28] Paper records are stored in different types of equipment. Filing cabinets work well for small files, compressible files work well for medium and moderately active files, and open-shelf files work well for large, active files.
- Filing systems can be either centralized or decentralized and use one of the three common filing methods: alphabetical filing, straight numerical filing, or terminal digit filing.
- File folders for paper records should be chosen after considering the size of the average record, the usage rate of the record, and the type of filing equipment used to store the record. Filing efficiency can be enhanced by choosing colored folders or by adding color coding to a plain folder.
- Manual record-tracking systems use outguides, requisitions, and transfer notices as their primary tools. Outguides mark the spot where a record was removed; requisitions list the patient identifiers and requester; transfer notices alert the file personnel that a record has been moved to a new location.
- Automated record-tracking systems hold the requisition and transfer information in a database. They allow computerized requesting of records and on-line inquiry regarding the current record location.
- Paper-based systems require large amounts of storage space. As records become less actively used, the format or medium is often changed to reduce the storage space they

require. Image-based systems, such as micrographic and optical imaging systems, are considered an acceptable alternative. Paper records may also be moved to off-site storage facilities.

- Micrographics programs offer the different microform options of roll microfilm, jacket microfilm, microfiche, CAR-roll microfilm, and CAR-jacket microfilm. Computer output microfilm can also be used to store computer output in a miniaturized form.
- Facilities must choose between completing the micro-filming process in house and using a contracted microfilm service bureau. In-house microfilming requires the purchase of a camera, developer, and jacket loader as well as management of the staff to complete the process. A service bureau charges for its work at a negotiated price per 1000 film images.
- An imaging system uses special disk platters that are written and read by a laser beam. Other system components include a scanner, workstation, file server, jukebox, and printer.
- An imaging system can be costly, but the cost can be justified by considering the space savings, productivity gains, multiuser access, on-line availability of information, and increased system security.
- The legality of imaged and fully electronic records as admissible evidence in court is determined differently in each state, and opinions should be obtained from the facility attorney.
- Retention and retrieval of records in various formats must be part of the initial planning for any system. Although microfilm, imaging, and electronic record systems all provide reasonable means to store and organize patient records, the HIM manager must continually balance access, retrieval, and retention schedules to make the stored information available over time in a manner that meets the needs of the patients, the organization, and other users. Constantly changing technology creates retrieval challenges in microfilm, imaging, and electronic record systems. Technology in use today may not be in use 5, 10, or 20 years from now, so continual planning for data access and retrieval as systems change and are upgraded is critical.[29]

REFERENCES

1. Skurka M: *Health information management in hospitals: Principles and organization for health record services,* Chicago, 1994, American Hospital Publishing.
2. Estep B, Kirk R: Relocating a medical record department: "a moving experience," *J Am Med Records Assoc* 57:22, 1986.
3. Bertrand M: Moving a medical record department: a case study, *Topics Health Record Manage* 6:65, 1985.
4. Johnson M, Kallaus W: *Records management,* 1982, Cincinnati, Southwestern Publishing.
5. Allen B, Barr C: The impact of automated medical record tracking systems on the ability to reduce staff—a research study, *J Am Health Inform Manage Assoc* 64:74, 1993.
6. Greenberg SP, Larsen EJ: An automated medical record ordering and tracking system at the Cleveland Clinic Foundation, *Med Rec News* 50:31-37, 1979.
7. Glass B, Mitchell S: The ambulatory care medical record: an administrative nightmare, *J Med Group Manage* 39:60, 1992.
8. Lach J, Longe K: Bar coding and the medical record manager, *J Am Med Records Assoc* 58:24, 1987.
9. Majerowicz A: Selection and implementation of a bar code–based record management system in ambulatory care, *J Am Med Records Assoc* 61:29, 1990.
10. Platz K, Thoman D, Craft T: Making tracks at the University of Iowa Hospitals and Clinics: design and implementation of a bar coded medical records tracking system, *J Am Med Records Assoc* 61:45, 1990.
11. American Health Information Management Association: Practice brief: retention of health information (2002): AHIMA.org. Accessed December 29, 2005.
12. American Hospital Association: *Preservation of medical records in health care institutions,* Chicago, 1990, American Hospital Association Institutional Practices Committee.
13. *Position statement issue: protecting patient information after a closure,* Chicago, 1994, American Health Information Management Association.
14. Buchanan S: Emergency management—Drying wet books and records, North Andover, 1994, Northeast Documentation Conservation Center.
15. Collen MF: The origins of informatics, *J Am Med Inform Assoc* 1:92, 1994.
16. Ball MJ, Collen MF, editors: *Aspects of the computer-based patient record,* New York, 1992, Springer-Verlag.
17. Trofino J: Voice recognition technology applied to nursing documentation, *Healthcare Inform Manage Syst Soc* 7:42, 1993.
18. Clayton PD, Pulver GE, Hill CL: Physician use of computers: is age or value the predominant factor? Proceedings of Patient Centered Computing, Seventeenth Annual Symposium on Computer Applications in Medical Care, American Medical Informatics Association, New York, 1994, McGraw-Hill.
19. Tunick D: Client server computing strategies for the 1990s, I: Industry services. Inside Gartner Group This Week Newsletter, July 28, 1993, p 2.
20. Lauersen N, Hochberg H, George M: Microfilm storage of fetal monitoring records: A practical solution, *Obstet Gynecol* 51:632, 1978.
21. McLendon K: Optical disk imaging—tomorrow's technology today for medical records, *J Am Med Records Assoc* 61:32, 1990.
22. Rhodes H, Dougherty M: Practice brief. Document imaging as a bridge to the EHR, *J AHIMA* 74:56A-56G, 2003.
23. Kahl K, Casey D: How to evaluate and implement office automation, *J Am Med Records Assoc* 55:20, 1984.
24. Little E: Starting up an imaging system: lessons learned, *J Am Health Inform Manage Assoc* 64:61, 1993.
25. Brick F: Running out of room for data. HIPAA requires healthcare organizations to re-assess data storage, *J AHIMA* 77:56-57, 64, 2006.
26. Continuity Data Incorporated: *Contingency and recovery plan,* Eugene, OR, 1999, Continuity Data Incorporated.
27. Mahoney M, Doupnik A: Health information department reorganization resulting from the implementation of optical imaging, *J Am Health Inform Manage Assoc* 64:56, 1993.
28. AHIMA e-HIM Work Group on Regional Health Information Organizations (RHIOs): Using the SSN as a patient identifier, *J AHIMA* 77:56A-56D, 2006.
29. Kohn D: When the writ hits the fan, *J AHIMA* 75:40-44, 2004.

section **111**

Health Care Informatics

chapter 8

Technology, Applications, and Security

Melissa Saul

 Additional content,
http://evolve.elsevier.com/Abdelhak/

 Review exercises can be found
in the Study Guide

Chapter Contents

Health Information Infrastructure, Technology, and Applications
Scope of Health Information Systems
    Components
Computers in Health Care—Past and Present
    Early Efforts, 1960s to 1980s
    Evolution of Hospital Information Systems: 1980s to Late
        1990s
    Late 1990s to Present
    Health Information Systems as an Emerging Discipline
Computer Fundamentals
    Hardware
    Terminals, Workstations, Personal Computers
    Network Computer
    Personal Digital Assistant
    Voice Recognition
Software
    Programming Languages
    Databases
    Database Models
    Network Technology
    Client-Server Platforms
    Interface Engine
Designing the User Interface
    User Interface Team

Key Words

Applets
Application gateway
Application software
ARDEN syntax
Ascension number
Authentication
Bandwidth
Biometric
Break Glass
Business rules
Cascading Style Sheets
Checksum
Clinical decision support systems
Data compression
Data mart
Data mining
Data repository
Database
Database management system
Database model
Decision support systems
Disaster Recovery
Encryption
Ethernet
Expert system
Extranet
Firewall

Frames
Granularity
Hardware
Hierarchical
Interface engine
Internet
Intranet
JAVA
Knowledge base
Lossless
Lossy
Mainframe
Malware
Medical informatics
Microcomputers
Middleware
Minicomputers
Network
Object
Object-oriented
Operating system
Order entry
Packet filter
Password aging
Phishing
Point-of-care system
Pointer

Point-to-point
Primary key
Protocols
Proxy server
Public key
Relational model
Results reporting
Servlet
Software
Store and forward
Symbology
Syndromic surveillance system
Tags
Templates
Terminals
Thick-client
Thin-client
Three-tier
Two-factor authentication
Two-tier
Token ring
Voice recognition
Wireless
Wi-Fi
Workstation

General Design Principles
  Needs of Users
  Selection and Sequencing of Items
  Instructions
  Guidelines for Designing Web Pages
  Screen Space
Computer Applications
  Administrative Applications
    Admission, Discharge, and Transfer System
    Decision Support Systems
  Clinical Applications
    Results Reporting
    Order Entry
    Computerized Provider Order Entry
    Clinical Decision Support Systems
    Point-of-Care Systems
Emerging Technologies
  Bar Coding
  Radiofrequency Identification Device
  Internet and Web Services
    Fundamentals
    Internet Tools
    JAVA
    Intranet
    Virtual Private Network
Telemedicine
  Fundamentals
  Implementation
Computer Security
  Authentication Tools
    Passwords
    Single Sign-On
    Tokens or Cards
    Biometric Devices
    Access Controls
  Reporting Capabilities
  Physical Security
  External Controls
    Firewalls
    Encryption
    Internet Security
    Malicious Software Protection
    Application Service Provider Models
Data Management Technology
  Data Mart
    Creating a Data Mart
  Data Modeling

Abbreviations

ADT—Admission, discharge, transfer

ANSI—American National Standards Institute

ASP—Application service provider

ASTM—American Society for Testing and Materials

ATM—Asynchronous transfer mode

CCOW—Clinical context object workstation

CGI—Common gateway interface

COBOL—Common business-oriented language

CODEC—Coder/decoder

CPOE—Computerized provider order entry

DOS—Denial of service

DTD—Document type definition

DMZ—Demilitarized zone

EIS—Executive information systems

ERP—Enterprise resource planning

FDDI—Fiber-distributed data interface

HTML—Hypertext markup language

HTTP—Hypertext transfer protocol

IEEE—Institute of Electrical and Electronic Engineers

IETF—Internet Engineering Task Force

ISO—International Organization of Standardization

JVM—Java virtual machine

LAN—Local area network

MUMPS—Massachusetts General Hospital Utility Multi-programming System

PDA—Personal digital assistant

RBAC—Role-based access control

RFID—Radio frequency identification device

SGML—Standardized generalized markup language

S-HTTP—Secure hypertext transfer protocol

SQL—Standard query language

SSL—Secure socket layer

TCP/IP—Transmission control protocol/Internet protocol

VPN—Virtual private network

W3—World Wide Web Consortium

WAN—Wide area networks

WEP—Wired equivalent privacy

WPA—Wi-Fi-protected access

WWW—World Wide Web

XML—Extensible markup language

Continued

HEALTH INFORMATION INFRASTRUCTURE, TECHNOLOGY, AND APPLICATIONS

The ideal scenario of a patient experience is one in which, on arriving at the physician's office, hospital, or other health care setting, the patient is quickly identified as someone who has been seen before. The patient's previous laboratory tests and imaging results are viewed through the Web browser on a hand-held device. Test results, combined with other historical and clinical data already collected into the computer system, are reviewed in minutes. If necessary, data are transferred through a network to a specialist for immediate feedback. The referring physician and the specialist view the information simultaneously while conferring by phone. New treatment is documented and automatically added to a central repository, from which the patient and other care providers can retrieve information in the future. Special reminders and flags that alert the physicians about special conditions that need to be investigated, such as abnormal laboratory results and new reports on patient allergies, are automatically presented when the patient's care information is retrieved. Even reminders for annual immunizations and screening procedures are generated with automatic notification to the patient. Also, claims for services are automatically processed through computerized systems and forwarded electronically for billing and reimbursement, and the laboratory results from the visit are posted to the patient's on-line personal health record. After the visit, the patient can access follow-up test results through a home computer. Scenarios such as this are becoming more accepted, addressing patient and provider expectations regarding health information systems (HISs).

We need more information in health care than ever before. We need to achieve better health care quality outcomes and cost-effectiveness in providing health services. We need to extend access to larger patient populations and health care information to more users. To meet these goals, we are applying new technology in information systems and communications to multiple business processes within the industry. Traditionally, the health care industry did not invest in technology as did other industries such as banking or retail. However, in the past few years, the health care information technology expenditures have been estimated to be from $17 billion to $42 billion annually.[1] This expenditure is expected to grow from 5% to 7% to 10% to 15% per year. The soar in interest in HISs comes from several factors. In 2003, health care information technology became part of the federal government's initiative at improving patient safety. To accomplish this, the Office of the National Coordinator for Health Information Technology was created to coordinate the adoption of information technology in hospitals and physician offices across the country.[2] (See Chapter 3 for more on this topic.) There is also an increasing demand from health care consumers to have more efficient and improved quality of health care. The purpose of this chapter is to describe the current HIS environment, the technology used, the key clinical applications, and the data management tools available. Health information professionals need to develop a greater appreciation of the role and potential of HISs.

The term *health information management system* serves as an alias for many types of information systems. These include hospital information systems, clinical information systems, decision support systems, medical information systems, management information systems, home HISs, and others. Lindberg, a pioneer in medical information systems, defined a medical information system as "the set of formal arrangements by which the facts concerning the health or health care of individual patients are stored and processed in computers."[3]

This chapter begins with a general discussion of the current overall picture of HISs, including some of their features, a review of their historical evolution, and what the typical HIS looks like today. The various technologies that support the information infrastructure are described. Computer security and the use of the Internet are discussed. Finally, the role of the health information management professional in using these technologies analytically is presented with examples of real-life scenarios. As health information professionals, we need to understand the environment in planning for the future.

Scope of Health Information Systems

It is important to determine the scope of an HIS and its components. Each of the components discussed in this chapter can be applied to almost any type of HIS. The scope includes the following:

Departmental—A system limited to a specific clinical or financial domain to serve the business functions of a department (e.g., respiratory therapy, social work)

Intradepartmental—A system that primarily serves the business function of one department but shares information and functions with other departments (e.g., laboratory, patient scheduling)

Hospital (or site of care)-wide—A system that focuses on the integration of the various departmental systems or, in the absence of integration, may provide the primary service for a clinical area

Enterprise-wide—The system that encompasses all the departmental systems throughout the health system, including hospitals, clinics, nursing homes, and other health facilities

External (cooperative)—A system that is shared among different health systems and primarily exists to report information required by regulatory agencies or as part of an information exchange for regional health information networks (RHIO)

Components

Comprehensive hospital information systems contain seven components:

1. Core applications such as patient scheduling and admission, discharge, and transfer (ADT) provide the central notification to the hospital of patient visits and form the initial database for many other applications.
2. Business and financial systems such as patient accounting, billing, and payroll provide data processing for the business activities of the organization.
3. Communications and networking applications including the Internet and Web applications transmit and manage messages among departments such as nursing and ancillary areas. Communications are used to notify these departments of patient admissions and provide for tracking orders and results.
4. Departmental systems such as pharmacy, radiology, and laboratory are designed to manage the clinical operations and connect data to institutional databases for results reporting, billing functions, and electronic health records.
5. Documentation systems are used to collect, store, and retrieve patient data. Applications in this category range from point-of-care bedside terminals for nursing documentation to transcription modules that capture and store clinical reports to direct clinician entry into electronic health records.
6. Reminder and advice functions assist health care providers in planning patient care activities. Such reminders can include messages to alert for significant test results, utilization criteria, and drug-drug interactions. This component includes monitoring of compliance with clinical guidelines and protocols.[4]
7. Surveillance and related systems that can detect disease at an earlier stage for public health surveillance. This type of system is generally referred to as **syndromic surveillance system** because it is designed to recognize outbreaks on the basis of the symptoms and signs of infection.[5] Because the data used by syndromic surveillance systems cannot be used to establish a specific diagnosis in any particular individual, syndromic surveillance systems must be designed to detect patterns of disease in a population.

In reality, hospital information systems can be viewed along a continuum from the first three major components to acquisition of all seven. Figure 8-1 is a schematic representation of the major categories in a hospital information system and shows examples of the components. Note that information needed at the time of registration is captured at one level and available at the next level. Components are connected through an interface engine, which is discussed in detail later. The organization relies on the HIS for daily processing activities, including patient care, research, administration, and educational initiatives.

Computers in Health Care—Past and Present

Early Efforts, 1960s to 1980s

Computers were introduced into the health care arena through punch card data processing. Early work in epidemiological and public health applications that performed statistical analysis on the incidence, distribution, and causes of diseases in society provided the early experience with

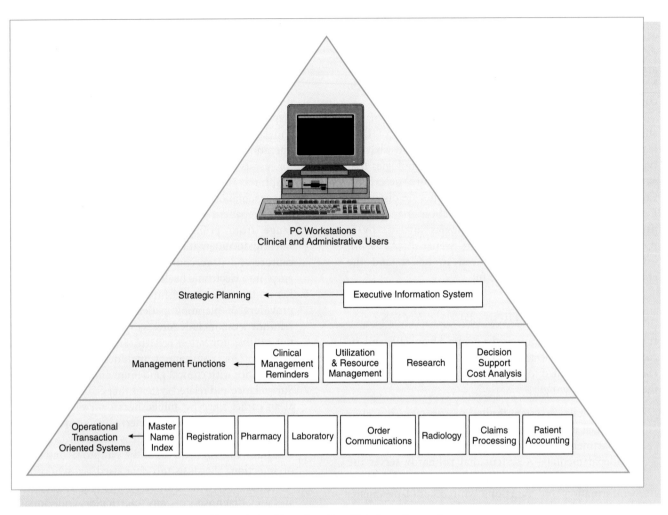

Figure 8-1 Hierarchy of health information systems.

computers. Although some of the early activities were focused on decision making for physicians, many developers worked on building total information systems for hospitals. Also, during the 1960s and 1970s, significant work was undertaken by Octo Barnett at Massachusetts General Hospital in the ambulatory care environment with the development of COSTAR (computer-stored ambulatory record system). The first patient care system that claimed to automate the patient record was initially marketed as the IBM Medical Information Systems Program in the late 1960s; it was sold until 1972. A number of other companies were involved in patient care information systems during this period, but only the system devised by Lockheed Aircraft—which became the Technicon Data System (TDS) and is now operated by the Eclipsys Corporation—is still in existence.[6]

During the 1970s, HISs were developed in several ways. Many hospitals approached information system development by creating financial information systems and using the same system or slightly modifying the database for clinical applications. Other hospitals adopted a goal of a single integrated system that was designed to use one large database that shared its resources among departments. In contrast,

other providers acquired versions of hospital information systems through departmental applications such as a clinical laboratory system to which custom features were later added. The intention was to create common data through a single shared database, but this proved difficult to achieve.[5] In large part, database structures and the tools needed to use them effectively were still immature during the 1970s. During this period, hospital databases were derived largely from discharge analysis of medical records. Many hospitals participated through contracts with external computer service organizations by submitting discharge abstracts to the service computer companies for processing and receiving printouts of hospital statistics. The most extensive program was maintained by the Commission on Professional Hospital Activities (CPHA). Its program brought health information professionals into the computer age as they worked with computerized data in new ways. Expectations were expanded as CPHA and others introduced more computing power and offered better ways to retrieve data and provide comparative reports.

As the technology grew to include minicomputers in the 1970s, more and more separate departments were able to acquire departmental systems that met their specific needs. Vendors began to offer packages of functions for hospital departments such as laboratory, radiology, and pharmacy. In addition, software tools emerged that reduced the mystery associated with computers, and clinicians became more interested in leading and participating in computing activities. Minicomputers provided computing power equal to or greater than that of the mainframe computers used previously.

At the end of the 1970s and into the 1980s, the introduction of the personal computer (PC) gave rise to additional empowerment and expectations of clinicians. In effect, technological advances produced computers that were reliable, small, and low in cost. Hardware became reliable and highly affordable. Computer and business communities recognized that the greatest cost involved in information systems development was in the software. Thus, software engineering emerged as a field dedicated to management of the software development process.[6] The three major computer characteristics of the 1970s were significantly improved reliability and computing power of hardware, availability of more functional software, and reduction in cost of ownership. All this laid a strong foundation for the work to come.

Evolution of Hospital Information Systems: 1980s to Late 1990s

In the 1980s, network technology emerged and expanded to enable the departmental systems that began in the previous decade to share and communicate with other systems within the organization. Demographic and associated information on patients who registered in clinics or were admitted to hospitals was now automatically sent to hospital departments so that the data could be incorporated in their database. Admission notices were communicated to dietary, housekeeping, laboratory, radiology, and other ancillary services electronically. In turn, order communications enabled physician orders to be sent from a nursing station directly to an ancillary area. In addition, significant gains were made in building computer networks that linked a variety of diverse applications together.[7]

In 1980, Ball and Jacobs[8] described HISs at three levels. A level I HIS included ADT application with bed and census reporting, order entry communications, and charge capture and inquiry functions for billing purposes. A level II HIS focused on systems that included part or most of the patient record. This provided fundamentally clinical databases and improved collection and use of clinical data within these systems. Level III described an HIS in which data were linked to knowledge bases that provided diagnostic support and actual intervention for patient care activities. In these systems, special alerts were made available that responded to specific data content and messages and notified providers through the system.

Late 1990s to Present

The prospect for developing health care information systems that are more effective and less costly greatly improved with advances in networking and computer technology. These advances include (1) the emergence of the Internet and World Wide Web (WWW); (2) the development of reliable, scalable servers; (3) the availability of low-cost PCs; (4) the introduction of the JAVA software development model; (5) the availability of free Internet browsers and utilities; (6) proliferation of data management tools to end users; and (7) the government's effort in promoting a national health care information technology program. This chapter focuses on the use of these advances for health care information systems in general. Chapter 5 includes an in-depth analysis of the electronic health record and the effect of emerging technology on its advances.

Health Information Systems as an Emerging Discipline

Health professionals from diverse backgrounds work together on medical computing in a variety of ways. Physicians, engineers, administrators, nurses, health information management professionals, software developers, and others have adopted new roles. The study of medical computing is referred to as the academic discipline of **medical informatics.** In 2001, Shortliffe and Perreault defined medical informatics as "the scientific field that deals with biomedical information, data and knowledge—their storage, retrieval and optimal use for problem-solving and decision-making."[4]

Postgraduate training programs are sponsored by the National Library of Medicine for physicians and other health care professionals interested in this field. Physicians usually spend several years after their residency to study medical informatics and to work on developing new health care applications and how biological sciences intersects with computer techology.[9]

Today, a number of professional organizations are active in advancing the study of medical and health care informatics. The Joint Health Information Technology Alliance (JHITA), the College of Health Information Management Executives (CHIME), the Health Information Management Systems Society (HIMSS), the American Medical Informatics Association (AMIA), and the American Health Information Management Association (AHIMA) all actively promote the advancement of HISs. Recently, the Department of Health and Human Services (DHHS) created a private-public collaboration called the American Health Information Community (AHIC). AHIC, composed of 17 members from the government and private sector, will make recommendations to the DHHS on how to ensure that electronic health records are interoperable while protecting the privacy and security of patient data. (See Chapter 3 for more on this topic.)

Computer Fundamentals

To deliver cost-effective and useful health information management systems, we must rely on information technology—hardware, software, and networking—to collect, store, manage, and transmit health information. The following section briefly reviews key concepts in these areas and illustrates their roles in health care information systems.

Hardware

Hardware is the physical equipment of computers and computer systems. It consists of both the electronic and mechanical equipment. The computer requires a central processing unit (CPU) with capacity to hold the data being processed and the equipment needed to carry out the system functions. Peripheral equipment including CD-ROMs and tape drives, data input devices such as workstations and PCs, and output devices such as printers and modems are also hardware. Computers come in mainframe, mini, and micro sizes. **Mainframe** machines have traditionally been used for large applications that need to support thousands of users simultaneously. Many different applications can run on one mainframe. Users interact with the mainframe through a terminal or terminal emulation software. The user input is transferred to the mainframe computer, where all processing occurs. **Minicomputers** are often used in departmental systems such as laboratory or radiology systems. They were popular in the 1980s and early 1990s. Minicomputers were less expensive than mainframes, so the cost of ownership was lower. They had some of the processing power of a mainframe and allowed devices and files to be shared. **Microcomputers** are based on small microprocessing chips found in individual PCs. They are used for desktop applications such as word processing and spreadsheets and, with the increase in computing power available on the PC, can serve as the hardware for a database management system.

The trend in the industry is to move from a thick-client environment to a **thin-client** one. Thick clients, which might include a desktop PC or a workstation, need a substantial amount of memory and disk space to perform functions that the application may require. Thin clients have minimal or no disk space; they load their software and data from a server and then upload any data they produce back to the server. Thin clients are devices that vary from a laptop computer to a hand-held network instrument.

Terminals, Workstations, Personal Computers

The most common devices for data retrieval are terminals or workstations. **Terminals** are connected to information systems and are used to enter and retrieve information. Terminals are sometimes referred to as "dumb" terminals because, without the connection to the information system, they cannot function. Although terminals are still found in HISs of all kinds, they have been giving way to the PC as a more sophisticated and powerful input device. A hospital information system may have terminals located at nursing units for data entry such as ordering patient services and retrieving information such as laboratory test results.

A **workstation** is a type of computer that requires a significant amount of computing power with highly specific graphics capabilities. It is well suited for applications that require more memory and disk storage than a desktop PC. Most workstations function as part of a hospital network. In the hospital setting, most intensive care unit (ICU) bedside computing is done on workstations because of the need for fast processing (from the monitoring devices) and the graphics resolutions for flow sheets and electrocardiogram (ECG) tracings. However, the differences between PCs and workstations can be a bit fuzzy. A PC with added graphics and memory capabilities might also be used as a workstation.

Network Computer

The network computer is a computer with limited memory and disk storage. Its basic function is to connect to the Internet. This device relies on the server to provide the data and processing power it needs. It is an attractive alternative to PCs and workstations because the hardware is less expensive and easier to install and maintain. Centralized applications reside directly on the server, not the client, so it is not as difficult to maintain the server as it would be for several hundred thick clients. These machines are also called thin clients because the client side of the software requirements is minimal.

Personal Digital Assistant

A **personal digital assistant** (PDA) is a hand-held device that combines computing, fax, and networking features. A typical PDA can function as a fax sender, e-mail retriever, or network device. These are devices that can be carried in the pocket. They have built-in communications and organizer software. Most PDAs use a special writing instrument rather than a keyboard for input. The PDA is capable of hand-writing recognition, so the user can write, using the special writing instrument, and store information in the PDA.

In the health care industry, one example of the use of PDAs is in home health organizations, in which visiting nurses use PDAs to record visit encounter data. Another example is the use of a pen-based device to document intravenous therapy data for hospitalized patients. In both examples, the devices are used for daily tasks and are plugged into a "dock" or receiving component that transfers the data to a larger computer system. As the capability of PDAs increases, more and more applications will be written for them. Another example is the use of the PDA as a resource for information. One clinic has loaded the PDA with basic clinical guidelines for treatment, drug formularies, and a *Physician's Desk Reference* (PDR) (Medical Economics, Montvale, NJ). This ready reference is portable. The goal is to offer a useful tool and gain some experience with hand-held devices before moving to more sophisticated applications.

Voice Recognition

A **voice recognition** system consists of both hardware and software. It is included in this section on hardware because it is primarily an alternative to a data input device. A voice recognition system can recognize spoken words. It is an attractive technology for health care applications because it offers the most efficient means for practitioners to incorporate data capture into their normal routines. Voice recognition means that the computer can record information that is being said. It still does not *understand* what is being said, and it is important to be aware of this distinction.

This technology has grown phenomenally over the past 10 years, particularly with continuous-speech systems. Continuous speech means that the user can use the system naturally and does not have to speak as slowly and distinctly as with previous systems. Most systems require an initial training session in which the software is taught to recognize the user's voice and dialect. Successful implementation of this type of system is heavily dependent on the user. An effective use of this technology is in emergency departments and radiology departments, where transcribed reports need fast turnaround. Sometimes the voice recognition software is combined with templates so that the user has to speak only to complete the blank spaces in a template and not the entire document. Software for voice recognition can exist on an individual PC or be a shared application across a network. Voice recognition is also being used to offer clinicians a way to immediately dictate, sign, and produce a report independently. In other settings voice recognition is turned on while an individual clinician dictates. The trancriptionist receives a draft document and the voice version and is more quickly able to complete the document and present it for signature.

Software

Software is the set of instructions required to operate computers and their applications. Software includes programs that are sets of instructions that direct actual computer operating functions, called the **operating system,** and sets of instructions used to accomplish various types of business processes, known as **application software.** Software written to process laboratory orders is application software. These instructions are combined to direct the overall functions of a given information system. The operating system directs the internal functions of the computer. It serves as the bridge to application programs. Without an operating system, each programmer would have to program all the detail involved in receiving data, displaying graphics on a screen, sending data to printers, and so forth. Operating systems contain all the standard routine directions that handle such tasks. Operating systems act as system managers that direct the execution of programs, allocate time to multiple users, and operate the input/output (I/O) devices and the network communication lines. With the increase in distributed computing, most operating systems are now able to run independently of the hardware platform. An example of an operating system is UNIX. UNIX, and flavors of UNIX, can run on mainframes and workstations. UNIX is capable of running a number of powerful utility programs to support Internet applications while allowing multiuser access and file-sharing capabilities.

Programming Languages

Programming languages refer to the various sets of instructions developed to operate applications and to generate instructions themselves. Software has developed significantly over the past 30 years, and the evolution of new generations of programming languages has enhanced the use and rapid development of computing power. Generally speaking, all instructions to computers are ultimately expressed in their native codes, known as machine language. This most basic level of programming refers to the system of codes by which the instructions are represented internally in the computer. To illustrate, a programmer writing in a computer's low-level machine language uses machine instructions (mostly all numbers) to address memory cells for storing data, accumulators to add and subtract numbers, and registers to store operands and results. Some codes represent instructions for the central processor, some codes move data from the accumulator into the main memory, some codes represent data or information about data, and some codes point to locations (addresses) in memory.

The second-generation programming languages built on machine codes by the invention of a symbolic notation called assembly language. Assembly language used key words to invoke sets of machine instructions instead of the numerical ones needed in the machine language. Terms such as "Add" or "Load" represented specific sets of key word machine instructions. All the assembly languages vary by type of machine or CPU. An assembly language program is written for a specific operating system and hardware platform. It needs to be rewritten for a new operating system. It is one step closer to human language than machine language.

Third-generation programming languages extended the efficiency of programmers by offering the capability to write programs in languages that were shorter and quicker to write. They combined more and more of the machine-level instructions to accomplish their tasks. This generation of language also introduced a new capability. Some could run on different operating systems. Examples of third-generation programming languages are FORTRAN (formula translator), COBOL (common business-oriented language), and C.

One third-generation programming language, MUMPS (Massachusetts General Hospital Utility Multi-Programming System), was established for specific use in health care applications. MUMPS was established in the late 1960s and is still used today in both health care and other industries. It has been renamed the M programming language. Both the Departments of Defense and Veterans Affairs have installed nationwide medical information systems using MUMPS as the primary language.[10]

Fourth-generation languages with even greater efficiencies enable programmers to use instructions at a higher level.

These types of programs are commonly known as 4GL. The concept is that program generators—sets of instructions that can be invoked as components when needed—are the foundation of the language. This allows the programmer to focus more on the logic of the program (application servers in the three-tier client server) and less on the instructions to the computer. In other words, the program generator is able to determine the lower level instructions needed to generate the output. 4GLs were designed for powerful data manipulation and the capability of developing code that can be reused in other applications. 4GLs are often proprietary to one vendor.

Databases

A **database** is a collection of stored data, typically organized into fields, records, and files. A **database management system** (DBMS) is an integrated set of programs that manages access to the database. Databases have evolved with advances of technology. The goal of the database is to represent the lowest level meaning of the data that allows users to retrieve and manipulate the data. A **database model** is a collection of logical constructs used to represent the data structure and the relationships between the data. The four major database models are as follow:

- Relational
- Hierarchical
- Network
- Object oriented

Database Models

Relational Model. The **relational model,** the most popular database model, was developed by E. F. Codd in 1970.[11] It is designed around the concept that all data are stored in tables with relationships among the tables. A relationship is created by sharing a common data element; for example, if two tables have a patient identifier, the patient identifier relates those tables. How the data are physically stored is not of concern to the user. The user needs to know only what the relationships are among the entities in the database.

Figure 8-2 shows an example of three tables in a relational database used in an ambulatory clinic. The rules for a relational database used in an ambulatory clinic are as follow:

1. Each patient has only one entry in the patient table and is identified by a unique identifier.
2. Each patient has one or more entries in the visit table.
3. Each patient in the visit table is linked to the patient table by the unique identifier.
4. Each working diagnosis entry in the visit table has a lookup entry in the diagnosis master file.

The rules listed in Figure 8-2 are defined as the associations among the data. There are three types of relationships to describe associations:

1. One to many—A patient may have many visits to the ambulatory clinic, but each visit is attributed to only one patient. A patient ("one") is related to the visits ("many"). A one-to-many relationship is sometimes identified as 1:M.
2. Many to many—A patient may have many physicians, and each physician may have many patients. A many-to-many relationship is referred to as M:M.
3. One to one—An ICD-9-CM (*International Classification of Diseases,* Ninth Edition, *Clinical Modification*) code has only one description, and the ICD-9-CM description has only one ICD-9-CM code.

There are several reasons for choosing the relational model for this ambulatory clinic application. First, we want to store the data only once. By creating a **primary key** for the unique patient identifier, we can eliminate storing the patient's name and other demographics in the visit table. We can always join the patient and visit table by patient

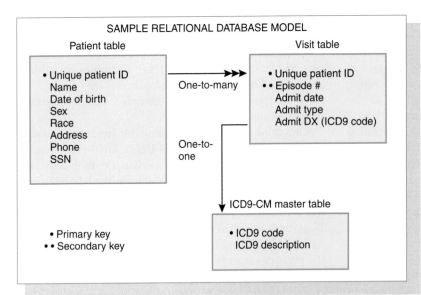

Figure 8-2 Sample relational database model.

identifier and report the data in both tables. Second, this application requires several master or look-up tables. Look-up tables enable data translations to be stored outside the visit and patient tables. In the preceding example, the visit table contains only the visit working diagnosis code (most often an ICD-9-CM code). The diagnosis look-up table stores two fields, the ICD-9-CM code and ICD-9-CM description. Each code and description is in the diagnosis look-up table only once. In this way, the ICD-9-CM description does not have to be stored in each visit record.

Structured Query Language. Structured query language (SQL) is the relational database model's standard language. It is pronounced "see-kwell" or as separate letters S-Q-L. It was originally designed in 1975 by IBM but has since been adopted by the American National Standards Institute (ANSI). SQL commands allow the creation and management of a database and provide a method of retrieval of data. All queries are based on the SELECT statement (see example of these queries).

Example of Queries Based on the SELECT Command

According to the relational database illustrated in Figure 8-2, the SQL query to list all the visits for a patient with patient identifier 663465 is

SELECT * FROM VISIT

WHERE PATIENTID='663465';

where * instructs all fields in the visit table to be printed. The output from the query would be

ID	Location	Doc	Date	Working DX
663465	CMED	Smith	02-Sep-99	428.0
663465	CRHE	Jones	13-May-99	714.0

Hierarchical Model. The **hierarchical** model differs greatly from the relational model. The hierarchical model supports a treelike structure that consists of parent (or root) and child segments. Each parent segment has a child. Each child segment can have only one parent segment. However, a parent can have more than one child. A user queries the database, and the search seeks the answer from parent to child. The answer to the query is found by matching the conditions by searching downward through the tree. Retrieving involves gathering the parent record and following a **pointer** to the record in the next lower level. This model is quite effective when the queries are predetermined and pointers already identified. It is not effective for ad hoc queries or when there is information only about the data contained in the child segment. This model requires the user to understand the physical and the logical structure of the database.

Because the logical model is replicated in the physical structure, it is difficult to change this structure. Many-to-many relationships (as described before) are difficult to represent in this model. It is also difficult to use the data for multiple purposes. If another type of query is needed, additional copies of the database need to be made so that the logical model can be changed to the copied database.

An example of a hierarchical database is found in hospital patient accounting systems. The system contains many patient accounts (parent) that in turn have many transactions (child). The total number of transactions is likely to be greater than 50. The rules would be as follow:

- Each patient account (parent) has at least one transaction (child).
- Each patient account can have many transactions.
- Each transaction can be defined as a debit or credit, so the relationship between parent and child is fixed.

A common user query would be to determine a patient's total charges. This model would easily handle that because the patient account (parent) is known. It would identify the parent and then trace the pointers to each of the transactions (child). However, it would be difficult in this model to determine all of the patients who had a specific transaction during the past year.

Network Model. The **network** model is similar to the hierarchical model except that a child can have more than one parent. In a network database, the parent is referred to as an owner and a child is referred to as a member. In other words, it supports the many-to-many relationship. It does not, as the name might suggest, refer to the physical configuration of the computer where the database resides but instead describes the logical arrangement of the data.

Object-Oriented Model. This model has had a surge in popularity as a result of the use of JAVA and other programming tools. The database is one that embraces the concept of an object. An object-oriented database is a collection of objects. Objects support encapsulation and inheritance. Encapsulation is the technique by which an object, such as a patient, is defined with certain characteristics. The user does not need to know how the characteristics are stored, just that the object "patient" exists and has certain attributes. Inheritance means that one object can inherit the properties of another object. For example, a physician is defined as an object with certain characteristics (a name, a specialty, an office address). A resident is defined as another object with certain characteristics, with the first characteristics being those of a physician. Therefore, the resident inherits the properties of the physician object. There are no primary keys in an object-oriented model. Access to data can be faster because joins are often not needed as in the relational model. This is because an object can be retrieved directly without a search, by following pointers.

Network Technology

Network technology is used within individual organizations to connect the PCs, workstations, printers, and storage devices to the organization's network and the entire outside world. It has evolved from the basic terminal to mainframe computer connection to local and wide area networks and the client-server technology. A **local area network** (LAN) connects multiple devices together by communications and is located within a small geographic area. An example of a LAN environment is a patient scheduling system at a primary care clinic in which seven PCs are connected to a server. Each of the PCs is able to execute its own programs (e.g., word processing, spreadsheet applications) but is also able to access data and devices anywhere on the LAN. This allows all users of the LAN to share hardware such as laser printers and scanners and to share patient files. Users can also use the LAN to communicate with each other by e-mail or to share schedule and appointment books. LANs are capable of transmitting data at a high rate, making access to the LAN resources seem transparent to the user. However, there is a limit to the number of computers that can attach to a single LAN.

The most widely used LAN network topology in use today is **Ethernet.** Developed at Xerox in 1976, Ethernet is a standard defined by the Institute of Electrical and Electronics Engineers (IEEE) as IEEE 802.3. This standard defines the transmission speed of data traveling across the LAN as either 10 million bits per second (Mbps) or 100 Mbps. The topology is designed with messages that are handled by all computers in the LAN until they reach their final destination. The disadvantage of this technology is that a failure in one segment of the network affects the entire LAN. Another type of LAN technology is **token ring.** Token ring (IEEE 802.5) means that the transmissions travel from one computer to another until they reach their final destination. This allows a single computer to be added to or disconnected from the network without affecting the rest of the computers on the LAN. Token ring transmission speeds vary from 4 to 16 Mbps.

Wide area networks (WANs) are used for extensive, geographically larger environments. They often consist of two or more LANs connected through a telephone system, a dedicated leased line, or a satellite. The Internet is an example of a WAN. WANs are usually found in organizations that need to connect computers across an entire health care delivery system. For example, the hospital, the long-term care facility, and the physician office all have an internal LAN in their own areas, and the LAN is connected to the backbone of the WAN.

The most widely used WAN technology today is the **fiber-distributed data interface** (FDDI). FDDI provides transmission at a higher rate than Ethernet or token ring. It is run with fiberoptic cable. There are hundreds to thousands of smooth, clear, thin, glass fiber strands bonded together to form fiberoptic cables. Data are transformed into light pulses that are emitted by a laser device. Current fiberoptic technology can transmit data at speeds of up to 2.5 gigabits per second, much faster than Ethernet or token ring.

A very popular type of network found in health care today is a **wireless or WiFi™** network. This type of network enables computers and other hand-held devices to communicate with the Internet and other network servers without being physically connected to the network. Wireless networks use the IEEE 802.11 standard, which was ratified in September 1999. There are several versions of the 802.11 protocol in use, with the most commonly used being 802.11g.

Each wireless network has a service set identifier (SSID). This is a code attached to all packets on a wireless network to identify each packet as part of that network. The code consists of a maximum of 32 alphanumerical characters. All wireless devices attempting to communicate with each other must share the same SSID. SSID also serves to uniquely identify a group of wireless network devices used in a given service set. For security purposes, it is important to change the default, factory-assigned SSID for each wireless network. The default SSID will identify your network location and potetially permit others to access your network.

To secure wireless networks, protocols were created to encrypt and protect wireless transmissions. One of the first protocol systems developed is the **wired equivalent privacy (WEP)** system, which is part of the IEEE 802.11 standard. It provides an encryption scheme so that the information transmitted over a wireless network is protected as it is sent from one device to another device. Because of some weakness in the WEP protocol, **Wi-Fi–protected access (WPA)** is the most popular method of securing wireless networks. Data are encrypted as they travels over the wireless network as with WEP, but the method of securing the network is greatly improved over WEP. A major improvement is the requirement that the authentication code used dynamically changes as the system is used. In previous versions, the same code was used with each transmission, so once the code was known by the outside, the network was compromised.

Wi-Fi's greatest strength is also a weakness. Every action that is made during a wireless network connection is broadcast to any other network within a certain distance. Therefore, it is important to secure each wireless network with encryption. Encryption is discussed in a later section in this chapter. Table 8-1 illustrates the differences between wired and wireless networks.

Several **protocols** are available for communicating across networks. A protocol is a specification or algorithm for how data are to be exchanged. It is similar to the telephone system, which expects an area code as part of the phone number. Two of the more popular network protocols are TCP/IP and ATM. TCP/IP is the acronym for transmission control protocol/Internet protocol. This protocol is the standard used to connect Internet sites. TCP/IP can run on various platforms and can connect hardware systems of different types as long as both systems support TCP/IP. It divides each piece of data that is to be sent across the network into packets, and the packets are then sent to the destination by the most available route at the time of transmission. TCP/IP allows packets to be rerouted if the network is particularly busy at one site. ATM is the acronym for asynchronous transfer mode. ATM creates a fixed path

Table 8-1 WIRED VERSUS WIRELESS COMPARISON

	Ethernet (Wired)	Wi-Fi (Wireless)
Advantages	Very secure; reliable transfer of data; data transfer speeds up to 94 Mbps	No cables to connect to device; minimal installation costs; allows for access to the network from any location
Disadvantages	Does not permit mobility; installation costs can be high for cable routing	Extra process required to secure network; some areas may not be reachable by wireless; data transfer rates are slower than Ethernet
Cost	Network cards, cables, and labor costs of installation	Network cards (although some PCs have technology built in)

between the source and destination. The packets are of a fixed size. The benefit of this type of network is that a single packet does not overload the network and very fast transmission is supported. It can relay images, sound, and text at very high speeds.

Client-Server Platforms

The client-server architecture was developed in the early 1990s. The concept is to have most of the processing occur on the server.[12] It reduces network traffic by providing a query response rather than total file transfer. It is also referred to as a **two-tier** architecture. The user interface is located on the user's desktop, and the database management application and data tables are stored on a database server. The server is a much more powerful PC or workstation than the individual desktop model. This type of architecture is found in smaller environments with fewer than 50 users.

An example of a two-tier client-server application would be found in the cancer registry department. The database would be located on a server. Each registrar would have client software applications residing on his or her PC. When the registrar issues a query to the database, the client requests the data from the server. The server processes the request and returns the data to the client. The client machine is then responsible for the display and graphics.

There are several obstacles to implementing the two-tier architecture approach. The client software needs to be replicated on every PC on the network, which can be expensive to administer and maintain. It is difficult to change the database structure because the client software also has to be reconfigured. In addition, because it is difficult to scale up to more users, the application depth is somewhat limited.

A three-tier architecture has become very popular.[13] The **three-tier** configuration is a type of client-server architecture that has three components:

1. User interface
2. Application server
3. Database server

The difference between this configuration and the two-tier one is the introduction of the application server. The user interface is the software that runs on the user or client machine, and it can be customized to the needs of the client. The application server processes the data. The logic behind the database queries is hidden from the user. An example of this would occur if certain utilization review coordinators were responsible for receiving a specific set of patient claim authorizations. The logic or rules of how to process the data would be included in an application server. The logic might contain items such as "if patient is enrolled in an HMO, then display the names of both the patient and the subscriber. If the patient is not enrolled in the HMO, only require that the patient's name be displayed." The database server is the physical location where the database resides and serves as the connection for the application server to process the logic.

Many health care applications that were written with the two-tier approach are being rewritten with the three-tier approach. Developers are discovering that health care requires a huge amount of application processing and that having three distinct layers to the product makes it easier to change the application piece. Changes to the application server do not have to affect the entire system. Health information systems need to change to reflect the changing business requirements of the industry. The choice of architecture is a critical one in deploying applications. (See example of three-tier configuration in the example below.)

Example of Home Health Care Data System

The home health division needs a system to provide case management services to its existing population and to identify current inpatients who may need home health services after discharge. Because the case managers are dispersed over a wide geographical region, including some in their homes, they cannot implement a system that requires a specialized PC configuration requiring daily maintenance. The database, which resides on the database server, contains all the patient information. However, not all home health case managers need to view all the data in the database on their PCs. Each case manager may have separate data requirements. The geriatric case managers and maternity case managers need different sets of queries and reports.

These rules are commonly known as **business rules.** These are the rules that determine the user interface and database services that may be required. The business rules reside on the application server. Other items that may reside on the application server include a data retrieval engine and formulas for medication administration. Examples of business rules in this scenario are (1) display laboratory values only if they are not within the normal range, (2) require patient date of birth on input, and (3) set reminder for next month to check blood pressure.

Interface Engine

Another technology component that is being used in HISs is an **interface engine.** An interface engine is considered a piece of **middleware**—software and hardware that serve as a bridge between applications. An example of middleware in the previous section on client-server technology would be found in a three-tier architecture model. The application server in the three-tier model is considered middleware.

An interface engine allows two applications to exchange information without having to build a customized interface for each application. Before the implementation of an interface engine, most interfaces between applications were **point to point.** Point to point refers to the method of connection. If the radiology system requires ADT information, then a point-to-point interface is created by the information system programmers to exchange this information between radiology and ADT. If the laboratory system requires the same ADT information, another interface is created to send ADT data to the laboratory system. The ADT data now exist in multiple copies. This is inefficient for three reasons:

- Separate programs need to be written for both the sending and receiving applications to agree on the protocol for the transmission and define the frequency of transmissions, error handling, and so forth.

- Duplication of data requires additional network traffic.
- It is difficult to support and maintain because each interface requires customization and monitoring.

Figure 8-3 illustrates how an interface engine may function for an HIS. Each of the HIS applications sends data to the interface engine, which then reroutes the data to the appropriate destination. The sending or source application initiates a network connection with the interface engine, usually by using the TCP/IP protocol. The interface engine can then reformat the data in a structure suitable for the target or receiving application. Reformatting might be necessary, for example, if the source application contains laboratory test codes from an outside laboratory. The target application may be expecting to receive only test codes that exist in the hospital laboratory system. The interface engine would be the translation service for both applications. Health Level 7 (HL7) transactions may be received and reformatted in the interface engine. Interface engines might also house the master patient index (MPI) service for an enterprise. The source applications from all the various systems throughout the enterprise could route their data through the interface engine. The interface engine could reference the MPI and assign the enterprise MPI identifier to the data before the data arrive at the target application. This is an alternative to having the MPI value collected and stored within each application.

DESIGNING THE USER INTERFACE

The user interface or computer view refers to the screen format for both data entry and output display. The power of database management systems allows flexibility in which views are created for data capture and data displays, including still and moving images, sound, and text and

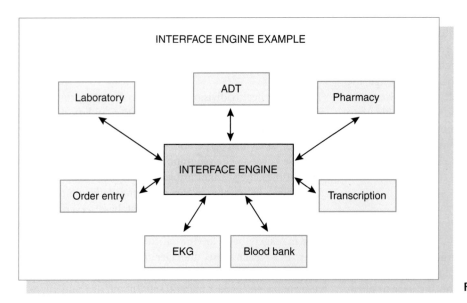

Figure 8-3 Interface engine example.

graphs. Computer views require menus of alternatives to be developed and screen or window formats that may include a variety of input formats and output formats including monitors, PDA screens, mobile telephones, and so forth. It is helpful to remember that standards such as those of the American Society for Testing and Materials (ASTM) are only a foundation from which to begin the process of selecting data items. Once captured, the data elements may be retrieved in new configurations to meet the needs of many different user groups. For example, a physician may want to view graphs that show the trends of laboratory data along with a menu of therapy options with costs, supported by a reference from a linked database. A social worker developing a discharge plan may select a summary of the patient's functional level, living arrangements, and insurance benefits to compare with services provided and prices charged by local home health care providers. This flexibility lends to both the promise and the problems of designing computer views.

When computer **views** (information on screens) are well designed and controlled, they enhance technology by providing a smooth link in the communication process. They permit recording of varying data without recopying constant information. This reduces clerical work, decreases the number of errors, and increases efficiency. In this section when we refer to a "view" we are primarily referring to "information on screens"; however, many of the design issues associated with views also apply to paper forms. (See Chapter 4 for additional discussion of forms design.) When views are well designed, they assist in actual direct patient care. For example, a well-designed nursing assessment view will enable the nurses collect the data related to the patient assessment process in the same way each time.

As with data collection and technology, user interface design should emphasize the needs of users. It is the responsibility of each health care facility to develop its own user interfaces. Accrediting and regulatory bodies such as The Joint Commission and standards organizations such as ASTM do not recommend particular views with which to collect their required data elements, nor do professional organizations such as the American Hospital Association (AHA) and AHIMA, although some standards organizations and the federal government are very interested in offering templates and core document structures in health care to facilitate the exchange of data. Large health care organizations often have enterprise-wide standards for screen displays (views and templates) so that all facilities within the organization use the same one. Before a project involving view redesign is started, it is recommended to research any existing standards or policies which may exist within your organization.

Well-designed screen views for data entry make it possible to:

- Organize the data entry fields in logical format
- Include field edits
- Include passwords to add, delete, or modify data

- Allow simultaneous entry or updating in many tables at one time
- Include brief instructions on the screens or provide more lengthy help screens
- Make the screens easy to navigate through the use of color, lines, borders, and hyperlinks
- Use default values in a field to eliminate the need to key repeated data between entries (e.g., the date field could be automatically set up to add today's date without the need to key the characters)
- Allow automatic sequential numbering (e.g., accession register numbers)
- Show data on the screen from a different table when the key field is entered (e.g., for the MPI screen form, when the physician's number is entered, the physician's name, address, and so on can automatically appear on the screen)
- Develop or customize menus or submenus to add, delete, or change data

Windows-style user interfaces provide menus that pull down from choices shown on a tool bar at the top of the screen. A menu is an important component of a computer interface because it is central to ease of navigation. Therefore, a carefully constructed sequence of menus is part of a comprehensive design.

User Interface Team

The creation and management of the user interface is a collaborative process. Members of the views and templates team include representatives from the following services in a hospital environment. A different environment might modify the team membership to represent its needs:

- Health information management
- Information systems
- Materials management
- Patient care services
- Quality improvement
- Medical staff leadership

The HIM professional plays a leadership role by providing knowledge of rules and regulations related to health record content, the flow of data throughout the facility, and the information needs of the health care delivery system. The views or templates design and control process also benefits from the involvement of an information systems manager who is responsible for the software application which will house the view, a materials or purchasing manager who is responsible for inventory and ordering paper forms, a patient care professional who represents clinical needs, a quality improvement professional to provide input regarding views or templates created to address quality issues, and physician representatives who will be using the views. It is extremely important to have physician and other clinicians involved in this process. The team's charge may be to work on administrative and patient information applications and to become involved in the selection of data collection technology. The team forwards its patient-related recommendations to the clinical information committee for approval, and its administrative recommendations follow the organizational chain of command.

General Design Principles

Needs of Users

The needs of both internal and external users must be considered when views or the user interface are designed. It is important to remember that users are not only the patient and providers but also the administrative, financial, and legal staff of the facility. External users collect data from many locations, and the data are combined or aggregated. These may be local, state, and federal agencies and other planning and research groups. Collecting enough of the right type of data to satisfy this range of users means clearly defining the purpose of the view.

Selection and Sequencing of Items

When the purpose of the view or template is established, the next step is to construct a list or grid of required data to ensure the collection of all essential items and the elimination of unnecessary or redundant items. Effective and efficient sequencing of the view or template should follow the traditional pattern—from left to right and top to bottom—permitting a continuous operation whether reading or entering data on the computer. The flow should be logical and take into consideration the order of data collection. (See Chapter 4 for additional discussion of designing forms.)

Another aspect of view design that promotes consistency is the development of a master format or template. The placement of data in the same sequence on similar forms or views with similar layouts facilitates rapid entry and retrieval.

Although this aspect is often overlooked, the organization should discuss how the printout from electronic views will be presented. There will be occasions when the entire electronic health record or major portions of the record will need to be printed to fulfill a request for information. The record may also be released electronically, but again, some plan must be in place to create a compact disk (CD) or other means of organizing the information.

Instructions

Instructions should briefly identify who should complete the data items and should provide any additional guidance that is necessary. Computer views typically provide this information on introductory screens and as needed throughout data entry.

Guidelines for Designing Web Pages

Designing a view/form to appear on a Web page provides more flexibility and options for improved usability. Consideration of type styles, or fonts, when well chosen, contributes to readability. Items of similar importance should be equal in size and type, and the overall number of different fonts used should be low. Italics and boldface characters should be used to maintain the effect of emphasis only. Style considerations may include the requirement to use a specified font type that is identified with the name and logo of the organization.

A Web-based user interface allows the form to contain **hypertext links** between documents. A hypertext link is an embedded object within the Web page that enables direct access to another related Web page. Often, reference materials are not included directly on the Web page, but rather there is a hypertext link so that, if the user wishes to go to the reference page Web site, it is only a click away.

It is important that each screen within the Web application follow the same "look and feel." This includes having clear and consistent icons to let the user know where to find items on the screen. For example, it is important to have the icon to print located near the top right corner of the screen. Users expect the icon to be in that location. Second, the user should always be able to return the home or main page of the application. The link to return to the main page should always be in the same location on the screen for each web page.

A well-designed screen will offer feedback for every required action. For example, if during data entry the user does not complete all items, there should be a message to alert the user to complete the missing information. Likewise, the screen should permit the user to undo the last action. This enables the user to feel free to navigate throughout the screen.

Users want to get information in the fewest possible steps. This means that the design of menus must be an efficient hierarchy of information to minimize steps through menu pages. Studies have shown that users prefer menus that present at least five to seven links and that they prefer a few very dense screens of choices to many layers of simplified menus. As a general rule, the screen should be designed so that the user has complete control over the system.

Screen Space

The use of **cascading style sheets** (CSS) can help the user interface optimize the use and appearance of the Web page.[14] With CSS-styled pages, users can easily apply personalized formatting to Web documents. A page with red text against a green background, for example, presents a problem for users with red-green color blindness: the contrast between text and background may not be great enough for the text to be distinguishable. If the colors are set according to a style sheet, users can set their browser preferences to override settings and can apply their own style sheet to the page instead. With CSS-styled pages, the user can transform Web content into a format that addresses their requirements for accessibility.

A Web page design should be checked to ensure that all navigation and content areas fit well within the display screen (usually 800 × 600 pixels). The use of frames within the Web page can assist in optimizing the screen space. Frames are vertical or horizontal lines that structure the form on the screen. They may vary in style but serve to divide the form into logical sections and to direct data entry length and location. If several people have areas to complete, the data sets each person is to document should be presented in the order of completion. Different colors or shading can help to separate sections of the form visually. Horizontal frames on the screen are desirable for long sections of the forms that require free text. Vertical and horizontal frames should be aligned as much as possible to make the form less "busy" visually. Box titles or captions should be located to the upper left of the boxes in small font sizes. Check boxes (or radio buttons) and drop-down boxes are other time savers that conserve space. When check boxes are used, there should be consistency throughout the form, whether the boxes or lines are to the immediate left or immediate right of the caption. These should be aligned vertically when appropriate. The box or line to check should be very close to the caption so that the person performing the documentation checks the correct line or box.

If data are to be entered on a computer screen and then printed on a preprinted paper form (e.g., billing form, patient care plan form), refer to the vendor or machine specifications for correct data placement. If the form is not designed appropriately, data will not be printed in the exact locations required on the form. Discussing such specifications with a printer or the purchasing department is important in all aspects of form design.

COMPUTER APPLICATIONS

In this section, several examples of administrative and clinical applications that are typical components of HISs are reviewed. Health care organizations today are heavily involved in acquiring or developing these applications and bringing them together in the electronic health record.

Administrative Applications

Administrative applications include those that operate the daily business functions in the organization. These typically include an MPI; an ADT system; the business functions carried out in health information management departments such as abstracting, release of information management, coding/ grouping and chart tracking; and enterprise resource planning (ERP) systems. ERP is the term given to a variety of applications that support materials management, general ledger, accounts payable, grants accounting, and payroll. In addition, decision support or executive information systems (EISs) are considered integral to the administrative domain.

Admission, Discharge, and Transfer System

The ADT system is an example of a core administrative system. A basic module contained in both inpatient and outpatient HISs, this application collects the initial set of data that is used to establish a "record" of a new visit in all affected hospital departments, to establish and update the MPI, and to modify and track the patient until discharge. It serves as an interface to almost all other departmental systems, so it is important to understand how the data are captured and stored in the database. The HL7 standard has defined a series of transactions to identify the types of action that can be used to create, update, or delete records from the ADT database. Some of the basic HL7 functions that are defined for an ADT system are as follows[15]:

- A01—Admit a patient
- A03—Discharge a patient
- A04—Registration
- A08—Update patient information
- A13—Cancel discharge

The ADT system houses most of the patient demographics, including financial information that will be needed to create the patient's entry into other applications. Typical data included in an ADT system are shown in Table 8-2.

In addition to basic demographic information such as name, address, and telephone number, the ADT system collects information on the patient's insurance coverage, the emergency contact for the patient, and, most often, the admitting diagnosis or chief complaint.

Table 8-2 EXAMPLES OF ADMISSION, DISCHARGE, AND TRANSFER DATA

Demographics	Insurance Information	Visit Information
Patient name	Name of insured	Patient ID (medical record number)
Patient Social Security number	Relationship to patient	Attending physician
Date of birth	Primary insurance	Referring physican
Sex	Subscriber ID	Financial class
Patient address	Plan code	Admit date and time
Marital status	Secondary insurance	Discharge date and time
Patient account number	Subscriber ID	Service location
Emergency contact	Plan code	Patient visit type

The ADT system can be used to accomplish the following functions:

- Create and update the institutional MPI
- Generate census displays
- Notify transcription services of the patient's status (for report distribution)
- Indicate insurance authorization for precertification
- Pass demographic data collected on a previous visit to outpatient scheduling systems to facilitate clinic appointments
- Notify and send visit data to local applications such as cancer registries

At the point of discharge, it generates similar notification to the necessary departments so that the information for that case can be closed. Notifications initiated for new activities such as room setup and materials ordering begin when the patient is discharged. The same notice generated from ADT can activate record-tracking modules and quality monitors for follow-up action in the health information management area.

Decision Support Systems

Decision support systems are information systems designed to support planning functions of an organization. They range from simple analysis of cost per patient for specific departments or clinics to high-level strategic analysis, marketing, and policy development. They draw from multiple databases to analyze the day-to-day business activities of the organization. The data found in an administrative decision support system consist mostly of feeds from financial, ADT, and medical record abstract systems. In the last section of this chapter, an example of a decision support system is presented in the form of a data mart.

EISs are a subset of decision support systems. An EIS is a system that extracts data from institutional databases; the data are then analyzed, reorganized, and reformatted for presentation in summary format. Designed so that administrators and senior executives can view a "snapshot" of summary and trend data, these systems focus on financial "readings" that allows both summary and trend data views and the options of drilling down to detail. Some examples of reports that would be contained in an EIS include the following:

- Average length of stay (LOS) for the past 12 months
- Average daily census
- Average number of recovery days for accounts receivable
- Net revenue and expenses by financial class for the past two quarters
- Number of same-day surgery procedures by day for the past quarter
- List of latest patient satisfaction survey results by nursing unit
- Geographically represented map of all of the acquired physician practices

Clinical Applications

A clinical system is any system that is involved either directly or indirectly with patient care. Table 8-3 lists some of the types of clinical systems either within a department or throughout the enterprise. Clinical systems are not currently regulated by the Food and Drug Administration (FDA), but continuing debate and legislation suggest that they might be regulated in the future.[14]

It is important to understand the specific capabilities of each type of clinical system. This section presents results reporting, order entry, clinical decision support, and point-of-care systems as some examples. Understanding the functionality of these applications will enable us to arrive at

Table 8-3 EXAMPLES OF CLINICAL APPLICATIONS FOUND IN A HEALTH INFORMATION SYSTEM

Laboratory	Radiology	Pharmacy
• Chemistry	• Diagnostic	• Orders
• Hematology	• Scanner services	• Medical administration record
• Microbiology	• Special procedures	• Discharge summary
• Immunopathology	• Nuclear medicine	
• Blood bank		
• Pathology		
• Cytology		
• Autopsy		

Cardiology	Nursing	Operating Room
• Echocardiograms	• Documentation	• Scheduling
• Electrocardiograms	• Assessments	• Resource utilization
• Nuclear cardiology	• Discharge orders	• Anesthesia notes
• Cath lab	• Progress notes	
• Cardiac rehabilitation	• Material management	

better technological solutions. Some of these solutions are discussed in the next section.

Results Reporting

Results reporting applications are modules designed to retrieve diagnostic test and treatment results from feeder systems such as laboratory, radiology, and other departmental settings such as transcription and present them directly on inquiry to the care provider. Results reporting usually includes a **graphical user interface (GUI)** for viewing laboratory results, ECG results, and other reports with use of graphics displays such as flow sheets. Results reporting is often the hospital's first attempt at providing electronic health record functionality or an initial comprehensive clinical information system. Implementing a successful results reporting system as the first phase of an electronic health record system can greatly assist in further EHR implementation. Physicians, nurses, and other care providers must see results that are timely and dependable if they are to develop an allegiance to computer-based data in general.

A results reporting system should include patient demographics (sent from the ADT system); a list of results available, usually sorted by date; and some minimal information to identify the report further. For example, it would be preferable if the first screen presented the patient's name, medical record number, attending physician, ordering physician, date of test or treatment, and a brief description of the test or treatment. It could include whether the laboratory test was done in the hematology or microbiology laboratory or whether the radiology report refers to a chest x-ray study or a computed tomographic (CT) scan.

There must also be a method for identifying corrected or revised results in the results reporting module. This becomes extremely important for data integrity. The results reporting module will almost replace the typical telephone call to the laboratory for a result or a paper review of a chart. Usually, most laboratory tests are stored with an **ascension number.** This is a unique identifier that identifies the specimen. Several tests can have the same ascension number because the same specimen is used to run various types of tests. However, the ascension number can be used to record the result in the results reporting system, and when a correction is received, it can overwrite the display of the previous result. Without a unique identifier, it would be difficult to identify the result that is to be modified in the results reporting system.

Order Entry

Order entry systems are designed to organize and communicate order processing functions to all personnel involved in the care of a patient. Originally driven by and connected to charge capture, they have evolved significantly and currently include order management functions, clinical event detection, and managed care initiatives support. In an HIS, **order entry** refers to on-line entry of orders for drugs, laboratory tests, and procedures, usually performed by nurses or unit clerks.[3] Most health care organizations are now implementating computerized physician (or provider) order entry (CPOE) systems, particularly for medication orders. This type of system will be discussed later in this section. In most facilities, the orders are initiated at the nursing unit (usually by physicians) for diagnostic tests and treatments. However, the order can be transcribed several times—once by the physician writing the order, once by the unit secretary to transcribe it on an approved hospital form, and then again by the pharmacist when the order is received in the pharmacy. The goal of the order entry system is to capture the order electronically only once.

In the interim, until the perfect world is achieved, many systems have adopted order entry systems used by nurses and unit clerks. They have been quite successful. See example of how an order entry system may function.

Example of Order Entry System

An order for a diagnostic radiology examination is entered through an order entry system in a hospital. The order is transmitted to the radiology system that will ultimately house the result (or report) for this test. Data noting date, time, patient demographics, and any special conditions are imported into the radiology system. The radiology system does not have to re-enter any of the information that was already collected from the patient when the order was initiated. All orders for a given day may emerge on a worksheet for the radiology department personnel to follow as they set up and execute a day's schedule. Once the work is completed, the result of the test is recorded locally and then transmitted back to the ordering source so that hospital personnel can view the status of the order and either see a result directly or follow up if appropriate. The result may be a message that an examination is complete and will be available at a specified time, or it may be the actual report. At the same time, the necessary charges for services provided to the patient are captured.

Now the basic function of order entry can be extended to include order management features. For instance, some order management systems also have an "autocomplete" function that allows the user to type the first few letters of a word that matches the desired order name. The system then searches for potentially matching terms from the possible choices and provides the user with a "pick list" of order names, from which the user can select. This is a feature that is borrowed from word processing software and e-mail systems, which also have this capability. For example, typing "potass" into an order system would return a list of possible choices including "potassium."

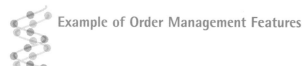

Example of Order Management Features

An order placed for a thyroid-stimulating hormone (TSH) test is received by the laboratory system and compared with data already collected for that patient in the laboratory system. The comparison shows that the same analysis was completed recently. The system invokes a standard message to the ordering location; the unit clerk may call the physician to reconsider the need for the order. This example is one of adding intelligence to the order entry system to avoid overuse of laboratory services. In fact, the current focus on such systems is to build them so that such interventions are standard features.

Computerized Provider Order Entry

In the ideal situation, a provider would place the order through the order entry system, and a clinical decision support system would validate the order and send it to the receiving service. If any clarification is needed, the provider can respond immediately. This is often termed a computerized provider order entry or CPOE system. CPOE refers to a variety of computer-based systems that share the common features of automating the ordering process and that ensure standardized, legible, and complete orders. It was shown as early as 1998 that a system like this can serve as an intervention tool to prevent adverse events such as medication errors.[16]

A CPOE system functions by having the user log in in with a user name and a password. After the CPOE application is initiated, a patient is selected. The user enters and modifies orders by using an electronic "notepad" that holds orders but does not deliver them immediately to the ancillary department. The user then reviews and edits the pending orders on the "notepad" and accepts the orders, and the order is sent to the ancillary department. There is no paper generated during this process. CPOE systems are usually designed with a hierarchical selection of orders with departments (i.e., pharmacy, radiology, laboratory) being the first level of entry. The second level of entry is the type of test or medication that needs to be ordered, such as a chemistry test or an intravenous medication. The third level of entry would then be the specific test or medication found in the second level. The process is designed to guide the user to making the correct selections for each order.

CPOE systems require a data dictionary that contains all the valid ordering selections and components. Each department maintains its own data dictionary and coordinates the entries with users in other departments. For example, the data dictionary contains an entry defined as "orderable" for an intravenous medication used for pain management. The user would select this medication from the list of orderable medications. However, within the data dictionary is a listing that defines what components are found in that medication. It is the individual components that are then sent to the pharmacy for dispensing. The CPOE system should not disrupt the usual workflow of how the clinician would perform the same order on a paper form.

Benefits of physician order entry include process improvement, cost efficiencies, clinical decision support, and optimization of provider time in many ways, including the following:

- Elimination of lost orders
- Elimination of ambiguities caused by illegible handwriting
- Check for potential drug-drug or drug-allergy interactions
- Alerts to physicians of high-cost tests and drugs before their actual use
- Access to on-line pharmacy and laboratory reference sources

Most important, these systems continue to serve can serve as an intervention tool to prevent adverse events such as medication errors.[17]

Clinical decision support features within CPOE systems can also promote implementation and enforcement of local hospital policies. The Regenstrief Medical Record System, a CPOE system developed by McDonald and colleagues at Indiana University, successfully used computer reminders to increase discussion about, and completion of, advanced directives (end-of-life, "do not resuscitate"—related orders).[19]

Clinical Decision Support Systems

Clinical decision support systems (CDSS) can be characterized as systems that provide diagnostic investigation tools and clinical guideline advice to patient care providers. Most CDSSs have become part of an existing system, such as the provider order entry system described in the previous section. Basic clinical decision support provides computerized advice regarding drug doses, routes, and frequencies, and more sophisticated CDSSs can perform drug allergy checks, drug-laboratory value checks, and drug-drug interaction checks and can provide reminders about corollary orders (e.g., prompting the user to order glucose checks after ordering insulin).

Another class of CDSSs is an automated alert system. This type of system notifies providers of potential adverse events. The intent of this type of system is to signal the physician that there is a potential problem and provide an opportunity for intervention. Generally, these systems have three different types of alerts: critical laboratory alerts, physiological alerts, and medication alerts. When an alert condition is detected, an application formats a message and transmits it by phone, pager, or fax to the medical team.

The transmission of these alerts is usually in the format of the Arden syntax. The **Arden** syntax language for medical logic modules (MLMs) allows encoding of medical knowledge (e.g., laboratory values, medication orders). The ASTM has adopted Arden as standard E31.15. It will be included in future implementations of HL7 as well.[19] See the following example of a CDSS.

Example of a Clinical Decision Support Alerting System

Each hour a list of patients who are receiving certain medications that are stored in the pharmacy database is queried against the laboratory system to determine whether any of these patients have abnormal laboratory values that may be caused by the use of the medications. The results of both the pharmacy and laboratory queries are then analyzed by a CDSS. Depending on the system, the physician who ordered the medication may receive an alert by pager or e-mail to log onto the HIS for a message. The idea of a decision support system is to provide guidance, not to actually make the decision in place of a physician.

Another class of decision support systems is an **expert system.** An expert system is a program that symbolically encodes concepts derived from experts in a field and uses that knowledge to provide the kind of problem analysis and advice that the expert might provide. Expert systems provide the capability to perform tasks that would be carried out by an expert in the field. The expert system is dependent on a **knowledge base** that is a collection of stored facts, heuristics, and models that can be used for problem solving. One example of an expert system is the software developed to help residents and interns move through steps designed to identify a specific diagnosis. The user is prompted to enter each of the patient's symptoms, and using the knowledge that it has already learned, the expert system suggests several working diagnoses for that patient. Identified as resources to strengthen the diagnostic investigation, evaluation, and treatment processes, these programs are seen as powerful tools for clinicians. At the same time, challenges arise in updating and maintaining the knowledge base needed for these types of systems to be successful.

Point-of-Care Systems

A **point-of-care system** is a system by which data are captured at the place where the care is provided. One of the most common examples is a bedside terminal system designed for patient data capture. These systems are located where the patient is receiving care, such as the bedside, or they are carried around by the caregivers, such as hand-held devices. As the use of hand-held and other devices expands, more options are available for entering data while in the presence of the patient.

Table 8-4 REPORT FUNCTIONS AVAILABLE IN A POINT-OF-CARE SYSTEM

1. Vital sign flow sheet with an overlay of medication history
2. Vital sign flow sheet identifying all caregivers who entered data on that patient showing date and time
3. View of the medical administration record
4. Detailed view of how a patient is following a specific protocol or clinical pathway
5. View of on-line nursing notes

In bedside terminal applications, nurses capture information about the patient directly—often through "smart" **templates** that prompt users to enter the information that is required for both documentation and coding. These systems are intended to minimize nursing data entry time and to ensure consistent and legible documentation.

Point-of-care systems also incorporate data read from bedside monitoring devices and transmitted into the computer directly. Examples would include data from ventilators, vital signs, and input and output balances (I/O). These systems can be found in ICUs, where a great volume of data is collected and monitored for each patient.

In an automated point-of-care system, the vital signs flow sheet, I/Os, fluid levels, and laboratory results are all calculated and recorded automatically on the patient's electronic chart. Table 8-4 lists some of the functions found in a point-of-care system. The tasks that can be automated in a point-of-care system include the following:

- Nursing assessments
- Nursing care plans
- Flow sheets
- Medication administration record (MAR)
- Data collection, calculation, and recording from bedside and home-based devices such as glucose monitoring devices

EMERGING TECHNOLOGIES

Bar Coding

Bar code technology is a replacement for traditional keyboard data entry. It requires that an identifier be converted to machine-readable identifier that that be printed on or attached to an item that can be read by a scanner and fed into a computer. Bar codes have been used in other industries, such as retail, for many years. Health care is a more recent user of this tool. The most common areas that bar codes are used in health care are in medication administration, materials management, and forms processing. Often, the forms contained in the medical record will contain a bar code to electronically scan the document into an optical disk system.

The application of this technology can be found in almost all departments. Examples of this include the following:

- Patient wristbands contain a bar code representing the patient identification (medical record number or name)
- Supplies used in diagnostic tests and operating room procedures that are consumed during the process can be scanned. This will enable inventory tracking and charge creation.
- Radiology films and laboratory specimens will contain bar codes for tracking of results delivery
- Medications given on the nursing unit have bar codes on each dose
- Patient invoices can have the bar code printed on the remittance portion of the bill to increase accuracy when posting patient payments
- Medical record forms contain a bar code to indicate the type of form (i.e., progress note, order sheet, discharge summary)

The format of the bar code is determined by **symbology.** Symbology is the term used to describe the font in which a machine-readable code is written.[20] Bar codes have printed bars and intervening spaces that define the output. The type and number of characters encoded, the print quality, and the amount of space available for the bar code determine which symbology is most appropriate. The two most common symbologies found in health care are code 39 and code 128. Code 39 produces a long bar code, whereas code 128 produces a denser bar code that will fit in smaller areas. Code 128 is the preferred symbology for patient wristbands, pharmacy packages, blood products, and laboratory specimens.

Bar codes always start with a special character, or symbol, that tells the machine scanning that bar code to start the reading process. The start character will also tell the reader what bar code symbology is being used. A bar code always ends with a special character, or symbol, called a stop character, that tells the reader that this is the end of the bar code. Some bar codes also require a **checksum.** A checksum is a special character that is added to the bar code. The checksum tells the bar code reader that the bar code is correct. The checksum character is read by the bar code scanner, but it is not passed along as part of the data. The checksum must be printed after the data and before the stop code.

Below is an example of a code 128 bar code for a patient with medical record number 000345 that will be placed on a discharge form numbered 06-996.

The pharmacy is heavily dependent on bar codes because the FDA has required all medications to have a bar code.[21] Contained in the bar code would be the National Drug Code (NDC), lot/control/batch numbers, and the drug expiration date. The regulation covers most prescription drugs and certain over-the-counter drugs. The rule also requires machine-readable information on container labels of blood and blood components intended for transfusions.

Radiofrequency Identification Device

A radiofrequency identification device (RFID) is a chip that is embedded in a plastic wristband or card. It is a means to store a greater amount of information locally that can travel with a patient. Currently, up to 1 megabyte of information can be stored on an RFID chip.

RFID tags contain antennas to enable them to receive and respond to radiofrequency queries from an RFID transceiver. There are three types of RFID tags: passive, semiactive, and active. A passive tag draws all its power from the radio waves transmitted by an RFID reader. A semiactive tag uses a battery to run the microchip's circuitry but not to communicate with the RFID reader. An active tag is powered entirely by battery to send and receive RFID information.[22]

RFID tags require a reader similar to bar code scanner, but the reader can read the chip content within 20 feet. There are no-line-of-sight requirements. The major advantage of the RFID chip is that is able to have write-many capability. Therefore it is feasible for a patient's allergy information to be contained on an RFID chip and, when this information changes, the RFID can be updated. Previous technologies were not able to handle changing information.

Internet and Web Services

The **Internet** has had a tremendous impact on the availability and accessibility of health care applications. There is no one central computer that runs the Internet. Rather, the Internet is equivalent to a network of networks. The Internet began in the 1960s when researchers began experimenting with linking computers to each other through telephone lines. This research was funded by the U.S. Defense Department Advanced Research Project Agency (DARPA). As the system, known at the time as ARPAnet, grew in size and volume, work was done to establish a protocol to transmit data among the networked computers. This is how the TCP/IP protocol was developed.

Today, the Internet is made possible through creation, testing, and implementation of Internet standards that determine how the network should function. These standards are governed by a nonprofit organization called the Internet Engineering Task Force (IETF) with oversight from the Internet Society.[23,24] This organization defines all of the technical aspects of the workings of the Internet. Further, the World Wide Web Consortium or W3 (*www.w3.org*) is responsible for managing the textual standards discussed in the next section.

Fundamentals

The workings of the Internet rely on software called a browser, which resides on the user's PC or workstation. Browsers are examples of client software. Examples of browser software are Microsoft Internet Explorer, Netscape Navigator, and Mozilla Firefox. The user of the browser does not have to know any technical details of where the data exist because the browser handles all the connections, display features, and security. Browsers can run on almost any type of operating system. This enables programs and data that might have been created on one computer and operating system to be displayed on a different computer with a different operating system. Web browsers are often found on thin-client devices because the requirements to run a browser on the client side can be programmed to be minimal.

The Internet adheres to the TCP/IP protocol for transmission of data, as discussed in the previous section. The IP component of the protocol refers to a unique network address that is assigned to each computer on the Internet. The specific algorithm assigned to the transfer of data through Web browsers is the Hypertext Transfer Protocol (HTTP).[25] HTTP determines how information is formatted and transmitted and what action browsers take in response to commands. S-HTTP is an extension of the HTTP protocol to allow data to be sent in a secure mode. S-HTTP was developed to transmit individual messages between the browser and the server. It does not secure the entire connection, just the transmission.

Internet Tools

Several tools are available for preparing documents to be viewed through a browser. The following are three types of Internet tools.

1. HTML—Hypertext markup language
2. SGML—Standard generalized markup language
3. XML—eXtensible markup language

HTML is the most common format used for structuring documents on the Web. HTML was created to give information on the Web an easy-to-read screen. It is designed to structure documents and makes the content accessible through a browser. HTML is well suited for distributing information such as on-line references because the content is displayed in the same style each time it is accessed.[26] A word processing document posted directly to the Web could not display properly any special structure such as titles, headings, and paragraphs. HTML makes use of *tags* that define the text that is contained in them. For example,

⟨B⟩ This will be bolded ⟨/B⟩

is the notation used to indicate that the text after the tag is to be displayed in boldface type until the closing tag. In the following example, a bold tag is given for the heading "History and Physical." Other examples of tags are as follow:

- ⟨P⟩ begins a new paragraph
- ⟨TITLE⟩ puts the name of document in the title bar
- ⟨img src="imagefilelocation"⟩ places an image in the document

Following is an example of a generic history and physical report as it would appear in HTML.

Example of a Generic History and Physical Report Appearing in HTML

⟨HTML⟩
⟨HEAD⟩
⟨TITLE⟩ ABC Physician Specialists⟨/TITLE⟩
⟨/HEAD⟩
⟨FONT SIZE=2⟩⟨ALIGN="CENTER"⟩ABC Physician Specialists⟨/P⟩
⟨P ALIGN="CENTER"⟩121 Main Street⟨/P⟩
⟨P ALIGN="CENTER"⟩Anytown, ZZ 12345-6789⟨/P⟩
⟨/FONT⟩⟨B⟩⟨FONT FACE="Times Roman" SIZE=4⟩⟨P ALIGN="CENTER"⟩History and Physical⟨/P;⟩
⟨P⟩ ⟨/P⟩
⟨/B⟩⟨/FONT⟩⟨FONT FACE="Times Roman"⟩
⟨P⟩NAME: John Doe⟨/P⟩
⟨P⟩UNIT#: 123456⟨/P⟩
⟨P⟩DATE: 12/01/2000⟨/P⟩
⟨P⟩DOC: Mary Brown, MD⟨/P⟩
⟨/FONT⟩⟨FONT SIZE=2⟩
⟨P⟩ ⟨/P⟩
⟨P⟩CHIEF COMPLAINT:⟨/P⟩
⟨/HTML⟩

During a document exchange, a browser requests a document from a WWW server and displays the document on the user's display device. If the first document contains a link to another document, the browser retrieves and displays the linked document.

A WWW server may receive and process an HTML form and then initiate a program to complete a specific action. This program that runs on the WWW server is called a common gateway interface (CGI) program. A CGI program is usually written in a scripting language such as Perl or a programming language such as C, C++, or BASIC. The CGI script is stored on the HTTP server so that when an HTML document is requested the server can tell that the file contains a program to be run, rather than a document to be displayed by the browser. When the program executes, it prepares an HTML document on the basis of the results of the CGI script. The HTML document is then sent to the browser in the usual fashion. CGI scripts are used extensively to integrate databases with the Web. Figure 8-4 illustrates

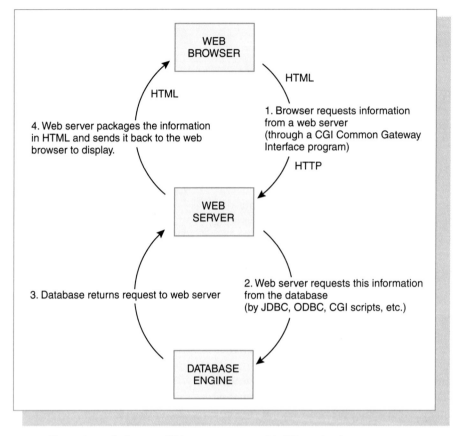

Figure 8–4   End user to Web server request with CGI mechanism.

how a WWW server running the HTTP protocol with a CGI script processes a user query.

HTML does have certain limitations. First, the language lacks expandability. The set of tags that can be used to identify text and images is limited. It is not possible to create additional tags to accommodate special formatting needs. Second, HTML treats the entire document as a single representation. In other words, HTML lacks any intelligence about items or fields in the document. It can process a form but not specific data elements that exist in the form. It does not make a distinction between forms and fields. Third, it lacks the ability to validate the information in the document. For example, HTML would not be able to process directly a request to view only inpatient data. That specific request would need to be handled in the CGI script. The CGI script would include commands to prepare the HTML document to be returned to the user. The HTML document, without the CGI script, could not understand how to filter data from the document. In summary, HTML is designed mainly as a presentation tool for information; it was not designed to process information.

HTML is actually a subset of SGML. SGML is a standard governed by the International Organization for Standardization (ISO)-8879. SGML is used more frequently to manage large documents that need to be printed in different formats. It is suited for documents that have the same content but are to be formatted for different purposes. It is built with a document type definition (DTD), a document describing its own grammar. In other words, the DTD allows the definition of specialized document type. For example, mailing addresses might have a DTD defined for an envelope and a separate DTD defined for printing on a sheet of labels. SGML was developed in the printing industry for editing and revising documents on a typesetter. It has many features that are not applicable to Web documents, which makes it somewhat difficult to use it for the Web.

Equipped with more Web functionality is **XML,** which is a language that is growing in popularity because of its advanced features.[27] XML still makes use of many of the HTML conventions but includes additional capabilities to enhance its functionality. XML is being used in the ASTM Standard for the Continuity of Care Record. This standard is intended to facilitate the transfer of certain data content among providers who are caring for a patient.

In a large EHR system with millions of patients, there is a great need for a single, easy-to-handle language capable of displaying only the patient's name and complete blood cell count. Likewise, this defined tag allows a result from a database query to be placed directly in the Web document at the proper location. XML allows a user to define new tag and attribute names. Tags can be invented to describe the type of information that resides within the tag. This enables a search to be done within the document to find only the patient's chief complaint. Using the preceding example, the XML version would be as follows:

⟨xml version="1.0"⟩
⟨LIST⟩
⟨PRACTICE____NAME⟩ABC Physician Specialists ⟨/PRACTICE____NAME⟩
⟨PRACTICE____ADDRESS⟩121 Main Street ⟨/PRACTICE____ADDRESS⟩
⟨PRACTICE____CITY⟩Anytown, ZZ 12345-6789 ⟨/PRACTICE____CITY⟩
⟨REPORT____TYPE⟩ History and Physical ⟨/REPORT____TYPE⟩
⟨PATIENT____NAME⟩ John Doe ⟨/PATIENT____NAME⟩
⟨UNIT____#⟩ 123456⟨/UNIT____#⟩
⟨DATE⟩ 12/01/2000⟨/DATE⟩
⟨PHYSICIAN⟩: Mary Brown, MD⟨/PHYSICIAN⟩
⟨CHIEF____COMPLAINT⟩ Shortness of Breath ⟨/CHIEF____COMPLAINT⟩
⟨/LIST⟩

JAVA

JAVA is a programming language introduced in late 1995 by Sun Microsystems.[28] It could have been discussed in the previous section on programming languages, but its purpose is more closely related to the Web. It is thought to be less complicated than the C programming language. The main objective of a JAVA program is to allow applications to be built as stand-alone ones that can be transferred across the Web and run independently on a client computer. JAVA is an object-oriented language that is compiled into a universal, non-machine-dependent format. Other programming languages such as COBOL or C++ require the compiled code to reside in the native mode for a specific processor. JAVA can run on any platform; it requires only that a JAVA compiler be resident on the client. A JAVA compiler is part of the browser software. JAVA applications are referred to as "write once, run anywhere."[29]

JAVA allows programs, called **applets,** to live on top of HTML pages. Applets, which run on the client side, are more efficient than CGI scripts. CGI scripts tend to run slower as the number of users accessing a Web page increases, which puts additional burden on the Web server. An applet might exist for a nursing unit to calculate the appropriate dosing for a medication given the patient's recent laboratory values. The JAVA applet would be available through the user's Web browser. After the user clicks on the submit button, the JAVA applet is downloaded to the user's machine temporarily and performs the calculations in real time. A device that is capable of running JAVA is also called a Java virtual machine (JVM). A network computer, as discussed in an earlier section, might be considered a JVM.

Another piece of JAVA is a **servlet or server-side scripting.** A servlet functions much like an applet but resides on the server side, not on the client. A servlet is much more efficient than a CGI script because it executes itself on the web server. It handles multiple requests simultaneously. Servlets functions by having the user's request run directly on the Web server to generate dynamic HTML pages. This technology is generally used to provide interactive Eeb sites that interface to databases or other data sources. The major advantage to servlets is the ability to highly customize the Web page on the basis of the user's access rights or database queries. Examples of server side scripting languages would be Active Server Pages (ASP) and PHP languages.

Intranet

An **Intranet** is like an Internet that runs exclusively within a network. It is accessible only by users who can be authenticated as being within a specific network. Intranets have become popular for communicating and sharing an organization's policies and procedures. For example, the corporate project tracking system might reside on the Intranet so that all the employees can update and view their project plans. The organization would not want this information available to users outside the organization. Another use would be to post the organization's employee handbook. This enables employees to have an updated reference manual with search capabilities, which would be difficult to obtain in a hard-copy form. There is no longer a need to publish and distribute these types of documents and be concerned with distributing updates to the employees.

Virtual Private Network

A **VPN** or **Extranet** is much like an Intranet, but it allows users outside the network to gain access to the network through a password. It would be equivalent to an access control list for a health care application. For example, a third-party payer might set up a Web site that contains information regarding claims processing but wants it to be available only to its current providers or those with whom it has a contract. The data should be available only to authorized and authenticated users.

Another component of a VPN is a demilitarized zone or **DMZ.** This is a network area that sits between an organization's internal network and the VPN. The DMZ allows outside organizations to access the area while protecting the network from possible intrusions into the internal network. Connectivity is allowed from the internal network to the DMZ, but no access is allowed from the DMZ to the internal network. Applications using a DMZ include mail and Web services as well as file transfers. Many of the outsourced medical record transcription services use a DMZ to transfer files to and from the dictation system to the transcription system.

TELEMEDICINE

Telemedicine is "the use of medical information exchanged from one site to another via electronic communications for the health and education of the patient or health care provider and for the purpose of improving patient care."[30] Telemedicine can refer to a diverse collection of technologies and clinical applications. The term "telehealth" was originally used to describe administrative or educational functions related to telemedicine. Now that physicians use e-mail to communicate with patients, and drug prescriptions and other health services are being offered on the Web, "telehealth" is generally used as an umbrella term to describe all the possible variations of health care services using telecommunications. The term "telemedicine" more appropriately describes the direct provision of clinical care by telecommunications—diagnosing, treating, or following up with a patient at a distance.

Examples of where telemedicine is used today include the following:

1. Providing a specialist referral service to geographical areas where there are not many medical specialists.
2. Performing patient consultations of audio or video to be exchanged between the patient and the physician. This consultation will take the place of a face-to-face visit.
3. Enabling remote patient monitoring for use in testing of blood glucose levels and measuring daily weights in home-bound patients.
4. Providing consumer health information to patients to participate in Web casts and other interactive video with experts in the field.

There are broad and different types of telemedicine technologies, which can include the following:

- Facsimile
- Audio
- Still images
- Full-motion video

Telemedicine is useful for situations in which physical barriers prevent the ready transmission of information between physicians or patients or the availability of information is key to proper medical management. Examples of telemedicine applications would occur in teleradiology, dermatology, pathology, behavioral health, and home health services. Telemedicine offers many benefits—better access for patients in rural and underserved areas, reduced travel time for health care providers, and improved techniques for medical education.

Fundamentals

One of the requirements of a telemedicine system is appropriate **bandwidth.** Bandwidth is a measure of how much information can be transmitted simultaneously through a communication channel. It is measured in bits per second (bps). The telemedicine system uses the available bandwidth to transmit the various forms of information that are necessary to complete the telemedicine interaction.

There are several different types of telemedicine interactions that vary in complexity. The simplest scenario might have the optical disk system at a hospital transmit images, text, and other data to a physician at home. The physician would require little bandwidth or specialized equipment. Second, a medical education course might be given from a hospital location to students who may be scattered throughout the region. A one-way video would enable the students to view the lecture; a two-way real-time video would enable the students to view and participate in the lecture. The instructor could transmit sound, video, text, images, and voice to multiple classrooms simultaneously. Minimum bandwidth for this type of interaction would be moderate to high.

Medical consultations are another service for telemedicine. The basic consultation could involve having a specialist review still images or video clips with text information. In this interaction, data could be transmitted on a low bandwidth because the data would be sent and then reviewed at a later time. This type of interaction is sometimes referred to as **store and forward** technology because the data are initially gathered and then sent at another time. The second type of consultation would incorporate real-time telephone voice interaction in addition to the images and video clips and would require greater bandwidth. Finally, the consultation could use real-time interactive video. This would be applicable to reviewing cardiology videos such as cardiac catheterizations or echocardiograms. It would require significant bandwidth.

Implementation

The use of telemedicine has increased with technologic advances, but there are still a few technical and administrative issues to work through for successful implementation. One of the obstacles for use in teleradiology is the size of the images that need to be transmitted. According to the American College of Cardiology's Cardiac Catheterization Committee, a 1-minute angiography image can range from 450 to 2700 megabytes, depending on the resolution.[31] Transmitting this amount of data, before data compression, could take hours to download the information.

Advances in **data compression** have greatly helped to overcome this barrier. Data compression is a mathematical technique that applies formulas to a file to produce a smaller file. Files are compressed by eliminating strings of redundant characters and replacing them with more compact symbols. If data compression is able to reproduce the original file exactly, the compression ratio is said to be **lossless.** If the compression causes some information to be lost in the translation, the compression is **lossy.** Depending on the amount of loss that the user is willing to tolerate in the output, typical compressions of 20:1 to 50:1 are possible.

Each multimedia file that is transmitted in a telemedicine application requires a utility that will both compress the file and decompress it on the receiving end. This is accomplished by using a mutually agreed on coder/decoder (CODEC). The operation of a CODEC is similar to the way a modem is used to connect to a personal communicator. It translates analog transmissions into digital ones and compresses the signals.

A second obstacle is the lack of bandwidth to transmit the image itself. A typical office LAN can support transmission at 10 Mbps, but that is usually not sufficient for a telemedicine application. Most telemedicine applications need to have fiberoptic or FDDI networks in place to deliver timely and sufficient data

Telemedicine faces several administrative barriers that are still undergoing regulatory review. The major issue today concerns the reimbursement of telemedicine services. In July 1997, Congress agreed to reimburse telemedical consultations for rural Health Personnel Shortage Areas (HPSAs) and those done with live two-way videoconferences.[32] Partial Medicare reimbursement for telemedicine services was authorized in the Balanced Budget Act (BBA) of 1997. Reimbursement expanded in 2000 with the Benefits Improvement and Protection Act of 2000 (BIPA). Store and forward consultations are currently not reimbursed except in Alaska and Hawaii. The Medicaid insurance project does not reimburse for telemedicine services; however, some states are authorizing the delivery of this service.

There is also an issue regarding physician licensing and medical liability. Because physicians are licensed by the state in which they practice, there is a question of what constitutes "practicing."[33] It is not clear whether providing telemedicine services from another state is considered practicing medicine. Physicians also need to review whether their malpractice insurance covers telemedicine services. Again, the increase in these regulatory constraints would make it difficult to attract and retain qualified physicians for a telemedicine program.

Finally, there is concern regarding patient confidentiality and security. From a security standpoint, it is a concern that the networks used to transmit patient data are not secure enough or do not have the proper encryption technologies to ensure patient confidentiality.

COMPUTER SECURITY

The substantial growth in the use of software, network technology, and the Internet has made it necessary to establish policies and procedures for protecting the data. This section discusses the technical approaches that are available for data security. This section presents three topics:

(1) technical components that are found in a secure information system, (2) the functionality required in an application to ensure proper data access, and (3) examples of organizational policies that can protect information systems from unauthorized use. Other examples of protecting the privacy of health information are found in Chapters 5 and 15.

The increased use of HISs has intensified both the amounts of data that are available electronically and the functionality to link the data to an identifiable person. The goal is to guard against inappropriate use without compromising the caregiver's "need to know." Often, the computerized version of the information is all that exists and denying access or making access impossible would have serious patient care consequences. Most systems that have tight security also have a "break the glass" option that allows a user who is not typically authorized to access a certain database or individual's record with that opportunity. When the "glass is broken," an automatic review of why the access took place is triggered. If there is a legitimate reason for access, no problem exists and there are no consequences to the individual who "broke the glass." There is a constant struggle for information system administrators to achieve a balance between protecting patient confidentiality and the cost of creating and implementing security mechanisms.

The costs of security can be viewed as both direct and indirect. Direct costs include the cost of purchasing and installing the security measures, which could be hardware or software or both. In addition, there is the cost of training and staff development of employees who are responsible for maintenance. Indirect (and harder to quantify) are the costs associated with the additional training of the user population to understand the security measures, the extra time required to modify the current operating procedures, and ultimately the cost of preventing access to an authorized user by mistake.

The National Library of Medicine asked the Computer Science and Telecommunications Board of the National Research Council to examine ways to protect electronic health information. The study began in 1995 and ended with the issuance of a report in 1997.[34] Some of the key practices that the committee recommended are as follows:

- Individual authentication of users
- Access controls
- Audit trails
- Disaster recovery
- Protecting of remote access points
- Protection of external electronic communication

The Health Insurance Portability and Accountability Act (HIPAA) of 1996 issued the Security Standards for the Protection of Electronic Protected Information.[35] The security standards were completed and promugated after the HIPAA privacy standards were completed and promulgated. The privacy standards are supported by the security standards. The security rule became effective as of April 2003, and most covered entities needed to be in compliance by April 2005.[36] This standard lists four general rules for security:

1. Ensure the confidentiality, integrity, and availability of all electronic protected health information the covered entity creates, receives, maintains, or transmits.
2. Protect against any reasonably anticipated threats or hazards to the security or integrity of such information.
3. Protect against any reasonably anticipated uses or disclosures of such information that are not permitted or required.
4. Ensure compliance with this regulation by its workforce.

Covered entity is defined as any group that transmits electronic protected health information. This includes health plans, health care billing companies, or health care providers. HIPAA applies to all covered entities, from the one-person physician office to the insurance company with thousands of employees. The security rule is organized into three categories, administrative safeguards, physical safeguards, and technical safeguards, containing 18 standards. The administrative safeguards require documented policies and procedures to protect electronic health information and the conduct of personnel handling this type of information. The physical safeguards relate to the protection of the physical systems, including hardware and software. The technical safeguards pertain to processes that control and monitor access to the information. Table 8-5 lists the elements of the HIPAA security rule.

The standards do not specify specific technology that the organization needs to implement. Instead, the regulation lists the capabilities that the organization needs to have in two categories—required or mandated and addressable or suggested. Mandated items include a risk analysis and management plan to assess and reduce potential risks and vulnerabilities, a sanction policy to handle violations of those who do not comply with the security policies, and an information system activity review. It also requires that the organization have a data backup plan, a **disaster recovery plan,** and an emergency mode operation plan.

It also requires that each system have a unique identification code for each user. In some instances, organizations previously used a shared login for access to systems.

The standard requires an emergency access procedure for obtaining necessary electronic protected health information during an emergency, such as if an emergency department physician's password did not function when needing to check a patient's electronic health record. This process is called a "break glass policy." **Break glass** (which draws its name from breaking the glass to pull a fire alarm) refers to a quick means for a person who does not have access to certain information to gain access when necessary. Systems containing primary source data (information) for treatment must develop, document, implement, and test *break glass* procedures that would be used in the event of an emergency requiring access to electronic information.

Authentication Tools

We examine in greater detail some of the authentication tools available. **Authentication** is the process of verifying or confirming the identity of a user who is requesting access to the information. This procedure has existed for many years in medical records departments with the paper version of the medical record. The user in need of the information has to present a valid form of identification to prove that he or she is entitled to receive the information. Authentication techniques need to be established in electronic form just as before the electronic age.

Authentication is usually based on various criteria:

1. Something that you know (password)
2. Something you have (a key, credit card)
3. Something that is a part of you (your fingerprint, DNA sequence)
4. Something indicating where you are located

Passwords

Passwords are a common part of everyday life. They exist for many types of operations from home security systems to access to library resources. Users, if not regulated or policed, tend to use common words or phrases for passwords. Passwords are sometimes shared among coworkers. However,

Table 8-5 SAFEGUARDS OF THE HEALTH INSURANCE PORTABILITY AND ACCOUNTABILITY ACT SECURITY RULE

Administrative Safeguards §164.308	Physical Safeguards §164.310	Technical Safeguards §164.312
Security management process	Facility access controls	Access control
Assigned security responsibility	Workstation use	Audit controls
Workforce security	Workstation security	Integrity
Information access management	Device and media controls	Person authentication
Security awareness and training		Transmission security
Security incident procedures		
Contingency plan		
Evaluation		
Business associate contracts		

technology can assist with certain steps to enforce proper use of passwords to keep them secure:

- Require the user to show photo identification to obtain the initial password or if the password is forgotten. Do not send passwords in the mail (electronic or United States) or provide over the telephone. For remote sites where providing photo identification might not be possible, a designated employee can be assigned at the site to be responsible for distributing the information to the user.
- Implement password aging on the operating system. **Password aging** is the term given to the process where users must change their passwords at a specific frequency (e.g., 30 days, 90 days). This enables the passwords to remain unique and identifies users who do not log in for a period of time.
- Install a password history file on the operating system. A password history file keeps a record of all of the previous passwords of a specific user. The physical file needs to be kept in an encrypted form so it can be viewed only by the system utilities.
- Allow only one log in per user identification at a time. The user should be allowed to log in to only one session. This helps to identify and monitor the sharing of passwords.
- Disable accounts after a maximum number of log in attempts. Failed log in attempts assist in identifying unauthorized uses of a password.
- Implement an automatic log out policy so that after a certain period of inactivity (e.g., 10 minutes, 30 minutes) the session is automatically disconnected from the system.

Single Sign-On

Many organizations are adopting the use of single sign-on technology for its clinical applications. This technology enables the user have one password to access multiple different systems. It is common for a health care worker to have five to ten different user names and passwords to access information. The goal of single sign-on is to only have one user name, usually the network sign on plus one password.

The most popular technique of implementing single sign-on is **CCOW** or Clinical Context Object Workgroup.[37] CCOW is a standard written and adopted by the HL7 group. It is vendor independent. The "clinical context" refers to having the information obtained by to CCOW to be of the same patient. In other words, a query of John Smith's pharmacy information on the pharmacy system will enable the user to obtain the laboratory results on the same John Smith. CCOW does not permit the user to view any other records on the secondary system, just the records that belong to the same patient that was accessed during the initial query on the initial application.

Tokens or Cards

A token is the size of a credit card and displays a number that changes each minute. Each user card generates a unique sequence of numbers and, through an algorithm, assigns the user access privileges for an application. The computer system incorporates the same algorithm in its authentication mechanism. Because the holder of the user card and the number sequence is unique, the number sequence is used as the session password for that computer system. If the number being generated is seen by an outsider, it needs to be synchronous with the holder of the card. There is discussion about using encoder rings instead of cards for the same purpose. The problem with cards is that they can be lost, stolen, or duplicated. The use of a token plus a password is called **two-factor authentication.** This authentication protocol requires two forms of authentication to access the system. This is also called strong authentication. A common example of this protocol is the use of a bank card to withdraw monies from an automated teller machine. The card is the physical item and the personal identification number (PIN) is something known only to the user. Deploying this technology requires that the organization's software applications have the capability to read the token sequence and the user password. Older applications are still written to accept only a user password.

Biometric Devices

A **biometric** is a unique, measurable characteristic or trait of a human being that can be used for automatic recognition or identity verification.[38] A biometric device is capable of analyzing human characteristics for security purposes. Examples would be fingerprints, retinal patterns of the eye, or speech scans. The primary advantage of using these types of devices for granting access to a computer system is that it is not possible to forge identity. The disadvantages are that the device may fail and prevent an authorized user from gaining access to the system. Because device failure has such serious consequences, implementing this type of security requires around-the-clock maintenance.

Access Controls

Each information system should have the ability to control which users can access the system and what a user can view. The term used to describe this is role-based access control (RBAC).[39] This type of control may also be referred to as a "need to know" basis. Usually, access is granted on the basis of two criteria:

1. The role of the user
2. The permitted roles for specific information access

The role of the user is usually defined by position or employee status. Table 8-6 shows an example of user roles found in a hospital information system. Within the access control, there are functions to determine the types of actions each user role can have. Usually these functions include (1) access to read the data, (2) access to write to the data, (3) access to change the data, (4) access to delete the data, and (5) access to change or override the access list itself. Table 8-6 also includes the permitted roles for each of the users.

Table 8-6 EXAMPLES OF ROLE-BASED ACCESS CONTROLS

Position	Hospital or Pharmacy System			
	Create	Modify	View	Authorize
Pharmacist	Y	Y	Y	N
Pharmacy technician	Y	N	Y	N
Nurse	N	N	Y	N
Attending physician	N	N	Y	Y
Consulting physician	N	N	Y	N
Home health nurse	N	N	Y	N
Social worker	N	N	N	N

Y, Yes; *N,* no.

The major obstacle to this type of implementation is developing a mechanism for a role that needs access on two different levels. For example, a unit nurse might need access to patients only at a certain location but on weekends might cover for the ICU nurse. The ICU nurse role is defined differently than the unit nurse role. The system needs a method for accommodating these special situations. In addition, the system should have the capability to override the standard settings in case of an emergency.

The creation and maintenance of RBAC lists is a difficult task. It requires collaboration among information security personnel, human resources, clinical administration, and others. Some organizations have a data protection officer to oversee these activities. Maintenance items include tracking when a user has changed roles or left the institution or when the role itself needs to be modified. Some RBAC utilities can receive a data file from the organization's payroll system that can aid in identifying users who might have changed positions or left the organization. Some users may have multiple roles, for example, a physician has a particular panel of patients that she is treating but she is also a member of the Quality Improvement Council (QIC). As a member of the QIC she is asked to review a set of clinical records and some administrative reports. The QIC role allows access to different data and information than the role associated with her panel of patients.

Reporting Capabilities

It is helpful for the information system to generate reports of user activity and role-based access lists for the various applications on a periodic basis. This helps to monitor and protect the system security. ASTM has a Standard on Audit Trails that provides some useful ideas for auditing and creating reports. Examples of security reports are as follow:

Examples of Security Reports

1. Show all users logged in and from what location or domain.

2. Show all users who have not logged into the system in the past 3 months.
3. Show all users who have access to delete records.
4. Show all users who have tried to log in unsuccessfully more than once.
5. Show all users who are defined in the role of "pharmacist."
6. Show all changes made to the role-based access lists and by whom.

Physical Security

Most networks have a central area where the servers, terminals, modems, and so forth are stored; access to this area must be controlled and the area must be locked at all times. Access cards should be granted to employees who maintain and support this hardware. There should also be a log of all employees who have entered the area.

When disposing of outdated computers, the data that reside on the disk should be entirely cleaned off by not only deleting the information but also cleaning the data from the disk. Files can be easily undeleted if they are not wiped clean. Similarly, dispose of all diskettes, tapes, and other storage devices properly. Again, the data protection officer should be able to assist in carrying out these functions.

It is also important to keep a detailed database of the inventory and configurations of the existing hardware. This information helps in identifying missing equipment and is useful if the internal configuration has been altered. An inventory consisting mostly of mainframe computers is fairly straightforward, but tracking individual PCs in various departments is a challenge. Users can easily add to or change the PC configuration without the knowledge of the information systems personnel. It is even more difficult to track the inventory for areas such as home health or patient education when most of the users work in remote locations. It is important to develop a policy and procedure for inventory control purposes to help prevent theft.

External Controls

Firewalls

The technology used to control access to the HIS network is growing in sophistication. Most of it is controlled by a **firewall**. A firewall is a system to prevent access to a private network from the outside or to limit access to the outside from within the network. Firewalls can be implemented by using hardware or software or a combination of both. The concept is basic—all data that enter or leave the organization's network must pass through the firewall. The firewall acts as a filter, providing a single point of entry to a network. Software can then analyze the incoming or outgoing data to determine whether they are appropriate and should be granted access to the network. A firewall is maintained by the system administrator, who is responsible for implementing the organization's policy on network access.

There are several types of firewall solutions:

1. **Proxy server**—Intercepts all messages entering and leaving the network so that the network address is hidden. A proxy server might be installed in an organization so that all outbound network traffic is sent and controlled through a central location.
2. **Packet filter**—Examines data entering or leaving and accepts or rejects the data on the basis of system-defined criteria. For example, all requests from an Internet address not associated with the organization could be denied.
3. **Application gateway**—Allows only certain applications to run from outside the network. This is applicable if an organization wants to prohibit outside entities from transferring files to its network. In this instance, the file transfer service would be restricted to users defined in the firewall software configuration.

See the example of firewall configuration and modification.

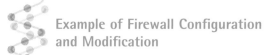

Example of Firewall Configuration and Modification

The hospital's outpatient dialysis clinic has been outsourced to a private, nonprofit organization. The organization has a computerized patient record system for the patients seen at its dialysis clinics throughout the country. The system physically resides in the corporate database at the main office in Tennessee. The patient care providers for these dialysis patients are still based at the hospital and need access to the computerized patient record in the corporate database. Currently, the dialysis organization does not allow network connections from outside the organization. To provide access to the clinical data, the system administrator at the dialysis clinic has modified the firewall configuration to accept connections from the hospital network. This type of example is a common one and is usually handled on a case-by-case basis.

Encryption

Encryption changes readable text into a set of different characters and numbers on the basis of a mathematical algorithm. Computers on either end of the transmissions must have keys to encrypt the information being sent and then decrypt the text at the receiving end into the original text. One of the most popular forms of encryption is a **public key.** A public key is a key that the user gives to anyone he or she wants to receive the message. Web servers often have a public key available to the requester of a Web document. A private key is one that the user maintains and never gives out. Together, these two keys scramble, send, and then unscramble an encrypted transmission.

The Internet makes use of public key encryption by the use of a certificate authority (CA). A CA acts like an electronic notary public and verifies and stores the sender's public and private encryption keys. The CA issues a digital certificate or seal of authenticity to the recipient (usually the system administrator for the Web site). The recipient includes a reference to the digital certificate on its Web server to enable encrypted communications. See the example of the use of the digital certificate.

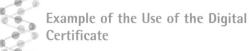

Example of the Use of the Digital Certificate

One of the local retail pharmacies would like to receive prescription orders and refills electronically. The new Web-based clinical information system in the ambulatory clinic has physician order entry capabilities, so the application is modified to include ordering to the retail pharmacy. However, the retail pharmacy needs to verify that the prescription was sent and authorized by the physician, and the physician needs to ensure that an authorized party received the order. In this scenario, the Web server in the ambulatory clinic would possess the digital certificate so that the retail pharmacy would be certain that the order came from a trusted source. The pharmacy would also access the Web server with a password to further protect access to the system.

Internet Security

To meet the need to provide encryption for connections to the Internet, the secure socket layer (SSL) protocol was initially developed by Netscape Communications Corporation.[40] Figure 8-5 illustrates how a Web server enables an SSL connection. An SSL connection allows the browser and the server of the Web transmission to authenticate identities and encrypt the data transfer. It ensures that the data came from the Web server it is supposed to have originated from and that no one tampered with the data while it was being sent. Web servers that support an SSL session have a Web address that starts with "https" instead of http. A remaining piece is left unsecured because the data are encrypted only during transmission between the two locations, and the data that reside locally on the client or server are still accessible in a nonencrypted format. HIPPA does require that all Internet transmissions containing patient data to be sent using, at a minimum, SSL to protect confidentiality. SSL works by using a private key to encrypt data that are being transferred.

Malicious Software Protection

HIPAA includes protection from malicious software (or **malware**) as one of the addressable components of the security regulation. The term "computer virus" is usually used to generalize malware, but computer viruses only represent one type of malware. Malware can be any unauthorized

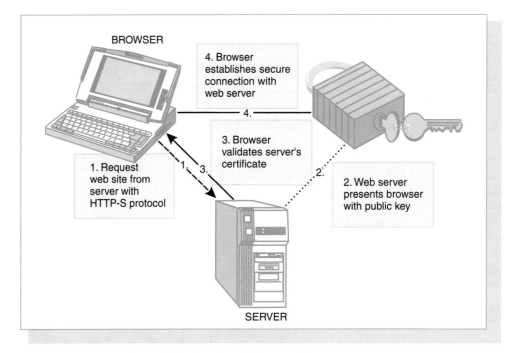

Figure 8-5 Example of SSL connection.

software that is found in an information system. Malware attacks often interfere with the computer's functionality and may cause loss or damage to software.

Types of malware include the following:

Masqueraders—Software that appears to be a part of the existing software but produces unwanted behavior. Examples of this software would be Trojan horses found in e-mail messages or macros that might be run in a word processing program. A masquerader could also be someone pretending to be the authorized recipient of sensitive data but who is not.

Incapacitation—The most common type of this software is a **denial of service** (DOS) attack. This occurs when the attacker overloads the targeted system by flooding it with data transmissions so that the target system becomes unavailable.

Corruption—A computer virus would be an example of corruption. If software is changed to perform a malicious activity without the user's knowledge, this would be a type of corruption. A recent development in this area is spyware. Spyware is software that is installed on a computer without the user's knowledge and that collects personal information from the user's computer and sends it to an unauthorized database.

Misuse—A computer worm will deliberately install itself on a computer connected to a network. The worm will then extend itself to every other computer on that network, either promoting DOS attacks or performing unauthorized acts. Worms can be found in e-mail

applications when a message is opened and automatically sends the worm to the e-mail server and then sends a second e-mail to every user listed in the mailbox directory.

It is critical that the organization have policies in place to deal with malware. Most organizations require that all computers run an antivirus software checker that screens all incoming email. Some e-mail servers will also run this software.

Viruses and worms typically infiltrate a PC by e-mail attachments or files downloaded from Web sites. Once they seize control of the computer, they can destroy critical files or disable the system. Some enable hackers to use the computer to send large volumes or spam or to attack specific Web sites. Viruses and worms have been known to spread by e-mailing copies of themselves to address book listings found in each PC.

Phishing is also considered a security threat. Phishing can be found in an e-mail message that appears to come from a legitimate business or organization requesting personal information such as an account number. The e-mail message contains a link to a Web site to submit the information. However, the Web site is not from the business or organization mentioned in the e-mail message but rather is a site designed to capture personal identifying information. These Web addresses often contain misspellings of business names or have logos or graphics similar to the business name. Once the user inputs his or her personal information, the phishers can use this information maliciously.

Application Service Provider Models

With the emergence of the Internet as a convenient way to access information from virtually any location, many health care organizations began using **application service providers** or ASPs. An ASP is a business that provides computer-based services to customers. The application software resides on the ASP network and is accessed by users through a Web browser. An ASP may offer functional services, such as billing and payroll management, to various types of businesses or may provide specialized services to a particular industry, such as medical transcription to a physician group. The health information management (HIM) professional will certainly be involved setting up the ASP operation as it relates to confidentiality and security of the organization's information.

General guidelines for using an ASP within the organization are as follow:

- The ASP owns and operates a software application.
- The ASP owns, operates, and maintains the servers that run the application. The ASP also employs the people needed to maintain the application.
- The ASP makes the application available to customers everywhere through the Internet.
- The ASP bills for the application either on a per-use basis or on a monthly/annual fee basis.

An ASP is an attractive option for medical transcription services. It is argued that it is more cost efficient to have an ASP operate the transcription system than to operate an in-house system. Economies of scale can be easily achieved because the software and hardware for transcription is a fixed cost. It usually costs the same whether five or fifty transcriptionists are using the system. Workforce shortages in this area also enabled organizations to go outside, even to other countries, to have transcriptionists working.

An organization's Web site could be run as an ASP model. Many ASPs provide Web hosting services that enable a customized Web site to reside on the ASP's Web server. This scenario is correct if the organization does not have full-time staff devoted to Web development or if the organization does not have the network bandwidth to support a busy Web site.

An advantage of an ASP is that there is a low cost to entry. There is no hardware or software to buy and the system can be operational rather quickly. There is no need to hire additional personnel to get a working system. The "pay as you go" model is also attractive for smaller organizations that cannot afford a large capital expenditure. Another instance where having an ASP would be beneficial is if the technology is highly specialized and the organization cannot support that. For example, if the technology requires an SQL database and the organization does not have the resources to hire a full-time SQL database administrator, it would be advantageous to have the ASP serve as the database administrator.

Some disadvantages to the ASP model is that the organization is making no investment in its own capital and resources. It is similar to leasing equipment when at the end of the lease period the leased equipment needs to be returned. There is also the possibility that the ASP could go out of business on short notice, leaving users without a working system.

It is important that the HIM professional be involved in selecting and negotiating the contract with an ASP. Because the information will be residing on the ASP network, it is critical that the ASP adhere to the organization's security and privacy policies. HIPAA requires that any ASP have a business associate agreement with the organization that clearly delineates the roles and responsibilities of the ASP's handling of protected health information.

DATA MANAGEMENT TECHNOLOGY

Throughout this chapter, descriptions of health care computer applications and technology were provided. The complex nature of health care almost always ensures that data will need to be integrated from various types of information systems. It requires substantial effort to provide effective data management that is useful to the health care organization. The effort requires expertise in database management, clinical data analysis, and technology assessment.

HIM professionals have an ideal skill set for directing and managing these types of projects. These projects require understanding of the technology, database management, and health care software applications and ensuring that the data are kept secure and are available only to authorized users.

This section explores two data management applications that are gaining popularity among most health care organizations—the data mart and data modeling or, as it is also called, data mining. Using an HIS for outcomes research can be a great tool, but a problem arises when the clinicians requesting the information lack the domain knowledge required for the specific databases.[41] Establishing a data mart removes some of the mystery of using databases for the health care providers. Figure 8-6 provides an illustration of how HISs interact with a data repository or data mart. Likewise, **data mining** encourages a broad view of all data for a set of patients to explore relationships among the data that might not be readily apparent during the initial hypothesis.

Data Mart

A **data mart** is a subset of data extracted from the larger database. It is not to be confused with the **data repository.** A data repository contains all or almost all the data in an information system. A data mart is a smaller application

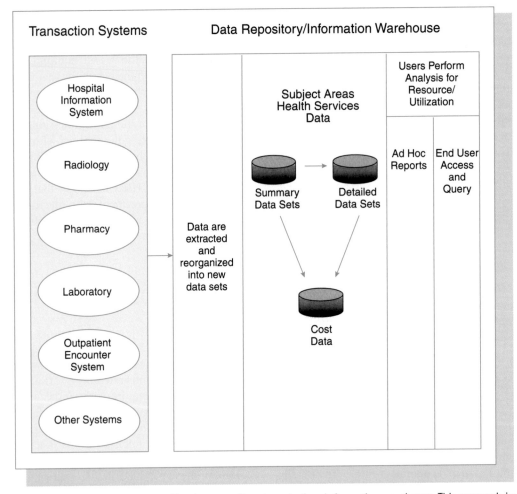

Figure 8-6 Feeding data for decision support. The data repository is part of an information warehouse. This approach increases the value of existing data stores and empowers end users to meet simple reporting needs through local workstations.

with a focus on a particular subject or department. A data mart has several advantages:

The unit cost of processing and storage is less than the unit cost of processing and storage in a large database.

The selection of a database model and technology can be tailored to the needs of a department.

The amount of historical data and level of granularity required for the data mart can be specific to the needs of the department.

Granularity is the term given to the level of detail in the data. For example, an ICD-9-CM code has finer granularity than a diagnosis related group (DRG). A DRG is a very broad category, and ICD-9-CM provides more specificity in the data.

BUSINESS CASE OF CREATING A DATA MART

The administrator for long-term care at a large health system is interested in tracking ancillary costs for all of the skilled nursing facilities in the system. The administrator currently receives monthly reports, but they do not allow

any further manipulation of the data or cannot incorporate outcomes data collected by the facility's case manager. In addition, the monthly report is not timely enough. The administrator would prefer weekly or perhaps daily uploads of the current data. The administrator and staff do not have the time to attend a week-long SQL class to learn how to query the data repository directly. There is also concern that the data capture methods for inclusion in the repository might be slightly different among the facilities. The administrator wants to be able to view the raw data and aggregate data as appropriate.

Table 8-7 contains a list of data elements that might be found in a data mart for a long-term care administrator.

Creating a Data Mart

Step 1. Define the scope. Determine, in collaboration with the end users, what purpose the data mart will serve and, just as important, what data analysis is outside the scope of the data mart. It is important to determine these in this step so

Table 8-7 EXAMPLES OF DATA ELEMENTS FOR A LONG-TERM CARE DATA MART

Cost Variables	Outcome Variables
Total cost	Mortality
Pharmacy cost	DRG
Physical therapy/speech therapy cost	LOS
Chemistry and hematology cost	Age
Medical procedures	Readmission to acute care
Room charges	Discharge disposition
Medical and surgical supplies	Ventilator dependent

that the project does not grow over time and result in the same functionality as the data repository. For instance, determine that the data mart will contain only inpatients discharged within the past 12 months. Analysis of outpatient activity will not be within the scope of this data mart.

Step 2. Perform a technology assessment to determine the selection of the most appropriate database model and architecture. As discussed earlier in the chapter, a relational database is the most commonly used model for data marts. This is because it is easier to add and modify the database structure and because several query language tools are already available to the end user. The architecture, however, requires some study. It needs to be determined whether it will be a small application that might be able to support a two-tier approach or whether the logic for the queries is complicated enough to warrant a three-tier approach and an application server. A hardware assessment within the user community also needs to be completed at this time. This helps to determine the parameters or size limitations that might have to be imposed on the application. It also enables decisions to be made about whether the client software is run as a thin-client or a thick-client application.

Step 3. Identify the data elements and best source. Analyze what types of data might be available initially and assess the data integrity. The data elements stored in the medical record discharge abstract might be more reliable and accurate than unstructured text captured on a form. It is important to document all of the decisions made at this point. It will be helpful to refer to this document as the project continues to develop.

Step 4. Develop and run the program for extracting the data elements. This procedure should be designed to run automatically at a given interval. It might be necessary to revise the run intervals if the data elements are collected from different sources. For instance, not all the financial data are available at the time of discharge. Several days are needed for late charges to clear. This type of special condition should be

noted when determining the extract schedule. Again, it is important to document and publish this as part of the project schedule.

Step 5. Perform any data cleansing or filtering. When data from different sources are combined, it is usually necessary to filter the data before it is imported to the data mart. The data might need to be converted to common units to support comparisons. For example, some incoming data might be expressed in hours and others for the same field expressed in minutes. Second, the end user of the data mart might not be interested in the lowest detail of data, so the data are aggregated and recoded if necessary. In a possible scenario, there are several ways to identify patients who died while in the hospital. In the data mart, there is only one field for mortality—a yes or no logical value. The data cleansing process will transform each of the coded elements in the hospital's database that represent died into the data mart logical value for mortality.

Step 6. Import the data into the data mart. This should be established as a routine procedure. After each import, quality control programs or queries need to be executed to ensure that the import was successful.

Step 7. Train the end users and solicit feedback on improvements or additional features.

Step 8. Maintain the data mart and establish a change-control form. The change-control form needs to be completed when any additions, deletions, or modifications to the data mart occur. This form provides documentation to the users and assists in any alterations that need to be made in the database structure.

Data Modeling

Another technique that the computer can assist with is identifying patient subgroups, a variation of data mining.[42] With a paper-based medical record, clinicians and other researchers were limited to analyzing the data that they knew about. For instance, an emergency department physician kept a log in the emergency department of patients treated for gunshot wounds. The physician's study was therefore limited to the cases that could be identified in the log.

Instead, a computer system can be used to identify the cases of interest. The first step is a broad definition of the study criteria, usually by ICD-9-CM code or some other structured data set. The researcher then reviews the cases and selects the final set of patients that meet the criteria. A statistical model is then constructed for the patient set and used to help locate additional cases. This cycle of modeling and classification continues until the user is satisfied that enough cases have been identified. See the example of a computer system identifying cases of particular interest.

Example of Computer System Identifying Cases of Particular Interest

A researcher is interested in the study of complications after kidney transplantation. The researcher is interested in all the things that happened to the patients after transplantation and wishes to determine whether any relationships exist among the patients. A query is written to identify all patients who received a kidney transplant procedure through the ICD-9-CM code (55.69). The first exclusion criterion is death on the same day as the transplantation. From the remaining cases, the computer generates a frequency distribution of the characteristics of these cases. Characteristics might include whether the patients received a certain drug, had an abnormal laboratory result, or received a blood transfusion. The researcher reviews the list and selects the characteristics that are important in identifying the proper set of patients with a complication. The data-modeling program will now restrict selection to patients meeting the revised criteria. The researcher adds characteristics to and deletes characteristics from the model after reviewing the on-line discharge summaries of the revised set of patients. The data-modeling program is run again to see how well the revised criteria performed in identifying the set. This cycle is repeated until an acceptable patient set is found. The model has retained the inclusion and exclusion criteria from the iterations so that, when presented with new cases, it will be able to recall lessons already learned.

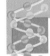

Key Concepts

- Why is the current focus on health information systems so strong? Will it affect the way work is accomplished? Quality and cost objectives drive information system development, and the rate of growth in health information systems is increasing. The computer has gone from being a tool to being a required part of any health care job. Users are demanding more sophisticated and faster tools for access and manipulation. More thought and planning are required to develop coordinated approaches that support new models of health information systems in the industry.
- What lessons have we learned from the past? History has provided key concepts for database models and information requirements of health care providers. Benefits of technology have been clearly demonstrated, and today major health information system components are geared to be used through tools largely targeted for widespread use.
- What knowledge will be required as we manage emerging technologies such as the Internet? Health information management professionals need to be well versed in the fundamentals of network technology, security, and Internet tools so that they can build on this knowledge as new technologies are introduced. Patient confidentiality

and medical record security issues will become more important as health information is stored in distributed environments rather than in one central location. Therefore, it is key that policies and procedures reflect the state of the technology environment. An understanding of how applications such as telemedicine are to be integrated into the work flow of the existing clinical information systems will be critical.

REFERENCES

1. Department of Health and Human Services: Health Information Technology Leadership Panel final report (March 2005): http://www.hhs.gov/healthit/HITFinalReport.pdf. Accessed November 11, 2005.
2. Department of Health and Human Services, Office of the National Coordinator for Health Information Technology: *http://www.hhs.gov/healthit/*. Accessed November 11, 2005.
3. Dick RS, Steen EB, editors: *Computer-based patient record—An essential technology for health care: Institute of Medicine report*, Washington, DC, 1997, National Academy Press.
4. Shortliffe EH, Perreault ME: *Medical informatics computer applications in health care and biomedicine*, New York, 2001, Springer.
5. Mandl KD, Overhage JM, Wagner MM, et al: Implementing syndromic surveillance: A practical guide informed by the early experience, *J Am Med Inform Assoc* 11:141-150, 2004.
6. Eclipsys Corporation: Eclipsys Corporate overview: http://www.eclipsys.com/About/PDFs/CorpFactSheet_GENERAL_WEB.pdf. Accessed November 11, 2005.
7. Dornfest S: History and impediments to progress in the development and implementation of the computerized patient record. Proceedings of the Health Information Management Systems Society, American Hospital Association, 1993, Miami Beach, FL.
8. Ball MJ, Jacobs S: Hospital information systems as we enter the decade of the 80s. *Proceedings of the IEEE Fourth Annual Symposium on Computer Applications in Medical Care*, New York, 1980, Institute of Electrical and Electronic Engineers.
9. Friedman CP, Altman RB, Kohane I et al: Training the next generation of informaticians: the impact of BISTI and bioinformatics—a report from the American College of Medical Informatics, *J Am Med Inform Assoc* 11:167-172, 2004.
10. U.S. Department of Veterans Affairs: VistA Monograph: http://www.va.gov/vista_monograph. Accessed November 12, 2005.
11. Date CJ: *An introduction to database systems*, ed 5, Reading, MA, 1990, Addison-Wesley.
12. oftware Engineering Institute: Client/server software architectures—an overview, 2004: http://www.sei.cmu.edu/str/descriptions/clientserver.html. Accessed November 11, 2005.
13. Software Engineering Institute: Three tier software architectures, 2004: http://www.sei.cmu.edu/str/descriptions/threetier.html. Accessed November 11, 2005.
14. Guidance for industry 21 CFR Part 11; electronic records, electronic signatures, electronic copies of electronic records: http://www.fda.gov/OHRMS/DOCKETS/98fr/03-4312.pdf. Accessed September 14, 2006.
15. Chapter 3 Admission, discharge transfer: http://www2.dmi.columbia.edu/resources/hl7doc/hl72.2/hl7chp3.html. Accessed November 11, 2005.
16. Bates DW, Leape LL, et al: Effect of computerized physician order entry and a team intervention on prevention of serious medication errors, *JAMA* 280:1311-1316, 1998.
17. Miller RA, Waitman LR, et al: The anatomy of decision support during inpatient care provider entry (CPOE): empirical observations from a decade of CPOE experience at Vanderbilt [electronic], *J Biomed Inform* October 21, 2005.

18. Dexter PR, Wolinsky GP, et al: Effectiveness of computer-generated reminders for increasing discussions about advance directives and completion of advance directive forms: a randomized, controlled trial, *Ann Intern Med* 2:102-110, 1998.

19. Arden syntax (March 2005): http://www.openclinical.org/gmm_ardensyntax.html. Accessed November 11, 2005.

20. Neuenschwander M, Cohen MR, Vaida AJ et al: Practical guide to bar coding for patient medication safety, *Am J Health Syst Pharmacy* 60:768-779, 2003.

21. Bar code label requirements for human drug products and biological products. 21 CFR Parts 201, 606, and 610. Docket No. 2002N-0204.

22. Federal Drug Administration: Radiofrequency identification feasibility studies and pilot programs for drugs (November 2004): http://www.fda.gov/ora/compliance_ref/cpg/cpgdrg/cpg400-210.html. Accessed November 11, 2005.

23. Overview of the IETF: http://www.ietf.org/overview.html. Accessed November 11, 2005.

24. Internet society mission statement (June 11, 1999): http://www.isoc.org. Accessed November 11, 2005.

25. Lee-Berners T: Hypertext transfer protocol design issues (1991): http://www.w3.org/protocols/DesignIssues.html. Accessed November 11, 2005.

26. Musciano C, Kennedy B: *HTML: The definitive guide,* ed 2, Sebastopol, CA, 1997, O'Reilly Associates.

27. World Wide Web Consortium: Extensible markup language (November 23, 2005): http://www.w3.org/XML/. Accessed November 24, 2005.

28. Sun Microsystems: New to Java center (2005): http://java.sun.com/learning/new2java/index.html. Accessed November 11, 2005.

29. Sun Microsystems: About the Java technology (2005): http://java.sun.com/docs/books/tutorial/getStarted/intro/definition.html. Accessed November 11, 2005.

30. American Telemedicine Association: Defining telemedicine: http://www.atmeda.org/about/aboutata.htm. Accessed November 11, 2005.

31. Singh M, Khandheria BK, Gura GM et al: Telemedicine links between developing and developed nations, *Ind Health J* 55:188-192, 2003.

32. Health Resources and Service Administration: Telemedicine reimbursement report: http://telehealth.hrsa.gov/licen/. Accessed November 11, 2005.

33. Wachter GW: Telemedicine liability: The uncharted waters of medical risk (July 2002): http://tie.telemed.org/articles/article.asp?path=articles&article=malpracticeLiability_gw_tie02.xml. Accessed November 11, 2005.

34. Committee on Maintaining Privacy and Security in Health Care Applications of the National Information Infrastructure, Commission on Physical Sciences, Mathematics, and Applications, National Research Council: *For the record: protecting electronic health information,* Washington, DC, 1997, National Academies Press.

35. Health Insurance Portability and Accountability Act of 1996, Pub L 104-191, 110 Stat. 1998, August 21, 1996.

36. Health Insurance Reform: Security Standards 45 C.F.R. § 160, 162, 164, 2003.

37. CCOW Information for the Health Care Industry: http://www.ccow-info.net/. Accessed November 20, 2005.

38. Biometric Consortium: Government applications and operations (1996): http://www.biometrics.org/REPORTS/CTSTG96. Accessed November 11, 2005.

39. National Institute of Standards and Technology: Role based access control: http://csrc.nist.gov/rbac/. Accessed November 11, 2005.

40. Onyszko T: Secure socket layer (July 22, 2004): http://www.windowsecurity.com/articles/Secure_Socket_Layer.html. Accessed November 11, 2005.

41. Coley KC, DaPos SV, Saul MI et al: Outcomes assessment in routine practice: use of an electronic medical records database, *Formulary* 34:52-57, 1998.

42. Cooper GF, Buchanan BG, Kayaalp M, et al: Using computer modeling to help identify patient subgroups in clinical data repositories, Proceedings of the AMIA Symposium, pp 180-184, Lake Buena Vista, FL, November 1998.

Information Systems Life Cycle and Project Management

Mary Alice Hanken
Gretchen F. Murphy

Additional content,
http://evolve.elsevier.com/Abdelhak/

Review exercises can be found
in the Study Guide

Introduction
  System Analysis, Design, and Implementation
    Initiation Phase
    Analysis Phase
    Design Phase
    Implementation Phase
    Evaluation Phase
The Players
  Role of the Health Information Management Professional
Project Management
System Life Cycles
  General System Life Cycle
  Information System Life Cycle
  Information System Life Cycles in the Organization
  Aggregate Information Life Cycle of the Organization
  System Obsolescence
Information System Development Life Cycle
  Principles for Systems Development
  Problem Analysis Basics
Analysis
  Tools and Aids for System Analysis
    Decomposition Diagrams—Hierarchy Chart
    Data Flow Diagrams/Process Modeling
    Data Dictionary
    Data Mapping
    Entity-Relationship Diagrams
    Computer-Aided Systems Engineering Tools
  Investigative Strategies for Analysis of Requirements
    Ways of Gathering Information
  Analysis Document
  System Design
    Logical and Physical Designs
  Design Principles
    Input and Output
    System Performance
Role of Prototyping in System Development
System Implementation
  User Preparation and Training
  Site Preparation
  System Testing and Conversion
    Test Phases
    System Conversion

Key Words

Benefits realization	General system life cycle	Prototype
Break-even analysis	Group decision support software	Request for information
Computer-aided software engineering	Hierarchy chart	Request for proposal
Cost-benefit analysis	Information system development life	Return on investment
Cost-effectiveness analysis	cycle	Scenario
Data dictionary	Information system life cycle	System design
Data flow diagram	Joint application design	System development life cycle
Data mapping	Logical system design	Use case
Discounted payback period	Payback period	
Entity-relationship diagram	Physical system design	

This is a revision of the chapter in the previous edition authored by Merida L. Johns.

Startup
    Abrupt Changeover
    Gradual Phase-In of Applications
System Evaluation and Benefits Realization
  Benefits Realization
  Cost-Benefit Analysis
    Break-Even Analysis
    Payback Period
    Discounted Payback Period
  Cost-Effectiveness Analysis
  Other Evaluation Methods and Techniques
Purchasing Process: Request for Proposal
  Request for Information
  Planning Steps Before Request for Proposal Preparation
  Analyzing System Requirements
  Development of System Specifications
  Development and Distribution of the Request for Proposal
    Disclaimer and Table of Contents
    Proposal Overview
    Enterprise Profile
    Conditions of Response
    Functional Specifications
    Technical Requirements
    Installation and Training Requirements
    Vendor Profile
    System Costs and Financing Arrangements
    Contractual Information, References, and Other Materials
    Distribution of the Request for Proposal
  Evaluation Criteria
  Demonstrations and Site Visits
    Demonstrations
    Site Visits
  System Selection and Contract Negotiation

Abbreviations

ADT—admission, discharge, transfer

ASP—application service provider

CASE—computer-aided systems engineering

CBA—cost-benefit analysis

CPOE—computerized provider order entry

CPT—Common Procedural Terminology

DFD—data flow diagram

EHR—electronic health record

EMR—electronic medical record

ERD—entity-relationship diagram

FTE—full-time equivalent

GDSS—group decision support software

HIM—health information management

ICD-9-CM—*International Classification of Diseases, Ninth Revision, Clinical Modification*

ICD-10—*International Classification of Diseases, Tenth Revision*

IT—information technology

JAD—joint application development

JRP—joint requirements planning

PERT—program evaluation and review technique

REG/ADT—registration/admission, discharge, transfer

RFI—request for information

RFP—request for proposal

ROI—return on investment

Objectives

- Define key words.
- Discuss similarities and unique characteristics among the various life cycles, including the general systems life cycle, information systems life cycle, and information systems development life cycle.
- Understand the impact on organizational resources of the juxtaposition of various information systems at different information system life cycle stages.
- Discuss the life cycle stages in Nolan's six-stage theory of information system development.
- Identify the three stages of the information systems development life cycle and the components of each.
- Apply techniques and tools, including hierarchy charts, data flow diagrams, data dictionaries, and entity-relationship diagrams, to perform information systems analysis and design.
- Understand and apply investigative strategy techniques for gathering information for system design and development.
- Evaluate information system interfaces from satisfying and efficiency perspectives.
- Describe the various techniques that are used to evaluate information systems, including benefits realization, break-even analysis, payback period, and discounted payback period.
- Describe the activities that take place during system implementation.
- Describe the purpose and content of a request for proposal.
- Describe the usual process that is followed in purchasing a vendor system.

INTRODUCTION

The manager of the clinical laboratory wants to replace the department's outdated information system to better manage information related to collecting specimens, tracking completion of laboratory tests, and reporting clinical test results. The radiology department director wants to install an information system that will help manage patient flow, track the completion of radiology tests, store transcribed radiology reports, and automatically retrieve patient demographic data from the hospital information system. The vice president for hospital human resources wants to purchase an automated system that will help manage information related to employee demographics, employment status, employee benefits, and salary administration. The director of health information management (HIM) plans to request the purchase or development of a system that will track the release of patient information and provide report generation capability.

The goal of all these managers is to use automation as an adjunct in helping them better manage information. Most of these systems will cost several thousands of dollars; the clinical laboratory and radiology systems may even cost millions of dollars. Considering the investment to be made, how can these managers be reasonably confident that the systems selected will meet the needs of their organizations and their various departments? If a stand-alone or special purpose system is considered, how will it be interfaced with existing and planned systems? Is it better to find a vendor who can offer an integrated system versus using many different vendors whose products each require an interface? How many vendors are using national standards to address interoperability questions? One strategy to help select appropriate systems is to follow a structured approach for analyzing user needs, identifying functional requirements that meet the user needs, choosing a system that has the required functionality, and implementing the system in an organized, well-thought-out manner.

Part of the health information manager's responsibility is to help analyze, design, select, and implement automated systems for patient-related and clinical data management on a departmental and an enterprise-wide basis. This chapter outlines a structured approach for accomplishing these tasks and provides tools to assist the health information manager to be successful in this process.

System Analysis, Design, and Implementation

Faced with the challenge of analysis, design, selection, or development and implementation of an automated system, the health information manager's primary goal is to provide a system that meets user or department needs and that also supports the strategic objectives of the enterprise. The basic system development life cycle is the process used to identify, investigate, design, select, and implement information systems. To assist in accomplishing this goal, the development process for an information system usually consists of five principal phases:

- Initiation phase
- Analysis phase
- Design phase
- Implementation phase
- Evaluation phase

Taken as a whole, these phases make up what is typically called the **system development life cycle.**

Initiation Phase

System initiation is the method by which organizations make decisions to invest in particular information systems. This leading effort is needed to understand what is involved in replacing existing information systems and in selecting new ones. Often performed in the context of the overall information technology strategic plan for the organization, the purpose of working through an initiation process supports an integrated approach to acquiring new products and ensures a clear identification of the project scope as a starting point. Goals, a budget, a schedule, and a statement of the problem as understood at this point are outlined. When the problem and the expectations are stated with an initial understanding, a baseline benchmark can be established against which the adjustments that always follow can be measured. The adjustments are tracked as the project progresses. Once agreement has been secured on the "problem" or the business opportunity to be addressed, then work can begin more definitively on the analysis phase. This phase affords early agreements with key users that will be valuable as the work progresses.

Analysis Phase

To provide an information system that meets user requirements, the health information manager must identify how an automated system can support the performance of user tasks. In fact, understanding the environment in which user tasks are performed is an essential part of the analysis phase and provides the context to formally identify user needs. Here, the business process and associated information are documented. The analysis phase lays the foundation and provides the map for **system design** and implementation. This is a detailed activity that includes the review of current practices, planned processes, and the associated functional requirements so that appropriate decisions can be made.

Several tools and approaches are available to help in the analysis process. Note that some of these tools may be used in a variety of management activities beyond a systems life cycle development process. Some of these are structured. Examples of structured development tools are graphic flow charts, decomposition charts, matrix tables, and data flow diagrams. These tools are useful in describing current practices, identifying problem areas, and mapping anticipated new processes. These tools are discussed in more detail later in the chapter.

Although the analysis process remains the underlying activity in developing and acquiring new applications, there are alternative approaches available. One of those approaches, a less-structured approach to identifying user needs, is the use of **prototype** systems. In this approach, a model or "draft" system is quickly developed to provide a preliminary model or early version application. Called a prototype, the system is presented to users and refined after initial use. Before the final product is achieved by use of this method, there may be several iterations of the prototype. On occasion, an off-the-shelf database program may offer sufficient capability to quickly put a prototype in place. Some organizations may use predesigned software that can be modified by in-house information technology (IT) staff. Others may contract with IT services. Another option is leasing packaged software from an application service provider (ASP). Health care organizations are making use of a variety of alternatives to keep pace with the demand for responsive information systems. The more structured process, however, is still the method of choice in most instances.

Design Phase

On basis of the findings or requirements that are identified in the analysis phase and on a decision to proceed, system design encompasses activities related to specifying the details of a new system. Typically, this includes making decisions about the logical and physical design of the system. Through the use of structured design tools such as **computer-aided software engineering** (CASE) programs, a systems blueprint is developed. This blueprint is analogous to an architect's blueprint and provides the basis for the physical system design. The physical design stage converts the system blueprint into specific detail so that computer code can be developed. In a health care setting, the traditional description of system design applies when the automated system is developed by a staff within the organization. However, in today's environment, health care organizations frequently purchase already designed systems from outside vendors. In these cases, the meaning of system design takes on a different perspective. It usually refers to the assessment of various characteristics of the design of the system rather than the development of the system itself.

Implementation Phase

System implementation involves making the system operational in the organization. Implementation characteristically covers a wide range of tasks including the following:

- System testing
- User training
- Site preparation
- Managing organization change and system impact

To achieve the primary goal of meeting user needs, the system must function efficiently and effectively. To minimize potential system defects and operational flaws, test data are constructed and entered into the system. The results of system testing are used to correct operational weaknesses and to make programming changes.

User training is an essential component for successful system implementation. If users are not proficient in system use, the effectiveness of the system is reduced. The element of user training is not always sufficiently emphasized, and plans for user training are often ill conceived and incomplete. Consideration needs to be given to how to organize the training effort, identifying and selecting the most appropriate training strategies for the task and users and developing the training materials or systems. In major implementations such as electronic health record (EHR) systems, user training is supported through available coaches who can serve as resource trainers around the clock as clinicians learn to work with new electronic tools. Also, "just in time" computer skills may be needed for clinicians and other staff who have limited experience with technology.

Evaluation Phase

The evaluation phase is important in any system development effort. Frequently, systems are developed and implemented but never evaluated to determine whether the original goals for implementation are met. Lack of evaluation can contribute to lack of realization of potential system benefits. Therefore, to achieve maximum benefits realization, all systems should be evaluated against predeveloped criteria and needs requirements.

THE PLAYERS

To proceed with a substantial information system project, a number of people need to get involved. Everyone in an organization from those who are in upper level positions who support the overall idea to those whose job may be substantially changed as the result of an implementation and, of course, those who will have a direct role in the project itself will be a player.

A project typically will have individuals who have an interest in the planned information system or perhaps in the existing information system. These individuals are called "stakeholders." A little closer to the project are those whose budgets fund the project and who must maintain it. These individuals or departments set priorities and policies and may also use the system and are called "owners."

The project will have a project manager who oversees the project. The project manager's role is using his or her knowledge and skills and the appropriate tools and people resources to bring the pieces together in a cohesive manner to meet the goals of the project. In an information system project the desired result is a functioning system that improves (more efficient, more effective) what it replaces and is completed within budget in a timely manner. There are excellent resources on project management and the typical responsibilities of a project manager.

The project is likely to have the following additional team roles assigned to individuals during the project phases:

Subject matter or "domain" expert—Provides information on what is actually happening or what should happen and the information needed in the process or product under development

Functional or "business" analyst—Captures the information from the subject matter experts, organizes it, and communicates it to the rest of the project team; lists requirements

Solutions architect—Converts the requirements into an architecture and design for the system being created

Development lead—Puts together the overall architecture on the basis of the work of the solutions architect and the developers

Developer—Translates technical specifications and algorithms into executable code

Quality assurance coordinator—Helps to develop cases and other means to test the system and verify that the system will meet the needs of the customers. The entry-level role is running test cases and scripts written by another quality assurance professional.

Deployment coordinator—Creates a program that can live in and work within a systems environment (i.e., configure changes, identify conflicting software, manipulate other components as needed); tests all the components to make the software work in an environment

Trainer—Creates the training materials for the users. Some of this training material may also be converted into help files and specific user instructions.[1]

The descriptions of these team roles are very brief, but they provide a clue to the skills and related tasks involved in each role.

Role of the Health Information Management Professional

Within a health care enterprise, the health information manager should be an advocate for use of appropriate strategies and tools that help ensure the development or selection of information systems that meet organizational needs. The health information manager usually chairs or serves on several information-related organization and department committees, including the following:

- Committees charged with enterprise-wide information management
- Information privacy
- Information security
- EHR systems
- Decision support systems
- Strategic planning for IT
- Departmental IT

As an advocate for effective system development or selection, the health information manager should assume a prominent role in the system development life cycle. Tasks assumed may vary from individual to individual, depending on specific job functions. For example, the director of an HIM department may assume overall responsibility for the analysis, design, and implementation of a departmental system. On the other hand, an HIM professional who has oversight for enterprise-wide clinical information systems may have responsibility for assisting clinical areas in carrying out the processes of the system development life cycle. The HIM manager may assume a more technical role and be responsible for direction and day-to-day operations of individual phases of the system development life cycle for a specific project. It is not unusual to see HIM managers leading project development teams for a variety of clinical and patient-related information systems. As noted in the list of project roles, the HIM professional could serve as a subject matter expert, as a functional analyst, as a quality assurance analyst, or as a trainer. Once again, the interests and specific background of the HIM professional will determine roles in any given project.

PROJECT MANAGEMENT

One of the crucial factors for ensuring the success of any project is the degree to which it is effectively managed. The systems development life cycle is no different from any other project. Success requires good planning, appropriate allocation of resources, and effective monitoring and control. Information system project managers may have a technical background or a management background.

The first step in project management is development of the project plan. One of the most crucial elements of the plan is the definition of the scope of the project. Identifying project scope identifies the boundaries of the project. For example, the scope of development and implementation of an order entry system would include considerations of interfacing with the laboratory, radiology, and pharmacy systems but would not include concerns with interfacing with a medical record chart tracking system. In the case of implementing a computerized provider order entry (CPOE) version of order entry, the team would also include physicians, nurses, and other care providers who would be users of the system.

A second crucial component of the planning phase is identification of project deliverables and activities. A deliverable is a tangible work product such as a computer code, documents, system specifications, a database design, and so on.

Once deliverables have been delineated, activities to support deliverable development must be identified. Good project management relies on breaking down the project into smaller and smaller activities. Frequently, a tool called the work breakdown structure is used to break the project into smaller and smaller activities. An example of a work breakdown structure appears in Table 9-1.

Table 9-1   SAMPLE WORK BREAKDOWN TABLE FOR DATABASE DELIVERABLE

Deliverable	Activity 1	Activity 2
Relational database	1.1. Data definition	1.1.1. Define data types
		1.1.2. Provide support for null types
		1.1.3. Provide support for primary keys
		1.1.4. Provide support for foreign keys
		1.1.5. Provide unique indexes
		1.1.6. Provide for multiple views
	1.2. Data model	1.2.1. Identify entity relationships
		1.2.2. Develop entity relationship diagrams
		1.2.3. Develop screen designs
		1.2.4. Develop extended entity relationship diagram
		1.2.5. Develop normal form relations
		1.2.6. Develop files
	1.3. Data dictionary	1.3.1. Define entities
		1.3.2. Define relations
		1.3.3. Define processes
		1.3.4. Define data stores
		1.3.5. Define data structures
	1.4. Backup and recovery services	1.4.1. Provide backup facilities
		1.4.2. Provide journaling facilities
		1.4.3. Provide recovery facilities
		1.4.4. Provide rollback of individual transactions
	1.5. Provide for security services	1.5.1. Password access
		1.5.2. Encryption
		1.5.3. View access

When activities have been identified, resources must be allocated to the project. Resources include budget, personnel, equipment, and materials. Part of resource allocation is identification of the project team and each team member's role and responsibilities. As is evident in the activities outlined in the database work breakdown structure, many different skill sets are needed to ensure that the project is efficiently completed. Individuals included as part of the team in this project would be systems analysts, database administrators, data administrators, system managers, technical writers, users, domain experts, and managers.

In addition to personnel, project resources include equipment, facilities, and materials. In the database project in Table 9-1, equipment would include computers, case tools, and printers. Facilities would include telephones and office and meeting space. Materials would include such things as office supplies and reference materials. Thus, a significant part of project planning includes identification of project deliverables, activities, and resources necessary for efficient project completion. These elements directly contribute to the development of the project budget.

Once deliverables, activities, resources, and budget are established for the program, a project schedule must be developed. The schedule incorporates project activities and personnel, identifying who will perform the activity and when the activity will be completed. Many computer-assisted tools have been designed to assist in development of the project schedule and overall management of project. Most of these tools include Gantt charts and various modifications of the program evaluation and review technique (PERT). These methods are described in other sections of this text.

When a project schedule has been completed, with deadlines, milestones, and personnel identified, the project manager can allocate resources to the project. This includes allocation of money, space, facilities, equipment, and people to the project. The project manager must ensure that there is appropriate resource leveling. This means that resources are appropriated only at the point in the project at which they are actually needed. Projects frequently exceed budget projections because personnel, equipment, materials, or facilities are allocated too far in advance of their need. On the other hand, project budgets can be exceeded when resources are allocated too late, thus holding up vital project activities.

Monitoring and control of the project are crucial components of the project manager's job. If the project is not adequately monitored and controlled, disastrous results may occur. Monitoring and control include tracking the schedule of the project and also include active intervention should the project either fall behind or exceed schedule. The project manager must be able to foresee problems and then readjust and allocate resources appropriately to ensure that deliverables are on time and within budget.

SYSTEM LIFE CYCLES

To appreciate fully the development of a system and its place within the organization, knowledge of the life cycle of systems is necessary. Like human beings, all systems go through a life cycle. Systems originate, develop, and, finally, decline. Several models have been developed that illustrate the concept of a system life cycle. In this section, four perspectives of system life cycles are discussed.

1. General system life cycle
2. Information system life cycle
3. Discontinuity of information system life cycle
4. Organization-wide information system life cycle

General System Life Cycle

Information systems are similar to biological, social, and political systems. All systems go through a system life cycle. All systems have a birth or development period, a period of growth, a period of maturity, and a period of decline or deterioration,[2] The following example demonstrates the four phases of the **general system life cycle.**

 Example of the Phases of the General System Life Cycle

BIRTH AND DEVELOPMENT (PHASE 1)
Ten years ago, the health information department of a community hospital implemented a system to track the release of information from patient records. The goal of the system was to allow health record employees to document the requests for information, the verification of those requests (as needed), and the description of the documents copied/released—to whom, why, when, and whether there was a charge associated with completing the request. The system was primarily a departmental system to meet the needs of this 300-bed facility.

GROWTH AND MATURITY (PHASES 2 AND 3)
In the intervening years, the hospital has formed several alliances that have broadened the scope of the services provided, and the laws related to release of patient-identifiable information have changed. Among the hospital changes is the expansion of outpatient services through acquisition of several clinics in the community, the addition of an outpatient surgery facility, and alliances with substance abuse, rehabilitation, and skilled nursing facilities. At first, the release of information tracking system was able to expand to keep pace with the institution's growing needs. However, as the hospital evolved into a health care enterprise, the needs for tracking and monitoring have changed. In addition, related laws have changed. For example, the Health Insurance Portability and Accountability Act (HIPAA) has specific regulations related to release of personally identifiable health information. In building the needed release of information tracking system, the organization will need to evaluate all the current and pertinent federal and state laws that apply to their particular organization. The HIM professional should take the lead in this endeavor.

DECLINE (PHASE 4)
The current release of information tracking system, which was designed primarily for internal departmental use, does not meet today's need for a more comprehensive, updated, enterprise-wide distributed system.

Information System Life Cycle

As the preceding release of information tracking example illustrates, information systems have a life cycle that is analogous to the general system life cycle. To be more definitive in describing what occurs at each phase in the **information system life cycle,** more descriptive labels are attached to each phase.[2]

- Design
- Implementation
- Operation and maintenance
- Obsolescence

For example, in the information system life cycle, the development phase of the general system life cycle is usually referred to as the *design* phase. This is the phase in which analysis of the requirements and design of the information system occurs. The general system life cycle growth phase is normally called the *implementation* phase. In this phase, development, testing, and implementation take place. The *operation/maintenance* activity of the information system life cycle is similar to the maturity phase of the general system life cycle. This is the functioning phase of the system in which activities to maintain, update, and operate the system occur. The fourth phase of deterioration or decline is identified in the information system life cycle as system *obsolescence.* Figure 9-1 shows a comparison between the phases of the general system and the information system life cycles.

The time over which each phase occurs varies from system to system. Large, complex systems may take months to years to design, whereas simpler, smaller systems may take a few weeks to design. The length of time over which a system can meet user needs depends on many variables. Sometimes these variables include a change in work volume, a change in strategic organizational objectives, or a change in the type of work performed. As the preceding release of information tracking system example illustrates, the system became obsolete because it could not accommodate a larger volume, different rules, and a broader range of users in a distributed environment.

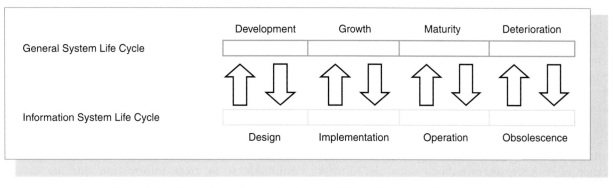

Figure 9-1 Comparison of general system and information system life cycle stages.

Information System Life Cycles in the Organization

An organization is composed of hundreds and perhaps thousands of interacting and interfacing information systems. For example, in a health care facility, there are information systems that support clinical functions, such as those that provide order entry, clinical monitoring, nursing care, dietary requirements, rehabilitation needs, and diagnostic testing. There are also information systems that support administrative functions, such as patient registration, billing, marketing, and human resources. All these systems use some type of IT to assist them in carrying out their functions. Given the number of information systems in any organization, it is easy to recognize that at any one time multiple information systems are in different phases of an information system life cycle. For example, the clinical laboratory system may be in the maintenance phase of the information system life cycle while the radiology information system is in the design phase of the information system life cycle. On the other hand, the HIM department tracking system for release of information may be in the implementation phase while the marketing information system is in the obsolescence phase. Thus, information systems throughout an enterprise are in a constant state of fluctuation (Figure 9-2).

It is unlikely that at any given time all organization information systems would be in a state of maturity. It is more likely that there will consistently be a significant level of variability in information system life cycles. Even when an organization purchases an integrated clinical and administrative system, the system will have a number of modules, and within the modules there may be basic and more advanced functionality. Therefore, the components of an integrated system may still be in different phases of the systems life cycle. Figure 9-2 shows the concept of information system fluctuation. It is important for the health information manager to recognize this variability because this phenomenon of discontinuity causes stress within the organization. This stress can be manifested in multiple ways. One aspect of stress is the competition for resources. There is competition for similar resources, including technical assistance (*people*) during approximately the same period (*time*) and use of the same hardware (*equipment*) resources.

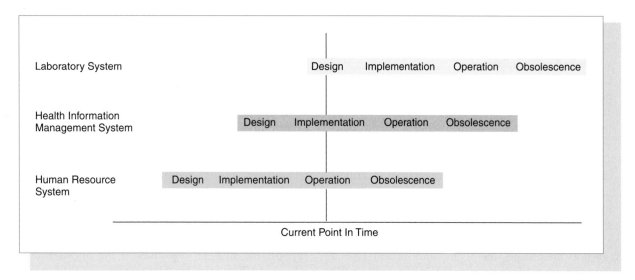

Figure 9-2 Comparison of departmental information systems at different life cycle stages.

There is also competition for financial allocation *(budget).* The HIM department needs technical assistance and training during the implementation stage of the release of information tracking system. The HIM department will then train other users in the organization. The clinical laboratory needs technical assistance in identifying system design. The human resources system requires technical expertise to perform the upgrade and may require a greater portion of the equipment resource. All systems bear some cost in regard to financial expenditure. Prioritization of needs and suitable allocation of resources are exceedingly important to meet organizational needs. It is, however, a significant challenge for the organization to balance the allocation of resources appropriately so that maximum benefit is realized.

Aggregate Information Life Cycle of the Organization

A logical question that might arise after the discussion of information system life cycles is whether the organization as a whole has a life cycle of its own. In other words, can a composite picture of an organization-wide information system life cycle be visualized if all information system life cycles are aggregated into a whole? This is an appropriate question because an organization's level of experience and sophistication with IT has an impact on how it manages the technology. For example, an organization that is just starting to automate its information functions would have a different emphasis in management of its technology than an organization in which most of the information functions were already automated.

Nolan[3] first described the concept of organizations that have information system life cycles. The view postulated by Nolan is that an organization at any given point in time is at a certain maturity or level of sophistication in deployment of IT. Nolan postulated the following stages in his organization-wide information system life cycle:

- *Initiation,* where the organization begins to automate information functions
- *Expansion* or growth of information automation, which is usually unplanned
- *Control,* where the organization tries to manage IT growth and control resources, primarily budget growth
- *Integration,* where the organization attempts to integrate distributed systems through organization-wide standards, policies, and procedures
- *Data administration,* where integrated databases are developed and information is considered a critical organizational resource
- *Maturity,* where growth of applications is focused on their strategic importance to the organization

At each of these stages, the organization usually takes a different approach to management of IT. For example, in the early stages of initiation and expansion, the organization is likely to assume a laissez faire attitude, allowing expansion of the technology with little or no organization-wide control. As the growth of technology expands, the organization becomes most concerned with budget, allocation of funds for technology expansion, and centralizing resources. In other words, the organization tries to gain control over the resources. As time goes on, the organization becomes more sophisticated in its management of the technology. The organization grows to realize the need for integration of technology and information management. In the stages of integration and data administration, the organization emphasis is to treat information and its associated technologies and management as critical to the survival of the organization. The main focus in these stages is to distribute functions but also to centralize standards for both technology and information management. In the final stage, maturity, the organization views information as a strategic resource and emphasizes development of applications that further the strategic advantage of the enterprise. At this point in development, the organization's IT planning will align with the business strategic plans.

Although it is important to understand that individual information systems have their own life cycles, it is equally important to recognize that an enterprise will also be at a certain stage of IT management maturity. Being able to identify an enterprise's point in its life cycle helps explain why certain policies exist or why specific strategies are deployed. For instance, if a health information manager works in an organization that is in the integration stage of the life cycle, the manager would likely have been part of developing centralized standards. This might be in areas related to the type of communication protocols, electronic signature tools, or documentation amendment approaches that are allowed. On the other hand, if the health information manager is employed in an organization in which technology is newly implemented, there may be few policies and procedures that help to direct information growth. Understanding at what stage of the information life cycle maturity an organization is helps the health information manager play a more effective role in the organizations system development process.

System Obsolescence

Information systems become obsolete for several reasons. A system may be obsolete because it uses older technology that cannot meet current information-processing demands. The use of older technology in itself does not necessarily mean that the information system is obsolete. Rather, it is whether technology meets required needs that determines obsolescence. Systems can also become obsolete because they cannot handle an increase in the volume of data or cannot handle more sophisticated data management tasks. Systems frequently become obsolete because they do not support the strategic objectives of the organization. The release of information tracking system described in the first part of this chapter is a good example. The strategic objective of the organization in that example was to provide a broader range of services at multiple, diverse sites. Because of the change in strategic objectives to include multiple distributed sites and the changes in the laws, the release of information tracking system could not meet the needs of the organization. Common examples of systems that quickly become obsolete are those in the area of administrative decision support. Decision support systems provide a variety of tools that help management in making decisions about semistructured and unstructured problems. Because the health care environment marketplace is changing at such a rapid pace, there is a need for accurate, reliable, and user-friendly decision support systems. Many decision support systems and their associated tools are not flexible enough to meet current demands for information access and analysis and quickly become outdated. Clinical decision support systems are also used to help make decisions about patient care. Some of these systems provide basic alerts, whereas others are very sophisticated. Again these systems require tending and rely on quality data. This is a growing area of health information systems, and today's expectations of EHR systems include the integration of real-time EHRs and clinical decision support tools. These decision support systems need to be updated regularly on the basis of determinations of quality-of-care profiles.

Sometimes information systems become obsolete because of a change in user expectations. For example, a hospital-wide information system may provide the necessary functionality for nursing care, but users expect the functionality to be enhanced in some way. The users might expect to be able to take their computer device with them, perhaps in their pocket rather than having to enter data at a central nursing station/terminal. As organizations work to advance health information exchange, new requirements for wide-area networks require a technology infrastructure that allows access from multiple external locations. Even a single user wants to be able to work from home or to use wireless technology to check on information. Many organizations have multiple work sites, and even if the organization itself does not have multiple work sites, health care providers are distributed. Care providers may be visiting a patient at home or simply working from an off-site location.

At the level of the user interface, another system improvement might elect to use color on the display screen to alert clinical providers to out-of-range laboratory values rather than using asterisks to mark such values. As users become more sophisticated about how information systems can help them perform their daily tasks more optimally and experience new ways to view data on workstations or on their hand-held devices, they are likely to expect system enhancements.

In addition to changes in technology, operational functions, strategic objectives, and user expectations, information systems may become obsolete because they simply wear out, in other words, break down. Mechanical failures with storage devices, input devices, output devices, or processing components are more likely to occur as the system grows older.

INFORMATION SYSTEM DEVELOPMENT LIFE CYCLE

Principles for System Development

The systems development life cycle is presented as a formal process. Everyone who undertakes a system development project wants to succeed. Therefore, discussions with colleagues and thorough research of existing systems—both highly successful and those that struggled, provide information for the planning and assessment process. Whitten et al[4] suggest eight principles to use with the systems approach and technologies. These principles are as follow:

1. Get the owners and users involved
2. Use a problem-solving approach
3. Establish phases and activities
4. Establish standards (documentation, quality, automated tools, IT)
5. Justify systems as capital expenses
6. Do not be afraid to cancel or revise scope (re-evaluate cost-effectiveness, feasibility, scope)
7. Divide and conquer (subsystems can be built into larger systems)
8. Design systems for growth and change

As a system project emerges, it is recommended that the first phase, the initiation phase, not be skipped or taken lightly. This phase is the opportunity not only to reaffirm that the project should go forward but also to carefully examine the problems, any significant reasons for proceeding and opportunities that occur as a result of having the system in place.[4] This is the time to set out project scope and objectives accompanied by a narrative to give context. Prepare a preliminary plan with an initial time table to be presented and negotiated. Assess the value of the project—the value may be monetary or it may be stated in other terms. This work should lead to a consensus related to the project, everything from "proceed to the next phase" to the "priority problems are...."

Problem Analysis Basics

Individuals may intuitively know that automating a problem will not fix it; therefore, business process redesign should be applied to address and resolve problems first, wherever possible, and then identify where the application of automation makes sense. Many of the quality improvement principles and tools can be used to make improvements to the processes in an organization before the formal systems design process. Doing the process improvement work first will help focus more clearly on how and where to apply automation to the problem.

After the initial phase the work proceeds to the next phase. Although there may be variation among authors about the names of these steps, the process usually encompasses the areas of analysis, design, implementation, and evaluation. Although the steps in the development life cycle are primarily concerned with new development efforts, they are equally appropriate with some modification for selection of already developed products from the vendor market. Because this chapter is concerned with the HIM professional's role in systems development, there is an emphasis on tasks associated with analysis, selection, implementation, and evaluation support activities and a de-emphasis on purely technical activities associated with each process. The focus in the design area is more conceptual than technical and concentrates on issues that relate to general system design principles and user interface concerns associated with input and output media. (Additional user interface information is contained in Chapter 8.)

Users tend to interact with the presentation layer of a software application, but in addition to the presentation layer there is a business logic layer and a data access layer. It might be helpful to think of the application as an iceberg and as the presentation layer the part of the iceberg that is visible above water. It may be the smallest portion of the iceberg because the business logic layer contains the programmed business rules and the data access layer contains the rules related to the storage and access of information along with the logic to navigate the database. The data access layer also contains the definitions of the data tables (Figure 9-3).

ANALYSIS

The development or selection of an information system can be an arduous and complex process. In the face of the challenge of information system development, a logical question that arises is "where should we begin?" The beginning of any development project effort usually starts with a perceived need or an effort to solve a problem. For example, a supervisor in the HIM department may recognize that a new information system for case mix analysis may

provide improved decision support capabilities. Or, a perceived need may arise when a current information system, such as the release of information tracking system, enters the obsolescence phase of the information system life cycle. The launching of the development process may also be initiated by users who believe that new technology is required to support their daily tasks. Whatever the reason for initiation, the goal of the analysis step is to build on the initial work and determine the feasibility of a new system and confirm the scope of the developmental or selection effort. In this context, the analysis will confirm or determine the following:

- Whether there is a need for a new system
- Whether the organization can afford a new system
- Whether sufficient technical expertise exists to develop or operate the new system
- What general functionality is expected
- What benefits are expected from system implementation

Tools and Aids for System Analysis

Health information professionals have many tools at their disposal to assist in determining the feasibility and scope of any new information system development effort. These tools are appropriate to use whether the system is being developed internally by the organization or whether the system will be purchased from a vendor. Several tools[4-6] are used in systems analysis, including the following:

- Action diagrams
- Context diagram (communication)
- Data analysis diagrams
- Data dictionary
- Data flow diagram/process model
- Data mapping
- Data models

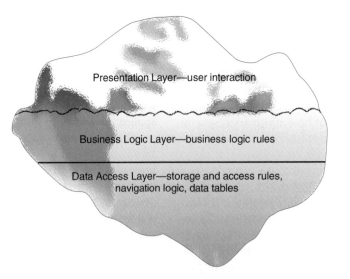

Presentation Layer—user interaction

Business Logic Layer—business logic rules

Data Access Layer—storage and access rules, navigation logic, data tables

Figure 9-3 "Iceberg" diagram showing architectural layers of software.

Table 9-2   STRUCTURED ANALYSIS TOOLS AND PURPOSE

Development Tool	Purpose
Data dictionary	Data modeling technique that is a repository for all primitive-level data structures and data elements within a system.
Data flow diagram/process modeling	Graphical representation of flow of data through a system. Can be a logical or physical data flow.
Decomposition diagram	Used to break down problems into smaller levels of detail. Usually depicted in a hierarchy chart similar to an organizational chart.
Entity-relationship diagram/data modeling	Data modeling technique that depicts the logical design of a database schema.
Use case	A description of how a component of system/process should work or how a component of a system/process is working now.

- Data navigation diagrams
- Data structure diagrams
- Decision trees and tables
- Decomposition diagrams
- Dialogue design diagrams
- Entity-relationship diagrams
- Fishbone (Ishikawa) diagram
- State transition diagrams
- Use case/scenario

The use of each of these tools depends on the desired output from the analysis and analyst preference. In this chapter, only selected tools are discussed. Table 9-2 lists selected tools and gives a brief description of their purpose.

Decomposition Diagrams—Hierarchy Chart

The **hierarchy chart** is a type of decomposition diagram. Its purpose is to break down problems into smaller and smaller detail. The hierarchy chart does this by identifying all the tasks in a process and grouping them into various hierarchical levels. The hierarchy chart is organized in a treelike manner. Each task in the chart is called a *node*. Each node, except for the uppermost node, has a single *parent node*. Each parent node may have none, one, or multiple *children nodes*. *Sibling nodes* are nodes that are all on the same level of the chart. The lowest nodes on each level of the chart (i.e., nodes that have no children) are called *functional primitives*. The functional primitive nodes are eventually translated into program modules that perform the work of the system.

To construct a hierarchy chart, the first step is to list all the tasks in the order in which they occur.

To develop a tree structure, it is necessary to assemble the processes together in functionally similar groups. Why would an HIM professional want to develop a hierarchy chart?

Whether the information system under consideration is to be developed in house or purchased from a vendor, a hierarchy chart of the system should be developed for the following reasons:

The process of developing the chart forces a review of the current process. Redundancies in work patterns can be identified and inefficiencies can be corrected.

The hierarchy chart can provide the foundation for building data flow diagrams (Figure 9-4).

The chart provides a means of communication with developers and can also be used to assess whether a vendor product will meet user needs.

Data Flow Diagrams/Process Modeling

Once tasks within a system are identified, it is necessary to expand this information into a data flow diagram. **Data flow diagrams** (DFDs) are used to track the flow of data through an entire system. They identify the data flow within a system, in essence providing a data map of what data go from an area, what data are received by an area, and what data are either temporarily or permanently stored in an area. In addition to tracking data flow, a DFD identifies transformations on data (processes) and data repositories (data stores).

There are four essential concepts related to DFDs: external entities, processes, data stores, and data flows. An *external entity* includes people or groups of people who interact with the system but are not internal to it. For example, a patient would be considered an external entity to a system of health care delivery. *Processes* are actions performed on data. *Data stores* are repositories for data. They may be either temporary or permanent storage areas. *Data flows* represent the movement of data through a system. Data move out of entities, to entities, between processes, and into and out of data stores.

Specific symbols are used to identify each DFD component. The external entity is represented by a square. Table 9-3 displays DFD symbols with examples of each. Like the hierarchy chart, DFDs are constructed by going from the complex to the simple. In other words, the system as a whole is first represented and successive levels represent more and more system detail. The method and construction rules for developing DFDs vary, depending on whose recommended process is followed. The description and construction of DFDs in this chapter follow general development rules. For readers with an additional interest in developing a greater depth of tool usage, appropriate references are provided.[4-6]

The context level of the DFD provides a relatively simple picture of the system under study. The context level identifies the major external entities, data transformation, data flows,

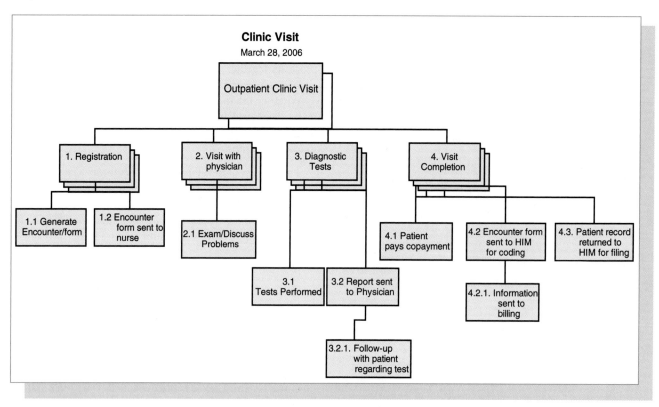

Figure 9-4 Hierarchy chart for an outpatient visit.

Table 9-3 DATA FLOW DIAGRAM SYMBOLS

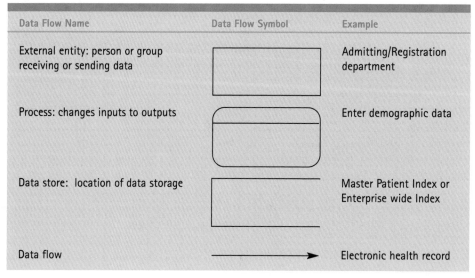

and data stores of the system (Figure 9-5). This diagram shows the relationship between the patient activities and the data that is part of the clinical activity of a visit. The data components is coded with a "D" and the process components are coded with a "P." Each major data and process component is numbered. This process begins with the patient

making an appointment and follows the process through registration, clinical service provision, collection and processing of the data needed to bill for service, the review and analysis of patient information, and updating of the patient's problems, allergies and immunizations. To understand the system fully, it is necessary to break down the

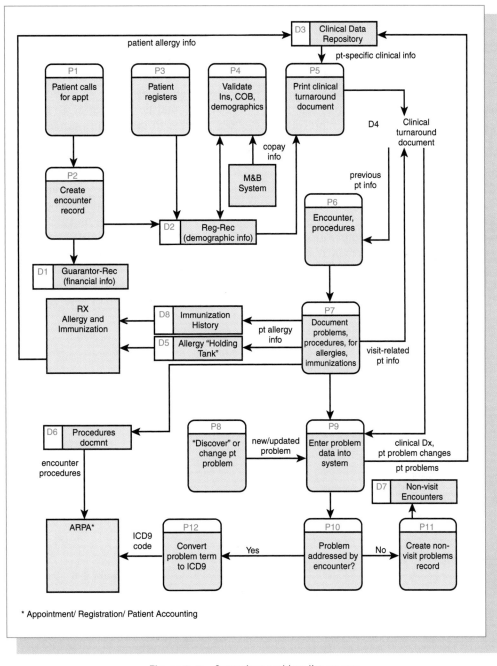

Figure 9-5 Outpatient problem list process.

process successively into more detailed parts. This is accomplished through explosion diagrams. Information contained in the hierarchy chart can be used to help construct the successive DFD explosions. Why should an HIM professional possess the skills to construct DFDs? Like the hierarchy chart, DFDs should be developed whether the system is to be developed in house or purchased from a vendor. An important aspect of HIM is the design of information systems to support organizational functions and strategic objectives. To design systems, processes must be systematically described at the level of detail provided by tools such as the DFD. The construction of DFDs provides an avenue to describe the following:

- Where data originate
- How data are transformed
- How data flow
- Where data are deposited

Without this level of detail, an information system cannot be adequately designed.

HIM professionals must be able to interact with users and assist them in systematically breaking down complex systems into smaller and smaller components. They frequently serve as intermediaries between users and system developers. The processes represented in DFDs are much easier for users and developers to understand than if the processes were described in narrative or prose form. DFDs often help to resolve discrepancies in perceptions of how something is done or should be performed. Using DFDs helps to avoid confusion, which is a critical element in any system design process.

Data Dictionary

The **data dictionary** describes all the primitive-level data structures and data elements within a system. It is the central repository for all information about the database and functions as a catalog for identifying the nature of all the data in a system. It provides the central resource for ensuring that standard definitions for data elements and data structures are used throughout the system. The typical data dictionary includes information about processes, data flows, data stores, and data elements in a system. For example, in a data dictionary, the data element "sex" used in a master patient index would contain information about the data element's data type, its length, its range, allowed values, and meanings. In this case, the data element "sex" would have a data type of alphanumerical, its length would be one character, and allowed values would be "F" and "M." The meaning would be included as a notation indicating that "sex" referred to the patient's gender and that "M" meant male and "F" female (Figure 9-6).

How is the data dictionary compiled? There are several ways in which a data dictionary can be notated.[2,7] The style used depends largely on the procedures established and the preference of individual information system departments. There is usually a unique notation for data structures, data processes, data flows, data stores, and data elements (Figure 9-7). The label is daily discharge list. The entry type is data flow. The description gives a more complete explanation of the data flow. There is no alias. Note that in this data dictionary entry there is no "values/meaning"

Project:	Master Patient Index
Label:	Sex
Entry Type:	Data Element
Description:	Patient gender
Alias:	None
Values/Meaning:	Length: 1 character Type: alphanumeric Value: M = male; F = female

Figure 9-6 Data dictionary element—sex.

Project:	Record Completion Review System	
Label:	Daily Discharge List	
Entry Type:	Data Flow	
Description:	Daily list of patients discharged from the hospital	
Alias:	None	
Composition:	Daily Discharge List 5	currentdate + medrecno + ptlname + ptfname + ptmidinital + ptdob + admitdate + dischgdate
Locations:	Context- and first-level explosions; second-level explosion of Process 1, Record Catalog	
	Data Flow → Daily Discharge List	

Figure 9-7 Data dictionary discharge list.

section. In its place is an area for noting the composition of the flow. In this case, the daily discharge list is composed of current date, medical record number, patient last and first names and middle initial, patient's date of birth, admission date, and discharge date. The location of the data flow is indicated in the last entry of this notation. This list can be generated from the hospital's REG/ADT system and stored as a report or printed as needed. A primary user of this report is the HIM department.

The Visible Analyst Workbench,[4] a CASE tool, provides a specific format for notation for data elements, data processes, data flows, data stores, and external entities. This notation includes identifying the following:

Project—Name of the project to which the element, process, flow, store, or entity is related

Label—Unique data name

Entry type—Type of data entity, such as data element, process, data store, external entity, data flow

Description—Used for more complete description of the data entity if the label is not self-explanatory

Alias—Other names by which the data entity is identified

Values and meanings—Notation depends on the data entity type

For a data element, the length, type, and values that the element can take on would be noted. For a data structure, such as patient account, all the data elements that compose

the patient account data structure would be noted. Additional categories such as Source or Location may also be part of a data dictionary.

Another data dictionary example is a data element used both for internal program evaluation and external reporting (Figure 9-8). A behavioral health organization contracts with managed care organizations to provide a variety of programs from residential services to outpatient counseling. One of the outcome measures used to review the attainment of objectives is the client's "residential arrangement" or where the client lives. This piece of data is collected when the client is admitted or registered for care, at review periods, and at discharge. For example, if a client is homeless at the time of registering for services and 6 months later is living independently in a stable housing setting then this is a positive outcome. Obviously this measure is combined with other measures such as a problem severity scale to determine whether the client has a reduction in symptoms from registration, to review points, and at discharge. See Figure 9-8 for the residential arrangement data dictionary reporting component and Figure 9-9 for a list of values associated with this data element.

Why is the development of a data dictionary important? One reason is that the data dictionary provides a central repository of standard terminology and the description of data used in all the information systems in the organization. The data dictionary helps to reduce data redundancy and

---

Data Dictionary

Residential Arrangement - used to report behavioral health care outcome

Project	: Outcome Reporting to Managed Care Provider
Label	: Residential Arrangement
Entry Type	: Data Element
Description	: An outcome measure that describes the residential arrangement of the client
Alias	: none
Values/Meaning	: Valid Codes: 10, 20, 22, 25, 26, 30, 41, 47, 50, 61, 62, 82, 83 (See Figure 9-9 for Code Definitions)
Process Description	: Collect and report data element after initial assessment and on change of residential arrangement and at discharge
Note	: Combine with action code of : Add = A, Change = C , Delete = D Combine with date: MMDDYYYY

Figure 9-8 Data dictionary element—residential arrangement.

Data Dictionary

Values for Residential Arrangement

Definition: This code describes the housing arrangement of the client on the date of the report.

Procedure: Reports are created after the initial assessment, at a change in residential arrangement and at discharge. For a change in residential arrangement report the date the client actually changed to a new residential arrangement.

Purpose: This is an outcome measure.

Type: text (2 digits)

Valid Codes	Definitions
	Type of Housing
10	Independent housing, alone or with others. Independent housing is defined as housing where no supervision is provided.
20	Supported housing alone or with others. Supervision by mental health staff is provided.
22	Adult family home – licensed as such by the State
25	Residential Drug/Alcohol treatment– treatment for 90 days or more. If the client is in treatment for less than 90 days, use the code for the living arrangements just prior to treatment.
26	Foster Care (for children)
30	Long-term Adaptive Services means a facility-based residential program with 24-hour nursing care and medical supervision, and mental health services which include: (a) Program and case consultation from a mental health professional (b) Individualized treatment, as appropriate (c) Staff training Types of facility include: Skilled Nursing/Intermediate Care Facility, Institute of Mental Disease (IMD), DD facility
41	Congregate Care Facility (CCF)
47	Group Care (children)

Figure 9-9 Data dictionary element values for residential arrangement.

50	Long Term Rehabilitative Services (LTR)
61	Jail/Juvenile Correctional Facility – Incarceration for 90 days or more. If the client is incarcerated for less than 90 days, use the code for the living arrangement just prior to incarceration.
62	Psychiatric Inpatient Facility – Voluntary or involuntary hospitalization for 90 days or more. Types of facilities include inpatient Psychiatric Hospital, Psychiatric Health Facility, Veterans Affairs Hospital, or State Hospital. If the client is hospitalizad for less than 90 days, use the code for the living arrangement just prior to hospitalization.
82	Homeless – Those persons of all ages who lack a fixed, regular and adequate nighttime residence including persons whose primary nighttime residence is one of the following: Emergency shelter (e.g., missions, churches) where residence is on a "night by night basis"; Living on the streets, in a vehicle, or abandoned building; Being discharged/discharged from an institution (e.g., jail, medical or psychiatric hospital) with no arranged residence; Temporary living accommodations by a voucher system (e.g., motel vouchers); Living in a public or private place not designated for, or not ordinarily used as, a regular sleeping accommodation for human beings; Children living in transitional housing
83	Temporary housing Temporarily or inadequately housed in a residence which is not their own (e.g., transitional housing, living with family or friends); Living in a temporary non-subsidized living arrangement (e.g., welfare hotel or motel)

Figure 9–9, cont'd   Data dictionary element values for residential arrangement.

increase the integrity of enterprise wide data. Without this standardization, it is unlikely that efficient and effective information systems can be created. When used with hierarchy charts and DFDs, the data dictionary helps to document an information system fully. This type of documentation can speed up the process of developing system programs. It also provides information that makes modification of programs and data easier. Without this type of documentation, system maintenance would be extremely difficult if not impossible. Like the development of DFDs, the development of a data dictionary helps to decrease confusion among users and analysts about the purpose and functions of a system.

Data Mapping

As health care organizations move to new systems they often have data in legacy systems. The legacy system is usually an older existing system that may either need to be interfaced into the new system and continue its unique function or it may be shut down in favor of a newer system. In either event, some or all of the data in the legacy system may need to be mapped to a new system. As decisions are made about purchasing a new system, it will be important to identify legacy systems data that will be needed in the new system environment. Data mapping and the data dictionary have relevance to one another in that the data dictionary may carry alias terms that help systems recognize that a term has several synonyms. For example, one system may call an individual who is receiving care a patient, another may call the individual a client, and another system may use the term resident. There are more complex mapping activities as well; for example, as health care organizations move from *International Classification of Diseases, Ninth Revision, Clinical Modification* (ICD-9-CM) coding to *International Classification of Diseases, Tenth Revision* (ICD-

10) coding, those diagnostic terms must be mapped. If an individual is pulling a research study, the authors of the study may have been using data from legacy systems. Older code "books" and references tend to disappear, so being able to use a map will help to identify the same diagnoses in both coding systems.

Entity-Relationship Diagrams

System hierarchy charts, DFDs, and data dictionaries are all important tools in the analysis and design process. Another tool frequently used to help describe the relations among data in an information system is the **entity-relationship diagram** (ERD). The ERD is used principally to illustrate the logical design of information system databases. This is accomplished by describing diagrammatically the relation between entities and by identifying entity attributes. ERDs are composed of three categories of items:

1. Entities
2. Relations
3. Attributes

Entities are objects such as people, places, things, or events that make up the data of a database. In the manual record completeness review system, entities include physicians (people), patient records (things), deficiency cards (things), and patient care areas (places). In an ERD, an entity is represented by a rectangle.

Relations are links or ties that exist between or among entities. In an ERD, a relation is represented by a diamond. An example of a relation in the manual record completeness review system is the relation between a patient record (an entity) and a deficiency card (an entity). In this relation, a patient record can have many deficiency cards (i.e., there are many physicians, each having a card, who can have a deficiency). Another example is the relation between a physician (entity) and a deficiency card (entity). In this relation, a physician can have many deficiency cards (i.e., have deficiencies for more than one record).

Attributes describe both entities and relations. Attributes may be thought of as the data elements that need to be captured to describe an entity fully. As an example, the attributes of the deficiency card in the manual record completeness review system include patient number, physician name, physician number, and list of deficiencies. The attributes of the entity "physician" would include physician number and physician name.

In an ERD, entity and relation symbols are connected by straight lines. In addition to indicating a relation among entities, it is important to indicate how frequently the occurrence can exist at any given point in time. In the preceding example, the relation between a patient record and deficiency cards can occur many times (i.e., a patient record can have more than one deficiency card at any given point in time). This relation is referred to as a one-to-many relation. Other examples of relations include many-to-many (m to m) and one-to-one (1 to 1).

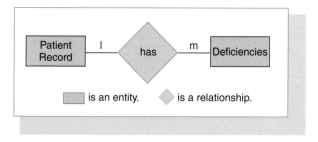

Figure 9-10 Entity-relationship diagram for deficiencies.

Figure 9-10 shows the use of a simple ERD, in this case the relationship between a patient record and a data deficiency. Note that both the entities (patient record and data deficiency) are represented by a rectangle. The relation "has" is represented by a diamond. The type of relationship (1 to many) is represented by the characters "1" and "m" on either side of the relationship symbol. This ERD is read in the following way: Each patient record can have more than one (or many) data deficiencies. The reverse of this is that each data deficiency can relate to only one patient record.

NOTE: In an EHR system the record deficiency data are posted as a "to do" list for the care provider and tracked by the HIM professional. The HIM professional also uses a related reporting function to aggregate individuals into clinical departments and identify the length of time involved in various deficiencies. Depending on the organization's rules, a clinical practitioner who does not respond to messages to remove deficiencies of documentation content or signatures may lose the privilege of admitting patients or an employee may receive organizational sanctions.

Another example of an ERD is shown in Figure 9-11. This figure shows the conceptual data model for an outpatient problem list. Starting at the left side, the diagram says that a panel of patients/consumers receives services/care events and that certain practitioners are responsible to manage the care for the patients/consumers in their panel. Once a consumer/patient receives a service the consumer's diagnosis or problem is placed on that individual consumer/patient's problem list. The problem list has a vocabulary table to help control and standardize the vocabulary use on problem lists. The problem vocabulary table is also used to categorize the types of problems and the risk factors associated with the consumers/patients in this managed care system. Each problem has the potential attributes of problem term modifier, status, practitioner after the problem, onset or entry date, and notes. This diagram also portrays other messages, for example, that a panel consists of many consumers/patients, that a consumer/patient can have many health concerns or complaints and many problems and receive many services.

Why is the ERD important? Development of ERDs should be done whether the system is to be developed in house or purchased from a vendor. In most system develop-

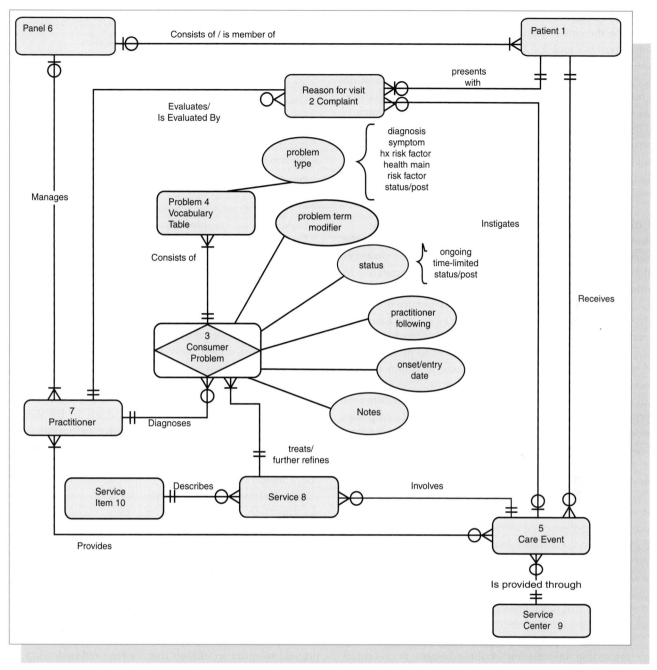

Figure 9-11 Conceptual data model for outpatient problem list.

Entity 1 = Patient. A patient is a person who has utilized or may utilize services from this provider. This provider must maintain specific information to conduct business. Entity 2 = Health Complaint/Presenting Problem. This is the reason for visit, the presenting problem which is the focus of attention for a particular visit or encounter. This statement can be made from the patient's point of view. Entity 3 = Problem. A patient problem is an incidence of a particular problem for a given patient. (the intersection table) Entity 4 = Problem Vocabulary Table. This table is a look-up table with vocabularies for defining clinical problems. Entity 5 = Care Event. This is an occurrence of care provided by a health care organization. A care event may be a visit, an encounter as an outpatient or it can be an inpatient or resident stay or episode of care or some other event such as a consulting nurse phone call during which health care services are provided. Entity 6 = Panel. A panel represents a relationship between practitioners/providers and patients. Some practitioners/providers have a specified group of patients for whom they are primarily responsible for providing care; this group is called a panel. Not all practitioners/providers have panels; not all patients are members of a panel. Practitioners/providers can treat patients who are not on their panel. Entity 7 = Practitioner/Provider. A practitioner/provider is a person who has met requirements, is authorized, and is directly engaged in the health care of patients. Entity 8 = Service. A service is an occurrence of a service item (procedure, visit, durable goods, etc.) for which the organization bills or records as a service. Corresponding documentation is expected in the patient clinical record. Entity 9 = Service Center. A service center is a place of business that provides services to patients. Entity 10 = Service Item. A service item is a procedure, visit, encounter, durable good or supply for which the organization bills, records in patient's health records.

ment projects, there are hundreds of complex ERDs that describe the entire system under development. The ERD is an important tool for the development of a logical data model of the system. The logical data model reflects a high-level, global view of information within the organization and forms the basis for the physical design of the database. As such, it prescribes physical database requirements such as a number of files, primary keys, and attributes. If the logical structure is badly designed, the databases are likely to be inefficient and ineffective. Therefore, a great deal of attention must be paid to the accuracy and completeness of the logical data model.

Computer-Aided Systems Engineering Tools

A logical question that should arise after studying the various structured analysis tools is "how are the products that are derived from each of these tools integrated?" In other words, how are the charts, diagrams, dictionaries, and tables tied together to derive a coherent picture of system design? Until recently, most of the work to develop hierarchy charts, data dictionaries, and DFDs was done by hand. This was a time-consuming process and tended to produce fragmentation in system development. These development tools have now been computerized to improve the efficiency, accuracy, and completeness of the system development process. These computerized systems are called computer-aided software engineering (also referred to as computer-aided systems engineering), or CASE, tools.

CASE tools provide a mechanism for the electronic development of systems analysis aids such as structure charts, DFDs, ERDs, and data dictionaries. Instead of developing charts and diagrams manually, the analyst can use a computer program with a graphic interface to assist in development. CASE tools do not automatically develop the various charts and diagrams. Rather, the designer interacts with the CASE program to select the appropriate symbols, connectors, and labels and electronically draw the proper diagram. All diagrams, graphs, tables, and dictionaries that are developed are stored electronically.

CASE tools help designers relate their work electronically by organizing information about a system in a central repository. The central repository may contain data models, logic definitions, functional models and may screen and report definitions. Once it is developed, designers can query the repository for information about the system. The physical design of databases and program code can also be generated from the repository by system developers. If new processes are added or current ones extended, previously developed models, graphs, tables, and dictionaries can be reused or easily updated.

Advantages of Using Computer-Aided Systems Engineering Products. There are many benefits of using a CASE product. An obvious benefit is convenience for system designers. CASE products provide an effective mechanism for development, storage, retrieval, and update of charts,

---

Box 9-1 ADVANTAGES AND DISADVANTAGES OF USING COMPUTER-AIDED SYSTEMS ENGINEERING PRODUCTS

Advantages
Convenient for system designers to use
Easy to alter existing charts and diagrams
Fast development of analysis tools
Increases productivity
Reduces design errors

Disadvantages
Expensive
Must purchase products from several vendors
Problems integrating products from different vendors
Decomposition diagram

---

tables, diagrams, and dictionaries.[4,5] Updates, enhancements, corrections, or extensions to already developed charts and diagrams can be easily accomplished with use of CASE products. CASE allows faster development of analysis tools. Data models can be efficiently developed and results shared with other design team members and users in a timelier manner than by using manual methods. Reduction of errors is another benefit of using CASE products in the design process. Because CASE products enforce organization of system details and contain automatic consistency checks, errors in design are reduced. CASE products also increase coordination within and among projects, resulting in better standardization. Standardization leads to better system documentation, which can be easily maintained and updated.

Disadvantages of Using Computer-Aided Systems Engineering Products. Although many advantages can be realized by using CASE products, some disadvantages also exist (Box 9-1). CASE products can be expensive. Training costs for updating the skills of designers and analysts must also be considered. Because one vendor does not usually provide an entire set of tools that are required to develop an information system, products from several vendors may have to be purchased. The use of several vendor products can increase costs and training time and can create problems with integration.

Investigative Strategies for Analysis of Requirements

In this chapter, information life cycles and the analysis of system requirements have been discussed. The importance of developing structured tools such as hierarchy charts, DFDs, and data dictionaries when describing a system has been addressed. However, these tools require the gathering of information before they can be constructed. A legitimate question to ask is "How is the information needed for input to these tools gathered?"

Various investigative strategies can be used to gather information during the analysis phase of system development. Among them are interviews with users, questionnaires, observation of tasks, and review of documents, forms, and procedures. This phase of the project is essential to successful systems design.[4] Because HIM professionals often serve as liaisons between system developers and the end-user community, it is important that they understand and become skilled in the techniques for gathering information.

Ways of Gathering Information

Interviews. Interviews are a common method for gathering information about system requirements. The use of the interview strategy has several advantages. First, it provides an opportunity for end users to feel as though they are co-owners in the design and development process. All too frequently, information systems are designed and selected without appropriate user input. The one-on-one interview process helps to break down barriers of user resistance by allowing the user to assume a vested interest in the process. If users are involved in the development and design of an information system, they are less likely to resist system implementation.

The type of questions asked during an interview process, the length of time that an interview takes, and the number of people to be interviewed depend on the system under development and the desired outcomes from the interview process. In general, the following factors can contribute to a successful interview process:

- Defining the target audience
- Identifying the objectives of the interview
- Developing appropriate interview questions and format
- Adequately analyzing and documenting responses

Target Audience
To be successful, the interview process must adequately identify the target audience—that is, which people are most familiar with system requirements on operational and strategic levels. For example, in the release of information tracking system presented earlier, several groups of people should be interviewed. Naturally, the HIM department staff members responsible for day-to-day release of information activities should be interviewed because they are direct users of the system. The interview process should also be expanded beyond direct system users and include those who are or might be remote users or secondary beneficiaries of the system. Secondary beneficiaries of the system often provide a different perspective and significant insights into system needs, in this case, employees and managers in inpatient and outpatient clinical areas and those responsible for oversight of the privacy and compliance areas. If the organization engages in research then a research representative should

also be included. If the organization offers specialty services such as long-term care, behavioral health, or home health, then representatives from those areas are candidates for the interview process. In this fact-finding process it will be important to identify any secondary record systems within the organization that contain patient-identifiable data, especially if those areas tend to release information outside the organization. It will also be important to identify events and people in the organization who might also be called on from time to time to respond to a request for patient-identifiable information and to document how they typically respond to those requests. It will also be required to check on mandatory reporting by the organization and to identify the current process. It is also important to identify the people in the organization who are political power brokers and whose support is essential for the system under development. For example, the director of the HIM department, who is knowledgeable about the federal and state regulations and current professional practices, would definitely be an important power broker in the successful development of a release of information tracking system and would be included in the roster of interviewees Often overlooked in the interview process are the people who have knowledge of the strategic uses of information in the organization. Too often, information systems are developed from only a day-to-day operational perspective. For example, a point-of-care nursing system might be selected by nurse users because of the system's interface and support of daily tasks. This system, however, may not support the organization's strategic objective of providing accessible data for continuous quality improvement. In this case, the system would support day-to-day operational tasks well but would be inadequate in supporting strategic information needs. Therefore, managers concerned with strategic information needs should also be included in the roster of interviewees when appropriate.

The potential number of people to be interviewed can grow to be quite large. Because the interview process can be time consuming (between 30 and 60 minutes), the interview audience should be selected carefully. All power brokers significant to the project should be interviewed. The managers who are knowledgeable about the strategic use of information in the organization should also be interviewed. Many times, it is not feasible to interview all end users. For example, in a 1000-bed hospital, it would not be cost-effective or efficient to interview all nursing staff to identify requirements of a nursing care information system. If it is not possible to interview all direct users, an appropriate sample from this group should be selected.

Interview Protocol
An interview protocol should be developed and field tested before the interview process is implemented. Because interview time is limited, the analyst often has only one chance to gather information from a person. Therefore interview questions must be appropriate, complete, and

unbiased. Interview questions can be structured or unstructured. Structured questions can elicit yes or no responses to a question, or they can present the interviewee with a list of options from which to choose. Examples of structured questions are "Which of the following data are important to you in your daily work?" and "Is the current system response time adequate in meeting your needs?" Because structured questions are asked the same way from interview to interview, they require limited interviewing skill by the analyst. Because there is a limited range of responses to structured questions, interviewers do not have to make judgments about what was meant in a response. Therefore, results from structured questions are usually easy to compile.

Unstructured questions allow more probing of end users than do structured questions. Unstructured questions may be tailored to each end user and allow a broad spectrum of response or opinion. Examples of unstructured questions might be "What are the three or four most important types of data required for you to get your job done?" and "What are the three to five most critical functions for a system to have to help you perform your daily tasks?" The responses to unstructured questions are more difficult to document, collate, and analyze. Therefore, the use of unstructured questions requires the analyst to be a highly skilled interviewer.

Scenarios/Use Cases

Scenarios and use cases can also be used in the interview process. With this technique, the end user is presented with a scenario or use case that represents an actual situation. The end user responds to questions posed by the scenario or use case. For example, the following scenario might be presented to an end user in a clinic.

Example of a Scenario Presented to End User at a Clinic

The clinic is losing reimbursement. Claims data are not being appropriately gathered. Physicians do not consistently complete encounter forms. When forms are completed, vague ICD-9-CM and Common Procedural Terminology (CPT) codes are often assigned. Frequently, encounter forms are lost or misplaced and bills are never generated.

After the scenario is presented, several questions are posed to the end user. The following questions might be used in this example: "What functions must a new information system support to eliminate these problems?" and "What characteristics of the current system make it difficult for physicians to complete encounter forms?"

The scenario or use case-centered interview is popular. One reason for this is that the end user can respond to questions in the context of a real environment. Relating responses to a current situation is thought to provide a more realistic perspective on the functionality required of a system. No matter which method of questioning is used, gathering responses from unstructured questions usually takes more time than gathering responses from structured questions. Therefore, to avoid lengthy interviews, there should be an appropriate balance between structured and unstructured questions.

Another related example is to present a scenario, such as the clinic scenario, to a small group and use the fishbone (Ishikawa) diagramming technique to better understand the problem. This has the advantage of identifying which components of the problem have nothing to do with building or purchasing an information system.

Scenarios and use cases are also helpful in presenting a narrative description of what happens in the context of an event or series of events. (Another example of a use case is presented later in this chapter as Figure 9-15.)

Before it is administered, the interview protocol should be field tested. A field test is a trial run of the questions in the protocol. Normally, the field test consists of posing the protocol questions to a sample group. Field testing is advantageous for a number of reasons.

- First, it allows the interview questions to be tried out on a sample group. The clarity, appropriateness, and completeness of the interview questions can be assessed during the field test process. It is much easier to make necessary modifications during the field test than after the interview process has begun.
- Second, the field test allows the analysts to determine how much time must be scheduled for interviews during the actual interview process. Because end users selected for the interview process are probably busy people, it is important to estimate accurately the time needed for each interview.
- Third, the field test gives the interviewers an opportunity to develop their interview skills and hone the interview process. The importance of training the interviewers should not be underestimated. The more skilled the interviewer, the better the results from the interview.

Format

Before any interview, the end user to be interviewed should be apprised of the interview's purpose. Advance notice of the interview goals gives prospective interviewees an opportunity to collect their thoughts and organize their opinions. Typically, advance notice is given by personal contact by the director of the interview team or through written communication. Adequate time for the interview should be allocated. Thirty to 60 minutes should be sufficient. If the interview drags on beyond 1 hour, results are usually nonproductive.

Although the interview format may vary from situation to situation, it usually has the following basic components:

- The number of interviewers usually consists of two or three persons. If two interviewers are present during the interview, one assumes responsibility for asking questions and the other serves as note taker.
- It is important that at least one interviewer be free from the distraction of note taking so that full concentration is devoted to the responses of the end user.

Documentation

After the interview is completed, the analysts should immediately review the interview notes. Immediate debriefing between the interviewers allows the analysts the opportunity to come to consensus on what the end user said and to add additional information to the interview notes. The interview notes should be organized into a report as soon as possible after the interview, preferably on the same day. The format for the interview documentation usually includes the following:

- Interview date
- Name and position of interviewee
- Names of interviewers
- List of questions posed
- Responses to questions
- Synopsis of the interview

In some cases, copies of the interview notes may be given to the interviewee to review. In this way, the end user provides formal confirmation of responses to the interview questions and has an opportunity to correct any errors.

After all interviews are completed, an overall analysis and synthesis are developed from all interview responses. This should include the following:

- Description of the method
- List of all interview questions
- List of all end users who were interviewed
- Synopsis of all facts and opinions
- General synthesis of interview material with recommendations

Questionnaires. Questionnaires are a popular method for gathering data. Questionnaire development and administration are less time consuming and less costly than the direct interview techniques. As opposed to the interview process, questionnaires can be distributed to a larger target audience. However, the benefits of using questionnaires can be severely diminished for several reasons. Questionnaires are frequently ambiguous, poorly constructed, and too long and have low response rates. To be effective, questionnaires should be used primarily to gather facts, not opinions. Questions should be of a structured nature, allowing yes or no responses or responses to lists of multiple choice options. If opinions are being gathered, a structured mechanism such as a Likert scale should be used.

Question Construction

Before any questions are prepared, the purpose and goals of the questionnaire must be defined. Only questions pertinent to the purpose of the survey should be included in the questionnaire. Questions are only as good as the degree to which they measure what they are intended to measure. Therefore, the purpose of any questionnaire must be clearly identified along with a list of measures that are anticipated. For example, a customer satisfaction survey would want to assess the satisfaction with the full range of customer services offered.

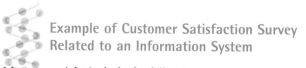

Example of Customer Satisfaction Survey Related to an Information System

Measures might include the following:

- Data about repair response times
- System downtime
- System response time
- Ease of navigation
- Degree of helpfulness of troubleshooting personnel
- Degree of availability of troubleshooting personnel

After the measures are identified, questions specific to each can be developed. In the customer satisfaction example, the following questions might be asked to measure repair response time:

- "In the past month, how often have you had to contact customer service for computer repair—one to two times, three to four times, more than four times?"
- "From the time you called the customer service unit, how long did it take a troubleshooter to respond—less than 15 minutes, 15 to 30 minutes, more than 30 minutes?"

Tabulation and compilation of survey results can be time consuming. Before any question is constructed, it is important to consider how responses to questions will be tabulated by the analyst. Responses can be nominal, ordinal, interval, or ratio data. The level of data used determines the type of tabulation and statistical techniques that can be applied to the data. As an example, nominal data refer to unordered categories. Types of nominal data include patient sex, patient third-party payer type, and patient employer. Nominal data can be tabulated by category, but sophisticated statistical tests cannot be used on nominal data. Ordinal data include people or events that are ordered or placed in ordered categories along a single dimension. Examples of ordinal data include responses to the following:

- "How would you rate your satisfaction with repair response time—very good, good, poor?"
- "How would you rate the degree of helpfulness of system troubleshooters—high, average, low?"

Ordinal data can be tabulated by category and can provide more opportunity for performing statistical tests. Interval and ratio level data are best if advanced statistical techniques are to be applied to the data. The level of data collected depends on what kinds of tabulation and measurement are desired outcomes of the survey.

It is important that the meaning of questions be clear to the survey respondent. A question should ask only one thing. Double-barreled questions that contain two or more concepts should be avoided. An example of a double-barreled question is "Are the daily discharge data you receive complete and accurate?" This question includes two concepts: completeness and accuracy. The data may be complete (include all data elements) but may not be accurate (the information associated with the data elements may be incorrect). It is also important that survey questions be nonbiased. Questions that lead the end user to a conclusion have no place on a questionnaire. An example of a leading question is "Don't you agree that the health information management department has poor customer service?" A better way to handle this question would be to ask "How would you rate the degree of customer service of the health information management department—excellent, good, average, poor, very poor?"

The meaning of questions should be clear to the end user. Many times, surveys include questions that are difficult to understand. The following is an example of an ambiguous question: "Do you favor or oppose health care legislation?" In this example, health care legislation can mean just about anything. Is it referring to a plan for national health insurance, legislation related to security of patient data, Medicare legislation, or some other type of legislation? The answer to this question cannot be interpreted without the analyst making assumptions about what the end user is thinking.

Questionnaire Construction

Having a set of good questions is the foundation for building a questionnaire. However, certain basic principles should be followed in the construction of the questionnaire if the survey is to be successful. A poorly constructed questionnaire, even if it contains good questions, can yield a poor response rate for a variety of reasons. A questionnaire should have a pleasing appearance to the end user, directions should be easy to understand, and the document should be easy to complete. If the survey is unattractive or too difficult or time consuming to complete, a low response rate is likely.

The following steps are guidelines for beginning questionnaire construction:

1. Choose a concise, suitable title for the survey document.
2. Clearly state the purpose of the survey in a brief paragraph at the beginning of the survey instrument, followed by simple, easy-to-follow directions.
3. Order the questions in a logical sequence.

Survey instruments usually begin with relatively easy-to-answer questions that help get the end user into the questionnaire. The questionnaire should flow easily. It is best to put questions referring to similar concepts together. This provides for easier survey completion and data tabulation. For example, in the customer satisfaction questionnaire, all questions related to troubleshooting might be placed together. Thought-provoking or sensitive questions are usually left to the end of the survey.

A consistent, clear, and attractive format should be decided on for the survey instrument. A practical step is to divide the survey into logical sections and assign titles and numerics or characters to each. For example, the section of a survey that collects data about the end user may be titled "A. Demographics," and all questions in that section are preceded by the character A—for example, A1., A2., A3.

The length of the survey varies, depending on its purpose and objectives. No questionnaire should take more than 30 minutes to complete. Therefore, it is important to select questions carefully, including only those that are directly related to purpose and desired measurements. Like the personal interview protocol, a survey document should be pretested. The pretest should be conducted on a small sample of people. Time estimates of survey completion should be gathered, and problems with question clarity, survey directions, format, and spelling errors should be identified in the pretest and corrected before general survey distribution.

Questionnaire Administration

Once the survey instrument has been developed and pretested, it is ready for general administration. A cover letter to the end user should accompany the questionnaire. The cover letter should be a vehicle for getting the end user excited about the survey. It should state the purpose of the questionnaire, what value the results will have to the end user, and how the results will be used. End users should be assured that their responses will be kept confidential. To facilitate follow-up, each questionnaire can be assigned a number. A master log of numbers with associated end-user names should be maintained. As surveys are returned, their numbers can be compared with the master list and the end users' names crossed out. If initial response is low, the master log can be consulted and users who have not returned their surveys can be sent a reminder notice or another questionnaire. To obtain a good survey response, follow-up cards or reminders usually have to be sent once or twice. The initial response rate to a survey is usually about 30%. Reminders significantly increase the response rate. Analysts should strive for a response rate of 60% or more to justify conclusions made from questionnaire results. Another option is to use an on-line questionnaire. The on-line questionnaire can be distributed to those individuals who are the target of the survey. Their response to the survey can be tracked by the system. Reminders can easily be sent to nonresponders. The survey can be structured to send responses to a database to assist in the analysis process.

Observation

Observation is an appropriate technique for collection of information about system requirements or identifying tasks performed by end users. Observation is usually used as an adjunct to interview and questionnaire techniques. The results of observation can be used to confirm or expand on information collected from interviews and questionnaires. Observation should not be distracting to the end users.

Conducting an observation takes a high degree of skill. It usually requires a structured technique for recording observations, the details of a system, or how users perform their tasks. When an observation is conducted, the subject of the review should be narrowed down. For example, in determining order processing needs for a hospital information system, the tasks of unit secretaries might be studied. Rather than observing all the tasks performed by a hospital unit support staff member, only one or a few tasks may be observed at a time. Because observation is tedious work, the analyst should not attempt to perform observations over extended periods. Because observations can also be distracting to the end user and disruptive to regular work flow, analysts should be unobtrusive. The maximum period for a single observation should be no more than 60 minutes.

Observation can also be used to confirm whether work tasks and workflow conform to written procedures. Procedure manuals are frequently a point of reference for information-gathering about system needs. However, they are often inaccurate or out of date. Therefore, observation of how a procedure is performed may be essential if incorrect assumptions about the process are to be avoided.

As with other information-gathering techniques, the purpose of the observation should be well defined. A structured observation protocol should be developed to facilitate easy note taking. For example, an analyst may observe how unit secretaries enter laboratory orders in the hospital information system. The purpose of the review may be to reduce duplication of work effort, ascertain whether procedure is being followed, or determine whether data entry flow is optimal. In this case, a list of tasks that make up the function could be compiled. As each task is observed, the analyst can note how many times the task was performed, who performed it, and how long it took to complete. Figure 9-12 is an example of an observation protocol for laboratory order entry by a unit support staff member. This example would change if the provider is creating the order at the time of the interaction with the system as in the CPOE process.

Laboratory Order-Entry Protocol for: ____________________

Unit Support Staff Member: (use all factors)
Provider Observation: (use factors 3-4, 6-11) Date: __________ Shift __________

Task Performed	MRN / Time	MRN / Time
1. Review provider's handwritten orders		
2. Check date and time or orders		
3. Log on to EHRS or Lab System		
4. Select patient		
5. Select provider		
6. Select lab test		
7. Check system messages, e.g., duplicate test order, and determine need to verify		
8. Order test		
9. Select schedule		
10. Select frequency of test		
11. Resolve or notify provider of any alert messages related to test order		
Total time		
Notes:		

Figure 9-12 Observation protocol for laboratory order entry.

One of the reasons for CPOE is to eliminate some of the steps, potential error opportunities, by having the care provider directly interact with the system. The care provider is also able to immediately respond to any alerts and decision questions presented during the order entry process.

Document and Forms Review. One useful method for gathering data about information needs is to conduct a document or forms review. Review of forms can identify what data elements are routinely collected by a facility. The forms review can also help to determine information flow by identifying form origination, distribution, and archival locations. Health care facilities are notorious for the number of forms they use to collect data. Forms review frequently helps to uncover duplication in work effort, variation in data meanings and use, rogue forms, and problems with data integrity.

Group Analysis and Design. Group analysis and design is often used in place of other traditional structured approaches to data gathering. This method is often referred to as **joint application design** (JAD) or joint requirements planning (JRP).[4] In JAD or JRP, a group of people spend a concentrated time together in determining system requirements. The group is usually composed of end users, managers, analysts, and others who may have an impact on or be affected by the system under study. The time spent together may range from several hours to several days, depending on the results desired. The group analysis process is led by a facilitator who uses various techniques to elicit facts and opinions. Brainstorming and nominal group methods are frequently used. If the facilitator is using nominal group technique, it is also possible to do the joint requirements planning or segments of it virtually. Everyone does not need to be gathered together in one room.

Group decision support software (GDSS) has been used to facilitate the JAD process. GDSS is usually a network of workstations or portable personal computers that are all located in a conference or meeting room. GDSS products typically include word processing and text and database manipulation. Other functions, such as electronic worksheets, graphics, and communication capabilities, are customarily included. With a trained facilitator, GDSS can be used to administer a survey or questionnaire to a group of people at the same time and to facilitate brainstorming or a nominal group technique. Group members can respond electronically and anonymously to survey questions or list ideas, participate in brainstorming, or answer questions posed by a facilitator through various GDSS features. The use of this kind of computer support allows anonymity of response, minimizes bias, and speeds up the deliberative process.

There are several benefits of using the JAD process. First, the use of JAD stimulates interaction between end users and analysts in a positive, nonthreatening environment. It facilitates the development of unbiased results through the use of structured processes such as brainstorming, Delphi, Nominal Group Technique, and group consensus techniques. Bringing individuals together in the same room also gives everyone the opportunity to meet and have informal discussions. The structured technique makes certain that the quieter members of the group are heard and that individuals have the opportunity to give their input while removing the influence factor of a showing of hands. The use of JAD usually produces results in a shorter time frame than other investigative techniques.

Analysis Document

When brought together, results from the various investigative strategies and details outlined in analysis tools depict what is required for the new information system. All this information is synthesized and documented in a *systems analysis document*. The systems analysis report presents a logical description of what was done during the analysis phase, how it was done, and what results were obtained. In addition to describing the analysis process, strengths and weaknesses of the existing system are documented. Any resource constraints that might preclude the acquisition or development of the new system should be identified and noted in the report. These constraints may include such things as time, budget, insufficient in-house technological expertise, lack of state-of-the-art technology, and external factors. Seldom does an organization possess all the resources needed to build or acquire the ideal system. Comparing constraints with the proposed ideal system helps the facility judge what is an affordable or appropriate system, given the current situation.

The content of the systems report varies, depending on the analysis team style and scope of analysis. Martin[2] suggests that the analysis report contain four major sections:

1. Analysis method
   - List of end users contacted
   - Description of analysis methods used
   - Procedures or processes observed or reviewed
   - Records, forms, reports analyzed
   - Strengths and weaknesses of method
2. Statement of user requirements
   - System objectives:
   - Output and report requirements
   - User training needs
   - Impact of system on end users
3. Statement of system constraints
   - Description of resource constraints
   - Impact of constraints
   - Description of realistic system, given constraints
4. Documentation
   - Data collection instruments
   - Analysis data (synopsis of interviews, tabulation of surveys)
   - Hierarchy charts, DFDs, data dictionaries, ERDs

Whitten et al[4] suggest an alternative report approach for those who want to read more from a results perspective and then stop reading when the report exceeds their level of interest in the detail. This administrative format would be organized as follows:

- Introduction
- Conclusions and recommendations
- Summary and discussion of facts and details
- Methods and procedures
- Final conclusions
- Appendixes with facts and details

A group might find that the information that has been gathered needs to be organized and presented in more than one way depending on the audience for the information. Key information and documents may also need to be prepared to be presented in meetings.

System Design

As mentioned in the introduction to this chapter, system design encompasses activities related to specifying the details of a new system. In the analysis phase, the needs and requirements of a system are specified. During the system design phase, these requirements are translated into specifications needed to build the system. During this stage, decisions about the logical and physical designs of the system are made.

In today's health care environment, major systems or integrated systems (i.e., laboratory, radiology, clinical record, order entry) are usually purchased from a vendor rather than developed by in-house systems personnel. Therefore the following processes are usually performed within the vendor domain, particularly the physical design phase. It is still important for the HIM professional to know about these processes and what the desired output alternatives are. Knowing both processes and preferred outputs helps the HIM professional better assess a vendor product.

Logical and Physical Designs

A specific sequence of events is used in the system design phase. This sequence usually consists of the **logical system design** and the **physical system design.** The logical design describes the functionality of the system and is sometimes called the functional specifications of a system. This is where the vision of system performance and its features are presented. In this section, the system conceptualization is stated in general rather than technical terms.

The format of the logical design section varies, depending on individual preferences of the design team and the scope of the project. Stair[7] provides a traditional list of logical design outputs:

Output design—Specifications, including format, content, and frequency, for all output such as forms, screens, and reports. An example of output is the display on the computer monitor of all current laboratory values with outlier values highlighted.

Input design—Specifications, including format, content, and frequency, for all input data. An example of input design for an order entry system is an automatic capability that flags drug contraindications whenever a pharmaceutical is ordered.

Processing design—Types of data manipulations required, such as calculations, comparisons, and text manipulations. An example of a processing design feature is the automatic calculation of the net fluid input and output for a patient with an intravenous line in place.

File and database design—Specifications of file and database capabilities. An example of a database capability is the real-time update of a patient file or record.

Controls and security design—Specifications for data access and backup. An example of security is that all users must use a log-on identification and password for entry to the system.

Another method of describing system functionality is to use a scenario-based format. This format was presented earlier in the discussion of investigative techniques. In that context, a scenario or use case was presented to an end user and questions were posed about how an information system could alleviate the problems presented. The same format is also a good mechanism for describing system functional requirements. The following is an example of the use case/ scenario format used for a nursing point-of-care system.

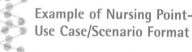

Example of Nursing Point-of-Care System Use Case/Scenario Format

The patient pushes the call button. The nurse goes to the patient's room. The patient requests pain medication and a beverage. The nurse logs on to the patient information system from a terminal at the patient's bedside. The nurse accesses the patient record and checks to see what medication can be administered and what beverages the patient is allowed to have.

A list of general goals and features usually accompanies the scenario-based format. In the preceding case, for example, the general goals might include the following:

- Present data at the bedside.
- Provide for data to be entered in one place and distributed appropriately.
- Provide different formats or views of the same data to accommodate a multidisciplinary team approach.

The physical system design section specifies all the characteristics that are necessary so that the logical design can be implemented. The physical design includes details about the design of hardware, software, databases, communications, and procedures and controls.

Design Principles

Both technical and functional characteristics must be considered during system design. In the technical arena, programmers and designers are interested in the degree of modularity a program has, its cohesion within a single module, and how independent each program module is. Included among other physical design characteristics are program accuracy, augmentability, completeness, consistency, efficiency, maintainability, reliability, and reusability. The HIM professional is commonly not involved in assessing these technical design characteristics. On the other hand, the professional is frequently called on to assess the functional qualities of a system and how they comply with good design principles.

What are basic design principles for system functionality? From an end user's perspective, system functionality usually involves three things: input, output, and system performance. The basic criterion that should be used to measure all three functionalities is "How well is each integrated into the daily work task of the end user?"

Input and Output

The goals of the input process are as follows:

- To make entry of data into an information system easy so that transactions can be quickly and accurately completed.
- To integrate the process to such a degree in the employee work flow that it is transparent to the end user; in other words, the input mechanism is unobtrusive. If nursing personnel must wait in line to access a computer terminal, then the input process is not satisfactory.
- To reduce duplication in work effort while ensuring a better-quality product. If a unit support staff member has to complete a source document and then re-enter the same data into the computer system, the input mechanism is duplicative and not satisfactory. On the other hand, if a unit support staff member has timely access to a computer terminal, can input data directly, and the system performs an automatic input consistency check, the input mechanism is more likely to be satisfactory.

The goals of the output process include the following:

- To assist the end user in retrieving appropriate data at the appropriate time in the appropriate format. As with the input mechanism, the end user should be able to retrieve data unobtrusively in the regular work flow pattern. Care providers will avoid accessing data from a computer terminal if it does not conveniently fit into their regular work flow process.
- To provide information that is accurate, timely, complete, and specific to the query. If a care provider queries a patient care system for all abnormal electrolyte results

during the past 48 hours but the system returns results of all laboratory tests, the output function is not satisfactory.

Screen Design

An important part of input and output is the design of the data display screen and its ease of use. Various interface elements can be used for data display. Among them are menus, windows, dialogue boxes, icons, color, and fonts. Menus present a list of options that users can browse and from which they can select a specific menu item. Menus can take several forms, including pull-down menus, hierarchic menus, and pop-up menus.

Windows can either be used as views to a document or provide utilities such as tools or commands for the user. For example, document windows contain user data and provide mechanisms for the user to interact with the data. Utility windows are usually smaller, accessory windows that provide additional tools to the user.

Dialogue boxes are a special application of a window. The purpose of a dialogue box is to elicit a response from the user. A common example of a dialogue box is a print options box that asks the user to specify which printer is to be used, how many pages to print, and how many copies of each page to print.

Icons are graphic representations of real-world objects that help convey to the user the purpose of a command executed through the icon. In other words, the icon presents a type of picture that graphically portrays the kind of function that is executed if the icon is selected. For example, a graphic display of a file cabinet may indicate that selection of that icon will open up a directory of files; a graphic display of an open book may indicate that the selection of that icon will initiate a thesaurus lookup function. A common representation in EHR systems is the use of tabs on the display that may be clicked to access specific locations within the electronic record. Examples are "tabs" for medications, progress notes, and discharge summary. Other icons may be used to represent pharmacy or laboratory. As data entry devices become smaller with hand-held devices, the use of icons helps streamline the visual identification and access to content in the patient record. Icons are useful devices in interface design because many end users recognize and understand pictures of things more easily than verbal commands of the same thing.

Color is an option that is often used in interface and screen display design. Although the use of color can make screen displays attractive to the user and often improve performance, there is also a danger of misuse. Color should be used conservatively, principally to enhance the identification of important data or draw the user's attention to important functions.

The HIM professional should remember that the development of data display screens is a complex process that involves knowledge of high-level theories and models from various cognitive sciences, including such disciplines as computer science, psychology, artificial intelligence, linguistics, anthropology, and sociology. It is important, therefore, that a computer interface engineer be involved in the development of data screen displays. User interface is important for HIM functions and for general organization functions. The HIM professional will benefit from working with the interface engineer as products are designed or modified for use by HIM staff members.

General Design Characteristics. Several general guidelines should be followed regardless of the type of screen or interface developed. A primary virtue of an interface is its degree of simplicity. Simple interfaces are easy to learn, easy to remember, and easy to use by a large target audience. A satisfying interface makes end users think that they are in control of the system. The system should be able to perform the following functions:

- Respond quickly to user commands
- Provide useful and simple messages
- Offer good navigation tools
- Provide adequate power to perform necessary tasks

Whitten et al,[4] Dennis et al,[5] and Kulak and Guiney[6] described several human-machine interface characteristics. Input and output interfaces should provide direction and learning. An end user should be able to interact with a system without extensive training. If the interface is designed to fit the normal work pattern of the end user, extensive directions are superfluous. Screens should be layered or windowed and good navigational tools provided. Users should be able to move within the system without getting lost in a maze of screens or commands.

Interfaces should provide the end user with a choice of style. As an example, a physician may want to review the 5-day trend in a patient's white blood cell count and compare it with the count after the administration of a chemotherapeutic agent over the same period. In this case, the system should be flexible enough to present the user with choices of a graphic, tabular, or other format for display.

Interfaces should be forgiving. This means that users should be able to recover easily from input or query errors. Error messages should be polite, meaningful, and informative. A flashing message "Error," for example, does not explain to the user what caused the error or how to recover from it. All interfaces should contain an escape feature. This allows the end user to interrupt a session at will or to recover from an error.

Another important part of an interface is the input device. Among input mechanisms are keyboards, light pens, touch-sensitive screens, voice recognition, pen-based systems, hand-held devices, bar code readers, and laser scanning. The measure of utility of these mechanisms is the degree to which each comfortably augments the normal work flow of the end user. No matter how attractive a technology is, its benefit is diminished if it disrupts rather than assists employees in their normal work. For example, the choice of voice recognition may seem like an attractive alternative to using a keyboard for input. However, the system should be easy to use and contain a medical vocabulary with spell check. The system should also be easy to train to one's voice and take a minimum of training time; otherwise, use of voice recognition would defeat the purpose of a robust interface.

System Performance

Besides input and output considerations, the system designer must think about system performance issues. From an end-user perspective, functional system performance indicators may include such criteria as degree of data accuracy, system response rates, system efficiency, system security, and ease of system use. The HIM professional should be involved in identifying functional performance criteria and thresholds and in developing plans for systematically auditing whether they are consistently met.

Criteria and thresholds for system performance vary depending on the application. For example, the response time in a clinical application may be more critical than in a billing application, or security issues may be more critical in situations that involve patient-identifiable information than in applications that deal with aggregate data. Because of this variability, system performance criteria should be developed with the application in mind. An example of functional system performance criteria for an order entry system for a unit staff member is presented in Table 9-4. These criteria would change with an order entry system for direct provider input. In this example, three performance issues are identified: accuracy, response rate, and efficiency. For each issue, subissues are identified. For example, under accuracy, issues related to input, transaction, and database accuracy have been noted. For each subissue, the criteria and methods for evaluation have been enumerated. In this order entry example, accuracy has been identified as a major performance issue and is divided into three components: input accuracy, transaction accuracy, and database accuracy. The evaluation of all three of these components is essential to determine the performance accuracy of the system. For example, orders may be correctly entered by unit support staff members, but there may be a transaction error (system error) in processing the order. In other words, the order could be correctly entered, but the order is not received by the recipient department, such as the pharmacy or laboratory. Although this type of error could occur for any number of reasons, it is nonetheless important to document the rate of such errors.

In the order entry example in Table 9-4 the criterion for measuring input accuracy is "entry error rate," and the method for evaluating this error rate is to compare the physician-written orders with the orders entered into the system by the unit support staff members. For transaction accuracy, the criterion for measurement is errors per time period and the method of evaluation is comparison of orders entered with orders received by the appropriate clinical department. In regard to database accuracy, the criterion for measurement is error rate per record and the method for evaluation is comparison of orders entered with the patient database.

Table 9-4 ORDER ENTRY SYSTEM PERFORMANCE CRITERIA

Accuracy	Criteria	Evaluation Method
Accuracy		
Input accuracy	Entry error rate	Compare physician orders with orders entered
Transaction accuracy	Errors per time period	Compare orders entered with orders received by department
Database accuracy	Error rate/record	Compare orders entered with patient database
Response Rate		
Input responses	No. of transactions per time period	Measure transactions per time period
Output response	Amount of time for one transaction	Transaction response rate
Down time	Down time minutes per time period	Down time rate
Efficiency		
Input efficiency	Errorless transactions per time period	Transaction error rate
System efficiency	Errors corrected per time period	Error correction rate

As this example illustrates, the development of system performance criteria is a nontrivial activity. It is important that every criterion important for system performance and specific to the application is identified and that appropriate methods for evaluation are established. One of the reasons for the emergence of CPOE is the recognition that removing steps in the order entry process and allowing the individual who created to the order to interact with the system's alerts and guidelines should reduce errors.

ROLE OF PROTOTYPING IN SYSTEM DEVELOPMENT

Within the information systems community there has been significant debate about whether the benefits of the system development life cycle outweigh the time and effort it takes to complete the process. One alternative to the system development life cycle is system prototyping. Prototyping a system usually has the following primary goals:

- To build a prototype of an information system quickly
- To involve the user heavily in the model development

Initially, the system prototype can be a preliminary model of the final system, but after several iterations of development, the prototype can evolve into the final system.

Although the prototype alternative involves investigating user requirements, it is not usually done at the depth required in the system development life cycle. The user is heavily involved in the requirements definition stage as well as all other stages of prototype development. After an initial requirements definition is compiled and analysis completed, a prototype design is developed. The first part of a prototype system is usually the development of on-line input and output screens and the generation of output document formats. At this stage of development, the prototype usually has little functionality. The purpose of this first step is to translate system requirements quickly into a format users can critique. The input and output mechanisms are evaluated and changed or enhanced as required.

After input and output prototyping is completed, system features are gradually added. The most important functions of a system are typically incorporated first. In a prototype of a master patient index, for example, the collection of patient data, data storage, and retrieval functions are incorporated at this stage. The end user continues to be involved in evaluation of the prototype. At this stage, there are opportunities to define information requirements further, refine system functionality, and correct defects.

The final stage of prototyping is generation of the completed prototype system. The prototype is tested and evaluated, and if changes to the prototype need to be made, the system is updated and evaluated again. If the test of the prototype is successful, it remains as the model for the final system. Prototype systems are usually developed in fourth-generation languages to speed up the development process. When this occurs, the final version of the prototype is usually recoded in a third-generation language for final system development.

Prototyping is gaining popularity for a number of reasons. First, prototyping provides immediate feedback to users in a format that has meaning to them. In the system development life cycle, a system may take weeks, months, or years to develop and the final product may still be unsatisfactory to end users. When the prototyping method is used, early in prototype development users assume responsibility for approval of design and function capabilities. Second, prototypes can simulate the dynamics of the real world. It is difficult in a DFD to assess the stress incurred by an emergency department physician and the urgency as she or he attempts to locate information about a drug regimen in a patient's file. Because the prototype can simulate real-world activity, issues related to input and output and data manipulation can be more easily identified. A final benefit provided by prototyping is faster delivery of products than that provided by the traditional method of systems analysis.

In addition to its apparent benefits, several other factors have contributed to the increased use of the prototype method. First, there has been an advance in technology that has made prototyping possible. In the past, mainframe computers and third-generation programming languages were incompatible with the concept of prototyping. Today, however, microcomputers have the power that only mainframes had a few years ago. This instant power and flexibility at the desktop have contributed to prototype increase. Second, there has been a growth in prototyping tools. Fourth-generation languages, screen generators, report generators, and interactive testing systems are but a few of the tools that today's analyst has that assist in prototype development. Additionally users have access to and experience with relational databases on their computers and may be able to do some initial design/use work to speed the formal process. Whitten et al[4] also suggest "time-boxing" as another way of getting a product to the user more quickly. In time-boxing the smallest subset of a system that, if implemented, will return immediate value is put into place and then every 6 to 9 months for a defined period versions are added to build the system to more fully meet the users' needs.

The prototyping process is not without its critics. Some believe that in the haste to develop a product quickly insufficient effort may be devoted to the analysis process. A quick-fix product may be developed that initially looks good but does not have the total functionality that is required.

Prototyping, however, can be integrated into the system development life cycle. In fact, the meshing of the traditional life cycle approach with prototyping can produce positive results. Through this process, the benefits of each strategy can be achieved, including a thorough analysis derived from the traditional approach with the rapid development of a model system from the prototype approach.

SYSTEM IMPLEMENTATION

System implementation usually refers to all the tasks associated with getting the information system installed and operating. Planning for implementation should occur as soon as feasible after the initial decision is made to go forward on the design or selection of a system. System implementation can be an enormous undertaking. The key to a smooth implementation process is planning and well-executed management. Many systems fail or encounter significant problems during installation because of inadequate planning or poor execution of plans. The steps in implementing a system may vary, given the project and the scope of installation, but the following activities are usually present to some degree:

- User preparation and training
- Site preparation
- System testing
- System conversion
- System startup

It is important to remember that the steps in system implementation are not necessarily linear. Rather, activities associated with two or more of the preceding categories may be occurring concurrently. For example, system testing and user preparation activities may take place in parallel. In fact, some of the implementation processes may also be occurring during the system design phase. For example, preparations for the site may be taking place at the same time as final system design.

User Preparation and Training

User preparation and training are probably among the most underestimated tasks in the implementation process. Users not only need to be trained how to use the system but also need to be educated about the system's purpose and benefits and how it supports the overall well-being of the organization. The implementation of a system should come as no surprise to end users if they have been appropriately included in the analysis and design phases.[8] Early in the implementation process, the system purpose, its general functionality, and its anticipated benefits should be reemphasized to end users, managers, and appropriate others. This can be accomplished through formal or informal presentations given by an implementation team member or through brochures, newsletters, seminars, and workshops. Users should be presented with a realistic view of the system. Although the system may have many benefits, these benefits should not be exploited so that unrealistic user expectations are developed.

The format, curriculum, and presentation materials for end-user training need to be carefully developed. The format varies given the type of end user and the complexity of the system. For example, the format for end-user training for physicians is likely to be different from that for unit support staff members. Format, such as time and place of training sessions, also varies. Format may consist of frequent, single sessions in small blocks of time (say, 60 minutes) or less-frequent, larger concentrated sessions. System training can take place in a structured training area or room, or it can be scheduled in the end user's area of work. For instance, it may be appropriate to conduct the initial training of nursing personnel in a classroom configured with a simulated system. Once nursing personnel have gone through the initial sessions, it may be more convenient to hold one-on-one sessions with personnel on a training computer located in the work area.

The curriculum needs to be configured differently for each type of end user. One size does not fit all. The content of the curriculum should correspond to the tasks that are normally performed by each end-user group. For instance, physicians do not need to know how to navigate through nursing pathways, and registration clerks do not need to know how to do order entry.

Curriculum content should begin with easy concepts and operations. As end users become proficient with each area, more difficult operations can be introduced. Competence testing is used to assess end-user proficiency at each level of the training. For example, in order entry training, users may be introduced systematically to different components (e.g., pharmacy, laboratory, radiology). Before an end user can proceed to the next module, a competence test is administered to assess mastery of the current section.

The presentation method for the curriculum must match the knowledge, skills, and availability of the end users. Among presentation options are demonstration, simulation, one-on-one training, on-line topic-based demonstrations, on-line interactive learning sessions, exercises, workbooks, and lecture and discussion sessions. Each of these methods has its benefits and drawbacks. The usage of each depends on the degree of skill to be developed, the scope of the system, the skill of the end users, and the need to provide just in time learning. For example, a demonstration might be used when the system is simple to operate and the end user does not have to possess a great deal of skill. On the other hand, a more complex system might require demonstration and simulation integrated with exercises and lecture and discussion sessions.

The development of self-paced training modules is an alternative to holding large classroom-style classes. Self-paced modules can be developed so that end users can use them with minimal assistance and they can be placed on-line. These modules can incorporate methods of lecture, exercise, simulation, and competence testing. They can be especially attractive in the health care environment, where employees work round-the-clock shifts and may not be available to attend training sessions scheduled during the usual daytime work period.

Scheduling of training sessions can be an enormous undertaking. Take, for example, the implementation of a hospital-wide information system in a 1000-bed facility. In this case, it is likely that as many as 2000 end users will need to be trained. If each training session averages 6 hours per person and competence testing consumes another 2 hours per end user, the total training hours would be 16,000 hours. The actual user training time needed would be calculated by determining how many end users would be in a class at one time, how many classes would be held per 8-hour shift, and how many days per week classes would be held. Hospital facilities operate around the clock and on weekends, and training scheduling must be flexible to accommodate all end users.

Another component of end-user preparation is the selection and training of the trainers. Few organizations have sufficient staff available to carry out the training efforts for a large-scale information system implementation. Therefore, consideration needs to be given to the selection of new staff, the number of staff required, and how these people are to be trained. Sometimes vendors or consultants are hired to develop and staff the training effort. The trade-offs of using in-house personnel versus outside contractual arrangements need to be assessed. Remember, though, that training is a continuing process and a training staff always needs to be available.

Site Preparation

The location of the system and its associated components needs to be planned well in advance of installation. If the system is small (i.e., microcomputer based), management of site preparation is minimal. With larger systems, however, installation site preparation is a major activity. For example, installation of a laboratory or total hospital information system may require special wiring or special wireless configuration planning, special room accommodations, special cables or boxes, and sufficient room for all components. If the system involves a wide area or a local area network, site preparation is likely to require facility-wide planning. For example, plans need to be developed for network backbone wiring, locations for wiring closets and hubs, and conduit for wiring.

Analysis of end-user space requirements should not be forgotten in the site preparation process. Too often, when system installation occurs, it is discovered that the allotted space for end-user terminals or computers is not adequate. Space may be too small, ill configured, or inconvenient to wiring, subject to wireless interference or not in an appropriate place to allow adequate access. This oversight can turn any installation process into a nightmare.

System Testing and Conversion

All systems must be tested to ensure that they perform in the way intended. It would be a disaster to install a system on an organization-wide basis and then have it fail in one or more transactions. Good system testing is a precursor to successful installation. The development of test scripts can be a tedious process. Therefore, development of tests will probably begin long before system installation. The adequacy of both the hardware and the software of a system must be assessed. Many manufacturers provide diagnostic routines to test major system components. These routines should be supplemented by organization-developed tests.

Test Phases

Several phases are used to test systematically the performance of software. First, each program is tested (*unit testing*) by providing test data or audit scripts that force the execution of all program statements. Total *system testing* is done to determine how well programs interact and execute in an integrated environment. Many times, a system may work well during a test situation in which limited amounts of data are used. Most production systems, however, operate in a data-intensive environment. Therefore it is important to determine how well the system works during actual production. This is accomplished through *volume testing,* in which large amounts of data are put through the system. Processing and response times can be more adequately assessed when volume testing occurs. Systems usually do not stand alone but are expected to interact with other systems. For example, the laboratory information system would be expected to interact with the admission and order entry systems. To determine how well interaction occurs, the new system is tested with other information system components. This is usually referred to as *integration testing.*

System Conversion

Before a new system is implemented, files from the old system often need to be converted from one medium to another. Sometimes this means the transfer of paper records to a computer format. For example, if the master patient index has been maintained manually, information in the index needs to be placed on a computer medium before the new system can be totally implemented. Conversion can take many forms. For example, it may involve converting from one computer medium to another, from one file structure to another, or from one operating system to another. The technical issues to be addressed during any conversion can be complex. When the transfer occurs, it is extremely important to have quality control procedures in place that ensure the integrity of data and transactions. The HIM professional should be part of the team that determines the criteria and methods for quality control during the conversion process.

Startup

System startup occurs when all activities leading up to installation have been completed. This includes activities related to user training, site preparation, hardware installation, testing, and conversion. The following approaches to the startup phase can be used:

- Abrupt changeover
- Gradual phase-in of applications in selected organizational units
- Gradual phase-in of applications organization wide

Abrupt Changeover

Abrupt changeover refers to the total rollout of a system across all organizational units at the same time. This approach is exceedingly risky unless the system is simple and does not affect a great number of organizational units. For example, an abrupt changeover may be appropriate for a utilization management system that affects a small number of people in one department. With larger, complex systems, however, abrupt changeover could prove disastrous. In an abrupt changeover, if problems occur, they are likely to affect the entire organization and potentially threaten mission-crucial operations. Debugging of system problems is usually difficult in an abrupt changeover because problem origin is difficult to isolate in a complex system.

Gradual Phase-In of Applications

Gradual phase-in of applications usually refers to bringing up one application at a time in selected units over a period of time. For example, three units in a hospital might initially bring up the order entry application. After a few weeks, the laboratory interface would be rolled out in the same units. Once the entire system was successfully operating in the selected units, organization-wide implementation would occur. This approach is risk adverse. If problems occur during the installation, the impact on end users and the organization is minimized. Debugging any problems that occur is also easier because each application is tested and debugged as it is implemented. Thus, at any one time, there are fewer modules to search for problem origin.

Systems can also be phased in application by application over the total organization. For example, the order entry application or the voice-activated history and physical application could be brought up at the same time in all patient care units throughout the facility. When the application is proved to be stable, the next module is brought on-line. This approach is not quite as risk adverse as the previous method. It does, however, provide more insurance than abrupt changeover does. Allowing all organizational units to be at the same point in system installation also has its benefits from both operational and training aspects, provided all system applications are problem free.

SYSTEM EVALUATION AND BENEFITS REALIZATION

Although system evaluation in this chapter is discussed at the end of the system development life cycle, this should not be construed to mean that the evaluation process begins only after system installation. In fact, planning for system evaluation and realization of benefits should start in parallel with the system design effort. What is system evaluation, and why is it important to begin the process early in the system development life cycle?

The purpose of system evaluation is to determine whether the system functions in the way intended. All too often, systems are installed but the degree of benefit derived from them is never measured. Organizations that fail to measure system benefits cannot systematically determine whether expenditures on system development or purchase were justified. As a result, such organizations have no method to determine what impact the time, effort, and expense of a system development or selection process has had on the organization. In today's environment of competition, continuous quality improvement, and cost justification, no organization can afford *not* to justify information system expenditures.

The following methods are used to evaluate systems:

- Benefits realization
- Cost-benefit analysis
- Cost-effectiveness analysis

Benefits Realization

In **benefits realization,** the criteria used for system evaluation evolve from the analysis and design sections of the development life cycle. Take, for example, a computerized release of information tracking system. Suppose that in the systems analysis document some of the goals of this system were as follows:

- Decrease response time to requests for information
- Easily track pending requests and due dates and reasons for pending requests
- Accurately document each release of information
- Accurately document the name of the staff member(s) responsible for the release of information
- Accurately document what is being released, when, why, how, and to whom
- Identify those releases made with patient/guardian consent
- Identify those releases required by law and not requiring patient consent
- Identify and track performance on those releases where local law may require notification of the patient to allow the patient to object to a mandatory release (subpoena) and the outcome
- Identify discretionary releases (where the laws are permissive)
- Identify the requests for information that were denied or not answered and the reason
- Reduce errors in the release of information to external entities
- Reduce employee time in documenting the release of information data elements
- Provide for reporting capability (i.e., releases of information made without the patient's consent)
- Calculate daily, weekly, and monthly work volumes
- Provide for retention of the database for a period of at least 6 years

In the evaluation of the release of information tracking system, these goals would be used as the basic criteria for determining the benefits of system installation. Using this method for evaluation of a system is usually referred to as benefits realization. In other words, has the system delivered the benefits that were anticipated? To determine the exact benefits derived from the system, good measurements must be established for each criterion. For example, the response time for responding to requests for information must be known before system implementation. If these and other data are not known, postimplementation benefits cannot be calculated. This points out the need for understanding and applying the necessary tracking of metrics. Consider the following examples of metrics or measurements that could be established for comparison in implementing EHR systems. Remember that before system implementation baseline data would need to be gathered to use as comparison data.

1. Increased number of patients seen per provider by reducing time spent on documentation.
   Reduce amount of time spent by physicians on clinical and administrative documentation
   Reduce amount of time searching for data/information in clinical record
   Allow more patients to be seen per day:

Measurements:

- Number of patient visits per clinic per hour
- Annualized patient visits per provider per clinic
- Current per clinic per physician patient revenue

2. Increased number of patients seen per provider by reducing wait time for clinical information.
   Reduce amount of time waiting for clinical data/information for drop in/same day patients

Measurements:

- Number of drop in/same-day patient visits per clinic per day
- Annualized drop in/same-day patient visits per provider per clinic
- Current per clinic per physician patient revenue for drop in/same-day patients

3. Increased efficiency in response to patient phone calls or written communication
   Reduce the amount of time involved in responding to a clinical phone call or written inquiry

Measurements:

- Number of clinical phone calls per day
- Number of written inquiries per day
- Amount of time involved in responding to clinical phone calls and written inquiries

4. Reduce nurse/support staff intake and nurse/other clinician clinical record documentation time
   Reduce time spent on patient intake information
   Reduce documentation time by automating collection of inpatient bedside monitoring devices
   Reduce documentation time by using templates to update clinical documentation

Measurements:

- Time spent by support staff gathering intake information
- Time spent by nurse (other clinician) documenting intake information
- per patient
- Current staff to physician full-time equivalent (FTE) ratio

5. Reduce transcription volume and costs related to transcribed documents

Reduce the volume of transcribed documents by encouraging clinicians to use voice-activated software

Reduce the volume of transcribed documents by providing easy-to-use on-line templates for certain types of clinical documentation

Reduce cost by reducing the complexity of integrating the transcribed documents into an EHR or electronic medical record (EMR) system

Measurements:

- Average lines of dictation per patient visit
- Average lines of dictation per patient hospitalization
- Change in productivity of transcriptionist(s) measured by lines of dictation or minutes of dictation
- Average cost of line of dictation (or minute of dictation) per patient visit (or hospitalization)
- Average cost of a report (could cost by report type) based on average number of lines or minutes
- Average cost of rework per day (tracking down information needed to complete a report or to match it to correct patient)

6. Reduce chart pulls for clinical records

Reduce the number of records pulled by HIM staff members to support direct patient care, research, release of information, coding, and other requests.

Measurements:

- Average cost of pulling a clinical record that is on site
- Average cost of pulling a clinical record that is stored off site
- Average number of clinical records pulled per day (can categorize by type of pull—clinic, readmission, emergency department, quality study, release of information, coding, etc.)

7. Identify new tasks associated with support of an EHR system and set up metrics to track associated time and costs[8]

For example, the electronic record system may need to accommodate some scanned documents. HIM staff reductions in the pulling and filing of clinical records may be redirected to scanning. Track the time and cost associated with this activity. The electronic record system will have errors in documentation that need correction. A small team of staff members need to be able to appropriately manage documentation errors that need to be addressed systematically and with approved policies and procedures.

The work of planning and accomplishing effective evaluation begins with a clear idea of what is to be improved by the new application. The case for purchasing or developing systems is made early on in project initiation and analysis phases and the foundation for future evaluation must be established and data collected for future evaluation collected before implementation. The examples given are related to processes; however, the organization could add other expected outcomes directly related to patient care improvement and patient safety, establish baseline data before implementation, and reassess. The reassessment findings might prove useful, although attributing changes solely to the implementation of a new system may not be possible.

Cost-Benefit Analysis

The benefits realization method is not usually economics based, although the potential costs in inappropriate release of information could be discussed. In other words, system benefits are not necessarily compared with an economic outcome. **Cost-benefit analysis** (CBA), on the other hand, attempts to measure benefits compared with system costs. Basically, the goal of CBA is to determine whether the information system decreases or increases benefits and whether it decreases or increases cost for the organization. Cost-benefit methods are frequently used before system development or selection of system alternatives. These methods are applied in an attempt to justify the selection of one alternative over another. For example, CBA would be used to justify selection of one vendor's product over another or to justify the purchase of a proposed information system.

The term "cost-benefit analysis" is used somewhat loosely in the information systems field as opposed to its use by economists. Basically, CBA uses microeconomic models to assist in making good decisions. In CBA, dollar values are assigned to the cost and benefits of a proposed information system. These dollar values are then compared to help make a decision between alternative systems. Several techniques are used to evaluate alternative solutions. Among them are break-even analysis, payback period, discounted payback period, return on investment, and internal rate of return. (These techniques are also discussed in the financial management chapter of this book.)

Break-Even Analysis

Break-even analysis is probably the simplest CBA technique. In break-even analysis, costs to operate the current system are compared with those to operate the proposed system. The point at which old system costs equal new system costs is called the break-even point. After the break-even point, the proposed system should begin to generate a positive monetary return compared with the old system. With this analysis, a set period is usually targeted ahead of time for monetary return (e.g., 2 to 5 years).

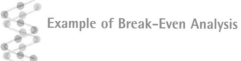

Example of Break-Even Analysis

The current software budget for the encoding system in the HIM department is $10,000 per year for licensing. Replacement and upgrades of hardware for the system cost $6000 per year. A new encoding system with added features is being considered. The HIM department plans to reconfigure the work area as part of this project with a one-time cost of $10,000. The new, more capable software will cost less. The subscription fee is $8000 per year, which will accommodate up to three new users. The department is budgeting a replacement/maintenance fee for hardware of $8000 per year. With the new expanded encoder, the department expects that it will increase reimbursement by at least $5000 per year. In addition, the new software should reduce coding and billing errors, which will improve the turnaround time from billing to collection, at least for some payers.

In this case, the current system is costing $16,000 per year. In the first year, the new system will cost $26,000, but reimbursement will increase by $5000. The net cost of the new system after the first year is $21,000, and the difference between the net cost of the new system and the old system in the first year is $5000. In the second year, the old system would continue to cost $16,000 to operate. The new system cost will also be $16,000 ($8000 license + $8000 maintenance). However, the new system will continue to increase reimbursement at $5000 per year. Thus, at the end of the second year, the break-even point has been achieved with the net cost of both systems being $16,000 each. Table 9-5 shows how the break-even point is determined.

Payback Period

Calculation of the **payback period** is often done to determine whether a new system will fully recover its investment (development) costs before the end of its life cycle. In the preceding encoding example, the investment cost was $10,000 (reconfiguring the work area) and the operating cost was $16,000. To determine the payback period, a comparison between total old system costs and total new system costs (including investment) is made. The difference between new system and old system costs is calculated on a year-by-year (cumulative) basis. When the difference between old system costs and new system costs reaches zero, the payback period has been reached. Table 9-6 shows the payback period calculation for the encoding example.

In year 1 of Table 9-5 the current system cost is $16,000. The new system cost is $26,000 ($10,000 + $16,000). The yearly difference in cost during the first year is a negative

Table 9-5 CALCULATION OF BREAK-EVEN POINT

Year	New System	Old System
Year 1		
Operation cost	$26,000	$16,000
Increase in revenue	+$5,000	0
Net cost	$21,000	$16,000
Difference in operation cost and net cost	$5,000	0
Year 2		
Operation cost	$16,000	$16,000
Difference in operation cost and net cost year 1	$5,000	0
Increase in revenue	$5,000	0
Net cost	$16,000	$16,000
Difference in operation cost and net cost	0	0

$10,000 ($16,000 – 26,000). Because this is the first year of calculation, the cumulative difference remains –$10,000. During the second year, the current system still costs $16,000. The new system costs $11,000 ($16,000 operating cost –$5000 increase in reimbursement). The yearly difference between the current and the new system costs is $5000 ($16,000 – $11,000). The cumulative cost difference is –$5000 (–$10,000 – +$5000). In the third year, the costs of the current system remain $16,000 and the costs of the new system remain $11,000. The yearly difference in costs is again $5000; however, the cumulative difference in costs has reached zero (–$5000 – +$5000). Thus the payback period has been reached after 3 years.

The encoding system problem illustrates the difference between the break-even point and the payback point. It is important to recognize how these different CBA techniques can be used to support different arguments to purchase or not purchase a system.

Discounted Payback Period

Another CBA technique uses the **discounted payback period.** In this method, an organization determines how much a system costs in future dollars. The basic concept underlying this approach is that today's dollars are worth more than future dollars. This is because an organization can usually invest today's dollars at a certain interest rate and receive a **return on investment** (ROI). Therefore future

Table 9-6 CALCULATION OF PAYBACK PERIOD FOR ENCODER SYSTEM

	Year 1	Year 2	Year 3
Current system cost	$16,000	$16,000	$16,000
New system cost	$26,000	$11,000	$11,000
Yearly difference in costs	$10,000	+$5,000	+$5,000
Cumulative difference in costs	($10,000)	($5,000)	0

dollars that are anticipated to be made by installing an information system are discounted in calculations used to determine the discounted payback period. For example, say a health care facility can invest $1 today at 8% interest. The value of that dollar next year will be $1.08. If it is projected that an information system will earn $5000 next year, that $5000 in future dollars would actually have less value than today's dollars (i.e., if the facility invested $5000 at 8% interest, the amount would be $5400 by next year). To illustrate how the discounted payback period is calculated, the encoding example discussed previously is used.

To determine the present value of today's dollar at any time in the future, the following formula is used:

$$1/(1 + ROI)^n$$

where ROI is the facility's expected return on investment and n is the number of years into the future. Let us assume that in the encoding example the facility expects an 8% ROI. Using the formula for present value, the discounted rate for years 1 through 5 after system startup has been calculated and is shown in Table 9-7.

Table 9-7 indicates that 1 year after project start the value of today's dollar is $0.93. The value of today's dollar after year 2 of the project is $0.86 and so on. Calculations to determine the discounted payback period for the encoding system appear in Table 9-8. Note that Table 9-8 is an extension of Table 9-5.

Table 9-7 indicates that the discounted payback period occurs some time between years 3 and 4. To interpret the table, the discounted difference is arrived at by multiplying the discount by the yearly difference in costs. For example, during year 1 the discount is 0.93 and the yearly difference in cost is −$10,000. Multiplying these figures yields the discounted difference in costs, which is −$9300 in year 1. All subsequent rows are calculated in the same way. To determine the cumulative difference in cost, the current year's discounted difference is subtracted from the cumulative difference. For example, in year 2 the discounted difference ($4300) is subtracted from the cumulative difference in year 1 (−$9300). This equals −$5000, which is the cumulative difference in costs between the current and new systems by year 2.

Table 9-7 CURRENT DOLLAR VALUE, YEARS 1-5

Years	Future Dollar Value
1	0.93
2	0.86
3	0.79
4	0.74
5	0.68

Cost-Effectiveness Analysis

As opposed to CBA, **cost-effectiveness analysis** attempts to evaluate certain beneficial consequences in nonmonetary terms. Therefore, in cost-effectiveness analysis, desirable benefits are not valued in monetary terms but are measured in some other unit. For example, what price could be placed on saving one life or making a patient's record available to a patient care unit more quickly? Or, can the investment in a new information system decrease medication errors or increase timelier drug administration? The determination of how much it is worth to decrease one medication error is a social question, not a technical or economic one. How much a nonmonetary item is worth is left for the specific facility to determine given current situations and constraints. There are and will be a number of organization-wide systems that do not meet monetary criteria but will still be necessary to build infrastructure and as business investments. Health care has been slow to recognize that investing in information systems is a continuing process and a regular budget item once a system is in place. As health care attempts to raise the level of consistency in the use of known quality performance in health care, it will be easier to quantify and attach dollars to the difference between high-quality care and mediocre care. The information systems such as the EHR will help in this endeavor.

It should be obvious from review of the previous methods why it is important for the health information manager to have an understanding of these various techniques. As the encoding system example demonstrates, statistics can mean whatever you want them to mean. To

Table 9-8 DISCOUNTED PAYBACK PERIOD FOR ENCODER SYSTEM

	Year 1	Year 2	Year 3	Year 4
Current system cost	$16,000	$16,000	$16,000	$16,000
New system cost	$26,000	$11,000	$11,000	$11,000
Yearly difference in costs	−$10,000	+$5,000	+$5,000	+$5,000
Discount (ROI = 0.08)	0.93	0.86	0.79	0.74
Discounted difference	−$9,300	+$4,300	+$3,950	+$3,700
Cumulative difference in costs	−$9,300	−$5,000	−$1,050	+$2,650

ROI, Return on investment.

evaluate the costs and benefits of a system objectively, a variety of analytic techniques should be used, including CBA and benefits realization.

Other Evaluation Methods and Techniques

In addition to the three previously discussed evaluation methods (benefits realization, cost-benefit analysis, and cost-effectiveness analysis), many other evaluation techniques can be used to assess the functional, technical, and economic outcomes of system implementation. Evaluation of computer systems should be approached in the same manner as any evaluation study. As a first step, the evaluation question(s) should be framed. For example, an evaluation question may be "Does the system work as it was intended to work?" In other words, does the system perform technically well? For an admission, discharge, and transfer (ADT) system, can the admitting clerk retrieve a patient's previous admission and discharge dates? Does the system provide the patient's medical record number and demographics? Can the admitting clerk update the demographic information?

Another type of evaluation question might be to assess whether the system is being used as it was intended. For example, who uses the system? What functions of the systems are being used most often? Which functions are being rarely or never used? Still another question for evaluation might be "What impact has the system had in the delivery of patient care?" For example, have medication errors been reduced since system implementation? Are laboratory results being reported faster? Are laboratory tests being processed faster? Is the waiting time in the emergency department or clinics significantly reduced? It is apparent that an infinite number of evaluation questions can be developed. The important point is that the evaluation questions must be narrowed to those that are deemed most important and critical to the enterprise.

After the evaluation questions have been chosen, the next step in the evaluation process is to choose a research method. The types of research methods that can be used include qualitative, survey, and experimental methods as well as mathematical and computer simulations and methods that use a combination of these approaches. Each of these methods has its own strengths and weaknesses. The choice of any method is directly dependent on the evaluation question(s) to be answered.

Qualitative research attempts to answer questions about how and why specific outcomes occur. This type of research frequently uses structured observation, focused interview of participants, and analysis of formal and informal notes and reports. A principal objective of qualitative research is to study a system in its natural environment or setting. Words, rather than numbers, are used to describe the results of the analysis. This type of research is particularly useful in studying the design, use, and implementation of health care information systems. For example, observing how clinicians actually use a system may provide better information about how the system facilitates ease of use than conducting a survey because it allows the evaluator to study the dynamics of a process. A drawback of the qualitative research technique is that it relies on the observation and interpretation of one or a few evaluators. This method may introduce bias into the evaluation results unless countermeasures are built into the evaluation process. The role of qualitative research is increasing in significance to answer questions that quantitative measurement does not answer. Freidman and Wyatt[9] note that the motivation of qualitative studies is to address what people really want to know, such as, "Is the information resource working as intended? How can it be improved? Does it make any difference? Are the differences beneficial? Are the observed effects those envisioned by the developers or are they different?" (p. 248-249). Like quantitative analysis, quantitative evaluation relies on a method to guide the process.

Survey methods are frequently used to study the outcomes of health care information systems. The type of survey conducted is dependent on the evaluation question selected for study. Survey evaluation can be used to assess the level of user satisfaction with a system and the level of user compliance. Survey data are also collected to describe the demographics of groups of system users or nonusers, identify the status of implementation or use of a system, measure attitudes toward computer use, and measure the degree of adaptation to computer usage. Survey evaluation is conducted by using a structured or standardized survey instrument or questionnaire applied to a population or sample of a population. Using a survey approach is usually an easier evaluation method then using a qualitative approach. A strength of survey research is that it is usually nonintrusive, easy to administer, and easy to compile data. A major drawback of survey research is that it cannot assess adequately the dynamics of how change occurs or assess the relationships between information systems and their external environment.

Experimental research methods can also be used to evaluate various aspects of information system implementation and use. However, these methods demand a much more rigorous environment and require the use of control groups. For these reasons, much of the experimental research conducted on health information systems has been performed in laboratory settings. Key requirements for an experimental research approach are random assignment of subjects to experimental and control groups and the manipulation of one or more independent variables. In addition, the evaluator must be able to control other independent and intervening variables that may affect the dependent variable under study and ultimately the outcome of the evaluation.

For the reasons cited, applying true experimental research design on health information systems is difficult. Therefore, a modification of the experimental design is often used. This is called a quasiexperimental or field design. In these situations, the evaluator frequently uses intact groups as opposed to randomly assigned groups. In addition, the evaluator does not have as much control over independent and extraneous variables. Although not as rigorous as the experimental design, the field evaluation does allow the study of an information system in its natural environment. As long as potential biases are recognized, the field design can be an important evaluation tool.

Mathematical and computer simulations are good strategies for studying the operational effectiveness of a computer system. For example, a computer simulation may be able to predict how an information system may affect the wait time of a patient being admitted to the hospital. Or it may be able to predict the throughput of laboratory tests and results given a certain volume of patients and laboratory tests. In one study, a computer simulation model of the order entry process was developed and used to perform computer simulation experiments to estimate the effects of two methods of order entry on several outcome measures.[2] The results indicated that the personal order sets for order entry could result in significant reduction of personnel and errors.

Once the evaluation question and the evaluation method have been chosen, the evaluation project must be managed in the same way as any other project. Resources must be allocated, including staff, equipment, money, and facilities, to carry out the evaluation. A project manager should be assigned to oversee the total evaluation process. Steps in the process must be identified. Responsibilities must be assigned and a time line developed. Monitoring of the project by the project manager must be a constant process to ensure that the project stays on time, has adequate resources, and is appropriately managed.

There is no one right question to ask, nor is there one right way to conduct an evaluation. The evaluation questions that are chosen and the methods used are highly dependent on the enterprise, its specific needs, and its individual context. What is important to one organization may not be important to another. Therefore, there is no "cookie cutter" or "one quick fix" approach to evaluation of information systems. It should be apparent, however, that evaluation of information systems should go beyond the technical aspects of the system. Because there is strong evidence that computer systems "affect the structure and functioning of operations, the quality of work life of employees within them, and ultimately the cost and quality of the goods and services they provide,"[3] each enterprise should have a rigorous program of evaluation. The program of evaluation should include study of how information systems affect the organization and functioning of the enterprise, the quality of work life of the employees, and the delivery and outcome of patient care.

PURCHASING PROCESS: REQUEST FOR PROPOSAL

Information system development for most health care applications is an enormous undertaking. Few health care facilities have the budget, expertise, or other resources needed to be able to develop most health care applications. Although every health care facility is unique, there are enough similarities across many functions to make the development of "vanilla" systems by vendors practical. These systems usually have general functionalities that can be modified to meet the needs of many health care facilities. For example, a health care facility would not usually develop a laboratory information system because this type of system is complex and the facility would probably not be able to justify the cost of development for benefit received. This type of system, on the other hand, is an ideal candidate for vendor development. Because most laboratories have similar functions, a general information system can be developed to meet the needs of many clinical laboratories. The cost of development, which is initially assumed by the vendor, can then be spread across many purchasers, making the individual cost to any one client less than if the client developed the system in house.

When a decision is made to purchase a system from a vendor rather than develop the product in house, a **request for proposal** (RFP) process is usually undertaken. An RFP is a document that details all required system functionality, including functional, technical, training, and implementation requirements. The document is distributed to a selected number of vendors, who are invited to respond to the proposal. The vendor response to the proposal indicates to what degree the vendor's product meets the proposed system requirements.

Request for Information

During the system specification process, the committee may issue a **request for information** (RFI) to vendors. Enough is generally known at this point about system capabilities so that an intelligent decision can be made about which vendor products are most likely to be competitive in a response to an RFP. The RFI basically solicits general information from vendors about their products. The RFI may state in general terms what the facility is looking for in system functionality. Vendors respond with information about their product lines and their experience in the marketplace and provide copies of their annual reports. The RFI is a good way for health care facilities to narrow down the field of vendors to whom an RFP will be sent.

Before an RFP is prepared, functional specifications for the new system must be generated. To produce the specifications, the same techniques used in the system development life cycle should be used. This includes development of hierarchy charts, DFDs, preliminary data dictionaries, and ERDs. Many health care facilities fail to do a thorough systems analysis when developing an RFP. This results in poorly drafted system specifications. When this occurs, the facility places itself in a vulnerable position. No RFP should be generated without a thorough analysis of user needs and projected system capabilities.

Planning Steps Before Request for Proposal Preparation

When the purchase of an information system is being considered, a steering committee is usually appointed to oversee the process. Membership of the committee is commonly multidisciplinary, including users, managers, and representatives from administration and information systems. The primary responsibility of the committee is to provide overall management of the system selection and implementation process. It is the committee's responsibility to develop a work plan and time table and ensure that the process is completed. Specific tasks of the committee vary from institution to institution but broadly encompass the following:

- Development of project work plan and time table
- Oversight of systems analysis
- Development of system specifications
- Determination of costs and benefits
- Compilation and distribution of the RFP
- Evaluation of responses to the RFP
- Selection of the system
- Conducting vendor negotiations
- Oversight of system implementation

Analyzing System Requirements

Although the decision has been made to purchase a system rather than develop a system, this does not obviate the need for an analysis effort. This process of identifying user requirements and determining system capabilities is essentially the same as in the system development life cycle. The steering committee may assign members of the committee analysis responsibilities, delegate these to in-house information system professionals, or contract with consultants to perform the function. No matter who is chosen to perform the function, the steering committee still has the final responsibility for the analysis process.

A detailed analysis document should be prepared. A benefits realization process should be identified and developed at this point, as well as the feasibility of the proposed system together with estimates of cost and benefits.

The results of analysis provide the foundation from which system functionality is determined. They also provide the basis for developing the function specifications of the RFP and the criteria by which vendor products are evaluated. Because of its importance, the analysis document should be complete and accurately reflect user requirements.

Development of System Specifications

System specifications include both the functional and the technical specifications of the system—the logical and physical descriptions of the system. Among logical system specifications are those related to output, input, processing, database, and security design. Physical specifications include details of hardware, database, communication, and control

needs. Training needs and implementation requirements are initially identified at this time. The details of system specification are later translated into the functional requirements section of the RFP document. Therefore, it is important that specifications be appropriate, complete, and accurate.

Development and Distribution of the Request for Proposal

After the analysis has been performed and system specifications identified, the RFP is prepared. The RFP is usually a lengthy document. Depending on the complexity of the system, an RFP can be several hundred pages long. Although format varies, an RFP usually includes the following sections:

- Proposal information and format
- Enterprise profile
- Conditions of response
- Functional requirements
- Technical requirements
- Training requirements
- Implementation requirements
- Vendor profile
- System costs

An RFP is a professionally prepared document. It is important that it be correct in all areas because sometimes it also functions as a legal document. Many times, the RFP and the response of the vendor who wins the bid are included in the final contract. Therefore, the importance of the accuracy of the RFP cannot be overemphasized.

Disclaimer and Table of Contents

An RFP usually begins with a disclaimer that the information contained in the document is considered proprietary and is to be considered in strict confidence and that no information contained in it can be disclosed without written permission from the organization issuing the RFP. A table of contents that functions as an index to the RFP is usually included. Figure 9-13 shows the table of contents of a typical RFP.

Proposal Overview

After the table of contents, an overview of the proposal is usually presented. Here the proposal format, time table, and requirements for proposal submission are detailed. One of the most important parts of this section is the proposal time table. Here, milestones of the process are listed with associated time frames. A typical time table is represented in Figure 9-14. The time frames in each proposal vary, depending on the complexity of the system being considered and on organizational constraints.

Enterprise Profile

The next section of the RFP usually contains a profile of the enterprise. This consists of a brief description of the organization and its demographic data. Statistics such

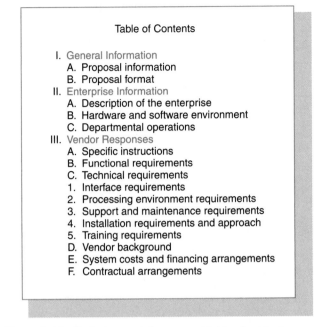

Figure 9-13 Typical request for proposal table of contents.

as bed size, occupancy rate, and number of admissions, discharges, procedures, and outpatient visits are frequently provided. These data provide the vendor with a perspective of the facility's volume of data and transactions. General information about the facility services and organization department operations is included. The current hardware and software environments are detailed in this section as well. This includes specifics about what type of hardware is in place, what applications are running, and who the developers of each application are. This provides vendors with important information to determine whether their products can easily interface with current applications or operate under the current hardware environment.

This section also includes a description of activities of all departments that are planning to use the proposed information system. These descriptions provide an overview of current departmental operations and usually include appro-

priate statistics related to work volumes that may affect system performance requirements.

Conditions of Response

In this section, guidelines to the vendors for response to the proposal are provided. This typically contains information about what format should be used, the date and time the response is to be submitted, detailed instructions for completing each section of the proposal, and the name and telephone number of the person to contact if questions arise.

Functional Specifications

The functional specifications together with the technical requirements section are the heart of the RFP. In this section, all system functionality is listed. Various formats are used to allow vendors to indicate whether their product has the desired functionality. The format of the response usually allows the vendor to indicate whether the feature is currently developed and operational, can be custom developed, is planned to be developed, or is not available. The length and areas covered in the functional specification section depend on the system under consideration. For example, if a total hospital information system is being considered, there will be a listing of hospital-wide systems such as the EHR and a subsection for almost every hospital department—for example, subsections for clinical laboratory, radiology, admission, HIM, and nursing. Functional specifications for a decision support system intended to support managerial personnel specifications would be limited to such areas as cost accounting, case mix, and budgeting. Functional specifications for a clinical decision support system would link strongly to the clinical components of the system and add features to support clinical decision making. Figure 9-15 provides a use case for electronic signatures as part of an EHR system and Figure 9-16 provides an example of the business rules associated with the electronic signature of a particular document (Consult) with the EHR system. Figure 9-17 provides sample functional specifications for a pharmacy module and Figure 9-18 shows samples specifications for an executive decision support system.

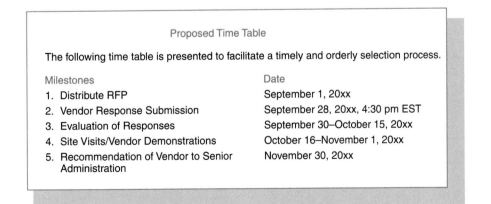

Figure 9-14 Time table for request for proposal process.

Organization: Community Behavioral Health Center

Use Case Name   : Electronically sign documents and entries in the EHRS
Date   :
Use Case #   :
Version # :

Iteration   : Focused

Summary: Only individuals authorized to create entries/documents in clinical records or authorized to review entries/documents in clinical records may sign the entries/documents. Each authorized signer must also be an authenticated user in the system. Signatures will be designated as required on certain clinical entries/documents. Certain individuals will require a cosigner on their clinical entries/documents. Certain individuals will have the authority cosign. Certain individuals will be able to sign independently.
This organization has a number of interns in their professional fields who will require cosignatures to demonstrate supervision of their work.
The organization will use the signature(s) as a means of finalizing and locking the entry/document so that it cannot be changed without invoking an amendment process.

Basic Course of Events:

1. Authenticated user who is also authorized to document in the clinical record enters the electronic health record system.
2. User finds correct client/patient, one that he/she is associated with as a caregiver or administrative contact.
3. User identifies correct category for documentation of entry/document.
4. User completes the entry/document the client/patient.
5. User electronically signs and locks the entry/document.
6. Entry document is made available in the system to all legitimate users.

Alternative Paths:

1. User clinician dictates the entry/document into the organization's dictation system.
2. Another user, designated as a transcriber, transcribes the document
3. The transcribed document is placed in a queue or electronic "to do" list for the user clinician to review and sign. If the clinician is satisfied with the document the path goes back to #5 in the basic path. If the clinician is not satisfied with the document it is routed back to the transcriber for revision and then the document is again listed on the "to do" list for review and signature.
4. If the entry or document needs a cosignature (and a cosignature may be for a variety of reasons) then at step #5 in the Basic Course the entry/document would be placed on the cosigner's "to do" list for review and signature.
5. The cosigner reviewer may change the entry/document and sign it or may send it back to the original author of the entry/document for revision. Once it is revised it would again go to the "to do" list of the cosigner reviewer for review and signature. Once signed by the reviewer the document is "locked" and the document is made available to all legitimate users.

Exception Paths: If entry remains unsigned for a period of time clinician is renotified through "to do" list. If entry remains unsigned for more than 2 weeks the clinician's manager is notified. If clinician is no longer available to sign (resigned, etc.) then the manager reviews entry, determines its appropriateness and may sign as the reviewer which allows the entry/document to be accessible to other legitimate users.

Extension Points:

Trigger: The user attempts to document in the EHRS and sign the entry/document.

Assumptions: The act of signing electronically signing the document "locks" the document when the authorized individual can sign independently or when a required reviewer signs.

Precondition: The EHRS is operational and the user has authorized access.

Postconditions: The signed entries are available to all authorized EHRS users.

Related Business Rules: Designation of who is authorized to document in the clinical record. Identification of which users or users types require cosignature. Amendments/corrections to locked documents.

Author:

Date:

Figure 9-15 Use case for electronic signatures.

Sample Business Rules for Electronic Consult Documents

1. An unsigned consult may be Deleted by a Provider who is also an Author/Dictator
2. An unsigned consult may be Deleted by a clinical student who is also an Author/Dictator
3. An uncosigned consult may be viewed by a Provider who is also an expected signer/Cosigner
4. An uncosigned consult may be Printed by a clinical student who is also an Author/Dictator
5. An uncosigned consult may be printed by a provider who is also an expected cosigner
6. An uncosigned consult may be edited by a provider who is also an expected signer/cosigner
7. An unsigned consult may be viewed by a provider who is also an Author/Dictator
8. An unsigned consult may be viewed by a clinical coordinator
9. A completed consult may be viewed by an authorized user
10. A completed consult may be viewed by a provider
11. A completed consult may be viewed by a clinical student who is also an Author/Dictator
12. An unsigned consult may be printed by a manager HIM
13. An uncosigned consult may be amended by a provider who is also an expected cosigner
14. An unsigned consult may be deleted by a manager HIM
15. An unsigned consult may be viewed by designated HIM staff
16. A completed consult may have its title changed by a manager HIM

Figure 9-16 Business rules for consultation.

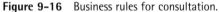

Pharmacy	Function Currently Available	Custom Modification Available	Planned Addition to Module	Function Not Available
1. Order may be entered on any terminal or approved device by authorized physician ARNP, PA, nurse, unit support staff or pharmacist				
2. System automatically notifies individual entering order if drug is not available in organization's formulary				
3. Formulary automatically provides link to relevant payer formulary				
4. All new drug orders are automatically screened against patient's drug profile for possible interactions				

Figure 9-17 Sample functional specifications: pharmacy system.

Application	Function Currently Available	Custom Available	Planned	Not Available
System allows for user-defined product lines.				
System stores a standard treatment profile for a product.				
System allows for online review and modification of standard treatment profiles.				

Figure 9-18 Sample functional specifications: executive decision support system.

A trend for describing functional specifications is to state requirements in a use case or scenario-based format. This format was discussed earlier in this chapter. One format of the use case/scenario-based description is to present the goal of the ideal system followed by a scenario of current problems. Vendors are asked to explain how their systems will support the general goal and how each will address the problems presented. The following is a brief example of such a format of a point-of-care RFP:

Example of a Point-of-Care Request for Proposal

Listed below are the goals and problems for our system. Please respond to each by indicating how your system would meet each goal and how it would address each problem.

> *Goal:* Deliver information to nurse caregivers at the patient bedside.
> *Problem:* Vital signs are taken at the bedside and then written down on a scratch pad by the nurse. The nurse then takes the data to the nursing station and rewrites the data onto the vital signs sheet. The data are then retranscribed and placed in the patient health record.

Technical Requirements

The technical requirements section of the RFP contains information about specifications for hardware, software, interfaces, processing environment, and communications. The following is an example of the technical interface requirements needed for a managerial decision support system:

Example of Technical Interface Requirements

1. Explain how your system accommodates the following interfaces:
- Accept payroll information from a personnel/payroll system
- Accept cost information from a general ledger system
- Update general ledger system with budget information
- Accept detail charge, payment, and patient information from patient billing, receivables, and registration systems
2. For those interfaces provided by you, describe the following:
- Who writes the interface
- Who maintains the interface
- Language used for the interface

In this section, vendors are expected to provide information about the performance of their systems. They may also be asked to submit samples of their system documentation, such as technical system, user, installation, and operations manuals. Support and maintenance details are also requested. For example, the RFP may ask the vendor to supply the following information:

- Indicate the location of personnel who would be assigned to the maintenance function.
- Describe the type of support the company is capable of providing on a continuing basis.
- Describe the means of support, such as hot lines, dial-up services, e-mail, and direct interactive support.
- Describe the procedure for requesting application software changes.

Installation and Training Requirements

In this section, vendors are requested to submit their installation work plans. Vendor responsibility, length of installation, customer responsibility, and skill level of installation personnel are described. Training requirements are also outlined in this section. Vendors are asked to describe the training they provide in areas of application usage, system operations, and continuing training. A description of training techniques and samples of training materials may also be requested. Vendors may be asked to describe what resources are needed for training (e.g., type of site), the number of people they will train, and the training time. All costs associated with training should be requested.

Vendor Profile

In any selection process, it is extremely important to ascertain the stability of the vendor. Too often facilities purchase systems only to have the vendor go bankrupt or be dislodged from the marketplace for some other reason. To minimize risk to the client, a thorough background analysis of the vendor should be done.

Information requested in the vendor profile includes demographic data, such as number of employees, number of support personnel, number of employees with installation experience, years the system has been available, and the number of systems installed. Vendor annual reports should be requested, including total revenues for several years, research and development expenditures, and systems contracted within the past few years. The facility may also want to ask whether a user group exists and, if so, how frequently it meets and how many members it has.

System Costs and Financing Arrangements

A system cost schedule should be prepared for both lease and purchase options. For each item in the schedule, the vendor should be requested to indicate the one-time cost, annual maintenance, and total cost over a certain period (e.g., 5 years). Among the categories in the cost schedule are hardware, software, software installation, software maintenance, custom development and interfaces, training, and consulting fees.

Contractual Information, References, and Other Materials

A sample copy of all contracts and addenda that are required for the facility to contract for the proposed system should be requested. It should be noted in the RFP that the facility reserves the right to negotiate the final terms and conditions of any resulting agreements. References for facilities that are using the vendor's product should be requested. The vendor should be asked to supply a list of all installations of their product, the contact person at each of these sites, and whether the site can be available for a visit. Any other manuals or references that the vendor may want to provide can be added in this section.

Distribution of the Request for Proposal

Once the RFP has been developed, it is ready for distribution to the vendors. Before distribution, a short list of vendors who probably have systems that will meet functionality specifications is identified. The short list is usually compiled from information received during the RFI process. Remember that for every RFP that is sent, a potential response is possible. Because responses tend to be longer than the RFP itself, review of these can be costly and time consuming. The facility will want to send out an RFP only to vendor candidates who are truly viable. The number of RFPs distributed depends on the vendor market, but no more than 15 are usually distributed. Once distributed, the RFP timetable is invoked and the process follows the time line prescribed in the RFP document.

Evaluation Criteria

Before distribution of the RFP, the steering committee develops evaluation criteria for analyzing and comparing vendor responses. Many methods are used for evaluation, and the type used depends on the system scope and individual preference of the facility. The following general categories of evaluation are usually considered:

- Hardware and software configuration
- Application functions and features
- Economic considerations
- Technical considerations
- Vendor considerations (Figure 9-19)

Some type of weighting scheme or priority measurement is assigned to each item within a category. One method of evaluation is to develop a weighting scale. The scale may range in value from 1 to 5. Each characteristic is then assigned a weight in relation to its importance. For instance, a hospital may consider security an extremely important item for its system. In this case, on a scale of 1 to 5, security may be assigned the weight of 5, which is the highest weight on the scale. On the other hand, management strength under vendor considerations may not be a highly valued characteristic, and this item may be assigned a lower weight of 2.

In addition to weighting each characteristic, each vendor's response can be evaluated by use of a Likert scale. This is usually referred to as scoring. For example, a scale of 1 to 3 might be used. If the vendor responded that the system currently had a required feature, then 3 points would be assigned for that option. If the vendor could custom configure the feature, then 2 points would be assigned. If the vendor has plans for the feature to be developed in the future, then 1 point would be assigned. If the system does not include the feature, then 0 points would be assigned. The weighted value of each characteristic is usually multiplied by the vendor's score for that feature, resulting in a weighted score for each characteristic. The weighted score is then added across all features to arrive at a final weighted score for each vendor. Table 9-9 shows how a weighted score would be calculated for the set of sample functional characteristics for a pharmacy system.

Table 9-10 compares the products of Vendor A with those of Vendor B. The calculations indicate that, overall, Vendor

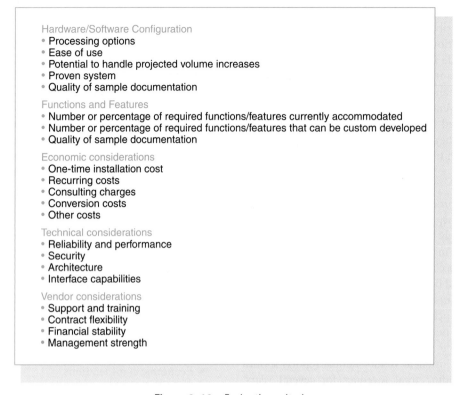

Figure 9-19 Evaluation criteria.

Table 9-9 WEIGHTED SCORES FOR PHARMACY INFORMATION SYSTEM VENDORS

		Score*	Score*	Weighted Score	
Functions	Weight†	Vendor A	Vendor B	Vendor A	Vendor B
Order may be entered on any terminal or approved input, device by physician, ARNP, physician's assistant, nurse, unit support staff member or pharmacist	5	3	3	15	15
System automatically notifies person entering order if drug is not available in organization's formulary	3	2	3	6	9
System automatically notifies person entering the order of match or suggested match with payer formulary	3	0	2	0	6
All new drug orders are automatically screened against patient's drug profile for possible interactions	4	2	3	8	12
Total weighted scores				29	42

*Score: 3, currently has; 2, can customize; 1, plans to have.
†Weight: 5, essential; 4, very important; 3, important; 2, somewhat important; 1, nice to have.

B's product appears to offer more functionality than Vendor A's product, given the pre-established weights.

There is no specific checklist of evaluation criteria that can be applied to every vendor product. Therefore, the categories listed in Figure 9-19 must be expanded or contracted depending on the system that is being evaluated. For example, if the product being evaluated were a laboratory information system, the specific functional requirements would include those listed in Table 9-10. However, if the system being evaluated were an encoder product, the vendor evaluation criteria would be entirely different.

There is not total agreement that the use of a weighting scheme such as that just described provides the best comparison method. For example, one vendor may score higher than all other contenders, but the product may in fact be mediocre in most categories. It is important, therefore, to

Table 9-10 SAMPLE FUNCTIONAL SPECIFICATIONS FOR LABORATORY INFORMATION SYSTEM

Functional Specification	Currently Available	Custom Design Available	Planned	Not Available, Not Planned
1. Order processing				
1.1. Test request with automatic accessioning				
1.2. Duplicate order checking				
2. Specimen collection				
2.1. Automatic generation of label				
2.2. Generation of specimen bar code labels at collection point				
2.3. Specimen location printed on label				
3. Result reporting				
3.1. Send report to EHR				
3.2. Print report on demand				
3.3. Result inquiry by patient name				
3.4. Result inquiry by patient EHR/EMR number				
3.5. Remote transmission of results to approved devices				
3.6. Remote query capability				
3.7. Trending of patient's lab results with visual presentation				

look at the scores of each criterion individually as well as the overall weighted scores. In reality, such a weighting method is only one input into the total decision process. The weighting process can also be helpful if individuals score the systems independently and then compare and discuss their reasons for the scoring. This should lead to more clarity and an opportunity to identify those vendors that are front runners in the selection process.

Use of a checklist of features and requirements against which vendors measure their own products has several drawbacks. One drawback of the checklist method is that frequently the scoring method of criterion evaluation does not ensure that the best product receives the highest score. Another drawback of the checklist method is that only the vendor's viewpoint is represented. Although this viewpoint is necessary, it may be biased.

Another shortcoming of the checklist method is that it is a static technique. This means that the features or requirements listed on the checklist might exist in the product, but there is no way to evaluate how these features work together. Therefore, demonstration use cases or scenarios are included in many RFPs to try to minimize the static nature of the checklist method. Demonstration **use cases** or scenarios are "stories" or simulations of processes that the system is expected to accommodate. For example, in a laboratory information system a demonstration use case/ scenario might describe processes for ordering test procedures, reporting test results, or printing work lists and reports.

Demonstrations and Site Visits

Demonstrations

After responses to the RFP have been reviewed, the steering committee culls the list of vendors. The vendors that come out highest in the evaluation process are invited to present demonstrations of their products. The demonstrations usually take place at the facility and, depending on system complexity, may last several hours to 1 to 2 days. Before the demonstration, the steering committee should have established a demonstration schedule. This schedule should include a list of all functions to be demonstrated and a schedule of end users who are to witness the demonstration. A set of evaluation criteria (e.g., apparent ease of use, interface flexibility, evaluation of inputs and outputs) should be developed by the steering committee. These criteria are then applied by the end users to evaluate the demonstration. Other methods, such as focus groups, can be used to debrief end users and gather their opinions about system functionality. All opinions and evaluations should be documented and evaluated by the steering committee. This evaluation will probably result in some vendors being eliminated from consideration.

Site Visits

After demonstrations have taken place, the steering committee usually schedules site visits to observe the vendor product in production mode. Site visits take place at facilities where the vendor product is installed. Usually 1 to 2 days are arranged for each site visit. The site visit team should have a visit protocol prepared in advance. The protocol should allow formal and informal observations of the system and discussion with end users at the selected site. This may be the only opportunity the team has to view the system in production mode. Therefore, it is extremely important that the site protocol be complete and affords the best possible opportunity for overview of the system and its management. After each site visit, the steering committee should be debriefed. Evaluations should be compiled. Discrepancies between what was reported in the vendor response to proposal and what was observed in production mode should be noted and investigated.

System Selection and Contract Negotiation

After all data have been gathered, demonstrations held, and site visits completed, the steering committee should be ready to select a vendor product. When a product has been selected, contract negotiations begin. The contractual process is extremely important because it lays down the rules by which the client and vendor are to operate. In complex installations, the vendor and health care facility are partners for months or even years. Therefore, it is important that the contract minimizes risk to both parties. Commonly, a special team is formed to carry out contract negotiation. Members of the team should have negotiation experience. Representatives from administration, information systems, legal counsel, and significant others are usually included in the facility negotiation team. It is important that the leaders of both the vendor and the facility teams be authorized to make decisions for their respective businesses.

The negotiation of a good contract is one of the most important elements in ensuring a successful system installation. The following items are usually part of any software contract:

- *Identification of products and services:* This should include detailed specifications for the software and support materials to be licensed.
- *License grant:* This includes the scope of rights to be transferred, the number of sites, and intellectual property rights.
- *Delivery terms:* This includes such things as time and date of delivery, method of delivery, schedule of delivery, and recourse for damages or slippage.
- *Installation:* This includes such items as site preparation, timing of installation, and training.
- *Warranties:* This includes such items as express and implied warranties, scope and term of warranties, and conditions on warranties.
- *Remedies and liability:* This includes such items as limitations on liability and types of liability.
- *Acceptance and testing:* This includes such items as how the system will be tested, timing of testing, and specifications for testing.
- *Price and payments:* This includes method of payment, such as lump sum or spaced payments, conditional payments, royalties, taxes, and prices for updates or modifications, service, or maintenance.
- *Term and termination:* This includes such items as effective date of agreement; notice of breach, insolvency, or bankruptcy; and termination for cause.
- *Support and maintenance:* This may include such items as training, documentation, maintenance, emergency and preventive maintenance, and access to source code.

It is important to remember that a contract is a binding document. Therefore software contracts should be negotiated by a team of people who have expertise in both legal and technological arenas. No matter how small the contract in monetary terms, the health care facility should always seek legal advice before signing any software contract.

Key Concepts

- Information systems have a life cycle that includes system design, implementation, operation and maintenance, and obsolescence. For each life cycle stage, different activities take place that have an impact on the resources of the organization.
- An organization is composed of hundreds and perhaps thousands of interacting information systems. Given this, the information systems in any organization are in different phases of individual life cycles. This discontinuity of life cycle phases causes stress within the organization. This stress can be manifested in multiple ways, including competition for resources such as personnel, hardware, and financial allocations.
- Each organization as a whole has its own information system life cycle. Nolan describes six stages of an organization life cycle with each stage manifesting a different approach to management of the information technology.
- A structured approach, called the information system development life cycle, is commonly used to develop new information systems. This life cycle has four steps: analysis, design, implementation, and evaluation. Structured techniques provide a tool kit for analysts as they perform system analysis and design.
- Prototyping is a technique that sometimes is used in place of the system development life cycle. This technique has been made possible because of advances in technology. The purpose of this method is to build a prototype or model of an information system quickly by involving the end user in repeated iterations of the design.
- System implementation is an enormous undertaking, and planning is a key to its success. Plans need to be developed that include user preparation and training, site preparation, system testing and conversion, and startup activities.
- Although often overlooked, system evaluation and development of a benefits realization process are extremely important parts of the system development life cycle. The purpose of system evaluation is to determine whether the system functions the way it was intended. Several techniques are used in evaluation. Among them are benefits realization, CBA, and cost-effectiveness analysis (CEA).
- When a decision is made to purchase an information system rather than develop it with in-house expertise, a

document called an RFP is usually prepared. The process for developing an RFP includes the analysis of user and system requirements and development of logical and physical system specifications. The process results in the compilation of the RFP, which includes information about the enterprise and functional, technical, training, implementation, and other requirements. An RFP is distributed to likely candidate vendors, and subsequent responses from vendors are reviewed and evaluated. Final system selection is made after careful review of RFP responses, vendor demonstrations, site visits to observe the product in a production environment, and negotiation of a satisfactory contract.

REFERENCES

1. Bogue R: Anatomy of a software development role: http://www.developer.com/img/articles. Accessed January 1, 2006.
2. Martin MP: *Analysis and design of business information systems,* New York, 1991, Macmillan.
3. Nolan RL: Managing the crisis in data processing, *Harvard Business Rev* 1979; (March-April).
4. Whitten J, Bentley L, Dittman K: *Systems analysis and design methods,* Boston, ed 6, 2003, McGraw-Hill.
5. Dennis A, Wixon BH, Tegarden D: *Systems analysis and design with UML, version 2.0,* Hoboken, 2005, Wiley & Sons.
6. Kulak D, Guiney E: *Use cases: requirements in context,* Boston, 2000, Addison Wesley.
7. Stair RM: *Principles of information systems: a managerial approach,* Boston, 1992, Boyd and Fraser.
8. Murphy GF, Hanken MA, Waters KA: *Electronic health records: changing the vision,* Philadelphia, 1999, WB Saunders.
9. Freidman CP, Wyatt JC: *Evaluation methods in biomedical informatics,* New York, 2006, Springer.

RESOURCES

Flynn DJ, Diaz OF: *Information modeling: an international perspective,* London, 1996, Prentice Hall.
McBride S, Gilder R, Davis R et al: *Data mapping:* http://library.ahima.org.
Whitten J, Bentley L: *Systems analysis and design methods,* ed 7, Boston, 2007, McGraw Hill.

chapter 10

Managing Electronic Health Record Systems: Collaboration and Implementation

Mary Alice Hanken
Gretchen F. Murphy

Additional content,
http://evolve.elsevier.com/Abdelhak/

Review exercises can be found
in the Study Guide

Chapter Contents

Value of User Perspective
  A Natural Dependence
Environmental Basics (Required for True Collaboration)
  Four Shared Environmental Basics
    Personal Commitment
    Trust
    Respect
    Policy Setting
  Four Unshared Environmental Basics
    Expectations
    Vocabulary
    Understanding
    Understanding Process
    Knowledge
The Tide Turns
Process Modeling
Database Design
Implementation Readiness
  User Processes and Procedures
  Plan Transition
  Training
  Prepare User Manual(s)
  Data Migration
  System Testing
  "Go Live"
System and Project Evaluation

Abbreviations

EHR—electronic health record
HIM—health information management
I/S—information systems
IT—information technology
MIS—management information systems

Key Words

Business data
Collaboration
Downtime
Project
Training Manual
Stakeholder
System life cycle
System testing
User
User manual

Objectives

- Develop a strong working relationship with information systems staff.
- Recognize the strengths of the health information management professional and the information systems professional in developing, selecting, implementing, and modifying health care information systems.
- Understand the difference between project activities and operational activities.
- Identify the skills needed to bring an information systems project to completion.

This is an adaptation of a chapter written by Ellen Anderson in *Electronic Health Records: Changing the Vision.*

- Describe the principles of collaboration between health information management and information systems that help projects be successful.
- Recognize the areas where health information management and information systems do not automatically share the same views or information or approaches to a project.
- Recognize the value of training in project success.
- Differentiate between a training manual and a user manual.
- Evaluate the success of systems projects.
- Identify both measurable metrics and organizational values addressed by a system.
- Recognize that systems projects move into an improvement phase after implementation.

VALUE OF USER PERSPECTIVE

The business community, or "user," perspective of systems projects can help business communities (1) understand the dependencies and the work effort involved in systems implementations, (2) hold realistic expectations of process and outcome, and (3) become a much more sophisticated partner in systems development and implementation.

A Natural Dependence

Collaboration Principle: There is a natural dependence between users and information systems (I/S) in the pursuit of definition, design, development, purchase, implementation, and usage of any EHR system.

Computer systems in the workplace are tools applied to business functions. They are the workhorses of business. On an equal plane, computer systems fail to perform if data structure and databases, operating systems, interfaces, and networks are not well planned, robust, and technically compatible. This business community/computer division dependence should be more than just recognized; it should be embraced.

Environmental basics is a term the author has created to define the "human elements" that exist as a natural part of humans composing work teams intended to accomplish specific tasks. The eight environmental basics covered in this chapter include personal commitment, trust, respect, policy setting to manage human behavior, expectations, vocabulary, understanding, and knowledge.

A **stakeholder** is any individual who has a stake or real interest in the computerization project and implemented electronic health record (EHR), regardless of department, position, or functional role in the company (Table 10-1).

The computer division of most organizations has a title that includes the word "information." This is true in health care organizations as well. A few examples are management of information systems (MIS), information technology (IT),

Table 10-1 USERS OF THE ELECTRONIC HEALTH RECORD

Physicians	Pharmacists
Nurses	Pharmacy technicians
Nurse's aides	Laboratory technicians
Physical therapists	Radiologists
Occupational therapists	Radiology technicians
Speech therapists	Data analysts
Health information staff	Quality improvement analysts
Medical records staff	Utilization review coordinators
Care/case coordinators	Business office personnel
Dieticians	Social workers
Decision support analysts	Mental health specialists
AND THE LIST GOES ON AND ON ...	

Table 10-2 PROJECTS VERSUS OPERATIONS

Projects	Operations
Peaks and valleys work flow	Steady stream of work
No direct authority, full responsibility	Full authority, full responsibility
Ad hoc teams	Business-aligned teams
Done once	Done repeatedly
Highly time dependent	Function dependent
Defined start and end dates	Not "start date" and "end date" dependent
Product/service driven	Business function/process driven

and information services or systems (I/S). The abbreviation **I/S** is used in this chapter when referring to either the department itself or the staff of individuals in this unit of work activity in any organization. It is not surprising to note that more than one work unit of an organization may use the word "information" in its title. Both the computer department and the health information department are in the business of managing information for the health care industry.

Webster's New Twentieth Century Dictionary of the English Language[1] defines **collaboration** as "to labor, especially in literary or scientific pursuits, as the associate of another or others." In this chapter the term is used to refer to the combined labor of users and I/S staff in the pursuit of EHRs. The important word here is, of course, together.

Project, in the context of this chapter, means a unit of work to acquire or build and implement a computer system (software, hardware, and all infrastructure) with a definitive start date, targeted stop date, steps, milestones, and outcome.

Project work is quite different from regular operations in any organization. Table 10-2 illustrates some comparisons. The nuances of projects make collaboration that much more important and that much more challenging.

ENVIRONMENTAL BASICS (REQUIRED FOR TRUE COLLABORATION)

The system "life cycle" has been used in describing computer system development for many years. Simply put, the stages of a system can be expressed in simple verbs: define, design, develop, do (or implement), and support. That system life cycle then recycles to redefine, redesign, and so forth, in a continuous fashion until the system is no longer used and another takes its place. (See Chapter 9 for more information on the system life cycle.)

Define, design, develop, implement, redesign, redevelop, and do are all action verbs that involve groups, and *lots* of them. Because EHR systems happen through groups, environmental basics that are group oriented must be in place *before* an EHR project is started. And all these environmental basics must be intact for project success. These same principles apply to a working relationship to improve and expand systems within an organization or in a community setting.

Four Shared Environmental Basics

Collaboration Principle: Personal commitment, trust, respect, and policy setting are four mandatory environmental basics shared between users and I/S for true collaboration.

Personal Commitment

Collaboration Principle:
Personal commitment builds computer systems champions.

Commitment is not easy when resources are tight, especially if the capital costs are high, the risks are great, and the resources are limited. Yet personal commitment to a project produces the political will to make the system happen. Nothing goes farther than a user who truly believes. Commitment needs to come, however, from all sides of the collaboration equation—from users *and* I/S. Personal commitment is more than verbalization. It is quite easy to verbalize commitment; it is quite another matter to stand behind that commitment.

If you are starting a major systems project, use focus groups, surveys, and interviews to assess the level of commitment. Study the positive and negative personal commitment feedback from all focus groups, surveys, or interviews. Is there a basis of personal commitment to this project? Is the perception warranted? Is it based on correct or incorrect facts? If incorrect, how can you correct them? Will correcting the facts change the degree of personal commitment? If correct facts have created a negative perception, can conditions be altered to raise the level of commitment? If users show strong personal commitment to the project, are they grounded in reality?

Grounded Champions. User managers make the best system and project champions. Sometimes, though, they need accurate resource information to be truly grounded in their commitment and genuine excitement. User managers can be very serious about the project but also blind to the resource commitment of their operational people and budget to ensure success. Test their commitment *before* beginning the project. They will usually underestimate resources in terms of both people and money—it is human nature to wish it done quickly and at a cost less than realistic.

I/S managers are another important group who must be personally committed to the project. They are faced with an overwhelming number of requests to automate or update existing automation from all business units within the organization. Setting a high I/S priority to a project is usually propelled by a combination of (1) a compelling business

reason and (2) the right technology fit and direction. For example, it makes no sense to automate a business function when the desired technology is not ready for general usage.

If I/S managers declare a project a high priority, you are half way there. Are there true capital dollars behind it? Is it assigned a budget? Is it a shared budget among a number of departments, including I/S? Is the budget "assigned" realistic? Does I/S appear ready with pen in hand to sign initial project documents if you moved forward immediately?

Trust

Collaboration Principle:
The worst of projects can succeed within a basis of trust, and the best of projects will likely fail without it.

It has been said that the worst of projects were successful because, even during the down and out periods, project members and business communities trusted each other. Together they pulled a project through the battles to victory. It has also been said that the best of projects and systems failed because no trust existed.[2] When no trust exists, each source of irritation or project component failure brings the project closer to its knees. A baseline level of trust must be in place as a project begins. Trust develops more completely as a project's work groups or teams grow comfortable in the natural dependencies between them. There are various levels of trust in any collective group of people— EHR systems are no exception. All levels within an organization must trust, and be trusted, for maximum use of group synergy.

Those who hold the corporate purse strings, or control the organizational finances, must trust the rest of the organization to be good stewards of the millions of dollars often required to get a system into production. They must also trust that the proposed budget reflects the true costs or costs as commonly computed within the organization. If they take the fiscal stewardship of the organization seriously, they will ask for a cost/benefit analysis or strong reasons about value to help in their prioritization of this capital expenditure relative to other capital expenditure requests.

Project Steering Committee members need to trust that their fight for the capital dollars will result in tangible computer systems. They also must trust that the people who will be empowered to select or create and implement the system have the talents and the will to do so. They may also trust that the potential system users have or will acquire the computer skills and aptitudes needed to use the system. Do they have these trusts?

User managers are the most trusting of all, especially if they are true champions of a potential system. They trust that the people above them will act on their commitment of resources. They trust that the users they supervise will embrace the system, or at least accept it and make it work. They trust that I/S staff knows how to implement and support the desired system, have budgeted appropriately, and will supply resources when needed.

If a system will be purchased, the organization must trust vendor representatives who provide sales information about the product, help to configure the system for use, and support implementation at time of going live. Do they trust that the vendor will deliver the promised system? Will the vendor work to fit their product to the client's environment or build only what sells in the marketplace?

The I/S staff must trust the user community to know what it wants and needs in system functionality. They must also believe that the users will deliver the human resources necessary to actively participate in the project that the user community will ultimately own. They must also trust that the business community stands ready to basically own and functionally support the system after implementation.

Users, then, must trust all of the above. Do users see the above groups as trustworthy? Do they perceive that the above groups will deliver? Is this particular project a "wise" use of the organization's dollars in their minds? Will the various departments really support users through initial training, implementation, *institutionalized* training and retraining, and system support?

Through the focus groups, interviews, and surveys, distrust may appear. Has I/S "let down" the user community in the past on the basis of technical promises not kept or a cost that is three times the estimate? Has the business community ill defined a system and "wasted lots of I/S dollars" trying to define it while in the middle of system development? These are two very common distrust statements. Neither contributes to future project success.

The potential list of double-sided "done me wrongs" could go on and on. This is truly only project background garbage and needs to be cleaned up before a good working relationship can develop in the dynamics of working groups and team efforts. Distrust does not contribute to positive group synergy.

Respect

Collaboration Principle:
Mutual respect breeds collaboration. Disrespect destroys it.

In computerization projects, the caste system that exists in most health care organizations can quickly disappear. The appointment clerk can be as important or more important than the physician in an appointment scheduling system implementation. This creates some interesting team membership. A baseline level of respect between project players can hasten the comfort level of multidiscipline, multibusiness unit project teams who have seldom worked side by side. Individuals need to feel respect, regardless of what role they play in the organization or in an automation project.

Equally critical factors in system implementation are two common problems with systems work: (1) resource tug-of-war and (2) timeline tag. Because there are so many components included with systems, planned people resources will likely get "shuffled" a lot, and unplanned resources will continually knock on managers' doors for staffing. For example, a user manager may have planned to have two of the staff "free" in May for 2 weeks for user testing, but the user testing will be delayed 3 weeks because of a delay in receipt of equipment. The staff is now needed in June, possibly not a good time from the business unit's perspective.

Using the delayed equipment example above, the project timeline has now leaped forward by at least 3 weeks. Project teams will be trying to play timeline tag to catch up or move the "go-live" date forward. If the "go-live" date is a "hard date" (which means it cannot be changed—perhaps it is a regulatory compliance date, for example), the pressure to play the tag intensifies.

Project teams and managers must be sensitive to user frustration resulting from this resource shuffling and the timeline movement, and the user community must be sensitive to what components of the project work are truly under the control of the project manager and teams.

It is also important to understand that the user community can cause the delays as well. Turning the tide, the user community can cause a delay because an operations activity suddenly "takes priority" or a consensus activity within the user community cannot be scheduled for when it was originally planned.

Gauge what mutual respect exists between the business units to be involved with the automation project and between the collective business units and the I/S staff. Does each appreciate the role and work effort of the other? Does each appreciate the time it takes to accomplish the designated work effort that contributes to the whole of the organization?

Policy Setting

Collaboration Principle: In the absence of clear policies and principles of information management, there will be internal conflict and civil war.[3]

It has been appropriately said that policies and principles manage human behavior. These directives for human behavior guide both system development and the project teams developing them. In large measure, data access, data use, data content, data standards, authentication, electronic signature, data exchange standards, data release, and data security are focused subjects for policies and principles directly guiding EHR systems. For example, patient confidentiality will remain a major concern until appropriate policies are in place that address patient identifying data running through FAX lines, internal messaging software, the Intranet, the Internet, and the World Wide Web, today's rapidly developing wireless technology, and, any other technology that develops in the future. The same concern appears as a data warehouse or clinical data repository project kicks into gear because data sare suddenly pulled from a transaction processing system where individuals have an easily established "need to know" and moves the data into the organizational hands of an entire enterprise. The warehouse or repository will create a need for new policies and procedures related to data access and use.

As the rate of technology advancement intensifies, policies and principles quickly become outdated and ineffective guides to human behavior amid exciting new automation. Project teams can become foes as one pushes ahead *with* no clear organizational directive while the other refuses to move *without* it. The users and I/S staff can quickly become antagonistic. *Before* this happens, the organization must create the appropriate behavioral framework for use in that organizational culture. Collaboration, then, is not hindered by lack of organizational directives for human behavior.

It takes real courage to develop such policies. Those who are pushing hard for the system can label policy makers a hindrance to automation because they anticipate that policy setting will result in a more complex system or a time delay. They may be right. Those who have this perception do not understand that this policy-setting work is as normal to system development as programming screens are. It is best to establish this policy through an enterprise-wide group that (1) takes the stewardship of data, especially patient identifiable data, to heart and (2) takes on the scope of "setting confidentiality criteria that would provide a basis for new applications and for new delivery system models."[4]

Four Unshared Environmental Basics

So far we have talked about four shared environmental basics. There are four other environmental basics; however, that will NOT be initially nor automatically shared between I/S and the user community.

> **Collaboration Principle:** Expectations, vocabulary, understanding, and knowledge are four environmental basics NOT common between the user community and I/S.

Work on these environmental basics because they will "make or break" a project.

Expectations

> **Collaboration Principle:** Perception is an individual's reality built on expectations. Individuals in the user community and individuals in I/S will NOT share initial project expectations.

Everyone has expectations. It's human nature. Users often "expect that the system would do" this or that. I/S developers often "expect that the user would use the system" this way or that way. Positive expectations are important because they have tremendous motivating power. User perception has a powerful influence on the success of EHR and other systems. In one very controlled man-machine study, "the most striking finding was that perceived usefulness was 50% more influential than ease of use in determining usage"[5] of new information systems. When the user community and I/S have shared expectations, then projects can embrace common goals and objectives built from those expectations. This builds the ultimate group synergy. If they do not share expectations (and its human nature that they will not), work needs to be done to bring them together.

All expectations, good ones as well as bad ones, must be "held in common." It is imperative that gathered expectations be brought to all stakeholders as a group and discussed. Shared expectations lead to project success, so work on group consensus. This defines project purpose. Powerful project goals and objectives depend on it.

Vocabulary

> **Collaboration Principle:** It is likely that NO common language exists between the user community and the I/S staff.

We don't speak the same language. Business buzzwords and I/S buzzwords abound. It's human nature to create them and then institutionalize them. Abbreviations are the mental shorthand for repeated communications of often-used words. Particularly since the age of the computer and data automation, codes now often replace words and abbreviations because codes are numerical and computer storage "friendly." They also consume less space on printed reports.

I/S staff especially needs to be consciously aware of the vocabulary blockade. Technology does not have to be discussed in terms unnecessarily technical. Highly technical language often results in the user member of the group sitting quietly, quite lost in the discussion. Technical-oriented staff members are often NOT comfortable communicators. It can, however, have little to due with personality. They may likely lack the communication skills to know how to simplify their terminology. They often face several big stumbling blocks. The first is their technical terminology anchorage. Once a new and important term is learned, it can be difficult for them to find another, more relevant term from a business function perspective that would be more successful in discussion. The second is detail. Once buried in detail, it can be tough to bring yourself to a higher, conceptual explanation of that detail. Yet the project team members often need and want the only concept. A good conceptual explanation is sufficient. Ask the I/S to explain and use analogies until the language is clear.

The user member, on the other hand, may use business jargon or abbreviations. The I/S individuals lose concentration and understanding in the midst of this jargon. If the terms are misunderstood, the I/S people can assume that they know the definition of business buzzwords, abbreviations, or codes and make faulty programming errors as a result. This can be very costly to the project and a real waste of organizational resources. Again, it is okay to ask questions and get clarification.

Vocabulary Blockade. Be proactive about vocabulary blockade. *Before* a group convenes, grasp the level of technical jargon a technical person intends to use in group settings. If you know that he or she will "lose the users" and will have difficulty in simplifying the terminology, suggest less technical terms that will get the message across without frustrating the group. After all, the listener usually will need only a conceptual understanding of the term used.

Encourage clarification through establishing and monitoring ground rules about vocabulary. "Don't interpret. Ask." should be a ground rule for all project groups. The project leaders should encourage a "no stupid questions" policy and then create a discreet procedure for stakeholders and project team members to submit questions if they are uncomfortable asking questions in a group setting. This gives team members a second, but indirect, way of obtaining clarification.

Keep It Simple. If you are in the middle of a group setting and the ill-prepared technical team member uses very technical words, again suggest simple terms to clear the communication early in the discussion. If that task seems too difficult for the technical team member, and no data definition role has been assigned to a team member, take a stab at your own nontechnical explanation through a simplified feedback statement. It can start as simply as, "If I understand correctly," or "I'd like to see if I could restate that in my own words." and end with a simplified explanation of the subject technology. This process clears the vocabulary blockade and keeps communications flowing. This is usually deeply appreciated by the user members and gives the technical person a clear message to simplify his or her vocabulary. Even the most complicated computer hardware configuration or network can be simplified dramatically so that users understand the basic concept.

The same holds true if you have a user member who uses lots of business buzzwords, abbreviations, or business codes. This often happens with front-line day-to-day operations personnel. Their world is very focused, and those shortened communication aids are second nature to them in their daily work. Ask what an abbreviation stands for or for a descriptive phrase or a word to help others in work groups understand. Sometimes even the manager of the department doesn't know the newest buzzwords or abbreviations. Clarification helps *everyone* on the team, not just the I/S members. The day-to-day operations personnel may not even know what an abbreviation or code means because they use it only in its shortened form. If so, record the term in question and get clarification after the session; then share it with the team.

Never lose the **"business balance"** in dealing with vocabulary. Ultimately, the system exists for **business** reasons, will use **business** data, and will be documented primarily in **business** terms. In a health care organization, this includes ALL aspects of the business, clinical as well as financial.

Understanding

Collaboration Principle: Much of understanding evolves around how people think. I/S people think in systems; users think in business tasks.

Ever hear the expression, "I never thought of it that way"? Understanding is dramatically affected by how we think. I/S people tend to think in systems. The business community tends to think in business tasks. For example, a physician may be describing the step-by-step process she uses to review critical laboratory test results and x-ray results, order additional laboratory work and pharmaceuticals, and finally refer the patient to home health care. The I/S person is interpreting her words in terms of systems—that laboratory system that feeds batch results to the clinical results reporting system twice a day that provides physicians with data to do orders that are entered at the time the laboratory or pharmacy order is placed, and so on. This different way of processing information allows varying views of the same material. Both brains need to work in their own thought process to maximize their skill sets in a successful implementation. The two styles should be encouraged. Problems can occur, however, if either type of thinking misinterprets the facts as presented by the other.

The team may be communicating through a mutually understood vocabulary but in very vague terms. Vagueness blocks understanding. Each team member can then interpret vague language to fit his or her own expectations and knowledge base. This hinders collaboration.

This is good time to discuss the differences between vagueness and concept and appropriate detail. We looked at concept versus detail in the previous discussion of vocabulary. Concept is most appropriate in "mixed" groups—those encounters where both user team members and various I/S technical team members are present. An example would be identifying the specific physical "closet" for server placement in the network architecture that will support the new system. (Because the user community may not recognize the term "closet" and "server," the technical team needs to make sure that the user community understands these terms as well.) Specific detail, rather than concept, is most appropriate in sessions where everyone in the room not only wants to but needs to understand even the smallest detail. Using the example above, the network team and the hardware team must know which wires in which specific closet will connect which specific server to which specific workstations and which specific printers, and so forth. Vagueness is the lack of enough fact in either of the above examples to clearly communicate your message. Suppose the project manager states that the server "will be placed in a closet in the facility" in a meeting with business unit leaders. Without understanding what is entailed in a closet from a computer network perspective, the user community may mentally and immediately place the server in the basement utility closet.

A clarification feedback exercise is also a helpful activity in team meetings when not all user community representatives are always present at every meeting. For example, one user member describes the desired process one way at a meeting on Monday and is absent at Friday's meeting. Her counterpart describes it another way on Friday. By listening carefully on Friday, you catch the different description. If you have a user facilitator in the meeting, he or she should catch this. Use the notes from the meeting on Monday, maybe even a model or flowchart or diagram or some visual way to show Monday's description, to verify the discrepancy. Ask that the group stop the discussion and clarify the discrepancy. Validate that clarification with the user member who was absent from the meeting. If there is a true inconsistency of belief between users, allow the whole team to understand that the inconsistency exists and that it needs resolution before moving on with project tasks. This can also work with user understanding of computer hardware layout for the office space or navigational demands on the user through network connectivity. Get the user members to explain their understanding of the configuration or navigational steps in simple language to the I/S people responsible for the placement. An amazing amount of understanding can result through this simple feedback and clarification technique.

Understanding Process

How many times in a work effort have you heard the phrase, "I don't have a clue what I'm doing"? If that statement is indeed true, that individual does not understand the process.

> **Collaboration Principle:** Team members must understand not only the content of the project and product but also, equally important, the process by which the team is obtaining the outcome.

Often project team members clearly understand *what* they are working toward. They "don't have a clue," however, about *how* they are getting there. If the process is clearly known; clearly communicate it for understanding. The effect on team members enables them to truly perform at their very best. If the process is not known, say so. At least give guidance about continuous work effort without a well-defined process. Do not leave project teams in process limbo. As process limbo increases, project team(s) morale decreases.

A word about the unknown is critical here. Many aspects of a project can be "unknown": unknown from an operations side (for example, a new procedure around a system that has never been in place for some new business functionality) and unknown from a technical prospective (for example, new sites are involved in the project or the volume estimated in the operational work expected on the system is much greater than volumes in other systems). The unknowns are constant and predictably there. To have true understanding from all team members, including the user members, project leaders must give members of the team the courtesy of knowing what aspects of the project are "unknowns." A project phenomenon then occurs. It can build incredible team unity, a "we are all on the same, uncharted waters together" camaraderie. It also identifies vulnerabilities that the team as a whole must embrace and work to minimize or mitigate. For example, if there is real concern on the part of I/S staff related to the volume of traffic over their lines with this "additional system," team members will want to take that into consideration in planning business procedures. Understanding the vulnerability *allows* the team members to do this planning and act. Lacking this knowledge and understanding leaves them in the dark, possibly unknowingly planning a use or activity that will have a negative impact on the system. This sets the project teams up for unnecessary conflict and possible collaboration failure.

Knowledge

> **Collaboration Principle:** I/S and the user community each initially have a knowledge base NOT well known to the other.

Another ground rule for projects should be "Never assume. Know." When a project starts, the user community has a knowledge base not well known to the I/S people. The I/S people have a knowledge base not well known to the user community. The knowledge that each member needs to support the project "rubs off" from other members as a natural part of communicating and understanding throughout the project's life. Each team member evolves into a teacher to the others. Each member also learns to absorb or filter out knowledge on the basis of their perceived need to know that information to function in their role.

Users should be aware of the knowledge base of today's I/S staff. It is never as good as it could be or should be because the speed and volume of today's knowledge in information technology is beyond the mental capacity of any I/S department or individual staff member. I/S staff tend to specialize to address the amount of information and its ever-changing complexity. The I/S staff will never know all that they could know about the desired database, operating system, network, workstations, and other components of the desired system's infrastructure. The question is do they know *enough* to make solid technical decisions? Probe the rationale for their potential choices to get clues about the supporting knowledge base.

It is frustrating for user communities when the I/S staff and users disagree over the "right" component to use in the new system. It may be based on different I/S staffers gaining different bases of knowledge that lead to differing conclusions. It might be based on the same knowledge base interpreted differently. Try to understand how much knowledge plays into the I/S decision making rather than, for example, a general preference toward a vendor or operating system, a likable sales representative, or price, or some other criteria in question. One of the legitimate computer-age questions that project teams often tackle is whether to go with an "older" but well-known system or component or strike out for the new, better but untested technology or perhaps an untested company. This dilemma will only get more complex as information technology leaps forward, rapidly outdating the technology known and used in today's health care world.

With all that said, users must still reply on I/S's knowledge for the physical infrastructure of the system through the design, development, selection, implementation, and support stages of the project. That does not preclude, however, users self-educating about these components through their own professional journals or other educational endeavors. As users read and explore this knowledge base, it is helpful for them to use I/S people as a sounding board to discuss their learning outside of the group sessions to clarify their understanding.

I/S units have another kind of knowledge that will be used during the development of a built system or the configuration of a purchased product and as problems are found in testing the system before implementation. This same knowledge spills over to support usage after the product is put into production. The I/S staff has a ready body of knowledge to draw on to "problem solve." When it could be "one of 10 possibilities," they will need to work their way through their problem-solving triage and knowledge bank to find the problem and then resolve it. There is no question that problem solving today is far more complicated than it was in the mainframe computer days when limited and isolated applications that rarely talked to other systems ran on a "tried and true" operating system.

The user community has no need to share this knowledge bank in detail. However, they will want to understand the general cause of the problem so that they can learn how to avoid the problem in the future, particularly if is it a "user error" problem. Users will also want to know the solution and have clear directions for what they should do if it occurs again. If triaging the problem and reaching solution involves "downtime" (time when the computer system is NOT available to the user community), that community also has a need *and* a right to know whether the resolution process could take an hour or several days. "Stretching" users from a promise of an hour that becomes several days of "downtime" destroys trust, although initially it may keep them quiet. The short-term peace is not worth the long-term price.

THE TIDE TURNS

What becomes an interesting twist is the knowledge advantage the user community gains over the I/S people as the system is implemented and then used over time. No one will know that system better than the user. Although I/S people will initially know the system better than the users do, they will become hard pressed to keep up with the learning curve of users who have incorporated the EHR system and other systems into their daily lives.

Users can get frustrated by the tendency of the I/S staff members to initially label reported bugs or problems found by the users as "user error" before true knowledge of the problem is unraveled. This is a dangerous practice because it can often be wrong—it is perhaps a programming error, network connectivity error, software incapability error, a client-server communications error, and so on. It also destroys

mutual respect because the users feel they are branded as incompetent in the eyes of I/S.

If you have a shared and well-defined proposal, built on relevant policies and principles that has been validated and driven by users and I/S staff who have a personal commitment to the project and its people on the basis of solid trust and respect that has solidified expectations through the beginnings of a common vocabulary and understanding of departmental knowledge bases, jump on this EHR project. We now have the environmental basics for moving ahead with collaborating EHR projects successfully.

PROCESS MODELING

Remember that the four components we must integrate in system design are technology, people, data, and business process. Events in a business environment trigger various kinds of transaction processing. Process has hierarchy too, much like data, to systems-thinking people. Process hierarchy has been identified as function, process, subprocess, and procedure. In an EHR system and in other systems, several challenges will need attention in modeling current process. First, workflow inconsistencies are possible if two or more persons perform the same subprocess. These inconsistencies may be *un*known to the user manager. Second, there may be multiple versions of the same subprocess within the business unit or whole organization, all sanctioned by multiple user managers. Documentation of "variance," sanctioned or unsanctioned, is important for understanding the old way of doing things and in planning and implementing new systems.

Although we are documenting the *current* work activity, this is a critical step in new system design. Some argue that focus on the "old" fosters a "stuck in a box" approach when they want a "new" visionary path. This visualization of current activity is detailed "baseline data," which becomes invaluable for (1) doing "what if" exercises to analyze the business impact of the new system in system design and implementation planning, (2) a powerful aid in discussions with vendors when buying a new EHR system that will be "retrofitted" to the business environment, and (3) a true measuring stick for "benefits" of new system once implemented. These models should be sanctioned by the business community before becoming working tools for new system design, development, and implementation. User team members are responsible for this. The finalized model should be documented in writing, possibly by using project method tools including visuals.

Once the current system is documented, the workflow for the new system is designed. User members should be visionary people, and the team must have the new data defined for the new system to guide new process definition. This will be a conceptual model of process that will change as constraints and opportunities present themselves down the development path as teams take the system design documents and breathe life into them.

New, unique system-oriented processes may be handled by the user community as the system is implemented and used. These might include system backup, system table maintenance, data purges and archiving, and so on. Today as computer systems become "friendlier," more and more system maintenance/support is being designed to be handled by the users—those who have the most stake in system reliability and integrity. Traditionally, these processes have been completed by computer operations/support staff.

Again, user members need to obtain user community acceptance of the conceptual workflow for the new system. The approval should be documented in writing, possibly through some project method document including visuals. Expect multiple queries from front end users at this time. Suddenly, they begin to understand the system plan and start assessing the personal impact because the proposed workflow directly includes them. They start seeing a living system rather than just plans. It is important for user members to work with user managers to address and honestly answer these queries now. Be honest about the unknowns: there are many of them in this design or conceptual stage of projects.

DATABASE DESIGN

We now move from design activities to development activities. The first of these is often the database design. Database designers and administrators take the conceptual model of data turned into a logical model for the new system and plan the physical database. The database administrator will likely plan the physical database somehow isolated from the user members, appearing infrequently to clarify or possibly to determine whether he or she might structure the database one way or the other, depending on the user's response to the database administrator's question about operations impact. This "plan" is usually a textual listing of database tables with "keys" (unique identifiers for the each of the subject tables) and component data and identified physical storage mode and location. This is not for user community usage. However, the user members of the teams that identified the desired data should understand and indeed formally accept the proposed physical structure of the new database. This requires a clear understanding of the proposed database presented by I/S staff.

Once the database plan is finalized, the database administrator builds it as a foundation for system feature and functionality. The programmers can dig in with actual screen planning and design, menu development, report planning and creation, and so forth.

The user team members usually enjoy this task very much. This is where all their prior work starts congealing. They will have defined their data and business rules, anticipated, and flow charted proposed new processes. If the "mock screen" technique was used in any of these earlier tasks, the users and the designers probably have a "gut feeling" for how many screens may work, how the screens would flow through the system, how much of the data would be chosen from "pop-up tables" versus entered as "free-form text," and so on. Find creative but patient people for the job—often a dichotomy. This task can be very time consuming.

Reach consensus on "seed" screens to be used in screen design sessions; there is no limit on number or versions. Screen ideas can be dropped quickly in these sessions, so multiple versions are actually a good idea. If the automated EHR has a data entry staff, plan some design sessions for data entry personnel only. If the system has a large number of data viewers from many departments or units, include them in design sessions. If the system has a lot of report functionality, do report design sessions that include supervisors and managers who request and read them.

Iterative design is the name of the game here. Avoid long time spans between sessions that allow (1) the programmers to get too far into a full-screen design and (2) the users too long to forget their prior creativity.

IMPLEMENTATION READINESS

System development will never go quite like project managers and teams expect. "Challenges" will surface as the teams attempt to "put it all together." A detail-oriented problem solver from the user community is the best choice to work through "challenges." This task can also be very time consuming and may require the user member or manager to muster resources quickly and without fanfare.

Users may need to get creative now. Sometimes solutions lay in choosing between a technical fix, a software fix, or a people fix, or among all three. For every system created or purchased, there are likely multiple "constraints" involved in implementation that will have a business impact. If environmental basics are solid, project teams and departments can work through constraints to a solution.

User Processes and Procedures

Users have plans for what operational workflow will likely change with the introduction of the new system. It is now time to review these plans and the system development and identify any changes to the plans. I/S staff will have very little to do with this task. A user or group of users will take on the sole responsibility of "process owner." It should be done in concert with the systems team members configuring the system and defining the database load. Include here direct business activities and also any system support activities that have been delegated to user's responsibility. This is a huge job but it is dramatically foreshortened with the planning aid. Poor process planning is generally one weak area for the user community, who do not comprehend the impact on implementation without carefully defined and orchestrated new workflow. User members should understand that the first go-round will not necessarily be totally functional. Thus, part of implementation is the iterative refinement of the workflow. It is also a helpful message to the user community who may be nervous about the impending implementation.

Plan Transition

Teams should know what the business unit is doing now and what is expected when the new system is in place, but the spatial move between systems can be wrought with bumps. The conversion from one system to another should be planned for a time least disruptive to the business operations. It may be a time, however, when other unautomated but important system rollouts are occurring. It may involve temporary staffing and their logistics or automated work activity to greatly foreshorten the task. Seasoned veterans of implementations are great resources for planning this work. User members need to work closely with the planning staff and the user managers to smooth the conversion path.

Users not only define the implementation process, they completely drive it. Do you want to implement the system throughout the organization, department or unit, or, "phase it in"? If it is phase-in, who goes first and why? Do others agree with that rationale? If the system is to be used by many disciplines, do you start with one, or a handful of many, and then spread out the implementation on the basis of your ability to train the users? When is the best time to implement? What other activities are occurring that might interfere with the implementation? Will you implement one module or the whole system at once? Is there space for more hardware in work areas? When can training be scheduled? How will you get appropriate security access for the system to the users? Users must drive these decisions to ensure workflow continuity.

Users will get lots of feedback from existing clients interviews/site visits about these decisions, often conflicting styles of implementation and conflicting opinions about their success or failure. For example, one client will have used only "champions" to begin implementation. Another may have used a mix of those computer proficient and those computer illiterate on the initially trained. The user member must be comfortable with decision making amid conflicting information from the past implementation experiences of others.

Training

The critical task of training is usually underfunded, understaffed, underscheduled, and often only concentrates on system functionality, forgetting process. Users are not interested, nor should they be asked, to separate learning the new system from learning the operational processes in place

to support the new system. This combination approach (new system supported by new processes) to training takes more energy if you buy a system because vendor manuals will be geared only to the system's features and functionality. When flexibility is part of the system's design, the flexibility will be discussed at length in the vendor's training materials. The chosen way the organization specifically configured the system to best meet the business needs of that particular organization will not be included. This leads to unnecessary system functionality information directed at the trainees, and the trainee may be lost or confused about how he or she is expected to take the new system and apply it to daily work activities. In other words, the training materials sold by the vendor must be applied to each client's environment.

Often user members on design/development teams make good trainers. The training plan may call for "train the trainer," in which case system developers or vendor trainers may train the user trainer who will go forth and train the rest of the user community. This is very tiring, repetitive work that can be frustrating if users are not grasping the important concepts or they seem very resistant to change. Sometimes trainers train the user community directly.

Lots of questions will need to be answered in planning training. How much is enough? Who needs it when? How will you backfill your staff with other employees who can do the work during the staff's training time? What prerequisites does the user community need? Do you need to survey their skills and knowledge? If system is purchased, did you "buy" training? If so, what training did you buy—train the trainer, train the users, and so forth? Does the vendor have a trainer? Do vendor's training materials—training agenda, training manual, goals, objectives, and evaluations—exist? Are they appropriate for users' needs? Who is going to put documented processes and procedures that support the new system into the training materials and curriculum? If vendor training materials do not exist (often the vendor offers only one "manual," which may not be suitable for training), then how do you get these materials? If you built the system, who will produce the training manual and training curriculum? Where can you do training and when? Is a training room temporary or can it serve continuing training needs? How can you "institutionalize" training and system trainers after implementation? How can you get a practice time and place for users between training and implementation and long after?

A word here about a training manual versus a user's manual. They are different, and they have different goals, as depicted in Table 10-3.

A training manual is intended to train: to teach concepts that serve as background to hands-on exercises that teach system functionality and outcomes. A user's manual should be a complete textural documentation of the system that includes all system features and functionality, complete rationale behind use of particular features, complete picture of system usage within organization or user environment, solutions to potential problems with usage, sources of help

Table 10-3 TRAINING VERSUS USER (REFERENCE) MANUAL

Training Manual	User (Reference) Manual
Training is objective	System knowledge reference is objective
Focuses on select, critical system functions	Encompasses documentation of entire system
Exposes trainees to select system features critical to usage of this unique application	Defines and describes all system features, which are available in the system design
Limits explanation of system logic to subject area being taught	Explanation of full system logic incorporated into format and text
Incorporates the adult learning principles of discuss, demonstrate, do, and evaluate	Lacks "exercises" and evaluation components in manual format
Outcome is satisfactory work performance	Outcome is self help in problem solving while accomplishing work tasks

for users, and so forth. One does not replace the other. Part of the plans for training entail securing (or creating) a useful training manual.

Try orienting a few users to the new system and then let them determine what would most help others in learning the system. Test any newly created materials on a few other users to gain valuable feedback. "Cheat sheets" are very helpful in the initial training and in the first month or two of system implementation. They come in many flavors and forms.

Prepare User Manual(s)

If you build the system, you are automatically forced to develop a user's manual that serves as a reference to system functionality, navigation and workflow to support the system. The user member may be asked to document the designed front-end user features and functionality of the system, whereas other members of the team write other appropriate chapters of the documentation. This will become the bible for the system, so this work must be done to accurately reflect the user's view. It then needs to be updated when system changes occur.

If you buy the system, you will need to carefully review the user's manual that is sold with the system for accuracy, completeness, and ease of use. It will only describe the features and functions of the system. It will not describe any of the processes the user community has put in place to support the new system. This will need to be added before training so that workflow can be learned along with the new

system. Include new workflow documentation in the user's manual, which will serve as a reference guide to the system once it is implemented.

Data Migration

If the decision has been made that data from an old automated system will migrate to the new system, programs must be written to accommodate this. Business units decide the need for such action and the structure of the data through migration, and they influence the timing of the migration. They then need to test for data availability and integrity. This data mapping activity forces users to assess the value of data in legacy systems.

System Testing

System testing is a BIG DEAL. It is often called the "user acceptance test" and it means just that. If this is an EHR application, I/S staff will set up a "test database" that consists of the full system features and functions complete with dummy patients supplied by users. This test database is isolated from the "production" database and made available to selected users who add fake data and then test the system's features and functionality. Performance is measured against test plan criteria established earlier. Does it work like you expected? Are you getting "strange messages"? What does it not do that you thought it would?

"Go Live"

Implementation is a time to be highly organized because things happen quickly. A response plan aids in focusing on the immediate tasks at hand. Identify what roles team members will play at "go live." Clearly and completely communicate to the user community the series of implementation events that are about to occur. Implementation teams can expect to do lots of hand holding on the initial days of "go live." There is a natural learning curve to every system, every user, and every I/S staff member involved in implementation. Everyone is learning: the user community, all of the I/S staff, the vendor representatives (if the system was purchased), *everyone*.

This is the time when the "unknowns" strike as problems and test the teams that designed, developed, and implemented the system for their patience and endurance. If you are supporting the system in any way during this time, you will be "going the extra mile"—probably putting in long hours in problem solving, helping users navigate through difficulties, supporting the user community through technical "snags," and so forth. It is an exciting and tiring time, and tempers can fly. Draw heavily on the environmental basics to sustain the teams and add humor whenever possible. Keep track of problems and issues that arise by using a formal log—these could need immediate attention or they could be fodder for system improvement or phase II work.

The implementation will not happen perfectly. The odds are against perfection with so many new variables in the pot. Be prepared to document and problem solve for at least the first several months of system usage. Keep a log that serves to track the problem, triage, and solution status because the volume identified soon overwhelms the human brain. Problem solving after "go live" is a continuation of major testing of the environmental basics in systems work.

SYSTEM AND PROJECT EVALUATION

In all the efforts that led up to system implementation, you should have accumulated some real figures to measure change or new business impact. Use these as a baseline to determine system implementation success or failure. Ask whether the system implementation is the only factor that has caused the change. Users will likely be asked to measure against these baselines because much of the data will be coming directly from their units. Once the changes to baselines are measured, it is time to review the implementation. Was it a success or failure? What made it so? If problems exist, can and should they be corrected now? Can some things wait until an identified "phase II"?

For example, the EHR system evaluation should evaluate how the system performs against both strategic values of the organization and value benchmarks.[6] Once electronic systems are in place, the sharing of episodes of care enhance the quality and continuity of care. The benefit may be stronger in ambulatory settings because of the longitudinal nature of care; however, all care settings should benefit. A number of opportunities to measure improvements are listed here:

- Improved access to medical history, allergies, and medications should reduce the number of adverse reactions from treatment.
- Improved access should reduce the amount of time spent in obtaining and reviewing patient history before ordering diagnostics or treatment, which should shorten the time it takes to provide care and should reduce the cost of care.
- Improved access should allow caregivers to place orders that are legible, timely, and screened for possible errors, which should result in fewer errors in the treatment process.
- Improved access to patient information should reduce the need to delay seeing drop-in or emergency care patients until a record is obtained from current or remote storage, which should reduce the amount of time patients spend waiting for this information to be available to the treating clinician.
- System prompts and reminders should reduce the possibility of adverse reactions to care.

- Use of electronic and embedded disease protocols should result in consistent comparison to an agreed on standard of care.
- Use of on-line formularies should save time for the ordering caregiver and result in lower medication costs.
- Use of electronic clinical decision support systems should improve the efficiency and effectiveness of care.
- Use of electronic systems should result in standardization of terms and data, which should allow comparison of both the quality and cost of care.
- Legibility is improved, which should reduce medication errors.
- Laboratory technicians can check and see when a medication was ordered/administered, which should allow better timing of specimen collections.
- Caregivers can complete their documentation without obtaining access to a paper record, which should allow more timely completion of documentation.
- Administrative access to clinical records for billing, coding, and release of information can be completed without access to a paper record, which should allow more timely completion of these functions.

Use of a value-based approach will help an organization assess both the financial and more intangible values associated with a major system, such as the EHR system (Table 10-4).

Use of value benchmarks will give an organization a broader view of measuring the potential value of an EHR system (Table 10-5). If the system is realizing a value benefit that translates into cost reduction, the most operationally valid benchmark is the "average cost per case."[4] Value benchmarks can help measure the achievement of objectives and expectations for an EHR system.

It is safe to say the quest for new and better ways to conduct business is an eternal one that continually requires collaboration between the user community and the I/S staff. Out of implementation and usage will come new desires for improving the system. This starts the project cycle all over again in search of new and better information systems.

Key Concepts

- We have spent considerable time studying project teams and tasks from the user community's perspective in this chapter. True collaboration is the thread that ties the teams and tasks together. Collaboration relies on a conducive environment. This requires the basics of personal commitment, mutual respect, and trust and the shared principles, common expectations, and learned vocabulary, knowledge, and understanding.
- The outcome is worth the effort. "By giving the people most directly affected by information management and

Table 10-4 ELECTRONIC HEALTH RECORD: STRATEGIC AND OPERATIONAL VALUE

Strategic Value	Operational Value
Improved patient satisfaction	Faster registration
Improved clinician satisfaction	Improved work flow
Improved data resources	Elimination of data entry
Better and safer patient care	Elimination of duplicate data storage
Enhanced decision support capabilities	Reduction of identification and billing errors
Improved ability to integrate into community care systems	Greater access to complete and accurate information
Improved standardization of information resource	Direct entry of orders by responsible clinician
	Clinical reminders and alerts
	Access to new sources of medical information
	Enhanced development and use of multidisciplinary clinical pathways/protocols
	Activity-based costing
	Standardization of quality of care measures
	Outcomes measurement

Integral components: Master Patient Index (MPI), Electronic Health/Patient Record (EHR), Clinical Data Repository (CDR).

Table 10-5 SAMPLE VALUE BENCHMARKS

Opportunity	Basis	Benchmark
Pharmacy		
FTE reduction	Improved efficiency	FTE/thousand pharmacy orders
Error reduction	Bar-coded inventory	Dispensing errors/per thousand orders
Improved drug utilization	Limited formulary	% Reduction in formulary
	Decrease in drug costs	Drug cost/patient day
		Drug cost/thousand covered lives
Enterprise Master Patient Index		
Reduction in denied claims	Improved eligibility verification	% Claims denied
		FTE/claim
Dollars saved	Improved cash flow	Days in AR
Increased revenue	Income growth from improved service	% Increase in net income
Enterprise Scheduling		
FTE reduction	Improved efficiency	Transactions/FTE
Increased revenue	Reduced no-shows and cancellations, improved service	% Increase in net income
Clinical Documentation		
Overtime reduction	Decreased shift overlap	% Nursing overtime hours
Full-time equivalent reduction	Improved efficiency	Nursing FTEs/AOB
		Nursing FTEs/thousand covered lives

Continued

Table 10-5   SAMPLE VALUE BENCHMARKS—cont'd

Opportunity	Basis	Benchmark
Health Information Management		
FTE reduction	Reduced manual chart processing	HIM FTEs/AOB
	Reduced storage costs	Total paper charts stored
		Health information management
		FTEs/thousand covered lives
Order/Results Management With Decision Support		
Reduced test volume	Guided ordering/protocols	Tests/unit of service
Reduced morbidity	Clinical rules	Adverse medical events
Reduction in length of stay	Results flags/alerts	Average length of stay
Enterprise-Wide Benchmarks		
Improved efficiency	Integrated systems	Cost/unit of service
		Cost/diagnosis-related group
		Cost/pathway

Adapted from Murphy G, Hanken MA, Waters K: *The electronic health record: changing the vision*, Philadelphia, 1999, Saunders/Elsevier.
FTE, Full-time equivalent; *AR*, accounts receivable; *AOB*, adjusted occupied bed.

trusting those people to carry out the process in a judicious manner, healthcare organizations can shorten the time and reduce the cost involved in selecting the new system, while increasing the probability that the new system will be accepted and employed successfully (p. 56)."[7]

- It is important to remember that not all tasks described in this chapter are included in all projects, that many varieties of these tasks exist, and, that new activities that lead to system creation or selection and modification will continually appear on the horizon.

REFERENCES

1. *Webster's New Twentieth Century Dictionary of the English Language*, unabridged, New York, ed 2, 1979, William Collins.

2. Goverman I: *Planning for success.* Presented at the Health Information Management Systems Society Northwest winter conference, January 23, 1997, Seattle, WA.

3. Kloss L: The politics of information system integration, *J AHIMA* 68:18, 1997.

4. Murphy G, Anderson E: An organizational model for data access and management—work in progress, *J AHIMA* 65:52, 1994.

5. Davis F: User acceptance of information technology: system characteristics, user perception and behavioral impacts, *IJMMS Int J Man Machine Stud* 38:475-487, 1993.

6. Murphy G, Hanken MA, Waters K: *The electronic health record:changing the vision*, Philadelphia, 1999, Saunders/Elsevier.

7. Ciotti V: Applying TQM/CQI principles to information system selection, *Healthcare Fin Man* 49:56, 1995.

Data Management and Use

chapter 11

Statistics

Valerie J. M. Watzlaf
Elaine Rubinstein

Additional content,
http://evolve.elsevier.com/Abdelhak/

Review exercises can be found
in the Study Guide

Chapter Contents

Overview of Statistics and Data Presentation
   Role of the Health Information Management Professional
Health Care Statistics
   Vital Statistics
   Rates, Ratios, Proportions, and Percentages
   Mortality Rates
      Gross Death Rate
      Net Death Rate
      Anesthesia Death Rate
      Postoperative Death Rate
      Maternal Death Rate
      Neonatal, Infant, and Fetal Death Rates
      Using and Examining Mortality Rates
   Autopsy Rates
   Morbidity Rates
   Census Statistics
Organizing and Displaying the Data
   Types of Data
      Nominal Data
      Ordinal or Ranked Data
      Interval Data
      Ratio Data
      Discrete Data
      Continuous Data
   Types of Data Display
      Frequency Distribution
      Bar Graph
      Pie Chart
      Histogram
      Frequency Polygon

Key Words

Alternative hypothesis	Incidence	Percentage of occupancy
Anesthesia death rate	Incidence rate	Pie chart
Autopsy rate	Infant death rate	Postoperative death rate
Average daily inpatient census	Inference	Postoperative infection rate
Average length of stay	Inpatient bed occupancy rate	Prevalence
Bar graph	Interval data	Prevalence rate
Bed turnover rate	Length of stay	Proportion
Census statistics	Level of significance	Random sample
Coefficient of variation	Maternal death rate	Range
Community-acquired infection	Mean	Rate
Comorbidity	Median	Ratio
Confidence interval	Mode	Ratio data
Contingency table	Morbidity rates	Regression analysis
Continuous data	Mortality rates	Sampling error
Direct method of age adjustment	Neonatal death rate	Standard deviation
Discrete data	Net death rate	Standardized mortality ratio
Dispersion	Nominal data	Stratified random sample
Fetal death rate	Nosocomial infection	Systematic sampling
Frequency distribution	Null hypothesis	Test statistic
Frequency polygon	Ordinal data	Tests of significance
Gross death rate	*P* value	Variance
Histogram	Pearson correlation coefficient	Vital statistics
Hypothesis	Percentage	Weighted mean

Statistical Measures and Tests
    Descriptive Statistics
        Measures of Central Tendency
        Measures of Dispersion
    Inferential Statistics
        Tests of Significance
        Interval Estimation
        Sampling and Sample Size

Abbreviations

AIDS—acquired immunodeficiency syndrome

ALOS—average length of stay

ANOVA—analysis of variance

CV—coefficient of variation

dfb—between-groups degrees of freedom

dfw—within-groups degrees of freedom

DRG—diagnosis related group

HIM—health information management

ICD—International Classification of Diseases

MSB—mean square between groups

MSW—mean square within groups

NCHS—National Center for Health Statistics

SMR—standardized mortality ratio

SSB—sum of squares between groups

SSW—sum of squares within groups

Objectives

- Compute health care statistics, including mortality and morbidity rates, autopsy rates, measures of central tendency, and dispersion, and determine the most appropriate use of these health care statistics in health information management.

- Organize data generated from health care statistics into appropriate categories, including nominal, ordinal, discrete, and continuous.

- Display data generated from health care statistics using the most appropriate tables, graphs, and figures, including frequency tables, bar graphs, histograms, Pareto diagrams, pie charts, and frequency polygons.

- Determine which tests of significance should be used to test specific hypotheses and which are most appropriate for certain types of data.

OVERVIEW OF STATISTICS AND DATA PRESENTATION

Health care organizations continuously generate health care data. These data are used internally by patients, medical staff, nursing staff, and physical, occupational, and speech therapists and externally by state and federal regulatory agencies, The Joint Commission, and insurance companies, to name just a few. No matter who the user may be, statistics and data presentation focus on answering the user's questions while complying with the standards of the health care facility. To accomplish this goal, various methods are used to calculate specific types of statistics. Different rates, ratios, proportions, and percentages are used to evaluate mortality, autopsy, and morbidity rates and census and vital statistics.

Organizing and displaying health care data are necessary. To choose appropriate methods of displaying and analyzing data the health information management (HIM) professional must identify the level of measurement (nominal, ordinal, interval, or ratio) for variables and determine whether data are continuous or discrete. Measures of central tendency (mean, median, mode) and dispersion (variance and standard deviation) and tests of significance are used to describe and analyze data. It is also important for the HIM professional to understand basic principles of sample size determination and to be familiar with commonly used statistical tests such as analysis of variance (ANOVA), correlation, and regression.

This chapter explains basic and advanced health care statistics that are used in the health care field. Each statistic is defined and the formula for calculating each statistic is provided along with examples of how each statistic is used. Various methods of displaying data are described and illustrated.

Role of the Health Information Management Professional

Now more than ever, health care data are being collected to serve many purposes. One primary purpose is to establish health care statistics to compare trends in incidence of disease, quality and outcomes of care, and management of health information departments; another primary purpose is to conduct epidemiological research. The HIM professional's goal is to collect, organize, display, and interpret health care data properly to meet the needs of the users. Data can be manipulated in many ways to demonstrate one result or another. HIM professionals need a broad base of knowledge to determine what data elements should be used and when data are being analyzed appropriately and inappropriately. To do this, an understanding of health care and vital and public health statistics is needed. Furthermore, knowledge of statistical analysis is necessary so that HIM professionals can be the forerunners in data analysis. Because HIM professionals oversee a vast array of health data, it is imperative that the interpretation of the analysis and results of health care data start with them.

The HIM professional should assume the lead in recommending and using statistical tests that promote improvement in the analysis, use, and dissemination of health care data. The HIM professional fills many diversified roles and responsibilities, such as clinical vocabulary manager, data miner, or clinical trials manager.

In each of these roles, understanding and applying the methods used to collect, analyze, display, interpret, and disseminate data are essential. Responsibilities undertaken in these roles may vary from person to person. For example, the clinical trials manager may play a clearly visible role in cancer research study analysis and interpretation of the data; the clinical vocabulary manager may play a key role in developing vocabularies and standards that can be effectively used in the design of the electronic health record; and the data miner may determine the appropriate databases to use when analyzing clinical and financial data.

The HIM professional may assume other managerial roles in which statistics are used to assess productivity in coding, transcription, correspondence, and record analysis. The HIM professional should have sufficient knowledge and skills to do the following:

- Collect quality health data.
- Organize the data into databases.
- Statistically analyze the data collected.
- Develop, generate, and interpret health care statistical reports.

HEALTH CARE STATISTICS

Vital Statistics

Vital statistics include data collected for vital events in our lives, such as births and adoptions, marriages and divorces, and deaths, including fetal deaths. Birth, death, and fetal death certificates are familiar reports to HIM professionals. Although each state can determine the format and content of its certificates, the National Center for Health Statistics (NCHS) recommends standard forms that most states have adopted. The purpose of the NCHS standard forms is to have a national uniform reporting system of vital statistics. These standard forms are revised periodically. The attending physician is responsible for the completion of birth, death, and fetal death certificates. The accurate completion of these certificates is supervised by the HIM department, and a copy of the birth or death certificate is kept in the medical record. A copy of the fetal death certificate is kept in the mother's medical record.

When the certificate is complete, the original is sent to the local registrar, who keeps a copy and forwards the original to the state registrar. At each of these stages, the certificate is checked by the registrar to make sure it is complete. Individuals can obtain from the state registrar certified copies of birth, death, and fetal death certificates. Each state sends electronic files of birth and death statistics to the NCHS. The death statistics are then compiled onto the National Death Index. The death index is a central computerized index of death record information used for research purposes by epidemiologists and other workers involved in health care research.[1] The natality, or birth, statistics are compiled onto the monthly vital statistics reports, and the data files are also available for purposes of research.

Refer to your state health data center or division of vital statistics to receive state-specific information on preparing and registering vital records.

Rates, Ratios, Proportions, and Percentages

A **rate** is defined as the number of individuals with a specific characteristic divided by the total number of individuals or, alternatively, as the number of times an event *did* occur compared with the number of times it *could* have occurred.

A rate contains two major elements: a numerator and a denominator. The numerator is the number of times an event did occur. The number of events under study, or the numerator alone, conveys little information. However, when the numerator is compared with the denominator or the population of people in which the event could have occurred, a rate is determined. The results of a quality improvement study showed that 20 patients with diabetes had a stroke while taking a certain medication. What does this tell you? Should this medication be discontinued in this population? The data provided here include only the numerator. To compute a rate, the denominator is needed, for this example, total number of patients with diabetes who are taking the medication. This particular example included a sample size of 1000 patients. The rate is 20 in 1000 or 2 in 100. A rate is normally expressed in the following manner: 20 in 1000, 2 in 100, 1 in 100,000, 10 in 1,000,000, and so on.

However, rates are also very commonly expressed as percentages by converting the rate into a decimal and then multiplying the decimal by 100. A **percentage** is based on a whole divided into 100 parts. In the preceding example, the rate could also be expressed as a percentage by taking $^{20}/_{1000} = 0.02 \times 100 = 2\%$ or by taking $^2/_{100} = 0.02 \times 100 = 2\%$. This tells us that 2% of the patients with diabetes (in the study) had a stroke while taking a certain medication. To express a fraction, such as $^1/_5$, as a percentage, the first step is converting the fraction into a decimal by dividing the numerator, 1, by the denominator, 5, to obtain 0.20. The decimal is then converted into a percentage by multiplying the decimal by 100, which can be accomplished by moving the decimal point two places to the right. The result of this process is 20%.

A **proportion** and a **ratio** are similar to a rate. A proportion, which is a part considered in relation to the whole, is normally expressed as a fraction—$^{20}/_{1000}$, $^2/_{100}$, $^1/_{100,000}$, $^{10}/_{1,000,000}$, and so on. A ratio is a comparison of one thing to another, such as births to deaths or marriages to divorces. A ratio is expressed as 20:1000, 2:100, 1:100,000, 10:1,000,000, and so on. The number of physicians relative to patients or teachers relative to students is normally expressed as a ratio. For example, if a physician group practice has 10 physicians and 1000 patients, the ratio is 10:1000, which reduces to 1:100.

Table 11-1 summarizes examples of rates, proportions, ratios, and percentages.[2,3]

Once percentages are calculated, they can be compared across different subgroups, as seen in Table 11-2. This table concisely shows differences among different geographic areas in the percentage of elderly people by age categories. It even allows a glance toward the future by projecting percentages for the years 2010 and 2025. Comparing percentages among different areas shows that Europe has the highest percentage of population aged 65 years or older (13.7% in 1990) and that it should remain the world leader for at least the next three decades. North America and Oceania also have relatively high percentages of elderly people, which are projected to increase substantially from 1990 to 2025.[4]

Mortality Rates

Mortality rates are computed because they demonstrate an outcome that may be related to the quality of the health care provided. There are many types of mortality rates. Table 11-3 provides definitions and formulas for the most commonly used mortality rates.[2,3]

Table 11-1   EXAMPLES OF RATIOS, PROPORTIONS, PERCENTAGES, AND RATES

Ratio	Proportion	Percentage	Rate (per 100,000)
1:100	1/100 = 0.01	1.0	1,000 in 100,000
3:10,000	1/10,000 = 0.0003	0.03	30 in 100,000
250:100,000	250/100,000 = 0.0025	0.25	250 in 100,000

Table 11-2 PERCENTAGE OF ELDERLY BY AGE: 1990-2025

Region	Year	Age 65 Years and Over	Age 75 Years and Over	Age 80 Years and Over
Europe*	1990	13.7	6.1	3.2
	2010	17.5	8.4	4.9
	2025	22.4	10.8	6.4
North America	1990	12.6	5.3	2.8
	2010	14.0	6.5	4.0
	2025	20.1	8.5	4.6
Oceania	1990	9.3	3.6	1.8
	2010	11.0	4.8	2.8
	2025	15.0	6.6	3.6
Asia	1990	4.8	1.5	0.6
	2010	6.8	2.5	1.2
	2025	10.0	3.6	1.8
Latin America, Caribbean	1990	4.6	1.6	0.8
	2010	6.4	2.6	1.2
	2025	9.4	3.6	1.8
Near East, North Africa	1990	3.8	1.2	0.5
	2010	4.6	1.6	0.8
	2025	6.4	2.2	1.1
Sub-Saharan Africa	1990	2.7	0.7	0.3
	2010	2.9	0.8	0.3
	2025	3.4	1.0	0.4

Source: U.S. Bureau of the Census: Center for International Research, International Data Base on Aging.
*Data exclude the former Soviet Union.

Gross Death Rate

The **gross death rate** is a crude death rate for hospital inpatients because it does not consider such factors as age, gender, race, and severity of illness, which also play an important part in death rates. The use of the gross death rate as a measure of quality in health care has been questioned because it does not take into account these factors. As long as the HIM professional is aware that other factors influence this rate and that they have not been taken into account in the calculation, the gross death rate can be a quick, useful means of analyzing mortality in hospital inpatients (see example of gross death rate).

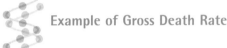 **Example of Gross Death Rate**

The discharge analysis report of Anywhere Health Care Facility shows 752 discharges (including deaths) for October 200X. Twelve deaths were also shown in the report.

Gross death rate:

$$= \frac{12 \text{ inpatient deaths}}{752 \text{ discharges (including deaths)}} \times 100$$

$$= 1.60\%$$

This means that 1.60% of total discharges from Anywhere Health Care Facility during October 200X ended in death or that the gross percentage of deaths, or the hospital death rate, for October was 1.60%.

Table 11-3 MORTALITY RATES

Rate	Formula
Gross death rate (hospital death rate)	$\dfrac{\text{Total number of inpatient deaths}}{\text{Total number of discharges (including deaths)}} \times 100$
Net death rate	$\dfrac{\text{Total number of inpatient deaths - Inpatient deaths <48 hours}}{\text{Total discharges (including deaths) - Deaths <48 hours}} \times 100$
Anesthesia death rate	$\dfrac{\text{Total number of anesthetic deaths}}{\text{Total number of anesthetics administered}} \times 100$
Postoperative death rate	$\dfrac{\text{Total number of deaths (within 10 days or surgery)}}{\text{Total number of patients who received surgery}} \times 100$
Maternal mortality rate	$\dfrac{\text{Total number of direct maternal deaths}}{\text{Total number of obstetrical discharges (including deaths)}} \times 100$
Neonatal mortality rate	$\dfrac{\text{Total number of neonatal deaths}}{\text{Total number of neonatal discharges (including deaths)}} \times 100$
Infant mortality rate	$\dfrac{\text{Total number of infant deaths}}{\text{Total number of infants discharged (including deaths)}} \times 100$
Fetal death rates	
Early fetal death (abortion) rate	$\dfrac{\text{Total number of early fetal deaths}}{\text{Total number of births (including early fetal deaths)}} \times 100$
Intermediate fetal deaths	$\dfrac{\text{Total number of intermediate fetal deaths}}{\text{Total number of births (including intermediate fetal deaths)}} \times 100$
Late fetal (stillborn) deaths	$\dfrac{\text{Total number of late fetal deaths}}{\text{Total number of births (including late fetal deaths)}} \times 100$

Note: The numerator and denominator in each formula must be for the same time period.

Net Death Rate

The **net death rate** is different from the gross death rate because it does not include deaths that occurred less than 48 hours after admission to the health care facility. The net death rate is useful because it provides a more realistic account of patient deaths related to patient care provided by a specific health care facility. For example, a 90-year-old patient arrives at the emergency department with shortness of breath, chest pain, and arrhythmia. After being evaluated, the patient is admitted, and it is determined that he has had a severe myocardial infarction (see example of net death rate).

About 24 hours later, the patient has cardiac arrest and dies. This particular death would be included in the gross death rate but not the net death rate because it occurred less than 48 hours after admission. Reporting agencies sometimes request net death rates because they may provide a more realistic reflection of patient care provided than gross death rates do. However, net death rates still do not take into consideration other risk factors that may also affect death, such as age, gender, race, and so forth. Therefore, an important note is that health care facilities are not necessarily responsible for deaths that occur more than 48 hours after patients are admitted; on the other hand, health care facilities are not necessarily free of responsibility for deaths that occur within 48 hours of admission. For this reason, some health care facilities do not make use of or report the net death rate.

Another consideration when computing any mortality rate is a health care facility must decide whether newborn inpatients will be included in these calculations. This decision is up to the health care facility; however, if a facility decides that newborn inpatient deaths will be included in the numerator, all newborn discharges must also be included in the denominator.

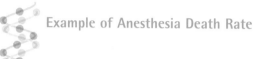 Example of Net Death Rate

Inpatient deaths at Anywhere Health Care Facility for 200X totaled 50. Inpatient deaths that occurred less than 48 hours after admission to the facility totaled 15. Total discharges (including deaths) were 15,546.

Net death rate:

$$= \frac{50 \text{ inpatient deaths} - 15 \text{ inpatient deaths} < 48 \text{ hours}}{15,546 \text{ discharges (including deaths)} - 15 \text{ inpatient deaths} < 48 \text{ hours}} \times 100$$

$$= 0.23\%$$

This means that 0.23% (fewer than 1%) of the deaths of discharges for 200X occurred more than 48 hours after admission to the health care facility, or that the net percentage of deaths or net death rate for 200X was 0.23%.

Anesthesia Death Rate

The **anesthesia death rate** can also be referred to as a cause-specific death rate because the death is determined by a physician or medical examiner to be due to a specific cause (e.g., an anesthetic agent). This rate indicates the number of deaths that are due to the administration of anesthetics for a specified period of time. If the recent anesthetic death rate is higher than the rate in previous periods, a focused evaluation may be necessary to determine why this is so (see example of anesthesia death rate).

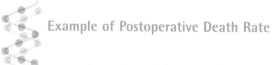 Example of Anesthesia Death Rate

Anywhere Health Care Facility performed 492 surgical procedures during November and administered 452 anesthetics. Deaths resulting from the administration of an anesthetic totaled two for the month.

Anesthesia death rate:

$$= \frac{2 \text{ anesthetic deaths}}{452 \text{ anesthetics administered}} \times 100$$

$$= 0.44\%$$

This means that 0.44% (fewer than 1%) of anesthetics administered resulted in a patient's death, or that the anesthesia death rate for November was 0.44%.

Postoperative Death Rate

The **postoperative death rate** may be considered a cause-specific death rate as well. This death rate indicates the number of patients who die within 10 days of surgery divided by the number of patients who underwent surgery for the period; therefore, it expresses the number of deaths that may have resulted from surgical complications. In both the anesthesia and the postoperative death rates, other risk factors, such as age, gender, race, and severity of illness, are not considered. Therefore, if it is found that these rates are higher in certain periods than in others, specific evaluations are necessary to determine whether the increase is truly due to the anesthesia or surgery or to other risk factors (see example of postoperative death rate).

Example of Postoperative Death Rate

Surgery was performed on 492 patients in the Anywhere Health Care Facility during November, and 27 of those patients died within 10 days of surgery.

Postoperative death rate:

$$\frac{27 \text{ postoperative deaths}}{492 \text{ patients having surgical procedures}} \times 100$$

$$= 5.49\% \text{ or } 5.5\%$$

This means that 5.5% of the patients who underwent surgery died within 10 days of the procedure or that the postoperative death rate for November was 5.5%.

Maternal Death Rate

Death rates are further categorized according to the type of service or department, such as the maternal mortality or death rate. A maternal death results from causes associated with pregnancy or its management but not from accidental or incidental causes unrelated to the pregnancy. The **maternal death rate** is the number of maternal deaths divided by the number of obstetric discharges. Again, like all the rates described previously, the maternal death rate does not take into account any other risk factors. The maternal death rate is useful because maternal deaths are rare. Therefore, if there is even one maternal death in a period, it is necessary to examine the cause of death in more detail (see example of maternal death rate).

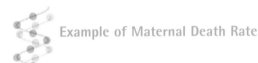

Example of Maternal Death Rate

Anywhere Health Care Facility had a total of 752 discharges for October, including 120 obstetrical discharges (including deaths) and 1 maternal death.

Maternal death rate:

$$= \frac{1 \text{ maternal death}}{120 \text{ obstetrical discharges (including deaths)}} \times 100$$
$$= 0.83\% \text{ or } 0.8\%$$

This means that 0.8% (fewer than 1%) of obstetrical patients discharged during October died, or that the maternal death rate for October was 0.8%.

Neonatal, Infant, and Fetal Death Rates

The formulas for these rates are given in Table 11-3. **Neonatal and infant death rates** are computed to examine deaths of the neonate and infant at different stages. A neonatal death is the death of an infant within the first 27 days, 23 hours, and 59 minutes of life. An infant death is death of an infant at any time from the moment of birth through the first year of life. Both of these figures are compared with the number of neonates and infants, respectively, who were discharged and died during the same period.

Fetal death rates are computed to examine differences in the rates of early, intermediate, and late fetal deaths. The definition of early, intermediate, and late fetal deaths may vary from state to state. These deaths are distinguished by the length of gestation or the weight of the fetus.

- Early fetal death (abortion) = less than 20 weeks of gestation or weight 500 grams or less

- Intermediate fetal death = 20 completed weeks of gestation but less than 28 weeks of gestation or weight 501 to 1000 grams
- Late fetal death (stillborn) = 28 weeks of completed gestation and weight more than 1001 grams

See example of neonatal, infant, and fetal death rates.

Example of Neonatal, Infant, and Fetal Death Rates

Anywhere Health Care Facility developed the following discharge analysis report for 200X. A segment of the report shows the following:

Live births	127
Neonatal discharges	115
Neonatal deaths (before 28 days)	2
Infant discharges	50
Infant deaths (before 1 year and at or after 28 days)	5
Intermediate fetal deaths	13

Neonatal mortality rate:

$$= \frac{2 \text{ neonatal deaths}}{115 \text{ neonatal discharges} + 2 \text{ neonatal deaths}} \times 100$$
$$= 1.71\% \text{ or } 1.7\%$$

This means that 1.7% of the neonates discharged/died or that the neonatal mortality rate for 200X was 1.7%.

Note: Because the intermediate fetal death rate is most commonly used, an example of that rate is given.

Intermediate fetal death rate:

$$= \frac{13 \text{ intermediate fetal deaths}}{127 \text{ live births} + 13 \text{ intermediate fetal deaths}} \times 100$$
$$= 9.29\% \text{ or } 9.3\%$$

This means that intermediate fetal deaths made up 9.3% of live births (excluding the live births at or before 20 weeks' gestation), or that the intermediate fetal death rate for 200X was 9.3%.

Infant mortality rate:

$$= \frac{5 \text{ infant deaths}}{50 \text{ infant discharges} + 5 \text{ infant deaths}} \times 100$$
$$= 9.09\% \text{ or } 9.1\%$$

This means that 9.1% of infants discharged died, or that the infant mortality rate for 200X was 9.1%.

Using and Examining Mortality Rates

Mortality statistics and trends are analyzed and used in many ways. When trends in mortality are examined, the possible reasons for differences in mortality rates should be considered. The influences can be grouped into three variables: time, place, and person. Changes over time include the following:

- Revisions in the rules for International Classification of Diseases (ICD) coding of death certificates
- Improvements in medical technology
- Earlier detection and diagnosis of disease

In relation to place, the following factors influence mortality trends:

- Changes in the environment
- International and regional differences in medical technology
- Diagnostic and treatment practices of physicians

Finally, the following characteristics of groups of people can also influence mortality:

- Age
- Gender
- Race
- Ethnicity
- Social habits (diet, smoking, alcohol intake)
- Genetic background
- Emotional and behavioral health characteristics

All these factors must be taken into consideration when mortality trends are examined within the health care facility or across health care facilities in relation to the quality of care provided.[5]

When examining mortality rates within a specific population as in the gross and net death rates, it is important to show age-specific rates or to adjust for age. Mortality rates are routinely adjusted for age because it is the most important influence in relation to death. As a person ages, the likelihood that the person will die increases. Age-specific rates can be used, but it becomes difficult to make com-

parisons of data with four or more age levels or categories. Therefore age adjustment is performed. Statistically, age adjustment removes the difference in composition with respect to age.[1]

Two methods can be used to perform age adjustment. One is the **direct method of age adjustment,** and the other is the indirect method of age adjustment or **standardized mortality ratio** (SMR). The calculations for these two methods are shown in Table 11-4.

The direct method uses a standard population and applies the age-specific rates available for each population. The expected number of deaths in the standard population is then determined. To use the direct method of age adjustment, age-specific rates must be available for both populations and the number of deaths per age category should be at least 5. The indirect method, or SMR, is used more often and can be used without age-specific rates and when the number of deaths per age category is small or less than 5. Standard rates are then applied to the populations being compared to calculate the expected number of deaths, which is compared with the observed number of deaths.[6]

Because the SMR is used in most national and statewide mortality reports, it is explained in more detail here. For example, in Table 11-5, hospitals across a state are examined for death rates associated with the diagnosis related group (DRG) 127–Heart Failure and Shock.

The actual or observed number of deaths in the hospital is compared with the expected number of deaths. The expected number of deaths is taken from a comparative national database adjusted for age and patient severity for each DRG. Table 11-5 shows a sample of the hospitals that treated patients included in DRG 127 and the actual and expected number of deaths. An SMR of 1 means that the number of observed deaths and the number of expected deaths are equal, and therefore the mortality rate is equal to what is expected from national norms. An SMR less than 1 means that the observed deaths are lower than the expected

Table 11-4   AGE ADJUSTMENT METHODS

Direct Method	Formula
Age-adjusted death rate (A)	$\frac{\text{Total expected number of deaths at population A rates}}{\text{Total standard population}} \times \text{Constant}$
Age-adjusted death rate (B)	$\frac{\text{Total expected number of deaths at population B rates}}{\text{Total standard population}} \times \text{Constant}$
Compare ages = adjusted death rates for populations A and B	
Indirect Method	**Formula**
SMR for population A	$\frac{\text{Observed deaths in population A}}{\text{Expected deaths in population A at standard rates}}$
SMR for population B	$\frac{\text{Observed deaths in population B}}{\text{Expected deaths in population B at standard rates}}$
Compare the two SMRs for populations A and B.	

SMR, Standardized mortality ratio.

Table 11-5 DRG 127 HEART FAILURE AND SHOCK

Hospital	Comments	Number of Patients	Average Admission Severity Score	Age 65 and over (%)	Deaths Actual Number	Deaths Expected Number	Deaths Statistical Rating	Medically Unstable During First Week: Major Morbidity Actual Number	Medically Unstable During First Week: Major Morbidity Expected Number	Medically Unstable During First Week: Major Morbidity Statistical Rating	Average Stay (Days)	Average Charge ($)
1	✔	268	2.5	85.1	23	21.03		35	25.12	–	7.9	15,420
2		412	2.4	87.1	30	33.08		61	36.66	–	9.2	8,149
3		201	2.2	87.1	17	12.16		9	14.52		9.4	7,645
4		208	2.6	64.4	8	16.56	+	24	21.52		7.7	15,669
5		471	2.5	89.0	40	40.31		40	44.18		8.3	8,193
6		90	2.6	78.9	9	7.49		12	9.35		9.0	14,766
7	✔	347	2.3	81.3	36	22.31	–	24	27.78		8.9	12,099
8		291	2.1	90.0	20	18.15		20	20.97		8.7	9,180
9		255	2.3	82.0	11	17.04		18	21.09		6.4	6.292
10		477	2.2	85.5	32	29.55		32	36.78		8.4	12,039

Hospital Effectiveness Report, Pennsylvania Health Care Cost Containment Council, Reporting Period January 1–December 31, 1991.

deaths, and therefore the mortality rate is lower than expected from national norms. An SMR of greater than 1 means that the observed deaths are greater than the expected deaths, and therefore the mortality rate is higher than expected from national norms (see examples of use of SMR).

Example 1: Use of Standardized Mortality Ratio

For hospital 1, an SMR of 1.09 means that the hospital had a 9% higher mortality rate for DRG 127 than is expected from national norms. This is calculated as follows:

$$SMR = \frac{23 \text{ actual deaths}}{21.03 \text{ expected deaths}} = 1.09$$
$$(1.09 - 1) \times 100 = 0.09 \times 100 = 9\%$$

Example 2: Use of Standardized Mortality Ratio

For hospital 4, an SMR of 0.48 means that the hospital had a 52% lower mortality rate for DRG 127 than is expected from national norms. This is calculated as follows:

$$SMR = \frac{8 \text{ actual deaths}}{16.56 \text{ expected deaths}} = 0.48$$
$$(1 - 0.48) \times 100 = 0.52 \times 100 = 52\%$$

The statistical rating column displayed in Table 11-5 is covered later in this chapter in the discussion of tests of significance.

Autopsy Rates

Autopsy rates are computed so that the health care facility can determine the proportion of deaths in which an autopsy was performed. This enables the facility to examine why a higher or lower autopsy rate may be seen from one month to another. Autopsies are performed to determine the cause of death, to better understand the disease process, or to collect tissue samples, as in patients with Alzheimer's disease. Autopsy rates can be further broken down to show the *gross autopsy rate,* or the rate of autopsies performed for total inpatient deaths; the net *autopsy rate,* or the rate of autopsies performed for inpatient deaths, excluding unautopsied coroner cases; and the *adjusted hospital autopsy rate* or the autopsy rate performed for all deaths of hospital patients whose bodies are available or brought to the hospital for autopsy (those *not* removed by coroners, medical examiners, and so on). Autopsies may be performed after the deaths of inpatients, outpatients, home care patients, skilled nursing care residents, patients who died at home, previous patients, and so on (see example of hospital autopsy rates). Table 11-6 presents the most commonly used autopsy rates.[3]

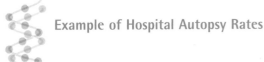

Example of Hospital Autopsy Rates

Anywhere Health Care Facility developed the following report regarding discharges, deaths, and autopsies during January 200X.

Table 11-6 AUTOPSY RATES

Autopsy Rate	Formula
Gross autopsy rate (ratio of inpatient autopsies to inpatient deaths)	$\dfrac{\text{Total inpatient autopsies}}{\text{Total inpatient deaths}} \times 100$
Net autopsy rate	$\dfrac{\text{Total inpatient autopsies}}{\text{Total inpatient deaths}-\text{unautopsied coroners' cases}} \times 100$
Hospital autopsy rate (adjusted)	$\dfrac{\text{Total hospital autopsies}}{\text{Number of deaths of hospital patients whose bodies are available for hospital autopsy}} \times 100$

Note: Numerators and denominators in each formula must be for the same time period.

Hospital Statistics

Discharges (including deaths)	1000
Total deaths	56
Inpatient (including two coroner cases)	52
Outpatient	2
Home care	2
Autopsies	13
Inpatient	10
Outpatient	1
Home care	2

Gross autopsy rate:

$$= \frac{10 \text{ autopsies on inpatients}}{52 \text{ inpatient deaths}} \times 100$$

$$= 19.23\% \text{ or } 19.2\%$$

This means that 19.2% of the hospital inpatients who died during January received an autopsy, or that the gross autopsy rate was 19.2%.

Net autopsy rate:

$$= \frac{10 \text{ autopsies on inpatients}}{52 \text{ inpatient deaths} - 2 \text{ unautopsied coroners' cases}} \times 100$$

$$= 20\%$$

This means that 20% of the hospital inpatients who died during January received an autopsy within the hospital, or that the net autopsy rate was 20%.

Hospital autopsy rate (adjusted):

$$= \frac{13 \text{ total hospital autopsies}}{52 \text{ inpatient deaths} - 2 \text{ coroner cases} + 2 \text{ out patients} + 2 \text{ home health care patients} = 54} \times 100$$

$$= 24.07\% \text{ or } 24.1\%$$

This means that 24.1% of all health care facility patients who died in January (inpatients, outpatients, and home care patients) received an autopsy within the hospital, or that the adjusted hospital autopsy rate was 24.1%.

Morbidity Rates

Morbidity rates can include complication rates, such as community-acquired, hospital-acquired or nosocomial, and postoperative infection rates. They can also include comorbidity rates and the prevalence and incidence rates of disease.

Hospitals use each of these rates to study the types of disease or conditions that are present within the health care facility and to examine the quality of care provided by the facility. These rates can aid health care facilities in planning specific health care services and programs. Table 11-7 provides a summary of the more common morbidity rates and the formulas used to compute them.[3]

Complications include infections, allergic reactions to medications, transfusion reactions, decubitus ulcers, falls, burns, and errors of medication administration. The complication rates for any of these complications can also be computed by using the formula for complication rates listed in Table 11-7.

One of the most common complications is infections. Infection rates are computed so that the health care facility can determine when infections developed and, therefore, how they may be prevented. A **nosocomial,** or facility-acquired, **infection rate** includes infections that occur more than 72 hours after admission.[7] Health care facilities may be more interested in this rate because it may show infections that occur as a result of the care that is provided in the facility. Further analysis of the nosocomial infection rate may show that other risk factors, such as age, compromising conditions such as cancer, the use of chemotherapy treatment, and the overall severity of the disease, may make an individual patient more susceptible to infection. Therefore, as with several of the mortality rates, other factors play a part in the development of the nosocomial infection. The postoperative infection rate is normally calculated to pinpoint how the infection may have developed. **Postoperative infection rates** are important to examine because the health care facility can determine which infections

Table 11-7 MORBIDITY RATES

Definition	Formula
Complication (condition that occurs during hospital stay that extends length of stay by at least 1 day in 75% of cases)*	$\dfrac{\text{Total number of complications}}{\text{Total number of discharges}} \times 100$
Nosocomial infection rate (infection that occurs >72 hours after admission to hospital)*	$\dfrac{\text{Total number of infections that occur >72 hours after admission}}{\text{Total discharges}} \times 100$
Postoperative infection rate*	$\dfrac{\text{Total number of postoperative infections}}{\text{Total number of discharges}} \times 100$
Community-acquired infection rate (infection that occurs in community or <72 hours of admission)*	$\dfrac{\text{Total number of community-acquired infections that occur <72 after admission}}{\text{Total number of discharges}} \times 100$
Total infection rate (includes both nosocomial and community-acquired infections)*	$\dfrac{\text{Total number of community-acquired and nosocomial infections}}{\text{Total number of discharges}} \times 100$
Comorbidity (preexisting condition that will, because of its presence with principal diagnosis, increase the length of stay by at least 1 day in 75% of cases)*	$\dfrac{\text{Total number of comorbidities}}{\text{Total number of discharges for a given period}} \times 100$
Prevalence (number of people with specific disease at specified period of time; number of existing cases of disease)	$\dfrac{\text{Number of cases of disease present in a population at specified time period}}{\text{Number of people in population at specified time period}} \times 100$
Incidence (number of people with disease during specified time period; number of new cases of disease)	$\dfrac{\text{Number of new cases of a disease occurring in population during a specified time period}}{\text{Number of people in population at specified time period}} \times 100$

*Numerators and denominators in each formula must be for the same time period.

occur after surgery and are probably a result of the surgical procedure.

Distinguishing between nosocomial and community-acquired infections is important because **community-acquired infections** are typically present less than 72 hours before admission to the health care facility. Health care facilities may be interested in this rate because it demonstrates the infections that patients probably had before admission to the facility. If the facility finds that their community-acquired infection rate is high, they may need to develop community-wide prevention programs, such as administering a vaccine for pneumonia. Health care facilities can benefit from analysis of their total infection rate (both nosocomial and community-acquired infections) to determine the additional cost, length of stay, and overall effect the infections have on the quality of care provided to the patient.

Comorbidities are pre-existing conditions, such as diabetes, hypertension, and osteoporosis. Analysis of the comorbidity rate is important because comorbidities can increase the length of stay and affect the outcome of care provided. Comorbidities include some of the other risk factors that affect mortality and morbidity rates.

Morbidity Data for Anywhere Health Care Facility During March 200X

Discharges (including deaths)	2000
Surgical operations	1543
Number of comorbidities	238
Number of complications	120
Nosocomial infections (includes postoperative infections)	22
Postoperative infections	8
Community-acquired infections	30

Complication rate:

$$= \frac{120 \text{ total complications}}{2000 \text{ discharges (including deaths)}} \times 100$$

$$= 6.00\%$$

This means that 6.0% of all discharges for March had at least one complication, or that the complication rate for March was 6.0%.

Nosocomial infection rate:

$$= \frac{22 \text{ nosocomial infections}}{2000 \text{ discharges (including deaths)}} \times 100$$

$$= 1.1\%$$

This means that 1.1% of all discharges for March had a nosocomial or hospital-acquired infection, or that the nosocomial or hospital-acquired infection rate for March was 1.1%.

Postoperative infection rate:

$$= \frac{8 \text{ postoperative infections}}{1543 \text{ surgical operations}} \times 100$$

$$= 0.52\%$$

This means that 0.5% of all those with surgical operations performed during March developed a postoperative infection, or that the postoperative infection rate for March was 0.5%.

Community-acquired infection rate:

$$= \frac{30 \text{ community-acquired infections}}{2000 \text{ discharges (including deaths)}} \times 100$$

$$= 1.5\%$$

This means that 1.5% of all discharges for March had a community-acquired infection, or that the community-acquired infection rate for March was 1.5%.

Total infection rate:

$$= \frac{52 \text{ total infections}}{2000 \text{ discharges (including deaths)}} \times 100$$

$$= 2.6\%$$

This means that 2.6% of all discharges for March had an infection, or that the total infection rate for March was 2.6%.

Comorbidity rate:

$$= \frac{238 \text{ total comorbidities}}{2000 \text{ discharges (including deaths)}} \times 100$$

$$= 11.9\%$$

This means that 11.9% of all discharges for March had at least one comorbidity, or that the comorbidity rate for March was 11.9%.

Prevalence and incidence rates are determined to examine the frequency of specific types of disease, such as cancer, acquired immunodeficiency syndrome (AIDS), and heart disease. **Prevalence** means the number of *existing* cases of disease, whereas **incidence** refers to the number of *new* cases of disease (see examples of prevalence and incidence rate determinants).

The **prevalence rate** is the number of existing cases of a disease in a specified time period divided by the population at that time. The quotient is then multiplied by a constant, such as 1000 or 100,000.

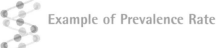

Example of Prevalence Rate

In a community of elderly people, the number of women alive with osteoporosis in the year 200X is 3593. The population of women in this community is 100,000.

Prevalence rate:

$$= \frac{3593 \text{ women with osteoporosis}}{100,000 \text{ women in population}} \times 1000$$

$$= 35.93, \text{ or } 36 \text{ osteoporosis cases per 1000 women in this community}$$

The **incidence rate** is the number of newly reported cases of a disease in a specified time period divided by the population at that time. The quotient is then multiplied by a constant such as 1000 or 100,000.

Example of Incidence Rate

In the same elderly community, the number of new cases of osteoporosis reported in 200X is 1113, and the population of women in the community at that time is 100,000.

Incidence rate:

$$= \frac{1113 \text{ new cases of osteoporosis}}{100,000 \text{ women in this community}} \times 1000$$

$$= 11.13, \text{ or } 11 \text{ new osteoporosis cases per 100,000 women in population}$$

To manage health care services effectively, the HIM professional should analyze prevalence and incidence rates of specific diseases that are prominent within a particular region or state. National sources of morbidity data include the National Health Care Survey. Originated in 1956, this survey is performed annually on a representative sample of 40,000 persons. Many subprograms are part of the National Health Care Survey, such as the National Hospital Discharge Survey, National Hospital Ambulatory and Medical Care Survey, and National Nursing Home Survey. Results of these surveys include incidence and prevalence rates of disease for specific geographic areas, length of hospital stays, cause of hospitalizations, and use of ambulatory care services.[1] The HIM professional should be aware that this information exists and can be used in conjunction with other morbidity rates to further analyze the distribution and effectiveness of health care services.

Characteristics similar to those that influence trends in mortality also influence trends in morbidity—time, place, person. For example, infectious diseases tend to occur more often at specific times of the year. The place of employment or geographic location can also increase susceptibility to disease. Age can influence the occurrence of infectious diseases; for example, diseases such as measles and chickenpox are more common in the young. Gender can influence morbidity trends, with differences in coronary artery disease for men and women. Race also influences morbidity trends, with hypertension being more prevalent in African Americans.[5]

Census Statistics

Ratios, percentages, and averages related to the length of stay, occupancy, bed turnover, and total number of patients present at a specified time within the institution can be useful both to health care administrators and HIM professionals. Such data can be used for the following purposes:

- To evaluate the current status of the health care facility
- To plan for future health care events
- To compare utilization of various units within a health care organization

The **census statistics** are extremely useful in the overall analysis of how much, how long, and by whom the health care facility is being used. Table 11-8 provides the formulas for the common census statistics[3] (see example of census statistics).

Example of Census Statistics

A 500-bed health care facility, during the month of June (30 days), had a total of 3600 discharges (including deaths), a total of 14,647 inpatient service days, and a total of 15,567 discharge days.

Inpatient bed occupancy rate (percentage of occupancy):

$$= \frac{14{,}647 \text{ inpatient services days}}{500 \text{ (beds)} \times 30 \text{ (Number of days in June)}} \times 100$$
$$= 97.6\%$$

This means that 97.6% of the available beds were occupied, or that the inpatient bed occupancy ratio was about 14,647:15,000, or that the percentage of occupancy was 97.6%.

Average daily inpatient census:

$$= \frac{14{,}567 \text{ inpatient service days}}{30 \text{ (Number of days in June)}} = 488$$

This means that the average number of inpatients during June was 488 or that the **average daily inpatient census** for June was 488.

Average length of stay:

$$= \frac{15{,}567 \text{ discharge days}}{3600 \text{ discharges (including deaths)}} = 4.3 \text{ days}$$

Table 11-8 CENSUS STATISTICS

Definition	Formula
Daily inpatient census (No. of inpatients present at census-taking time plus any inpatients who are both admitted and discharged after census-taking time the previous day)	Formula is presented as the definition.
Inpatient service day (unit of measure including services received by one inpatient in one 24-hour period). Synonyms: patient day, inpatient day, census day, bed occupancy day.	Formula is presented as the definition.
Inpatient bed count (No. of available inpatient beds [occupied and vacant] on any given day. *Note:* Not all beds are included in the inpatient bed count. These include beds in examination rooms, therapy, labor rooms, and recovery rooms as well as bassinets. Beds set up for temporary use are not included.)	Formula is presented as the definition.
Average daily inpatient census (average number of inpatients in a facility for a given period of time)	$\dfrac{\text{Total number of service days for a period}}{\text{Total number of days in that period}}$
Length of stay (for an inpatient, number of calendar days from admission to discharge). Synonyms: discharge days, duration of inpatient hospitalization, days of stay. **Total length of stay** (for all inpatients: total days in facility of any group of inpatients discharged during specified period). Synonyms: discharge days, total inpatients days of stay	Duration of hospitalization for one inpatient. Day of admission in not counted unless it is the day of discharge or the day of discharge is not counted unless it is the day of admission. Either method is correct if done consistently.

Table 11-8   CENSUS STATISTICS—cont'd

Definition	Formula
Average length of stay (average length of stay of inpatients discharged during specified period).	$$\dfrac{\text{Total length of stay (discharge days)}}{\text{Total number of discharges (including deaths)}}$$
Inpatient bed occupancy rates (proportion of inpatient bed occupied, defined as ratio of inpatient service days to inpatient bed count days in specified period). Synonyms: **percentage of occupancy,** occupancy percentage, occupancy rate.	$$\dfrac{\text{Total service days for a period}}{\substack{\text{Total bed count days in the period} \\ \text{(Bed count} \times \text{number of days in period)}}} \times 100$$
Bed turnover rate (number of times a bed, on average, changes occupants during a given period of time)	Direct formula: $$\dfrac{\text{Number of discharges (including deaths) for a period}}{\text{Average bed count during the period}}$$ Indirect formula: $$\dfrac{\text{Occupancy rate} \times \text{number of days in period}}{\text{Average length of stay}}$$

This means that patients stayed in the health care facility an average of 4.3 days during June, or that the **average length of stay** (ALOS) for June was 4.3.

Example of Census Statistics for Oncology Department

Discharges (including deaths)	1322
Hospital days for discharged patients	10,576
Patient A	Admitted June 18 and died the same day
Patient B	Admitted June 18 and discharged on June 19
Patient C	Admitted on June 19 and discharged June 25
Patient D	Admitted June 25 and discharged on August 8

Average length of stay for Oncology Department:

$$= \dfrac{\substack{\text{10,576 discharge days} \\ \text{for oncology patients}}}{\substack{\text{1322 discharges from} \\ \text{oncology department}}} = 8.0 \text{ days}$$

Patients in the Oncology Department stayed an average of 8.0 days during June, or the average length of stay for the Oncology Department for June was 8 days. The Oncology Department average length of stay (8 days) can then be compared with the overall facility length of stay (4 days) and determine why the Oncology Department length of stay is double that of the facility length of stay.

Length of Stay for individual patients

Patient A = 1 day because the patient was admitted and died on the same day

Patient B = 1 day because the patient was admitted one day and discharged the next

Patient C = 6 days by subtracting the date of admission from the date of discharge because the patient was admitted and discharged within the same month

Patient D = 44 days = 5 days in June + 31 days in July + 8 days in August

The individual patient lengths of stay can be compared with one another, especially if the patients received the same services or were from the same department.

Bed Turnover Rate:

Direct method:
$$= \dfrac{3600 \text{ discharges (including deaths)}}{500 \text{ beds}} = 7.2$$

Indirect method:
$$= \dfrac{\substack{97.6\% \text{ (percentage of occupancy)} \\ \times 30 \text{ days in June}}}{4.3 \text{ (average length of stay for June)}}$$

$$= \dfrac{0.976 \times 30}{4.3} = 6.8$$

This means that during June each of the hospital's 500 beds changed patients about 7.2 times according to the direct method and 6.8 times according to the indirect method—a small difference between the two methods.

ORGANIZING AND DISPLAYING THE DATA[8]

Types of Data

Before it is decided how to display data, it is important to recognize that different methods of display are appropriate for different types of data. Variables or data can be grouped into the following four categories on the basis of what kind of information or meaning the numbers convey:

- Nominal
- Ordinal
- Interval
- Ratio

Variables can also be classified as *discrete* or *continuous* based on how many possible values the variable can assume.

Nominal Data

The term **nominal data** is used to describe data collected on variables where qualitative (what kind) rather than quantitative (how much or how many) differences exist between individuals. Nominal data are also called categorical, qualitative, or named data. Examples of nominal variables include the gender and race of subjects in a research study. To facilitate tabulating and analyzing data, numerical values are often assigned to the categories of nominal variables. Using the variable gender as an example, the female category could be coded as "0" and the male category could be coded as "1." The variable employment status could be coded "10" for employed and "9" for unemployed, and so on. It is important to realize the numerical values used to represent nominal data only serve as labels for categories. The values or codes convey no quantitative (how much or how many) information. Therefore the choice of numerical values is arbitrary; gender could also be coded as 1 for female and 2 for male, and so forth. Table 11-9 shows nominal data of types of health insurance by gender.

Ordinal or Ranked Data

Ordinal data are data expressing rankings from lowest to highest according to some criterion. An example of the use of ordinal data is found in severity of illness scores used in assessing quality of care outcomes. Atlas, a severity of illness system, uses the following ordinal data to describe the severity of illness:

0 = no or minimal risk of vital organ failure
1 = low risk of vital organ failure
2 = moderate risk of vital organ failure
3 = high risk of vital organ failure
4 = presence of vital organ failure

Ordinal data can also include responses to questionnaires or interviews:

1 = strongly disagree
2 = disagree
3 = neutral
4 = agree
5 = strongly agree

Commonplace examples of ordinal data include class rank of graduating high school seniors and the ranking of sports teams within a league. A key feature of ordinal data is that the equal distances between ranks do not necessarily correspond to equal distances on the underlying criterion. For example the distance between class ranks of 1 and 2 is equal to the distance between class ranks of 3 and 4. However, when we consider the underlying criterion of grade point average, those of the students ranked as 1 and 2 may be closer to each other than are those of the students ranked and 3 and 4. See Table 11-10 for an example of ordinal data used in a frequency table explaining student perceptions of leadership characteristics.

Interval Data

Interval data convey more precise quantitative information than do ordinal data because it is assumed that equal differences between numbers correspond to equal differences in the trait or characteristic being measured. Examples of

Table 11-9   FREQUENCY TABLE—NOMINAL DATA: PRINCIPAL HEALTH INSURANCE COVERAGE BY GENDER

Health Insurance	Male (n = 50) Number (%)	Female (n = 50) Number (%)	Total (n = 100) Number (%)
Medicare	13 (26)	25 (50)	38 (38)
Medicaid	2 (4)	6 (12)	8 (8)
Blue Cross	25 (50)	10 (20)	35 (35)
Commercial	9 (18)	6 (12)	15 (15)
Other	1 (2)	3 (6)	4 (4)
Totals	50 (100)	50 (100)	100 (100)

From Watzlaf VJM, Abdelhak M: Descriptive statistics, *J Am Med Record Assoc* 60:37-41, 1989. Reprinted with permission from the American Health Information Management Association.

Table 11-10 FREQUENCY TABLE—RANKED ORDINAL DATA: STUDENT PERCEPTIONS OF LEADERSHIP CHARACTERISTICS

Leadership Characteristic Ranking	Management Clinical Internship (n = 35)	
	Before Number (%)	After Number (%)
1 Very weak	5 (14)	0 (0)
2 Weak	10 (29)	1 (3)
3 Moderate	15 (43)	5 (14)
4 Strong	2 (6)	12 (34)
5 Very strong	3 (9)	17 (49)

From Watzlaf VJM, Abdelhak M: Descriptive statistics, *J Am Med Record Assoc* 60:37-41, 1989. Reprinted with permission from the American Health Information Management Association.

Table 11-12 FREQUENCY TABLE—CONTINUOUS INTERVAL DATA: TOTAL CHARGES FOR 152 INPATIENTS IN A LARGE TEACHING HOSPITAL

Total Charges ($)	Frequency	Relative Frequency (%)
0-4,999	62	40.8
5,000-9,999	46	30.3
10,000-14,999	25	16.5
15,000-19,999	7	4.6
20,000-24,999	5	3.3
25,000-29,999	4	2.6
30,000-34,999	0	0
35,000-39,999	0	0
40,000-44,999	0	0
45,000-49,999	3	2.0

From Watzlaf VJM, Abdelhak M: Descriptive statistics, *J Am Med Record Assoc* 60:37-41, 1989. Reprinted with permission from the American Health Information Management Association.

interval data include scores on college examinations and scores on nationally administered tests such as the SAT (Scholastic Aptitude Test). If Student A received a score of 400 on the verbal section of the SAT, Student B received a score of 450, Student C received a score of 500, and Student D received a score of 550, it is assumed that the difference in verbal aptitude between Student A and Student B is equal to the difference in verbal aptitude between Student C and Student D.

Ratio Data

Ratio data share the property of equal differences with interval data. What is unique about ratio data is that the value of 0 represents the total absence of the trait or characteristic being measured. For example, if the speed of a car when it is stopped at a red light is 0, the value of 0 can be interpreted as the absence of speed; the car is not moving. Other examples of ratio data include height and weight of patients and length of stay at a hospital.

Discrete Data

Discrete data are data on quantitative variables that can only take on a limited number of values, typically only whole

numbers. Examples of discrete data include the number of medications a person is taking, the number of children in a family, or the number of records that are coded. See Table 11-11 for an example of discrete data used in a frequency table on hospital admissions by residence.

Continuous Data

Continuous data are data on quantitative variables that can assume an infinite number of possible values. Examples include height, weight, temperature, and costs or charges. See Table 11-12 for an example of continuous interval data for total charges for inpatients in a large teaching hospital.

Types of Data Display

Many methods are used to display data effectively (Box 11-1). Some methods of particular value to the HIM professional are frequency distribution tables, bar graphs, pie charts, histograms, frequency polygons, and Pareto diagrams.

Table 11-11 FREQUENCY TABLE—DISCRETE DATA: UNIVERSITY HEALTH CENTER HOSPITAL ADMISSIONS BY RESIDENCE

	City (n = 77) Number (%)	Suburbs (n = 38) Number (%)	Rural (n = 29) Number (%)	Total (n = 144) Number (%)
Hospital A	20 (26)	8 (21)	12 (41)	40 (28)
Hospital B	30 (39)	4 (11)	9 (31)	43 (30)
Hospital C	10 (13)	12 (32)	6 (21)	28 (19)
Hospital D	17 (22)	14 (37)	2 (7)	33 (23)
Total	77 (100)	38 (100)	29 (100)	144 (100)

From Watzlaf VJM, Abdelhak M: Descriptive statistics, *J Am Med Record Assoc* 60:37-41, 1989. Reprinted with permission from the American Health Information Management Association.

- Ask yourself what is the main message you wish to convey to the reader and then choose the type of graph that is most appropriate for the information you want to communicate.
- Be careful to choose a type of graph that is consistent with the type of data shown in the graph. For example, do not choose a histogram for nominal data.
- Create an effective graph that is visually attractive and numerically accurate.
- Aim for simplicity; unnecessary detail in a graph can be distracting to the reader.
- When applicable, give careful consideration to the scaling of the vertical axis (the minimum and maximum values displayed, and the number of units between consecutive labeled values).

Frequency Distribution

A **frequency distribution** table presents the number of times that each category of a qualitative variable or value of a quantitative variable is observed within a sample. When continuous variables that have a large number of possible values are represented, it is common for the frequencies of ranges or intervals of values rather than the frequencies of individual values to be reported. For example, a frequency table representing the age of patients could show the number of patients whose ages are between 20 and 29 years, 30 and 39 years, 40 and 49 years, and so forth. To allow comparisons to be made across samples of varying size, percentages that represent relative frequency are usually reported along with the frequency count. To compute these percentages the number of observations within a category is divided by the total sample size and the result is multiplied by 100. The frequency table should be self-explanatory and not show so much data that the table becomes un-interpretable. The table should be clearly labeled, the total sample size displayed, and units of measurement included. When intervals are used, the number of intervals should be not less than 5 and no more than 20 and of equal width, and the end points of the intervals are mutually exclusive and do not overlap. Tables 11-9 through 11-13 are examples of frequency distribution tables for nominal, ordinal, continuous, and discrete data, respectively.

Bar Graph

Bar graphs can be used to illustrate nominal, ordinal, discrete, and continuous data. The discrete categories are shown on the horizontal, or x, axis and the frequency is shown on the vertical, or y, axis. The purpose of the bar graph is to show the frequency for each interval or category. The scale of the vertical axis must begin at zero so that the heights of the bars are proportional to the frequencies. By using different colors or patterns of bars to represent different samples, bar graphs can be used to compare the frequency of categories or intervals in two or more samples. Figure 11-1 is an example of a bar graph using the data in Table 11-9. Other types of bar graphs are those shown in Figures 11-2 and 11-3. These graphs are still considered bar graphs but incorporate a line over the bars to show the total number of cases of salmonellosis (see Figure 11-2). Also, Figure 11-3 shows the incidence of meningococcal disease by age with use of a stacked bar graph.

Pie Chart

A **pie chart** is effective for representing the relative frequency of categories or intervals within a sample. It is constructed by drawing a circle, 360 degrees, and dividing that circle into sections that correspond to the relative frequency in each category. For example, if the relative frequency is 15%, then the slice of pie should span (0.15) × (360 degrees), or 54 degrees. Figure 11-4 is an example of a pie chart with use of the data in Table 11-9.

Histogram

The **histogram** is used to present a frequency distribution for continuous data. It is similar to a bar graph, but the horizontal axis of the histogram usually represents intervals of the continuous variable. Because theoretically there is no separation between the end point of one interval and the starting point of another, the bars of a histogram touch. The heights of the bars correspond to the frequency within each interval. Because intervals are usually of equal width, the width of all bars of a histogram is usually the same. If the areas (interval width × interval frequency) of all the bars are summed, the result should be equal to the total sample size multiplied by the common interval width. Figure 11-5 is an example of a histogram with use of data from Table 11-11.

Frequency Polygon

The **frequency polygon** is another method used to present a frequency distribution with continuous data. It is constructed by joining the midpoints of the tops of the bars of a histogram with a straight line. The total area under the polygon is equal to the sum of the areas of the bars in the histogram and therefore equal to total sample size multiplied by interval width. The frequency polygon is effective when comparing the distribution of a variable in two or more data samples. Figure 11-6 is an example of a frequency polygon using data from Table 11-11. Figure 11-7 is an example of a frequency polygon comparing two data sets.

The reader may find variations of these data presentation methods. For example, statistical process control, which is used in the quality improvement process, uses many of the graphs and figures displayed previously but may change them slightly or call them different things. For example, the Pareto diagram (Figure 11-8) is similar to the bar graph and the histogram and is used to order causes or problems from most to least significant. (See Chapter 13 for discussion of Pareto charts.)

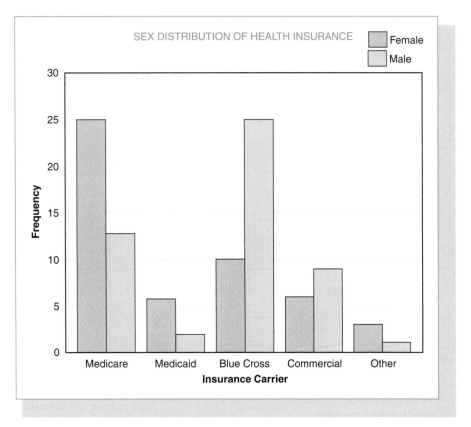

Figure 11-1 Bar graph. (From Watzlaf VJM, Abdelhak M: Descriptive statistics, *J Am Med Record Assoc* 60:37-41, 1989. Reprinted with permission from American Health Information Management Association.)

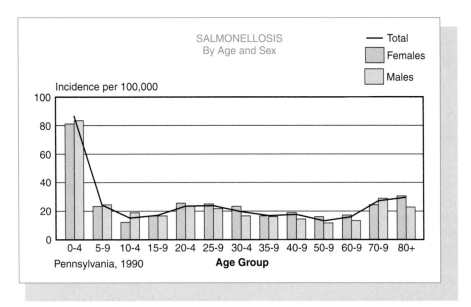

Figure 11-2 Bar graph and line graph. (From *Infectious Disease Epidemiology Report*, Pennsylvania Department of Health, Bureau of Epidemiology and Disease Prevention, 1990.)

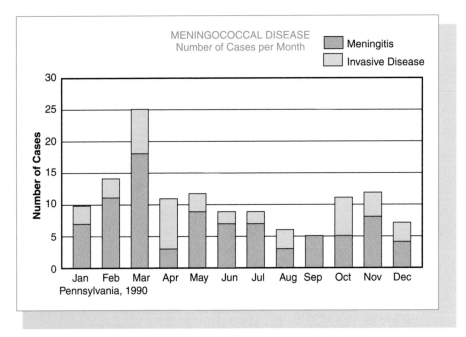

Figure 11-3 Stacked bar graph. (From *Infectious Disease Epidemiology Report,* Pennsylvania Department of Health, Bureau of Epidemiology and Disease Prevention, 1990.)

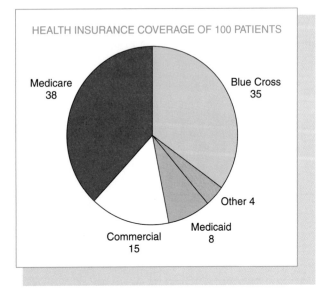

Figure 11-4 Pie chart. (From Watzlaf VJM, Abdelhak M: Descriptive statistics, *J Am Med Record Assoc* 60:37-41, 1989. Reprinted with permission from American Health Information Management Association.)

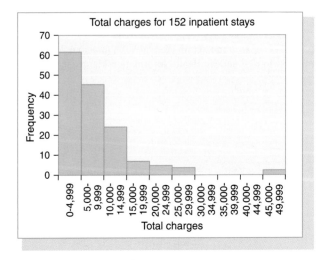

Figure 11-5 Histogram. (From Watzlaf VJM, Abdelhak M: Descriptive statistics, *J Am Med Record Assoc* 60:37-41, 1989. Reprinted with permission from American Health Information Management Association.)

STATISTICAL MEASURES AND TESTS

Descriptive Statistics

The following measures and methods are often referred to as descriptive statistics because the objective is to summarize and describe significant characteristics of a set of data.

Measures of Central Tendency

The common measures of central tendency are as follow:

- Mean
- Median
- Mode

These measures are used to locate the middle, average, or typical value in a data set. The selection of which one of

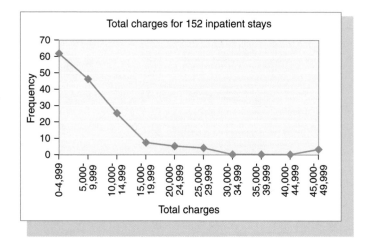

Figure 11-6 Frequency polygon/line graph. (From Watzlaf VJM, Abdelhak M: Descriptive statistics, *J Am Med Record Assoc* 60:37-41, 1989. Reprinted with permission from American Health Information Management Association.)

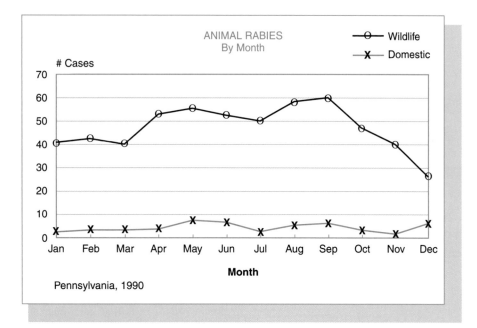

Figure 11-7 Frequency polygon comparing two types of data. (From *Infectious Disease Epidemiology Report*, Pennsylvania Department of Health, Bureau of Epidemiology and Disease Prevention, 1990.)

these measures is most suitable in a given situation depends on the type of data and the purpose for which the measure is being reported.

Mean. The **mean** is the most common measure of central tendency because it is easily understood by audiences and also because determining the mean is a step toward deriving other statistics discussed later, such as the variance and standard deviation. The purpose of the mean is to summarize an entire set of data by means of a single representative value. The mean or average is calculated by adding up the values of all the observations and dividing the total by the number of observations. Sometimes it is necessary to calculate an overall mean for a total sample when separate means are reported for different subdivisions of the sample. In this situation, a **weighted mean** can be calculated, as illustrated in the example on the following page.

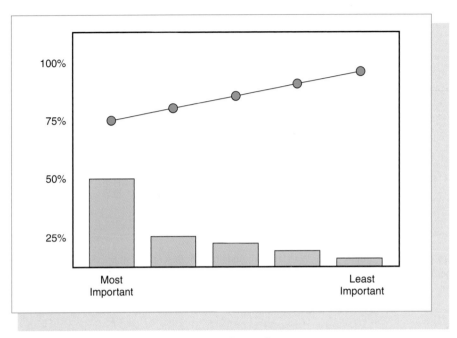

Figure 11-8 Pareto diagram.

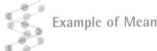 **Example of Mean**

The lengths of stay in the hospital for eight patients in a pediatric department are 6, 4, 2, 5, 20, 25, 18, and 4 days. The mean, or average, length of stay is calculated as follows:

Average length of stay (mean):

$$= \frac{6 + 4 + 2 + 5 + 20 + 25 + 18 + 4 \text{ (lengths of stays of each patient)}}{8 \text{ patients}}$$

$$= \frac{84}{8}$$

$$= 10.5 \text{ days}$$

Weighted Mean:

Department	Number of Patients	Average Length of Stay (days)
Internal medicine	40	6
General surgery	20	4
Pediatrics	5	2

If the average lengths of stay are 6, 4, and 2 days for three departments that have seen 40, 20, and 5 patients, respectively, the weighted mean, or average, length of stay is as follows:

$$= \frac{(40 \times 6) + (20 \times 4) + (5 \times 2)}{40 + 20 + 5}$$

$$= \frac{330}{65}$$

$$= 5.1 \text{ days}$$

Median. The **median** represents the middle value within a data set. When the values are arranged from lowest to highest, the number of values above the median is equal to the number of values below the median. For an odd number of observations, the median is the middle number in the ordered set of numbers; for an even number of observations, it is the mean of the middle two numbers.

The median is the most appropriate statistic to use for describing ordinal or ranked data because it allows for more meaningful descriptions of the data (e.g., the median response was between "strongly agree" and "agree"). It may also be useful to report the median for interval or ratio data when the data set contains extreme values, in other words, values that are much higher or much lower than the majority of other values. Although the mean can be strongly affected by extreme values, the median is not affected. Therefore, the median may provide a better representation of central tendency than the mean in some situations.

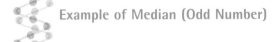 **Example of Median (Odd Number)**

Data: 1, 8, 6, 4, 2, 5, 9
Data after ordering: 1, 2, 4, 5, 6, 8, 9
Median = 5

Example of Median (Even Number)

Data: 16, 4, 21, 100, 7, 1
Data after ordering: 1, 4, **7, 16,** 21, 100 =

$$\frac{7 + 16}{2} \text{ (two middle numbers)}$$

Median = 11.5

Mode. The **mode** is the value that occurs most frequently in a given set of values. Some distributions do not have a mode, whereas others may have two modes (bimodal). The mode is the only measure of central tendency that can be used with nominal data. In Table 11-9, the modal health insurance is Medicare because it is the one that occurs most often.

Measures of Dispersion

When interval or ratio data in a sample are summarized, determining the amount of dispersion or variability within the data set is important. **Dispersion** or variability refers to the extent to which scores within a set vary from each other. Measures of dispersion describe the extent to which scores in a set are spread out (or clustered together) around the mean.

Range. The **range** is one way to measure dispersion because it is the difference between the highest and lowest values. The major disadvantage of the range is that it is concerned only with the most extreme values and ignores all other values. When the range is reported, the highest and the lowest values should be included as well as the difference between them. The following statistics show length of stay for patients with pneumonia and how the range is computed by taking the highest length of stay minus the lowest length of stay for both community-acquired and nosocomial pneumonia.

Example of Range

Length of Stay: Patients with Pneumonia

Community-Acquired		Nosocomial	
Medical Record Number	Length of Stay (days)	Medical Record Number	Length of Stay (days)
207658	20	123579	15
214592	10	275816	22
221459	7	254137	18
158645	14	321096	10
129876	8	153992	8
Mean	11.8	Mean	14.6

The range for the length of stay for patients with community-acquired pneumonia was as follows:

20 (highest value) – 7 (lowest value) = 13

The range for the length of stay for patients with nosocomial pneumonia was as follows:

22 (highest value) – 8 (lowest value) = 14

Variance and Standard Deviation. The variance and standard deviation demonstrate how values are spread around the mean. The calculation of these measures is based on deviations (differences) between the value of each score and the value of the mean. The **variance,** or s^2, is computed by squaring each deviation from the mean, summing the deviations, and then dividing their sum by 1 less than n, the sample size.[9] The **standard deviation,** represented by the symbol s is the square root of the variance. The reason for taking the square root is to express dispersion in terms of the same units as values of the variable. (If height is measured in inches, the variance of height would express dispersion in units of square inches, but the standard deviation would express dispersion in units of inches). Because of this property, the standard deviation is the most commonly reported measure of dispersion.

Example of Computation of Variance and Standard Deviation of Length of Stay of Patients with Pneumonia

Community-Acquired Pneumonia Variance:

$$s^2 = \frac{\begin{array}{c}(20 - 11.8)^2 + (10 - 11.8)^2 + (7 - 11.8)^2 \\ + (14 - 11.8)^2 + (8 - 11.8)^2\end{array}}{5 - 1}$$

$$= \frac{67.24 + 3.24 + 23.04 + 4.84 + 14.44}{4}$$

$$= \frac{112.8}{4} = 28.2$$

Standard Deviation:

$$s = \sqrt{28.2} = 5.3$$

Nosocomial Pneumonia Variance:

$$s^2 = \frac{\begin{array}{c}(15 - 14.6)^2 + (22 - 14.6)^2 + (18 - 14.6)^2 \\ + (10 - 14.6)^2 + (8 - 14.6)^2\end{array}}{5 - 1}$$

$$= \frac{0.16 + 54.76 + 11.56 + 21.16 + 43.56}{4}$$

$$= \frac{131.2}{4} = 32.8$$

Standard Deviation:

$$s = \sqrt{32.8} = 5.7$$

The greater the deviations of the values from the mean, the greater the variance. Therefore compare the variance of the length of stay of the patients with community-acquired pneumonia (28.2) and the variance of the length of stay of the patients with nosocomial pneumonia (32.8). This shows that there is greater deviation from the mean of length of stay values in the nosocomial pneumonia group than in the community-acquired pneumonia group.

The standard deviation for length of stay for patients with community-acquired pneumonia was 5.3. This means that, on average, observed length of stay values fall 5.3 units from the mean. The standard deviation for the nosocomial pneumonia group was 5.7, which means that, on average, observed length of stay values fall 5.7 units from the mean. Therefore, there is greater variation or dispersion in the length of stay for patients with nosocomial pneumonia than in the length of stay for patients with community-acquired pneumonia. The health care facility may want to examine this further to determine whether there are more outliers in the nosocomial group and to examine the outlier cases in more detail.

Coefficient of Variation. When two samples or groups have very different means, the direct comparison of their standard deviations could be misleading. Therefore, when two groups have very different means, it is best to compare their standard deviations expressed as percentages of the mean. The **coefficient of variation** (CV) is used to do this. The coefficient of variation can also be used to compare dispersion in variables that are measured in different units.

$$CV = \frac{s}{|\bar{x}|} \times 100$$

where

s = standard deviation
$|\bar{x}|$ = absolute value of mean

 Examples of Coefficient of Variation for Community-Acquired and Nosocomial Pneumonia

Coefficient of variation for community-acquired pneumonia:

$$= \frac{5.3}{11.8} \times 100 = 45\%$$

Coefficient of variation for nosocomial pneumonia:

$$= \frac{5.7}{14.6} \times 100 = 39\%$$

The CV was computed because it was important to determine whether the variation of length of stay values in the community-acquired pneumonia group was greater or less than the variation of length of stay values in the nosocomial pneumonia group. By using the CV, the variation can be computed exactly. The CV for the length of stay of the patients with community-acquired pneumonia was 45%, and the CV for the length of stay of the patients with nosocomial pneumonia was 39%. This means that the variation in the length of stay of the patients with community-acquired pneumonia was somewhat greater than that of the patients with nosocomial pneumonia.

Inferential Statistics

In almost all research studies, researchers can collect data from only a sample of the population of the cases about which they are interested in making conclusions. For example, a researcher interested in finding out whether the average salaries of entry-level HIM professionals differ across four geographical regions of the United States could not possibly collect data from *every* entry-level HIM professional in the country. However, through the use of a family of statistical tools known as inferential statistics it is possible to make **inferences** (or generalizations) about a population based on data collected from a sample. With inferential statistics, the generalizations are made that go beyond the known data. The domain of inferential statistics can be subdivided into two main areas: tests of significance and estimation of population parameters.

Tests of Significance

The purpose of **tests of significance** is to determine whether observed differences between groups or relationships between variables in the sample being studied are likely to be due to chance or **sampling error** or whether they reflect true differences or relationships in the population of interest. The term "sampling error" refers to the principle that the characteristics of a sample are not identical to the characteristics of the population from which the sample is drawn. Even if the average salaries of entry-level HIM professionals were equal across regions in the population, the sample means would still differ.

Although there are a number of different tests of significance, all are based on the same underlying logic and all involve a similar series of steps. The first step in carrying out a test of significance is to state the null and alternative hypotheses. A **hypothesis** is a claim or statement about a property or characteristic of a population. It indicates the nature of the difference or a relationship between characteristics. Each hypothesis can be expressed in two forms: as a null hypothesis or as an alternative hypothesis. The **null hypothesis** states that there is no difference or relationship in the population and the observations are the result of chance, whereas the **alternative hypothesis** states that there is a difference or relationship and that the observations are the result of the effect plus chance variation. In the example of the salaries of entry-level HIM professionals, here is how the null and alternative hypotheses could be stated:

Null hypothesis: There is no difference in the mean salaries of entry-level HIM professionals across geographical regions of the United States.

Alternative hypothesis: There is a difference in the mean salaries of entry-level HIM professionals across geographical regions of the United States.

The next step in carrying out a test of significance is computation of a statistic, sometimes referred to as the test statistic, which is based on the relevant data from the sample. The **test statistic** measures the size of the difference or relationship observed in the sample. In the example of the salaries of entry-level HIM professionals, the test statistic would reflect the size of the difference among sample means from the four geographical regions.

Once the test statistic is computed, the probability that the observed value of the test statistic could occur in the event that the null hypothesis is true is determined. This probability is known as a **P value** and can range from 0 to 1. The *P* value provides an answer to the following question: How likely is it that we could observe a difference or relationship of this size in the sample if, in reality, the difference or relationship did not exist in the population? A second way of posing the same question is: How likely is it that the observed difference or relationship is due only to sampling error? A third way of phrasing the question is: What is the probability that the observed difference or relationship could occur through chance alone? The smaller the *P* value, or closer it is to 0, the less likely the null hypothesis is true and the smaller probability that the observed difference or relationship could be due to chance or sampling error alone.

The availability of models of probability derived by statistical theorists makes it possible to determine the *P* value or probability associated with a given value of a test statistic. These models, known as theoretical sampling distributions, are discussed in greater depth in statistics textbooks. Commonly used theoretical sampling distributions include the normal, *t*, chi-square, and *F* distributions. Software programs that calculate test statistics also determine the associated *P* values as well.

The last step in carrying out a test of significance is to decide whether the *P* value is small enough to support making the decision to reject the null hypothesis. It is up to the researcher to choose the criterion or standard, which is known as the **level of significance.** The levels of significance that are most commonly chosen are .05 and .01. Setting the level of significance at .05 means that the decision will be made to reject the null hypothesis if the probability is smaller than 5 in 100 that the observed difference or relationship could be due to sampling error; setting it at .01 means the decision to reject will be made if the probability is smaller than 1 in 100. The recommended practice is for the researcher to choose the level of significance before carrying out the significance test.

When the *P* value is greater than level of significance either .05 or .01, the conclusion could be stated as either "accept the null hypothesis" or "fail to reject the null hypothesis." Whatever statement is used, this conclusion does not mean that the null hypothesis proved to be true. It does mean that the sample evidence is not strong enough to warrant rejection of the null hypothesis. This is a similar finding to when a jury determines there is not enough evidence to convict a suspect.

The choice of a level of significance depends on the maximum probability of incorrectly rejecting the null hypothesis (rejecting the null hypothesis when in reality the null hypothesis is true) that the researcher is willing to tolerate. Incorrectly rejecting the null hypothesis means concluding that there is evidence of a true difference or relationship when, in reality, the observed difference or relationship is due only to sampling error. The term for this type of incorrect decision is *Type I error.* It is also possible for a researcher to make a second type of incorrect decision: failing to reject the null hypothesis when in reality the null hypothesis is false. This second type of incorrect decision, known as *Type II error,* means concluding that the observed difference or relationship is due to sampling error when, in reality, a true difference or relationship exists in the population.

As stated previously, the maximum probability of Type I error, denoted by the Greek letter alpha, α, is set by the researcher. On the other hand, the probability of Type II error, denoted by the Greek letter beta, β, depends on several factors. One of these factors, the size of the sample, is within the researcher's control. The larger the sample size, the smaller the probability of Type II error. An important influence on the probability of Type II error is the size of the true difference or relationship in the population. This factor is not directly within the researcher's control. The larger the difference or relationship in the population, the smaller the probability of Type II error.

Type I error: Reject the null hypothesis when it is true, alpha (α)

Type II error: Accept the null hypothesis when it is false, beta (β)

The only way in which a researcher could know with certainty whether the null hypothesis is true would be to study the entire population, and this is hardly ever possible. When researchers make the decision to reject the null hypothesis based on the *P* value associated with a test statistic, they can never be absolutely certain that they have not made a Type I error. However, they can be assured that the probability of making a Type I error is very small.

Many different tests of significance are available to researchers. The choice of which test of significance to apply in a particular situation depends primarily on three factors:

1. What is the nature of the hypothesis? Does the hypothesis involve differences between groups, relationships between variables, or prediction?

2. What is the design of the study? How many groups are involved? Are the groups independent or matched on certain characteristics such as age or gender? Are data collected only at one time point or at two or more time points?

3. Which type of data (nominal, ordinal, or continuous) has been collected to measure each of the variables being studied?

Choosing the appropriate statistical method to test a particular hypothesis requires considerable knowledge of statistics. Therefore, it is recommended that HIM professionals consult a statistician as part of the process of planning a research study. The following sections describe several commonly used tests of significance.

Independent Samples *t* Test. Researchers are often interested in finding out whether a significant difference exists between two or more groups with respect to a quantitative variable. Examples of questions of this type include: Is the length of stay shorter with a new protocol compared with an old protocol? Are health care costs different across regions? Is patient satisfaction greater in teaching hospitals or nonteaching hospitals? When there are two groups and these groups are independent (not matched), a significance test known as the independent samples *t* test is applied. This test examines the differences between the means of the two groups and determines whether the difference is large enough to justify rejection of the null hypothesis. The decision of whether to reject the null hypothesis is based on the *P* value associated with a test statistic known as a *t* value.

The first step in performing an independent samples *t* test is to compute the mean and standard deviation for each group. Next, the standard deviations for the two groups are averaged, or pooled. Then a value of *t* is computed. Finally, it is determined whether the *P* value associated with the *t* value is smaller than the level of significance. Averaged/pooled standard deviation:

$$s_p = \sqrt{\frac{(n_1 - 1)s_1^2 + (n_2 - 1)s_2^2}{(n_1 - 1) + (n_2 - 1)}}$$

where

n_1 = number of cases within group 1
n_2 = number of cases within group 2
s_1^2 = variance of group 1
s_2^2 = variance of group 2

t value:

$$t = \frac{\bar{x}_1 - \bar{x}_2}{s_p \sqrt{\frac{1}{n_1} + \frac{1}{n_2}}}$$

$\bar{x}_1$ = mean of group 1
$\bar{x}_2$ = mean of group 2

n_1 = number of cases within group 1
n_2 = number of cases within group 2
s_p = pooled standard deviation

The data for the following example of an independent samples *t* test and the data for some subsequent examples were taken from the Hospital Effectiveness Report (Volume 5, Reporting Period 1992) published by the Pennsylvania Health Care Cost Containment Council in 1994. This report contains charge and treatment effectiveness information for acute care hospitals in Pennsylvania with more than 100 beds.

The hospitals making up the research sample in the following example include urban and suburban hospitals within the same metropolitan area. A researcher is interested in whether there is a difference between urban and suburban hospitals with respect to percentage of patients admitted for DRG 87, Pulmonary Edema and Respiratory Failure, who were aged 65 years and older. The researcher compiles the following information:

Example of Independent Samples *t* Test

	N	Mean	Standard Deviation
Urban	11	55.00	15.75
Suburban	11	74.05	13.40

$$s_p = \sqrt{\frac{(11 - 1)(15.75^2) + (11 - 1)(13.40^2)}{(11 - 1) + (11 - 1)}}$$

$$= \sqrt{\frac{(10)(248.06) + (10)(179.56)}{10 + 10}}$$

$$= \sqrt{\frac{2480.6 + 1795.6}{20}} = \sqrt{213.81} = 14.62$$

$$t = \frac{55.00 - 74.05}{(14.62)\sqrt{\frac{1}{11} + \frac{1}{11}}}$$

$$= \frac{-19.05}{(14.62)(.43)} = -3.06$$

In this example, the *t* value is computed as −3.06, and the associated P value is found to be .006. At a significance level of .05, the null hypothesis is rejected. There is evidence that a difference exists between urban and suburban hospitals with respect to the percentage of patients admitted with DRG 87 who are aged 65 years and older.

One-Way Analysis of Variance. When there are three or more groups, a significance test known as one-way analysis of variance (ANOVA) is applied to test for significant differences among group means. In this test, variability among subjects' scores is analyzed by dividing it into two components: variability between groups as reflected in differences among the group means and variability within groups as reflected in differences among the scores of subjects who belong to the same group. The logical principle underlying ANOVA is that, if true differences among group means exist, then between-group variability must be greater than within-group variability. As an application of this logical principle, the procedure for carrying out a one-way ANOVA involves three main steps.

Step 1 is to quantify the amount of between-groups variability, in other words, to evaluate how different the group means are from each other. Step 1 entails three substeps. In the first substep, a measure known as sum of squares between groups (SSB) is computed.

$$SSB = \Sigma\, n_j(\bar{X}_j - \bar{X})$$

where

n_j is the number of cases within the "jth" group
$\bar{X}_j$ is the mean of the "jth" group, and
$\bar{X}$ is the grand mean.

In the second substep, the between-groups degrees of freedom (dfb) are computed.

$$dfb = J - 1$$

where

J = the number of groups

In the third substep, the mean square between groups (MSB) is computed.

$$MSB = \frac{SSB}{dfb}$$

The second main step is to quantify the amount of within-groups variability—in other words, to evaluate the size of differences among the scores of subjects that belong to the same group. The substeps of step 2 parallel the substeps of step 1. In the first substep, the sum of squares within groups (SSW) is computed.

$$SSW = \Sigma\, (n_j - 1)s_j^2$$

where

n_j is the size of the "jth" group and
s_j^2 is the variance of the "jth" group.

In the second substep, the within-groups degrees of freedom (dfw) is computed.

$$dfw = N - J$$

where

N = the total sample size
J = the number of groups

In the third substep, the mean square within groups (MSW) is computed. Like the pooled variance that is computed when carrying out an independent-samples *t* test, the MSW represents the average amount of within-groups

variance. Notice the similarity between formulas for dfw and MSW and the formula for the pooled standard deviation.

$$MSW = \frac{SSW}{dfw}$$

The third main step is to compute the *F* ratio, the ratio of between-groups variability to within-groups variability. To reject the null hypothesis, the *F* ratio must be large enough; in other words, between-groups variability must be sufficiently greater than within-groups variability. The larger the *F* ratio, the smaller the associated *P* value will be.

$$F\text{-ratio} = \frac{MSB}{MSW}$$

Drawing again on the data related to DRG 87 in the Hospital Effectiveness Report, suppose a researcher is interested in comparing the average length of stay for three groups of hospitals: urban hospitals, suburban hospitals within the same metropolitan area, and hospitals outside the metropolitan area in surrounding counties. The steps in carrying out a one-way ANOVA are illustrated in the example computations below. Notice that the grand mean is computed as a weighted mean of the three group means (see the example of a weighted mean earlier in this chapter).

Example of ANOVA Computation

The researcher compiles the following information:

	N	Mean Length of Stay	Standard Deviation
Urban	11	7.43	2.98
Suburban	11	8.92	2.34
Outside	13	8.83	2.35

$$\bar{X} = \frac{(11)(7.43) + (11)(8.92) + (13)(8.83)}{11 + 11 + 13}$$
$$= \frac{81.73 + 98.12 + 114.79}{35} = 8.42$$

$$\begin{aligned}SSB &= (11)(7.43 - 8.42)^2 + (11)(8.92 - 8.42)^2 \\ &\quad + (13)(8.83 - 8.42)^2 \\ &= (11)(.98) + (11)(.25) + (13)(.17) = 15.74\end{aligned}$$

$$dfb = 3 - 1 = 2$$

$$MSB = \frac{15.74}{2} = 7.87$$

$$\begin{aligned}SSW &= (11-1)(2.98^2) + (11-1)(2.34^2) \\ &\quad + (13 - 1)(2.35^2) \\ &= (10)(8.88) + (10)(5.475) + (12)(5.52) \\ &= 88.80 + 54.75 + 66.24 = 209.79\end{aligned}$$

$$dfw = 35 - 3 = 32$$

$$MSW = \frac{209.79}{32} = 6.56$$

$$F = \frac{7.87}{6.46} = 1.20$$

The *F* ratio is computed as 1.20 and the associated *P* value is found to be 0.314. Because the *P* value is larger than the selected significance level of .05, the null hypothesis cannot be rejected. The researcher concludes that the three groups of hospitals do not differ with respect to the average length of stay for patients within DRG 87.

Pearson Correlation Coefficient. Many questions investigated in research studies are concerned with the relationships between variables. Different tests of significance are used to evaluate relationships depending on the type of data involved.

A statistic known as the **Pearson correlation coefficient** is used to assess the direction and degree of relationship between two continuous variables. The direction of the relationship between two continuous variables can be either positive or negative. In the following explanation of positive and negative relationships, the first variable is designated as X and the second variable is designated as Y. When the relationship between X and Y is positive, high scores on X tend to be associated with high scores on Y; as X increases, Y increases. When the relationship between X and Y is negative, high scores on X tend to be associated with low scores on Y; as X increases, Y tends to decrease. The relationship between HIM professionals' length of experience in the field and their current salaries would be expected to be positive; professionals with more experience would be expected to receive higher salaries. On the other hand, the relationship between the amount of stress experienced on the job and job satisfaction would be expected to be negative. As job-related stress increases, job satisfaction would be expected to decrease.

Values of the Pearson correlation coefficient for positive relationships can range from 0 to +1; values for negative relationships can range from 0 to −1. The closer the value is to +1 for positive relationships or to −1 for negative relationships, the stronger the relationship. The closer the value is to 0, the weaker the relationship. General guidelines for interpreting Pearson correlation coefficients suggest that values less than 0.30 may be considered to indicate weak relationships, values between 0.30 and 0.59 may be considered to indicate moderate relationships, and values of 0.6 or higher may be considered to indicate strong relationships. Because the procedure for calculating the Pearson correlation coefficient by hand is quite time consuming, computation is almost always done by computer. Readers interested in learning about the computational procedure are encouraged to consult an elementary statistics textbook.

When the Pearson correlation coefficient is computed, a related significance test is performed. This test determines the probability that the observed value of the correlation coefficient could occur through sampling error alone. If the *P* value is smaller than the predetermined level of significance, there is evidence that a true relationship exists in the population. At this point, a word of caution is in order: a statistically significant relationship is not necessarily a strong relationship. Sample size has a great influence on the outcome of the test for the significance of a correlation coefficient. When sample size is very large, a very weak relationship can be significant. Therefore, in interpreting results it is essential to consider the value of the correlation coefficient as well as the *P* value.

Returning once more to data related to DRG 87 in the Hospital Effectiveness Report, a researcher hypothesizes that a positive relationship exists between the average illness severity score of patients admitted to a hospital and the average length of stay for patients at a hospital. In the Hospital Effectiveness Report, the average illness severity score is reported on a scale from 0 to 4, with 0 indicating the least severe and 4 the most severe illness. The researcher reasons that patients whose condition on admission is more severe will tend to stay in the hospital longer than patients whose condition is less severe. Therefore, the researcher expects data compiled at the hospital level to indicate that, when the average admission patient severity score is relatively high at a given hospital, the average patient stay will be relatively long at that hospital as well. The researcher finds that the value of the Pearson correlation coefficient is 0.46 and the associated *P* value is .003. Therefore, there is evidence of a true positive relationship between average severity and average length of stay.

Regression Analysis. Regression is a statistical method closely linked to correlation that has many useful applications in HIM. The purpose of **regression analysis** is to learn to what extent one or more explanatory variables can predict an outcome variable. Extending the correlation example discussed before, the researcher might be interested in finding out how well average admission severity score predicts average length of stay. The single most important result of regression analysis is a statistic known as R-squared (also written as R^2), which can range from 0 to 1. R-squared represents the squared correlation between the explanatory variable(s) and the outcome variable. Although correlation coefficients can be negative, R-squared can never be negative because squaring a negative number generates a positive number. The value of R-squared indicates the proportion of variability in the outcome that is explained by the predictor variable(s). The closer the value of R-squared is to 1, the better or stronger the prediction. The *P* value associated with R-squared indicates the probability that the observed value of R-squared could occur through sampling error alone. When there is only one explanatory variable, R-squared may be computed by simply squaring the value of the Pearson correlation coefficient.

Regression analysis produces another important result known as a regression equation. The regression equation is a formula for calculating a case's predicted score on the outcome variable based on that case's score(s) on the predictor variable(s). Regression equations can be very useful in making decisions in situations in which data have been collected on the predictor variables but data on the outcome variable are not available. When there is only one explanatory variable, the regression equation takes the form of the formula for a straight line. As readers may recall from high school algebra, a straight line is determined by only two numerical values, the value of its slope and the value of its intercept. The slope is defined as the amount of change in Y per unit change in X and the intercept is defined as the value of Y when X is equal to 0. The general form of a regression equation when there is only one predictor is shown in the following formula:

$$\hat{Y} = bx + c$$

where

$\hat{Y}$ = the predicated value of Y
b = the slope
c = the intercept

The values of the slope and the intercept for a specific regression equation can be computed according to the following formulas:

$$b = r \left(\frac{s_y}{s_x} \right)$$
$$c = \bar{Y} - b\bar{X}$$

where

b = slope
c = intercept
r = value of the Pearson correlation coefficients
s_x = standard deviation of x
s_y = standard deviation of y

When a regression analysis is carried out on the data for DRG 87 using average length of stay to predict average charge, R-squared is computed as 0.46 squared or 0.21, and the associated *P* value is found to be .0004. Therefore, there is evidence that average length of stay is useful as a predictor of average charge. The following demonstrates computation of the values of the slope and intercept for the regression equation.

	Mean	Standard Deviation
Average severity score (X)	2.80	0.20
Average length of stay (Y)	8.42	2.58

Pearson r = 0.46

$$\text{Slope (b)} = 0.46 \left(\frac{2.58}{0.20} \right) = 5.93$$

$$\text{Intercept (c)} = 8.42 - [(5.93)(2.80)] = -8.18$$

Based on the values of the slope and intercept computed in the above equation, the following regression equation can be used to compute a hospital's predicted average length of stay for patients admitted under DRG 87:

Predicted average length of stay
= [(5.93)(Average severity score)] + (−8.18)

Suppose the average severity score at a particular hospital was 2.6. By substituting the value 2.6 into the regression equation and carrying out the arithmetic, the predicted average length of stay is found to be 7.24 days.

Chi-Square Test. The significance tests described up to this point are appropriate only for quantitative data. Many variables of interest to HIM professionals are nominal or qualitative rather than quantitative. The chi-square test is one of the most commonly used tests of significance that is appropriate for qualitative data. It can be applied to assess the degree of relationship or association between two qualitative variables or to determine whether there are differences between two or more groups with respect to a qualitative variable. The data used in computing a chi-square test are frequently displayed in the form of a **contingency table,** a table that displays the joint frequencies of the two variables. Table 11-13 displays the joint frequencies for smoking status and outcome of an experimental surgical procedure, coded as success or failure.

Certain terms are commonly used in referring to the parts of a contingency table. The variable whose categories define the rows is known as the *row variable,* and the variable whose categories define the columns is known as the *column variable.* In Table 11-13, therefore, smoking status is the row variable and surgical outcome is the column variable. The sum or total of frequencies within a row is known as the *row total,* and the sum or total of frequencies within a column is known as the *column total.* The sum or total of frequencies across all rows (or all columns) is known as the *grand total.* The grand total is equal to the total number of subjects or cases. The "square" within a contingency table that is formed by pairing a single category of the row variable with a single category of the column variable is known as a *cell.* Table 11-13, therefore, has four cells: nonsmoker, success; nonsmoker, failure; smoker, success; and smoker, failure.

From the data in Table 11-13, it can be seen that the overall success rate was 50% (13 of 26 patients).

Table 11-13 FREQUENCIES FOR SUCCESS AND FAILURE OF SURGICAL PROCEDURES

Smoking Status	Surgical Outcomes		Total
	Success	Failure	
Nonsmoker	9 (75.0%)	3 (25.0%)	12
Smoker	4 (28.6%)	10 (71.4%)	14
Total	13	13	26

However, for nonsmokers the success rate was 75% per cent (9 of 12 patients), whereas for smokers the success rate was 28.6% (4 of 14 patients). Is this difference significant? To answer this question, the chi-square test evaluates differences between observed and expected cell frequencies. Observed cell frequencies are the frequencies actually observed; expected frequencies are the frequencies that would be expected to occur if there was no association between the two variables. Subscripts are commonly used to identify cells within a contingency table. The first of the two numbers forming the subscript identifies the row and the second number identifies the column. For example, O_{11} stands for the observed frequency within the cell located in the first row, first column of the table; O_{12} stands for the observed frequency within the cell located in the first row, second column, and so forth.

The formula below is applied to compute expected frequencies for cells within a contingency table, and the example computation demonstrates the computation of expected cell frequencies for Table 11-13.

$$E_{ij} = \frac{(\text{Row total})(\text{Column total})}{\text{Grand total}}$$

Example Computation for Expected Frequency

$$E_{11} = \frac{(12)(13)}{26} = 6$$

$$E_{12} = \frac{(12)(13)}{26} = 6$$

$$E_{21} = \frac{(14)(13)}{26} = 7$$

$$E_{22} = \frac{(14)(13)}{26} = 7$$

We learn from the expected cell frequencies that, if the null hypothesis of no association between smoking status and surgical outcome were true, the success rates for nonsmokers and smokers would be equal to the overall success rate. In other words, the outcome of success would be expected for six nonsmokers (50% of the 12 nonsmokers) and seven smokers (50% of the 14 smokers). Likewise, the outcome of failure would be expected for six nonsmokers and seven smokers. After the expected cell frequencies have been computed, the chi-square statistic is then computed by applying the following formula:

$$\chi^2 = \sum \frac{(O - E)^2}{E}$$

where
O = Observed or actual
E = Expected

The following example computation illustrates computation of the chi-square statistic based on the observed cell frequencies shown in Table 11-13 and the expected cell frequencies computed in the preceding example.

Example Computation for Chi-Square Test

$$\chi^2 = \frac{(9-6)^2}{6} + \frac{(3-6)^2}{6} + \frac{(4-7)^2}{7} + \frac{(10-7)^2}{7}$$
$$= 1.50 + 1.50 + 1.29 + 1.29$$
$$= 5.58$$

The P value associated with the chi-square value of 5.58 is .018. Therefore the null hypothesis is rejected at the .05 level of significance, and it is concluded that surgical outcome is associated with smoking status.

Interval Estimation

Significance tests constitute an important and useful set of data analysis techniques. However, they can be appropriately applied only in situations where there are hypotheses to be tested. In some situations, the researcher's primary interest is in making use of data obtained from a sample to estimate the characteristics of a population, for example, in using the value of a sample mean to estimate the value of the population mean. It would be an extremely rare occurrence for the mean of a single sample to be exactly equal to the population mean. Furthermore, the means of multiple samples drawn from the same population would not all be the same but rather would vary from one sample to another. However, statistical theory has proved that when all possible samples of the same size are drawn from a given population and a mean is computed for each sample, the average of the sample means is equal to the population mean. Furthermore, statistical theory has demonstrated that as sample size increases, the average difference between the sample mean and the population mean decreases. In the long run, means of large samples will be closer to the population mean than means of small samples.

The application of statistical theory makes it possible to construct a **confidence interval** for the population mean based on the value of the sample mean. A researcher chooses a level of confidence, which is usually 95% but sometimes 90% or 99%. Like the choice of a level of significance, the choice of a level of confidence depends on the maximum probability of error a researcher is willing to tolerate. The probability of error is 100% minus the level of confidence. The interpretation of a 95% confidence interval is that there is a 95% probability that the population mean falls between the lower and upper limits of the interval (and consequently a 5% probability that the population mean does not fall within the interval).

The steps in constructing a confidence interval for the population mean include computing the mean and standard deviation of the sample and looking up the appropriate critical value (based on the level of confidence and sample size) in a table of the t distribution. The following formula is applied to compute the lower and upper limits of a confidence interval for the population mean:

Lower limit = Sample mean - [(Critical value)(Sample standard deviation/Square root of sample size)]

Upper limit = Sample mean + [(Critical value)(Sample standard deviation/Square root of sample size)]

The following example computation of confidence interval illustrates computation of a 95% confidence interval for the population mean based on data for average length of stay of patients admitted under DRG 87.

Example Computation of Confidence Interval

Sample mean = 8.42
Sample standard deviation = 2.58
Critical value of t for a 95% confidence level = 2.03
Sample size = 35
Square root of 35 = 5.92
Lower limit = 8.42 − (2.03)[2.58/5.92] = 7.54
Upper limit = 8.42 + (2.03)[2.58/5.92] = 9.30

There is a 95% probability that the mean average length of stay in the population for patients admitted under DRG 87 falls between 7.54 and 9.30 days.

Sampling and Sample Size

Because most populations under study are fairly large, researchers usually choose to study samples of those populations. Results obtained by studying a sample can be generalized to the population from which the sample is drawn as long as the sample is representative of the population. When a sample is representative, the characteristics of the sample do not differ from the characteristics of the population in any systematic or consistent way. For example, if a researcher wished to select a sample of hospitals within a certain state and selected only urban hospitals, the sample would not be representative of the population of *all* hospitals in the state. The best way to ensure that a sample is representative is to apply random sampling. A **random sample** means that:

- Every member of the population has the same chance of being included in the sample and
- The selection of one member has no effect on selection of another member-independent selection.[10]

Types of Random Sampling. In the current computer age, simple random sampling is usually carried out with randomization programs. Such programs are available either through statistical software packages or through stand-alone procedures available through the Internet. Simple random sampling can also be conducted with a table of random numbers. For example, if the population consists of 50 patient records and you would like to obtain a random sample of 20 of those, you can assign each patient a number or use an existing medical record number. Then refer to a table of random numbers, randomly pick a page to start on, and go up, down, or across, looking at the first two digits. If the first two digits are in the number assigned to the patient record, then that patient record should be included in your sample. Continue this process until your sample of 20 is met.

A **stratified random sample** is obtained by dividing a population into groups or strata and taking random samples from each stratum. This is done to assure that the sample is representative of the population. For example, when studying a group of college students that was 60% female and 40% male, the population would be divided into groups by gender and the selected sample would reflect the same ratio as to total population. Another example is when studying coding accuracy, medical records could be grouped by the most common principal diagnoses and selected to reflect the percentage as would be found in the whole population of records coded.

Because both simple and the stratified random sampling are time consuming without the aid of computer software, researchers have sometimes chosen another sampling method known as **systematic sampling.** With this method, the researcher must first decide what fraction or proportion of the population is to be sampled. If a researcher decided to sample one tenth of the population, the researcher would first randomly choose a starting point on a list of the population and then select every tenth record beginning with the designated starting point. Strictly speaking, systematic sampling can only be considered a random sampling method if the list itself is in random order.

Determining Sample Size. How do you know how many records or patients or subjects to include in the sample? This question is pondered by people completing performance improvement studies, epidemiologic research studies, or studies of any kind in which a sample is being taken. There is no easy answer to this question. Different approaches to sample size determination are taken depending on whether the researcher's purpose is interval estimation or hypothesis testing.

When the researcher's purpose is interval estimation, an important factor in sample size determination is the amount of error the researcher is willing to accept. Another way of thinking of the amount of error is in terms of how accurately or precisely the researcher wants to estimate the relevant population parameter, such as the population mean or proportion. The less error there is, the more accurate or precise the estimate is. The size of the sample increases the smaller the desired level of error and greater precision.

To illustrate this concept, suppose that a researcher wanted to estimate a population proportion. For example, a health care researcher wants to conduct a survey to determine the proportion of patients who were satisfied with the health care services they received. The population for this facility includes 1000 patients who were discharged within the past year, and interviewing all of them would take an unreasonably long time. Therefore, because no prior information is available to estimate p (the population proportion), the P value is set at .5. (This is the best guess when no information is available.) Also, the researcher decides that an acceptable amount of error is 0.05. This means that the researcher wants the sample proportion to differ from the population proportion by no more than 0.05. N is the population size and n is the sample size. Therefore the following formula can be used:

$$n = \frac{Npq}{(N-1)D + pq}$$

Where

p = estimated population proportion
B = acceptable amount of error
N = the size of the population
n = sample size
$D = \dfrac{B^2}{4}$
$ = \dfrac{(0.05)^2}{4}$
$D = 0.000625$
$q = 1 - p = 1 - 0.5$
$q = 0.5$

If we insert the information from the example, the formula is as follows:

$$n = \frac{(1000)(0.5)(0.5)}{(999)(0.000625) + (0.5)(0.5)}$$
$$= \frac{250}{0.874375}$$
$$= 285.9 \text{ or } 286$$

Therefore, for this example, the total sample needed in which only 5% error would be due to sampling variability is 286. Many other methods are used to estimate the appropriate sample size, depending on the sampling method chosen (simple random, stratified random, systematic). It is highly recommended that sample size selection be researched in more detail by using sampling books. *Elementary Survey Sampling* is an excellent book that clearly describes sample size and methods of selection.[10]

If the researcher's purpose is hypothesis testing, sample size determination is closely related to the concept of **power**, which is defined as the probability of correctly rejecting a false null hypothesis. Power is equal to 1 minus the probability of Type II error. The three factors that determine power are alpha (the level of significance set by the researcher), sample size, and **effect size** (the size of the difference between means or the strength of the relationship between variables in the population). Large effect sizes require smaller samples; small effect sizes require larger samples. To find the appropriate sample size it is necessary for researchers to arrive at an estimate of effect size. Effect size is defined differently, depending on the specific statistical method (i.e., *t* test, correlation, regression, etc.) to be used. Researchers often consult with statisticians regarding necessary sample size for hypothesis testing because of the number of factors that must be considered.

Key Concepts

- Health care statistics are necessary to evaluate a specific health care system or facility and should be calculated properly and used appropriately.
- For research statistics to be understood, clear and organized data presentations in tables, graphs, and diagrams should be used.
- There are several statistical tests that should be used for certain research studies. Knowing which statistics to use and when is extremely important and has a great impact on the results.
- Significance tests constitute an important and useful set of data analysis techniques. However, they can be appropriately applied only in situations in which there are hypotheses to be tested.
- Statistical theory has demonstrated that as sample size increases, the average difference between the sample mean and the population mean decreases. In the long run, means of large samples will be closer to the population mean than means of small samples.

REFERENCES

1. Kuzma J, Bohnenblust S: *Basic statistics for the health sciences*, ed 5, New York, 2005, McGraw-Hill.
2. Skurka MF: Statistics. In *Health information management in hospitals* (pp. 141-146), Chicago, 1994, American Hospital Publishing.
3. Hanken MA, Water K, editors: *Glossary of healthcare terms*, Chicago, 1994, American Health Information Management Association.
4. U.S. Bureau of Census: International population reports. In *An aging world II* (pp. 25, 92-93), Washington, DC, 1992, U.S. Government Printing Office.
5. Lilienfeld D, Stolley PD: *Foundations of epidemiology*, ed 3, Oxford, 1994, Oxford University Press.
6. Slome C, Brogan D, Eyres S, et al: *Basic epidemiological methods and biostatistics: a workbook*, Belmont, CA, 1986, Jones & Bartlett.

7. Watzlaf VJM, Kuller LH, Ruben FL: The use of the medical record and financial data to examine the cost of infections in the elderly, *Topics in Health Records Management* 13:65-76, 1992.

8. Watzlaf V, Abdelhak M: Descriptive statistics, *J Am Med Record Assoc* 60:37-41, 1989.

9. Shott S: *Statistics for health professionals,* Philadelphia, 1990, WB Saunders.

10. Scheaffer R, Mendenhall W, Ott L: *Elementary survey sampling,* ed 3, Boston, 1986, Duxbury Press.

chapter 12

Research and Epidemiology

Valerie J. M. Watzlaf

Additional content,
http://evolve.elsevier.com/Abdelhak/

Review exercises can be found
in the Study Guide

Overview of Research and Epidemiology
Role of the Health Information Management
  Professional
Designing the Research Proposal
  Hypothesis and Research Questions
  Review of Literature
  Methodology (Draft)
  Research Plan
    Specific Aims
    Significance (Review of Literature and Preliminary Research)
    Methodology
    Human Subjects
    Literature Referenced
    Budget Development
    Appendix Design
    Additional Considerations
Validity and Reliability
  Validity
  Sensitivity and Specificity
    Analysis and Discussion
  Reliability
Biases
  Confounding Variables
  Sampling Variability
  Ascertainment and Selection Bias
  Diagnosis Bias
  Nonresponse Bias
  Survival Bias
  Recall Bias
  Interviewer Bias
  Prevarication Bias

Key Words

Analytic study	Focus groups	Period prevalence rate
Bias	Generalizability	Point prevalence rate
Case	Historical prospective study	Prevalence rate
Case-control study	Hypothesis	Prevalence study
Case finding	Incidence rate	Prospective study
Case studies	Incidence study	Qualitative research
Censored	Incident case	Relative risk
Clinical trial	Independent variable	Reliability
Close-ended questions	Interobserver reliability	Response rate
Cohort study	Intraobserver reliability	Research question
Community trial	Institutional review board	Retrospective study
Confounding variables	Life-table analysis	Risk factors
Control	Literature review	Sensitivity
Correlation coefficient	Methodology	Specific aims
Cross-sectional study	Nosocomial	Specificity
Dependent variable	Odds ratio	Subject blind
Descriptive study	Open-ended questions	Survey design
Double blind	Outcome measures	Triple blind
Epidemiology	Participant observation	Validity
Experimental epidemiology	Peer-reviewed journal	
Exposure characteristics	Pilot testing	

Epidemiologic/Research Study Designs
  Descriptive Study
    Cross-Sectional or Prevalence Study
    Survey Research
    Qualitative Research
  Analytic Study Design
    Case Control or Retrospective Study Design
    Prospective, Cohort, or Incidence Study
    Historical-Prospective Study Design
  Experimental Epidemiology
    Clinical and Community Trials
    Life-Table Analysis
Use of Computer Software in Research
Outcome Studies and Epidemiology
  Study Procedures
  Data Analysis

Abbreviations

ADL—activities of daily living

AHIMA—American Health Information Management Association

ALOS—average length of stay

ASTM—American Society for Testing and Materials

BMI—body mass index

CAD—coronary artery disease

CAI—community-acquired infection

DRG—diagnosis related group

EHR—electronic health record

FN—false negatives

FP—false positives

HIM—health information management

ICD-9-CM—*International Classification of Diseases, Ninth Edition, Clinical Modification*

IR—incidence rate

IRB—institutional review board

JCAHO—Joint Commission on Accreditation of Healthcare Organizations (now The Joint Commission)

K—Kappa statistic

NI—nosocomial infection

PHR—personal health record

r—correlation coefficient

RR—relative risk

SPSS—Statistical Process for Social Sciences

TN—true negatives

TP—true positives

Objectives

- Explain the steps necessary for designing a research study or grant proposal.

- Given a specific hypothesis, design a research study to test the hypothesis.

- Given examples of research studies conducted in health care settings, detect and describe the different types of biases that occur within these research studies.

- Determine the most effective methods to use to test validity and reliability.

- Given an explanation of different epidemiologic research study designs, state the advantages and disadvantages of each and the health care statistics that should be used or generated from each design.

- Explain how each epidemiologic research study design can be used in health information management.

- Demonstrate knowledge of the most applicable computer software to use when applying epidemiologic research study design principles.

- Recognize outcome measures and discuss how epidemiologic study designs can facilitate executing outcome studies.

Epidemiology and health information management (HIM) are two fields that complement each other. Validity and reliability of the data managed by HIM professionals are essential to the soundness and integrity of epidemiologic research studies. The epidemiologic research techniques provide a basis for HIM professionals to take part in designing and conducting research studies that examine several clinical, financial, and administrative areas. Epidemiologic techniques aid the HIM professional not only in conducting clinically based research studies but also in the study of specific HIM department functions, such as whether concurrent coding is more beneficial and cost-effective than coding performed at discharge or whether productivity standards developed for HIM employees are effective.

Because HIM professionals oversee a vast array of health data, it is essential that all epidemiologic methods known to examine these data be used. **Epidemiology** is the study of disease and the determinants of disease in populations; however, it is also the study of clinical and health care trends or patterns and the ability to recognize trends or patterns within large amounts of data. When HIM professionals master the basic epidemiologic techniques, they become premier detectives seeking out the most prominent, logical, and important trends in the data. This is not an easy task and takes a great deal of practice and thought. However, when the epidemiologic techniques are known, used, and understood, the HIM professional becomes more competent.

future research are explained and discussed. HIM professionals who are actively involved in analysis, interpretation, and complex research study design should continuously supplement their knowledge through coursework, seminars, and in-service training in these areas as well as work closely with a statistician and an epidemiologist.

Familiarity with research study protocol (Figure 12-1), including formulating a hypothesis, reviewing and analyzing the literature, developing specific aims, determining the significance of the research, and defining the methodology for collecting and analyzing the data, is necessary for the HIM professional. When the steps of the research design are well formulated and understood, then the data, statistics, and data display are easier to interpret.

Familiarity with the different types of epidemiologic research study designs is necessary to determine whether the health care data generated from a research study are accurate and appropriate. The different epidemiologic research study designs to be examined are the **descriptive study** (cross-sectional or prevalence), **analytic study** (case-control or retrospective, cohort or prospective, and historical-prospective), and experimental study (clinical and community trials). The selection of the study design depends on the hypothesis or research question.

HIM professionals should recognize that every research study involves some degree of bias or error. This may be due to sampling variability, methods of data collection, or confounding variables.

OVERVIEW OF RESEARCH AND EPIDEMIOLOGY

Leadership in the field of HIM begins with knowledge. Research provides knowledge. It enables individuals to learn something valuable about their profession. Research also provides new ideas to be shared, new methods and systems to be tried, and new infrastructures to be constructed. The purpose of research is to discover or learn something new about a specific area that was not known before. It enables one to take a question, review the literature related to that question, collect data related to that question, analyze the data collected, and then formulate answers to the question. Research is not formulating answers to your question from your own opinions or perceptions without the collection of new data.

This chapter introduces the reader to research methods and epidemiology. It also includes the types of statistical tests that are most appropriate to use when certain types of epidemiologic studies are conducted. This chapter discusses the relationship between epidemiology and outcomes studies and provides an example of an epidemiologic study that is also a clinical outcomes study. The actual database, methods of data collection and data analysis, and areas of

ROLE OF THE HEALTH INFORMATION MANAGEMENT PROFESSIONAL

Medical Language and Classification Expert and Domain Manager are two roles that are included in the *Report on the Roles and Functions of the e-Health Information Management* by the American Health Information Management Association (AHIMA).[1] Do you feel capable of taking on these new roles? Becoming a leader in research in the HIM field and using epidemiologic principles to enhance that research could help you get there.

Becoming a leader in research[2] should be a goal of every HIM professional because research leads to advanced knowledge and advanced knowledge leads to advancement of issues that directly affect patient care. The research process can be difficult, and it sometimes takes years before results are established and used. Nevertheless, research enables an individual to test an idea and to determine whether an association between two variables exists. Sometimes this idea has been tossed around for years but, because of priorities given to other aspects of the HIM department, has not been studied. It is important that every HIM professional take the time to perform research on topics that are of interest and relevant to the HIM field.

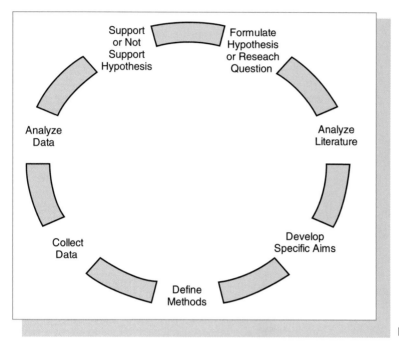

Figure 12-1 Cyclical nature of research.

Healthy People 2010[3] is a prevention agenda for the nation that identifies the most significant preventable issues related to health and focuses public and private sector efforts to address those issues. It is a comprehensive agenda organized into two major goals that are monitored through 467 objectives in 28 focus areas with 10 leading health indicators. Some of the goals, objectives, and leading health indicators most related to HIM are shown in the following example.

Example of *Healthy People 2010:* Goals, Objectives and Health Indicators Related to Health Information Management

Goal 1: Eliminate Health Disparities—One factor in eliminating health disparities includes improving data collection methods used to assess accurately the health status for specific populations, especially small ones. Also, to reduce health disparities empowering individuals to make informed health care decisions is important. One way to reach this goal is through the development and use of the personal health record (PHR) that is on the forefront of the HIM profession and will have a direct impact on public health.

Objective 2: Determinants of Health—This objective examines biology, behaviors, social and physical environment, and policies and interventions. Determinants of health not only includes services received through health care providers but also health information received through other venues in the community. The HIM professional can work toward developing effective tools so that accurate health information is received either through the electronic health record (EHR), the Internet, or other clinical databases or registries. In *Healthy People 2010,* goals focus on preventing illnesses on a population basis. The HIM professional, through work with the EHR, PHR, or with other clinical databases and registries, has a direct impact in the prevention of diseases.

Health Indicator: Access to Health Care—There are many barriers to access, such as financial, structural, or personal barriers. Personal barriers include cultural or spiritual differences, language barriers, not knowing what to do or when to seek care, or concerns about confidentiality or discrimination. The HIM professional should be the primary researcher in the area of privacy and confidentiality of health information. By doing this he or she can work to break down the personal barriers that affect access to health care.

These are national priorities that, when examined through research studies, could make a difference that may affect the world. More specific research goals could also be examined and may include determining the prevalence of specific HIM functions across the country through observation and surveys, determining a national coding accuracy rate, or studying the performance (work) satisfaction levels of HIM employees in different health care settings.

All the areas described are examples of potential research projects. However, choose one that is of extreme interest to you and proceed. The HIM professional is a leader, and as a leader, he or she should strive to advance the profession. Research provides the avenue for that advancement.

DESIGNING THE RESEARCH PROPOSAL

Several steps should be taken when a research or grant proposal is designed that will make the entire process interesting, rewarding, and fulfilling.[4] These steps include the following:

1. Identification of a research hypothesis or question
2. Review of the literature
3. Draft of research methods
4. Development of the research plan or study design
   - Specific aims
   - Significance and preliminary research
   - Experimental design and methods
   - Human subjects (when human subjects are involved the researcher must seek approval of the institutional review board [IRB])
   - Literature cited
5. Development of the research budget
6. Design of the appendix

Hypothesis and Research Questions

A **hypothesis** or **research question** identifies the goal of the research. The hypothesis is an educated guess about the outcome of the study. It poses an assertion to be supported and may predict a relationship between two or more variables; a research question asks a question to be answered. A hypothesis is not an opinion or value judgment. For example, the statement that every American has the right to health care is a value judgment that can be proved neither right nor wrong. Some statements that seem like an opinion on the surface can become a hypothesis with definition of the concepts. The statement "The poor do not have access to health care" can become a testable hypothesis by defining the concept of poor by income level, adequacy by the average in the United States, and health care by the number of physician office visits within a specified period of time. Research questions are used in a new area when not much is known about the topic. Answers to the question will help determine the relationships.[5]

The concepts in the hypothesis are the **variables**, which are either **independent** or **dependent**. The variable that causes change in the other variables is called an independent variable. A variable whose value is dependent on one or more other variables but that cannot itself affect the other variables is called a dependent variable. The hypothesized relationship between the variables of interest determines their category. The dependent variable is the variable we wish to explain, and the independent variable is the factor that we believe may explain it. In a causal relationship, the cause is an independent variable and the effect a dependent variable. For example, because smoking causes lung cancer, smoking is an independent variable and lung cancer a dependent variable.[5]

Suppose a researcher wanted to test whether the medical record would prove to be a useful collection tool for factors suspected of being associated with ovarian cancer. Previous research has found that at least 20 factors may be associated with this disease. However, few studies used the medical record alone to collect data pertaining to these factors. Ovarian cancer is a devastating disease that defies early detection. If a link could be made to one or more specific factors, then preventive measures could be taken by women with the factors to decrease the risk of developing ovarian cancer. This study has the following research question:

Is the medical record a useful tool for collecting data pertaining to factors suspected of being associated with ovarian cancer?

and the following hypothesis:

An association exists between risk factors suspected of being linked with ovarian cancer. The ovarian cancer is the dependent variable and the risk factors are the independent variables.

How do you propose an effective hypothesis or research question? Many times a researcher proposes a hypothesis or research question on the basis of ideas that are generated from reading the literature. Other times a researcher has an idea that is generated from personal experiences and then through the review and analysis of the literature develops an insightful hypothesis or research question. Either way, an extensive review of the literature is needed.

Review of Literature

Once the hypothesis or question is established, the second step of a sound research study design is to conduct an extensive **literature review** (Figure 12-2). A review must be conducted to determine the research that has already been performed in this area. The best way to accomplish this task is to conduct a literature search. Most librarians can conduct a literature search by entering key words and phrases into a computer that then searches through journals, books, and other publications. How far back in time to search must also be specified. A literature search can also be performed independently by searching the Internet or by using other on-line sources such as MEDLINE. Depending on the type, the search will produce a list that includes the title, author's name, and journal title and an abstract, if one is available, summarizing each article.

The key words and phrases that are used can make or break the literature search, so they should be chosen with care. If there is uncertainty about which key words to choose, the wording should be discussed with the reference librarian. For example, the key words chosen for the ovarian cancer study included *epithelial ovarian cancer, risk factors, epidemiology,* and *medical record.* The Internet is also an excellent resource for conducting the literature search; however, care should be taken because some articles that are

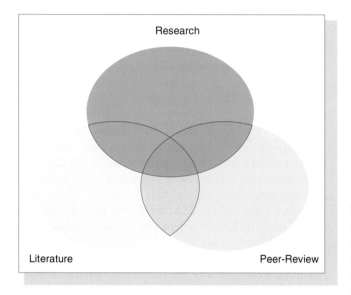

Research

Literature   Peer-Review

Figure 12-2 Relationship between peer-reviewed journal, research articles, and professional literature.

found through the Internet may not be peer reviewed (see below). Even so, the Internet can link you to many peer-reviewed articles through MEDLINE, Ovid, and other excellent on-line searches. Ovid is an international resource of electronic medical, scientific, and academic research information. It supports researchers, students, and others by providing methods on how to search for specific information relevant to a specific research topic.

When the literature search is concluded, it must be carefully examined and any articles of interest should be collected and reviewed. An important step here is to determine whether a particular article is valuable for your research study. For example, the type of journal should be examined. Some journals are **peer reviewed** and others are not. Peer reviewed means that peers within the specific research area have extensively reviewed the article and provided comments and feedback to the authors to incorporate into their revision of the article before publication. Some journals, editorials, government reports, and so forth may not be peer reviewed, and although the information in the report may still be important and useful, it did not go through the extensive review process just described.

A critical review of a research article through a peer-review process normally focuses on the following areas:

1. Content is of value, interest, and importance to the reader
2. Hypothesis or research question is clear and appropriate
3. Review of the literature supports the study
4. Study design chosen is appropriate for the hypothesis/research question
5. The methods are appropriate and support the specific aims

6. Statistical analysis is appropriate for the study design
7. The discussion and conclusions are appropriate on the basis of the results
8. Writing, illustrations, tables, and so forth are clear, well organized, and accurate
9. Replication of the methods described could be performed by the reader
10. Qualitative comments including an overall impression (accept or reject) and any major problems and suggested revisions.

It is also important when collecting information for the literature review to distinguish among the citations, references, and bibliographies that are contained in some research articles. Citations provide information about the source of the written material in the body of the article. The citation, which is usually depicted as a number or author's last name, depending on the style manual used, does not provide much information by itself. You need to go to the reference list or bibliography to get the exact title, author, journal name, and so forth. The reference list is usually at the end of the article and includes only the articles cited within the body of the article. The bibliography is like a list of references; however, it includes additional articles and books not cited in the text but that were reviewed to prepare to write the article and are included for further reading. Therefore, the bibliography may contain many more articles and books than are cited in the article itself.

The purposes of the literature review are:

- To develop a solid foundation in the particular field through study of that topic
- To become an expert through reviewing past literature to determine how one's hypothesis is different from previous research studies
- To determine what it is about one's idea or hypothesis that makes it worth carrying out
- To find gaps or problems with existing studies and begin thinking about how to design a study to fill those gaps

Another important task to incorporate into the literature review is to organize all the articles selected into a table that includes the following:

1. Title of the article and journal, book, or report
2. Author(s)
3. Publisher, date, and so on
4. Summary of the article
5. Advantages of the article specific to study design for your research topic
6. Disadvantages of the article specific to study design

By developing a table such as this, the researcher will be better able to determine the gaps of previous research studies and will then know where to better focus your research study design.

Methodology (Draft)

At this point, the researcher should begin to think about how to design the study so that the hypothesis can be properly tested. The **methodology** can be the most difficult task and, therefore, should be started as soon as possible. The methodology should include a step-by-step process of what is done in the research study and why this process is necessary to test the hypothesis properly. A rough draft of the methodology should be developed to determine whether the study is feasible. It also allows the researcher to realize how much is known about the subject matter and to think about what the research involves.

Research Plan

When a draft of the method has been written and the feasibility of the study confirmed through the literature review, the research plan should be written. It includes the following:

- Specific aims or objectives
- Significance (review of literature or preliminary research)
- Research design and method
- Population under study—sample selection
- Time frame
- Place of study
- Data collection process
- Application to the IRB
- Analysis of the data
- Human subjects (if applicable)
- Literature cited

Specific Aims

The **specific aims** should briefly describe the project's goals or objectives. The goals, objectives, aims, or purposes should be enumerated for better clarification. The list should include both short- and long-term goals. For example, the specific aims in the ovarian cancer study are as follows:

- To determine whether the medical record is a useful tool for collecting data pertaining to risk factors and other health history information (short-term goal)
- To narrow the number of factors suspected of being linked to ovarian cancer by providing evidence that a potential risk factor is found more in the **cases** (women with the disease) than in the controls (women without the disease) (short-term goal)
- To identify groups of women who may be at high risk for development of ovarian cancer and work toward designing and implementing preventive measures to control the disease (long-term goal)
- To benefit future researchers who examine chromosomal markers and ovarian cancer so that they begin to incorporate risk factors in the analysis of their data (long-term goal)

Significance (Review of Literature and Preliminary Research)

This section should detail the importance of the research project by including a review of past research studies on the same subject (literature review) and preliminary research or pilot studies (if any) performed by the researcher. It should state why the research study must be done, how it is different from previous research studies, and who the research will benefit. This section should also demonstrate the researcher's knowledge by including a discussion of existing research that has been performed in the same area and showing the gaps in that research. When these deficiencies are discussed in detail, this part of the plan should reveal how the current research will address these deficiencies.

The key to this section is to be succinct, clear, and organized to convey why the research is important. If the preliminary research is brief, it can be included in the significance section, particularly if it adds to the study's importance. If the preliminary research is extensive, it should be included in a separate section titled "Preliminary Studies" or "Preliminary Research."

An excerpt of the significance section is shown in the example to demonstrate how the preliminary research is used to show the importance of the proposed study.

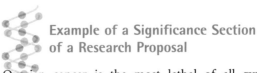

Example of a Significance Section of a Research Proposal

Ovarian cancer is the most lethal of all gynecological cancers. It is an almost-silent disease in a deep-seated organ that defies early detection. In fact, the appearance of vague, nonspecific symptoms (pelvic pain, low back ache, aching legs, bloating, nausea) may already be a manifestation of advanced disease. Epithelial cancers predominate (incidence rate of ovarian cancer is approximately 20,000 cases per year and epithelial ovarian cancer makes up about 65% of that amount), and except for a minority in which torsion or hemorrhage occurs, the majority of patients are asymptomatic. At present, ovarian cancer is responsible for half of the deaths related to female genital malignancy, and although mortality rates for gynecologic cancers are declining, those for ovarian cancer are slowly increasing.[2,3]

A number of risk factors are suspected of being linked to epithelial ovarian cancer. These include nulliparity, infertility, menstrual tension, abnormal breast swelling, marked dysmenorrhea, early menopause (50 years), irradiation of pelvic organs, exposure to talc, high socioeconomic status, smoking, alcohol use, breast cancer, cervical fibroids, endometrial cancer, obesity, oral contraceptive use (inverse relationship), use of fertility drugs, history of colorectal cancer, white ethnicity, age older than 40 years, and family history of ovarian cancer.[4,6-12]

A research study has been performed through a small grant from the School of Health Related Professions'

Research and Development Fund in which risk factors in 20 ovarian cancer cases and in 40 randomly selected age-related controls were evaluated. Interpretation of the data has been limited because 30% of the risk factors were not found in the medical record for the cases or controls. These results may be due to the small sample size and collection of data from only one hospital.

The proposed project will be able to analyze effectively the large number of risk factors suspected of being linked to ovarian cancer by evaluating the disease at an earlier stage and by incorporating an improved method of epidemiologic assessment. By examining the risk factors in incident cases and in age-matched control subjects from the medical record and from telephone interviews, we will be able to pinpoint the risk factors cited immediately after diagnosis and follow-up with a telephone interview to add any risk factors not collected from the medical record. This proposed project would enable us to remedy inadequacies of the past study and, therefore, determine a risk factor truly linked to the development of epithelial ovarian cancer. This identified risk factor will lead to the identification of women at high risk for development of ovarian cancer. Future prospective studies can be designed to follow women with and without the risk factor to determine whether ovarian cancer develops.

(Footnotes/references are not provided because this is an example of the significance section.)

Methodology

The method should include a research design in relation to time, place, and persons. It should consist of the following:

- *Time frame.* This should state exactly when the study will be conducted and why it is necessary to conduct the study for this specific time period.
- *Place of study.* This section should explain where the study will be conducted and whether it will include one facility or multiple facilities and why.
- *Population under study.* This includes which subjects will be in the study, how they will become part of the study, why these specific subjects will be part of the study, whether a representative sample of the population will be used and why, and how sample size will be determined.

The method should also include a step-by-step plan of how the study is to be performed. This is called the "Procedures" and can include the following:

- *Data collection process.* This section should reveal how the data will be collected (by questionnaire, interview, abstracting techniques); what data will be categorized and why; how the data will be categorized and why; who will collect the data; whether training techniques will be needed and, if so, what the training will consist of; where the data will be stored; whether the data will

include patient identifiers and why; and how the data will be accessed. A separate paragraph or statement regarding how the confidentiality of the subjects will be protected should be included.

- *Application to the Institutional Review Board (IRB).* The methodology section should state that the study will be submitted for approval to an IRB. An IRB, or research and human rights committee, is part of most health care facilities and meets at least quarterly. Some boards may meet more often, depending on the number of applications they receive. The aim of any IRB is to protect human subjects or patients from research risks and invasion of privacy. The IRB reviews all research studies that involve subjects or patients, including experiments, interviews, and questionnaires, and any study that collects data from a patient's medical record. The scientific merits of a proposal are considered in the context of assessing the risks and benefits of the proposed research.
- *Analysis of the data.* This section should describe how the data will be analyzed and the types of statistical tests that will be performed (e.g., frequency distribution, chi-square, confidence intervals, and assessment of validity and reliability, to be addressed later in this chapter). The researcher must be sure to describe why this type of statistical analysis will be used.

An excerpt from an actual methodology section is described in the example.

Example of a Methodology Section of a Research Proposal

Objective/Time Frame: The current research will evaluate the relationship between epithelial ovarian cancer and characteristics suspected of being linked to the disease in a population of individuals newly diagnosed with epithelial ovarian cancer over a 1-year period.

Place of Study: New or **incident cases** of a particular disease will be ascertained from several hospital-based cancer registries. Incident cases will be used because the medical record provides a more complete past history of medical information when a patient is newly diagnosed with a condition. Also, if the patients are well enough and willing, telephone interviews will be performed. Telephone interviews can be performed with family members, physicians, and so on, if the patient is unable to provide information.

Population Under Study: The controls will be randomly selected from a population of women undergoing surgery or hospitalization for reasons unrelated to cancer. Each control will be matched with the case on age (within 5 years), admission date (within 1 week), and hospital. The number of cases with epithelial ovarian cancer will be 150. The number of controls will be 300.

Procedures—Data Collection Process: The 150 cancer cases will be categorized by stage, histologic grade, metastases, demographic data, and risk factors as listed in the significance section. The 300 controls will be categorized by risk factors and demographic data.

Application to Institutional Review Board: The hospitals will be notified and the study will be explained and submitted for approval by their IRBs. Consent to participate in the study will be obtained from the cases and controls by mail 1 week after discharge.

Data Collection Process: The hospital will notify the research team whenever a patient with ovarian cancer is admitted. The research team will match the case with the control and after discharge will abstract data from the medical record using a pretested data collection instrument (see the sample questionnaire in Figure 12-3). The abstractors will be trained so that each one is certain about where to find specific information in the record when a risk factor or characteristic is not applicable, not documented, or not present in the case or control.

Once the data are collected, a telephone interview will be performed using the pretested data collection instrument to collect any data not found in the medical record and to assess the validity of the data in the medical record.

Analysis of the Data: The data will be entered into a personal computer, and statistical analysis will include frequency distribution, chi-square, and odds ratios. Because the examination of risk factors from medical records may vary from one abstractor to another, various members of the research team will repeat the abstracting of another member,

levels of agreement will be determined, and a kappa (κ) statistic will be computed.

Human Subjects

The human subjects section is necessary only if human subjects are used in the research or if there are any risks to a human subject. The following should be included in this section:

- Demographic description of the subject population, including age, percentage of males and females, race
- How informed consent will be obtained
- If necessary, how confidentiality (risk of privacy) will be safeguarded
- Potential risks and benefits of the study to the people enrolled
- Any letters validating IRB approval should be placed in this section to show that the facility where the research will be conducted has approved the study methodology.

Literature Referenced

All literature discussed or reviewed in any section of the research proposal should be numbered or cited in that section and a full reference listed at the end of the proposal. Different formats for references are used depending on the preference of the funding agency. Use the format that the funding agency specifies. The general format for a journal

Sample of Ovarian Cancer Questionnaire (Abstracted from 119 Total Elements)

1. Do you know of any blood relatives in your family who have or have had any type of cancer?

_____ Yes   _____ No   _____ ND*

If yes, what relation?

_____ Mother   _____ Sister
_____ Father   _____ Brother
_____ Aunt   _____ Grandfather
_____ Uncle   _____ Grandmother
_____ Niece   _____ Nephew

Other _____

_____ ND*   _____ NA*

If yes,   _____ Lung   _____ Liver   _____ Lymphomas
what type: _____ Brain   _____ Breast   _____ Colon
                 _____ Skin   _____ Pancreas   _____ Blood-related (leukemia)
                 _____ Other: _____
                 _____ ND*   _____ NA*

2. Do you smoke cigarettes? _____ Yes   _____ No   _____ ND*

If yes, how many cigarettes do you smoke each day?

_____ 1/2 pack or less   _____ 1 pack
_____ 1 to 2 packs   _____ More than 2 packs
_____ ND*   _____ NA*

*ND = Not documented

*NA = Not applicable

Figure 12-3 Excerpt of ovarian cancer questionnaire.

reference includes the author(s), year of publication in parentheses, title, name of journal, volume, and page numbers. For a book, it generally includes the author(s), year of publication in parentheses, title, and place and name of publishing company.

Budget Development

A detailed budget is necessary to determine the actual costs of the research project and is required for most funding agencies. The budget can include the following:

- Salary and fringe benefits for personnel
- Equipment
- Supplies
- Travel
- Patient care costs—if applicable to the research problem
- Contractual costs such as including another agency or organization to assist with the study
- Consulting costs
- Telephone or fax costs
- Internet access
- Paper
- Computer usage
- Equipment maintenance

Justification is essential in the budget and should include the specific functions of the personnel, consultants, and collaborators. At times, incentives to study subjects may be necessary to encourage them to participate in the research study. If that is done, the amount of dollars or the specific health care benefit should be listed in the budget as well.

An outline of the budget for the ovarian cancer study if it were carried out today is shown in the example.

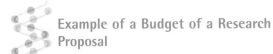

Example of a Budget of a Research Proposal

Secretarial Salary   **Total: $1056.00**
Duties include typing study protocol for review by IRB at hospitals and universities, copying the study protocol, preparing envelopes for mailing, typing preliminary and final results of study.

80 hours × $10.00/hour = $800.00
Fringe benefits: $0.32 × $800.00 = $256.00

Research Assistant Salary   **Total: $5220.00**
Abstractors (Each abstractor will review 450 records to determine agreement levels. Total of three abstractors will be used.)

450 records × 0.30 hours/record × 3 = 405.00 hours
    × $8.00/hour = $3240.00

Abstractor for data entry

450 records × 0.25 hours/record = 112.50
    hours × $8.00/hour = $900.00

Telephone interviews

450 interviews × 0.30 hours/interview = 135
    hours × $8.00/hour = $1080.00

Travel to Hospitals   **Total: $2141.40**
To decrease the amount of travel, visits can be made to hospitals at the end of the month because more cases will be available. Because 78 cases were available from three hospitals, six hospitals can be used with 33 visits.

33 visits × 3 abstractors × 20 miles × $0.33
    per mile = $653.40
Parking = 33 × 3 = 99 × $10.00 = $990.00

Travel will also include visits by principal investigator to each of the hospitals initially and throughout the study.

5 visits × 6 hospitals = 30 visits × 20 miles
    × $0.33/mile = $198.00
Parking = 30 × $10.00 = $300.00

Supplies   **Total: $2100.00**
Photocopying, postage, disks, paper, fax, telephone costs
Total Budget   **$10,517.40**
There will be no costs or payments made to or from the subjects.

Appendix Design

The appendix can comprise tables, figures, laboratory tests, data collection forms, and letters of support. It can include anything that is important and relative to the research study or that better clarifies a topic described in the study but that may be too voluminous to include in the body of the proposal. Information such as research articles reviewed or a sample of a database from a preliminary study is not pertinent to the research project and should be excluded. For the ovarian cancer study, the data collection instrument was included in the appendix section of the grant application.

Additional Considerations

Most research proposal guidelines have page-length limitations for each of the sections just discussed. It is important to adhere to any page limitations or any other instructions because failure to do this may make the research application ineligible for review by the funding agency.

VALIDITY AND RELIABILITY

Validity

Validity assesses relevance, completeness, accuracy, and correctness. It measures how well a data collection instrument, laboratory test, medical record abstract, or other data source measures what it should measure. Validity can assess, for example, whether a thermometer truly measures temperature or whether an IQ test really measures intelligence.

It is crucial that the HIM professional be aware of validity problems in specific types of studies. The data collection instrument and the method of data collection have a great impact on the validity of data. To determine whether the validity of a research study is upheld, specific methods should be used. One such method includes gaining confirmatory information from different sources to determine whether the information collected for the study is correct. For example, information recorded in the medical record regarding the patient's method of payment or insurance carrier can be validated by further examining financial records, physicians' office records, and pharmacy records. Brief interviews with family members can further confirm or validate the accuracy of correctness of the insurance type.

Sensitivity and Specificity

Validity also refers to correct measurement or correct labeling. Assessments of methods used to test whether a person has a disease are considered tests of validity regarding the correctness of measurement or labeling. Two measures of this are **sensitivity** and **specificity**. To use sensitivity and specificity, one must know the following definitions:

- True positives (TP) correctly categorize true cases as cases—valid labeling.
- False negatives (FN) incorrectly label true cases as noncases—not valid.
- True negatives (TN) correctly label noncases as noncases—valid.
- False positives (FP) incorrectly label noncases as cases—not valid.

Sensitivity is the percentage of all true cases correctly identified—TP/(TP + FN) or TP/Total positives (or total cases).

Specificity is the percentage of all true noncases correctly identified—TN/(TN + FP) or TN/Total negatives (or total noncases).[6,7]

Analysis and Discussion

Table 12-1 shows the accuracy of a specific blood test in detecting prostate cancer. The specificity rate of 91% suggests that this blood test correctly labels noncases as noncases 91% of the time and misses the noncases 9% of the time. The sensitivity rate of only 83% suggests that the blood test misses 17% of the true cases, or patients with prostate cancer. This blood test could pose serious health problems when true cases may be missed, and therefore diagnosis and treatment may be delayed or missed. Each researcher must determine when the sensitivity and specificity levels are accurate enough to use the test.

Coding validity is a major area of research in the field of HIM. However, there is a paucity of literature in the area

Table 12-1 SENSITIVITY AND SPECIFICITY: ACCURACY OF BLOOD TEST TO DETECT PROSTATE CANCER

Test	Prostate Cancer	No Prostate Cancer
+	TP (100)	FP (20)
–	FN (20)	TN (200)
Totals	TP + FN (120)	FP + TN (220)

Sensitivity = TP/TP + FN = 100/100 + 20 = 100/120 = 83.3%
Specificity = TN/TN + FP = 200/200 + 20 = 200/220 = 90.9%

of coding accuracy or validity of HIM professionals. Often it is difficult to assess the validity of a principal diagnosis, ICD-9-CM (*International Classification of Diseases*, Ninth Revision, *Clinical Modification*) code, or diagnosis related group (DRG) because the basis of the categorization may be subjective. However, the accuracy or validity of coding can be established when a "gold standard" is determined. The gold standard is used as the correct code when conducting research studies. However, one must be aware of the limitations in using such a standard and must strive to lessen the error. The correct diagnosis, code, or DRG can be determined on the basis of coding standards and agreement by expert coders. For example, the validity of coding quality can be determined by having the coding supervisor recode a random sample of records of patients with a principal diagnostic code of coronary artery disease (CAD) (Figure 12-4). Two coders—coder A and coder B—did the coding. The recoding performed by the coding supervisor can be considered the gold standard. The validity (sensitivity and specificity) could then be recorded as shown in Figure 12-4. Coder B's coding is more accurate than coder A's in accurately coding true cases of CAD (100% versus 60%) and in accurately coding noncases as noncases (80% vs 73%).

Specific factors cause incorrect or inaccurate labeling. In the coding example, these factors can include inexperience and lack of knowledge regarding the disease (CAD), ICD-9-CM coding principles, and proper review and analysis of the medical record. Other factors may be related to the equipment, such as outdated coding books. Also, it is obvious that validity is influenced by the gold standard that is selected. When results of such studies are assessed, it is important to consider the subjectivity of the standard.

Reliability

Reliability refers to consistency between users of a given instrument or method. In many research studies, more than one research assistant collects the data. For example, in the ovarian cancer study, an abstract was used to collect the information from the medical records for both cases and controls. Because different research assistants were used to abstract the medical records to collect the data, the classification of the results might differ from one assistant to another. Reproducibility or **reliability** between more than

CODING SUPERVISOR/VALIDATOR		
Coding Status	True Case CAD	True Noncase No CAD
Coder A		
CAD (+)	9 (TP)	4 (FP)
No CAD (-)	6 (FN)	11 (TN)
Totals	15	15
Coder B		
CAD (+)	15 (TP)	3 (FP)
No CAD (-)	0 (FN)	12 (TN)
Totals	15	15

	Coder A	Coder B
Sensitivity = True positives (TP)/ All true cases (Total)	9/15 = 60%	15/15 = 100%
Specificity = True negatives (TN) / All non cases (Total)	11/15 = 73%	12/15 = 80%

Figure 12-4   Recoding of a random sample of patent records with a principal diagnostic code of coronary artery disease (CAD).

one research assistant or observer is called **interobserver reliability**. However, even one individual observer's response may vary over time. Reliability within one research assistant or observer is called **intraobserver reliability**.

To test for the reliability of risk factors that were collected from the medical record between research assistants in the ovarian cancer study (described in more detail later in the chapter), each medical record was abstracted three times to determine levels of agreement. Levels of agreement ranged from 71% to 100% for all the characteristics or risk factors collected for the study. A κ statistic was also calculated. This statistic enables the researcher to determine whether the agreement levels that are seen are real or to the result of chance. A statistic can range from 0.00 to 1.00. After deliberation with our statistician and review of the literature, a statistic of 0.60 was chosen as the standard level for this study; therefore, anything below 0.60 was determined not to be real and caused by chance or sampling variability. Therefore, the usefulness of the agreement levels for those risk factors could be limited.

Another method of testing interobserver reliability when interviewing is to use different research assistants on the first and second interviews of the same subject. One can then measure consistency of recall and variations of response to different research assistants. To measure intraobserver reliability, the same research assistant can be used at different times while measuring consistency of the subject's response.

Sometimes reliability is measured and reported in the form of a **correlation coefficient** *(r)* rather than a proportion or percentage. A correlation coefficient is a statistic that shows the strength of a relationship between two variables. A correlation coefficient, when used to measure degrees of reliability, can range from −1 to +1. The closer *r* approaches −1 or +1, the stronger the reliability or the relationship between two variables. The closer r approaches zero, the weaker the relationship or reliability.[8] For example, if an HIM professional was interested in the correlation between the number of health care providers attending medical record documentation seminars and the number of complete medical records received in the HIM department on discharge of the patient 1 week after the seminar was conducted, a correlation coefficient can be used. A high positive score, such as 0.91, means that as the number of health care providers attending the seminar increased, the number of completed medical records at discharge increased. A high negative score, such as −0.91, means that as the number of health care providers attending the seminar increased, the number of completed medical records decreased.

BIASES

No research study is perfect. No matter how well designed a research study is, there is always some type of error or **bias**. Therefore, it is imperative that researchers be aware of the types of bias that can occur and the methods used to decrease the amount of bias. The following are examples of common types of error or bias.[9]

Confounding Variables

If other characteristics such as age or sex are known to be associated with both the independent (risk factor or exposure characteristic) and the dependent (disease) variables, these confounding **variables** should be controlled so that they are not the reason an association is seen. Methods to control for age, for example, include matching (discussed later in this chapter) cases and controls on age or performing age adjustment when analyzing the data.

Sampling Variability

The results of a study may be false because of improper sample size and selection. It is important to obtain an effective sample so that the results of the research study can be generalized to the population under study. Sometimes this is difficult but very necessary because, when the sample is large enough, random, and truly represents the population under study, the results can be generalized or extrapolated to the entire population under study. This is discussed in more detail in Chapter 11.

Ascertainment or Selection Bias

When selecting subjects, researchers are more likely to choose people who are frequently under medical care. If a disease or condition is asymptomatic or mild, it may escape routine medical attention and may have an impact on the condition under study.

In addition, volunteers and paid subjects may be very different from the general population. Volunteers may volunteer to be in a study because they are very healthy or because they have a special interest in the study.

Diagnosis Bias

Certain diseases are not easy to diagnose, and different health professionals may offer different opinions. For example, when the stage and grade of certain types of cancers are determined, a standard review of slides by one or more pathologists who are unaware of the specimens' origin can be used. This method may provide more clarity in assessing an accurate diagnosis, which can be extremely important when obtaining cases and controls for a study.

Nonresponse Bias

Subjects who refuse to participate in a study may be different from the subjects who do participate. The solution is to collect basic demographic characteristics on participants and nonparticipants to see whether the characteristics are similar. In this way, the researcher can determine whether the study participants represent the general population and are not different in relation to health or risk characteristics.

Survival Bias

Survival bias occurs with cross-sectional studies because only those who have lived long enough to be in the study are examined. The solution is to use incident or new cases to relieve this bias.

Recall Bias

Recall bias can be attributed to faulty memory or to subjects who tend to remember certain types of information because of the exposure or disease. Before the study begins, list possible biases and ways to reduce them. For example, mothers of children with anomalies or complications tend to remember more about their deliveries than do mothers of healthy children. Mothers of children with anomalies are the cases, whereas controls can be mothers of children with a different type of anomaly or adverse pregnancy outcome. Mothers with healthy children could be yet another comparison group. In this way, recall bias should be reduced because cases and controls would be similar in recalling specific events relevant to their children because both groups would have children with anomalies.

Interviewer Bias

Interviewers tend to ask questions differently or may probe more if they know which subjects have the characteristic of interest. To reduce interviewer bias, the solution is to standardize the interview form and to provide intensive training for the interviewers, stressing that they must be consistent when performing the interview.

Prevarication Bias

Prevarication bias occurs when an individual tends to exaggerate a response in an interview or questionnaire. A worker who receives disability compensation might exaggerate his or her exposure. The solution is to use several independent raters and several sources of data to validate the information collected.

EPIDEMIOLOGIC/RESEARCH STUDY DESIGNS

An important step in designing a research study is to choose the most appropriate study design to test the hypothesis. The HIM professional can appropriately choose the study design to use if he or she is aware of the many designs that exist. Because epidemiology is so closely related to the HIM field, the study designs described in this chapter include epidemiologic research study designs. Epidemiology is the study of the distribution and determinants of disease or events in populations. The results of the study are used to prevent and control public health problems. The most common types of study designs are described in detail here and summarized in Table 12-2. Examples of each design are provided, and common statistics that are generated from these studies are described.

Descriptive Study

The descriptive epidemiologic study describes the frequency and distribution of diseases in populations. It is usually the first study design chosen when little is known about the disease or health characteristics. Qualitative studies or exploratory studies also describe or explore a new area of study and will also be explained later in this section. First, let us look at a cross-sectional design.

Cross-Sectional or Prevalence Study

The **cross-sectional** or **prevalence study** is one type of descriptive study; it concurrently describes characteristics and health outcomes at one specific point or period in time. The cross-sectional or prevalence study cannot answer questions regarding cause and effect or whether the health characteristic came before the disease. This study design is used to *generate* hypotheses, not to test them. For example, a health care facility may be interested in examining the prevalence of community-acquired pneumonia in elderly people. Pneumonia is debilitating and increases the cost and length of stay when pneumonia develops in an elderly person who is hospitalized for another condition. The cross-sectional or prevalence study can be used to determine the prevalence of pneumonia in the region within the elderly population. To do this, the condition under study (i.e., pneumonia) needs to be defined.

Specific criteria related to the type of pneumonia are needed along with any other criteria necessary to define the condition further. Positive results of culture and sensitivity and chest x-ray studies and clinical symptoms such as fever and malaise can be used as criteria to define pneumonia. This can be further validated by the DRG and ICD-9-CM codes for pneumonia and a review of the medical record by an infectious disease physician or epidemiologist. Further clarification of the pneumonia should specify that it is community acquired and not **nosocomial** (developing 72 hours after hospitalization).

Then the **prevalence rate** is determined as shown in the following example.

Table 12-2 TYPES OF EPIDEMIOLOGIC RESEARCH STUDY DESIGNS

Study Design	Description
Descriptive studies—cross-sectional or prevalence study	Examine the distribution of disease or health characteristics in populations at one point in time. Used to generate hypotheses.
Analytic studies Case-control or retrospective Cohort or prospectives Historical—prospective	Examine a disease to determine whether certain health characteristics are causing the disease.
Experimental studies Clinical trials Community trials	Modify the health characteristics that are found to cause the disease by using health care interventions that control progression of the disease or prevent the disease from occurring.

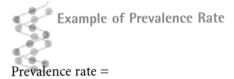

Example of Prevalence Rate

Prevalence rate =

$$\frac{\text{Number of people aged 65 years or older with community-acquired pneumonia in a in a specific region during 200X}}{\text{Number of people aged 65 years or older in a specific region during 200X}} \times 1000$$

Once the prevalence rates are determined, they can be compared across certain groups. For example, further defined prevalence rates for pneumonia may be calculated for people younger than 65 years and a comparison of the two groups can be made. One cannot determine from this study design that being elderly (age 65 years or older) causes an increase in pneumonia incidence. However, one can make statements of associations; that is, older age has a greater association with the development of community-acquired pneumonia. One can then develop a hypothesis such as that community-acquired pneumonia is more prevalent in individuals aged 65 years and older than in those younger than 65 years and conduct further studies to determine whether the hypothesis is true or false.

Prevalence rates can facilitate **case finding,** assist health care administrators in planning for diversified health care facilities and special care units, aid health planners in developing appropriate health programs, and assist HIM professionals in further describing morbidity rates within the health care facility. Case finding includes targeting individual cases that have a particular disease or exposure so that health care services can be provided for them.

Prevalence rates can be categorized into two types: **point prevalence rates** and **period prevalence rates.** Point prevalence refers to evaluating a health condition at a specific point in time. Therefore, each study participant is assessed only *once at one point* in time, although the actual point prevalence study may take months or years to conduct. Period prevalence refers to evaluating a health condition over a *period of time,* such as 1 year. Study participants are counted for period prevalence even if they die, migrate, or have a recurrence of the disease during the period.[6] Figure 12-5 demonstrates the difference between point and period prevalence when examining specific cases within a study.

Advantages and Disadvantages. Table 12-3 indicates the advantages and disadvantages of the cross-sectional or prevalence study design. It is a useful study design when time and resources are limited. Using the cross-sectional design is appropriate when little is known about the health characteristics or disease under study. This study can provide new or beginning information on a multitude of conditions with modest effort and time. Analysis of this new information will stimulate the researcher to develop hypotheses that would motivate further testing and the use of more extensive study designs. Because the cross-sectional

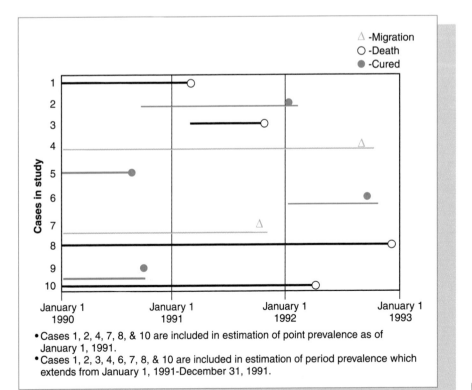

- Cases 1, 2, 4, 7, 8, & 10 are included in estimation of point prevalence as of January 1, 1991.
- Cases 1, 2, 3, 4, 6, 7, 8, & 10 are included in estimation of period prevalence which extends from January 1, 1991-December 31, 1991.

Figure 12-5 Chronology of cases in a community to measure prevalence.

Table 12-3 ADVANTAGES AND DISADVANTAGES OF CROSS-SECTIONAL OR PREVALENCE STUDY DESIGN

Advantages	Disadvantages
Takes less time than other studies before results are seen	Describes only what exists at the time of the prevalence study; does not answer whether the health characteristic or the disease came first
Inexpensive	Examines only survivors and those alive to be found as cases.
Helpful in case finding, program planning, planning of health care facilities or special units, and sample size determination	Not good for rare conditions or diseases
Stimulates new ideas or hypotheses	Given a health characteristic, fails to identify future likelihood of developing the disease

or prevalence study may be considered a descriptive study, its intent is not to show cause-and-effect relations between, for example, a characteristic such as alcohol intake and a disease such as breast cancer. Analytic and experimental study designs, which are discussed later in this chapter, can assess the cause-and-effect relation. Unlike the analytic and experimental study designs, the cross-sectional design cannot assess the risk or likelihood for development of a disease. Other limitations of the cross-sectional design include dealing only with survivors, not being effective in studying rare conditions because a large sample is necessary to obtain cases, or missing an epidemic because it may occur and end within a short period.[6]

By becoming familiar with the cross-sectional or prevalence study design, the HIM professional can better assess how prevalence rates are determined, determine whether this study design is the most appropriate one to use, and evaluate whether cross-sectional studies performed within the health care facility have formed appropriate conclusions (i.e., not cause-and-effect relations).

Survey Research

Other types of descriptive study designs include the **survey design**. Here, the research focuses on collecting data with a survey instrument such as a questionnaire or interview guide. When surveys are constructed, there are certain elements to pay particular attention to. These elements include the following:

- Framing of questions—Include questions that collect data to answer the research question or address the study's specific aims.
- Wording—When constructing the survey instrument, think about your audience or recipients and write so that it is clear to them. Also, work with an expert in survey design, who can help formulate effective questions that are clear and appropriate for the particular audience.
- Cover letter—The cover letter that will accompany the survey is very important. It should briefly describe the study, identify

the research sponsor and the researcher's qualifications, ask for the recipient's participation, stress that responses will be kept confidential, list the date when the survey should be returned, and state that a copy of the results will be provided once the study is completed. Incentives related to completion of the survey can also be included to increase the response rate. (See example of cover letter on the following page.)

- Mail, fax, e-mail, Web—Choose the medium to present the survey. With the wide distribution of the Internet and its related technologies, on-line questionnaires have become a rational carrier of survey investigation compared with traditional methods such as mail, fax, or phone surveys.[10] The commonly cited advantages include easy access, instant distribution, and reduced costs. In addition, the Internet allows questionnaires and surveys to reach a nationwide or even worldwide population with minimum cost and time. Other reported benefits include the graphical and interactive design on the Web. The automated storage of data from the Web server into the database at the backend, after the responder submits the form, can save the time of tedious data entry and create less data entry errors. Also, it can prevent the responder from sending inappropriate data by using certain programming restrictions. Additional features that may help the respondents complete the survey include the help button, as in the following example. In the study by Schleyer and Forrest,[10] the authors state that the Web-based survey will be more economical than the mail survey when the sample size is more than 275. Recognize the bias in using the Internet—those without access are eliminated from participating.
- Length—Most surveys should be limited to a maximum length of two to three pages so that they will most likely be answered. In the EHR study described below, the Web-based survey totaled 13 pages and, although the authors thought this would still work because it was Web based, it was too long for effective response and data collection.
- Question ordering—It is important to think about the order of specific questions. Normally, the demographic

questions are listed first, then the more content related questions, and then the open-ended questions.

- Open versus closed questions—**Open-ended** or unstructured format questions are those that ask a question and do not provide a list of responses to choose from, similar to an essay question. It enables the recipient to write out his or her thoughts in free form. **Close-ended** or structured format questions are those that ask a question and do provide a list of responses to choose from, similar to multiple-choice questions, dichotomous or yes/no questions, or questions based on level or measurement or ranking. In the EHR study both closed-ended and open-ended questions were used. We decided to add the open-ended or unstructured questions so that richer data could be obtained.
- Pilot testing—Every survey should be pilot tested with a small sample of the potential recipients. The recipients should go through the survey as if they are going to answer the questions and provide feedback on any changes or additions to the survey. Once the feedback is received by the research team, the survey should be changed to meet the feedback received, where applicable.
- Sample size (one can choose to use the following available lists)
  - Faculty/student lists
  - Insurance lists
  - Clinic/hospital list
  - Organization list
  - Society list

Once it is decided who will be surveyed, it is easy to choose a systematic sample from an existing list. For example, once the sample size of 100 is decided and your recipients are members of AHIMA who joined in the past year, a list of the recipients can be obtained and then a systematic random sample can be taken from this list.

- **Response rate**—Researchers always strive for a very high response rate. Wyatt states that to have valid results from survey studies a response rate of at least 80% should be obtained.[11] However, this can be quite difficult to obtain and extensive follow-up techniques are needed. After 2 weeks, if the facility/respondent does not respond, a follow-up e-mail and or phone call should be made to the facility asking them to complete the survey, reiterating the importance of the study and its results, and asking if they have any questions regarding the survey. Also, including different types of survey medium and follow-up e-mails or phone calls are essential in obtaining a high response rate.
- Low response—Do not be that alarmed if the intended response rate is not reached. If it is found that the recipients who did respond are similar in demographics to all the intended recipients, then this allows the researcher to state that the responses received, although lower than expected, are similar to what can be expected from the entire sample. Because the list of intended recipients is available, the demographic information can be obtained from the list provided and compared with the recipients who did respond.

- Coding survey and data entry—Once all data are received from the survey, they should be coded and then entered into an appropriate statistical software package for analysis. If a Web-based survey is used, then the coding and data entry does not have to be performed because this is completed when the survey is designed. Data entry is automatic because, as the recipient responds, the data are automatically downloaded to a database management system for data quality checks and statistical analysis. See Figure 12-6, which outlines how the survey is built on the Web and sent to the respondent through the Internet, where it can be automatically reviewed by the researcher as it is being stored on the database server.

Provided below is an example of a descriptive/prevalence study with a Web-based survey focus. The purpose of the study was to measure the awareness of individuals of the American Society for Testing and Materials (ASTM) standards for content and structure of the EHR.[12] The examples include the cover letter and part of the Web-based survey (Figure 12-7) used to collect data.

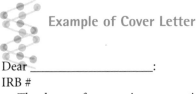 **Example of Cover Letter**

Dear _____:
IRB #

Thank you for agreeing to participate in the research study entitled "Standards for the Content of Electronic Health Records" sponsored by the American Health Information Management Association (AHIMA).

As we described to you previously, your participation in this study is extremely important because your responses could lead to the uniform data standards for the electronic health record (EHR), which HIPAA is recommending.

As we described to you previously, the focus of this research is the American Society for Testing and Materials (ASTM) E1384 Standard Guide on Content and Structure of Electronic Health Records and the corresponding ASTM E1633 Coded Values for Electronic Health Records. We are investigating the level of awareness and measuring the extent of usage of the standards for the content of the EHR. We are also attempting to collect feedback on how the standards for EHR content meet users' needs.

Your prompt participation is extremely important and will aid in the next revision of the standards. For your efforts in completing the survey, we are offering an opportunity for your name to be entered into a drawing to win $200.00! There will be two $200.00 prizes awarded from the pool of people completing the survey!

In addition, you will receive the overall results of the study and a complimentary copy of the most recent edition of the *Journal of the American Health Information Management Association (JAHIMA)* or, if you already receive that journal, another comparable AHIMA journal of your choice.

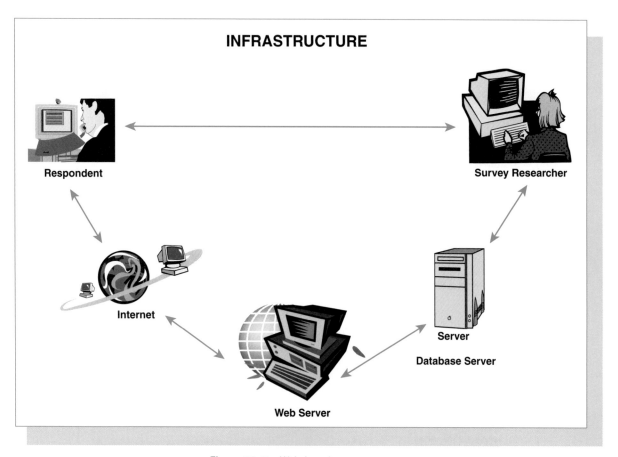

Figure 12-6 Web-based survey process.

Your responses will be kept completely confidential and will only be reported in aggregate form. Completion of the survey will take approximately 20 minutes. Please click here to access the survey.

Once you access the Web site, please follow the directions included in the survey. Please provide your responses to us not later than _____ to be eligible for the drawing.

Your responses will be kept completely confidential.

If you have any questions or concerns regarding completion of the survey, please contact Valerie Watzlaf or Patti Firouzan at _____.

Thank you very much.

Sincerely,

Valerie J. M. Watzlaf
Patti Firouzan

Qualitative Research

Qualitative research is another type of descriptive study design that is used when little is known about a specific topic. It is quite effective and popular in HIM research because much of what is studied within the HIM context

has not been examined before. Qualitative research designs provide a foundation for larger quantitative studies. It also provides richer information than can be obtained from quantitative-based studies alone. It is most appropriate to use in examining attitudes, feelings, perceptions, or relationships, but it can also be used to obtain more extensive information than what can be collected with quantitative methods. For example, in the obesity and breast cancer recurrence study by Katoh et al,[13] quantitative methods were used to collect the data. So, when data were examined in relation to survival, for example, the length of survival was collected but not the quality of life. This is one variable that could have been collected through a qualitative design by asking the study participants about their quality of life through focus groups or interviews. Sometimes, a mixed-methodology design can be used in which quantitative methods and qualitative methods are used together to collect the data.

There are three main types of qualitative research: **participant observation, focus groups,** and **case studies.**

The first, participant observation, is where the researcher is immersed into the subject's environment to learn what the subject experiences first hand. The researcher pays special attention to the physical, social, and human environment as well as formal and informal interactions and unplanned activities. The researcher can choose to be disguised or

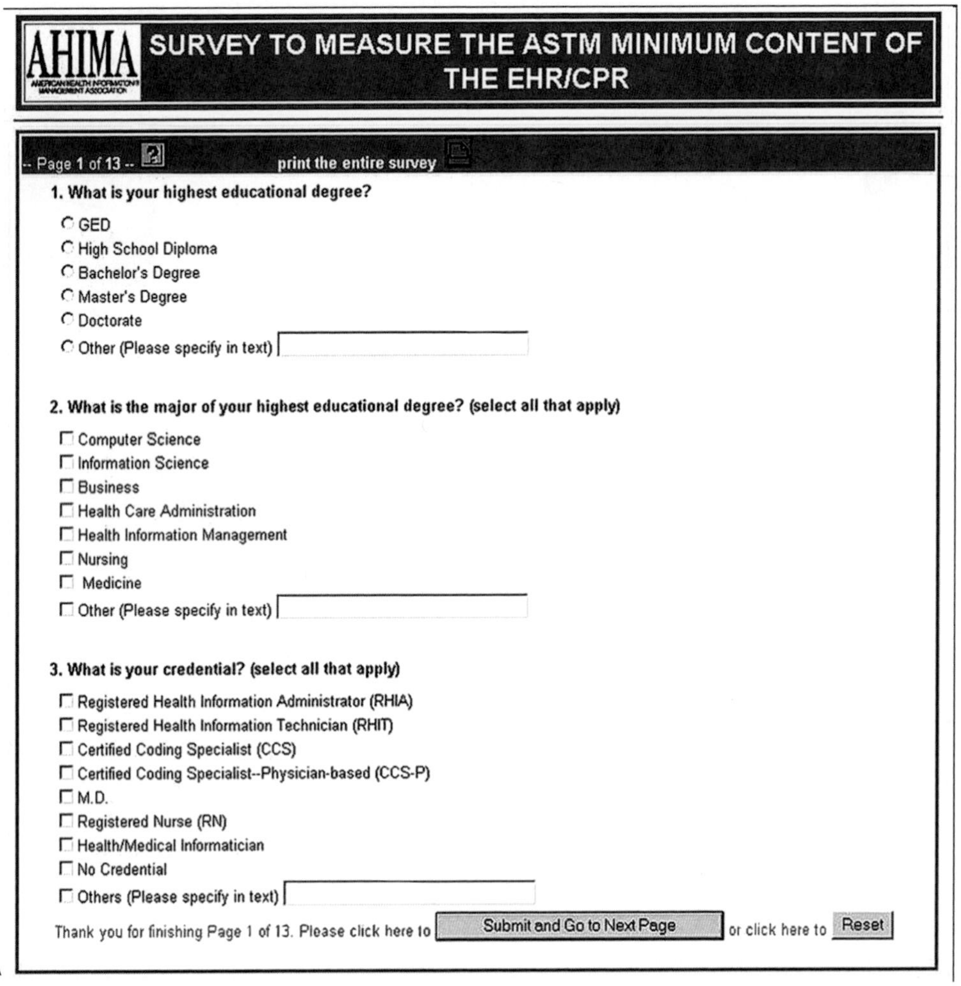
AHIMA SURVEY TO MEASURE THE ASTM MINIMUM CONTENT OF THE EHR/CPR

-- Page 1 of 13 -- print the entire survey

1. What is your highest educational degree?

- GED
- High School Diploma
- Bachelor's Degree
- Master's Degree
- Doctorate
- Other (Please specify in text)

2. What is the major of your highest educational degree? (select all that apply)

- Computer Science
- Information Science
- Business
- Health Care Administration
- Health Information Management
- Nursing
- Medicine
- Other (Please specify in text)

3. What is your credential? (select all that apply)

- Registered Health Information Administrator (RHIA)
- Registered Health Information Technician (RHIT)
- Certified Coding Specialist (CCS)
- Certified Coding Specialist--Physician-based (CCS-P)
- M.D.
- Registered Nurse (RN)
- Health/Medical Informatician
- No Credential
- Others (Please specify in text)

Thank you for finishing Page 1 of 13. Please click here to Submit and Go to Next Page or click here to Reset

A

Figure 12-7 A-C, Sample on-line survey. (Used with permission from the American Health Information Management Association.)

undisguised and is basically there to describe a problem to outsiders on the basis of the understanding of the insider's perspective.[5] For example, participant observation in HIM may include observing employees' perceptions and interactions after an EHR system is implemented in their health care facility. The researchers should focus their observations on activities surrounding the use of the EHR and how well the activities are carried out when using the EHR; who is in command or control of using the EHR for HIM functions, the channels of communication when the EHR is in use, and how effective the communication is. The participant observation experience should help to address the why's and how's of the research questions.

Focus groups or focus group interviews include a small group of people (usually experts in the field or people whose opinion on the topic is being sought—for example, a study in Nebraska of the uninsured and underinsured involved focus groups of those individuals who fit the category—and what living without insurance was like) that are brought together to answer and discuss specific questions. Here the study participants can discuss issues, hear one another's viewpoint, and comment on those views. It enables the researcher to learn more about the topic because a group of experts is brainstorming. It also provides the researcher with the ability to examine interactions among members of the group. There is usually a moderator and a recorder, and sometimes the focus group is videotaped. Also, more than one focus group can frame a particular study. For example, in a study examining the effectiveness and efficiency of public health reporting with ICD-10-CM and ICD-10-PCS, a group of experts in ICD-10 and public health would be solicited to form a focus group to answer questions related to information accumulated from the first three study parts and to make recommendations on where changes need to be made. Some questions may include the following:

1. After review of the public health diagnoses and procedures reportable list, are there any diagnoses or procedures that you believe should be added, deleted, or changed? If so, please explain.
2. Based on the information provided to you, what recommendations do you have to improve the ICD-

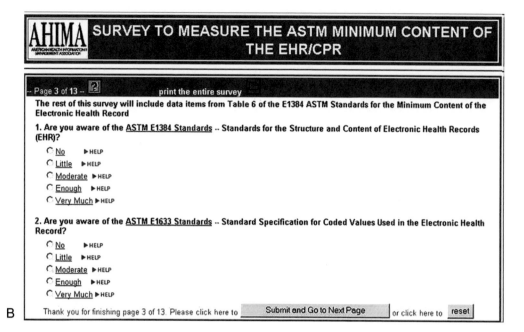

Figure 12-7, cont'd A-C, Sample on-line survey. (Used with permission from the American Health Information Management Association.)

Continued

10-CM and ICD-10-PCS coding systems for public health reporting?

Notice how the questions are framed to elicit discussion. The focus group interview is flexible and is usually of low cost because in just one setting data from six to twelve individuals can be gathered. The focus group data can be difficult to analyze and control and can sometimes be difficult, however, a good moderator can diminish the negative effects.

Case studies seek to provide a richly detailed portrait of an individual, program, event, department, time period, culture, or community.[5] For example, case studies can be conducted on health care facilities by use of report cards on their clinicians to determine their effects on the quality of patient care and outcomes. Extensive interviews can be carried out with physicians and other health care providers, patients, administrators, and other staff to determine their perceptions of the use of the report cards and their thoughts on how it has affected patient care. Then, additional sources can be used to substantiate and complement what was found, such as medical records, report card databases, and observations of relevant quality management committee meetings.

One of the most difficult parts of conducting qualitative research is making sense of the data that have been collected. Sometimes the data are extremely voluminous, leading to hours of organization and analysis. However, the researcher can examine qualitative data quite effectively if the following questions are examined:

1. What patterns and common themes emerge from the data collected?

2. Can these patterns or themes be narrowed to three or four basic themes in which data can be categorized?

3. Can data matrices be developed to answer the research questions?

Based on the study described above on report cards and quality, one example of a matrix describing common themes may look like this:

Report Cards	Quality	Cost	LOS	Outcomes
Clinicians				
Management				
Staff				

One of the major weaknesses of qualitative research is its lack of **generalizability** or extrapolation of the results. This is because the sample size is usually very small and cannot be taken as representative of the population under study. Also, the reliability of the results is another problem because the collection and analysis of the data can be quite different across different researchers. However, when one wants to obtain more comprehensive information in an inexpensive and less-time-consuming way, and when one is exploring new areas, it is an excellent design to use.

Analytic Study Design

Case-Control or Retrospective Study Design

In an **analytic study**, a disease or health condition is examined to determine possible causes. Intensive research related to the disease is necessary to determine characteristics that may cause the specific disease. These characteristics are also referred to as **exposure characteristics** or

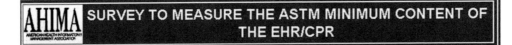

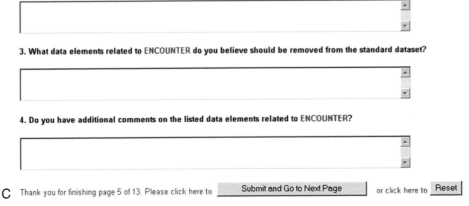

SURVEY TO MEASURE THE ASTM MINIMUM CONTENT OF THE EHR/CPR

-- Page 5 of 13 --   print the entire survey

1. Below is a list of data elements related the to ENCOUNTER entity for the CPR/EHR. ENCOUNTER entity captures the facts relating to the events that took place in the health care environment. Certain information that characterizes the time, place and circumstances of the initiation of the encounter are required.

Please indicate which of those elements you already include or will include in your existing system. Click ▶ HELP for detailed explanations.

Elements of Encounter Data	Already Included/will include in CPR/EHR?		
	Yes	No	Not Applicable
Date time encounter/admission ▶HELP	○	○	○
Treatment facility name ▶HELP	○	○	○
Encounter type	○	○	○
Episode ID ▶HELP	○	○	○
Episode diagnosis (es) ▶HELP	○	○	○
Disposition date time ▶HELP	○	○	○
Disposition type (master table) ▶HELP	○	○	○
Disposition destination ▶HELP	○	○	○
Disposition patient instructions ▶HELP	○	○	○
Text of note/report ▶HELP	○	○	○
Authentication /signature ▶HELP	○	○	○

2. What other data elements related to ENCOUNTER do you believe are needed to be included in the standard dataset?

3. What data elements related to ENCOUNTER do you believe should be removed from the standard dataset?

4. Do you have additional comments on the listed data elements related to ENCOUNTER?

C   Thank you for finishing page 5 of 13. Please click here to   [Submit and Go to Next Page]   or click here to [Reset]

Figure 12-7, cont'd A-C, Sample on-line survey. (Used with permission from the American Health Information Management Association.)

risk factors because they may increase the risk for development of the disease. The exposure characteristic or risk factor may also be referred to as the independent variable and the disease under study as the dependent variable. The **case-control** or **retrospective study** is one type of analytic study design. The researcher collects data on the cases (those who have the disease that is under study) and controls (those who are similar to the cases but do not have the disease that is under study) by looking back in time. For example, in the ovarian cancer study described earlier in this chapter, the cases included patients with epithelial ovarian cancer and the controls included patients with other diagnoses who were admitted to the same hospital during the same time period as the cases. The cases and controls were also similar in age. Specific exposure characteristics

(possible risk factors) were collected for both groups by retrieving the data from medical records and through personal interviews.

When conducting a case-control or retrospective study, the following design issues must be considered:

0. Randomly select cases by using incidence or prevalence rates, and obtain information on the patients' past history of exposures or risk factors. Specify criteria for the cases (i.e., epithelial ovarian cancer, ICD-9-CM code of 183.0, pathology reports, and slides indicating that the case truly is a case and does have the disease under study).

1. Randomly select controls similar to the cases in characteristics such as age and sex but without the disease and obtain a past history of their exposures. Select controls

from populations such as hospitals and other health care facilities and residents of a community and neighbors, friends, or siblings of the cases. Cases and controls should come from similar populations to demonstrate that those who have the disease under study are similar to other people in the community except for the disease of interest. For example, if the cases are hospital patients, controls should also be hospital patients but with a different disease or illness from the one under study.

2. Determine whether matching will be used. Some studies match on variables such as age and sex because these variables affect both the independent variables (exposure characteristic or risk factor) and the dependent variables (disease). When variables affect the dependent and independent variables, they are referred to as confounding variables. In the ovarian cancer study, cases and controls were matched on age within 5 years because age is related to several of the risk factors, such as use of birth control pills and nulliparity and incidence of ovarian cancer.

3. Design the research instrument. To collect the data, the research instrument should be developed. The following are the different types of research instruments that may be used in a case-control study:
   - Interviewer-administered questionnaire (in person or by phone)
   - Self-administered questionnaire through the mail or on the Internet
   - Worksheet to collect data abstracted from medical records
   - Data collection worksheets for recording data from slides, laboratory tests, observations from physical examinations, and so on

The following list provides steps used in the design and development of the research instrument:

1. List all variables to be measured.
2. Develop the data collection instrument. Precode each variable on the data collection form with a number. When the data are entered into the computer for analysis, each variable will be recognized. Use closed-ended questions because they are easier to code. Use of pictures and lists will improve the subject's recall.
3. Pilot test the data collection instrument to verify collection of the variables.
4. Select the data sources so that comparable details for cases and controls are provided.

An example of some sections of the research instrument used in the ovarian cancer study is presented in Figure 12-3, sample of ovarian cancer questionnaire.

Hypothetical Example of How Subjects Are Selected into a Case-Control Study. Figure 12-8 is a hypothetical example of how subjects are selected from a health care population into a case-control study. In this example, the independent variable (exposure characteristic or risk factor) is alcohol use and the dependent variable (disease) is breast cancer. The cases are subjects with breast cancer separated into alcohol users and nonusers. The controls are subjects with other diseases, such as heart disease, separated into alcohol users and nonusers. In most research studies, a larger number of controls than cases are chosen to better determine differences between the cases and controls.

Determining the Odds Ratio. The **odds ratio** is an estimate of the **relative risk** a person has if he or she is exposed to a certain characteristic. One should use the odds ratio only with case-control studies, when the disease is rare, and when cases are true representatives of all cases and controls are true representatives of all controls.[6]

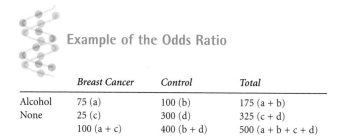

Example of the Odds Ratio

	Breast Cancer	Control	Total
Alcohol	75 (a)	100 (b)	175 (a + b)
None	25 (c)	300 (d)	325 (c + d)
	100 (a + c)	400 (b + d)	500 (a + b + c + d)

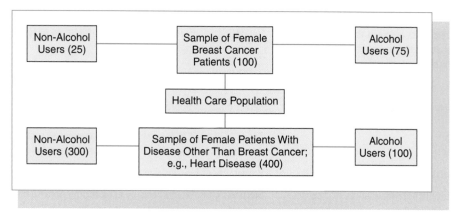

Figure 12-8 Example of case-control study population.

a = Subjects with the independent variable (alcohol) who have the disease (breast cancer)

b = Subjects with the independent variable (alcohol) who did not have the disease (breast cancer)

c = Subjects without the independent variable (alcohol) who have the disease (breast cancer)

d = Subjects without the independent variable (alcohol) who did not have the disease (breast cancer)

If a disease is rare, then a/(a + b) is about equal to a/b because a is small relative to b. Also, c/(c + d) is about equal to c/d. Therefore, by assuming that a + b is about equal to b and that c + d is about equal to d, the formula for the odds ratio is as follows:

$$\frac{(a/b)}{(c/d)} = \frac{ad}{bc}$$

Therefore, in the hypothetical case shown before:

$$\frac{(ad)}{(bc)} = \frac{(75)(300)}{(100)(25)} = \frac{22,500}{2500} = 9$$

This means that a person who drinks alcohol is nine times more likely to get breast cancer than a person who does not drink alcohol. Further refinement of this odds ratio could include defining alcohol levels to the actual amount a person drinks. Then 2 × 2 tables (such as the table used in the preceding example) could be constructed to examine levels of alcohol intake, and odds ratios could be developed and compared. Other confounders for the development of breast cancer, such as age, are not addressed here. More advanced statistical analysis beyond the scope of this chapter would be necessary to examine the risk of alcohol intake and breast cancer while controlling for confounding variables.

Advantages and Disadvantages. Table 12-4 summarizes the advantages and disadvantages of the case-control study design. Like the cross-sectional or prevalence study design, it is useful when time and resources are limited. The intent of the researcher is to establish some association between the disease and the exposure characteristic. This study design does have drawbacks because it relies on recall or past information from the subjects, making validation of that information somewhat difficult. Also, obtaining an appropriate control group for the case-control study to be valid is difficult. It is recommended that four controls be obtained for each case. Finding that large a control group while matching for specific characteristics such as age and sex can be difficult. Another major limitation of the case-control study is that the true relative risk cannot be determined; it can only be estimated by using the odds ratio. However, when one wants to determine quickly and inexpensively whether an association exists between a health condition and a characteristic, the case-control method is an appropriate route to take.[6]

The HIM professional can perform research with the case-control study design when directing a disease registry, such as a cancer or trauma registry, and when performing departmental and facility-wide performance improvement studies. Also, performing and aiding researchers in carrying out this study design is an important role of the HIM professional.

Prospective, Cohort, or Incidence Study Design

The **prospective study** design does something that neither the cross-sectional nor the case-control method can do. It determines whether the characteristic or suspected risk factor truly preceded the disease or health condition. The prospective study design is the best method for determining the magnitude of risk in the population with the

Table 12-4   ADVANTAGES AND DISADVANTAGES OF THE CASE-CONTROL DESIGN

Advantages	Disadvantages
Well suited for rare diseases or those with a long latency period, such as cancer and heart disease	Relies on recall or records for information on past exposures of certain factors; accuracy may be difficult to obtain
Takes less time before results are seen than the prospective or cohort study but more time than a cross-sectional or prevalence study	Validation of information collected difficult to obtain
Inexpensive	Occurrence of exposure obtained from selected cases and controls
Requires comparatively few subjects	Selection of an appropriate control group may be difficult
Uses existing records	Rates of disease in the exposed and unexposed subjects cannot be determined because the subjects are not being followed over time
Minimal risk to subjects	Probability of bias may be greater than in the cohort study
Allows a study of multiple potential causes of disease	Supports causal hypothesis by establishing an association but does not prove it.

characteristic or suspected risk factor. A prospective study typically includes the following steps:

1. Identify subjects with the characteristic under study who are free from the disease
2. Identify subjects without the characteristic under study who are free from the disease. These subjects are considered the comparison group.
3. Follow both groups forward in time to determine if and when they develop the disease or health condition under study

The initial assessment to determine who should be included in the prospective study is the same as that for a cross-sectional or prevalence study. In both designs, the researcher must identify cases and noncases and determine whether they have the characteristic under study. However, when the the disease under study begins to develop in subjects in the prospective study, incident cases or new cases are collected. Prospective study participants are usually volunteers. They are examined to make sure they do not have the disease at the beginning of the study. To do this, the researcher collects data related to their occupations, medical histories, and social status. Physical examinations and laboratory tests may also be needed to ensure that the subjects do not have the disease.

Some prospective or **cohort studies** begin in a community or an industrial setting or within a hospital. The subjects are separated into two groups on the basis of their exposures or health characteristic and then are followed forward to determine whether the disease develops. A hypothetical example would be subjects who are asked to participate in a prospective study to determine whether at any time after delivery they have postpartum depression. The hypothesis for this study is that women with babies who spend some time in the neonatal intensive care unit may have a higher incidence of postpartum depression than women whose babies do not spend time in the neonatal intensive care unit. Data on prenatal care, history of depression, family history of depression, and family life after delivery of the baby are collected from both groups. The women in both groups are then followed forward in time to see whether postpartum depression develops.

Another common example is comparing a group of people in the community who have certain social habits, such as comparing a group of people who exercise with a group of sedentary people. In this example, both groups receive physical examinations and laboratory tests to be certain that they are not hypertensive. Interviews to collect data on family and personal histories are also conducted. Both groups are then followed to determine whether they become hypertensive. The hypothesis for this study is that people who exercise have a decreased incidence of hypertension compared with those who do not exercise. Data on specific types, amounts, and levels of exercise also need to be collected and analyzed.

To determine whether one group does have an increased risk for development of a disease as a result of health habits or characteristics, incidence rates must be determined. As stated previously, an **incidence rate** (IR) is as follows:

$$\frac{\text{Number of new cases over a time period}}{\text{Population at risk (those free of disease at start of study)}} \times 1000$$

For the preceding examples, the IRs would be as follows:

$$\frac{\text{Number of postpartum depression cases during a time period}}{\text{Women who delivered babies in hospital during a given time period}} \times 1000$$

$$\frac{\text{Number of new cases of hypertension during a time period in a specific community}}{\text{Population (both sedentary and those who exercise) in the specific community during a given time period}} \times 1000$$

To determine which groups have a greater risk for development of the disease under study, the relative risk (RR) is determined according to the following formula:

$$RR = \frac{\text{Incidence rate exposed (IRe)}}{\text{Incidence rate unexposed (IRo)}}$$

By using the data displayed in Table 12-5, one can calculate the RR. The IR of the group who does not exercise is 145 and the IR of the group who does exercise is 50. The RR for this study is $^{145}/_{50} = 2.9$. Therefore, the people who do not exercise are about three times more likely to have hypertension develop than are the people who do exercise.

Although there are more advantages than disadvantages to using the prospective study (Table 12-6), a major benefit of this design is that it accurately determines whether the characteristic was present before the disease developed.[6] Because the IRs and RRs can be calculated, the researcher can determine the number of cases that can be prevented if a specific characteristic or exposure is controlled. This is a major advantage over the study designs discussed earlier.

Table 12-5 DETERMINING THE RELATIVE RISK: INCIDENCE RATE PER 1000 OF HYPERTENSION BY LEVELS OF EXERCISE

	Population	Cases	Incidence Rate
Exercise	1000	50	50
No exercise	1000	145	145
Total	2000	195	97.5

Table 12-6 ADVANTAGES AND DISADVANTAGES OF PROSPECTIVE, COHORT, OR INCIDENCE STUDY

Advantages	Disadvantages
Describes what came first—the characteristic or the disease	Not good with rare diseases because it take so long to follow them
Relative risk is determined, not established	Subjects are lost during follow-up because of death, withdrawal, migration
Analytically tests the hypothesis of cause and effect	Long time to see results
Decreases the amount of bias caused by recall or memory	Expensive
Subjects tend to participate less because of the amount of time they must spend in the study	Unexpected changes in environment or social habits may influence the health outcome

Historical-Prospective Study Design.

In the **historical-prospective study** design, past records are used to collect information regarding the exposure characteristic or risk factor under study. Then, over the next 10, 15, or 20 years, medical records, death certificates, and so on are monitored to determine the number of cases of a particular disease that have developed. The time of the actual study and the end of the follow-up period happen some time in the future. IRs and RRs are then calculated for the exposed and unexposed groups.

The purpose of the study illustrated in Figure 12-9 was to examine the association between obesity using body mass index (BMI) levels and recurrence and mortality in breast cancer. The risk factor or independent variable is obesity and the dependent variable is recurrence of breast cancer or mortality with breast cancer as the primary cause of death. Both the obese and nonobese cohorts were identified some time in the past (1977 through 1985) from medical records, an existing database from the oncology department, and cancer registry data. The study required all subjects to be free of a breast cancer *recurrence* from 1977 to 1985. The groups were stratified on the basis of their BMI levels. They were followed by use of both the cancer registry and medical

record to determine their rates of breast cancer recurrence and mortality caused by the breast cancer.

Advantages and Disadvantages. The major advantages of this study design compared with the prospective study design are that less time and effort are expended and the cost is lower. All other advantages and disadvantages listed in Table 12-5 for the prospective design hold true for the historical-prospective design, except that the RR is really an estimate of risk similar to an odds ratio.

Experimental Epidemiology

Clinical and Community Trials

Two types of studies are referred to in **experimental epidemiology**. They are the clinical trial and the community trial.

The **clinical trial** and the **community trial** are similar to the prospective study in that they comprise two groups that have different exposures and that are followed to determine their outcomes. In this design, a certain medication or treatment is given to a group and their outcomes are compared with those of a control or comparison group (subjects who

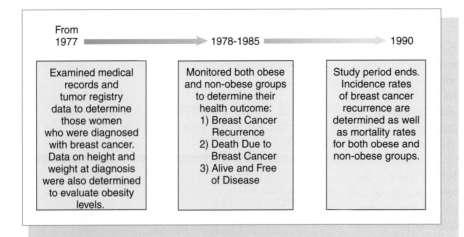

Figure 12-9 Historical-prospective study design.

do not have the intervention). In the clinical or community trial, the researcher provides the "exposure" in a controlled environment by providing some intervention procedure (e.g., medicine, education, surgical procedure). The researcher decides what the intervention will be and which subjects will receive it and which will not.

Before beginning the trial, the researcher must obtain informed consent from subjects and IRB approval to conduct the study and select the methods that will be used to randomize subjects into specific groups.

The researcher must also consider the following when conducting a clinical or community trial:

- How will adverse reactions and other complications be recorded and addressed?
- What criteria will be used to exclude and include subjects?
- Will the study be **single blind** (subject blind as to which group he or she is in), **double blind** (subject and observer blind), or **triple blind** (subject, observer, and statistician blind)?

- Ethical considerations: If the treatment group responds favorably to treatment, should the study be stopped and the treatment offered to both groups?

The difference between a clinical trial and a community trial is that the clinical trial usually begins in a clinical setting and the intervention medication, treatment, or procedure is tested on selected subjects. In a community trial, the intervention medication, treatment, or procedure is tested on a group of subjects as a whole within a particular community, outside a clinical setting.[6]

Comparison. Selection of the study design will greatly affect the results of the research. Table 12-7 compares the various research designs discussed in this chapter.

Life-Table Analysis

Life-table analysis is most appropriate for prospective studies or experimental studies when the researcher has a loss of subjects as a result of follow-up or the study ends before recurrence or death has occurred in some subjects.

Table 12-7 EPIDEMIOLOGIC RESEARCH

| Type | Descriptive Cross-Sectional Prevalence Study | Analytic Studies | | | Experimental Studies: Clinical and Community Trials |
		Case-Control Retrospective	Cohort Prospective, Incidence	Historical-Prospective	
Description	Examines the distribution of disease or health characteristics in populations at one point in time. Useful when little is known about the disease or characteristics under study.	Examines a disease to determine whether certain health (risk factor) characteristics are causing the disease.			Modifies the health characteristics that are found to cause the disease by using health care interventions that control progression of the disease or prevent the disease from occurring
Outcomes	Hypotheses Further research Case finding Program planning Planning of health care facilities or special units Determining sample size Morbidity rates within a health care facility	Studies of multiple potential causes of diseases Supports causal hypothesis by establishing an association but does not prove it Odds ratio	Describes what came first: the characteristics or the disease Determines relative risk (not estimates) Analytically tests the hypothesis of cause and effect	Outcomes are the same as in the cohort study except that the relative risk is really an estimate of risk that is similar to an odds ratio	Compares changes in a disease over time in a treatment and control group Life-table analysis is used to compare survival times in the two groups Determines whether an experimental intervention is effective

Continued

Table 12-7 EPIDEMIOLOGIC RESEARCH—cont'd

| Type | Descriptive Cross-Sectional Prevalence Study | Analytic Studies | | | Experimental Studies: Clinical and Community Trials |
		Case–Control Retrospective	Cohort Prospective, Incidence	Historical–Prospective	
Time	Takes less time than other types of studies	Take less time before results are seen than the prospective or cohort studies but more time than the cross-sectional or prevalence studies	Requires a great amount of time on part of subject (subjects may participate less because of it) because they must be monitored to determine whether they develop the disease	Takes less time than the full prospective study but somewhat more time than the cross-sectional or case-control study	Time varies depending on the type of trial that is being performed; most experimental studies take longer than the cross-sectional, case-control, and historical prospective
Financial resources	Uses modest effort and financial resources	Inexpensive; uses existing records	Expensive because of the time needed to follow the subjects	Less expensive than the full prospective study but more than the case-control or cross-sectional studies	Expenses vary depending on type of intervention and length of time of the trial but can be very high
Sample size	Large sample size is necessary, so does not work well with rare conditions	Requires comparatively few subjects. Well suited for rare diseases or those with a long latency period, such as cancer and heart disease	Large random sample is always better to truly represent the population under study	Same as prospective	Sample sizes vary and may be small depending on the type of intervention and the appropriateness of the subjects who receive it
Limitations	Fails to identify future likelihood of developing the disease. Does not answer the questions whether the health characteristic or the disease came first. Does not assess risk or likelihood of developing the disease. Examines only survivors and those alive found as cases. Misses an epidemic that may only be present for a short period	Because of reliance on subjects' recall or records for information of past exposures to risk factors: • Accuracy may be difficult to obtain • Difficult to validate information Selection of appropriate control group may be difficult. Rates of disease in the exposed and unexposed subjects cannot be determined because the subjects are not being followed over time	Subjects are lost during the study period from death, withdrawal, and migration. Not good with rare diseases because of the length of time needed for following the cases. Unexpected changes in the environment may influence the health outcome	Same as prospective study except that subjects lost to follow-up may be fewer because of the shorter time period to follow them	Adverse reactions. Ethical considerations. Loss of subjects through death, withdrawal. Compliance of subjects

Life-table analysis examines survival times of individual subjects. Survival time includes the time subjects are free of disease after diagnosis or the time to recovery or improvement after the start of a specific intervention medication, treatment, or procedure. Subjects tend to enter a study sample at different times as they enter for treatment. Each subject is followed until death, and during that time a subject may be lost to follow-up because the researcher is not able to locate the subject and, therefore, cannot determine whether death has occurred. Also, some subjects may withdraw from the study because they do not want to participate in it or because it has ended. When a survival time is **censored**, this means that the subject is alive at the time of analysis or was alive when last seen. Survival times are flagged with a + to indicate that they are censored.[14]

Life-table analysis operates on a premise called the person-time denominator. This is a special denominator that must be used in calculating rates for small study groups when subjects in the study are not all observed for the entire study period because of withdrawal, death, or loss to follow-up.

Assumptions for use of the life table analysis are as follow:

- The risk of the outcome event (death) should not be different if a patient enters the study during the first year of the study versus the second or third year.
- The rate of the outcome event should not be higher at the end of 2 years of observation than at the end of 1 year.
- The rate of the outcome event is as similar among subjects lost to follow-up and among subjects who remain under observation.

One type of life-table analysis is the Kaplan-Meier product limit method, which is appropriate for both small and large sample sizes. The result of the Kaplan-Meier product limit method is a survival curve.

The following is a hypothetical example of subjects in a clinical trial and how the Kaplan-Meier product limit method is calculated.

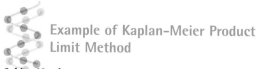

Example of Kaplan–Meier Product Limit Method

Subject Number	Survival Time (months)
1	47
2	40+
3	37
4	34
5	48+
6	41
7	41
8	45
9	23
10	43

+, censored observations, withdrawn alive or lost to follow-up.

Survival Time (1)	Rank (2)	Uncensored Rank (3)	Proportion Surviving (4)	Cumulative Proportion Surviving (5)
23	1	1	$^9/_{10} = 0.90$	0.900
34	2	2	$^8/_9 = 0.889$	0.800
37	3	3	$^7/_8 = 0.875$	0.700
40+	4	—	—	
41	5	5	$^5/_6 = 0.833$	0.583
41	6	6	$^4/_5 = 0.80$	0.466
43	7	7	$^3/_4 = 0.75$	0.350
45	8	8	$^2/_3 = 0.667$	0.233
47	9	9	$^1/_2 = 0.50$	0.117
48+	10	—	—	

(1) Survival time (t_i) months; (2) rank; (3) uncensored ranks (r_i); (4) proportion surviving $(n - r)/[(n - r) + 1]$; (5) cumulative proportion surviving s(t).

Column 1 lists all survival times, both censored and uncensored, in order from smallest to largest. (Uncensored observations are listed first if censored and uncensored observations have the same survival times.)

Column 2 lists the rank of each observation shown in column 1.

Column 3 lists the rank of uncensored observations only, where $t(r) \geq t$.

Column 4 shows the estimated proportion of subjects in the sample who survive longer than *t*. To calculate the proportion of subjects surviving through each time interval, *n* is sample size (10) and *r* is the uncensored rank, compute $(n - r)/(n - r) + 1$. Therefore $9/10 = 0.90$ means that 90% of the subjects in the sample have survived longer than 23 months.

In *Column 5*, all values in column 4 up to and including *t* are multiplied for each survival time. For example, $9/10 = 0.900$; $9/10 \times 8/9 = 0.800$; $9/10 \times 8/9 \times 7/8 = 0.700$, and so on.[15]

An example of the Kaplan-Meier curve for obesity and breast cancer survival is shown in Figure 12-10. This figure shows that about 80% of both groups survived about 58 months, or 4.8 years. At about 110 months, or 9.2 years, about 68% of the nonobese group had survived, whereas only 54% of the obese group had survived.

USE OF COMPUTER SOFTWARE IN RESEARCH

Because most research studies generate large amounts of data, a variety of computer software is used to sort and analyze the data, depending on the type of statistics that are generated. An initial database can be constructed with any spreadsheet or database software or statistical software such as SPSS (Statistical Process for the Social Sciences, SPSS, Inc., Chicago, Ill.). Then further statistical analysis can be performed using software to perform frequency distributions, tests of significance, or life-table analysis.

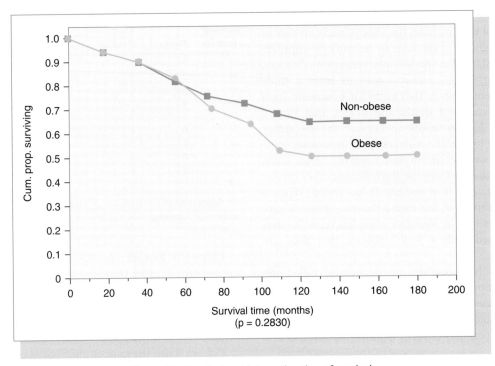

Figure 12–10 Kaplan-Meier estimation of survival.

For example, the HIM professional in conjunction with risk management personnel has been collecting data on the number of falls by both patients and employees that have occurred within the health care facility. Data collected include where and how the fall occurred; the type of injury that was sustained; the cause of the fall; and the age, sex, and race of the patients and employees who fell. The data have been coded and entered into an electronic spreadsheet. Further analysis is necessary to determine a frequency distribution on the total number of falls and the number of falls per nursing unit. Spreadsheet software can determine these distributions and can generate graphics to display the data. However, using spreadsheet software to determine more extensive statistical analysis may not be the most efficient route to take. To determine whether there is a significant association between a specific nursing unit and the number of falls, correlation coefficients and tests of significance may be necessary. These types of statistics may be more easily generated with statistical software. Further analysis to examine health outcomes 1 month, 6 months, or 1 year after the fall may include life-table analysis with SPSS software.

The HIM professional should know the types of software that are available to perform certain statistical tests. Statisticians should be consulted to aid in this process and in the interpretation and explanation of the data. Remember that the computer software or statistical analysis performed is only as good as the data that are collected and entered into the computer. It is up to the researcher to determine whether the results make sense and, therefore, how they should be applied and interpreted.

Other types of statistical software can aid in the collection of the data for a research study by assisting in the development of the questionnaire or data collection instrument. One example of such software is EPIINFO (Centers for Disease Control and Prevention, Atlanta, Ga.). This software, which can be obtained at a low cost, not only aids in constructing the data collection instrument but also includes features such as SPSS to perform basic and advanced statistical analysis of the data.

Many types of computer software and statistical analysis applications are available. It is beyond the scope of this chapter to discuss all of them. However, the HIM professional should be aware of the computer software available to assist in database development and analysis of data

This may be the most important step the HIM professional takes when conducting research studies in the health care environment.

OUTCOME STUDIES AND EPIDEMIOLOGY

Today more than ever before, health care facilities, managed care organizations, federal and state governments, and the like are focusing on the outcomes of care and designing and carrying out outcomes studies. The HIM professional will be able to conduct unique, thorough, and sound outcomes research with a thorough understanding of epidemiologic research methods and the specific **outcome measures** that are being studied. In the beginning of this chapter the epidemiologic study designs were explained and discussed, and the design of a research proposal or plan was explained. Now, the outcomes measures are briefly explained and an outcomes study that was performed by the author and colleagues is discussed in relation to how it applies to outcomes research.

Outcomes research can focus on several different measures. In the past, its main focus was on mortality rates. Now, because health care facilities are interested in knowing many other things about the end results of care and The Joint Commission and the ORYX initiative require health care facilities to provide clinical outcome measures, the HIM professional must think of many different ways to study outcomes. The outcomes may focus on causation, efficiency (cost), treatment impact, or more generic measures such as morbidity, mortality, satisfaction, physical function, pain, emotional function, social function, cognitive function, vitality, and overall quality of life. Disease-specific measures are also quite common and require intense design and analysis to find accurate results.

The outcomes study that was performed by the author and colleagues[16] is a descriptive epidemiologic study that used a cross-sectional study design. Past research demonstrated that the medical record alone is not always an effective epidemiologic research tool when data are collected on specific risk factors associated with ovarian cancer.[17,18] However, when the medical record, as well as financial data and physician input, was used to study the cost of infections in an elderly population, an effective database emerged. This pilot study was designed to analyze noninstitutionalized elderly patient hospitalizations for type of diagnosis and procedures, DRGs, and infections. The hypothesis tested was that the elderly patient hospitalized with an infection has an increased length of stay and cost compared with those hospitalized without infections.

Study Procedures

All Medicare patients who were participating in the "Good Health Study" and admitted to a hospital in Pittsburgh, Pennsylvania, from July 1, 1986, through December 31, 1987, were studied.

The Good Health Study[19] examined noninstitutionalized elderly individuals for incidence rates of clinical infections, organisms responsible for infection, patterns of transmission, and the outcome of the infections measured by mortality, morbidity, and the adverse effects of treatment. This free-living elderly population is representative of the elderly in general. Comparisons of the Good Health Study population for health habits, living arrangements, medical conditions, and activities of daily living (ADLs) were consistently similar across three other studies of elderly persons in Boston, Massachusetts; New Haven, Connecticut; and Iowa.[20] Medicare patient hospitalizations (n = 165) were analyzed by abstracting the medical records to determine the principal and secondary diagnoses and procedures. Diagnoses and procedures were recorded if they appeared anywhere in the medical record, including the discharge summary, progress notes, operative reports, and data on laboratory and clinical findings. The criteria for infections used in the Good Health Study were used to determine whether the symptoms, signs, and laboratory findings documented in the medical record reflect an infectious disease.[21] Any infections recorded that differed from what was recorded by the hospital were reviewed by an infectious disease physician to determine whether the differences seen were accurate. An infection was considered to be nosocomial if it developed after 72 hours of hospitalization and community acquired if it developed 72 hours before admission.

The diagnoses and procedures were coded according to ICD-9-CM. The age, sex, disposition, admission and discharge dates, diagnosis, and procedure codes were entered into a DRG grouper system (same software used by the hospital for past DRG groupings). This step enabled computation of a final DRG and relative weight. Data such as total charges, cost, DRG payment, total payment, and whether there was a gain or loss for the hospital were obtained from the financial department at the hospital. With this information, the total payment for the abstracted hospitalizations could be calculated.

An example of sections of the database used to analyze some of the study data can be found on the Evolve Web site. Patient hospitalizations without infections are listed first followed by those with infections. The format of the database works very well with Access and Excel software for performing data analysis.

Data Analysis

Because this was a descriptive, pilot outcome study, basic statistical analysis was used. To determine whether there were differences in cost, length of stay, and reimbursement for hospitalizations with and without infections, the average length of stay (ALOS), average DRG payment, average total payment, and the difference between the average total payment and average cost by specific weight categories were analyzed. This was done in the following ways:

1. ALOS, cost, DRG, and total payment by relative weight for patients with and without infections (Table 12-8)
2. ALOS, cost, DRG, and total payment by relative weight for patients with community-acquired infections (CAIs) and patients without infections (Table 12-9)
3. ALOS, cost, DRG, and total payment by relative weight for patients with nosocomial infections (NIs) and patients without infections (Table 12-10)

The weight of the DRG must be controlled to determine whether the differences seen in Tables 12-8 through 12-10 are due to the infection. This was analyzed in the following ways:

1. Average cost and total payment per weight for patients with and without infections by low and high relative weights (Table 12-11)

Table 12-8 AVERAGE LENGTH OF STAY, COST, DRG, AND TOTAL PAYMENT BY RELATIVE WEIGHT FOR HOSPITALIZATIONS WITH OR WITHOUT INFECTIONS

DRG Weight	Total Hosp.	Infection							No Infection						
		n	ALOS	Acost	Adrg	Atot	Diff.		n	ALOS	Acost	Adrg	Atot	Diff.
<0.70	39	12	6.8	4260	2263	3629	−631		27	5.5	3487	2388	3632	145
0.7-0.89	42	20	8.9	5032	3191	4548	−484		22	6.1	4258	2788	4300	42
0.9-1.19	36	12	5.5	3298	3483	4607	1309		24	5.7	3588	3677	4986	1398
1.2-1.9	22	10	10.8	6635	5599	7907	1272		12	9.1	5875	5032	7187	1312
2.0-2.9	21	11	29.4	40,819	9344	26,483	14,336		10	22.3	15,957	9277	13,088	2869
Without outlier	19	10	20.5	18,448	9216	15,546	−2902		9	13.8	10,815	9240	12,838	2023
≥3	5	1	13.0	7669	12,167	14,918	7249		4	14.7	16,733	15,465	20,940	4207

Hosp., hospitalization; *ALOS*, average length of stay; *Acost*, average cost; *Adrg*, average DRG payment; *Atot*, average total payment; *Diff.*, average total payment − average cost.

Table 12-9 ALOS, COST, DRG, AND TOTAL PAYMENT BY RELATIVE WEIGHT FOR HOSPITALIZATIONS WITH CAIS AND HOSPITALIZATIONS WITHOUT INFECTIONS

DRG Weight	Total Hosp.	Community Acquired Infection							No Infection						
		n	ALOS	Acost	Adrg	Atot	Diff.		n	ALOS	Acost	Adrg	Atot	Diff.
<0.70	38	11	6.3	3728	2065	3270	−458		27	5.5	3487	2388	3632	145
0.7-0.89	40	18	8.4	4659	3242	4481	−178		22	6.1	4258	2788	4300	42
0.9-1.19	32	8	5.9	3493	3965	5259	1766		24	5.7	3588	3677	4986	1398
1.2-1.9	22	10	10.8	6635	5599	7908	1273		12	9.1	5875	5032	7187	1312
2.0-2.9	17	7	31.1	53,363	9780	33,257	20,106		10	22.3	15,957	9277	13,088	2869
Without outlier	16	6	16.6	18,170	9640	16,158	−2012		9	13.8	10,815	9240	12,838	2023
≥3	4	0	—	—	—	—	—		4	14.7	16,733	15,465	20,940	4207

Hosp., hospitalization; *ALOS*, average length of stay; *Acost*, average cost; *Adrg*, average DRG payment; *Atot*, average total payment; *Diff.*, average total payment − average cost.

Table 12-10 ALOS, COST, DRG, AND TOTAL PAYMENT BY RELATIVE WEIGHT FOR HOSPITALIZATIONS WITH NI AND HOSPITALIZATIONS WITHOUT INFECTIONS

DRG Weight	Total Hosp.	Nosocomial Infection							No Infection						
		n	ALOS	Acost	Adrg	Atot	Diff.		n	ALOS	Acost	Adrg	Atot	Diff.
<0.70	29	2	9.5	6081	2360	4443	−1638		27	5.5	3487	2388	3632	145
0.7-0.89	24	2	13.5	8390	2742	5151	−3239		22	6.1	4258	2788	4300	42
0.9-1.19	29	5	9.4	5136	3672	5402	266		24	5.7	3588	3677	4986	1398
1.2-1.9	13	1	12.0	7564	6987	9741	2177		12	9.1	5875	5032	7187	1312
2.0-2.9	17	7	39.0	57,904	9222	33,981	23,923		10	22.3	15,957	9277	13,088	2869
Without outlier	15	6	25.8	23,467	8989	17,002	−6465		9	13.8	10,815	9240	12,838	2023
≥3	5	1	13.0	7669	12,167	14,918	7249		4	14.7	16,733	15,465	20940	4207

Hosp., hospitalization; *ALOS*, average length of stay; *Acost*, average cost; *Adrg*, average DRG payment; *Atot*, average total payment; *Diff.*, average total payment − average cost.

Table 12-11 AVERAGE COST AND TOTAL PAYMENT PER WEIGHT FOR HOSPITALIZATIONS WITH AND WITHOUT INFECTIONS BY LOW AND HIGH RELATIVE WEIGHTS

DRG Weight	Total Hosp.	Infection				No Infection			
		n	Cost/wt	Tpay/wt.	Diff.	n	Cost/wt.	Tpay/wt.	Diff.
<1	90	34	6073	5546	−527	56	5368	5587	219
>1	75	32	7629	6574	−1055	43	4263	4969	706
Without outlier	73	31	4972	5296	324	42	3800	4948	1148

Hosp., Hospitalization; *Cost/wt*, average (cost/weight); *Tpay/wt.*, average (total payment/weight); *Diff.*, average (total payment/weight) − average (cost/weight).

2. Average cost and total payment per weight for patient hospitalizations with CAI and patient hospitalizations without infections by low and high relative weights (Table 12-12)
3. Average cost and total payment per weight for patient hospitalizations with NI and hospitalizations without infections by low and high relative weights (Table 12-13)

Length of stay also had to be controlled. This was done in the following way:

1. Average cost and total payment by length of stay (≤1 week and >1 week) for hospitalizations with and without infections (Table 12-14)
2. Average cost and total payment per day (<1 and >1) per weight for hospitalizations with and without infections (Table 12-15)

The results are described as follows:

1. The average cost and ALOS were higher in hospitalizations with infections than in hospitalizations without infections.
2. When the DRG and length of stay were controlled simultaneously, however, lower average costs per day per weight were seen for hospitalizations with infections.
3. Similar results (lower average costs per day per weight) were found when comparisons were done to separate infection types NI and CAI.
4. Sixty-eight percent of all NIs developed on or after day 5, and the risk of infection increased in hospitalizations with longer lengths of stay.

Two models were developed to explain the results. In the first model, individuals have an increased length of stay

Table 12-12 AVERAGE COST AND TOTAL PAYMENT PER WEIGHT FOR HOSPITALIZATIONS WITH COMMUNITY-ACQUIRED INFECTIONS AND HOSPITALIZATIONS WITHOUT INFECTIONS BY LOW AND HIGH RELATIVE WEIGHTS

DRG Weight	Total Hosp.	Community-Acquired Infection				No Infection			
		N	Cost/wt	Tpay/wt.	Diff.	n	Cost/wt.	Tpay/wt.	Diff.
<1	86	30	5791	5452	−339	56	5368	5587	219
>1	67	24	8102	6899	−1203	43	4263	4969	706
Without outlier	65	23	4542	5190	648	42	3800	4948	1148

Hosp., Hospitalization; *Cost/wt*, average (cost/weight); *Tpay/wt.*, average (total payment/weight); *Diff.*, average (total payment/weight) − average (cost/weight).

Table 12-13 AVERAGE COST AND TOTAL PAYMENT PER WEIGHT FOR HOSPITALIZATIONS WITH NOSOCOMIAL INFECTIONS AND HOSPITALIZATIONS WITHOUT INFECTIONS BY LOW AND HIGH RELATIVE WEIGHTS

DRG Weight	Total Hosp.	Nosocomial Infection				No Infection			
		N	Cost/wt	Tpay/wt.	Diff.	n	Cost/wt.	Tpay/wt.	Diff.
<1	61	5	8954	6454	−2500	56	5368	5587	219
>1	56	13	13168	8981	−4187	43	4263	4969	706
Without outlier	54	12	6768	5879	−889	42	3800	4948	1148

Hosp., Hospitalization; *Cost/wt*, average (cost/weight); *Tpay/wt.*, average (total payment/weight); *Diff.*, average (total payment/weight) − average (cost/weight).

Table 12-14 AVERAGE COST AND TOTAL PAYMENT BY LENGTH OF STAY FOR HOSPITALIZATIONS WITH AND WITHOUT INFECTIONS

Length of Stay	Total Hosp.	Infection				No Infection			
		N	Cost/wt	Tpay/wt.	Diff.	n	Cost/wt.	Tpay/wt.	Diff.
<1 week	81	26	731	1533	802	55	771	1294	523
>1 week	84	40	667	625	-42	44	697	712	15
Without outlier	82	39	627	611	-16	43	698	725	27

Hosp., Hospitalization; *Cost/wt*, average (cost/weight); *Tpay/wt.*, average (total payment/weight); *Diff.*, average (total payment/weight) − average (cost/weight).

Table 12-15 AVERAGE COST AND TOTAL PAYMENT PER DAY PER WEIGHT FOR HOSPITALIZATIONS WITH AND WITHOUT INFECTIONS

DRG Weight	Total Hosp.	Infection				No Infection			
		N	Cost/wt	Tpay/wt.	Diff.	n	Cost/wt.	Tpay/wt.	Diff.
<1	90	34	883	1328	445	56	1031	1344	313
>1	75	32	424	563	139	43	474	769	295
Without outlier	73	31	413	568	155	42	479	785	306

Hosp., Hospitalization; *C/d/wt.*, average [(cos/day)/weight]; *T/d/wt.*, average [(total payment/day)/weight]; *Diff.*, average [(total payment/day)weight] − average [(cost/day)weight].

leading to the development of the NI, which then further increases length of stay with attendant increased costs. In the second model, there may be sicker individuals who have an increased risk of infection, which leads to a longer length of stay and therefore higher cost.

This outcome study demonstrates what can be accomplished when the medical record and financial data are used. By using the medical record as well as financial data and input from the infectious disease department, a detailed analysis of infections in an elderly population in relation to cost and length of stay (two important efficiency outcome measures) was completed. This outcome study also enabled the hospital to determine the types of studies that should be done in the future. Performance improvement studies that examine the effectiveness of infection control procedures over time, the importance of examining both CAIs and NIs, and the differences that severity of illness may have on cost and length of stay are all areas that have been identified as needing further study. Future outcome studies in this area and other areas will continue to use the medical record. However, the data obtained from the medical record should not be examined alone. The data should be analyzed along with data from other sources such as severity of illness data, financial data, quality improvement data, infection control data, and risk management and patient safety data to examine epidemiologic trends over time. Only when several data sources are used together to investigate a particular aspect of care can that aspect of care be thoroughly and completely examined. The EHR may be the key to bring all of these data sources together. As research in these areas moves forward, it will inevitably promote the advancement of the EHR. What a major breakthrough research can provide for HIM and health care in general.

Key Concepts

- Several research study designs can be used to assess disease occurrence or the risk of getting a disease. Knowing when to use which study design is important and should be examined carefully.
- Every research study has specific steps that should be followed, such as developing a hypothesis, specific aims, significance, methodology (sample size, how data will be collected, data sources), and analysis.
- Every study has within it some type of bias or error, and the researcher should be aware of these biases and discuss their impact when writing up the results.

REFERENCES

1. e-Health Task Force of the AHIMA: *Report on the roles and functions of e-health information management*, April 2002.
2. Watzlaf VJM: The leadership role of the health information management professional in research, *Top Health Inform Manage* 15:47-58, 1995.

3. U.S. Department of Health and Human Services: *Healthy People 2010: understanding and improving health,* ed 2, Washington, DC, 2000, U.S. Government Printing Office.

4. Watzlaf VJM: The development of the grant proposal, *J Am Med Rec Assoc* 60:37-41, 1989.

5. Shi L: *Health services research methods,* Albany, NY, 1997, Delmar Publishers.

6. Slome C, Brogan D, Eyres S et al: *Basic epidemiological methods and biostatistics: a workbook,* Belmont, CA, 1986, Jones & Bartlett.

7. Lilienfeld A, Lilienfeld D: *Foundations of epidemiology,* ed 2, New York, 1980, Oxford University Press.

8. Kuzma J: *Basic statistics for the health sciences,* Mountain View, CA, 1998, Mayfield Publishing.

9. Schlesselman JJ: *Case-control studies—design, conduct, analysis,* New York, 1982, Oxford University Press.

10. Schleyer TKL, Forrest JL: Web-based survey design and administration, *J AMIA* 7(4), 2000.

11. Wyatt JC: When to use Web-based surveys [editorial comment], *J AMIA* 7, 2000.

12. Watzlaf VJM, Zeng X, Jarymowycz C et al: Standards for the content of the electronic health record, *Perspect Health Inform Manage* 1:1, 2004. http://www.ahima.org/perspectives.

13. Katoh A., Watzlaf VJM, D'Amico F: An examination of obesity and breast cancer survival in post-menopausal women, *Br J Cancer* 70:928-933, 1994.

14. American College of Surgeons: *Module 14—Statistics fundamental tumor registry operations,* 1991, Commission on Cancer, Chicago.

15. Kramer S, Jarrett P: *Biostatistics and epidemiology for the tumor registry professionals,* Harrisburg, PA, 1984, Pennsylvania Department of Health and Pennsylvania Tumor Registrars Association.

16. Watzlaf VJM, Kuller LH, Ruben FL: The use of the medical record and financial data to examine the cost of infections in the elderly, *Top Health Rec Manage* 13:65-76, 1992.

17. Watzlaf VJM: Is the medical record an effective epidemiological data source? Proceedings of the National Center for Health Statistics Public Health Conference on Records and Statistics, Washington, DC, July 1989.

18. Watzlaf VJM: The medical record as an epidemiological database, *Top Health Rec Manage* 7:61-67, 1987.

19. Ruben FL, Dearwater SR, Norden CW et al: Clinical infections in the noninstitutionalized geriatric age group: methods utilized and incidence of infections. The Pittsburgh Good Health Study, *Am J Epidemiol* 141:145-157, 1995.

20. National Institute of Aging: *Established population for epidemiologic studies of the elderly: Resource data book,* Bethesda, MD, National Institutes of Health Publication No. 86:2443, 1986.

21. Mandell GL, Douglas RG, Bennett JE, editors: *Principles and practice of infectious disease,* New York, 1979, Wiley.

chapter **13**

Performance Management and Patient Safety

Patrice Spath
Donna J. Slovensky

Additional content,
http://evolve.elsevier.com/Abdelhak/

Review exercises can be found
in the Study Guide

The Big Picture and Key Players
  Federal Oversight Agencies
  Accrediting Bodies
    The Joint Commission
    National Committee for Quality Assurance
  National Quality Awards
  Purchasers
  Consumers
  National Health Care Quality Measurement Priorities
Performance Measurement
Structure, Process, and Outcome Measures
  Structure Measures
  Process Measures
  Outcome Measures
  Developing Performance Measures
  Collecting Measurement Data
Performance Assessment
  Reports for Analysis
  Performance Goals and Targets
  Use of Comparative Data
Performance Improvement
  Performance Improvement Models
    Rapid Cycle Improvement
    Six Sigma
    Lean Thinking

Key Words

Accreditation	Fishbone diagram	Performance assessment
Adverse event	Flowchart	Performance measure
Affinity diagram	Focused review	Performance measurement
Aggregate data	Force field analysis	Physician advisor
Bar chart	Health plan employer data and	Potentially compensable event
Benchmarking	information set	Practitioner profiles
Brainstorming	Healthcare integrity data bank	Privilege delineation
Case management	Histogram	Retrospective review
Cause-and-effect diagram	Incident report	Quality improvement
Checksheet	Indicator	Quality improvement organizations
Clinical practice guidelines	Intensity of service/severity of illness	Rapid cycle improvement
Concurrent review	Lean thinking	Reliable
Conditions of Participation	Leapfrog Group	Report card
Control chart	Licensure	Risk
Correlation analysis	Line graph	Root cause analysis
Credentialing	Matrix	Run chart
Credentials registry	Mishap	Sentinel event
Credentials verification organization	National Practitioner Data Bank	Six Sigma
Data sheet	Nominal group technique	Statement of work
Discharge planning	Pareto chart	Statistical process control
Electronic health record	Patient advocacy	Threshold
Evidenced-based medicine	Patient safety improvement	Utilization management
Failure mode and effects analysis	Patient safety indicators	Valid
Federal Register	Pay for performance	Value chain

Process Improvement Tools
    Idea-Generating Techniques
    Data Organization
    Data Analysis and Presentation

Patient Safety
  Safety Measurement
  Patient Safety Databases
  Safety Improvement
  Root Cause Analysis
  Proactive Risk Assessment

Risk Management
  Loss Prevention and Reduction
  Claims Management

Utilization Management
  External Requirements
  Program Components
    Prospective Review
    Concurrent Review
    Discharge Planning/Case Management
    Retrospective Review
  Plan and Program Structure

Credentialing
  External Requirements
  Credentialing Program Components

Role of Managers

Abbreviations

AHA—American Hospital Association

AHRQ—Agency for Healthcare Research and Quality

CABG—coronary artery bypass graft

CDC—Centers for Disease Control and Prevention

CMS—Centers for Medicare and Medicaid Services

COP—*Conditions of Participation*

CVO—credentials verification organization

DEA—Drug Enforcement Agency

DMAIC—definition, measurement, analysis, improvement, and control

EBM—evidenced-based medicine

EHR—electronic health record

FDA—Food and Drug Administration

FLEX—Federal Licensing Examination

FMEA—failure mode and effects analysis

HACCP—hazard analysis and critical control point

HCO—health care organization

HEDIS—Health Plan Employer Data and Information Set

HIM—health information management

HIPDB—Healthcare Integrity and Protection Data Bank

HMO—health maintenance organization

IOM—Institute of Medicine

ISMP—Institute for Safe Medication Practices

IS/SI—intensity of service/severity of illness

JCAHO—Joint Commission on Accreditation of Healthcare Organizations (now The Joint Commission)

LIP—licensed independent practitioner

MBHO—managed behavioral health care organization

MCO—managed care organization

MDC—major diagnostic category

MSO—medical staff organization

NCQA—National Committee for Quality Assurance

NGT—nominal group technique

NIST—National Institute of Standards and Technology

NPDB—National Practitioner Data Bank

NQF—National Quality Forum

P4P—Pay for Performance

PCE—potentially compensable event

PDCA—Plan, Do, Check, Act

PPO—preferred provider organization

PSI—patient safety indicator

QI—quality improvement

QIO—quality improvement organization

RCI—rapid cycle improvement

SIP—surgical infection prevention

SOW—statement of work

SPC—statistical process control

UM—utilization management

UR—utilization review

URAC—Utilization Review Accreditation Commission

Objectives

- Define key words.
- Identify key societal and regulatory drivers for quality and safety initiatives in health care organizations.
- Identify legislative mandates and oversight agency requirements for performance of management activities in health care organizations.
- Identify key stakeholders and their primary objectives for performance management and patient safety in health care delivery.
- Differentiate among structure, process, and outcome measures of performance.
- Discuss various approaches used by health care organizations to improve performance through process improvement.
- Describe and apply statistical tools frequently used in problem analysis and performance management.
- Describe the process of conducting a root cause analysis.
- Describe the process of conducting a risk assessment.

Most people expect quality in the delivery of health care services. Consumers expect to receive the right medical interventions, achieve good outcomes, and to be satisfied with personal interactions with caregivers. Additionally, consumers expect the physical facilities where care is provided to be clean and pleasant and to have the "best" technology available. Each of these characteristics is a part of quality; none is the whole. The way a health care consumer defines quality may differ from what providers or purchasers view as important quality attributes.

Without question, "quality" is expected to be an integral component of all health care services. Despite this universally accepted belief, how to measure performance and what constitutes an acceptable level of quality continue to be greatly debated. Scholars and researchers, health care providers and payers, and individual consumers of health care all bring different perspectives into the debate.

In the past few years, the public has become increasingly concerned about the safety of health care services. Media reports about errors made in the delivery of patient care have raised consumer awareness of the potential for medical mishaps. In November 1999, the Institute of Medicine (IOM) released the report, *To Err is Human: Building a Safer Health System*.[1] The report purported to show, for the first time, the extent to which medical errors may cause preventable deaths in the United States. It was estimated that between 44,000 and 98,000 deaths occur each year in hospitals as a result of medical errors by physicians, pharmacists, and other health care providers. The lower estimate, 44,000 deaths, places medical errors as the eighth leading cause of death in the United States, whereas the higher estimate, 98,000 deaths, places medical errors as the fifth leading cause of death in the United States. The IOM report suggested that most medical errors are a result of the complexity of health care services, not incompetent individuals.

In the 2001 IOM report, *Crossing the Quality Chasm: A New Health System for the 21st Century*,[2] the Committee on Quality of Health Care in America identified six key dimensions of health care quality:

- *Safe*—avoiding injuries to patients from the care that is intended to help them.
- *Effective*—providing services based on scientific knowledge to all who could benefit and refraining from providing services to those not likely to benefit (avoiding underuse and overuse, respectively).
- *Patient centered*—providing care that is respectful of and responsive to individual patient preferences, needs, and values and ensuring that patient values guide all clinical decisions.
- *Timely*—reducing waits and sometimes harmful delays for both those who receive and those who give care.
- *Efficient*—avoiding waste, including waste of equipment, supplies, ideas, and energy.
- *Equitable*—providing care that does not vary in quality because of personal characteristics such as gender, ethnicity, geographic location, and socioeconomic status.

THE BIG PICTURE AND KEY PLAYERS

Although health care providers have numerous internal incentives for improving the quality and safety of the services delivered in their organizations, the details for accomplishing these activities are often influenced by external mandates. Some requirements are grounded in law; others are stipulated by agencies with which a health care organization (HCO) interacts on a voluntary basis. Purchasers and consumers also play a role in influencing performance management in health services. This section focuses on the key players and how these groups affect health care quality and patient safety.

Federal Oversight Agencies

Because most HCOs provide services to Medicare or Medicaid beneficiaries, the regulations of the Centers for Medicare and Medicaid Services (CMS) have a significant impact on the "what" and "how" of performance improvement activities at the provider level. Regulations governing providers of services to Medicare beneficiaries are detailed in the **Conditions of Participation** (COP). These regulations require that providers develop, implement, and maintain an effective organization-wide, data-driven quality assessment and performance improvement program. The specifics of the regulations vary according to the provider setting. For instance, hospitals must measure, analyze, and track quality indicators, including adverse patient events, and other aspects of performance that assess processes of care, hospital service, and operations.[3] Revisions and addenda to these regulations are published in the **Federal Register**, a Monday-through-Friday publication of the National Archives and Records Administration that reports regulations and legal notices issued by federal agencies, presidential proclamations and executive orders, and other documents as directed by law or public interest.

CMS also conducts nationwide health care performance measurement and improvement initiatives, contracting at the state level with **quality improvement organizations** (QIOs) to direct and oversee these initiatives. Requirements for QIOs that contract with CMS are outlined in comprehensive triennial documents, the QIO **Statement of Work** (SOW) numbered consecutively beginning in 1983. The Eighth SOW, encompassing October 1, 2005, through September 30, 2008, includes initiatives related to hospital reporting of quality measures, improvement of surgical care and management of medical patients, and improvement of hospitals' readiness to adopt information technology systems (computerized order entry, bar coding or telehealth). The current SOW is available on the CMS Web site.

Accrediting Bodies

Many health care organizations voluntarily participate in national accreditation programs. **Accreditation** is a credential given to an organization that meets a defined set of standards, some of which relate to performance management. Only organizations seeking accreditation must comply with these mandates.

The Joint Commission

The most common health care provider accreditation programs are those sponsored by The Joint Commission. The Joint Commission is a not-for-profit, nongovernmental entity that offers voluntary accreditation programs for all types of health care facilities. It provides education, leadership, and objective evaluation and feedback to health care organizations in the quest for health care quality and patient safety.

Although The Joint Commission does not specify a particular method for performance management, some standards applicable to measuring and evaluating health services and clinical care are prescriptive in orientation. The Joint Commission utilizes a comparative performance measurement project that involves the collection and analysis of data from accredited organizations. In July 2002, hospitals began collecting core measure data on four initial areas: acute myocardial infarction, heart failure, community-acquired pneumonia, and pregnancy and related conditions. The results of these performance measures are one of the elements taken into consideration by the The Joint Commission when accrediting an organization. As with all regulations in health care, The Joint Commission standards are subject to change. Current performance measurement and improvement initiatives, accreditation issues, and other information are available on The Joint Commission's Web site.

National Committee for Quality Assurance

The National Committee for Quality Assurance (NCQA) is a private, not-for-profit organization established in 1991. NCQA accredits a variety of organizations from health maintenance organizations (HMOs) to preferred provider organizations (PPOs) to managed behavioral health care organizations (MBHOs,) and each accreditation program has distinct performance management requirements.[4] The NCQA accreditation method is similar to that of The Joint Commission. NCQA also sponsors the Health Plan Employer Data and Information Set (HEDIS), which is a comparative performance measurement project that evaluates an organization's clinical and administrative systems. These data are made available to purchasers and consumers to assist them in making choices about health care providers.

NCQA accreditation and participation in HEDIS is voluntary, but many large employers require or request accreditation or HEDIS reporting for the health plans they make available to their employees. Additional information about the NCQA's programs and activities is available on their Web site.

National Quality Awards

Some health care leaders seek to advance performance improvement by voluntarily participating in quality award programs at the state and national levels. An example of such a program is the Baldrige National Quality Award, established by Congress in 1987 to recognize organizations for their achievements in quality and business performance and to raise awareness about the importance of quality and performance excellence as a competitive edge. The Baldrige Healthcare Criteria for Performance Excellence, first published in 1998, provide a systems perspective for managing an HCO to advance performance excellence. The Baldrige Criteria are designed as an interrelated system of 19 items that address 32 areas. The items are organized into seven categories or management disciplines[5]:

- Leadership
- Strategic planning
- Focus on patients, other customers, and markets
- Measurement, analysis, and knowledge management
- Staff focus
- Process management
- Organizational results

The Baldrige Criteria help HCOs to stay focused on improvement goals and to align all activities to achieve these goals. The criteria are the basis for many national quality award programs sponsored by professional organizations. An example is the American Health Care Association's Quality Award that addresses the key requirements of performance excellence in long-term care facilities. The criteria for the American Hospital Association's Quest for Quality Prize cover many of the concepts found in the Baldrige Criteria.[6] Information about the Baldrige Award and the criteria underpinning the award is available on the National Institute of Standards and Technology (NIST) Web site.

Purchasers

Federal and state governments are by far the largest purchasers of health care services. The quality of these services is regulated by the COP and by state health department regulations. There are also many private health insurance companies, and employers that purchase health insurance for their employees that have a vested interest in health care quality. Like federal and state governments, these purchasers want to receive good value for the dollars they expend on health care services. In response to the rising cost of health care, nongovernment health care purchasers are taking a more assertive role in advancing quality and patient safety. The **Leapfrog Group,** a collaboration of large employers, came together in 1998 to determine how purchasers could influence the quality and affordability of health care. The Leapfrog Group identified four hospital quality and safety practices that are the focus of its health care provider performance comparisons and hospital recognition and reward. The quality practices are computer physician order entry, evidence-based hospital referral, and intensive care unit staffing by physicians experienced in critical care medicine. More information about the Leapfrog Group initiatives can be found on their Web site.

Some health plans have initiated payment systems that financially reward providers who achieve specific quality or patient safety goals. These initiatives are commonly called **Pay for Performance** (P4P). The fundamental principles of Pay for Performance are (1) common performance measures for providers (usually represent a balance of patient satisfaction, prevention, and long-term care management) and (2) significant health plan financial payments on the basis of that performance, with each plan independently deciding the source, amount, and payment method for its incentive program.

Consumers

Consumers do not have the power to mandate specific health service performance management activities; however, they do influence what is required by federal regulations and accreditation standards. This influence occurs in many different ways. There are numerous consumer/patient advocacy groups that work in partnership with legislators, providers, and purchasers to promote health care quality and patient safety improvements. Often one or more consumer representatives serve on the governing board or advisory groups of accreditation organizations to provide the "public perspective" when accreditation standards are revised. Individual consumers and consumer groups have the opportunity to comment on proposed changes in the Medicare COP, which are published in the publicly available *Federal Register.*

Patient advocacy services may be available in individual HCOs as a proactive approach to ensuring patient satisfaction with the process and outcomes of care episodes. In addition to responding to individual patient complaints, patient advocates may monitor overall patient satisfaction with the facility and with staff interactions by use of written questionnaires or telephone surveys. The patient advocacy program also may encompass patient education. Information brochures, videotapes, public service broadcasts on an internal television network, and other media facilitate communication between the patient and medical and professional staff. Better-informed patients who participate in their own care are more compliant with treatment and achieve better outcomes.[7] Patients who are informed

about their treatments and prognoses and who are involved in decision making are more satisfied with their care providers. The American Hospital Association (AHA) has published and disseminated a statement of patient rights and responsibilities. The AHA brochure with this statement or a similar pamphlet is often provided to consumers during inpatient admission procedures as evidence of patient advocacy.

National Health Care Quality Measurement Priorities

During the 1990s great emphasis was placed on the need for public accountability of providers and insurers to furnish comprehensive, high-quality health care at an acceptable cost.[8] In effect, the charge was to ensure value for health care expenditures. Within this context, value is reflected by maximized health outcomes and satisfaction in concert with optimal use of resources. "Public accountability" is assumed to be achievable through published reports, or **report cards**, reflecting provider or health plan performance on critical indicators of cost, clinical outcomes, and consumer satisfaction.

In 1999 the National Quality Forum (NQF), a not-for-profit membership organization, was created to develop and implement a national strategy for health care quality measurement and reporting. The NQF includes representatives from a diverse group of national, state, regional, and local organizations, including purchasers, consumers, health systems, health care practitioners, health plans, accrediting bodies, regulatory agencies, medical suppliers, and information technology companies. The mission of the NQF is to improve American health care through endorsement of consensus-based national standards for measurement and public reporting of health care performance data that provide meaningful information about whether care is safe, timely, beneficial, patient centered, equitable, and efficient.[9] The specific goals of the NQF are as follows[10]:

1. Promote collaborative efforts to improve the quality of the nation's health care through performance measurement and public reporting
2. Develop a national strategy for measuring and reporting health care quality
3. Standardize health care performance measures so that comparable data are available across the nation (i.e., establish national voluntary consensus standards)
4. Promote consumer understanding and use of health care performance measures and other quality information
5. Promote and encourage the enhancement of system capacity to evaluate and report on health care quality

At this time, the NQF has endorsed several condition-specific performance measure sets that address the quality of patient care across the continuum. For instance, sets of measures that can be used to evaluate the quality of hospital care cover conditions such as the following:

- Acute coronary artery syndrome
- Cerebrovascular disease
- Heart failure
- Pneumonia
- Pregnancy/childbirth/neonatal conditions

Many of the condition-specific measures in the NQF measure sets are being used by CMS, The Joint Commission, NCQA, and other accrediting and regulatory groups to evaluate the performance of HCOs. Information about the work of the NQF and the measure development and dissemination process can be found on the NQF Web site.

Although there are numerous factors influencing health care performance management and differing stakeholder incentives and priorities, the fundamental elements are constant: performance measurement, assessment, and improvement. These are the basic building blocks of performance management. To promote a systematic organization-wide quality management approach, providers may have a written performance management plan. This plan describes the organization's structure and processes for measuring, assessing, and improving performance.

As the health care delivery system struggles to achieve a balance between costs and access, performance management and clinical outcomes become increasingly important. HCOs and other players in the industry will inevitably compete in terms of quality. Orme[11] succinctly describes the goals of **quality improvement** (QI) efforts in health care as "to improve the processes of delivering care and thereby increase customer satisfaction with the quality of care (service outcomes), to improve the functional health of patients (clinical outcomes), and to reduce the costs of providing care."

As Collopy[12] noted, "the constant dilemma in the health care industry as opposed to industry in general is that of maximizing versus optimizing: clinicians must aim for the best outcome of care and health care managers at the 'macro' level are constrained, by a limitation of resources, to aim for an optimal level of care." Goldsmith[13] argued that "the real issue… is not quality per se, but value." Here again, a consensual definition of "value" may not be achievable between recipients and providers. Enmeshed in this ambivalent environment, medical and administrative leaders in HCOs strive to integrate performance measurement processes, to ensure consistent achievement of desired performance standards, and to communicate a genuine consumer orientation through patient-centered care.

to the materials or resources used in a process, such x-ray film and the radiographer's time. Output is the product of a process, such as a transcribed record document or a completed diagnostic test. Outcome is the end results of a process, such as a "complete" health record or a patient's satisfactory physical condition after a surgical procedure. Efficiency refers to "doing things right," or using an acceptable ratio of resources used to output or outcome achieved. Five ruined films before an acceptable diagnostic image is achieved would not be considered efficient! Effectiveness refers to "doing the right thing." For example, using only the appropriate diagnostic tests to establish a treatment plan that returns a patient to a state of wellness is effective.

In recent years medical professionals have increasingly relied on **evidence-based medicine** (EBM) to select the "right thing" to do for patient. EBM involves the use of current best research evidence in making decisions about the care of individual patients. This research is incorporated into **clinical practice guidelines**—statements of the right things to do for patients with a particular diagnosis or medical condition. Hundreds of examples of evidence-based clinical practice guidelines can be found on the Internet at the National Guideline Clearinghouse sponsored by the Agency for Healthcare Research and Quality.

Performance measures are composed of a number and a unit of measure. The number provides the magnitude (how much) and the unit is what gives the number its meaning (what). For example, "100% of all patients undergoing hip replacement surgery will receive prophylactic antibiotics as specified by the treatment protocol" is an example of a performance measure. Performance measures are often described as "indicators." As implied by the general usage of the term, an **indicator** is an indirect measure. It describes events or patterns of events suggestive of a problematic process or behavior. The Joint Commission defines an indicator as "a quantitative instrument that is used to measure the extent to which an organization or component thereof carries out the right processes, carries out those processes well, and achieves desired outcomes as a result of carrying out the right processes well."[14] An example of an indicator is having a history and physical examination documented in the health record before surgery. Records can be screened to determine when the history and physical examination was documented and compare the timing with the date/time of surgery. **Performance measurement** is a strategic process used to assess accomplishment of goals and objectives. The process of performance measurement involves review of many different performance measures or indicators·

PERFORMANCE MEASUREMENT

Performance measure is a generic term used to describe a particular value or characteristic designated to measure input, output, outcome, efficiency, or effectiveness. Input refers

STRUCTURE, PROCESS, AND OUTCOME MEASURES

Avedis Donabedian's early work in the definition and assessment of health care quality resulted in one of the most widely acknowledged and conceptually sound models for measuring quality in health care. As a prelude to defining quality, Donabedian dichotomized "care" into technical and interpersonal domains.[15] The technical domain encompasses the science and technology components of medicine ("science"); the interpersonal domain refers to social and psychological interactions between the practitioner and patient ("art"). He further acknowledged an element of care he called "amenities," or what might be generally called satisfiers. Amenities include such features as comfortable and clean surroundings, good food, and personal convenience items. Donabedian used these domains to conceptualize quality as a property of and judgment about some definable unit of care.

Under Donabedian's model, technical quality is quantified as the degree to which the benefits of using medical science and technology are maximized and associated risks are minimized. Defining quality in the interpersonal domain is more nebulous because measures of values, norms, and expectations are less well defined. Most measures attempt to quantify expectations and the degree to which expectations were met. Donabedian did not attempt to quantify the amenities element of care but considered it a notable contributor to patient satisfaction with interpersonal interactions.

Expanding on the domain definition of care, Donabedian defined three approaches to assessing quality of care indirectly by using measures that examine structures, processes, and outcomes associated with the delivery of health care. Table 13-1 defines the approaches and provides examples of measures frequently used to evaluate the quality of care or services provided by individuals and organizations.

Structure Measures

Structure measures indirectly assess care by looking at certain provider characteristics and the physical and organizational resources available to support the delivery of care. Structure measures essentially look at the capability or potential for providing quality care. By their nature, structure measures are static: the organization or individual is evaluated at a unique point in time. The organizational structure of a facility, operational policies and procedures, technological capabilities, compliance with safety regulations, and competency assessment at the time of initial use all are examples of structure measures.

Process Measures

Process measures focus on the interactions between patients and providers. Process-oriented measures examine an individual health care professional's decision-making processes as they direct a patient's course of treatment or, at the organization level, investigate the procedures that guide operational decisions. Examples of process measures include peer review of patient records indicating problems with patient care or documentation, compliance with discharge planning procedures, and patient waiting time in the emergency department before triage. Process measures are often used to evaluate compliance with clinical practice guideline recommendations.

Outcome Measures

Outcome measures look at the end results or product of the patient's encounter with the system. One of the most commonly used outcome measures in acute health care settings is patient mortality rates. Although the mortality rate is certainly an important measure, other variables may be necessary to examine the quality of care provided to patients. For instance, what if the patient's diagnosis is terminal metastatic carcinoma? Would death suggest poor quality care for this patient? Measures such as adequate pain control and adherence to living will requirements might be more appropriate. Other examples of outcome measures that address categories of patients rather than individual patient outcomes include comparison of patient lengths of stay with regional norms, infection and complication rate review, and the number of transfers to another inpatient facility.

Table 13-1   DONABEDIAN'S MODEL OF STRUCTURE, PROCESS, AND OUTCOME

	Individual	Department	Organization
Structure	Professional certification Credential review	Staffing analysis Equipment safety	Licensure Fire safety inspections
Process	Peer reviews Performance evaluations Productivity monitors	Review of performance indicators Flow process analysis	Infection surveillance Review of utilization data
Outcome	Practice profiles Rework required	Error/complication rate analysis	Mortality rates Quality sanctions

We want to know: For patients recovering from surgery, is the patient's pain assessed and documented every 2 hours while awake for the first 24 hours following surgery?

Raw data needed: The number of patients whose pain was assessed and documented every 2 hours while awake for the first 24 hours following surgery.

Performance measure:

$$\frac{\text{\# cases meeting criteria}}{\text{\# surgery cases (total)}} \times 100$$

Data collection strategy: Records of consecutive surgery patients will be reviewed and results reported monthly.

Figure 13-1 Example performance measure.

Developing Performance Measures

The choice of performance measures is an important consideration for an HCO because it is impossible to measure all aspects of patient care and services. Several factors must be considered when performance measures are selected. These factors include the following[16]:

- External accreditation and regulatory requirements
- National quality measurement priorities
- Clinical importance
- Strategic priorities of the HCO
- Available resources
- Reporting techniques and analytic tools

The measures chosen by many HCOs often are those developed by national groups that sponsor comparative performance databases. For instance, CMS has several health care measurement projects involving hospitals, home health agencies, skilled nursing facilities, and other providers. For instance, the CMS and the Centers for Disease Control and Prevention (CDC) are working together to conduct a national health care quality improvement project aimed at preventing postoperative infections. The project's goal is to improve the selection and timing of administration of prophylactic antibiotics, both important factors in effective prophylaxis. Surgical procedures studied for the surgical infection prevention (SIP) project include coronary artery bypass graft (CABG), cardiac procedures, colon procedures, hip and knee arthroplasty, abdominal and vaginal hysterectomy, and selected vascular surgery procedures. The performance measures for this project are listed in Table 13-2.[17] Details about the performance measures in the CMS quality improvement projects and in the comparative measurement projects sponsored by other regulatory agencies, accreditation bodies, and professional groups can be found on the Agency for Healthcare Research and Quality Web site.

Development of a performance measure involves three basic steps:

1. Identifying what you want to know.
2. Identifying the raw data necessary for creating the measure.
3. Defining a data collection strategy.

These steps are illustrated in Figure 13-1 for a measure of postoperative pain management.

Performance measures are typically classified as one of two types: important single events or patterns of events evident in **aggregate data**. Aggregate data are related primary data that have been compiled into meaningful categories to facilitate analysis and understanding. An important single event is an infrequently occurring undesirable happening of such magnitude that each occurrence warrants further investigation. Examples are unexpected obstetrical death, severe transfusion reaction, and surgery on the wrong body part. When an important single event occurs, there is an immediate investigation to determine the cause and to initiate corrective actions to prevent the event from recurring. These events, often referred to as sentinel events, will be discussed in greater detail in relation to patient safety.

The second type of measure (patterns evidenced in aggregate data) reflects performance that, although un-

Table 13-2 EXAMPLE OF SURGICAL INFECTION PREVENTION PROJECT PERFORMANCE MEASURES

Performance Measures in the Surgical Infection Prevention Quality Improvement Project

- Proportion of patients who receive antibiotics within 1 hour before surgical incision
- Proportion of patients who receive prophylactic antibiotics consistent with current recommendations
- Proportion of patients whose prophylactic antibiotics were discontinued within 24 hours of surgery end time

desirable, is less dramatic or injurious than an important single event and can reasonably be expected to occur with some frequency. For example, hospital meal trays delivered late or delayed administration of medication are undesirable events but can be expected to occur in the normal course of operations. Typically, these types of events are monitored until the occurrences reach a predetermined **threshold** that triggers a **focused review** to initiate corrective action. For instance, a hospital monitoring compliance with the postoperative pain assessment measure illustrated above might set a threshold of 95% or less. When the measurement result falls below 95%, a focused review is conducted to determine the cause of the less-than-desired performance.

To achieve their potential value, performance measures must be **valid** and **reliable**. Validity refers to the following[18]:

- Degree to which all items in the measure relate to the performance being measured
- Extent to which all relevant aspects of performance are covered
- Extent to which the measure appears to measure what it is intended to measure

A reliable measure is stable, showing consistent results over time and among different users of the measure. A reliable measure has low levels of random error. For example, a properly calibrated scale will measure an individual's weight accurately each time he or she steps on the scale no matter who reads the weight value. A coding skills test would be valid if it accurately distinguishes between high-performing coders and low-performing coders. It would be reliable if the distinction is made each time the test is administered, even if the grader changes.

Collecting Measurement Data

Two types of paper-based forms are commonly used to gather performance measurement data. A **checksheet** is a form specially designed so that the results can be readily interpreted from the form itself. This form of data collection is ideal for capturing data concurrently (during actual delivery of patient care or services) because the employee can interpret the results and take corrective actions immediately. A **data sheet** is a form designed to collect data in a simple tabular or column format. Specific bits of data (e.g., numbers, words, or marks) are entered in spaces on the sheet. As a result, additional processing is typically required after the data are collected to construct the performance measure. Illustrated in Figure 13-2 is a data sheet used to capture information about the occurrence of specific events that might take place during a patient's hospitalization. One form is completed for each patient record reviewed. Although the example shown is a paper form, the data could be captured in an electronic form or simply entered into a spreadsheet or database application. Those tasked with performing the data collection should understand the data definitions (the exact intended meaning of the variables being collected), have the necessary forms at hand, and be trained in the data collection process such as where in the record this data item should be collected.

With the growth in electronic health records (EHRs), data that were previously gathered manually will likely be available in electronic format. This will reduce, but not totally eliminate, the need for manual data gathering. Even when an HCO has a central data repository for information about patients and their health care experiences, it may be necessary to gather information from other sources. Data warehouse systems provide consolidated and consistent historical data about patient care activities; however, careful planning is necessary to ensure that the information supports performance measurement activities.

A vital element of data collection is the need for accuracy. Inaccurate data may give the wrong answer to questions about performance. One of the most troublesome sources of error is called bias. It is important to understand bias and to allow for this during the development and implementation of any data collection system. Well-designed data collection strategies and processes can reduce bias. Some types of biases that may occur include the following:

- Some part of the process or the data has been left out of the data collection process.
- The data collection itself interferes with the process it is measuring.
- The data collector biases (distorts) the data.
- The data collection procedures were not followed or were incorrect or ambiguous.
- Some of the data are missing or not obtained.
- The time period or frequency selected for data collection distorts the data, typically by missing significant events or cyclical occurrences.

The role of health information management (HIM) professionals in ensuring valid and reliable data collection is significant. From the front-end capture of data to back-end reporting of measurement results, no nonclinical department has greater influence.[19] As coordinators of data quality, HIM professionals can influence consistent recording and capture of data that later becomes performance measurement information that can assist in monitoring data quality.

PERFORMANCE ASSESSMENT

Performance assessment (sometimes called evaluation, appraisal, or rating) involves a formal periodical review of performance measurement results. If the data collection strategy has been carefully planned, the HIM professional should end up with data that provide a good understanding of performance. Once the performance data have been verified for accuracy, it is time for the assessment phase.

SAMPLE HOSPITAL

Unexpected Outcomes
Occurrence Screening Report

INDICATOR	PRESENT
1. Unexpected transfer to another acute facility.	
2. Unscheduled return to operating room.	
3. Unplanned organ removal/repair subsequent to or during surgery.	
4. Neurological deficit not present on admission.	
5. Patient fall resulting in injury.	
6. Nosocomial infection.	
7. Hospital-acquired decubitus.	
8. Unscheduled admission following outpatient surgery.	
9. Patient discharged against medical advice.	
10. Post-surgical death.	
11. Medication error or adverse drug reaction.	
12. Transfusion error or transfusion reaction.	
13. Return to intensive care unit within 24 hours of transfer to nursing unit.	
14. Abnormal physiological findings documented without further investigation or resolution.	
15. Complications attributed to anesthesia.	

Figure 13-2 Generic quality screens.

However, before the results can be analyzed, the information needs to be assembled and presented in a meaningful way. The performance data should help people answer the following questions:

- What is the current performance?
- Is there a trend over time?
- Should we take any action? What kind of action?
- What contributes the most to undesirable performance (the vital few)?
- Are we focusing on the highest priority actions?

Reports for Analysis

To facilitate performance assessment, data must be presented in a format that makes it easier to draw conclusions. This grouping or summarizing may take several forms: tabulation, graphs, or statistical comparisons. Sometimes a single data grouping will suffice for the purposes of performance measurement. Where larger amounts of data must be dealt with, multiple groupings are essential for creating a clear base for analysis. Spreadsheets and databases are useful for organizing and categorizing performance measurement data to show trends. Performance measurement reports may take many forms. Some of the more common graphical presentations are histograms, bar charts, pie charts, line graphs, and control charts. These presentation formats are described in greater detail later in this chapter.

At the assessment stage, the objective is to transfer information to the responsible decision makers. Reports will likely consist of sets of tables or charts of performance measurement results, supplemented with basic conclusions. Before actually presenting any performance information, it is beneficial to evaluate and understand a few key factors:

- Who is the audience?
- What is the intended use of the data? Will it be used to support decisions and take actions or is it just to monitor performance?
- What is the basic message you want to communicate (here is where we are and how we are doing)?
- What is the best presentation format (report, brochure, oral presentation, etc.)?

The image provided by a well-constructed graph or table is often the most compelling way to communicate performance measurement data. Statistical tools can elaborate on the story told by the graphs or tables and provide validation for the information displayed on the graph or table. Two fundamental concepts are important in statistics: *summarizing* numbers and *distributions*. Summarizing numbers condenses information from many numbers into one meaningful number (e.g., mean, median). Distribution is an association between different values of a variable and a summarizing number that quantifies that association (e.g., range, standard deviation).

Performance Goals and Targets

In years past, HCOs judged their performance one patient at a time. It wasn't until 1917, when the American College of Surgeons developed minimum hospital standards, that hospitals began to look more closely at performance in the aggregate (e.g., mortality rates, complication rates). In 1953, when The Joint Commission took over the Hospital Standardization Program from the College of Surgeons, new performance measurement requirements were gradually added. However, even then performance assessment was still done in a vacuum. A provider evaluated its current data and compared the results with its own past performance; asking questions such as the following: Is our mortality rate going up or down? Have complications decreased over the past years' performance? Before the mid-1980s it was rare to find a provider that assessed its performance on the basis of what other providers were able to achieve. For the most part, comparative health care performance data was hard to come by. Today, instead of evaluating performance on the basis of past performance alone, HCOs have all kinds of tools at their disposal for assessing the quality and safety of clinical services.

HCOs may use their own historical performance rates to establish thresholds and comparative data from other providers to establish targets for performance rates. The threshold is the minimum acceptable quality, based on the organization's historical performance. The target is the "stretch goal" based on comparative data. If there is no significant variance from thresholds or targets, then data collection continues. If there is a variance between the performance goal and the measurement results, then the magnitude is evaluated. If it is significant, corrective action may be warranted. In many cases, "significance" is defined statistically. For example, the mean value for length of stay between two calendar quarters may differ in raw numbers but be accounted for by random variation. Thus, the difference would not be statistically significant. Significance may also be "practical," in the sense that the difference "matters," even if not statistically significant. Performance variation related to patient safety issues may be addressed even if the variation is not statistically significant.

Use of Comparative Data

Benchmarking, or comparing an organization's performance against organizations that have been identified as excellent, once was thought of as a costly and time-intensive venture undertaken only for processes critical to successful operations. As the health care environment becomes increasingly competitive and cost conscious, benchmarking is becoming a commonly used tool for gathering data and identifying ways to improve processes and initiate change at all operational levels. Most benchmarking processes are derived from the model developed by Xerox in the early 1980s. Organizations adapt, modify, and rearrange various steps to fit their goals. A generic model is shown in Figure 13-3.

Basically, three types of benchmarking are used to stimulate the improvement process. *Internal benchmarking* compares performance between functional areas or departments within an organization. The goal is to decrease or eliminate errors in existing processes or to improve the efficiency of the process. A health care organization might use this approach to decrease patient wait time in departments or work units where diagnostic tests are conducted. Time and money investment is minimal.

Competitive benchmarking, sometimes called performance benchmarking, is used to close the gap between an organization's performance and that of its industry competitor(s). Such efforts often examine safety, vendor or supplier relationships, and operational cost controls. Data collected from public sources or databases may be helpful for analyzing trends or identifying performance patterns.

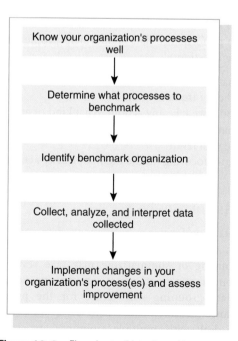

Figure 13-3 Flowchart of benchmarking process.

Sharing information with noncompeting organizations, or strategic benchmarking, can have very good returns for limited investment of time and money. However, getting the type and amount of the data required to understand a competitor's process well enough to replicate it may be difficult.

Comparative benchmarking involves examining a process in another industry to apply the principles that make it effective to a similar process. For example, an HCO might examine the ticket sales and itinerary planning process in the airline industry to improve its patient registration and scheduling processes.

PERFORMANCE IMPROVEMENT

A profusion of published literature is available describing problem-solving approaches, promoting a plethora of tools and techniques for data collection and analysis, and touting critical success factors to implementing performance improvement in an organization. The sheer volume and diversity of information available can be overwhelming. Most HCOs currently use integrated, organization-wide systems to ensure conformance to standards of performance and continual improvement.

Performance Improvement Models

An improvement model is a description of the steps required to achieve better performance. Most performance models are essentially variations on the scientific method (i.e., controlled, systematic investigation of empirical evidence). The most commonly used model of performance improvement is the Plan-Do-Check-Act (PDCA) method developed in the 1920s by Walter Shewhart and popularized in Japan by Deming (Figure 13-4).[20]

The PDCA improvement model is not written in a straight line for a reason. It is intended to be a model that is applied through recurring improvement cycles, as described below.

1. **Plan** for improvements. How is the process performing? What are the constraints to improvement? What are you trying to accomplish? Develop improvement actions on the basis of the evidence. A question to be answered during the plan stage: How will you know if a change is improvement? Select process measures that correlate with expected results and make predictions of how the changes will affect performance.
2. **Do** the improvement actions. On a small scale, perhaps a pilot test in one area, implement the process changes that are expected to achieve better performance. Collect data that can be used to accurately assess the effect of these process changes.
3. **Check** the results of improvement actions. Compare the effects of the process changes with the predicted

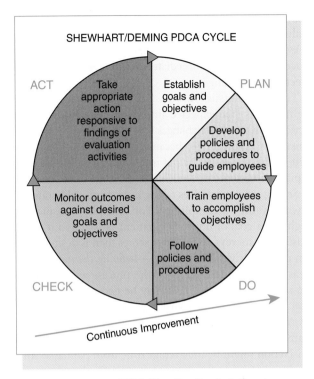

Figure 13-4 PCDA (Plan, Do, Check, Act) cycle.

outcomes. When expectations are realized the theories about what will work (the plan) has been supported and the changes are implemented on a wider scale. When expected performance is not realized, the theories about what would work are wrong (not validated).

4. **Act** on the evidence. Make the changes permanent, run new trials, revise improvement actions, or whatever is appropriate to the findings. Share the learning from the project with other people in the organization—the specifics of the process improvements and the general change principles—so that others may benefit from the lessons learned. Sharing is key to organizational learning and continuous improvement.

HCOs are also implementing performance improvement models, derived from the PDCA cycle, that been shown to be effective in business and manufacturing applications. Some of the approaches that have made the transition to health care well include **Rapid Cycle Improvement, Six Sigma,** and **Lean Thinking**.

Rapid Cycle Improvement

Rapid cycle improvement (RCI) has been successfully applied to improving both the operational aspects of health care delivery and clinical patient care processes. RCI is based on the PDCA model,[20] using an accelerated method (usually less than 4 to 6 weeks per improvement cycle) to collect and analyze data and make informed changes based on that analysis. This is then followed by another improvement cycle to evaluate the success of the change. RCI relies on small process changes and immediate, careful measurement of the effect of these changes.

The model entails four steps: set the aim (the goal), define the measures (the expected improvements), make changes (action plan); and test changes (the solution). The process is considered "rapid cycle" because it focuses on small, concrete changes that can be put into action quickly, usually in a "pilot" situation.

Setting the aim involves taking a clear and deliberate look at what is to be accomplished. For example, a hospice unit might set a goal of improving patient satisfaction if patient satisfaction surveys reveal lower scores than is desirable. The aim or goal drives the next step—*defining the measure*. The measure should describe what the process will accomplish if a solution is successful. It may be necessary to set more than one measure for a goal, and the focus should be on key measures that address the goal as directly as possible. For example, a measure to meet the goal of improving patient satisfaction might be the average time from pain assessment to administration of appropriate medication.

The third step is to *select process changes* that are expected to achieve the aim. Although many organizations search relevant literature for ideas for process changes, frontline staff and project team members can be invaluable sources. Possible processes to investigate for the example presented

might be those related to medication ordering and administration.

The last RCI step is to *test the changes* using a rapid-cycle PDCA process. Evaluating the solution in a very short time is a key factor. If the changes do not work, iterative PDCA cycles are initiated until a workable solution is found. Repetition of the improvement cycles leads to continuous improvement and facilitates creation of internal performance benchmarks.

Many health care improvement initiatives use the RCI model, including the breakthrough projects sponsored by the Institute for Health Care Improvement and the Medicare quality improvement initiatives sponsored by the CMS and overseen by the state Quality Improvement Organizations.

Six Sigma

Like many other quality and performance improvement approaches, **Six Sigma** has its roots in the manufacturing industry. In recent years, health care organizations have begun using the tools of Six Sigma with good results (Figure 13-5). In the late 1980s Motorola began an initiative to eliminate defects and improve the efficiency of their operations. Their overall goal was to reduce defective work so that they could deliver their products at a lower cost while offering superior customer service. Motorola's approach came to be known as Six Sigma, derived from the Greek symbol sigma (σ), used by statisticians to denote the measure of standard deviation of a population. Standard

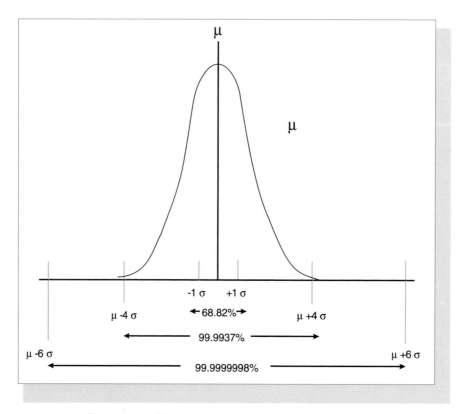

Figure 13-5 Diagram of a distribution illustrating Six Sigma.

deviation is a measure of variability. In a normal distribution, approximately 99% (more precisely, 99.99966%) of all events or observations will fall within + three standard deviations from the mean ("six sigma").

In Six Sigma terminology, results that fail to meet performance standards are called "defects," typically reported as defects per million opportunities. Six Sigma is the performance level attained when a process yields only 3.4 defects per million opportunities. The goal is to achieve an almost perfect level of quality (defect free). This requires understanding and eliminating defects in a process to move continually closer to the goal of "six sigma."

Six Sigma projects follow a highly structured process of five sequential steps: defining the problem, measuring the problem, analyzing the data, improving the system, and controlling and sustaining the improvement. Taking the first letter from each of these steps creates an acronym, DMAIC (pronounced as *dee-MAY-ick*), that is typically used to label the method.

Problem definition requires knowing the customers of the process and their requirements (both output and service). Once customer wants are known, it is possible to *measure performance* against these requirements. Measuring and sampling systems are required to know what is actually happening in the processes. The data collected are used to calculate a Six Sigma score for the process. *Analysis of the information and hard facts* obtained through measurement activities leads to prioritizing the potential causes of the problems being investigated. At this time, an initial hypothesis of the cause should be formulated. Further information analysis is conducted until the root cause of the problem has been identified. Potential solutions should be assigned a priority on the basis of the probability of solving the problem and the ease and cost of implementing them. After *a solution for improvement has been implemented*, the Sigma score for the process should be calculated to quantify the improvements made. Performance measures should be established to capture deviations from standards and to predict future problems before they occur and to *sustain the improvement.*

Lean Thinking

In the 1980s Japanese success in the global marketplace brought QI philosophies and techniques to international attention. Although initially applied in the manufacturing sector, these principles are now gaining popularity in the service sectors, including health care. One example is the Toyota Production System, also called "lean manufacturing" or "lean thinking."[21] Often, lean thinking is a natural complement to Six Sigma. For example, the data gathered while analyzing a process flow can be used to identify high priority/high impact areas for Six Sigma projects. In general, the principles of leaning thinking are as follow:

- Eliminate waste and retain only value-added activities
- Concentrate on improving value-added activities

- Respond to the voice of the customer
- Optimize processes across the organization.

The central tenet of lean thinking is value—providing "perfect" value to the customer by using only value-adding processes and eliminating waste. Value-adding activities are those steps in a process that contribute to the organization's overall goals and business objectives. In short, value is defined by those processes and activities where outcomes are meaningful to the customer and lead to their purchase decisions.

In health care, this means that every process should add to the value of the services provided to patients, their families, and other customers. Although activities such as diagnostic testing are of obvious value, others are more difficult to "see." For example, clerical services may seem unrelated to the patient's view of the care they received. At the structural level, however, clerical inefficiencies may compromise the organization's ability to provide excellent patient care.

Applying lean thinking techniques requires viewing every activity in the organization as supporting a customer, either directly or indirectly. Those activities that do not support customers are not value adding. Eliminating waste and non-value-adding activities requires a focus on the entire value chain of a process or linked processes. Health care managers must concentrate on optimizing the flow along the entire **value chain** and forego manipulation of separate tasks and activities in their efforts to improve performance.

Cursory reviews of process elements and quick fixes rarely produce long-lasting performance improvement. Adequate data collection and process analysis based on facts, not opinions, are essential to success. The amount of data required depends on the nature and condition of the processes. Optimizing the process flow comes from having the right data and knowing how to use it.

Fundamentally, "going lean" is a process improvement method that involves two primary techniques:

1. Analyzing each step of the process to determine which steps add value and which do not. This requires asking such questions as:
   - Does this step create value for the customer?
   - Is it capable of producing a good result every time?
   - Is it able to produce the right result at the right time?
   - Is the capacity adequate so that wait time is not excessive, or is there too much capacity?
2. Linking the value-added steps to optimize process flow and eliminate the unnecessary steps. This requires asking such questions as:
   - Do all the steps in the process occur in a tight sequence with little waiting? Does the information flow smoothly?
   - Does each step only occur at the command of the next downstream step, within the time available?
   - Are demand signals filtered to remove unnecessary variation and leveled to smooth the workload?

Process Improvement Tools

Often people confuse performance improvement models with the tools and techniques used during application of the model. Although an HCO uses clearly defined steps for performance improvement initiatives, such as the PDCA model, during the life of an improvement project many different tools may be used. As performance management practices have evolved, greater emphasis has been placed on using structured analytical and evaluation techniques to measure and improve performance.

Although the list of available performance improvement tools is extensive, it can be collapsed into four general types of techniques:

- *Idea-generating* techniques generally use tools such as brainstorming, affinity diagrams, and other methods for capturing divergent thinking.
- *Data organization* methods usually involve tools such as matrices, cause-and-effect diagrams, and force field analyses.
- *Data evaluation* and *data presentation* methods include the use of tools such as histograms, run charts, Pareto charts, control charts, and correlation analysis.

Idea-Generating Techniques

Brainstorming is a structured but flexible process designed to maximize the number of ideas generated. It is primarily used in the exploratory phase of problem analysis and solution development.[22]

Brainstorming requires a leader who serves primarily as a facilitator and recorder and a team of six to ten persons brought together to generate ideas about a relevant issue.

The issue is defined, a time limit for discussion is set, and ideas are recorded for all team members to discuss. All ideas should be expressed vocally, and criticism should be avoided. The goal is to examine a large number of options. Brainstorming has become an integral part of performance management in response to emphasis on worker empowerment and the need to solicit various opinions from all levels of workers within an organization. A **nominal group technique** (NGT) is similar to brainstorming but uses silent generation of ideas and a sequential reporting approach to ensure participation by all group members.

Affinity diagrams may be used to bridge the gap between idea generation and data organization. After the initial brainstorming session, affinity diagrams often are used to organize and prioritize information into clusters or categories (Figure 13-6). Affinity diagrams are particularly useful when dealing with large amounts of complicated information. This technique reduces what may be considered an unmanageable amount of information into a smaller number of homogeneous groups. In addition to organizing information, affinity diagrams may be used effectively to generate new ideas and in solution planning. By organizing data into homogeneous groups, teams may begin to prioritize action according to importance, need, or resources for a particular issue. As in the case of brainstorming, time limits should be set to facilitate action and keep the amount of new information generated manageable.

Data Organization

Flowcharts are graphic representations of a specific sequencing of steps in a process. A flowchart can be an outline or schematic drawing of the actual process that

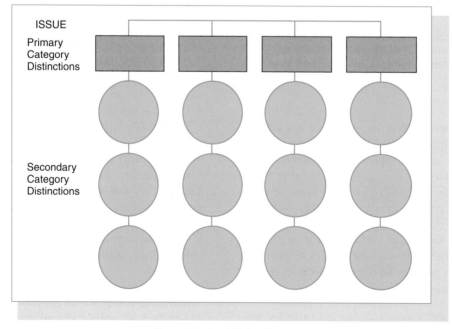

Figure 13-6 Affinity diagram.

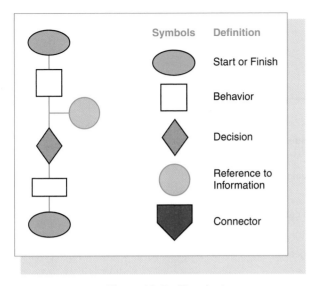

Figure 13-7 Flowchart.

needs improving or a picture of the *ideal* process once improvement actions are taken. A flowchart consists of a series of connected symbols that represent actual or expected process steps (Figure 13-7). Flowcharts are used during an improvement project to help people:

- Agree on the steps of a process and the order in which they occur
- See some of the duplicated effort and other non-value-added steps that might be lurking in a process
- Clarify working relationships between people and organizations
- Target specific steps in the process for improvement

Flowchart analysis begins by deciding on the starting and ending points. Tasks are sequentially arranged and decision-making points identified. The ultimate goal of flowchart analysis is to portray real-life situations accurately in an ordered and understandable format.

The **matrix** is a multidimensional tool that may be used to organize, categorize, and reduce information into a more usable form. As an organization and data reduction tool, the matrix may be used in the decision-making process by weighting information or in the evaluation of performance over an extended period. In addition to focusing on internal processes, the matrix may be used to examine influences of external factors (e.g., economic conditions). To use the matrix, first identify the information to be collected. After the information is collected, develop relevant categories that may be maintained over time. The matrix is used in conjunction with both qualitative and quantitative methods to store and retrieve data for performance evaluation or in various aspects of the decision-making process. The matrix allows for a quick reference to information over time by synthesizing and integrating ideas into manageable structures. For example, a decision matrix would be useful to compare various characteristics of information systems to determine which one is the best fit with established criteria.

Cause-and-effect diagrams are useful tools for solving complicated problems by helping people consider many factors and the cause-and-effect relationships between those factors. They are also called **fishbone diagrams** because they look something like fish skeletons (Figure 13-8). Cause-and-effect diagrams are particularly useful in the plan phase of the PDCA cycle. Constructing a fishbone diagram requires only a few simple steps. First, an outcome variable or goal is placed on the right side of the diagram at the end of the horizontal causal line. Second, major causes are directly linked to the causal line in an ordered sequence. Finally, minor causes are linked to each of the major causes along the time line. Often brainstorming is used to generate a list of major and minor causes. The completed diagram provides a

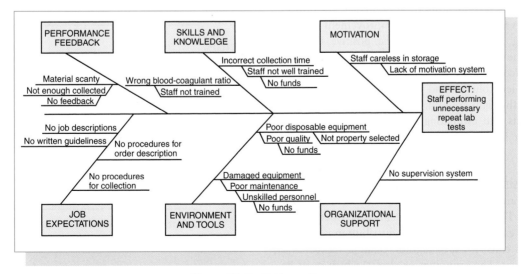

Figure 13-8 Fishbone diagram.

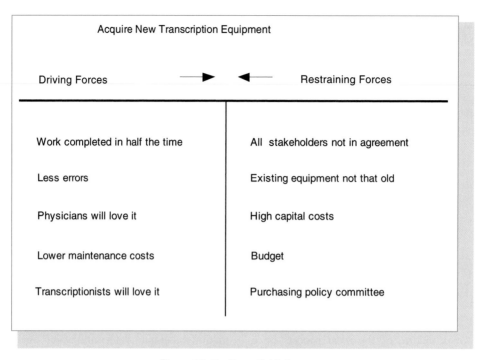

Figure 13-9 Force field diagram.

focus for identification of root causes and development of plans for improvement.

Force field analysis is similar to fishbone analysis in that it connects process variables to outcomes. In addition to identifying the causal order, force field analysis estimates the relative effect of each process variable (such as the number of available trained workers) on an outcome variable (such as increasing the number of outpatient visits). Force field analysis is used to identify the variables that help and variables that hinder reaching the desired outcome or solution to a problem. It depicts the situation as a balance between two sets of forces: one that tries to change the status quo and one that tries to maintain it (Figure 13-9). This tool is particularly useful during the Plan stage of the PDCA cycle when it is often important to reduce the impact of process variables hindering improvement plans. Brainstorming is used to identify the positive (driving forces) and the negative (inhibiting forces) to achieving a particular outcome. Expected positive effects (drivers) are placed in the left column, and negative effects (inhibitors) are placed in the right column. By identifying positive and negative effects and estimating the relative effect of each variable, both helping and hindering factors are visually identified.

Data Analysis and Presentation

Histograms are graphic representations of frequency distributions. They are useful for identifying whether the variation that exists in the frequency distribution is normal or skewed. To construct a histogram, create a vertical and a horizontal axis. The groupings or classes, which must be *continuous* data, are shown as contiguous bars placed on the horizontal axis. The frequency of occurrence for each class is plotted on the vertical axis, with the height of the bar representing the count. A **bar chart** is used to report count values of *categorical* data, such as the number of outpatient visits for each day of the week. The categories are labeled on the horizontal axis with the frequency count plotted on the y-axis (Figure 13-10). This may seem similar in appearance to a histograms; however, the bars are separated as the x-axis is a label, not a continuous variable.

Run charts and **line graphs** provide a simple, yet highly graphic, visual method of monitoring trends over time. A run chart can illustrate performance trends and standards

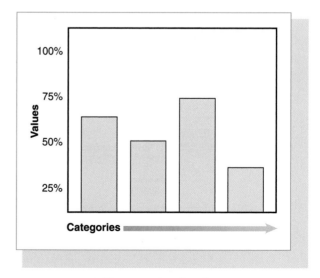

Figure 13-10 Bar chart.

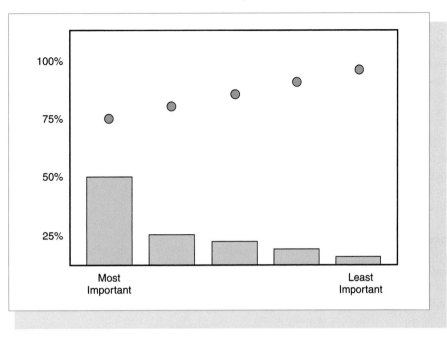

Figure 13-11 Pareto chart.

of evaluation over a long time period. First, decide the time period for which data are to be collected and analyzed (e.g., continual or time restricted). Second, draw a graph with a vertical and a horizontal axis. Here, the horizontal axis indicates increments of time, and the vertical axis indicates increments of measurement. Finally, plot the data points and evaluate any trends evident in the data.

Pareto charts are similar in form to bar charts and histograms. The primary difference is that occurrences plotted on a Pareto chart are ordered from the largest or most frequently occurring category (and presumably most important) to the smallest or least frequently occurring category (Figure 13-11). First, select the types of causes and conditions to be studied. Second, determine the standard for comparison (i.e., frequency, cost, or amount). Third, draw the vertical and horizontal axes. Label the vertical axis with standards used for comparisons and the horizontal axis with categories. Finally, draw bars that represent the frequency of each factor according to a predetermined rank ordering. Pareto charts often are used in conjunction with brainstorming as a visual aid to demonstrate where attention to specific problems should be focused. A second y-axis may be used to plot a cumulative frequency curve as an additional visual tool to establish the relative magnitude of a class.

Control charts are data display tools used to monitor performance (Figure 13-12). Although control charts may look similar to run charts or line graphs, they add another dimension to performance analysis—that is, the ability to determine whether a process is statistically in control. To do that you need a control chart. In the 1920s Walter A Shewhart, a physicist, was charged with improving the

quality of telephones in Bell Laboratories. Shewhart developed a theory of process variation which forms the basis of **statistical process control** (SPC).[23] The critical feature of Shewhart's theory of variation is that it categorizes variation according to the action needed to reduce it. To reduce common cause variation, one must act on the process. To reduce special cause variation, one must find and act on the special cause(s). Common cause variation is due to routine, random events. For example, a clerk assembles 10 records the first hour. However, the second group of records contains more documents than the first group and the clerk only assembles eight records in the second hour. Special cause variation is not random and is due to an unusual event. For example, a clerk can routinely photocopy documents at an average rate of 50 pages per minute. If a paper

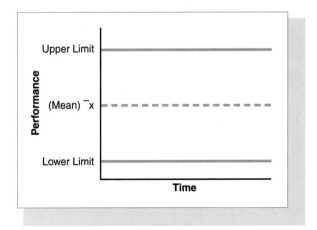

Figure 13-12 Control chart.

jam occurs, the time taken to correct the jam and reset the documents will extend the average rate of production. To help distinguish between these two kinds of variation, Shewhart devised the control chart. Control charts have three important lines. The central line is the mean or median, and the upper and lower lines are termed control limits. Data points outside the control limits (or unusual data patterns) indicate a special cause that should be found and eliminated.[24]

The simplest control chart is the *individuals chart*. This chart is used for processes that produce one value in each time frame. An example of this might be daily output from coding staff. To use this kind of chart, the data should have a normal distribution. To create an individuals control chart (Box 13-1), 20 or more data points are needed. Fifteen is the absolute minimum.

If all the values plotted on a control chart are within the control limit lines and there are no trends or tendencies that indicate otherwise, the process is considered in control. *In control* means that only *common cause* or chance variation is affecting the process. If a process is in control, it is possible to predict what future performance will be without improving the process. Processes are predictable only if they are *in control*, that is, unaffected by extraordinary or *special cause variation*. The usefulness of the control chart is enhanced when it is integrated with other performance improvement tools such as cause-and-effect diagrams, Pareto charts, and flowcharts.

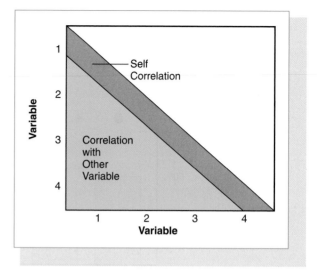

Figure 13-13 Correlation table.

Correlation analysis determines the strength, direction, and statistical significance of a relationship between one or more performance variables (Figure 13-13). Correlation coefficients provide an exact interpretation of the relationship noted on the run chart. In correlation analysis, scores range from -1.0, signifying a perfect negative relationship, to 0.0, signifying no relationship, to 1.0, signifying a perfect positive relationship (See Figure 13-13). To use correlation analysis, first select variables with relationship of interest. Second, set the acceptance level of significance. Finally, examine the coefficients to determine significance, direction (positive or negative), and strength of association. Correlation analysis provides easily interpretable numbers and a straightforward method of examining relationships between various performance measures. Figure 13-14 lists the steps of an improvement project and the tools that may be used during each of these steps.

PATIENT SAFETY

Driven by media attention and growing concerns about the costs associated with medical mistakes, patient safety improvement has become a national imperative. Although some believe that purchasers and consumers are having the greatest influence on patient safety improvement activities, a recent study found that The Joint Commission has been the primary driver of hospitals' patient safety initiatives.[25] Professional and market initiatives have also facilitated improvement, but hospitals report that these have had less impact to date. The National Patient Safety Goals issued by The Joint Commission each year have strongly influenced adoption of safer patient care practices in all provider sites.

Starting in 2003, The Joint Commission published National Patient Safety Goals to promote specific

---

Box 13-1   STEPS TO CREATE A CONTROL CHART

1. List the data points in time order.
2. Determine the range between each of the consecutive data points. The range is the absolute difference between two consecutive data points. The range is always positive, even if the next data point is lower than the one being compared with. There will be one less range value than there are data points.
3. Find the mean range. To do this, total the ranges and divide by the number of range values. The symbol for the mean range is $\bar{R}$.
4. Find the mean or average of the data point values. To do this, total the values of all the data points and divide by the number of data points. The symbol for the mean data value is $\bar{X}$.
5. Calculate the control limits. [2.66 $\bar{R}$ = 3σ.] Upper Control Limit = $\bar{X}$ + (2.66 $\bar{R}$) Lower Control Limit = $\bar{X}$ - (2.66 $\bar{R}$)
6. Draw a solid horizontal line representing the data mean. Label the line and write the actual mean value next to it.
7. Draw two dotted horizontal lines representing the upper and lower control limits. Label the two control limit lines and write the actual upper and the lower limits next to them.
8. Plot the data points in time sequence. Connect each point to the next point in the sequence with a line.

Performance Improvement Tools and Techniques	Performance Improvement Steps				
	Identify opportunity	Analyze the process	Generate solutions	Implement solutions	Evaluate results
Brainstorming	X	X	X		
Norminal group technique	X	X			
Affinity diagram	X	X			
Flowchart	X	X	X		
Matrix	X	X			
Cause and effect diagram		X			
Force field analysis			X	X	
Histogram	X	X			X
Bar chart	X	X			X
Run chart/ line graph	X	X			X
Pareto chart	X	X			X
Control chart	X	X			X

Figure 13-14 Example tools used in performance improvement.

improvements in patient safety. Accredited organizations are evaluated for continuous compliance with the specific requirements associated with these goals. For example, one of the 2006 goals applicable to all accredited organizations is to improve the accuracy of patient identification. Providers are expected to use at least two patient identifiers (neither to be the patient's room number) whenever administering medications or blood products; taking blood samples and other specimens for clinical testing, or providing any other treatments or procedures. The current National Patient Safety Goals can be found on The Joint Commission Web site.

It can sometimes be difficult to differentiate between patient safety improvement and other types of health care performance management activities. In truth, there is no clear-cut distinction. For the purposes of this text, **patient safety improvement** is defined as the actions undertaken by individuals and organizations to protect health care recipients from being harmed by the effects of health care services.

Patient safety improvement involves the familiar performance management building blocks: measurement, assessment, and improvement. Many of the same process improvement tools described earlier in this chapter can also be used to improve patient safety. Some concepts that are unique to patient safety improvement are detailed in this section.

Safety Measurement

Information about patient incidents is obtained primarily from **incident reports.** These are paper-based or electronic reports completed by health care professionals when an incident occurs. Common categories of reportable patient incidents are listed in Table 13-3. Incident reports have been used in health care organizations for many years. Health care facilities require the staff fill out an incident report when a variance has occurred from the usual process of patient care or when a mishap or injury occurs involving a patient, staff member, or visitor. These reports are meant to be nonjudgmental, factual accounts of the event and its consequences, if any. Incident reports are prepared to assist the organizations in identifying and correcting problem-prone areas and in preparation for legal defense. Incident reports are *not* incorporated into the health record at any time. They are properly considered administrative documents prepared to facilitate intervention to minimize potential adverse effects of an undesirable event. Most HCOs use procedures to routinely submit the incident report form to their legal counsel to invoke the attorney-client privilege and provide protection from discovery in the event of litigation. Incident reports should not be photocopied or prepared in duplicate. Strict adherence to procedures for preparing and routing incident reports directly to the attorney is critical to achieving protected status.

Obtaining reliable information about patient incidents is not without its challenges. An individual's willingness to report an incident is strongly linked to the organizational culture and how the information is used. If the involved staff member is blamed for the event and disciplined or dismissed by management because of his or her involvement, it is unlikely people will voluntarily incriminate themselves or their colleagues by completing incident reports. Experience

Table 13-3 EXAMPLES OF REPORTABLE PATIENT INCIDENTS IN A HOSPITAL

Suicide gesture: Suicidal behavior that does not meet the definition for suicide attempts.
Suicide attempt: Suicidal behavior that is either medically serious or psychiatrically serious.
Suicide: Act of taking one's own life voluntarily and accidentally.
Alleged patient abuse: Includes acts of physical, psychological, sexual, or verbal abuse.
Rape/attempted rape: Sexual assault with or without penetration.
Homicide: Death of a patient or staff caused by a patient or death of patient caused by another individual.
Patient-on-staff abuse: Physical injury, intentionally striking staff.
Patient-on-patient abuse: Patient injured or assaulted by another patient.
Falls: All patient falls whether observed or not observed regardless of whether there is injury.
Blood transfusion error: Blood or blood products erroneously administered to wrong patient, therapy not ordered, administered wrong blood product, error in typing/cross-matching, with or without any reaction or evident adverse effect.
Medication error: A dose of medication that deviates from the physician's order as written in the patient's chart or as written on an outpatient prescription or from standard medical center procedures. Except for errors of omission, the medication dose must actually reach the patient; a wrong dose that is detected and corrected before administration to the patient is not considered a medication error.
Medication reaction: Anaphylaxis or other adverse reactions seriously affecting the well-being of patient.
Idiosyncratic reaction to blood or blood products: Reaction to blood or blood products that has been properly typed/cross-matched and administered.
Surgery-related death: Includes death in operating room, recovery room, during induction of anesthesia, and death within 48 hours of surgery.
Unexpected death: Includes events such as death during or after procedures such as cardiac catheterization, biopsy, radiological procedure, endoscopy; cause of death unknown; death reportable to local medical examiner or coroner; death from previously unknown problem or diagnosis; death from misadventure such as respirator malfunction, medication error, failure to diagnose, or failure to treat appropriately.
Patient involved in fires: Patient sets the fire, is involved in a fire, is burned, or is exposed in smoke of fire (i.e., smoke inhalation).
Inaccurate counts in surgery: Needle, sponge or pad counts.
Other: Any incidents that result or may result in significant patient disability or disfigurement.

has shown that when caregivers are provided protection from disciplinary actions they are more willing to report incidents.[26]

The value of collecting patient incident data is in the knowledge that can be gained from analysis of the data. Figure 13-15 illustrates a patient safety report created from incident data. The report provides information about the number of patient falls that have occurred each month. It also details the common causes for these falls and alerts caregivers as to what can be done to reduce the incidence of falls in the future. Collection, analysis, and reporting of patient incident data are often responsibilities assigned to the quality or risk management department.

Patient Safety Databases

A number of groups are gathering and analyzing information about patient incidents that occur at many different facilities to identify the error-producing factors in repeat mishaps. This analysis provides important learning opportunities for health care organizations. Some examples of these patient safety database projects are listed below:

- The American Society of Anesthesiologists' Closed Claims Project is an in-depth investigation of closed anesthesia malpractice claims designed to identify major areas of loss, patterns of injury, and strategies for prevention.

- The Pediatric Perioperative Cardiac Arrest Registry sponsored by the American Academy of Pediatrics' Section on Anesthesiology and the Committee on Professional Liability of the American Society of Anesthesiologists is an investigation of cardiac arrests and deaths of pediatric patients during administration of or recovery from anesthesia. The registry is designed to identify the possible relationship of anesthesia to these incidents.

- The Institute for Safe Medication Practices provides an independent review of medication errors that have been voluntarily submitted to the Medical Errors Reporting Program sponsored by the *United States Pharmacopeia*. Information about the common factors causing medication errors and how to reduce such errors is distributed to health care facilities by the Institute for Safe Medication Practices through their biweekly *Medication Safety Alert* newsletter and various other educational offerings.

- The Joint Commission has been collecting data about sentinel events since 1996. The findings of these review activities are regularly summarized and shared with the health care community on their Web site by sentinel event alerts. The alerts also serve as the basis for development of National Patient Safety Goals.

- The Food and Drug Administration (FDA) collects and analyzes data about patient incidents involving medical device failures. Through the FDA's Medical Products Reporting Program, MedWatch, information about

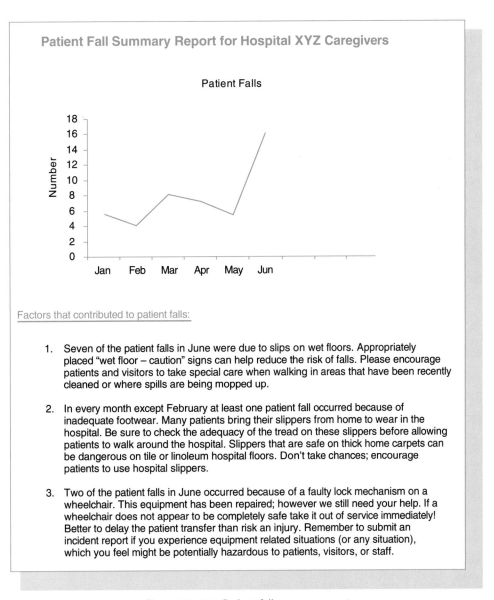

Figure 13-15 Patient fall summary report.

product safety problems is rapidly communicated to the medical community, thereby improving patient care.

- The Vaccine Adverse Event Reporting System is a cooperative program for vaccine safety of the FDA and the CDC. Health care professionals and the public are encouraged to report incidents of adverse events or side effects after vaccine administration.

Health care systems are also creating their own **mishap** databases. Here are just a few examples:

- In 1996 the Harvard Medical System formed a Risk Management Incident Collaborative for the purpose of developing a comparative database using consistently defined incidents. The database is being used by participating facilities to: identify best practices, implement quality improvement initiatives, continually measure performance, and reduce incidents.

- In 1997 the Veterans Health Administration began creating a system-wide database of adverse events. Included in this database is information about (1) the frequency with which particular care delivery systems have been problematic so managers know where the best opportunities for improvement exist, (2) system redesigns that should be adopted throughout the network or nationally, (3) needed changes in network and national policies and procedures, and (4) lessons learned.

In December 1999 the patient safety panel of the IOM recommended that hospitals and other health care providers be required to report to a nationwide reporting system medical errors that lead to a serious patient injury or death.[27] Data compiled from the reporting system could be used to learn how to prevent future occurrences. The panel also endorsed the development of voluntary reporting systems for less serious errors to detect system weaknesses that may ultimately lead to serious patient harm. Several states already require that health care facilities report certain types of patient incidents to the state health department.[28] Right now, the federal government is debating the need for and usefulness of a nationwide reporting system. Federal legislation is already in the works that will eventually mandate health care facilities to report serious patient incidents.

In March 2003 the Agency for Healthcare Research and Quality (AHRQ) published a set of **patient safety indicators** (PSI).[29] These measures can be used with hospital inpatient discharge data to provide a perspective on patient safety. Examples of these indicators are found in Table 13-4. Specifically, PSIs screen for problems that patients experience as a result of exposure to the health care system and that are likely amenable to prevention by changes at the system or provider level. Although quality assessments based on administrative data cannot be definitive, the measures can be used to flag potential patient safety problems that require further investigation.

Safety Improvement

Ensuring patient safety involves the establishment of operational systems and processes that minimize the likelihood of errors and maximizes the likelihood of intercepting them when they occur.[30] Techniques for establishing safer health care systems and processes are similar to any performance improvement initiative. First, the process to be improved is identified. The process is analyzed to determine where improvements are needed. Then actions intended to achieve desired improvement goals are implemented.

Patient safety improvement projects initiated after a serious patient incident are considered reactive. The impetus for starting the project is an undesirable event that needs to be investigated. These projects are often called "root cause analyses." Some patient safety improvement projects are proactive. These projects are initiated prospectively for the purpose of avoiding an undesirable event. These projects are often called "proactive risk assessments."

Table 13-4 EXAMPLES OF AGENCY FOR HEALTHCARE RESEARCH AND QUALITY PATIENT SAFETY INDICATORS

Indicator	Definition
Complications of anesthesia	Cases of anesthetic overdose, reaction, or endotracheal tube misplacement per 1000 surgery discharges. Excludes codes for drug use and self-inflicted injury.
Death in low-mortality DRGs	In-hospital deaths per 1000 patients in DRGs with less than 0.5% mortality. Excludes trauma, immunocompromised, and cancer patients.
Decubitus ulcer	Cases of decubitus ulcer per 1000 discharges with a length of stay of 5 or more days. Excludes patients with paralysis or in MDC 9, obstetrical patients in MDC 14, and patients admitted from a long-term care facility.
Failure to rescue	Deaths per 1000 patients having developed specified complications of care during hospitalization. Excludes patients age 75 years and older, neonates in MDC 15, patients admitted from long-term care facility, and patients transferred to or from other acute-care facility.
Foreign body left during procedure	Discharges with foreign body accidentally left in during procedure per 1000 discharges
Iatrogenic pneumothorax	Cases of iatrogenic pneumothorax per 1000 discharges. Excludes trauma, thoracic surgery, lung or pleural biopsy, or cardiac surgery patients and obstetrical patients in MDC 14.
Selected infections resulting from medical care	Cases of secondary ICD-9-CM codes 9993 or 00662 per 1000 discharges. Excludes patients with immunocompromised state or cancer.
Postoperative hip fracture	Cases of in-hospital hip fracture per 1000 surgical discharges. Excludes patients in MDC 8, with conditions suggesting fracture present on admission and obstetrical patients in MDC 14.
Postoperative hemorrhage or hematoma	Cases of hematoma or hemorrhage requiring a procedure per 1000 surgical discharges. Excludes obstetrical patients in MDC 14.
Postoperative respiratory failure	Cases of acute respiratory failure per 1000 elective surgical discharges. Excludes MDC 4 and 5 and obstetric admissions.

Source: *AHRQ quality indicators—guide to patient safety indicators,* Version 2.1, Revision 3, (January 17, 2005), p. 19, Rockville, MD, 2003, Agency for Healthcare Research and Quality, AHRQ publication No. 03-R203.
MDC, Major diagnostic category.

Root Cause Analysis

Root cause analysis is a systematic investigation process that occurs after a complication or adverse event that resulted in a patient injury caused by medical management rather than by the underlying disease or condition of the patient.[31] The Joint Commission uses the term **sentinel event** to describe serious patient incidents that should have a root cause analysis. Listed below are examples of sentinel events:

- Any event that results in an unanticipated patient death or major permanent loss of function, not related to the natural course of the patient's illness or underlying condition
- Suicide of a patient in a setting where the patient receives around-the-clock care, treatment, and services (for example, hospital, residential treatment center, crisis stabilization center)
- Unanticipated death of a term infant
- Infant abduction or infant discharge to the wrong family
- Hemolytic transfusion reaction involving administration of blood or blood products having major blood group incompatibilities
- Surgery on the wrong patient or wrong body part

Simply stated, a root cause analysis is a process designed for investigating what, how, and why something happened and for determining how to prevent the same thing from happening again. Understanding why an event occurred is the key to developing effective improvement recommendations. Imagine you find that one of the people in the HIM department is not documenting release of information requests as required by the procedure. Typically, the manager might conclude that the cause of this mistake is a non-compliant employee. However, stopping here in the investigation only tells the manager what happened and how it happened. If the manager does not probe deeper to understand the reasons for the mistake then preventing its recurrence will be difficult. Mistakes do not just happen. They can often be traced to some root causes. In this case the manager might ask, "Why didn't they follow the procedure?" "Is the procedure clear, understandable, easy to follow?" "Am I asking the employee to do something that is beyond the scope of his or her training?" "Are there incentives for not documenting each release of information, such as productivity bonuses?" "Do the employees have someone to answer their questions?" "Are any other employees having the same issues?" Each question leads to more questions. This constant questioning, asking "why" "why" "why," will help determine the root causes so that meaningful corrective actions can be designed.

Root cause analysis is a four-step process. The first step is to collect the data. Generally a team of individuals is brought together to review what happened, when it happened, and how it happened and to begin to explore why it happened. This may include participants or witnesses to the events, individuals who are expert in various aspects of the event (clinicians, human resources, technicians, etc.), and organizational leaders who can clear away barriers that may impede process improvements. The second step is to identify the causal factors. Causal factors are events or conditions that collectively, with other factors, increased the likelihood of an incident. By themselves the causal factors may not have caused the incident, but when they occurred concurrently the probability of an incident increased.

Step three is to identify the root causes. These are the causes that, if corrected, would prevent recurrence of this and similar incidents. Root causes are fundamental factors that address underlying system issues rather than single problems or factors. Root causes can include system deficiencies, management failures, inadequate competencies, omissions, nonadherence to procedures, and inadequate communication. This step may involve the use of a cause-and-effect diagram. This diagram can be used to structure the inquiry process by helping people consider all the reasons why a particular causal factor exists. For example, you may find that the HIM department procedure for recording in the release-of-information log is too cumbersome (a causal factor). To discover the root cause of inadequate or missing log entries, you would consider all the reasons why the procedure is too cumbersome. Eventually, through this questioning process, you would get to the root cause of the problem.

The final step of a root cause analysis is to generate recommendations for corrective action. Actions can fall into three categories: eliminate the chance for error, make it easier for people to do the right thing, and mitigate the effects of the error after it has occurred. Process changes may be needed, staff may need some additional training, or any number of actions may be taken. The goal is to reduce or eliminate the root cause of the event so that future similar events do not occur. The completed root cause analysis is documented and shared with appropriate staff, physicians, and leaders in the organization.

Students can review actual serious patient incidents and the investigations of these events on the Morbidity and Mortality Rounds Internet Web site sponsored by the AHRQ. The case studies on this site illustrate the importance of tracking down the causes of sentinel events and significant "near-miss" events so that health care processes can be changed to prevent similar occurrences in the future.

Proactive Risk Assessment

In addition to improving patient safety by use of traditional performance improvement techniques, in July 2001 The Joint Commission began to require that accredited organizations conduct proactive risk assessment projects. In the context of an HCO, a **risk** is any event or situation that could potentially result in injury to an individual or financial loss to the HCO. Many organizations are meeting this requirement by using a method known as **failure mode and effects analysis** (FMEA). FMEA is a risk analysis technique used in manufacturing, aviation, computer software design, and other industries to conduct safety system evaluations. It is now being used in HCOs to analyze existing systems and to evaluate new processes before implementation. It is a technique that promotes systematic thinking about the safety of a patient care process in terms of:[32]

- What could go wrong?
- How badly might it go wrong?
- What needs to be done to prevent failures?

During a FMEA the people involved in the process work together to objectively answer these questions. The fundamental purpose of the FMEA is to take actions that reduce the likelihood of a process failure.

The first step in conducting a FMEA is to define the process to be analyzed. Because these projects can be labor intensive, it is best to select a process that is high risk or known to be problematic. For example, FMEA is a good tool for health care facilities to use in analyzing various medication administration processes because these activities have been shown to be at high risk for errors.[33,34]

Once the process has been selected, a multidisciplinary team is convened consisting of subject matter experts and people representing various viewpoints. The team members include both management and staff level positions. The team starts out by creating a flowchart of the process. Next, for each process step the team determines how that step might fail. For example, at the step of ordering medication, the physician may order the wrong medication or the wrong dosage. The physician may write an illegible order or use abbreviations that can be misinterpreted by the pharmacist. The team brainstorms all possible failures that can occur at each step in the process.

For each possible failure, the team defines the effect of the failure by answering several questions[35]:

- What would likely happen if this failure occurred?
- How serious would it be if this failure occurred?
- What are the chances that this failure will actually happen?
- What are the chances that this failure will be detected and corrected before patients are harmed?

Determining the effect of each failure is as important as defining the failure itself. The process improvement actions ultimately recommended by the team will be directly toward the "vital few" failures that will cause the greatest harm to patients should they occur. The next step in the FMEA is to identify the causes for the failures. For each significant failure, a "mini" root cause analysis is done. Although the failure is theoretical, the team tries to identify the factors that could contribute to or cause the failure. Recommendations for improvements and corrective actions are then developed to prevent the significant failures. Just as the team would do in any type of performance improvement project, the corrective actions are pilot tested to ensure they are effective and do not introduce new problems into the system. If effective, the corrective actions are fully implemented and monitored to ensure continuing effectiveness. Other than the demand on human resources and time, the main limitation of FMEA is that it deals with process failures one at a time. In most cases, adverse events are typically the result of multiple failures and preexisting hazardous conditions.[36]

A variety of other prospective risk assessment tools and techniques are available to HCOs. One technique that is gaining popularity for improving patient safety is simulation. Simulation is a technique to replace or amplify real-life experiences with guided experiences that evoke or replicate substantial aspects of the real world in a fully interactive manner.[37] This technique is helpful in preparing people for error-prone, high-risk, or unusual situations. By simulating possible adverse events, people learn to recognize problems and understand the effects of their responses in a safe environment. Simulation forces people to review processes on a very detailed level, which can help to improve patient safety. Typical results of simulations include changing the process flow, reducing process times, changing material handling methods, reassigning functions, bringing in new technologies, updating information processing methods, and adding or replacing resources. These changes, when appropriate, can help to improve patient safety.

The fundamental purpose of all proactive risk assessment techniques is to recommend and take actions that reduce the likelihood of a process failure. Any process can be chosen for a risk assessment; it does not have to be a process involving direct patient care. Proactive risk assessment techniques can be applied to the work activities in the HIM department to help reduce mistakes and improve efficiency of services.

RISK MANAGEMENT

In the context of an HCO, a **risk** is any event or situation that could potentially result in an injury to an individual or in financial loss to the HCO. The definition of injury as used in legal terms is more encompassing than its general definition of physical harm. In the legal sense, harm or injury may be defined as any wrong or damage done to a person or to a person's rights or property. As social welfare agents, HCOs hold a public trust. Risk management programs acknowledge accountability to the public for a safe physical environment and adherence to accepted standards of clinical practice.

Risk management encompasses all policies, procedures, and practices directed at reducing risk and subsequent liability for injuries that occur in the organization's immediate environment. The specific policies and procedures that constitute a risk management program are developed in collaboration with the HCO's legal counsel because judicial interpretation of statutory law in the court system is a continually evolving process. In general, risk management activities are intended to minimize the potential for injuries occurring, ensure prompt and appropriate response to injured parties, and anticipate and plan for ensuing liability when injuries occur. Activities are specifically directed at preventing or reducing financial loss, allocating funds for compensable events, and diminishing negative public image resulting from injury claims. Although malpractice litigation often captures public visibility with large monetary awards for death or personal injury resulting from medical treatment, the organization's administrative and governance bodies must be concerned with potential injury to all people who enter the facility or its grounds for any reason. These potential claimants include patients, employees, visitors, contractual and business affiliates, and members of the medical staff.

Risk management documentation must be created and maintained in strict accordance with legal guidelines to prevent discoverability. Attorney-client privilege cannot be invoked for records maintained in the ordinary course of business or in provision of patient care.[38] Therefore, information about specific incidents or individual patients should be documented only as private communications between the risk manager or HCO leadership and the legal counsel. This communication may serve as the basis for administrative decisions or action plans to respond to an identified risk or **potentially compensable event** (PCE). A PCE is an adverse occurrence, usually involving a patient, that could result in a financial obligation for the HCO.

Claims resolved through the court system often require defensive legal action over a period of several years. A finding against the HCO results in a monetary award to the claimant usually paid out several years after the injury occurred. Substantial costs associated with the defense are incurred whether the courts find for or against the HCO. Financial planning to ensure adequate resources to meet future legal obligations requires accurate, complete information from the claims management program. Many claims by injured parties are settled without legal action. The insurance carrier or the organization may determine that settlement is preferable to trial for several reasons, including insufficient information for adequate defense, risk of greater financial loss than the settlement amount, and adverse impact on public image.

Loss Prevention and Reduction

The best protection against injuries and ensuing financial liability is prevention. Prevention requires identifying and monitoring high-risk and problem-prone processes and physical plant locations. Historical aggregate data on injuries, identified hazards, complaints, and claims can be helpful to define risk indicators. Monitoring efforts may be directed at individual behaviors (wearing gloves to administer intravenous medications), physical safety (prominently displayed signs to indicate wet floors), personal security (functional locks on employee lockers), or some other aspect of corporate risk. Action to correct identified problems and follow-up to prevent recurrence are critical to the risk prevention process.

Loss reduction focuses on a single incident or claim and requires immediate response to any adverse occurrence. Injured people should receive prompt medical attention. Investigation of the incident should include examining the site and interviewing witnesses immediately after the occurrence to collect all pertinent facts. If the incident is considered potentially compensable, a claims representative for the liability insurance carrier should be contacted to ensure that all necessary information has been collected and appropriate responsive action taken. In many cases, prompt, sincere efforts to correct the problem can avert a claim for financial damages.

Claims Management

Claims management refers to the administrative and legal procedures initiated when adverse events are identified. For individual cases, these procedures may include the following:

- An internal audit of the charges billed
- Examination of the health record for completeness
- Sequestration of financial and health records
- Interrogatories
- Settlement negotiations
- Preparation for trial
- Tracking of the status of claims
- Profiling of aggregate claims and losses
- Objective use of resulting information to improve individual and organization performance

Aggregate data generated through facilitywide monitoring and evaluation activities, hazard surveillance, infection control, and other medical staff review activities are properly integrated into performance and patient safety improvement and peer-review functions. Information is thus available to achieve the following objectives:

- Improve system processes
- Increase patient and employee satisfaction
- Improve clinical outcomes
- Decrease risk factors

Students may find it helpful to compare and contrast performance improvement, utilization management, and risk management on several dimensions to distinguish elements unique to each. A brief comparison is provided in Table 13-5.

Table 13-5 COMPARISON OF PERFORMANCE IMPROVEMENT, UTILIZATION MANAGEMENT, AND RISK MANAGEMENT

	Performance Improvement	Utilization Management	Risk Management
Purpose	Improve quality of care and services	Efficient and effective use of resources	Avoid or manage financial liability
Reference population	Cohorts of similar cases	Individual patients	Individual patients, employees, visitors, and professional staff
Process used	Criterion-referenced documentation review	Individual patient needs/characteristics compared with criteria to determine need for health care services	Review causes of single events or occurrences and patterns of events
Tools/techniques	Statistical analysis	Discharge planning case management	Occurrence screening
Primary question(s)	Can the outcome of care or service be improved?	Can the necessary treatment or service be provided elsewhere more cost-effectively or equally effective by use of a less-invasive approach?	Could the occurrence have been prevented? Can we minimize the loss?
Actions	Revise policies, procedures, or processes	Approve or deny patient access to or payment for diagnostic services and clinical treatments	Revise processes; change environment; allocate financial resources
Key external driver	Accrediting and regulatory agencies, MCOs, and payers	MCOs and payers	Liability insurers

MCO, Managed care organization.

UTILIZATION MANAGEMENT

Health care in the United States is in the midst of a revolution that is sure to continue until the costs level out and there is broad consensus that national economic and health care goals are being met. Health care has experienced unparalleled escalation in costs brought on by a series of factors. Suffice it to say, health care cost increases have led to widespread public outcry and to intense pressure to contain the costs. **Utilization management** (UM) activities are intended to ensure that facilities and resources (both human and nonhuman) are used appropriately on the basis of the health care needs of patients. Both underutilization (unmet patient needs) and overutilization (provision of care or services not medically necessary) are undesirable outcomes. Wickizer and Lessler[39] estimate that 50% to 60% of patients are subject to some form of UM.[39] In certain regions of the country where managed care is prevalent, this percentage is likely to be much higher. HCOs, providers, and health plans are all involved in UM activities.

The goal of UM is to maintain or increase quality of care and to improve access to timely and quality care for those who need it through the efficient provision of resources. UM involves the three familiar building blocks of performance management:

- Measurement of how organizations and providers are using resources;
- Assessment of how well resources are being used
- Improvement of resource use

UM encompasses the dual objectives of cost containment and quality of care. Although UM activities are often independent in an HCO, these activities are interdependent with performance and patient safety improvement functions.

External Requirements

The Medicare COP includes requirements for utilization management activities. For example, hospitals must have a process for reviewing services furnished by the institution and by members of the medical staff to patients entitled to benefits under the Medicare and Medicaid programs. These review activities include an analysis of the medical necessity of hospital admissions, continued hospital stays, and the professional services furnished. Medical necessity means that a patient's clinical condition, as documented by a diagnostic test or physical finding, warrants services that can be provided only as an inpatient.[40] Hospitals are required to have a committee that oversees the UM functions. At least two members of the committee must be doctors of medicine or osteopathy.

For the most part, The Joint Commission standards are silent on the topic of UM. The Joint Commission standards are designed to ensure that HCOs design and implement processes to evaluate the appropriateness of interventions and continuing treatment and the appropriateness, clinical necessity, and timeliness of diagnostic and treatment services. For instance, the Provision of Care standards include performance expectations related to ensuring continuity of care for patients transitioning from the hospital to another care setting or to home. Data collected during these activities should be integrated with the organization's overall performance improvement activities. Leadership is charged with responsibility for allocation of resources necessary to ensure the effectiveness of UM activities.

The UM activities of health plans are governed by CMS regulations (for federally funded beneficiaries) and state insurance commission regulations. Health plans accredited by the National Committee for Quality Assurance (NCQA) or the Utilization Review Accreditation Commission (URAC) must comply with prescriptive UM standards that are similar to the CMS and state regulations. Organizationally, UM may be a program area within a health plan or it may be a service provided by a third-party vendor (stand-alone UM company outsourcing company). Health plans may delegate UM for different aspects of health care to different organizations. For example, UM for behavioral health, pharmacy services, and medical review may be provided by separate entities. Many health plans and stand-alone UM companies offer purchasers multiple medical management programs and often share staff and data systems among the program areas.[41]

Program Components

Review of health services utilization is intended to reduce unnecessary or inappropriate medical care by making medical necessity determinations. The UM function involves four activities: prospective review, concurrent review, discharge planning/case management, and retrospective review.

Prospective Review

The prospective review process is initiated before a patient actually receives health services. If the patient's health plan requires utilization review (UR), the provider or facility contacts the UM company or health plan for approval of the services on behalf of a patient. UM nurses at the health plan collect clinical information and use criteria to determine whether the health services are medically necessary. These criteria are often supplied by a commercial entity such as Milliman or InterQual. The InterQual criteria are referred to as IS/SI criteria—**intensity of service/severity of illness**—because they measure a need for health care services that can be provided only in an inpatient facility or define a degree of

acute physical impairment that requires inpatient medical intervention.

Cases that meet criteria are approved for payment by the health plan. Cases that do not meet criteria undergo additional review. Additional review may include gathering of more detailed clinical information, clinical consultation between physicians, or review by a specialist. The health plan's final determination of medical necessity is communicated to the provider or facility, often in an electronic format. All health plans have some type of appeals process that can be initiated by patients if there is disagreement about the medical necessity of planned services.

Concurrent Review

Even when not required by health plans to precertify admissions, a hospital may elect to determine medical necessity for all admissions as a matter of policy. Typically, these reviews are conducted within 24 hours (or 1 working day) of admission and use the same procedures as preadmission certification. Admission justification conducted in this manner and evaluations to determine the necessity for continued inpatient stay are termed **concurrent reviews** because need is assessed simultaneously with provision of care and services. InterQual IS/SI criteria are often used for both admission and continued stay reviews. The intent of these reviews is to determine the point at which the maximum benefits of inpatient care have been achieved. Discharge is indicated when information in a patient's health care record no longer conforms to the IS/SI criteria. As with any criteria or guideline, the recommendations are not considered hard-and-fast rules. The final decision regarding appropriateness of admission and continued stay is left up to the attending physician. A flow chart of the utilization review process is shown in Figure 13-16.

Most hospitals use a two-stage review process with nonphysician personnel conducting the initial review. The staff screen patient health records (or information submitted by the admitting physician for prospective reviews) for documentation to establish compliance with predetermined criteria. If documentation is sufficient and criteria are met, admission or continued stay is deemed justifiable. If criteria are not met, the admitting physician may be asked to provide additional information or the case will be referred to a physician advisor for peer review and discussion with the admitting physician. If documented compliance with the criteria cannot be achieved, the health plan may withhold reimbursement for services provided.

Cases that meet the criteria are monitored for continued compliance. Problematic cases, those with inadequate documentation to judge compliance or with evidence of noncompliance, are identified for administrative and clinical intervention.

The information needs may be met through more comprehensive admitting or progress notes, documentation of physical findings, or reports of diagnostic test results. If

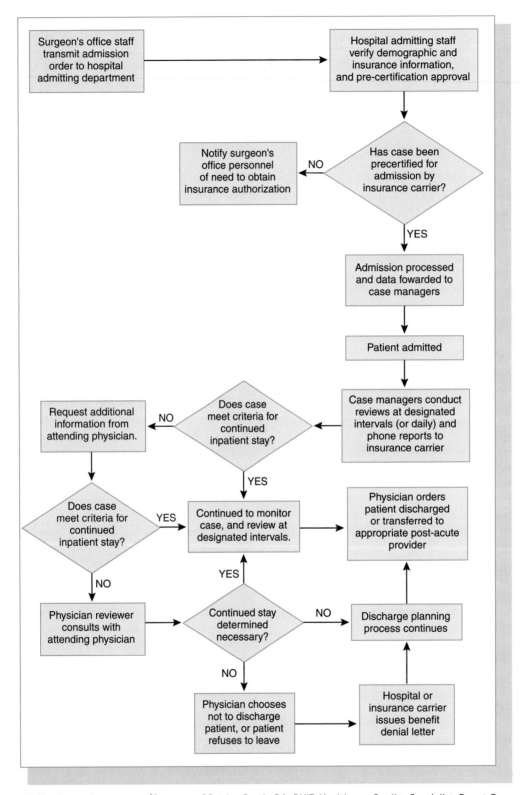

Figure 13-16 Utilization review process. (Courtesy of Patrice Spath, BA, RHIT, Healthcare Quality Specialist, Forest Grove, OR. Used with permission.)

medical necessity still is not evident after additional information has been provided, the reviewer should refer the case for peer evaluation by a physician advisor.

If, after review of the health record and discussion with the admitting physician (and sometimes examination of the patient), the UR physician advisor cannot verify compliance with criteria, the case is deemed an inappropriate admission or continued stay. When a patient's admission or continued stay is not considered medically necessary, the hospital may notify the patient of probable noncoverage by the patient's health plan. After receipt of the notice detailing the review process and outcome, the patient is expected to assume personal responsibility for payment of hospital charges incurred beyond the date specified in the letter. In most cases, the patient is discharged promptly. For many reasons, including the loss of community good will, the hospital prefers to avoid this type of review outcome.

Health plans often conduct concurrent review to authorize continued hospital stays after expiration of the initial approved stay. Concurrent review may also be done by the health plan to authorize selected diagnostic and surgical procedures. Health plans may conduct concurrent review remotely, with the hospital providing information about patients by phone or electronically (fax or secure e-mail). Some health plans employ UM nurses to go on site in a facility to review records of patients currently hospitalized.

Discharge Planning/Case Management

Discharge planning is a UM function designed to assist patients in transitioning from one level of care to another. Often UM staff conduct an initial discharge assessment but will refer patients in need of intensive **discharge planning** to case management services. **Case management** is patient focused and provides additional care coordination for patients with complex medical needs or in need of posthospital health care services. Case managers, often registered nurses or social workers, interact with patients and providers to optimize efficient and timely care. Unless postdischarge needs are identified and planned for, a patient's inpatient stay may be prolonged beyond the point of medical necessity. The Medicare COP requires that hospitals have a process that identifies patients in need of discharge planning and ensures that appropriate arrangements for posthospital care are made before discharge.[42]

Retrospective Review

Retrospective review occurs after care has been rendered. Examples of cases where a health plan might conduct a retrospective review include an emergency department visit for care out of network or after a claims submission for services that were not precertified. Medical necessity and appropriateness of care also may be investigated by an HCO after services have been rendered to a patient. Appropriateness of care means that services provided to a patient are consistent with their clinical needs. For example, an elderly patient may require rehabilitation services after hip replacement. Although retrospective review offers no opportunity to control inappropriate utilization for patients, the reviews can provide valuable information about patterns of undesirable practices that can be used to improve future performance.

In HCOs retrospective review often involves an analysis of resource use to determine where there are opportunities for improving the efficiency of care or decreasing costs. Figure 13-17 is an example of the type of utilization report that would be useful for retrospective review in a hospital. The report shows the hospital's average costs in ten different revenue centers for patients in DRG 174 (gastrointestinal hemorrhage with comorbidities or complications) compared with the average costs at other hospitals in their market area. In five of the ten revenue centers, the hospital has higher average costs compared with other hospitals. Physicians and other caregivers investigate the cause of these higher costs and initiate improvement actions on the basis of what they find. The data in the figure originated from the Medicare MEDPAR files and the comparative analysis was provided by Solucient, a health information vendor.

Plan and Program Structure

HCOs and health plans have a utilization management plan. The purpose of this plan is to define the structure and processes that support measurement, assessment, and improvement activities. The plan identifies authority and responsibility for the UM process, accountability and reporting structures, the role of physician advisors, the review mechanisms, and mechanisms for handling review decisions and payment denial appeals.

In a hospital the UM activities are overseen by a distinct UM committee or the task may be assigned to another medical staff committee. Although UM committee membership may vary according to whether it is a separate group or part of another, the committee is primarily composed of staff physicians representing all clinical departments. This includes representatives from surgery, family practice, internal medicine, psychiatry, pediatrics, obstetrics, and the other specialties. Nonphysician members of the committee may include the director of case management or utilization management, a senior leader from hospital administration or nursing, the performance improvement director, the director of HIM, and a representative from the finance department. The primary responsibility of the UM committee is to review utilization data and to make recommendations for change in patient care practices and health care delivery processes.

Staffing of the UM function in an HCO will vary depending on the size of the facility. In many smaller HCOs the person responsible for UM wears a number of other hats. UM coordinators often have a clinical background. Many UM departments also have a pool of data abstracters and information management consultants to assist with retrospective review activities.

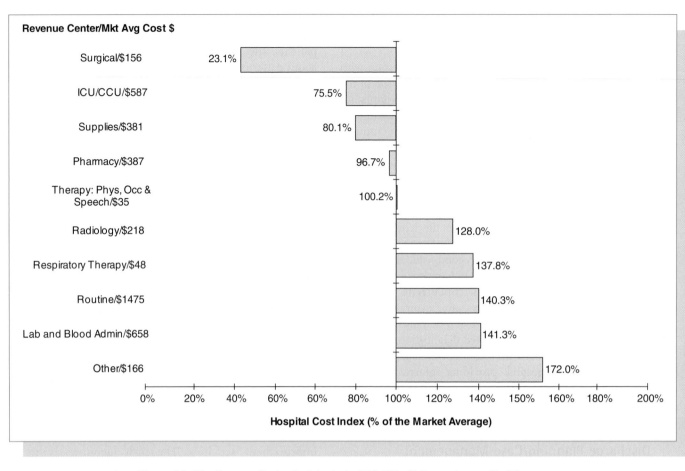

Figure 13-17 Revenue Center Cost Analysis: DRG 174- GI Hemorrhage with CC.

Physician input into the UM process is critical. Health plans have a designated medical director to oversee UM activities. HCOs often appoint one or more **physician advisors** to serve as support to the UR process. Some hospitals have a rotating schedule assigning each physician a time in which he or she functions as physician advisor. Others have permanent physician advisors that are full time and paid. A growing trend is to use the title "medical advisor" rather than "physician advisor" although the responsibilities are essentially the same.

CREDENTIALING

Credentialing refers to any process by which practitioners are evaluated with the intent to affect control over their professional practices. More specifically within HCOs, the term refers to the policies and procedures used to determine the membership category and clinical privileges to be granted to each member of the professional staff. As with the obligation for ensuring a safe environment, the social welfare responsibility attributed to HCOs requires assurance of the technical competence of those who practice their professions under the auspices of the organization. The professional staff credentialing process is an objective mechanism used by the governing body to demonstrate accountability for professional staff practice behaviors and associated clinical outcomes in a proactive manner. In the simplest sense, the credentialing process serves as a performance appraisal of medical staff members. Data collected are used to assess professional staff members' productivity, efficient and effective use of organizational resources, and quality of intervention outcomes.

The primary objective of professional staff credentialing is to ensure that professional staff members perform only procedures and services for which they are qualified through education, training, and experience. Failure to verify an applicant's credentials in the appointment and privileging process places the HCO at risk of liability for injuries resulting from practitioner incompetence. The courts consistently have held HCOs accountable for the governing body's responsibility to know about the competence of practitioners or professionals granted privileges.

Results of medical staff peer review activities are pivotal to evaluating the competence and performance of individuals who provide patient care within the health care organization. In general, certain care processes (such as medication usage, blood usage, and operative procedures) are monitored routinely to ensure that practice patterns are within established standards and expectations. These reviews examine aggregate data and evaluate groups of patients or providers. (See The Joint Commission standards for specific requirements.) When problems are identified or undesirable events occur, a focused evaluation of a single instance of care or evaluation of a single provider's practice pattern should be initiated. This type of peer review is directed at improving the practitioner's performance and generally is not disciplinary in nature.

Professional staff membership and clinical privileges ultimately are awarded at the discretion of the governing body, although in most cases decisions for physician applicants are based on the recommendations of the active medical staff (or its credentials committee) through an executive committee. Nonphysician members of the professional staff, such as licensed independent practitioners (LIPs), must be appropriately evaluated and their privileges specifically defined as well. LIPs are individuals who are qualified by education, training, and experience to perform their professional services without supervision by a physician. Examples include dentists, psychologists, podiatrists, and others permitted by the scope of their professional license to practice independently. Midlevel providers such as physicians' assistants and nurse practitioners undergo the credentialing process as well.

External Requirements

As with other systems and processes to ensure health care quality, accrediting bodies such as The Joint Commission and the NCQA are key players in establishing guidelines for credentialing professional staff. From its inception, The Joint Commission has emphasized physician credentialing as a key factor in the accreditation process and has consistently maintained the position that privilege delineation is entirely within the purview of the individual facility and that credential reviews conducted by other facilities or agents should not be automatically accepted.

Similar to the standards of The Joint Commission, the NCQA standards specify categories of information that must be verified in the credentialing process. Credentials files should document verification of the following information as appropriate to the type of health care professional seeking membership or privileges:

- Licensure
- Hospital privileges
- Drug Enforcement Agency (DEA) registration
- Medical education or specialty board certification
- Malpractice insurance

- Liability claims history
- National Practitioner Data Bank queries
- Medical board sanctions
- Medicare/Medicaid sanctions
- Application for membership and privileges

Operating as agents of the state, the duty of licensure boards is to ensure that professionals are qualified to practice with reasonable skill and safety. The boards are thus empowered to award, deny, limit, suspend, or revoke a person's license and to invoke disciplinary actions specific to practice behaviors under the scope of the license granted. Graduate physicians seeking **licensure** in any state must pass either a sequence of examinations conducted by the National Board of Medical Examiners or the Federal Licensing Examination (FLEX) to qualify. Additional information about medical licensure examinations is available from the National Board of Medical Examiners and the Federation of State Medical Boards Web sites.

Credentialing Program Components

Medical staff appointment or reappointment assigns qualified applicants to an existing unit of the medical staff organization (MSO) and designates a membership category and assignment to a department or clinical service. Department or service members carry out organizational duties that may include committee service, peer review, recommendations to the organization's leaders, and other activities that ensure accountability for department operations. Each membership category carries different responsibilities and privileges, which are specified in the organization's MSO bylaws.

Privilege delineation refers to the process of determining the specific procedures and services a physician or other professional is permitted to perform under the jurisdiction of the HCO. At the time of initial appointment and each subsequent reappointment, the applicant formally requests specific privileges. Any award of privileges must be supported with documentation of training, education, and other evidence of qualification or competence. For example, a clinician requesting privileges to perform laser procedures would submit certification of training in using the laser and perhaps copies of operative reports describing procedures performed.

Credentials verification is primarily an administrative process to determine that an applicant has provided all required documents for review pursuant to staff appointment. Specific documentation requirements and application procedures for appointment and privileges vary among HCOs, but requirements are documented and made known to all applicants. At a minimum, all organizations should require proof of:

- Education and training
- Liability insurance coverage

- Current licensure
- Clinical competence
- Satisfactory health status

In addition, hospital medical staffs considering applications for membership (either initial appointment or reappointment) or requests for clinical privileges *must* query the **National Practitioner Data Bank** (NPDB) to identify any available adverse quality-of-care information about the applicant. A similar database of practitioner-specific information is available only to managed care organizations. This information source, known as the **Healthcare Integrity and Protection Data Bank** (HIPDB), contains the same practitioner-specific data that is in the NPDB and civil judgments, criminal convictions, and actions taken by licensing agencies.

Because verifying the validity of documents and statements attesting to professional credentials is a time- and resource-consuming process, many HCOs outsource the document verification process to an external agent. These entities, referred to as **credentials verification organizations** (CVOs), make the contacts necessary to verify an applicant's education, training, experience, and professional licenses and certifications through primary source agencies. HCOs that use a CVO should contract only with accredited agencies. CVOs may be accredited by the NCQA, by the URAC, or by both agents. URAC's primary focus is the HCO's operational process for credentialing. NCQA, which has been accrediting CVOs since 1996, verifies compliance with NCQA professional staff credentialing standards.[43]

A **credentials registry**, on the other hand, provides a document management service to individual professionals. The registry organization maintains an individual's credentials verification documents and releases copies of the file or selected relevant documents to HCOs at the individual's request when they seek appointment or clinical privileges.

Practitioner profiles frequently are used as a mechanism to integrate information compiled from performance improvement activities into the credentialing process. A physician's unique profile incorporates findings from all required review functions, summaries of participation in MSO committees, pertinent judgments from external review agencies such as the QIO or licensure board, and clinical activity information such as number of patients admitted. Many hospitals also include such data as the number of meetings attended and the continuing medical education credits earned at hospital-sponsored programs. Specific profile data are determined by MSO policies and procedures for credentialing (Figure 13-18). These profiles provide a concise summary of information crucial to objective credentialing of professional staff. When properly prepared and exploited, the profiles contribute to objectivity in credentialing decisions. The inclusion of comprehensive profile documents in credentials files demonstrates the administrative mechanism used to integrate performance improvement data into the MSO appointment and privilege delineation processes.

ROLE OF MANAGERS

Performance management and patient safety improvement cannot simply be delegated to staff. To create and sustain an environment that promotes continual improvement, it is necessary for senior leaders and managers to set the tenor, provide support, and clear away barriers. Improving performance takes some investments. People must receive some training in problem solving, process improvement tools, and team building. Although training can be a substantial expenditure in terms of financial and human resources, it is one of the better investments that can be made.

Performance management and patient safety improvement also require patience and discipline. Experience demonstrates that positive changes do not come as quickly as one would like. There are some false starts. People may be threatened by process changes or increased employee involvement in decision making. A temptation is to accept quick-fix process "tweaks" rather than commit resources to sustainable process redesign and system enhancements. It is no coincidence that W. Edwards Deming's first principle of total quality management is "Practice Constancy of Purpose."[44] Deming, one of the early leaders in performance improvement in manufacturing, made a profound impact on quality management in all industries through the application of statistical principles.

Financial and human resources are expended on improvement projects and processes are undergoing almost constant redesign. Yet, familiar problems seem to creep back into the system to disrupt the performance of key processes. The chapter's key concepts offer some suggestions for achieving lasting performance improvements.

Key Concepts

- **Change things and behaviors**. Often performance improvement efforts focus on standardizing or streamlining work steps, and unfortunately the human part of the process is overlooked. Modifying attitudes and behaviors is important. Otherwise people will lapse into the old way of doing things without giving the new process a chance to become a habit. Empowerment, delegating responsibility to permit employees to make decisions and institute needed changes in their work processes, requires the employees to be adequately trained and competent to make those decisions.
- **Train people**. Educating people in the use of the performance improvement skills they need to get the job

```
                    CREDENTIALS COMMITTEE REVIEW SHEET
                    PRACTITIONER REAPPOINTMENT PROFILE
                     REAPPOINTMENT PERIOD 1998–1999

     1          AAEXAMPLE    DOCTOR              DPT      CATEGORY    SPECLTY

  BASIC HOSPITAL STATISTICS:

  DISCHARGES:                 123        INPATIENT DAYS:               1234
  CONSULTS:                   123        OUTPATIENT ADMISSIONS:        123
  INPT PROCEDURES:            123        HOSPITAL DEATHS:              123
  OPT PROCEDURES:             123

  * * * * * * * * * * * * * * * * * * * * * * * * * * * * * * * * * * * * * *

  THE FOLLOWING FINDINGS MUST DEMONSTRATE ACCEPTABLE PERFORMANCE FOR REAPPOINTMENT

  * * * * * * * * * * * * * * * * * * * * * * * * * * * * * * * * * * * * * *

    BYLAW REQUIREMENTS:       1          GS-MTG   1      DEPT-MTGS  12   CME

  * * * * * * * * * * * * * *PERFORMANCE FROM QUALITY REVIEW MONITORS* * * * * * * *

    MEDICAL RECORDS:          1          SUSPENSIONS          1     DELINQUENT
                             12          RECORDS REVIEWED

    MEDICAL PEER REVIEW:     12          REVIEWED            12     JUSTIFIED

    SURGICAL PEER REVIEW:    12          REVIEWED            12     JUSTIFIED

    CRITICAL CARE QI:         1          REVIEWED             1     JUSTIFIED

    MORTALITY REVIEW:        12          DEATHS REVIEWED     12     JUSTIFIED

    BLOOD UTILIZATION:       12          REVIEWED            12     JUSTIFIED

    DRUG UTILIZATION:        12          ORDERS CLARIFIED     0     LETTERS SENT

    UTILIZATION REVIEW:       1          DENIALS              0     LETTERS SENT

    PEER REVIEW COMMENTS:       QI COMMENTS FOR UNJUSTIFIED REVIEWS
  _____

  * * * * * * * * * * * * * * * * * * * * * * * * * * * * * * * * * * * * * *

  BASED UPON REVIEW OF THIS INFORMATION, THE FOLLOWING IS RECOMMENDED:
  (   ) NO   (   ) YES   ADJUSTMENTS TO CLINICAL PRIVILEGES REQUESTED
  (   ) NO   (   ) YES   ADJUSTMENTS TO STAFF CATEGORY_____
  (   ) YES  (   ) NO    RECOMMEND REAPPOINTMENT


  _____        _____
  For the Department                    Credentials Committee Chairman

  Hospital Statistics/Quality Review Monitor Information given is for January 1998–June 1999.
  Citizenship Information and General Staff Meeting Attendance is for January 1998–October 1999.
```

Figure 13-18 Practitioner reappointment profile. (Courtesy of The Children's Hospital, Birmingham, AL.)

done is critical. Everyone should know how to apply the organization's fundamental improvement model and, at a minimum, how to use basic improvement tools.

- **Test redesigned processes.** An important way to ensure that improvements are sustainable is to test possible process changes with a small subset of activities. Quantitative and qualitative data should be collected during the pilot phase for the purpose of learning what effect specific changes in a process will have on related processes and systems.
- **Do not order change and ignore support.** For health care services to get better every day it takes knowledge, diligence, effort, focus, and resources. You can't give employees

training about performance improvement, tell them which processes to improve, and then turn and walk away. Managers must take an active role in steering the improvement efforts of the department.

- **Process management is a dynamic activity.** Regulations and incentives that guide performance measurement, assessment, and improvement activities in health care organizations are constantly changing. HIM professionals must keep abreast of the latest changes to be ready to meet the current information needs of health care leaders.
- **Focus on results and creating value.** Performance measurements of health care activities need to focus on key results. The results are used to create value for the key

stakeholders: patients and their families, employees, payers, and the community at large. By creating value for key stakeholders, the organization builds loyalty and contributes to public good.

- **Manage information assets.** The contemporary operating environment in health care organizations is challenging. To survive, everyone needs to be well informed. Health care organizations must continually measure and analyze performance. Many types of data and information are needed for performance management to support organizational decision making and operational improvement. HIM professionals have an important role in providing physician leaders and the senior executive team with information on the organization's current performance and the direction it is heading.

- **HIM involvement is crucial.** Collection and analysis of performance data is expensive in terms of monetary and human resources. Inadequate planning can result in misdirected endeavors—causing wasted efforts or, worse yet, incorrect patient care decisions. The HIM professional's advice, support, and expertise are crucial to the success of health care performance management. Regardless of how often regulations change or accreditation standards are revised, there is always one certainty: valid, reliable and timely information about organizational performance will always be needed by managers and caregivers.

REFERENCES

1. Kohn LT, Corrigan JM, Donaldson MS, editors: *To err is human: building a safer health system,* Washington, DC, 2000, National Academy Press: http://www.nap.edu/catalog/9728.html.

2. Committee on Quality of Health Care in America, Institute of Medicine: *Crossing the quality chasm: a new health system for the 21st century,* Washington, DC, 2001, National Academy Press: http://www.nap.edu/catalog/10027.html.

3. Department of Health and Human Services, Centers for Medicare and Medicaid Services: 42 CFR Part 482 Medicare and Medicaid Programs: Hospital Conditions of Participation: Quality Assessment and Performance Improvement (effective on March 25, 2003), Sec. 482.21 Conditions of participation: Quality assessment and performance improvement program. Washington, DC, 2003, Department of Health and Human Services.

4. Accreditation programs: http://www.ncqa.org/Programs/ Accreditation/accreditation.htm. Accessed August 2005.

5. National Institute of Standards and Technology: *Malcolm Baldrige criteria for health care 2004,* Washington, DC, 2005, National Institute of Standards and Technology.

6. Spath PL: *Leading your healthcare organization to excellence: a guide to using the Baldrige criteria,* Chicago, IL, 2005, ACHE Management Series/Health Administration Press.

7. Spath PL, editor: *Partnering with patients to reduce medical errors,* Chicago, IL, 2004, American Hospital Association Press.

8. Spath PL, editor: *Provider report cards: a guide for promoting health care quality to the public,* Chicago, 1999, American Hospital Association Press.

9. National Quality Forum: *A national framework for healthcare quality measurement and reporting,* Washington, DC, 2002, National Quality Forum.

10. National Quality Forum: Mission: http://www.qualityforum.org/ mission/home.htm. Accessed July 2005.

11. Orme CN: Customer information and the quality improvement process: developing a customer information system, *Hosp Health Serv Administration* 37:197-212, 1992.

12. Collopy BT: Do doctors need Deming? *Qual Assur Health Care* 5:3-5, 1993.

13. Goldsmith J: A radical prescription for hospitals, *Harvard Business Rev* May-June 67:104-111, 1989.

14. Joint Commission on Accreditation of Healthcare Organizations: Agenda for change Q & A: indicators and the IMS, *Joint Commission Perspect* 12:9, 1992.

15. Donabedian A: *Explorations in quality assessment and monitoring,* vol 1, The definition of quality and approaches to its assessment, Ann Arbor, MI, 1980, Health Administration Press.

16. Spath P, Stewart A: *From quality to excellence: using comparative data to improve health care performance,* Forest Grove, OR, 2002, Brown-Spath & Associates.

17. Surgical Infection Prevention Improvement Project: http://www.qipa. org/pa/medical_professionals/hospitals/scip.aspx. Accessed October 2005.

18. Agency for Health Care Policy and Research: *Using clinical practice guidelines to evaluate quality of care,* vol. 1, Issues, Washington, DC, 1995, U.S. Department of Health and Human Services, AHCPR Pub. No. 95-0045.

19. Hjort B: The HIM role in patient safety and quality of care (AHIMA Practice Brief), *J AHIMA* 76:56A-56G, 2005.

20. Langley G, Nolan K, Nolan T et al: *The improvement guide: a practical approach to improving organizational performance,* San Francisco, 1996, Jossey-Bass.

21. Womack J, Jones DT, Roos D: *The machine that changed the world: the story of lean production,* New York, 1990, HerperPerennial.

22. Huber G: *Managerial decision making,* Glenview, IL, 1980, Scott, Foresman.

23. Shewhart WA: *Economic control of quality and manufactured product,* New York, 1931, D Van Nostrand (reprinted by American Society for Quality Control, Milwaukee, WI, 1980).

24. Kelly DL: *How to use control charts for healthcare,* Milwaukee, WI, 1999, American Society for Quality, Quality Press.

25. Devers KJ, Pham HH, Liu G: What is driving hospitals' patient-safety efforts? *Health Affairs* 23:103-115, 2004.

26. Bagain JP, Lee C, Gosbee J et al: Developing and deploying a patient safety program in a large health care delivery system: you can't fix what you don't know about, *Joint Commission J Qual Improv* 27:522-532, 2001.

27. Kohn LT, Corrigan JM, Donaldson MS, editors: *To err is human: building a safer health system,* Washington, DC, 1999, National Academy Press: http://www.nap.edu/catalog/9728.html.

28. Aspden P, Corrigan JM, Wolcott J et al, editors: *Patient safety: achieving a new standard for care,* Washington, DC, 2004, National Academy Press: http://books.nap.edu/books/0309090776/html.

29. *AHRQ quality indicators—guide to patient safety indicators,* Rockville, MD, 2003, Agency for Healthcare Research and Quality: AHRQ publication No. 03-R203: http://www.qualityindicators.ahrq.gov.

30. Hurtado MP, Swift EK, Corrigan JM, editors: *Envisioning the national health care quality report,* Washington, DC, 2001, National Academy Press: http://www.nap.edu.catalog/10073.html.

31. Brennan TA, Leape LL, Laird NMet al: Incidence of adverse events and negligence in hospitalized patients: results of the Harvard Medical Practice Study I, *N Engl J Med* 324:370-376, 1991.

32. Spath PL: Using failure mode and effects analysis to improve patient safety, *AORN J* 78:16-37, 2003.

33. Thomas, EJ, Stuodert DM, Burstin HR et al: Incidence and types of adverse events and negligent care in Utah and Colorado, *Med Care* 38:261-271, 2000.

34. Barker KN, Flynn EA, Pepper GA, et al: Medication errors observed in 36 health care facilities, *Arch Intern Med* 162:1897-1903, 2002.

35. Institute for Healthcare Improvement. Failure modes and effects analysis tool: http://www.ihi.org/ihi/workspace/tools/fmea/. Accessed June 2005.

36. Croteau RJ, Schyve PM: Proactive error-proofing healthcare processes. In Spath PL, editor: *Error reduction in healthcare: a systems approach to improving patient safety,* p. 189, San Francisco, 2000, Joeey-Bass/AHA Press.

37. Gaba DM: The future vision of simulation in health care, *Qual Safety Health Care* 13:12-110, 2004.

38. Pozgar GD: *Legal aspects of health care administration,* ed 9, Gaithersburg, MD, 2004, Aspen.

39. Wickizer TM, Lessler D: Utilization management: Issues, effects and future prospects, *Annu Rev PublicHealth* 23:233-254, 2002.

40. Department of Health and Human Services, Centers for Medicare and Medicare Services: Part 482—Conditions of Participation for Hospitals, Sec. 482.30 Condition of participation: Utilization review. October 1, 1999.

41. Greenberg, L., Carneal G. Hattwick M: Trends and practices in medical management: 2001 industry survey. Washington, DC, 2001, URAC.

42. Department of Health and Human Services, Centers for Medicare and Medicare Services: Part 482—Conditions of Participation for Hospitals, Sec. 482.43 Conditions of participation: Discharge planning. October 1, 1999.

43. Nelson P: The elements of provider credentialing, *J AHIMA* 70:34-39, 1999.

44. Deming W: *Out of the crisis,* Cambridge, MA, 1986, Massachusetts Institute of Technology, Center for Advanced Engineering Study.

Data Analysis and Use

Jennifer Garvin

Additional content,
http://evolve.elsevier.com/Abdelhak/

Review exercises can be found
in the Study Guide

Data Uses
Registries Overview
  Case Definition and Eligibility
  Case Finding
  Abstracting
  Registry Quality Control
  Confidentiality and Release of Information
Cancer Registries
  Hospital Cancer Registries
  Population–Based Cancer Registries
  Cancer Registry Abstracting
  Cancer Registry Coding
  Cancer Registry Staging
  Quality Management of the Cancer Program and Registry
    Data
  Use of Cancer Registry Data
  The Cancer Registrar Profession
Birth Defects Registries
  Birth Defects Case Definition and Coding
  Quality Control of Birth Defects Registry Data
  Use of Birth Defects Registry Data
Death Registries
Diabetes Registries
  Diabetes Registry Case Finding
Implant Registries
Immunization Registries
  Immunization Registry Case Finding and Data Use
Organ Transplant Registries
  Transplant Case Registration and Data Use
Trauma Registries
  Trauma Registry Case Finding and Data Use
Research and Use of Data
  Health Services Research

Key Words

Abstracting	Data warehouse	Passive case
Accessioned	Differentiation	Pay-for-performance
Active case ascertainment surveillance	Entities	Population-based registry
Attribute	Epidemiologic case definition	Primary data
Bioterrorism	Etiology	Record
Case	Field	Reference date
Case eligibility	Follow-up	Secondary data
Case finding	Grading	Stage
Clinical case definition	Incidence	Surveillance
Clinical decision support	Logical data model	Table
Comorbidity	Major birth defects	Topography
Core measure	Metadata	Value/coding
Data dictionary	Morphology	
Data element	Outcome	

This is a revision of the chapter in the previous edition authored by Sue Watkins, RHIA, CTR.
Significant portions of Chapter 14 related to data dictionaries and decision support were adapted from chapters by Maida Herbst and Kathleen Aller in
Electronic Health Records: Changing the Vision.

Medical Research
   Role of a Data Broker in Research
Public Health
Planning and Assessment
Data and Health
Performance Management
Outcomes
   Outcomes Data and Information Systems
   Outcomes Data Use
   Outcomes and the Electronic Health Record
   Outcome Indicators
   Outcomes and Coding Issues
   Desirable Outcome Systems
Clinical Decision Support
Data Dictionary
   Data Dictionary Definitions
   Purpose of the Data Dictionary
   Scope of the Data Dictionary
   Meta-Content of the Data Dictionary
   Building the Data Dictionary
      Step 1: Inventory of an Existing Enterprise
      Step 2: Identifying New Data Content Needs
      Step 3: Consensus Development
   Criteria for Data Element Inclusion
   Cataloging Standards

Abbreviations

AAFP—American Academy of Family Physicians
ACG—Adjusted Clinical Group
ACIP—Advisory Committee on Immunization Practices
ACS—American College of Surgeons
ACSCOT—American College of Surgeons Committee on Trauma
AIS—Abbreviated Injury Scale
AJCC—American Joint Committee on Cancer
ANSI—American National Standards Institute
APACHE—Acute Physiology, Age, and Chronic Health Evaluation
APR-DRG—All Patient Refined DRGs
ASTM—American Society for Testing and Materials
CCS—Clinical Classification Software
CDC—Centers for Disease Control and Prevention
CMS—Centers for Medicare and Medicaid Services
CoC—Commission on Cancer
CPT—Current Procedural Terminology
CODES—Crash Outcomes Data Evaluation System
CTR—Certified Tumor Registrar
DCE—Distributed Computing Environment
DCG—Diagnosis Cost Group
EHR—Electronic health record
EMS—Emergency medical system
FIGO—International Federation of Gynecology and Obstetrics
HEDIS—Health Plan Employer Data and Information Set

HIM—Health information management
HIS—Health care information system
HISPP—Healthcare Informatics Standards Planning Panel
HITSP—Healthcare Information Technology Standards Panel
HL7—Health Level 7
HOI—Health Outcomes Institute
ICCS—International Classification of Clinical Services
ICD-9-CM—*International Classification of Diseases, Ninth Revision, Clinical Modification*
ICD-10-CM—*International Classification of Diseases, Tenth Revision, Clinical Modification*
ICD-O-3—*International Classification of Diseases for Oncology, Third Edition*
IDDM—insulin-dependent diabetes mellitus
IWG—Informatics Working Group
JCAHO—Joint Commission on Accreditation of Healthcare Organizations (now The Joint Commission)
MACDP—Metropolitan Atlanta Congenital Defects Program
MHCA—Mental Health Council of America
NAACCR—North American Association of Central Cancer Registries
NCDB—National Cancer Data Base
NCI—National Cancer Institute
NCQA—National Committee for Quality Assurance
NCRA—National Cancer Registrars Association, Inc.
NIDDM—Non-insulin-dependent diabetes mellitus
NOTA—National Organ Transplant Act
NTDB—National Trauma Data Bank
NVAC—National Vaccine Advisory Committee
OPTM—Organ Procurement and Transplantation Network
OSF—Open Systems Foundation
ROADS—*Registry Operations and Data Standards*
SEER—Surveillance, Epidemiology, and End Results
SQL—Standard Structured Query Language
TNM—Tumor, lymph node, and metastases
UNOS—United Network for Organ Sharing
WHO—World Health Organization
XML—Extensible markup language

Objectives

- Define key words.
- Describe various registries and their purposes.
- Discuss the uses of registry data.
- Describe and develop data collection methods.
- Discuss how health care data can be used for registry development, research purposes, administrative analysis, outcomes research, and consumer decision making.
- Delineate the content and infrastructure of an outcomes information system.
- Discuss the importance and methods of formulating a data dictionary for a health information system.

DATA USES

Health care data are created by health-related events and are used by many different people, organizations, and agencies for multiple purposes. Users of health data range from the individual patient, the health care providers, and organizations to epidemiologists, researchers, health care payers, grant funding organizations, politicians, and public agencies. The uses vary as much as the users. The primary purpose of health care data is obviously for the care of the patient. Secondary uses, including validating reasons for reimbursement by health care payers, evaluation and planning related to health care services, tracking and preventing disability and disease, health policy analysis, tracking outcomes of treatment, and assisting individuals and communities in achieving better health, have grown in importance.

Health care data are often in the form of coded data that translate narrative prose into numerical or alphanumerical codes (numbers and letters). This information can be recoded or translated into other coding schemes beyond the original through a mapping process. Coded data are discussed in depth in Chapter 6.

Given the importance of these data, attention to quality is paramount. The accuracy of data is based on how well the codes match the information they represent. The quality of the data can be affected by several factors, including how it is generated, the training of the individuals who are assigning the codes, and the supporting reference material that is available. Coded data are aggregated from individual health encounters into large databases. Within databases, it is possible to generate a variety of descriptive reports, including the number of each type of diagnosis patients have during a given time period, the number and type of procedures, and provider statistics and demographics. These summary reports are indices of the types of diagnoses treated, procedures performed, and providers who treated the patients in a given setting during a given time period.

The information contained in the actual patient record is considered **primary data,** whereas the information that is generated from the record is considered to be **secondary data**. Both primary and secondary data can compose the information in databases. This chapter will cover the many uses of data beginning with registries and discussion of outcomes research and development of data dictionaries and standards.

REGISTRIES OVERVIEW

A registry is a systematic collection of data specific to a type of disease (e.g., cancer, acquired immune deficiency syndrome [AIDS]), exposure to hazardous substances or events (such as Agent Orange), or trauma and treatment (such as implanted medical devices). The data collected, methods of data collection, reports generated, and their use vary with the kind of registry. They provide **surveillance** (collection, collation, analysis, and dissemination of data) mechanisms and, for some, **incidence** (occurrence) measures. A registry can be established for any disease; an overview of the characteristics of some of them will be provided in this chapter. Registries can also vary by location or type of agency. Some are specific to an organization such as a hospital.[1] Others are operated by a governmental agency and collect data about a geographic area such as a city, county, or state.

Case Definition and Eligibility

A **case** is defined as a person with a given disease or condition that will be included in the registry. Criteria are established to determine who should be included. Whether a person has the disease is established through a set of criteria. Some definitions are set as reportable conditions by the Centers for Disease Control and Prevention (CDC) as **epidemiologic case definitions.** These are of diseases that must be reported to a public health agency. Epidemiologic analysis is then undertaken on the basis of the specific issues of interest regarding the disease being studied.

A **clinical case definition** may be established as well. A clinical definition is a list of signs and symptoms that establish a clinical diagnosis. A clinical case may be reported as a reportable disease if it meets the epidemiologic case criteria. In addition to the clinical diagnoses, other criteria may need to be met for the condition to meet the epidemiologic definition. A patient may have the clinical signs and symptoms requiring treatment and yet may not meet the strict definition for reporting designated by the CDC.[2]

Case definitions are provided for all reportable diseases, and the case definitions for specific types of registries are discussed later in applicable sections of the chapter.

Case Finding

Case finding is the method by which all the eligible cases to be included in the registry are identified, accessioned into the registry, and abstracted. Case finding mechanisms should be redundant and include multiple methods to identify all the cases. This may mean that the same patient is found more than once; care should be taken to only include the patient once in the database. For example, receiving information from multiple data sources such as the pathology department or laboratory, an applicable section of the disease index from the health information management (HIM) department, the radiology department, the operating suite, and outpatient departments that may interact with the patients who are served by the registry will likely result in identifying several episodes of care for the patient.

Depending on the type of registry, the various treatments will be denoted for the patient or the patient is simply accessioned, and the abstract is done and sent (reported) to the registry involved.

Abstracting

Generally, a set of predetermined data is obtained from the patient record and related sources through a process called **abstracting**. These data items are collected because of their relevance to the disease or condition addressed in the registry. Abstracts are prepared for each case and then form the information included in the database. **Abstracting** this information provides a succinct summary characterizing various issues including demographic information about the patient, diagnostic information, treatment data, outcome of treatment, and **follow-up** information.

Registry Quality Control

Visual and computerized checks on data entered into the database should be performed by the personnel responsible for the database of the registry. This may be required by the organization external to the registry or simply to ensure that the database has consistent, complete, accurate data. Accuracy and completeness of data are important to ensure data integrity. The value of registry data is directly related to the validity of the data collected. Generally, to ensure data validity, a systematic quality control sampling of 5% to 10% of all cases in the registry should be reviewed for data quality.[3] The linkage of computerized information may allow cross-referencing of data to ensure that all cases have been included and that the data elements in the records match other records.

Confidentiality of Registry Information

Registries contain patient-identifiable information that is derived from primary patient record information. All information in the registry must be kept confidential. Confidentiality policies and procedures are required in all phases of registry operations and should address protection of the privacy of individual patients, facility information, and the privacy of the physicians and health care providers who report the cases. They should also provide public assurance that the data will not be abused and that all confidentiality-protecting legislation or administrative rule(s) will be enforced.

CANCER REGISTRIES

Cancer registries are described in this chapter in more detail than other registries are because they are the most common type of registry. They are located in hospitals of all sizes and in every region of the country. In addition, all states have central or population-based cancer registries. Understanding the fundamentals of cancer registries provides the reader with an excellent foundation for developing other types of registries. The collection, retrieval, and analysis of cancer data by cancer registries are important to physicians, epidemiologists, and researchers concerned with assessing cancer incidence, treatment, and end results.

The purpose of the hospital cancer data system is to collect and maintain information on every patient with cancer from the initial date of diagnosis or treatment until death. The information collected furnishes the health care team with outcome data that enable them to see the results of their diagnostic and therapeutic efforts and provide them with the tools to improve patient care.

Hospital-based cancer registries or their equivalents have existed in the United States for many decades. Reports on cancer experience were issued in the late 1800s from such institutions as the American Oncologic Hospital in Philadelphia, the General Memorial Hospital in New York City, the Johns Hopkins Hospital in Baltimore, and Charity Hospital in New Orleans.[4] In the 1920s, the American College of Surgeons (ACS) asked its members to submit information on living patients with bone cancer. Subsequent requests were made later in the same decade for data collection on cancer of the cervix, breast, mouth and tongue, colon, and thyroid. In 1930, the ACS's Commission on Cancer developed standards for hospital cancer clinics and began surveying facilities. By 1937, there were 240 approved cancer clinics, but it was not until 1956 that a cancer registry providing life-long follow-up of cancer patients became a requirement for an approved cancer program.[5]

The first central registry was established in Connecticut when a group of New Haven physicians began compiling data that showed a steady increase in the cancer rates in their community. The physicians proceeded to start cancer clinics in their hospitals and to maintain uniform records. The Connecticut Medical Society formed a Tumor Study Committee and was instrumental in getting legislation passed that created the Division of Cancer and Other Chronic Diseases in 1935. In 1941, statewide cancer surveillance began when a team from the division visited each hospital and abstracted data from the records of all patients with cancer for the period 1935 through 1940.[5]

The National Cancer Act of 1971 mandated the collection, analysis, and dissemination of data for use in the prevention, diagnosis, and treatment of cancer. This mandate led to the establishment of the Surveillance, Epidemiology, and End Results (SEER) Program, a continuing project of the National Cancer Institute (NCI). The SEER Program operates *population-based cancer registries* in various geographic areas of the country covering about 14% of the U.S. population. The selection of demographic areas is based primarily on the areas' epidemiologically significant subgroups to provide a sampling of the U.S.

population. Trends in cancer incidence, mortality rates, and patient survival in the United States are derived from this database.[6]

With the passage of the Cancer Registries Amendment Act (Public Law 102-515) in 1992, a national program of population-based cancer registries was created. Funding of $16.83 million was allocated by Congress for 1994 to set up statewide registries in states where none existed and to enhance existing registries. Today, there are more than 2000 hospital-based cancer registries and all states have population-based registries. The categories of cancer registries are generally defined as hospital based or population based.[5]

Hospital Cancer Registries

The primary goal of hospital-based cancer registries is to improve patient care. The cancer registry provides a system for monitoring all types of cancer diagnosed or treated in an organization. The data collected are used to optimize care for patients with cancer, to compare the institution's morbidity and survival rates with regional and national statistics, to determine the need for professional and public education programs, and to help allocate resources.[1]

Hospital-based registries may be in single-institution or multi-institution settings, military hospitals, managed care programs, or free-standing treatment facilities. The patient care–oriented goal usually dictates the type of data collected. Data items collected include patient identification and demographic information, cancer diagnosis, treatment rendered, prognostic factors, and outcome.

A hospital cancer registry is one of the components of a cancer program approved by the ACS Commission on Cancer (CoC). The latest edition of the Cancer Program Standards, available on the CoC's Web site, delineates the total program requirements.

Hospitals are required by law to report cancer cases to a state registry but not to have an ACS-approved cancer registry. A hospital-based registry may be associated with a population-based registry (such as a registry operated by the state government); the latter often supports and facilitates the hospital's efforts as a major source of its data. Support from the population-based registry may consist of analyzing data, generating reports that allow comparison of data, providing data collection software, assisting in quality improvement activities, and providing professional training to the hospital cancer registry staff.

The **case eligibility** for most cancer registries is defined by all the organization's patients diagnosed (clinically or histologically) or treated for active diseases on or after the **reference date** or beginning of the registry are eligible for inclusion. For example, patients who were diagnosed and are being treated at the hospital, patients diagnosed at autopsy, patients who were diagnosed elsewhere and are receiving all or part of their first course of therapy or whose therapy was planned at the hospital, and patients who were diagnosed at

the hospital and are receiving all their first course of therapy elsewhere should be included in the registry. The cancer manual for each registry will define specifically the types of cases to be included.

When patients are determined eligible and added to the registry, they are said to be **accessioned** into the registry.

The ability to identify every reportable case of cancer is essential to the success of a cancer registry system.[7] The case finding system must include all points of service from when patients enter the health care delivery system for diagnostic or therapeutic services for the management of cancer.[8] The primary case finding sources are the pathology, HIM department information, and outpatient departments. As a key resource, cancer registry personnel examine the reports from the pathology department for all pathologic diagnoses of cancer. The types of reports include surgical specimen, autopsy, bone marrow, hematology, and cytology reports. The second most common source is the organization's database of diagnosis codes. Logs of patients seen in radiation therapy and other outpatient departments are also examined to ensure all cancer patients are identified for inclusion in the registry.

Population–Based Cancer Registries

There are three types of **population-based cancer registries**. These include incidence only, cancer control, and research. Most incidence-only registries are operated by a government health agency and are designed to determine cancer rates and trends in a defined population. Monitoring cancer incidence is legislatively mandated in most states. The mandate usually outlines the duties of the registry system and the data to be collected, targets the sources from which data are to be obtained, details the confidentiality policies of the system, provides protection from any liability, and in many states defines the penalties for noncompliance. Data collected are typically limited to patient and cancer identification.

Cancer control population-based registries serve a broader function; often combining incidence, patient care, and end results reporting with various other research and cancer control activities, such as cancer screening and smoking cessation programs. Their data set is often the same as that of their reporting hospitals, including treatment and outcome data and incidence-only information.

Many universities operate research-oriented registries to conduct epidemiologic research focused on **etiology** (study of the causes of disease). Research requirements commonly include rapid case ascertainment so that patients can be identified and contacted as soon as possible after diagnosis. Research data are typically defined and collected on a project-specific basis by an ad hoc mechanism of chart review, patient contact, or some other special procedure. For example, a study of the incidence of cancer in twins may include sibling identification, chart review of a twin with cancer, and patient and family interviews. Another study may be conducted to determine the risk factors of women younger than age 30 years with breast cancer (a population with a low incidence of this disease).

Conversely, a cancer-control type of registry is operated primarily to support the targeting and evaluation of control programs, such as cancer screening for early detection and education. The registry may be limited to specific types of cancer for which distinctive intervention strategies have been established. The data collected are limited to what is needed for an intervention strategy or to evaluate the intervention effect. Data are used to assess areas of high risk, plan education programs, and focus resources aimed at reducing or eliminating the incidence of cancer. Information is shared with public officials and health care providers and often published in medical and research journals.

Many population-based registries are, in effect, combinations of all three types. The legislative mandate and funding sources normally dictate the effort expended in any one particular area—incidence monitoring, research, or cancer control.[5]

The case definition for cancer registries consists of neoplasms that are to be reported to the registry. The best classification system for developing a reportable list for a cancer registry is based on the *International Classification of Diseases for Oncology,* Third Edition (ICD-O-3).[6] This publication includes coded data that is based on the anatomical site and the behavior of the tumor. The ACS requires that all tumors with a morphology behavior code of 2 or higher, indicating an in situ or a malignant tumor in the ICD-O-3, be included for approved cancer programs.[1] The medical or research staff associated with the registry may request that other cases be included (e.g., nonmalignant meningiomas, villous adenomas of the colon, benign liver tumors).

Central registries that collect data for the states in the United States each have a cancer registry manual that describes the case definition and case eligibility. For example, in New Jersey all cases of cancer that were diagnosed after October 1, 1978, are reportable. The exceptions to this requirement are skin cancers that are localized. In addition, benign and borderline tumors of the brain and central nervous system are also reportable.

Cancer Registry Abstracting

The cancer abstract must permit recording of all relevant data in a logical and uniform manner. Abstracting guidelines are provided in the *Self Instructional Manual for Tumor Registrars,* Book 5, SEER Program,[9] and the *Registry Operations and Data Standards* (ROADS), CoC, American College of Surgeons, 2004.[8] In addition, most state and regional registries have established abstracting requirements. The amount of data collected is dictated by the CoC for approved cancer programs, policies established by the cancer committee, and the limitations inherent in a specific computer software system (see CoC Data Set). A sample abstract is shown in Figure 14-1.

Cancer Registry Coding

The coding scheme traditionally used by cancer registries is the ICD-O-3, published by the World Health Organization (WHO). This coding scheme is recommended by the CoC[1] and is used by the National Cancer Registrars Association, Inc. (NCRA) in its annual certification examination.

The ICD-O-3 represents a more detailed extension of the *International Classification of Diseases,* Tenth Edition, *Clinical Modification* (ICD-10-CM) chapter on neoplasms. ICD-O-3 permits coding of all neoplasms to include **topography** (site), **morphology** (cell structure and form), **grading** (variation from normal tissue), and **differentiation** (another term for variation from normal tissue).[7]

Cancer Registry Staging

The extent of the spread of cancer or **stage** at the time of initial diagnosis and treatment is recorded for every case included in the registry. Numerous staging systems have been developed for use by the medical community. Some are site specific (e.g., Dukes A-D Stage Grouping for Colorectal Cancer) or system specific (e.g., International Federation of Gynecology and Obstetrics [FIGO] classification for gynecologic sites). Others are general and may be applied to almost all sites.

Historically, the staging system most commonly used was developed in 1977 by the SEER Program of the NCI, *Self Instructional Manual for Tumor Registrars,* Book 6, or the *Summary Staging Guide.* This system is used to stage cases as in situ, localized, regional spread to lymph nodes or adjacent tissue, or distant spread to lymph nodes in other areas of the body or distant sites. In addition, the CoC requires that all sites, excluding pediatric tumors, be staged according to the current edition of the American Joint Committee on Cancer (AJCC) *Manual for Staging of Cancer.*[1,10] Registries have the option of using either the AJCC staging scheme for pediatric tumors or nationally accepted protocol staging systems. In the AJCC staging system, the extent of disease is categorized according to tumor size (T), lymph node involvement (N), and metastases (M). Frequently referred to as the TNM system, it brings together information on staging of cancer at various anatomic sites in cooperation with the TNM Committee of the International Union Against Cancer. The proper classification and staging of cancer allow physicians to determine appropriate treatment, evaluate results of case management, and compare outcome with worldwide statistics reported from various institutions on a local, regional, state, and national basis.

Although the TNM system was designed for use by physicians, in some hospitals staging is done by the registry staff.[7,11] A working knowledge of both the SEER and the AJCC staging systems is necessary.

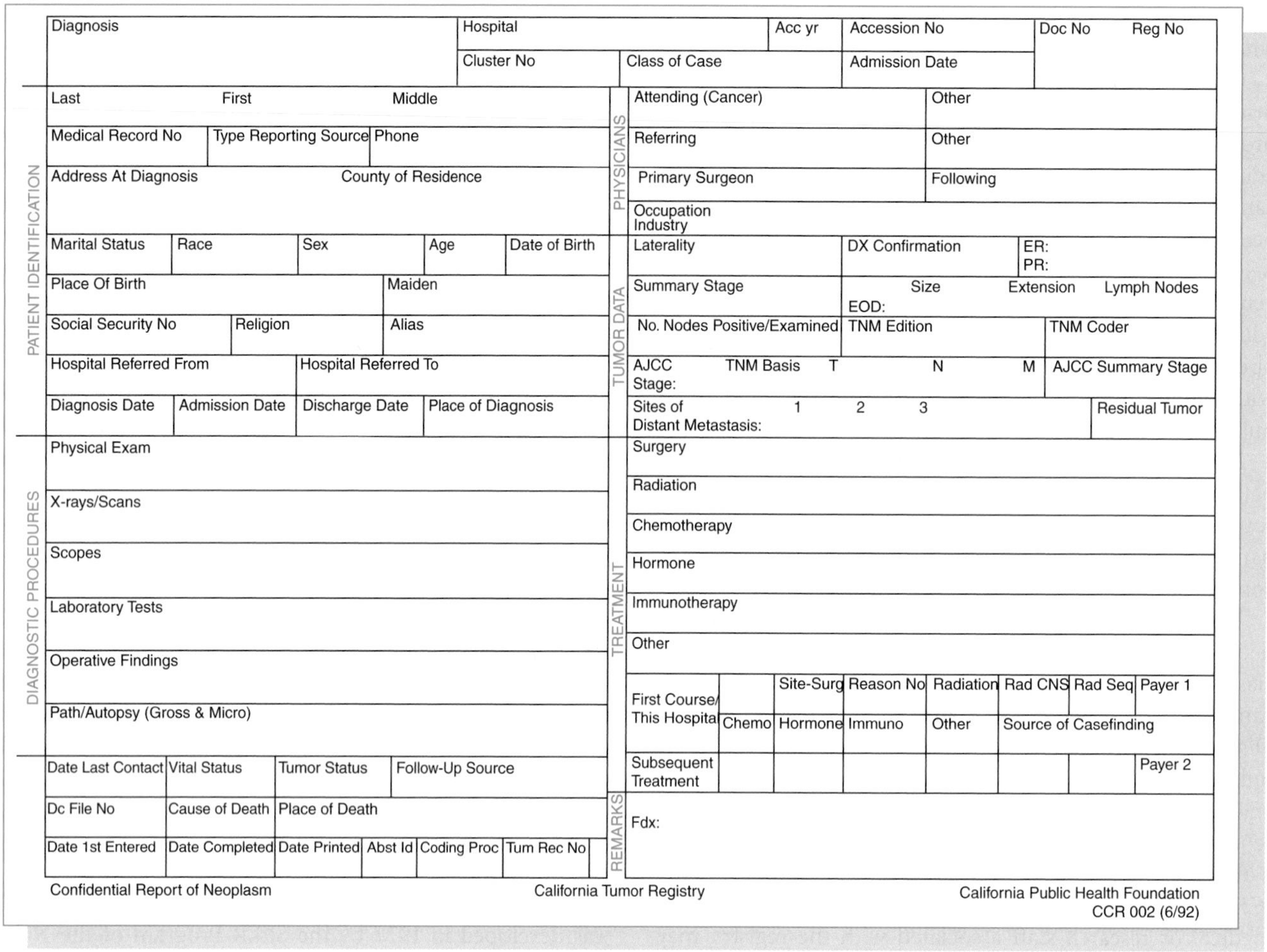
Diagnosis | Hospital | Acc yr | Accession No | Doc No | Reg No
Cluster No | Class of Case | Admission Date

PATIENT IDENTIFICATION
Last | First | Middle
Medical Record No | Type Reporting Source | Phone
Address At Diagnosis | County of Residence
Marital Status | Race | Sex | Age | Date of Birth
Place Of Birth | Maiden
Social Security No | Religion | Alias
Hospital Referred From | Hospital Referred To
Diagnosis Date | Admission Date | Discharge Date | Place of Diagnosis

PHYSICIANS
Attending (Cancer) | Other
Referring | Other
Primary Surgeon | Following
Occupation Industry

TUMOR DATA
Laterality | DX Confirmation | ER: PR:
Summary Stage | Size | Extension | Lymph Nodes | EOD:
No. Nodes Positive/Examined | TNM Edition | TNM Coder
AJCC Stage: | TNM Basis | T | N | M | AJCC Summary Stage
Sites of Distant Metastasis: | 1 | 2 | 3 | Residual Tumor

DIAGNOSTIC PROCEDURES
Physical Exam
X-rays/Scans
Scopes
Laboratory Tests
Operative Findings
Path/Autopsy (Gross & Micro)

TREATMENT
Surgery
Radiation
Chemotherapy
Hormone
Immunotherapy
Other
First Course/This Hospital | Site-Surg | Reason No | Radiation | Rad CNS | Rad Seq | Payer 1
Chemo | Hormone | Immuno | Other | Source of Casefinding
Subsequent Treatment | Payer 2

Date Last Contact | Vital Status | Tumor Status | Follow-Up Source
Dc File No | Cause of Death | Place of Death
Date 1st Entered | Date Completed | Date Printed | Abst Id | Coding Proc | Tum Rec No

REMARKS
Fdx:

Confidential Report of Neoplasm | California Tumor Registry | California Public Health Foundation CCR 002 (6/92)

Figure 14-1 Cancer registry abstract.

Quality Management of the Cancer Program and Registry Data

To be effective, the quality management program must be multidisciplinary and must include four components: quality planning, measurement, evaluation, and improvement. The quality management plan details the roles and responsibilities of the cancer committee and members of the health care team. Some of the outcomes assessed in a quality management program include appropriate and timely diagnosis, appropriate and timely consultations and referrals, accessibility of available health care services, evaluating patient outcomes, and absence of clinically unnecessary diagnostic or therapeutic procedures.

The cancer committee is responsible for establishing the quality improvement priorities of the cancer program and for monitoring the effectiveness of quality improvement activities.[1] The cancer committee is required to identify at least two important issues related to cancer patient care to evaluate annually. At least one priority should be related to site-specific patient survival rates. Sources to be used in selecting quality improvement priorities include comparison of local experience with regional and national survival and outcome data. This benchmarking provides insight into whether the care given at the hospital meets or exceeds that given elsewhere. These measures should be used to evaluate compliance with treatment. The cancer committee evaluates the results of the measurement activities to assess current performance and to evaluate the need for interventions aimed at reducing or eliminating poor performance.

The usefulness of the data collected by a registry depends on the quality of the data. Quality control procedures are important to ensure the completeness, accuracy, and timeliness of the data collected. The CoC places accountability for quality control of registry data with the cancer committee because it is responsible for the overall supervision of the cancer registry.[1]

It is the policy of many registries to perform visual inspection on 100% of their cases. In large registries, a review or reabstracting of a portion of the cases by another member of the registry staff ensures consistent recording and interpretation of information. In the latter instance, the two abstracts are compared and discrepancies are noted and discussed.[7]

Computerized registries have quality management tools for edits and computer-assisted coding. Registry staff must not rely solely on the electronic tools for quality management because, as of yet, computers are unable to read the documentation to determine completeness, accuracy, and support for the coded data.

The data collection component encompasses the data items required by the CoC for approved hospital programs. Optional data fields might include hospital-specific, financial, and The Joint Commission clinical indicators. Other features available from some vendors consist of multiple-user networks, hospital mainframe interface, expanded statistical applications, and graphics. Some hospital software vendors maintain national databases that contain aggregate data submitted by their users. The Tumor Registry Software Checklist presented at the 1993 annual meeting of the National Cancer Registrars Association, Inc., can be used by hospitals to evaluate cancer registry software (Figure 14-2).

The North American Association of Central Cancer Registries, Inc. (NAACCR) has developed a national standard for data exchange. The NAACCR Record Layout provides a common standard record layout that can be used for the electronic exchange of data.[12] The NAACCR Record Layout has been used by the ACS Commission on National Cancer Data Base (NCDB) Call for Data. Participation in the NCDB became a mandatory standard of the ACS Approvals Program beginning with the 1996 data year.

Use of Cancer Registry Data

Cancer registry data are used for performance improvement projects, cancer conferences, administrative reports, and marketing. Hospitals with ACS-approved cancer programs are required to publish and distribute an annual report. Approved cancer programs are also required to document the use of cancer registry data through the use of a request log.[1]

The Cancer Registrar Profession

The Council on Certification of the NCRA approved the definition of the cancer registry field:

- Individuals working in or supervising cancer registry and organizations or companies that actively support cancer registration. Cancer registration involves the management and analysis of cancer incidence data for all of the following purposes:
  - Research
  - Quality management/improvement
  - Cancer program development

- Cancer prevention and surveillance
- Survival and outcome data
- Compliance of reporting standards
- Development of accreditation standards for cancer registration[11]

Cancer registrars are dedicated to providing quality data with the goal of improved treatments and, ultimately, cures for cancer. The significant demand for cancer registrars extends to every level of the cancer surveillance community, including regulatory agencies, accrediting organizations, researchers, pharmaceutical firms, software vendors, and contract services providers.

The NCRA is a nonprofit, professional organization representing the cancer registrars. The NCRA promotes education, credentialing, and advocacy for cancer registry professionals. The Council on Certification of the NCRA certifies the professionals who meet the eligibility requirements and are successful on the national examination as Certified Tumor Registrars (CTR).

HIM professionals have historically been one of the major areas for career progression into the cancer registry field. Their education and experiences makes them uniquely qualified to transition into the field of cancer registration with minimal additional training.

BIRTH DEFECTS REGISTRIES

Birth defects are the leading cause of infant mortality in the United States, and genetic diseases account for about one half of pediatric hospital admissions.[13] In addition, birth defects are the fifth leading cause of years of potential life lost and contribute substantially to childhood morbidity and long-term disability. Major birth defects are diagnosed in 3% to 4% of infants in the first year of life.[14] Population-based birth registries have operated since the 1920s, with the earliest being in the state of New Jersey. In the early years, birth registries strictly used vital records to identify malformations. The Birth Defects Prevention Act of 1998 requires that data are collected and analyzed, epidemiologic research is undertaken, and information and education efforts with the aim of preventing birth defects are facilitated. Birth defects surveillance systems are characterized as either active or passive case reporting systems.

Active case ascertainment surveillance systems identify cases in all hospitals, clinics, or other medical facilities through systematic review of patient records, surgery records, disease indexes, pathology reports, vital records, and hospital logs (obstetrical, newborn nursery, neonatal intensive care unit, postmortem) or by interviewing health professionals who may be knowledgeable about diagnosed cases.

Passive case ascertainment surveillance systems rely on reports submitted to the registry by hospitals, clinics, or

This checklist can be used to evaluate cancer registry software

Functional and Technical Requirements	Commission on Cancer Requirements	Software _____
Overall software		
Menu-driven		
User-friendly		
Network capability (single or multiple users, one or several locations)		
Case identification		
Suspense file/system	●	
Interface with other databases (pathology, disease index, outpatient visit/charge file) to assist in casefinding		
Flags for special populations, eg, cancer screening		
Combined with master patient file		
Patient Data Collection		
Data sets		
Commission on Cancer	●	
State registry		
SEER		
Hospital specific		
Other data items, such as The Joint Commission clinical indicators, financial		
English text space		
Data entry		
Capability to add/change/delete cases		
Retention of follow-up information		
Ease in changing previously entered materials		
Assistance in coding		
Duplicate record detection	●	
Verification of data entry	●	
Edit checks (valid codes and interfield/relational edits)		
Editing of new data and changed data		
Help screens to assist in coding		
Reporting		
Flexibility in selecting data elements	●	
Interface with any "canned," ad hoc report, or follow-up listing		
Accurate and useful reports	●	
Reports displayed on screen as well as printed		
User-designed reports		
Statistical analysis (cross tabulations, summary analysis, & survival analysis by life-table or actuarial method)	●	
Administrative reports (printouts and on-screen displays)		
Alphabetic patient listing (patient index file)	●	
Numerical listing of patients (accession register)	●	
Abstract or case summary	●	
Primary site list by year (abstract file)	●	
Suspense list (file)	●	
Staff productivity report (cases abstracted, follow-up posted, suspense cases added, etc, by each staff member)		
Other reports		

● Required, ☐ Preferred

Source: Suzanna Hoyler, CTR, Washington Hospital Center, Washington, D.C. 1993 NTRA Annual Meeting, 5/6/93

Figure 14-2 Cancer registry software checklist.

other facilities, supplemented with data from vital statistics. In some states, staff submits reports voluntarily, but, in general, reporting requirements are established by state legislation. One example of a passive surveillance system is the national Birth Defects Monitoring Program. Newborn hospital discharge summaries are obtained from electronic health information systems, and investigators have no opportunity to review the rest of the patient record.

Many state and regional birth defect registries are modeled after the Metropolitan Atlanta Congenital Defects Program (MACDP), which is the first active case ascertainment system in the United States. The MACDP criteria include cases in which the infant has a serious or major structural defect that can adversely affect health and development and cases of live-born infants and stillbirths, 20 weeks of gestation or more, weighing 500 grams or more. Pregnancies with birth defects prenatally diagnosed and terminated before 20 weeks of gestation are ascertained whenever possible, but because of incomplete ascertainment, the records are kept as separate data.[16]

Birth Defects Case Definition and Coding

In all birth defects registries the goal is to capture data about specific types of congenital anomalies and conditions. However, the goals vary by the type of case surveillance system (active vs passive) used. These anomalies are identified and coded with *International Classification of Diseases,* Ninth Revision, *Clinical Modification* (ICD-9-CM) codes that fall within the range 740.0 to 759.9.

In 70% to 80% of cases, birth defects occur as isolated defects. Attempts are being made to classify infants with multiple birth defects according to biologically meaningful categories to assist in identifying etiological and pathogenetic mechanisms. Birth defects can also be classified as major or minor; **major birth defects** are those that affect survival, require substantial medical care, or result in marked physiological or psychological impairment.

The CDC has defined a set of core data items to be included in a birth defects registry. Some of the items include syndrome identification, demographic data, pregnancy history, birth-related data, cytogenetic and laboratory data, family history, and etiological information.

Quality Control of Birth Defects Registry Data

To evaluate the completeness and accuracy of data collection, reabstracting procedures similar to those used by cancer registries are often followed. The linkage of computerized discharge summary indexes with prenatal records is another quality control procedure that is used. The abstracts are reviewed by clinical geneticists, who evaluate them for accuracy and completeness of the diagnosis as well as for defect coding.[15]

Use of Birth Defects Registry Data

The analysis of birth defects surveillance data allows health care planners and epidemiologists to monitor the birth defect rates in different areas as well as changes in the rates. The data are monitored by statistically evaluating the difference between observed and expected numbers of specific defects or defect combinations for a specified time in a defined area. Comparisons may lead to the identification of clusters of birth defects. Investigation of such clusters may yield useful etiologic information. The goal of many birth defects registries is to provide health care providers and policymakers with information necessary to plan, develop, and implement strategies for the treatment and prevention of serious congenital malformations.[16]

Because individual birth defects are rare, researchers have difficulty in obtaining enough cases for etiological studies. Data for population-based state systems are an important source of information to improve knowledge and understanding of birth defects and to further prevention and intervention. The CDC funds some state and regional birth defects registries.

Other examples of the uses of registry data are illustrated by reports provided by the Illinois Department of Public Health at their Web site. Issued by the Illinois Department of Public Health's Adverse Pregnancy Outcomes Reporting System, the reports include information on the prevalence of birth defects in Illinois. For example, the prevalence of birth defects among Illinois and Chicago neonates from 1999 to 2001 is presented with graphs reporting quarterly data since 1989. Some of the other reports address neural tube defects, birth defects resulting from maternal diabetes, and prenatal exposure to controlled substances.[17]

DEATH REGISTRIES

Mortality statistics are considered part of the vital statistics kept by the National Center for Health Statistics. These statistics are used to develop reports that are available to the public and to researchers. Examples of reports are tables of life expectancy, fetal death rates, and causes of death.

The causes of death from the death certificate are translated into medical codes through use of the classification contained in the applicable revision of the ICD, published by the WHO. These coding rules make statistics useful by giving preference to certain categories by consolidating conditions and by systematically selecting a single cause of death from a reported sequence of conditions. The single tabulation requires that the underlying cause of death be reported.[18]

DIABETES REGISTRIES

The detection and management of diabetes can result in significant improvement in health and in morbidity rates. Diabetes registries' surveillance data are used to identify high-risk groups, target intervention programs, evaluate disease prevention and control activities, and establish an infrastructure for community-sponsored disease prevention programs.[19,20] Population-based registries provide an excellent foundation for family studies of autoimmune disease.[19] Monitoring diabetes at a regional, state, or national level is crucial to identifying where diabetes is the greatest problem so that resources can be allocated for primary and secondary prevention. Moreover, registries are useful for evaluating the effectiveness of prevention programs.

The types of diabetes that are monitored include the following:

- Insulin-dependent diabetes mellitus (IDDM) or Type 1
- Non-insulin-depended diabetes mellitus (NIDDM) or Type 2
- Gestational diabetes
- Maternal diabetes

The rates of complications and the methods by which they develop are important aspects of diabetes. Complications of diabetes include severe eye disease (e.g., blindness), amputations of the lower extremities, and end-stage renal disease. Diabetes also places the patient at an increased risk for cardiovascular disease. IDDM aggregates in families. Cumulative risk estimates for first-degree relatives range from 3% to 6% by age 30 years compared with less than 1% for the general population. Other autoimmune diseases, such as rheumatoid arthritis and autoimmune thyroid disease, are also frequently observed in IDDM families. NIDDM is almost ten times more common than IDDM. Increased life expectancy, along with changes in lifestyle, has resulted in an increasing prevalence of NIDDM in many geographic areas.[20]

Diabetes Registry Case Finding

Case finding sources include hospital admission and discharge logs, pharmacy records, dietary records, emergency department logs, and physician surveillance and reporting. For example, a large registry operated by the Kaiser Foundation in northern California identifies new cases by using a passive surveillance system. The sources of information include pharmacies (prescriptions for diabetic medications), laboratories ($Hb_{A1c} = 7.0\%$), and outpatient, emergency department, and hospitalization records listing a diagnosis of diabetes.[21]

Medical and demographic data are obtained by reviewing hospital patient records and data reporting forms submitted by physicians and pharmacies or by populating the registry from other databases. For example, a registry that is maintained by a health care insurer can populate a registry with information from all relevant encounters. Data variables include patient demographics, diagnoses, reasons for admission, treatments, medications, diabetic education, attending physicians, complications, and lengths of stay.

No uniform software system is used by all diabetes registries. Software is usually designed by and for the registry and is tailored to meet its needs. The Indian Health Service, an agency of the U.S. Public Health Service, encourages each of its clinics and hospitals to maintain a diabetes registry. (American Indians and Inuits have one of the highest known prevalence rates of type 2 diabetes.) Although the registries may be maintained in a manual or electronic format, integration of the diabetes registry with the hospital clinical information system is recommended.[22]

IMPLANT REGISTRIES

In 1988, the International Implant Registry was started by the MedicAlert Foundation, a nonprofit emergency alerting organization. The main objectives of the registry were to track patients so that their whereabouts are known and to facilitate timely, accurate communication between manufacturers, health care providers, and patients.[23]

Millions of patients have medical devices implanted in or on their bodies. These devices include pacemakers, heart valves, artificial joints, ocular lenses, defibrillators, breast implants, insulin pumps, and other devices. Although these medical devices have improved the quality of life for many people and have saved the lives of countless others, numerous safety alerts and voluntary manufacturer recalls have been issued for these devices. These safety alerts and recalls have raised procedural questions with life-threatening implications: Who is responsible for notifying the patients? Through the International Implant Registry, physicians are notified when important safety information needs to be communicated. If the physician cannot be contacted, patients are notified directly to contact their physicians or the manufacturers of their devices.

The voluntary registry efforts begun by the MedicAlert Foundation were taken a step further with the passage of the Safe Medical Devices Act of 1990, which was effective in November 1991. This law requires manufacturers to register and track certain implantable medical devices and to notify recipients regarding important safety information. It also requires hospitals, ambulatory surgical facilities, nursing facilities, and outpatient diagnostic or treatment facilities other than physicians' offices to file reports with the Food and Drug Administration or device manufacturers when there is a probability that a device caused or contributed to a death, serious illness, or serious injury.[24] Hospitals may choose to keep internal implant registries to identify patients and answer manufacturer recall or other research questions. Maintaining this information in a retrievable mode facilitates current and future requests for data on these patients.

IMMUNIZATION REGISTRIES

Immunization registries collect vaccination information about children within a geographic area. Registries provide a central location to collect vaccination records of children from multiple providers and also to generate reminders and recall vaccination notices. They can also provide official vaccination forms and vaccination coverage assessments. Immunization registries are a useful tool in achieving one of the national health objectives for Healthy People 2010 discussed in Chapter 1. This objective sets as a goal that 95% of the proportion of children aged less than 6 years participate in fully operational population-based immunization registries by 2010. A "fully operational" registry is defined as one that includes 95% enrollment of all area children less than 6 years of age with two or more immunization encounters administered within the geographic area. This definition is described in a 2002 report from the Advisory Committee on Immunization Practices (ACIP) and the American Academy of Family Physicians (AAFP) that provides recommendations regarding the provision of immunizations.[25]

Children are entered into the registry through a variety of mechanisms including linkage with electronic birth records and by a health care provider at the time of a child's first immunization. Immunization registries also can be used to enhance adult immunization services and coverage.

Immunization Registry Case Finding and Data Use

Functionally the registry stores data electronically on the basis of all National Vaccine Advisory Committee (NVAC)– approved core data elements. These data elements are used to establish a registry record within 6 weeks of birth for each child born in the geographic area. This enables access to and retrieval of immunization information in the registry at the time of the patient encounter. The registry should receive and process immunization information within 1 month of vaccine administration and must have safeguards and policies to protect the confidentiality and security of medical information. The software must exchange immunization records according to Health Level Seven (HL7) standards and automatically determine the routine childhood immunization(s) needed, in compliance with current recommendations of the ACIP, when an individual is seen for a scheduled immunization. The registry should also automatically identify individuals who are due or late for immunization(s). This requires enabling the production of reminder/recall notifications. By virtue of the registry data, immunization coverage reports can be automatically produced according to providers, age groups, and geographic areas. The registry is also required to be able to produce official immunization records as needed. The CDC National Immunization Program provides useful information about national and statewide registry systems.[26]

ORGAN TRANSPLANT REGISTRIES

The first successful organ transplantation operations were performed in 1954. Thanks to medical advances, today's technology makes transplantation a recognized and accepted mode of treatment for patients with organ failure. The success of transplantation and the scarcity of organs have raised many ethical, legal, and economic issues.[27]

The National Organ Transplant Act (NOTA, Public Law 98-507) was passed by Congress in 1984. The NOTA called for a national task force on organ transplantation that was charged with conducting an in-depth study of transplantation and making recommendations about medical, ethical, legal, economic, and social issues pertaining to human transplantation. In 1986, the task force recommended the establishment and operation of a national scientific registry. In October 1986, the United Network for Organ Sharing (UNOS) was established. It is a nonprofit, scientific, educational organization that administers the nation's only Organ Procurement and Transplantation Network (OPTN). Through the OPTN, UNOS does the following:

- Collects and manages data about every transplant event occurring in the United States
- Facilitates the organ matching and placement process with use of UNOS-developed data technology and the UNOS Organ Center
- Brings together medical professionals, transplant recipients, and donor families to develop organ transplantation policy[28]

UNOS members include transplant centers, independent procurement organizations, tissue-typing laboratories, consortia, public members, and voluntary health and professional associations.

Transplant Case Registration and Data Use

All UNOS member institutions and organizations involved in organ procurement, tissue typing, and organ transplantation are required to submit comprehensive data concerning transplant activities. To place a patient on the waiting list, the transplant center submits information that contains such patient information as address, race, ethnicity, education level, cause of organ failure, and number of previous transplants and whether the patient's name appears on any other lists.

The registry collects data through the whole transplant process from before transplant until graft failure or death. Transplant centers and organ procurement organizations enter data into the OPTN database through the Internet by using the secure Web-based application UNet.

The on-line database system UNet is used for the collection, storage, analysis, and publication of all data pertaining to the patient waiting list, organ matching, and transplants. Launched on October 25, 1999, this system contains data regarding *every* organ donation and transplant event occurring in the United States since 1986. UNet enables the nation's organ transplant institutions to register patients for transplants, match donated organs to waiting patients, and manage the time-sensitive, life-critical data of all patients before and after their transplants.

Data regarding transplants can be used by the government, the scientific community, and the public. Uses include the development of health care policy regarding reimbursement, performance standards, and public health research, and patients and their families can also assess their treatment options. Data from the UNOS database are currently used to monitor the efficacy of the organ allocation process. Data recorded on the potential recipient form are especially useful for this purpose. These data, combined with waiting list information, can be used to determine retrospectively the patient with highest priority to receive each organ.[29]

The quality assurance department at UNOS provides training for data coordinators and related personnel on data collection and offers assistance to members when they have questions or concerns about reporting requirements.

TRAUMA REGISTRIES

Traumatic injury, both accidental and intentional, is the leading cause of death in the first four decades of life according to the National Center for Health Statistics. Trauma typically involves young adults and results in the loss of a great number productive work years. Traumatic injury kills more people between ages 1 and 34 years than all other causes combined. The loss of productivity and the cost of health care costs the general public billions of dollars a year.[30]

Regional or statewide trauma systems of emergency trauma centers and emergency medical systems (EMS) have been shown to reduce mortality and morbidity rates and the loss of productivity from traumatic injuries. The evidence to support this claim has been based on data from hospital-based trauma registries. The data in these independent registries vary in their content and structure, thus impeding comparisons.[30]

In response to this concern, the ACS Committee on Trauma (ACSCOT) with funding from the federal government developed the National Trauma Data Bank (NTDB) and the associated data dictionary. The data dictionary spells out inclusion criteria and uniform registry variables to be used in all trauma registries. Annually, local, regional, or state registries are encouraged to report a subset of these variables to become the National Trauma Registry.[30]

Trauma registries gather data about patients who are injured. These registries can be hospital based or population based. The registry contains demographic information, data collected by EMS personnel before hospitalization, and medical information based on the patient hospital record. The medical information will be used to determine injury severity measurement. Injury measurements can be based on ICD codes (ICDMAP) or anatomical descriptors of tissue damage caused by the injury (Abbreviated Injury Scale [AIS]). The injury severity measurement is also included in the trauma registry.[31, 32]

Trauma Registry Case Finding and Data Use

Case finding is performed by reviewing emergency department logs, admitting department face sheets, patient records, and the disease indices—injury codes 800 to 959.9 and E codes listed in the ICD-9-CM. After appropriate cases are identified, information is abstracted from the record. Data elements that are important in trauma registry include patient-specific and demographic information, place of accident, cause of injury (E code), site of injury, condition of patient at the scene of the accident, transport modality, prehospital interventions, vital signs on admission, consciousness status, blood transfusions, procedures and treatment, total days in the intensive care unit, complications, discharge recommendations, and other information.[33]

Both the AIS scores and the Injury Severity Scale scores are routinely documented. The Glasgow Coma Scale is required by the ACS Trauma Registry on admission to the emergency department.[34]

RESEARCH AND USE OF DATA

Many areas of research use the data generated from the HIM-related data gathering processes. As discussed above, data from registries can be used at the organizational or the population levels to prevent disease or mitigate disability. Further, the data can form the basis for the need for new health care programs or to substantiate funding a research project. In addition to the use of registry data, the coded data that is generated for reimbursement is also used for health services research, medical research, and public health.

HIM professionals have access to a vast amount of information that can be used in research. The research can evaluate clinical services provided or government policy. They can also provide data for clinical studies or be used to analyze HIM practice. For all these uses, the key issue for the HIM professional is to identify the correct data that an individual or group would like to have to answer the research question that underlies the study.

Coded data can be used in many applications as described above, but to compare populations the data must be risk adjusted. Several methods have been used to accomplish this, including the Elixhauser comorbidity measurement,[35] the All Patient Refined DRGs (APR-DRGs),[36] Diagnostic Cost Groups (DCGs), and Adjusted Clinical Groups (ACGs),[37] to name a few. These methods use coded data to derive a way to risk adjust groups.

According to Petersen et al,[37] health-based risk adjustment is the means by which the disease risk is evaluated when determining payment rates, assessing outcomes, researching variation in the use of health services, and performing other comparisons of patient populations. The variables that constitute the method of risk adjustment can also be used to predict outcomes in some cases. For example, the Elixhauser Comorbidity Measurement[35] uses approximately 30 ICD codes to predict increased length of stay, inpatient mortality rates, and charges. Another recent development is the creation of Clinical Classification Software (CCS),[38] which can be used in lieu of ICD codes to predict outcomes. These means of risk adjustment are readily derived from the coded data that HIM professionals generate.

Health Services Research

Health services research is an applied field that encompasses many disciplines. The focus of research is generation of knowledge through scientific inquiry about how resources, organization, financing, and policies relate to the provision of health services. There are two main area of research. The first focuses on the organizational level and the second on the policy level. Major areas of interest include social and economic determinants, organizational design of health services at the population level, and the consequences of health policy.[39]

HIM practice is intertwined with the research interest areas of health service researchers. This is primarily due to the impact the HIM department has on the reimbursement process. Further, HIM professionals have intimate knowledge of the structure and organization of health care. Because of this, HIM professionals may be especially well suited to work in health services research and to contribute to the data needs of researchers in this area. An example of research is health care financing and health outcomes. A summary of research using discharge databases can be found in the report entitled *The Value of Hospital Discharge Databases*. Studies cited involve evaluating the effect of market competition on hospital costs, studying the effect of insurance status and intensive care unit resources, and the relationship between nurse's educational level and surgical outcomes, among others.[40]

Medical Research

Comorbidity is a condition that is in addition to a primary condition and that affects the course or treatment of a condition. Comorbid conditions can be used in health services research to adjust for the effect of secondary conditions. Typically they can be used in clinical research related to inpatient care, but as research continues, outpatient comorbid conditions could also be developed. The outcomes of interest can vary by usually involve one or more of the following: mortality, cost of health care, and length of stay.

To assist in determining the impact of comorbid disease, a variety of tools have been developed. For example, Anne Elixhauser developed one that uses ICD codes.[35] In a study that predicted mortality in the intensive care unit, comorbid disease measured by the 30 Elixhauser conditions was more predictive than was the Acute Physiology, Age, and Chronic Health Evaluation (APACHE) method.[41]

Role of a Data Broker in Research

To facilitate the research process, a structured interview model has been developed by Teslow et al[42] in the article "Asking the Right Questions: Connecting Users and Data through a Formal Interview Process." The changes in the HIM profession allow a redefinition of traditional practice as it transforms to meets the needs of the users of health information. The Health Information Services Interview can help to facilitate discussion of health information needs.

PUBLIC HEALTH

Many states have used the data from discharges to increase public safety and to research injuries. For example, North Carolina uses hospital data to track suicide and suicide attempt rates, Rhode Island has evaluated hospitalizations of patients with spinal cord injury to determine the demographic characteristics and discharge dispositions of this patient group, and several states use inpatient data as part of the Crash Outcomes Data Evaluation System (CODES), which is used to monitor motor vehicle crashes.[43] The incidence of disease is also estimated by some states through the use of hospital discharge data. For example, Vermont estimates the incidence of Guillain-Barré syndrome, and in 2000 Massachusetts used hospital discharge data to investigate a tularemia outbreak.[43] In addition to disease registry data, hospital discharge data are used for public health research, planning, and evaluation.

PLANNING AND ASSESSMENT

As was discussed earlier in the chapter, information from the various disease registries can be used by organizations to assess services and quality of care as well as to assist in planning. For example, ACS-approved cancer programs publish an annual report that provides summary information about the treatment provided to cancer patients and how that care compares with the care in other ACS-approved programs throughout the country. The data from the annual analysis can also help determine future patient needs for expansion of facilities and services.

Similarly, hospital discharge data can be used for strategic planning and outcome analysis. For example, the Intermountain Heath Care System, a nonprofit integrated health system in Salt Lake City, uses statewide data to compare itself with other organizations. Further, the New Hampshire Hospital Association develops an annual market share report. This allows hospitals to evaluate their market position and to determine how to position themselves and reallocate resources in a way that is both beneficial to the institution and to the patient population it serves.[40]

DATA AND HEALTH

Surveillance systems use coded data to monitor possible **bioterrorism**. In the case of syndromic surveillance, the main objective is to identify illness clusters before diagnoses are confirmed and to report the clusters to public health agencies so that a rapid response can occur that mitigates morbidity and mortality. The CDC recommends that, before the use of ICD-9-CM codes is implemented in syndrome monitoring systems, health care providers must assess how the use of these codes will help accomplish the goals of the system. Time is important in the effort to transmit the clusters of symptoms immediately. Before initiation of this type of surveillance program, the organization or unit that is expected to report should be evaluated to ensure that the range of reportable conditions are known and that the system is in place to accept the codes.[43]

Consumers can also use data available to select providers who provide good quality of care. The Rand Corporation undertook research, titled the Community Quality Index Study, which assessed the extent that recommended care was provided to a representative sample of the U.S. population. The research showed that patients receive 55% of recommended care and that this performance was similar across the country in the areas studied. Of note, those with the chronic conditions of diabetes and hypertension received 45% and 65% of recommended care.[44]

In this context it is not surprising that consumers seek information to make informed decisions about choosing a health care provider. Several Web sites are available to help consumers make educated choices. A section of the Centers for Medicare and Medicaid Services (CMS) Web site and those of several commercial vendors such as—Health Grades—provide information about the quality of care in hospitals and nursing homes. Both of these sites used coded data to evaluate the facilities. By providing this type of information to consumers, educated choices can be made with regard to selecting a nursing home.

Further, health care payers are using financial incentives to improve practice. The primary mechanism is through initiatives that reward good-quality care with financial reward. One of these programs is called **pay for performance** whose main goal is to improve patient safety and to increase the methods for management of chronic disease.[44] Included in this program is the incentive to stimulate implementation of the electronic health record (EHR) in physician offices.

PERFORMANCE MANAGEMENT

The Joint Commission uses data to describe the **core measures** quality improvement process. The data are transmitted to The Joint Commission from the accredited health care organizations. After transmission and evaluation, the quality data are provided to the public. It is also used to assess The Joint Commission accreditation, and by health care organizations to internally analyze areas that can be improved.[45] Performance measurement is used by health care organizations to evaluate and support performance. It is also used externally, to show accountability to consumers, payers, and accreditation organizations. It provides statistically valid, data-driven information. This enables a health care organization to evaluate itself. This type of information is particularly beneficial to consumers, enabling them to make critical decisions about where to seek quality health care.

For example, a section of The Joint Commission Web site discusses the derivation and reporting of core measures. The Specifications Manual for National Implementation of Hospital Core Measures, Version 2.0, provides information about how the care provided for patients with acute myocardial infarction, heart failure, pneumonia, pregnancy and related conditions, and surgical infection prevention are measured. Information about these areas are continuously monitored and reported to The Joint Commission. The statistics derived from these data is one area of focus that The Joint Commission uses to prepare for an accreditation visit. Medicare is also using core measures to monitor the quality of care for its beneficiaries.

The Joint Commission's Web site has a section called "quality checks" where anyone can find the accreditation status of accredited organizations. Consumers can search for accredited organizations to find information about the services provided and the organization's performance on the basis of various measures, including the core measures.[46]

OUTCOMES

Patients, purchasers, payers, and providers are clamoring for objective information about what really works in health care. The term **outcome** refers to an indicator of the results of a process. Although that process may be of almost any type, typically it is related to the content and delivery of health care.

Those whose primary concern is with quality of life may look for very different outcomes than those interested in years of life or others more concerned with costs. Although there are certainly instances where all indicators point to the same conclusion, often it is necessary to balance quality, cost, or other considerations to some degree.

Many lists of outcomes variables have been assembled. For those looking to develop outcomes information systems, a more straightforward approach to the data issue may be to recognize that nearly all health care information can be considered some component of outcomes data, segmented along the dimensions of:

- Administrative: Demographics, billing events, cost and payment models, etc.
- Patient perceptions: Physical health status, mental health status, access, satisfaction, etc.
- Clinical: Interventions, observations, conditions, results, etc.
- Life domains: Employment, housing, community supports, etc.

Researchers obtain access to large sets of claims data, sometimes supplemented with paper medical records. Claims data include data from insurers, the CMS, and regional data sets. Claims data contain some limited number of coded data elements representing clinical condition, procedures or treatments, discharge disposition, and possibly some other indicator of how the case was resolved. This information source represents a large, fairly uniform set of data that is readily available in coded form, on-line, and theoretically ready for use. It can be combined into a longitudinal record and analyzed for specific conditions and patient populations, as depicted in Figure 14-3.

Unfortunately, claims data tend to provide a limited clinical picture, are often fragmented, and usually contain inaccuracies such as mismatched patient identifiers. It may also have been distorted as a result of coding practices that are driven more by reimbursement requirements than by a

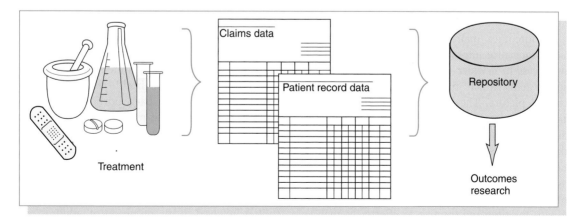

Figure 14-3 Outcomes research. (From Murphy GF, Hanken MA, Waters KA: *Electronic health records: changing the vision,* Philadelphia, 1999, Elsevier.)

concern for clinical accuracy. One study found that claims data failed to identify as many as half the prognostically important clinical conditions found in a clinical information system.[47]

Outcomes Data and Information Systems

Those with some right to the data from a large number of organizations include insurers or benefits managers, regulatory or watchdog groups, and private health care data base developers. Like the academic researchers, this group must confine itself to the set of coded data submitted, so the scope of its work is limited. However, it is often in a position to specify the content of the data submitted to it, so it is able to focus on specific areas of interest, usually through the periodic submission of defined indicators. For example, the National Committee for Quality Assurance (NCQA) has defined a set of indicators for the Health Plan Employer Data and Information Set (HEDIS). This set is limited, but it permits comparison of health plans across a large, consistent data sample. Performance measurement is intended to lead to quality improvement within participating provider organizations by highlighting trends and offering comparisons to similar organizations. Likewise, most insurers have available large case samples with common data elements from a diverse group of providers that help them to identify organizations and practices they wish to encourage.

Outcomes Data Use

Outcomes may also be presented in terms of life domains and being able to return to the activities of living. Some managed care systems include information on life domains. This information is usually important when care spans a period of time. For example, on entry into the care process the individual was not able to work or live independently because of his or her condition. After completion of the treatment process, the individual is able to return to work and to an independent living situation.

Intraorganizational outcomes teams use their own data and are more likely to focus on local processes. Their goal tends to be outcomes management through profiling, guidelines, performance improvement, and the like. These teams have access to a wider range of data elements and information systems, which may provide a more comprehensive clinical picture. They may also be able to make modifications to the data collection systems to allow them to expand their data sets to reflect specific interests and to address data quality issues. Intraorganizational outcomes teams generally have cleaner, more comprehensive data sets available to them, but the sample size is often too small to be significant. Further, few provider organizations have personnel with the time and training to effectively analyze and interpret outcomes data.

Outcomes and the Electronic Health Record

In the absence of both a comprehensive EHR and true outcomes information systems, all these groups have had to make do with the information systems available to them. General health care information systems (HIS) are operational systems that work with the transactional data on a single patient at a time. Although they may have a comprehensive information set, it is usually not readily accessible across patients or time. Patient survey data management and analysis products aggregate data across time and patients but tend to lack core operational data necessary to the analysis. Health care decision support packages are also strong in the aggregation and analysis components but have historically lacked the comprehensive data set desired. Generic databases and statistical packages are excellent tools, but lack health care domain knowledge and require the users to build their own data model.

It is imperative that EHRs explicitly support these requirements. In simplified form, they may be diagrammed as seen in Figure 14-4.

That is, comprehensive data drawn from clinical and operational management systems must be warehoused in a format that allows necessary indicator data to be transmitted to those who need the data. The data must be supplemented with other relevant information such as benchmarks or standards of care. Health care–specific applications need to operate over the combined data to support analysis and reporting needs for outcomes research and management.

This ideal record is a complete, longitudinal picture of all health-related activities from birth to death, including occupational, physical fitness, nutritional, and other relevant lifestyle data. With it, the researcher can look for correlations between treatments, prior conditions, lifestyle, and long-term outcomes. Further, it allows groups of related health care events to be grouped together into episodes of care. This ideal record is a logical whole, not necessarily a single physical record. It might be stored on many different computers but is entirely on-line, and the components can easily be linked together when needed.

Figure 14-5 shows the reality of an encounter-based record, distributed across multiple providers. Actual health care records are often discontinuous and impossible to integrate. The patient is identified differently in each piece and there is little or no health-related information apart from formal encounters. Large portions of the record are not on-line at all. There are many reasons for this. Some are inherent in the structure of the health care industry, others in the history of health care information systems, and still others in the nature of the data itself.

The health care industry is still characterized by large numbers of autonomous or semiautonomous business entities involved in the provision of, administration of, or payment for, care. These organizations are linked in an

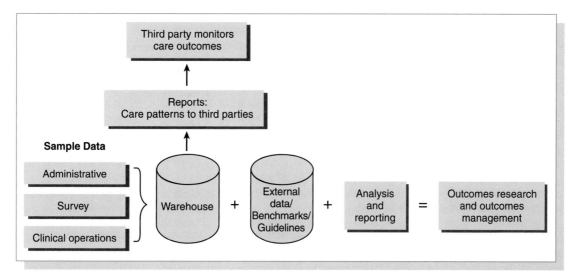

Figure 14-4 Outcomes information systems requirements. (From Murphy GF, Hanken MA, Waters KA: *Electronic health records: changing the vision*, Philadelphia, 1999, Elsevier.)

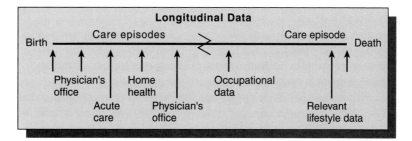

Figure 14-5 Longitudinal data. (From Murphy GF, Hanken MA, Waters KA: *Electronic health records: changing the vision*, Philadelphia, 1999, Elsevier.)

intricate network of relationships, but each has its own data set. The standard concerns of any business regarding proprietary data apply to health care organizations and are compounded by the uniquely confidential nature of health care data.

Providers involved with many managed care organizations cannot possibly use all these different information systems and may not have the resources and expertise necessary to generate each of the data sets requested by the organizations. Even if they can, differing data definitions, and the encounter-based orientation of most provider data, may seriously limit analysis at the level of the managed care organization. There may be gaps where systems are entirely absent or where key types of information, such as clinical data or critical specialty information, are not available. finally, it must be acknowledged that no matter what the structure of the health care system, there is no current way to routinely capture complete data about such issues as patient participation in or compliance with a treatment regimen.

Within a given health care enterprise, there is no guarantee that the computerized data that does exist can be linked into a coherent longitudinal record of care. Many large providers, such as hospitals, have a number of different information systems. These often come under the ownership of individual departments, each with differing priorities and data definitions. The systems may or may not communicate with each other effectively, making it difficult to link the records of a single patient across systems (see Figure 14-6).

Outcome Indicators

Outcome measures are still in the early development stage. Most outcomes are condition or process specific, making it difficult to identify a single, simple set of outcomes data. Various groups have developed indicators such as blood transfusion or maternal deaths to monitor outcomes of specific events. Others have relied on diagnosis and procedure codes, discharge status, length of stay, and proxy measures such as cost. Within a health care organization, researchers can collect data such as unplanned returns to surgery, but they are often limited to data from a single encounter and cannot track long-term outcomes if the patient receives future care outside the organization.

Actual Healthcare Record

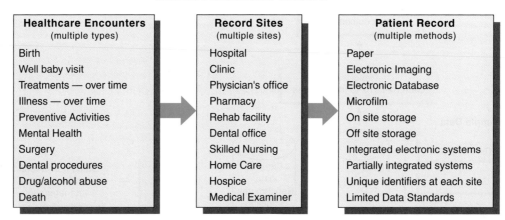

Healthcare Encounters (multiple types)	**Record Sites** (multiple sites)	**Patient Record** (multiple methods)
Birth	Hospital	Paper
Well baby visit	Clinic	Electronic Imaging
Treatments — over time	Physician's office	Electronic Database
Illness — over time	Pharmacy	Microfilm
Preventive Activities	Rehab facility	On site storage
Mental Health	Dental office	Off site storage
Surgery	Skilled Nursing	Integrated electronic systems
Dental procedures	Home Care	Partially integrated systems
Drug/alcohol abuse	Hospice	Unique identifiers at each site
Death	Medical Examiner	Limited Data Standards

Figure 14–6 Current Health Records. Current health records describe multiple types of treatment and preventive activities from birth to death in an often fragmented delivery system. The records themselves are also in transition, and in individual's records may be stored at multiple sites in a variety of formats and media. (From Murphy GF, Hanken MA, Waters KA: *Electronic health records: changing the vision*, Philadelphia, 1999, Elsevier.)

One major area of research and development within this field has been in the development of survey instruments to measure health status, access to care, and satisfaction, as reported by the patient. Much of the effort has gone into the development of standard, easy-to-complete instruments that can be readily incorporated in the patient care process and that provide a comparable set of data across health care providers. Some of the best known health status measures are the SF-36 and SF-12 from the Medical Outcomes Trust, and the HSQ and HSQ-12 from the Health Outcomes Institute. Mental health has standard client satisfaction surveys as well, notably one from the Mental Health Council of America (MHCA) and Telesage.

Survey data have not traditionally been incorporated into the clinical information system as a part of the patient care process but are a critical component of the complete outcomes data set. The need for better and more comparable outcome indicators has spawned a myriad of indicator development, cataloging, and standardization efforts. For example, the Health Outcomes Institute (HOI), which was spun off from Ellwood's initial outcomes work, promotes the development, dissemination, and use of public domain outcomes measures. In 1996 it worked with the American Medical Group Association on a software package known as the Outcomes Data Conversion Utilities. The utilities provide access to a database of standardized survey questions for developing survey instruments and also translate existing indicators into standard equivalents for comparative purposes.[48] Good indicators reflect outcomes over which caregivers have some degree of control. They are also readily collected, thoroughly tested, and widely accepted so that they can be used for comparative purposes.

Outcomes and Coding Issues

There has been considerable incentive for payers to standardize medical coding and for providers to code medical activities. A number of researchers have developed coding systems for nursing diagnoses and care, but there is to date no one standard model. (Coding and vocabulary issues are discussed in more depth in Chapter 6.) From an outcomes research standpoint, this is disastrous because a significant component of care is lost to handwritten textual notes or organization and vendor-specific coding schemes. A similar, even more pronounced situation holds for other allied health professions.

Coding schemes may also differ by setting. Thus, if one wishes to compare inpatient and outpatient surgery outcomes, it has been necessary to look at both Current Procedural Terminology (CPT)–4 and ICD-9-CM codes to identify all similar procedures. These coding systems may not be useful when looking at outcomes for specialty care such as mental health or drug treatment. Different settings typically capture differing levels of detail within the record as well. For example, in the inpatient hospital setting, it is common for information systems to store 15 or more diagnosis codes, whereas in a physician office setting there are generally only four. Once again the reasons may be traced to billing and payment issues. Furthermore, these are U.S. standards. Comparisons across national boundaries may require that other coding schemes such OPCS4 (United Kingdom) for procedures or ICD-10 for diagnoses be incorporated in the analysis.

The coding issue is important and extends beyond coding data to identify diagnoses and procedures because uncoded textual data are difficult to analyze in any comprehensive, automated fashion given today's information systems technology. Although there are limitations inherent in all coding systems, they do provide a structured approach to storing comparable data. Data that are coded according to organization-specific coding schemes such as billing or service codes can be analyzed locally, but, unless it is mapped to some universal scheme or cross walk, it cannot be compared across organizations. Given that a typical acute-care hospital has thousands of service codes, this is a formidable task. An example of a universal coding scheme is the International Classification of Clinical Services (ICCS), originally developed by Stan Mendenhall at the Commission on Professional and Hospital Activities in an attempt to standardize descriptions of treatments and to provide more clinical data within codes.

Finally, it must be acknowledged that some of the most important elements of care can never be coded. The intangibles of a sunny room, a cheerful smile, or an empathetic listener may affect outcomes but cannot be quantified or captured within the clinical record. It should be noted that mental health systems do include items that are often not included in other aspects of health care. For example, the client has and uses his or her natural support system (family or friends) to help address the problem.

Desirable Outcome Systems

It is desirable that data collection systems be available wherever care is rendered, whether in an office, at a bedside, in a home, or at a remote location and that the data be entered by the person first acquiring it.[49] This is important, too, in that we want not only to gather information, but to provide it back to the caregiver in such a manner as to influence care in a positive way.

Ideally, the outcomes **data warehouse** will be structured around persons, not the patient—that is, it will include information on a population of people who have either received care in the past or who may receive care at some time in the future. This larger population is helpful for indicator denominators, for example, x% of women of childbearing age within our sample received regular Papanicolaou smears. It is also important for modeling future patient populations, and it can help us to understand why some people become patients and others do not. If there are nonpatients for whom we have some responsibility (e.g., as a capitated provider or as a payer) and about whom we have specific demographic or survey data, these should be included. Information about the larger community may not be as detailed but can still be descriptive of demographics, use rates, risk factors, and so forth. It is also beneficial to include comparative or benchmark data on treatment approaches, resource allocation, and outcomes of particular interest. In recent years, there have been many public and private regional and national data pools created. These should provide ready access to comparative data. They may also provide large enough data samples for statistically valid studies.

It should be noted that the need for a master identifier is just as critical for caregiver records as it is for patients because we cannot hope to do effective provider profiling unless we can accurately identify the care rendered in many different locations by the same individuals. The national provider identifier will help in this regard.

To understand what contributed to an outcome, it is beneficial to know the entire course of care, from the onset of symptoms to full recovery, which implies the presence of a mechanism to identify all the components of an episode of care. On the surface this seems straightforward, but automating the process for huge numbers of patient records poses both theoretical and processing challenges. For example, where does one episode end and another begin? What do we do if services rendered during a single encounter apply to more than one condition? How do we categorize similar episodes for comparative purposes? This process is complex enough for relatively straightforward disease processes. Where there are chronic or comorbid conditions it becomes far more so. Further, we should also be able to identify preventive care as an episode in and of itself. The whole concept of episodes of care, in the context of data management, is still in its infancy. A few providers have begun tagging encounter records with an episode at the outset of care for administrative purposes. This is problematic because a visit that initially appears to be for one condition may ultimately be seen to be the result of some other condition entirely, or, a part of more than one concurrent episode of care.

Episodic groupers are a fairly recent development in health care information processing. These have been developed by companies that process millions of health care claims a year for benefits management firms, payers, and managed care plans. Although each episodic grouper uses proprietary logic to assign claims events to a condition and an episode, the groupers all have certain points in common:

- Clinical groupings—Each episodic grouper begins by categorizing individual claims by medical condition, usually on the basis of proprietary groupings of ICD-9-CM diagnosis codes that represent some level of clinical or treatment homogeneity. There are usually several hundred conditions within a given model.
- Assigning events to episodes—Where services are clearly linked to a single diagnosis on the claim, the grouper is able to assign them to an episode fairly easily. Other services can only be assigned with use of clinically based logic that takes into account expected time frames, concurrent episodes, and sophisticated data reconciliation processes.
- Determining the end of an episode—Groupers use either discrete time periods or a window of time during which there are no services for a condition to decide when an episode is at end. Each approach has some drawbacks. Under the discrete time period approach, all appropriate services during the expected duration of the episode are included. If actual care exceeds this time period, the grouper may end up counting too many episodes for the same condition because a new episode would start when the time period expires. Under the clear window approach, the end of the

episode is determined by the absence of treatment for defined periods of time. This may result in counting too few episodes where a new instance begins during the expected window and is assumed to be part of the previous episode.

Early generations of episodic groupers were limited to claims data and focused on ambulatory and physician billing data. As they begin to move into the provider and acute care arena, we can expect to see increasing sophistication in the modeling process. Over time, these systems should prove invaluable to the outcomes movement.

The data warehouse relies on internal codes to provide comprehensive analytical functionality. Whether these codes are user defined or standard, data from multiple source systems will need to be interpreted and mapped to the codes. There are now powerful, commercially available mapping engines that can assign codes, compute event durations, fill in gaps within records and generally scrub and reconcile data as they are fed into a warehouse. More experimental are processors to read and interpret text so that it can be stored in a format useful for analysis. At the same time, clinical information systems are becoming better at guiding the user through structured text entry in a way that allows data to be stored behind the scenes in code but presented to the user as text.

The data warehouse must be complemented by a robust set of tools designed and built with an understanding of health care and outcomes information requirements. These allow information to be derived from the outcomes warehouse and interpreted. At a minimum, this tool set needs to include functionality for the following:

- Data sampling—Identifying the characteristics and volume of records to be included in a given analysis. Some data sampling tools allow records to be selected by number or value (e.g., include all records in DRG 50 or exclude abnormal white blood cell counts). Others look across records to allow such samples as the physician who treated the fewest cases during the month of July or the diagnosis with the highest variable cost per case.
- Grouping—Continuing analysis requires that data be segmented into meaningful subsets. Grouping functions allow the creation of subsets based on flexible criteria that may be as simple as age/gender cohorts or complex combinations of diagnoses, interventions, and outcomes.
- Tabular and graphical reporting—Reporting functionality runs the gamut from rigid, standardized reports in flat, tabular formats to flexible ad hoc reports that allow the user to drill through increasing layers of detail, shift perspectives, resort, and present the information in a variety of graphical formats. Reporting functionality also varies widely in its usability and its efficiency. Some "user-friendly" report writers may be

simple to use but offer limited functionality or they may be downright unfriendly. Standard Structured Query Language (SQL)–based reporting functions have no "knowledge" of health care so require considerable expertise to perform such functions as properly counting cases where each uses multiple services. Even well-designed, health care–oriented reporting tools require that the user have knowledge of the data model to use them effectively, so a strategy of offering tiered reporting tools for power users versus the occasional or casual user is perhaps most realistic.
- Modeling—Changes in treatment patterns, resource mix, staffing, and so forth are all of interest.
- Indicator reporting functions—Performance measurement requires the collection and dissemination of indicators both internally and to third parties such as the NCQA and The Joint Commission. These should be automatically gathered from within the warehouse and formatted for the necessary review and transmission.
- Benchmarking/comparative reporting capabilities— All these tools should be able to operate over both detailed internal data and external comparative data.

For outcomes management, it is also beneficial to have specific functionality for process improvement studies and for the development and use of standards of care such as pathways and guidelines. One other function that deserves mention is data mining. This is another term with a range of connotations, depending on the source. The idea is to extract gems of information from mountains of data. Data mining software is intended to facilitate the review of large volumes of data for insights, trends, patterns, and hypotheses. This can be done by using a basic set of sampling and reporting tools. It can also be pursued with more experimental software designed to identify patterns and relationships in raw data. The latter have not yet achieved broad acceptance for general health care applications but show promise for outcomes research purposes.

Information dissemination requirements are dependent on the audience and the purpose. Audiences with an interest in outcomes information include the following:

- Caregivers and provider organizations
- Patients and consumer groups
- Health care purchasers
- Regulators and accrediting bodies
- Researchers

Each of these audiences has its own perspective on what may be the same information. Although a patient may want outcomes data to assist in deciding on a provider and a course of treatment, he or she will probably want that information highly processed in an explanatory format. The researcher, on the other hand, is likely to want data in their raw form. The information dissemination approach will also be affected by the purpose of the data; for example, purposes may include the following:

- Education
- Behavior modification
- Quality optimization
- Resource management
- Evaluation
- Research

From an information systems development standpoint, this means that no single information dissemination module will be designed, coded, and implemented. Instead, information dissemination must be a function of the entire system. Table 14-1 gives examples of strategies that may be effective for selected audiences and purposes.

The results of outcomes research should be available to caregivers in a variety of forms: through on-line bibliographical tools, through guideline lookups, and through the clinical decision support functions provided within the workstation. This last will include reminders, alerts, order sets reflecting the results of outcomes research, and detailed analytical tools for the caregiver who is also a researcher.

Some of the most significant trends of benefit to the outcomes movement include the following:

- Standard data definitions and interchange mechanisms for health care data. The work of standards developers and promoters such as HL7, American Society for Testing and Materials (ASTM), and the American National Standards Institute's Healthcare Informatics Standards Planning Panel (ANSI HISPP) and ANSI Healthcare Information Technology Standards Panel (ANSI HITSP). This work is intended to break down barriers between information systems caused by differing data definitions. This not only allows the information systems from various newly affiliated health care organizations to exchange data, but also allows the often-incompatible systems within single organizations to exchange data.
- Open systems, including communications and data base standards. These remove the technical barriers to systems integration, just as standard data definitions remove the data barriers. Common data base access formats such as SQL mean that data can be retrieved easily from a number of sources and combined to build up a complete picture of conditions, interventions, and outcomes. This approach should allow the merging of local organizational data with state, regional, and national public databases and with proprietary data sets from specialty companies. Common methods of identifying data between systems, such as that used by extensible markup language (XML), are also helpful.
- Security. Network-based security standards such as the Open Systems Foundation's (OSF) Distributed

Table 14-1   SAMPLE INFORMATION DISSEMINATION STRATEGIES

Audience	Purposes	Strategies
Caregivers	Quality optimization	Guidelines and other references available as look-ups within the clinical information system.
	Behavior modification	Alerts, reminders, and standard order sets incorporated within data collection systems for real-time impact on care.
	Resource management	Profiles generated and disseminated on-line but reviewed in person with a peer.
	Education	
Patients	Education	Customized patient education materials generated on-line and printed for the patient.
	Behavior modification	Reminder notices generated through triggers on patient data and mailed, e-mailed, or automatically planned to the patient (or to nonpatient members).
		Web page look-up of guidelines for self-care with an e-mail connection to the caregiver.
		Triggers to case managers to prompt in-person follow-up.
Purchasers Caregivers/providers Patients	Evaluation	Report cards, profiles, and other performance measures generated from the analysis system and distribution in printed and electronic formats.
Purchasers Regulations/accrediting bodies	Performance measurements Benchmarking	Electronic transmission of indicators and other outcomes to data banks on predefined formats.

From Murphy GF, Hanken MA, Waters KA: *Electronic health records: Changing the vision,* Philadelphia, 1999, Elsevier.

Computing Environment (DCE) provide vehicles for controlling system and data access, whereas field definitions within databases guard specific data elements from inappropriate usage. Data security and confidentiality is a major concern of health care consumers. The ability to ensure it is critical to the public's acceptance of outcomes data sharing.

- Local and wide area networking, with and without wires. Not only do networks enhance communication, but they also make it possible for everyone to "work off the same page." That is, caregivers in many locations can have access to the same applications and information at the same time, thus increasing the uniformity and integrity of the data set. Without networks, each caregiver accesses and enters data on a separate, local computer system, duplicating some, misspelling others, and leaving some out entirely, making it difficult to ever build up a single, comprehensive record of care. Wireless networks provide the additional benefit of allowing the computer to move with the caregiver.
- Graphical user interfaces. These make information systems more approachable and easier to use, thereby helping to expand the user community to caregivers and even patients. This in turn should enable the capture of a richer, far more complete information set for outcomes analysis. It should also improve the accuracy of the data by moving health care data capture to the point of care.
- High-powered, commodity hardware. Inexpensive and interchangeable hardware makes it feasible to collect data at the point of care, wherever that may be. Powerful hardware makes it feasible to work with distributed data, enormous databases, and huge transaction volumes. This supports not only the data collection effort but the manipulation of large data sets for analysis purposes.
- The Web, the Internet, and Intranets. These are significant information dissemination vehicles. They also provide a platform for the rapid and relatively low cost development and deployment of distributed applications.

Most acute-care hospitals have some type of case mix analysis capability. Even a fairly simple system should permit a general analysis of such proxy outcome measures as length of stay and discharge status by type of case. This information can be used to develop guidelines, critical pathways, or other process improvement approaches. For example, you might look at reducing the length of stay for total hip replacement cases. Using the case mix system, you can examine the characteristics of cases with differing outcomes, in this example, length of stay, and develop a plan to adopt a similar pattern of care on the basis of the characteristics of the cases with the lower length of stay.

This plan can be loaded into existing clinical systems, to the extent those systems can support it. For example, if you have nursing care plans on-line, the new plan can be incorporated in those. If you have an order entry system with standard order sets, the new plan can be set up as a standard order. As you begin to collect data on patients treated under the new plan, you will be going back to your case mix system to assess the impact of the change and possibly to fine tune it.

Simultaneous with the change in clinical process, you will want to consider how to enhance your existing systems to further support this change. You might want to add additional data elements to better measure outcomes within your case mix system. You might want to implement system modules you have purchased but not yet installed. You may want to purchase additional modules for systems you already have, such as advanced nursing functions. Or it may be time to begin moving forward with major new components of your long-term information systems strategy and architecture. Both sides of the process, the analysis and systems implementation and the modification of clinical processes and ways of thinking, are iterative. The goal is to discover how much outcomes data are already available to you and how best to use the data while moving forward with your long-term plan. As new system components and data elements are put in place, the outcomes information and functionality available will expand, enabling you to reap the benefits of the outcomes movement. This will help support clinical decision making as well.

CLINICAL DECISION SUPPORT

Clinical decision support is typically presented as a system that brings knowledge to caregivers to assist them in making decisions about patient care. The system may generate an alert for an abnormally high laboratory test result or for a patient is taking two medications that may interact negatively. The caregiver is then given the opportunity to review the situation and determine the appropriate course of care. The system can also automatically provide time-based reminders (i.e., this patient is due to have a routine bone density screening). Another feature of clinical decision support systems is to link the caregiver to other resources. These resources may be clinical guidelines or reference materials that can be accessed online. The overall objective to bring knowledge resources to the caregiver in real time during the care process. Again a clinical decision support system includes a controlled vocabulary, a central data repository with appropriately structured clinical data, a knowledge representation scheme, an inference engine, and output mechanisms such as the EHR.

DATA DICTIONARY

An understanding of data dictionaries is useful to better understand all types of data, to enhance the ability to analyze data, and to use the data appropriately to assess outcomes and support clinical decision making.

The **data dictionary** is as critical to the EHR as the English dictionary is to other forms of communication. The data dictionary conceptually is no different from any other dictionary except that it must be more precise and complete in its definitions.

Data Dictionary Definitions

- **Metadata**—The term "metadata" is defined as "data about data."[50] It defines the structure that will be used to define all of the characteristics about data so that different individuals looking at characteristics of a data element would arrive at the same conclusion as to what the data means and how it is to be used. Properly created, the metastructure of data allows for a clearer understanding of the meaning and greater reliability of the quality of information that is part of any electronic record.[51]

- **Data element**—The data element is the atomic level of information.[25] It is best described as a single question that demands a singular defined response. For example, the data element "gender" implies a question about the gender of a person. It demands a defined response that may include "male," "female," or "unknown." The data dictionary describes the nature of the data element sufficiently so that any user of the system will understand what the question and the response means, what it does not mean, and the limits of what it can express.

- **Field**—A field is a physical term that refers to the place in a computer system in which a data element might reside. It is best described as the container for the data. The field container may accommodate the data element in terms of data size or data type, or it may impose limits on how the data element can be defined

because of the limits of the system. In many instances, the term "field" and "data element" have been used interchangeably.[25]

- **Entities**—An entity (or subject) represents a higher level than the data element.[52] It refers to a subject of information that may be a thing, a concept, or a process. The entity may contain many data elements that act as attributes, or descriptors of the entity, and are used to identify the nature of an instance of the entity. For example, the entity "physician" might have many data elements that define the gender, age, address, license number, and so forth, of the instance of a physician.

- **Table**—A table is the physical representation of the entity. Like the field, it is the container that has the data elements that will describe many instances of the entity in the manner established by the logical data model (see Table 14-2).

- **Record**—A record is a row within the table. It contains the data elements within fields that will provide sufficient data to identify a unique instance of the entity. For example, a record in the table that represents the entity "physician" would contain an identifier number and the age, gender, address, and other information about an individual physician to record him or her in the table as a unique instance of the entity "physician."

- **Attributes**—An attribute is a data element that describes the entity. It is generally represented as a column in a table (e.g., city).[53]

- **Domain**—The domain represents the type of value that is allowable for a specific element.[52] For example, an alphabetical character cannot be included in the of the data element "date of birth." The domain might specify that 01/01/1997 is acceptable, but Jan 1, 1997, is not.

- **Value/coding**—The value or coding for a data element represents a more specified way that values may be returned to the data element question. In general, it represents a tighter leash on the domain of the element by specifying more specifically what the answer to the data element question can be. For example, the definition for data element "gender" might specify that

Table 14-2 COMPARISON OF CORE HEALTH DATA ELEMENTS

PhyID	Lst_nm	Fst_nm	Addr	City	State	ZIP
239879	SMITH	TOM	234 GREEN ST	SEATTLE	WA	98104
234098	WHITE	MARY	234 LINCOLN AVE	TACOMA	WA	98234
239487	BROWN	JAMES	256 TENDAL PL	PUYALLUP	WA	98398

From Murphy GF, Hanken MA, Waters KA: *Electronic health records: changing the vision*, Philadelphia, 1999, Elsevier.

only the characters "M," "F," or "U" are acceptable values and that "M" equals "male," "F" equals "female," and "U" equals "unknown."

- **Logical data model**—The logical data model represents the structure of the relationship of data elements and entities within an information system. The logical model is crucial to the proper function of any system within an enterprise.[53] The logical model allows for elegance in system design so that the system is adaptable to the changing information needs of the enterprise. The data dictionary is important to complete a good logical data model, but the dictionary should not be dependent on the logical model. By use of the data dictionary to define elements independent of the model, different systems with different logical models will be able to share data that are defined precisely and independent of the manner in which the data elements are structured in different logical models.

Purpose of the Data Dictionary

The data dictionary is a critical part to any information system design. To really understand this significance, it is important to first understand the context in which the data dictionary should operate. An information system is not computer hardware, software, or even paper forms. It is a consensus among individuals to share information in a specified way so that all participants derive the same meaning from the content and all participants contribute content in a manner that expresses the intended meaning of the contributor.[54] The data dictionary is a point of consensus that institutionalizes the structure and meaning of the individual elements of the information system. EHRs are tools that support this consensus and allow for a more efficient sharing of the information. Because most computerized information systems are less tolerant than nonelectronic information systems, they help enforce the rules and definitions that have been established. The more effort put into the establishment of the data dictionary, the greater the quality of the information product of the system.

The development of the data dictionary does not occur by default. A great deal of effort and forethought is required to create a data dictionary that will consistently provide for a meaningful information system. Many institutions have failed to see the value of a formal effort to establish a common enterprise wide data dictionary and have paid the price in systems that will not integrate and reports and analysis that are worse than meaningless. It is surprising how many sophisticated institutions are relying on invalid or inconsistently defined data that leads to decisions based on misinformation. Many simply assume they understand the meaning of their data or the calculations associated with those data.

Scope of the Data Dictionary

The data dictionary should include all the elements that are required for a person or institution to make key business decisions. In building toward an EHR, institutions will need to map out the foundation data and agree on a strategy to address it. A great deal of effort is necessary to define the functional requirements of an information system that supports decision making. Further effort is necessary to define the structure or logical data model that will support those requirements. Once this is understood, then the logical model will dictate what data elements are necessary to support these functional requirements. These elements will form the scope of the dictionary. The scope of the information systems frequently expand beyond their intended boundaries. The process of building the data dictionary and defining the logical data model can bring criteria and discipline to help control this "scope creep."

Meta-Content of the Data Dictionary

The data dictionary must have a meta-content that defines the attributes that will be included in the data dictionary for each element.[25] The authors recommend the following attributes should be included for each data element:

- *Logical name*—A long name given to the element on the basis of a naming convention. For example, a name that proceeds left to right from the broadest (largest granularity) to most specific (smallest granularity) term, such as [hospital_department_admit_phone_number].
- *Physical name*—A short name given to the element limited by the size of the physical database system. This name will be the name that is identified by the computer as the data element in the physical data base, for example, [adm_ph_no].
- *Category*—The dictionary should attempt to categorize the element in a broad category such as demographic, health history, symptom, physical sign, and so forth.
- *Definition*—The definition of the data element.
- *Type*—The data type (character, numerical, date, logical, calculated, free text/memo, etc.)
- *Length*—The size of the field required to hold values for the data element
- *Decimal*—A description of the number of decimal places that might be required in a numerical field
- *Domain*—The description of the allowed values for the data element, including the rule for exclusion of invalid data.
- *Coding*—A description of coded values if they are required for the data element.
- *Reference*—A reference for the source that was used to define the data element in the dictionary, if applicable.

This might be a standard such as ANSI X12, ASTM, or HL7.

Building the Data Dictionary

Most information systems do not start de novo in health environments. In most instances, health institutions have had multiple systems for recording a great deal of information. Each application uses a set of definitions appropriate to the application or department. Thus radiology systems would have items such as "gender," "date of birth," "height," "weight," and so forth, whereas the laboratory or admission department might have similar elements that are defined differently in "their" systems. The problem is intensified when different institutions wish to compare their data.[55] As institutions try to integrate new systems or automate paper systems, they begin to grapple with the decision support functions they require. Many of these institutions simply layer on new data elements and structures rather than reassess or overhaul their existing systems. Although some institutions make a valiant effort to integrate and upgrade their information environment, they quickly identify the cost and complexities involved in replacing old systems and cultures. The process of building a fully integrated information structure appears so daunting at times that many institutions just give up, or put off system's integration for a "sunny" day.

There is a solution to the dilemma, however, if the process of building a new data model and data dictionary is done intellectually, systematically, and with an eye to the future. This process cannot be driven by vendors, but rather should be used to drive vendors response to the institutional needs.[56]

Step 1: Inventory of an Existing Enterprise

The first step in building the data dictionary for any information system is to inventory the content of the existing system. To do this appropriately, all aspects of the enterprise-wide data collection process must be analyzed. Every form and every computer input screen must be reviewed so that data elements that are collected by the institution are catalogued. Similar elements need to be grouped, and the source and purpose of each needs to be recorded. Once all data elements are assembled and grouped, a meticulous and time-consuming effort must be undertaken to analyze each element and to identify those elements that are synonymous.

Step 2: Identifying New Data Content Needs

The process of identifying new data content is very complex and requires a great deal of planning and discipline to accomplish appropriately. This process falls into the realm of logical data modeling, which is outside the scope of this chapter. The processes for logical data modeling and data dictionary development are intimately linked and

must occur together. The data dictionary provides the structured container for the product of this process and represents one piece of the overall data design of any enterprise.

Step 3: Consensus Development

As described previously, information systems are totally dependent on a consensus of the users about the definition and management of all the atomic (cannot be further divided) bits of information within an enterprise. Without a solid consensus, the information system is severely compromised. The ability to build an EHR requires that users of the system understand and buy into the definitions of elements that will be used in the system. Otherwise the data will lack validity and integrity.

Box 14-1 shows an example of a process for developing that consensus through the use of an informatics work group that is given a specific work plan to accomplish its goal.

Criteria for Data Element Inclusion

Each data element to be included in the data dictionary should be evaluated to see whether it is appropriate for inclusion on the basis of a set of criteria. The following are our recommendations for criteria to apply to proposed data elements.

- The element should belong to the enterprise under development.
- The element should be a variable used to *make decisions* important to the enterprise.
- The element should be obtainable as a normal part of the transactions that occur within the enterprise.
- The element must be unique and clearly definable.
- Each element must have only one defined value response that may include a prescribed set of coded values (e.g., acceptable gender options) or any other single response type allowed by the database management system.
- Collection of the data element should not produce an undue burden on the data reporter.
- In general, the value returned for a data element should not contain more than one meaning. For example, an alphanumerical member number might have buried within the string, a number of attribute values such as member date of birth, plan type, risk type, program type, or any other variables about the member, any or all of which might change over time might be less than desirable.

Cataloging Standards

Standards are nothing new to most health care practitioners. Their relevance and importance in many areas of health delivery are well understood and appreciated. Few organi-

Box 14-1 DEVELOPING A DATA DICTIONARY THROUGH CONSENSUS BY USING AN INFORMATICS WORK GROUP

Phase 1: Data Gathering

1. The Informatics Working Group (IWG) meets to present the members with the goals and background of the data dictionary structure. Each member receives the following:
   - A process consensus document
   - Guidelines and procedures
   - An example of data dictionary elements
   - A copy of the data element worksheet
   - A review of the database program used to store and retrieve the elements.

2. The IWG accepts its work charge that specifies the content area selected to be addressed. This content area might have a number of specific elements already listed to include as part of the charge, or it might be left fairly open to the IWG to identify elements within that content area. Examples of content areas are demographic data, plan and coverage data, and encounter data.

3. IWG members provide comment on existing elements and begin reviewing other data elements to consider for further discussion.

4. All proposed data elements are evaluated to see whether they are appropriate for inclusion on the basis of a defined set of criteria.

5. The IWG confirms the initial set of elements for data dictionary development.

6. Data element general descriptions are compiled by project staff.

7. IWG members submit additional elements, with preliminary coding and definition recommendations from respected sources, to the staff for investigation as additions to the set under development. Elements with defined definitions and coding should be referenced by individual group members supplying the data elements. The governing board appoints a task force to serve as a resource to the content area and connect to the IWG to assist in content, definition, and coding in specialty areas.

8. All work is documented in the data dictionary software and appropriate documentation is prepared.

Phase 2: Organization and Task Completion

1. Staff compiles the list supplied by the task force and begins research through as many sources as possible (including members of the task force) to complete specific definitions and coding of the elements. Each element is also assessed to see that it meets basic criteria for inclusion. Each element is evaluated to see if whether could be used in a logical data modeling process.

2. Staff prepares documentation on each data element that notes the following:
   - Data element definition
   - Data element source (where the element came from [e.g., form, person, contract requirement])
   - Data element priority (significance to users for billing, clinical needs)
   - Data element references (who requires the element for what purposes)
   - Data element code references where appropriate
   - Data element inclusion within a data model
   - Category (content area?) in which the data element most commonly resides

3. The IWG is delivered the first iteration of the data element definitions and coding. When the task force reconvenes, its members review the current product; critique the elements' definitions and coding; suggest changes, additions, or deletions; and specify any additional follow-up required.

4. Staff perform follow-up tasks and return the product to the IWG for final review.

5. The IWG reviews one more iteration of the definition content product to that point and makes additional changes. Final recommendations are secured by consensus.

Phase 3: Validation

1. The reconciled product of the IWG is submitted for a 30-day review and comment process by stakeholders or any interested party. All comments are summarized from a questionnaire tool. Both objective ratings and written comments are requested.

2. Comments are returned to the staff and organized for an initial review by the IWG.

3. The IWG provides preliminary recommendations for action to the governing body where specific changes are recommended.

4. The governing body reviews recommendations from the IWG along with the feedback from the questionnaire and makes a final determination on data element changes.

5. Revisions on content are added to the existing data dictionary and disseminated to stakeholders and interested parties through the established dissemination process carried out by the staff.

Phase 4: Maintenance

1. The value of the dictionary will grow over time. Changes that need to be made will be considered for compelling clinical/business reasons. All modifications to the dictionary will follow a prescribed protocol that includes the following steps.

2. As new standards are developed or modified nationally and the need for new content areas develop, any health care entity can submit a request for modification of existing elements or addition of new elements to existing elements within the data dictionary.

3. Where changes occur, pointers to reference archive data and original documentation will be maintained to support continuity and accuracy of data over time.

4. The governing body reviews requests, determines when changes should be considered, and refers proposed changes to the IWG to be considered by the standard process identified in this work plan.

zations are not subject to measurement against standards established by The Joint Commission, the NCQA, and other accrediting bodies. Manufacturers of medical devices, particularly those companies that produce patient monitoring and life-sustaining equipment, must comply with very specific standards set forth by government regulatory agencies.

In many disciplines, standards of practice are international and universally recognized. For example, the notations and intonations associated with the standard musical scale are used by musicians throughout the world. Thus, listeners of Beethoven's fifth symphony as performed by the Vienna Philharmonic orchestra should be capable of identifying the same piece when it is delivered by a local high school orchestra (though the quality of its delivery might vary). Likewise, agencies within the European Economic Council have decreed that the dimensions of door hinges produced by hinge manufacturers in any member country must adhere to mutually agreed standards. This enables a French housing contractor to purchase door hinges from a low cost supplier in Belgium for use in constructing homes in Portugal.

The standards of music and European door hinges are well documented and catalogued. However, the highly variable and complex nature of health care information renders it much more difficult to standardize. However, as noted previously, this variability is often the source of confusion when clinical data recorded by one practitioner are later interpreted by another practitioner. Similarly, if the content and attributes of a broadly used patient identifier (i.e., the enterprise medical record number) are not uniform within various departmental-based systems, the ability to merge these data for various analyses is thwarted.

Once standards of data capture and retention are instituted and incorporated into the enterprise data dictionary, they must be catalogued and distributed to all users of the dictionary. The source of these standards can vary. Whenever possible, standards ordained by broadly acknowledged agencies and parties should be adopted. Thus, ICD-9-CM or ICD-10 would be referenced as the approved means of recording diagnoses in light of its general acceptance as a disease classification scheme.

Intraorganizational standards should also be acknowledged and referenced by the data dictionary. If a "customized" approach to calculating patient acuity has been developed within an acute-care hospital, only those scores resultant from its use should be cataloged. It would be futile to reference the format and content of a commercially available severity scoring system if it is not used in nursing practice.

Ideally, the format and content of a corporate-wide data dictionary are defined before the design and development of automated systems. However, most organizations, particularly health care entities, do not have the luxury of "scrapping" extant applications and rebuilding them from "scratch." Hence, data dictionaries are often implemented *after* many organizational systems have been implemented and are in broad use.

Even if a "start-up" health care facility possessed the opportunity to construct its data dictionary, there are no national or international standards that dictate and direct its complete design. The complexity of our health care delivery system has produced a more fragmented approach to the design and standards. These have typically arisen from specialty organizations or cooperatives that are associated with a particular specialty (the American College of Radiology's standards for image archiving) or function (the use of the American Medical Association's CPT-4 for the coding of various types of procedures).

Lacking any nationally recognized composite data model, health care organizations should strive to pursue and implement standards for specific types of information (such as those mentioned above) wherever possible. With the increased demand for the exchange of clinical information among providers, government agencies, payers and other parties, the need to adhere to recognized standards is obvious. Use of established taxonomies and guidelines greatly enhance the "exchangability" of medical data as well as reducing administrative costs.

Key Concepts

- The health information and informatics professional provides expertise in the areas of data collection and analysis. This information is used for a variety of purposes and, because of this, it is of the utmost importance that the data be accurate and complete. Further, as the EHR becomes prominent, more and more information may be coded through automated mechanisms. This allows the population of registries and databases. HIM professionals are poised to capitalize on emerging technology as the nation implements electronic health information.

- Data are used as a surveillance mechanism for specific disease processes or incidence to monitor the impact of using medical devices and to assess the health issues surrounding exposures to hazardous substances. The need for such information has led to the development and implementation of numerous registries and databases.

- Registries and other databases vary in mission, design, size, use of technology, and regulations. Regardless of the type, registries and databases track patient patterns, assess care through follow-up and quality assessment activities, and provide data for administrative planning of resources and for identifying health care needs. They also provide data that affect the development of health policies.

- Regardless of the type of registry or database, the patient record is a primary source of information and EHRs offer a more useful resource.

REFERENCES

1. American College of Surgeons: *Standards of the Commission on Cancer, cancer program standards,* Chicago, 2004, American College of Surgeons.

2. Centers for Disease Control and Prevention: *Case definitions for infectious conditions under public health surveillance,* Atlanta, Centers for Disease Control and Prevention: http://www.cdc.gov/epo/dphsi/casedef/case_definitions.htm. Accessed November 4, 2006.

3. American College of Surgeons: Trauma registry. In *Resources for optimal care of the injured patient: 1993,* chapter 17, Chicago, 1993, Committee on Trauma, American College of Surgeons.

4. Kraybill WG, editor: *News from the Commission on Cancer, vol 4,* No. 2, Chicago, 1993, American College of Surgeons.

5. Menck HR, Smart CR, editors: *Central cancer registries: Design, management and use,* Bethesda, MD, 1994, American Association of Central Cancer Registries.

6. *Cancer statistics review, 1973-1987,* NIH Publication No. 90-2789, Institute Division of Cancer Prevention and Control Surveillance Program, Bethesda, MD, 1990, U.S. Department of Health and Human Services.

7. Watkins S, editor: *Tumor registry management manual,* ed 4, Santa Barbara, CA, 1992, Tumor Registrars Association of California.

8. *Standards of the Commission on Cancer,* volume 2, *Registry operations and data standards (ROADS),* Chicago, 1996, rev 1998, rev 2004, American College of Surgeons: http://www.facs.org/cancer/coc/roads.html.

9. Shambaugh E, editor: *Self-instructional manual for tumor registrars,* book 5,. SEER Program, Biometry Branch, Bethesda, MD, 1993, National Cancer Institute, 1993: http://seer.cancer.gov/training/manuals/. Accessed September 26, 2005.

10. American Joint Committee on Cancer: *Manual for staging of cancer,* ed 6, New York, 2002, Springer-Verlag.

11. National Tumor Registrars Association, Council on Certification: http://www.ctrexam.org/eligibility/index.htm#status. Accessed August 17, 2006.

12. American Association of Central Cancer Registrars: *National standard for cancer data exchange, record description,* Bethesda, MD, 1993, American Association of Central Cancer Registries.

13. Cordero JF: Registries of birth defects and genetic diseases, *Med Genet* 39:65, 1992.

14. Lyndberg MC, Edmonds LD: Surveillance of defects program: Surveillance of birth defects. In Halpern W, Baker EL, Monson RR, editors: *Public health surveillance,* pp. 157-177, New York, 1992.

15. Khoury MJ, Edmonds LD: Metropolitan Atlanta congenital defects program: Twenty-five years of birth defects surveillance at the Centers for Disease Control, presented at the Italian Association for Study of Malformations, International Symposium, December 1992.

16. Murray AL: *1988-1990 North Carolina birth defects registry report,* no 74. Raleigh: State Center for Health and Environmental Statistics, 1993.

17. Illinois Department of Public Health, Adverse Pregnancy Outcomes Reporting System: http://www.idph.state.il.us/about/epi/aporsrpt.htm. Accessed August 18, 2006.

18. Centers for Disease Control and Prevention: Mortality data from National Vital Statistics System: www.cdc.gov/nchs/about/major/dvs/icd10odes.htm. Accessed September 28, 2005.

19. Schaubert DS: Role of registries in diabetes prevention and control: a perspective from North Dakota. Presented at Multi-purpose diabetes registries: innovation in research and practice, Berkeley, CA, June 1993.

20. Bruno G: Application of capture-recapture methodology, an approach to diabetes registries, presented at Multi-purpose diabetes registries: Innovation in research and practice, Berkeley, CA, June 1993.

21. Kaiser Permanente, Division of Research, Diabetes Registry: http://www.dor.kaiser.org/studies/diabetes/Diabetes-06.shtml. Accessed August 20, 2006.

22. Mayfield J: Diabetes registration within the U.S. Indian Health Service, presented at Multi-purpose diabetes registries: Innovation in research and practice, Berkeley, CA, June 1993.

23. Nichols DG: Millions benefit from the Safe Medical Devices Act (SMDA) of 1990, *J Am Health Inform Manage Assoc* 63:60-62, 1992.

24. Bryant LE: Health law: Medical record implications of the Safe Medical Devices Act of 1990, *J Am Health Inform Manage Assoc* 63:17-18, 1992.

25. Kendall KE, Kendall JE: *Systems analysis and design,* ed 3, Englewood Cliffs, NJ, 1995, Prentice Hall.

26. National Immunization Program, Centers for Disease Control and Prevention: http://www.cdc.gov/nip/registry/Default.htm. Accessed August 20, 2006.

27. Hearington DK, Ettner BJ, Breen T, White R: National Scientific Registry of Organ Transplantation: Data needs and uses, *Top Health Rec Manage* 11:1-12, 1990.

28. United Network for Organ Sharing: Who we are: http://www.unos.org/whoWeAre/#ref. Accessed August 20, 2006.

29. United Network for Organ Sharing: www.unos.org/data/about/collection.asp#def. Accessed August 20, 2006.

30. American College of Surgeons: Trauma programs: www.facs.org/trauma. Accessed August 20, 2006.

31. Centers for Disease Control and Prevention (2005): http://www.cdc.gov/nchs/data/injury/DicussionDocu.pdf. Accessed September 26, 2005.

32. Ehlinger K, Gardner MJ, Nakayama DK: The trauma registry: An administrative and clinical tool, *Top Health Inform Manage* 11:43-48, 1990.

33. Ackerman MA, Peterson FV, Manni PJ et al: Evolution of a hospital-based trauma registry, *Top Health Inform Manage* 11:49-58, 1990.

34. News from the American College of Surgeons: National Trauma Registry is initiated by the American College of Surgeons, press release, Chicago, March 1993.

35. Elixhauser A, Steiner C, Harris D et al: Comorbidity measures for use with administrative data, *Med Care* 36:8-27, 1998.

36. *What are APR-DRGs? An introduction to severity of illness and risk of mortality adjustment methodology,* 2003, 3M.

37. Petersen L, Pietz K, Woodard L et al: Comparison of the predictive validity of diagnosis-based risk adjusters for clinical outcomes, *Med Care* 43:61-67, 2005.

38. Agency for Healthcare Research and Quality, CCS Software: http://www.hcup-us.ahrq.gov/toolssoftware/ccs/ccs.jsp.

39. Williams S, Torrens P: *Introduction to health services,* ed 5, Albany, 1999, Delmar.

40. Schoenman J, Sutton J, Kintala S et al: *The value of hospital discharge databases,* Salt Lake City, UT, 2005, National Association of Health Data Organizations.

41. Johnston J, Wagner D, Timmons S et al: Impact of difference measure of comorbid disease on predicted mortality of intensive care unit patients, *Med Care* 40:929-940, 2002.

42. Teslow M, Mueller I, Schmidt K: Asking the right questions: Connecting users and data through a formal interview process, *J AHIMA* 76:42-45, 2004.

43. American Health Information Management Association: Homeland security and HIM, *J AHIMA* 76: 56A-D, 2004.

44. Kerr EA, McGlynn EA, Adams J et al: Profiling the quality of care in communities: Results from the Community Quality Index Study, *Health Affairs* 23: 247-256, 2004.

45. Quality Net: http://www.qualitynet.org/dcs/ContentServer? pagename=QnetPublic/Page/QnetHomepage 50.

46. Joint Commission on Accreditation of Healthcare Organizations: www.jcaho.org.

47. Jollis JG, Ancukiewicz M, DeLong ER, et al: Discordance of databases designed for claims payment versus clinical information systems, *Ann Intern Med* 119:844-850, 1993.

48. Association jumps into outcomes software game, *Health Data Network News* 5:4, 1996.

49. American Health Information Management Association: *Automated coding software: development and use to enhance anti-fraud,* Chicago, 2005, American Health Information Management Association.

50. Inmon WH, Hackathorne RD: *Using the data warehouse,* New York, 1994, John Wiley.

51. Tobias D: *Meta-dictionary: A system for data administration,* Washington, DC, 1989, IEEE Computer Society Press.

52. Brackett M: *Data sharing, using a common data architecture,* New York, 1994, John Wiley.

53. Simsion G: *Data modeling essentials,* Boston, 1994, International Thompson Publishing.

54. Batini C, DiBattista G, Santucci G et al: *Design of data dictionaries,* Amsterdam, 1992, IOS Press.

55. Clayton C, Genton S: Health information managers and clinical data repositories: A natural fit, *J AHIMA* 67:48-51, 1996.

56. Institute of Medicine: *The computer-based patient record,* Washington, DC, 1991, National Academy Press.

chapter 15

Privacy and Health Law

Jill Callahan Dennis

Additional content,
http://evolve.elsevier.com/Abdelhak/

Review exercises can be found
in the Study Guide

Chapter Contents

Why Are Legal Issues Important to Health Information Management Professionals?
Fundamentals of the Legal System
Sources of Law
    Constitutional Law
    Federal and State Statutes
    Rules and Regulations of Administrative Agencies
    Court Decisions (Case Law)
The Legal System
The Court System
    Federal Courts
    State and Territory Courts
    Roles of the Key Players: Court Procedures
Cases That Involve Health Care Facilities and Providers
    Malpractice and Negligence
    Intentional Torts
    Products Liability
    Contractual Disputes
    Antitrust Claims
    Crimes and Corporate Compliance
    Noncompliance with Statutes, Rules, and Regulations
Legal Obligations and Risks of Health Care Facilities and Individual Health Care Providers
    Duties to Patients, in General
    Duty to Maintain Health Information

Key Words

Advance directive	Deidentified	Power of attorney
Alternative dispute resolution	Deposition	Precedent
Antitrust	Designated record set	Pre-empt, or pre-emption
Arbitration	Discovery	Preponderance of evidence
Assault	Due process	Privacy
Authentication	Durable power of attorney for health	Privileged communication
Authorization	care	Protected health information
Bailiff	Emancipated minor	Proximate cause
Battery	Evidence	Qui tam
Best evidence rule	False imprisonment	"Reasonable man" standard
Breach of contract	Fraud	Regulation
Burden of proof	Health care operations	Res ipsa loquitur
Business associate agreement	Hearsay rule	Respondeat superior
Case law	Incident report	Restraint of trade
Charitable immunity	Informed consent	Right of privacy
Clerk of the court	Institutional review board	Satisfactory assurance
Common law	Intentional tort	Security of health information
Complaint	Interrogatory	Slander
Confidential communications	Invasion of privacy	Standard of care
Consent	Jurisdiction	Stare decisis
Contemporaneous documentation	Libel	Statute
Contract	Living will	Statute of limitations
Corporate negligence	Malpractice	Subpoena
Court order	Minimum necessary	Subpoena duces tecum
Court reporter	Motion to quash	Tort
Covered entity	Negligence	Whistleblower
Credentialing	Occurrence report	Workforce
Defamation	Plaintiff	
Defendant	Pleading	

Duty to Retain Health Information and Other Key
    Documents and to Keep Them Secure
    Error Correction
    Addenda
    Authentication and Authorship Issues
    Validity of Health Information as Evidence
    Retention of Other Records and Information
Duty to Maintain Confidentiality
    Privacy Act of 1974
    Freedom of Information Act
    Regulations on Confidentiality of Alcohol and Drug Abuse
        Patient Records
Internal Uses and External Disclosures of Health
    Information
General Principles Regarding Access and Disclosure Policies
    Health Information Ownership
    Resources on Releasing Patient Information
    Authorizations for Disclosure of Patient Information
    Disclosure for Direct Patient Care
    Disclosure for Performance Management and Patient Safety
    Disclosure for Educational Purposes
    Disclosure for Research
    Uses for Administrative Purposes
    Disclosure for Payment Purposes
    Disclosure to Attorneys
    Disclosure to Law Enforcement Personnel and Agencies
    Disclosure to Family Members When the Patient Is a Minor
    Disclosure to Family Members When the Patient Is an
        Emancipated Minor or an Adult
    Disclosure to Family Members in Cases of Incompetence or
        Incapacity
    Patient Access to Personal Health Information
    Other Patient-Directed Disclosures
    Rediclosure Issues
    Disclosure to Outsourcing Firms Handling Health
        Information Functions
    Disclosure to the News Media
    Disclosure Pursuant to Legal Process
    Health Information Management Department Security
        Measures to Prevent Unauthorized Access
Duty to Provide Care That Meets Professional Standards
Duty to Obtain Informed Consent to Treatment
Duty to Provide a Safe Environment for Patients and
    Visitors
Duty to Supervise the Actions of Employees and the
    Professional Staff
    Medical Staff Credentialing Process
    Accessibility of Credentials Files and Quality Profiles
    Legal Risks
Contract Liability Issues and the Health Information
    Management Department
Legal Resources for Health Information Management
    Professionals

Abbreviations

AHA—American Hospital Association

AHIMA—American Health Information Management Association

CFR—Code of Federal Regulations

CMS—Center for Medicare and Medicaid Services

DHHS—Department of Health and Human Services

DRS—designated record set

EMTALA—Emergency Treatment and Active Labor Act

FOIA—Freedom of Information Act

HIM—health information management

HIPAA—Health Insurance Portability and Accountability Act

HIV—human immunodeficiency virus

IIHI—individually identifiable health information

IRB—institutional review board

JCAHO—Joint Commission on Accreditation of Healthcare
    Organizations (now The Joint Commission)

MIB—Medical Information Bureau

NPDB—National Practitioner Data Bank

OIG—Office of the Inspector General

PHI—protected health information

Objectives

- Define key words.
- Explain why health information management professionals
  must be knowledgeable about medicolegal issues.
- Distinguish between confidential and nonconfidential
  information within a health information system.
- Describe general legal principles governing access to
  confidential health information in a variety of circumstances.
- Distinguish proper or valid requests for access to health
  information from improper or invalid requests.
- Have a basic understanding of the federal and state court
  systems.
- Describe the four components of negligence.
- Distinguish between properly executed consents and
  authorizations and incomplete or improper consents and
  authorizations.
- Identify major resources for locating information on laws,
  rules, regulations, and standards related to health
  information.

WHY ARE LEGAL ISSUES IMPORTANT TO HEALTH INFORMATION MANAGEMENT PROFESSIONALS?

At this moment, personal information about the health care or health status of millions of people is being collected, recorded, reviewed, analyzed, transmitted, used, and even misused. For every person who goes to a physician, clinic, hospital, or other treatment provider, somewhere there is a data set related to that visit or treatment. There is a record of all births, every operation, every treatment episode, every test result.

Health information management (HIM) professionals design and manage the information systems that hold these vital records. Earlier chapters discuss some of the reasons these records are kept. Scores of people and organizations want and need health information. As a result, health care providers are required by law to maintain these records. *HIM professionals must ensure that the information systems they manage, run, or design meet these obligations.* This chapter discusses some of those obligations.

Some requests for health information are legitimate. Others are not. How do HIM professionals decide which requests are valid and which are not? And for the requests that are granted, how do HIM professionals decide what can be disclosed and what cannot? HIM professionals are called on to make these decisions every day. In a health care facility, the HIM professional is the resident expert on these questions. Legal counsel is not always readily available. To make wise decisions—decisions that appropriately protect the confidentiality of health information—HIM professionals must be aware of the rules, **regulations,** and laws that govern access to health information. A large part of this chapter is devoted to access issues. The rules that govern access to and disclosure of health information are fluid and often thorny. For many HIM professionals, these issues are among the most interesting they encounter in their career.

Why are legal issues so important to HIM professionals? It is because HIM professionals are relied on by the following to understand these issues:

- Patients or clients whose health information they manage
- Health care organizations in which they are employed
- All users of health information, such as public health officials, who track communicable and other disease patterns, and government agencies responsible for setting health policy.

HIM professionals must take this trust seriously. By gaining a good understanding of legal issues, HIM students and professionals can be worthy of that trust.

Fundamentals of the Legal System

In civilized societies, laws guide actions. These laws set forth principles and processes for our actions and for handling disputes over those actions. Laws govern both our *private* relationships (the relationships between private parties) and our *public* relationships (the relationships between private parties and the government).

Private law consists of two types of actions: **tort** actions and **contract** actions. In a tort action, one party alleges that another party's wrongful conduct has caused him or her harm. The party bringing the action to court seeks compensation for that harm. In a contract action, one party alleges that a contract exists between himself or herself and another party and that the other party has breached the contract by failing to fulfill an obligation that is part of that contract. The party bringing the contract action seeks either compensation for the breach or a **court order** to force the breaching party to fulfill that obligation.

Public law is composed of rules, regulations, and criminal law. Congress has charged various governmental agencies with the responsibility for overseeing various aspects of many of our nation's most important industries, including health care. These agencies, acting under the authority of state and federal **statutes,** issue rules and regulations that touch every department of every health care organization. They cover diverse subjects, such as laboratory safety, incineration of medical waste, employment policies, confidentiality of peer review records, and mandatory reporting of medical device failures or problems. Failure to follow these rules can involve monetary penalties as well as criminal penalties. In addition to these rules and regulations, public laws include a body of criminal law—laws that bar conduct considered being harmful to society—and set forth a system for punishing "bad acts."

Sources of Law

Laws that affect the health care system come from four main areas:

- Federal and state constitutions—the supreme law of the nation and state, respectively
- Federal and state statutes—laws enacted by Congress and state legislatures, respectively
- Rules and regulations of administrative agencies—acting under powers delegated to them by the legislature
- Court decisions—decisions that interpret statutes, regulations, and the Constitution and, where no such statutes or regulations are applicable, that apply **common law** (the large body of principles that have evolved from prior court decisions).

Constitutional Law

The U.S. Constitution grants certain powers to the three branches of the federal government: executive, legislative, and judicial. It also grants certain powers to the individual states. Powers granted by the Constitution may be either express or implied. Express powers are those specifically stated in the Constitution, such as the power to tax and the power to declare war. Implied powers are not specifically listed in the Constitution. They are the actions considered "necessary and proper" to permit the express powers to be accomplished.

The Constitution also limits what federal and state governments can do. For example, the first 10 amendments to the Constitution—the Bill of Rights—protect the rights of citizens to, among other things, free speech, freedom of religion, and due process before deprivation of life, liberty, or property. In a public health care facility (which is considered a governmental unit, as opposed to a private nongovernmental facility), a physician's appointment to the medical staff is considered a property right. Therefore, before that appointment could be terminated or rejected, the hospital would be obliged to provide **due process** to that physician, such as by a full hearing.

Another constitutional right important to the health care industry is the **right of privacy,** although that right is not an express one. What is the right to privacy? Generally, it is considered to be a constitutionally recognized right to be left alone, to make decisions about one's own body, and to control one's own information. In the court decision of *Griswold v. Connecticut,* the U.S. Supreme Court recognized a constitutional right of privacy.[1] This right limits the government's power to regulate abortion, contraception, and other reproductive issues. The constitutional right to privacy has also been interpreted as permitting the terminally ill (or their legal guardians) to make decisions regarding the termination or withholding of medical treatment to prolong life.

It is important to note that the Constitution is the overriding, or highest, law in the United States. If lower laws (e.g., state or federal laws) conflict with principles in the Constitution, the Constitution overrides the conflicting law. When a law has been struck down because it is "unconstitutional," that means that the lower law conflicts with the Constitution and is thus invalid.

Federal and State Statutes

Laws enacted by legislatures, be they Congress, state legislatures, or local city councils, are another important source of laws that affect health care facilities. One federal law that dramatically affects health care facilities as well as other business is the Americans with Disabilities Act.[2] This law not only affects the hiring and employment practices of businesses but also forces public facilities to remove or modify physical plant characteristics that may serve as access barriers for the disabled. The Safe Medical Devices Act is another federal statute that affects all health care facilities.[3] It requires that certain incidents that involve medical devices and equipment be reported to a national data bank.

When federal and state laws conflict, valid federal laws supersede the state laws. When state laws and local laws conflict, the valid state law controls.

Rules and Regulations of Administrative Agencies

Among the powers delegated to administrative agencies and departments of the executive branch by legislatures is the power to adopt rules and regulations to implement various laws. These rules and regulations provide instruction in how to comply with the law. Some of the most important agencies and departments at the federal level that affect health care are the Department of Health and Human Services (DHHS) and its Centers for Medicare and Medicaid Services (CMS), the Food and Drug Administration, the Internal Revenue Service on tax matters, the Department of Justice and the Federal Trade Commission on **antitrust** issues, and the Department of Labor and the National Labor Relations Board on labor and employment issues.

The rules and regulations of these bodies are valid only if they are within the limits of authority granted to them in their charter. Congress, in passing legislation creating these bodies, decides the broad areas in which these federal agencies may regulate, just as state legislatures do for state agencies. In promulgating their rules and regulations, federal agencies and many state agencies must follow administrative procedure acts passed by the legislature. These acts set forth the steps that administrative agencies must follow in issuing new rules and regulations and deciding disputes about those regulations. The Federal Administrative Procedure Act and most of the states' acts provide for advance notice of proposed rules and opportunity for public comment. Many federal agencies must publish both proposed and final rules in the daily *Federal Register.* An HIM professional should be familiar with the *Federal Register* and with how to scan it for notices of proposed rule making. By doing so, a facility can have early warning of upcoming changes that may affect facility operations. By commenting on proposed rules, the facility can also influence the language of the final rule.

Court Decisions (Case Law)

When cases are brought before them, federal and state courts interpret statutes and regulations, decide their validity, and follow or create **common law** (also referred to as **case law**) when no statutes or regulations apply. In deciding cases, courts generally adhere to the principle of **stare decisis** (let the decision stand). This can be described as following **precedent.** By referring to similar cases that have been decided in the past and by applying the same principles, courts generally arrive at the same ruling in the current case as in similar previous cases. Sometimes, however, even slight factual differences can result in departures from precedent. Sometimes courts decide that the precedent no longer adequately serves society's needs. One of the most important examples of this from a health care standpoint was the elimination of the doctrine of **charitable immunity,** which had until the early to mid-1960s protected nonprofit hospitals from liability for harm to patients. Courts now permit harmed patients to sue hospitals for their wrongful

Box 15-1   FACTS OF THE DARLING CASE

In the *Darling* case, a college football player fractured his leg during a game. He was taken to the emergency department of a community hospital, where the physician on emergency department duty was a general practitioner who had not treated a major leg fracture for several years. The physician ordered a radiograph, which revealed a fracture of the tibia and the fibula. The physician reduced the fracture and applied a cast that extended from the patient's toes to just below his groin. Shortly after the cast was applied, the patient began to complain of pain, and he was admitted. The physician split the cast and visited the patient frequently while he was an inpatient. Complaints of pain continued. No specialist consultation was called.

After 2 weeks, the patient was transferred to a larger hospital and placed under the care of an orthopedic surgeon. The surgeon found much dead tissue in the fractured leg and over the next 2 months removed increasing amounts of tissue in an effort to save the leg. Finally, it became necessary to amputate the leg eight inches below the knee.

The patient's father filed suit against the physician and the first hospital, alleging negligence. The physician settled out of court, but the hospital chose to go to court. Darling alleged that the hospital was negligent in its failure to provide enough trained nurses for bedside care of all patients at all times. In this case, Darling claimed that the nurses should have been capable of recognizing the progressive gangrene in the leg and should have called it to the attention of the medical staff and hospital administration so that adequate consultation could have been obtained. The hospital argued that its liability as a charitable corporation—if there was liability at all—was limited to the amount of its liability insurance.

Judgment was eventually returned against the hospital in the amount of $100,000. The court decided that the doctrine of charitable immunity should no longer apply. On appeal, the Illinois Supreme Court agreed, stating: "We agree that the doctrine of charitable immunity can no longer stand …[A] doctrine which limits the liability of charitable corporations to the amount of liability insurance that they see fit to carry permits them to determine whether or not they will be liable for their torts and the amount of liability, if any."[4]

acts. The landmark case on this point is *Darling v. Charleston Community Memorial Hospital* (Box 15-1).[4]

As a result, hospitals are held liable for the negligent acts of their employees and, in some circumstances, their physicians. Health care organizations' liability is discussed in more detail later in the chapter.

Not all disputes, however, are resolved by courts. In health care, for example, health care facilities sometimes avoid the need to resort to the courts by participating in mediation or **arbitration,** also described as **alternative dispute resolution,** in which a neutral party or panel hears both sides of a dispute and renders a decision, or by settling claims against them by negotiating a direct payment to the parties bringing the claim in exchange for the claimants' dropping the claim.

THE LEGAL SYSTEM

The Court System

Federal Courts

The federal court system and many state systems have three levels of courts: trial courts, intermediate courts of appeals, and a supreme court. The federal trial courts are called U.S. district courts. They cannot hear just any case. To be eligible to hear a case, a court must have **jurisdiction.** To be heard in a federal court, a case must involve either a federal question or diversity of jurisdiction. Federal question cases involve questions of federal law, such as possible violations of federal law or violations of a party's federal constitutional rights. Diversity cases—cases that involve citizens of different states—are heard in federal courts, but rather than use federal law, federal judges apply the laws of the applicable states in deciding these cases. In many of these diversity cases, a minimum of $10,000 must also be involved.

Appeals from federal trial courts (U.S. district courts) go to a U.S. court of appeals. The United States is divided into 12 circuits. These courts are typically referred to as the U.S. Court of Appeals for the First (Second, Third, Eleventh, or D.C.) Circuit.

The U.S. Supreme Court is the nation's highest court. It decides appeals from any of the U.S. courts of appeals. It may also hear appeals from the highest state courts if those cases involve federal laws or the U.S. Constitution. In some instances, if a U.S. court of appeals or the highest state court refuses to hear an appeal, the case may be appealed directly to the U.S. Supreme Court. The U.S. Supreme Court need not and could not possibly hear all cases. Because the Court's time is limited and the volume of cases is large, the Supreme Court picks and chooses most of the cases it hears. There are no cut-and-dried criteria for which cases are chosen, but the Court attempts to hear the cases involving the most important questions of law or having the greatest potential impact on society. With a few exceptions, the Supreme Court may decide not to review an appealed case. This does not mean that the Supreme Court necessarily approves of the lower court's decision; it merely means that it chooses not to review the decision.

State and Territory Courts

In some states, trial courts are divided into special branches that hear certain types of cases. Probate court, traffic court, juvenile court, and family and divorce courts are examples. In addition to these special branches, there are trial courts with general jurisdiction—the power to hear all disputes not otherwise assigned to one of these special branches or not otherwise barred from state courts by law.

The job of the trial court is to hear the facts, review the applicable law, and decide the outcome. Sometimes there are no factual disagreements, but the parties to the lawsuit simply disagree over what the law provides. At other times, there may be no disagreement over the law, but the facts are in dispute. Often a case involves questions of law and facts.

Most states also have an intermediate appellate court that hears appeals from state trial court decisions. These appellate courts do not hold a new trial and hear new evidence; they generally limit their review to the trial court record to determine whether proper procedures were followed and whether the law was correctly interpreted.

Every state has a single high court, usually called the supreme court.* A state supreme court hears appeals from the intermediate appellate court or, if no intermediate court exists, the state trial courts. The high court often has other duties as well, such as formulating procedural rules for the lower state courts to follow.

Roles of the Key Players: Court Procedures

The **plaintiff** is the party who initiates the lawsuit. Plaintiffs initiate suits by filing a **complaint,** petition, or bill with the **clerk of the court.** This complaint is a written statement by the plaintiff that states his or her claims and commences the action. Plaintiffs sue one or more **defendants,** the party or parties from whom relief or compensation is sought. The defendant then files an answer to the complaint, which may also be called a responsive **pleading.** In this answer, the defendant denies or otherwise responds to the plaintiff's claims. If the case is not immediately settled, it proceeds into a process of **discovery.** Sometimes HIM directors are involved in the discovery phase of lawsuits by providing certain information used in the discovery devices described next.

During discovery, each party seeks to discover important information about the case through a pretrial investigation. It includes obtaining pertinent testimony (through **depositions,** sworn verbal testimony, and through **interrogatories,** sworn written answers to questions) and documents that may be under the control of the opposing party. For example, a patient who is suing a clinic for negligent care of an infected cut needs to obtain copies of the clinic's patient records that describe the care that was provided to the patient.

The purpose of the discovery phase is to encourage early out-of-court resolution of cases by acquainting all parties with all pertinent facts. If the case cannot be settled out of court, it proceeds to trial. Evidence properly uncovered during the discovery phase is available in court. The judge is in charge of deciding which laws are applicable and also uses the state or federal rules of evidence (as applicable to the setting) in deciding whether certain pieces of evidence are admissible at trial. Not all evidence produced during the discovery phase is admissible. Often, certain evidence is judged to be unfairly prejudicial to one side or the other or is subject to certain protective laws (such as the laws that pro-

tect peer review information in health care organizations). The judge examines the evidence, hears arguments on both sides of the question, and then uses the applicable rules of evidence to decide whether the information can be fairly used at trial.

The judge also keeps order and makes decisions necessary to facilitate a fair, impartial trial. If the case involves a jury, the jury's job is to determine the facts as presented in court, at least in part by deciding which witnesses and which evidence to believe, and to apply the law as instructed by the judge.

Even when a jury is present, the judge has substantial influence over the trial result. If he or she finds that insufficient evidence has been presented to establish an issue for the jury to resolve, the judge may in various circumstances refuse to send the case to the jury, dismiss the case, or direct the jury to decide the case one way or another. In civil cases, even if the jury has already rendered a verdict, the judge may decide in favor of the other side, setting aside the jury's verdict. This is called a judgment n.o.v.—judgment non obstante verdicto (notwithstanding the verdict).

Some of the other players involved in trial proceedings are the clerk of the court, **court reporter,** and **bailiff.** The clerk of the court is the administrative manager of the court and handles the paperwork associated with lawsuits. Complaints are filed with the clerk, as are other pleadings and documents. The court reporter is responsible for creating a verbatim transcript of court proceedings. Bailiffs are courtroom personnel who are present to assist in keeping order, administering oaths, guarding and the assisting the jury, and performing other duties at the direction of the judge.

Cases That Involve Health Care Facilities and Providers

Malpractice and Negligence

Among the most frequent types of claims made against health care facilities and individual providers are claims of **negligence** or **malpractice** (professional negligence). Negligence is conduct that society considers unreasonably dangerous because "first, the [individual or party] did foresee or should have foreseen that it would subject another or others to an appreciable risk of harm, and second, only the magnitude of the perceivable risk was such that the [individual or party] should have acted in a safer manner."[5]

At this point, some readers may ask, "How can hospitals be held accountable for actions when they are simply the bricks and mortar within which people work?" Two theories of negligence are used to hold hospitals and other health care organizations accountable for their conduct. Under the first theory, **respondeat superior** (meaning "let the master answer" for the actions of the servant—the doctrine of "agency"), the legal system imputes the negligent actions of the organization's employees or agents over whom it has

---

*In some states, the terminology is quite different. In New York, the highest court is the New York Court of Appeals, and the trial courts are called supreme courts.

control to the health care organization itself. Using this theory, courts hold employers responsible for the acts of their employees or agents that are performed within the scope of employment. For example, a hospital can be held responsible for the actions of its nurses while they are acting within the scope of their employment (e.g., when they are performing some aspect of their job assignment), but a hospital would not be held responsible for the actions of a nurse in its employ while the nurse is grocery shopping after work.

Under the second, more current theory of **corporate negligence,** courts can hold health care organizations liable for their own independent acts of negligence. This theory holds organizations responsible for monitoring the activities of the people who function within their facilities, whether those people are employees or independent contractors, such as physicians, and for complying with appropriate industry standards, such as accreditation (The Joint Commission) standards, licensing regulations, and *Conditions of Participation* issued by Medicare. Health care organizations are no longer considered to be merely physicians' "workshops." They retain some responsibility for all who are authorized to function within their facilities (see examples of situations that can lead to malpractice claims against health care organizations and providers).

Examples of Situations Leading to Malpractice Claims

- Failure to properly diagnose a condition, such as cancer
- Failure to properly treat a condition—for example, not cleaning a wound before stitching it up
- Failure to monitor or supervise a patient's condition and take appropriate action; for example, in the *Darling* case described earlier in the chapter, the nurses failed to note and report the leg's worsening condition
- Failure to credential medical staff members properly (e.g., granting a physician privileges to perform some types of surgery for which the physician is not qualified)

Malpractice claims are not the only kind of claims against health care organizations and providers. The following are some of the other types of claims that HIM professionals may encounter in their professional careers.

Intentional Torts

Intentional tort claims that may be brought against health care facilities include **assault** and **battery, false imprisonment, defamation** of character, **invasion of privacy, fraud** or misrepresentation, and intentional infliction of emotional distress.

When one thinks of assault and battery, one often thinks of a mugging or an attack of some sort. But an assault is simply a deliberate threat, coupled with the apparent ability,

to do physical harm to another person without that person's consent. No contact is required. For example, if a nurse stood over a patient with a syringe, stating that he or she was going to inject the patient with a strong sedative regardless of whether the patient agreed to it, that would constitute an assault if the patient was aware of the threat. If the nurse proceeded to inject the patient, that would constitute a battery. A battery is nonconsensual, intentional touching of another person in a socially impermissible manner. Awareness of the victim is irrelevant. An unconscious patient who has surgery performed without express (actual) or implied consent (such as when a patient is brought to the facility for life-saving treatment) is the victim of a battery.

Could assault and battery ever really happen in a health care facility? In *Peete v. Blackwell,* a nurse was awarded damages after a physician with whom she was working struck her and cursed at her while ordering her to turn on suctioning equipment.[6] Although there were no lasting injuries, the jury awarded $1 in compensation and $10,000 in punitive damages.

The laws concerning battery are one of the prime reasons behind the requirement to obtain the patient's written consent to treatment. Allegations of battery against health care facilities most often involve situations in which improper or no patient consent was obtained before a surgical procedure. Regardless of whether the procedure helps or harms the patient, unconsented-to invasions of the patient's person entitle the patient to at least nominal damages.*

False imprisonment is unlawful restraint of a person's personal liberty or the unlawful restraining or confining of a person. Physical force is not required; all that is required is a reasonable fear that force will be used to detain or intimidate the person into following orders. How could this apply to a health care facility? If a facility tried to prevent a patient's departure from the facility until the patient's bill was paid, this could qualify as false imprisonment. The use of physical restraints to keep a patient in bed for no other reason than inadequate staffing available to monitor patients could also qualify.

False imprisonment issues can be complex. For example, if an intoxicated driver involved in a motor vehicle accident is treated for minor cuts in an emergency department and now wants to be discharged to drive home but is still extremely intoxicated, must the facility release that patient or may he or she be restrained until capable of driving safely? Statutes in some states permit intoxicated or mentally ill people to be detained by a hospital if they are dangerous to themselves or others. This is one example of why it is so important for the staff in health care organizations to be

---

*See, for example, *Perna v. Pirozzi,* 457 A.2d 431 (N.J. 1983) in which the supreme court of New Jersey held that a patient who consents to surgery by one surgeon but who is actually operated on by another has grounds for an action for battery!

familiar with state laws. In judging reasonableness of a health care provider's actions in detaining a patient, documentation in the patient record is often vital.

Defamation of character is oral (**slander**) or written (**libel**) communication to a person (other than the person defamed) that tends to damage the defamed person's reputation in the eyes of the community. To succeed in a defamation action, the defamed person must show that there was communication to a third party. Truth of the statements is a defense, as is privilege. If the defamation occurs during a **privileged communication**—such as during **confidential communications** between spouses or in a talk with a priest or minister—defamation is not found as long as the statements are made without malice (evil intent). Defamation cases in health care are unusual but they do occur, especially in the context of medical staff credentialing and granting of privileges, when the defamed party argues that the defamatory remarks were made with malice. Professionals who are called incompetent in front of others generally have a right to sue to defend their reputation. If the person making the remark cannot prove that the comment is true or that some other privilege applies, he or she may be held liable for damages. For that reason, it is generally wise to refrain from making disparaging remarks about other health professionals and colleagues.

Invasion of privacy is an intentional tort with which HIM professionals must be concerned. By the very act of submitting to treatment, patients give up some privacy. However, negligent disregard for patients' privacy can and does result in actions against health care providers and organizations, and it can also result in regulatory penalties such as fines for violations of those regulations, which is discussed later in this chapter. Because HIM professionals and other health professionals work with sensitive information on an almost constant basis, it is easy to become callous to privacy issues. Readers who have visited friends or family members in the hospital and overheard staff members talking casually about patients and their conditions in hallways, elevators, and the cafeteria have witnessed what may have been an invasion of privacy or breach of confidentiality. Health care providers who divulge confidential information from a patient's record to an improper recipient without the patient's permission have invaded the patient's privacy and breached their duty of confidentiality. A great deal of this chapter is devoted to identifying what health information is confidential and who is a proper or an improper recipient. HIM professionals must learn these principles well and become expert in applicable state and federal laws so that they not only avoid violating patients' privacy themselves but also can help other health professionals understand how to respect patients' privacy and confidentiality rights.

Fraud is a willful and intentional misrepresentation that could cause harm or loss to a person or the person's property. In addition to fraud associated with improper billing for procedures not performed (criminal fraud), fraud can occur in health care facilities when a physician promises a certain surgical result, although he or she knows that the result is not so certain. For example, a physician who promises that there is no chance of a complication resulting from plastic surgery, although such complications can occur, is guilty of misrepresentation.

Intentional infliction of emotional or mental distress can also result in claims against health care facilities. In a 1975 case, a court found that a physician and hospital (through its employees) were guilty of intentional infliction of emotional distress. In this case, the mother of a premature infant (who died shortly after birth) had gone to her physician for a postpartum checkup.[7] She noticed a report in her medical record stating that the child was past 5 months' gestation and therefore could not be disposed of as a surgical specimen. On questioning her physician about what had happened to the body, the physician told his nurse to take the mother to the hospital. At the hospital, the mother was taken by a hospital employee to a freezer. The freezer was opened, and the mother was handed a jar containing her baby. The mother was awarded $100,000 damages, upheld on appeal. The cases are not always so dramatic. In 1985, a Georgia court found a physician guilty of intentional infliction of emotional distress for yelling at a patient and her husband.[8]

Products Liability

Products liability cases sometimes involve health care facilities. Products liability is the liability of a manufacturer, seller, or supplier of a product to a buyer or other third party for injuries sustained because of a defect in the product. The injured party may sue the seller, manufacturer, or supplier. If, for example, a hospital improperly processes or stores blood in its own blood bank, it may be liable to any patient who is harmed as a result. If the staff of a research hospital designs a new type of medical equipment that is tested on patients, any harm resulting from product defects can result in product liability claims. Products liability is a complex subject beyond the scope of this chapter. It is included here simply as a reminder that there are many potential sources of liability for today's health care organizations.

Contractual Disputes

Breach of contract is a common claim in litigation that involves health care providers and organizations. Typically, the claims arise when one party to a contract fails to follow the terms agreed to in the contract. Interestingly, courts have been willing to enforce ethical standards prohibiting breach of confidentiality (such as the American Hospital Association's [AHA's] patient right's statement entitled *The Patient Care Partnership: Understanding Expectations, Rights and Responsibilities,* and ethical standards of the American Medical Association) as part of a contractual relationship between health care providers and their patients. Thus, improper disclosure of health information can give rise to a breach of contract claim and an invasion of privacy or breach of confidentiality claim. (Invasion of privacy and breach of confidentiality claims are discussed later in this chapter.) In an important case on this subject, *Hammonds v. Aetna Casualty and Surety Co.*, the court found that a physician breached an implied condition of his patient-physician contract when he disclosed health information to a hospital's insurer without the patient's authorization.[9]

Antitrust Claims

Although such claims have decreased in recent years, health care providers and organizations have been targets of antitrust claims. Most of these claims revolve around mergers and acquisitions and alleged anticompetitive behavior in medical staff **credentialing** activities. For example, if the obstetricians on the medical staff of a local hospital seek to remove an obstetrician's staff privileges so that there is less competition for patients, that hospital may find itself entangled in an antitrust suit. These suits usually do not directly involve the HIM department or service, but sometimes HIM professionals are involved to the extent that they support the medical staff's peer review and credentialing functions.

Crimes and Corporate Compliance

Criminal activity can take place in any health care facility. A nurse practicing in a hospital is probably able to tell of mysterious discrepancies in narcotic counts (counts done on each unit that stores narcotics to ensure that no drugs are missing). Angel-of-death murder scenarios have been sensationalized in books and television, but they have their basis in actual events in which the weak and ill have become prey for criminal or deviant behavior by facility employees. For example, in 2004, Charles Cullen, a registered nurse, pled guilty to the murder of 29 patients he had cared for at various health care facilities. Patient abuse and sexual improprieties are also terrible phenomena that can occur in health care facilities. In addition, falsification of business or patient records (e.g., by billing Medicare for patients not seen or services not performed) may be grounds for criminal indictment.

Concerns about improper billing practices have led to the passage of laws and regulations targeting health care providers who submit false claims, engage in fraudulent coding practices, and otherwise fail to comply with statutory and regulatory mandates. The Health Insurance Portability and Accountability Act of 1996 (Public Law 104-191) (HIPAA), the Balanced Budget Act of 1997 (Public Law 105-33), and even the Federal False Claims Act (1863, with 1986 amendments) and its subsequent interpretation by the DHHS are examples of laws imposing penalties—up to and including criminal sanctions—against health care providers who engage in fraudulent practices.

The growth in prosecution against health care providers has led to a profound interest (and need) among provider organizations in developing corporate compliance plans with the goal of preventing, detecting, and resolving wrongdoing in health care organizations. Ideally, the compliance program not only discourages unlawful activity but also promotes a culture in which suspected problems can be safely raised internally, preventing the need for "whistleblowers" to go to outside regulatory bodies to raise concerns. These **whistleblower**-based prosecutions, called "**qui tam**" prosecutions, have been particularly attractive to employees (disgruntled or otherwise) because the whistleblower is entitled to a share of the government's winnings in these cases. Health care leaders have recognized the sense of solving suspected problems internally and rapidly.

The health care organization's compliance plan should focus on all areas of regulatory compliance, with special emphasis on preventing fraudulent coding and billing practices. The Office of the Inspector General (OIG) of the DHHS has issued model compliance plans for various types of health care organizations (such as clinical laboratories and hospitals), which provide organizations with a logical starting point in developing their own corporate compliance plans. The OIG also issues periodic advisory opinions and fraud statistics to show their prosecutorial priorities, which is useful to health care organizations in planning their own fraud prevention efforts. In addition, the American Health Information Management Association (AHIMA) has published numerous articles on the subject, a model Health Information Management Compliance Program, and a practice brief that is available on AHIMA's Web site. Common to all compliance programs is the need to address internal standards of conduct, education of staff on compliance, auditing of coding and billing practices regularly, continual monitoring of practices, and methods of further developing and updating the organization's plan.

Issues germane to the HIM professional take center stage in these compliance plans. Not only must HIM professionals be concerned with accurate coding and billing, they must also focus on other areas of regulatory compliance, such as ensuring the confidentiality and security of health information. HIM professionals must also guard against outside contracts with vendors containing terms that may lead to risks of noncompliance.

Noncompliance with Statutes, Rules, and Regulations

As mentioned earlier, health care organizations that fail to follow government-imposed mandates run the risk of a variety of potential penalties, including monetary or criminal penalties, removal from participation in the Medicare program, and even loss of licensure.

With this information as a backdrop, the remainder of this chapter looks at the most common legal obligations and risks that face health care facilities, health care providers, and HIM professionals in particular. First, which legal obligations and risks involve HIM professionals most directly?

LEGAL OBLIGATIONS AND RISKS OF HEALTH CARE FACILITIES AND INDIVIDUAL HEALTH CARE PROVIDERS

Duties to Patients, in General

Patients have numerous rights associated with their health care. Some of these rights are discussed in detail in this section. Laws, rules, or regulations establish some rights; others are based on ethical codes and even the federal Constitution. Beyond the specific rights discussed in the following, HIM professionals should be aware of patient rights granted in the AHA's patient rights statement discussed earlier, the Ethics, Rights and Responsibilities chapter of the accreditation manuals issued by The Joint Commission, and specific laws governing access to care, such as the Emergency Medical Treatment and Active Labor Act (EMTALA) (42 USC 1395 dd). The EMTALA imposed new obligations on health care facilities to provide medical screening examinations and stabilizing treatment to patients before transferring them to other facilities. The purpose of the law was to reduce inappropriate transfers (such as those done primarily for financial reasons when the patient has no insurance) that put the patient at risk of harm. The net effect of these various bills or rights, codes of conduct, and laws has been to alert patients to their rights and to provide remedies when their health care providers fail to respect those rights. We are entering the era of empowered health care consumers. This should lead to more interaction between patients and the HIM department as patients seek more information about their care and treatment.

Duty to Maintain Health Information

One of the most fundamental duties that involve HIM professionals and their health care facility employers is that of maintaining health information about patients. This duty is imposed explicitly by state and federal statutes and regulations as well as accreditation standards. In some states, the hospital licensing statutes specify not only that a medical record must be kept for every patient but also what that record must contain at a minimum. Failure to meet the requirements of these licensing statutes could subject a facility to loss of licensure and closure. The law and regulations setting forth the *Conditions of Participation* in federal payment programs such as Medicare also require that medical records be kept, and they outline in broad terms what those records must include.[10] Accreditation standards of the JCAHO also require accredited facilities to maintain medical records, and the HIPAA privacy rule also speaks to what documents must be maintained for patient access and use as part of a "**designated record set**." (DRS)—defined in that rule as a group of records maintained by or for a **covered entity,** as follows:

- The medical records and billing records about individuals maintained by or for a covered health care provider
- The enrollment, payment, claims adjudication, and case or medical management record systems maintained by or for a health plan or
- Used, in whole or in part, by or for the covered entity to make decisions about individuals

Patients must be able to access that information for at least 6 years, and even longer if state or other federal laws require longer retention periods.

The duty to maintain health information is also implied in other laws. For example, vital statistics laws require the reporting of births and deaths. Under federal and state statutes, health care facilities must report to various data banks certain disease conditions and medical events, such as the treatment of gunshot wounds, suspected child abuse, elder abuse, industrial accidents, certain poisonings, abortions, cancer cases, and communicable diseases.

Mandatory reporting requirements vary from state to state. These statutes have in common that reporting is required and the authorization of the patient is generally not needed. In fact, even if the patient expresses the wish *not* to have information released, the health care organization must comply with the reporting requirement. This tension between the reporting statutes and confidentiality often arises with state requirements for reporting actual or suspected child abuse. Reports made in error admittedly cause much pain and embarrassment for the family involved. Many states, recognizing the natural reluctance of people to make such reports when the abuse is not proved, have exempted the party making the report from liability for erroneous reports as long as the report is made in good faith (in other words, without malice or evil intent).

The reporting statutes attempt to encourage reporting in another important way. For example, failure to report child abuse can result in liability for injuries a child later sustains when discharged home to the suspected or actual abuser.

The problem becomes even stickier when mandatory reporting statutes conflict with other laws, such as state laws that bar disclosure of mental health treatment records and federal laws that bar disclosure of substance abuse treatment. If in the course of therapy a child or an elderly person indicates that he or she has been abused, what must the therapist do? Some court decisions have permitted the protection of these confidentiality laws to be circumvented, but only to the extent necessary to fulfill the requirements of the reporting statute.[11] In addition, some state confidentiality laws permit exceptions in cases of imminent harm, in which the child or abused party is in immediate danger. Other statutes, however, do not provide convenient solutions to this problem. HIM professionals who face such a situation should consult legal counsel, who may seek direction from the court in reconciling all the interests involved.

These examples illustrate why compliance with mandatory reporting statutes is not always as simple as it may seem. HIM professionals must determine their state's requirements and how those requirements may conflict with other confidentiality obligations so that appropriate reporting procedures are in place.

Duty to Retain Health Information and Other Key Documents and to Keep Them Secure

Just as there are requirements to create patient records, there are also requirements to retain that information. Health care facilities take guidance from federal and state record retention laws and regulations and from state **statutes of limitations** in setting their own record and information retention policies. Facilities must also take into account the uses of and needs for that information, the space available for hard copy storage, and the resources available for microfilming, creating optical disks, or electronic storage. (See the discussion of record retention in Chapter 7 for more factors to consider and AHIMA's Practice Brief on the *Retention of Health Information*.) But remember, record retention regulations are just a baseline; in other words, facilities must meet these minimum retention periods but may establish longer retention schedules if desired.

It is not enough just to keep these records. HIM professionals must ensure that the records are kept in a way that minimizes the chance of their being lost, destroyed, or altered. Plaintiffs have won negligence suits against facilities that failed to safeguard their records from loss or destruction.[12] **Security of health information** has taken on new and more complex dimensions as more and more health information is stored in various electronic and other media. Medical records security used to be a simple matter of controlling access to the file area and having adequate safeguards against physical threats such as fire, flood, and severe weather. Now, with each new form of data storage and retrieval technology, HIM professionals must be alert to the new security threats that may accompany those technologies.

HIPAA security regulations, which went into effect in 2005, will assist in avoiding those security threats. In 1996, Congress passed the act commonly referred to as HIPAA. As part of that act, Congress added a new section to Title XI of the Social Security Act, entitled "Administrative Simplification." The purpose of the Administrative Simplification amendment was to improve the efficiency and effectiveness of the health care system by stimulating the development of standards to facilitate electronic maintenance and transmission of health information. The act directed the Secretary of DHHS to adopt standards for electronically maintained health information and standards for electronic signatures and other matters such as unique health identifiers and code sets.

The standards, which went into effect in April 2005, apply to health care providers, health plans, and health care (data) clearinghouses.

Certain administrative procedures, physical safeguards, and technical security services and mechanisms are required under these regulations. See Chapter 8 for an in-depth discussion of security safeguards.

The regulations apply to all electronically maintained health information in health care organizations, and it is important for HIM professionals to become familiar with the final standards.

Health information is valuable only if it is accurate, complete, and available for use when needed. Therefore, HIM professionals must design safeguards that not only protect the information from loss or destruction and prevent the corruption of electronically stored data from power losses or surges but also protect the integrity of the information itself. In other words, the information must be protected from inappropriate alteration.

Why would anyone want to alter health information or documentation in a patient's record? In some situations, such as when a health professional is sued for malpractice, he or she may be tempted to alter the record to make the documentation appear more complete than it originally was. Some health professionals have not yet learned the importance of thorough **contemporaneous documentation** (i.e., documentation made while care is being provided, while the information is fresh in the care provider's mind), and as a result, when the time comes to defend the provider's actions, the record may not reflect the care of the patient in a positive light. HIM professionals must guard against inappropriate alterations to health information by controlling access to records with extra precautions for records that are involved in litigation. If presented with a request to make a change to a patient record involved in litigation, an HIM professional should refer that request to the facility's defense counsel. Rather than "improving" the documentation, a health professional who makes later alterations often ends up harming the case because the plaintiff's attorney may have already gotten a copy of the original, unaltered record from the patient before filing suit. Imagine how it might appear to a jury if the plaintiff's attorney can show that the defendant altered the record when the suit was filed and that the health facility took no steps to protect the record from alteration.[13] For these reasons, it is wise to supervise all access to patient records that are involved in litigation. By doing so, the integrity of the record can be maintained while appropriate access is permitted.

Falsification of records can lead to other problems as well. In some states, it is a crime if it is done for the purpose of cheating or defrauding and may lead to sanctions against health professionals' licenses.

Error Correction

Errors that are made in documenting information must be corrected as soon as they are detected with use of proper error correction methods. These methods should be outlined in the facility's policy and procedure manual and taught to all people who document patient health information.

Generally, the person who made an error should correct the error. If the correction is a major one (e.g., erroneous laboratory results were entered on the record and resulted in a problem in the patient's care), the person making the correction should consult the HIM manager, risk manager, and perhaps even facility legal counsel to ensure that the correction method complies with facility policy and that all appropriate steps that need to be taken are followed. Most corrections are not so dramatic. A nurse begins to chart patient A's information on patient B's record but instantly realizes the error. Or, in the course of making up a new medication administration record, the unit clerk misspells the name of a medication and the nurse who double-checks the record quickly catches it. In situations that involve paper-based health information, the person making the error should simply draw a single line through the incorrect entry, enter the correction and initial it, and note the time and date of the correction (Figure 15-1). Under no circumstances should the original entry be erased, scribbled over, or hidden, because an obliteration can raise suspicion in the minds of jurors about the original entry and whether it is an attempt to cover up a major problem.

Error correction methods are different for electronic health record systems. A system's procedures should clearly specify how errors are to be handled. Errors that are caught immediately at the time they are made can simply be changed, with no need to preserve the original entry. Errors that are caught after the point in time when someone has relied on the erroneous information pose a problem; the system must provide some way to save the original entry and show the new entry and the date and time it was made. Health information systems software varies, and procedures differ with each system. HIM professionals should insist that the system they use permits appropriate error correction and addendum procedures so that the integrity of the information is preserved.

Addenda

In some circumstances, simple error correction methods are insufficient. For example, if a substantial portion of a patient's history and physical examination was left out of the original dictated report, it would be impossible to squeeze in the missing information on the original typed report. When new information is being added to a record, an addendum is used. The person making the addendum should enter a reference to the addendum near the original entry or information (e.g., "1/3/06—See addendum to H&P"—signature) and then file the addendum.

Sometimes, after they have reviewed their health information, patients ask that their records be amended. The Privacy Act (discussed later in the chapter) permits such amendments, but it applies only to health care organizations operated by the federal government, such as Department of Defense health care facilities, Veterans Administration health facilities, and Indian Health Service facilities. HIPAA's privacy rule also permits such requests and requires covered entities to consider those requests. In fact, there are very few circumstances under which a facility may deny an amendment request under the HIPAA privacy rule Requests for amendment may also arise in the context of mental health therapy, when patients have said something during therapy that they later wish they had not said. Facility policy should outline how these requests are to be handled. Ordinarily, requests for amendments should be discussed with the

					NURSES NOTES	
					Date: _8/18/0x_	
Time	B. P.	Temp.	Pulse	Resp.	Treatments-Procedures Special Medication P.R.N. Medication	Remarks
1900	150/70		76	24		Sleeping-arouses easily. Oriented to name only. Other neuro assessment unchanged. _____ Reynolds
1930	142/88		104	24	error 8/18/0x WBJ	Oriented to name and place. Vest restraint applied.
2000	132/84		96	24		Neuro assessment unchanged.
2030	130/80		94	24		Earlier assessments unchanged.
2100	134/82		96	24		
2200	136/84		104	24		Remains very sleepy. Arouses easily. Side rails up.

Figure 15-1 Correcting errors in documentation.

attending physician or the health professional who authored the original entry that is in dispute, if that is the reason for the amendment. If the physician believes that the request is inappropriate, and his or her reasoning falls under one of the permissible reasons under the HIPAA privacy rule for denying an amendment request, he or she should discuss the matter with the patient. Otherwise, the patient's amendment should be handled as an addendum to the record without change to the original entry and identified as an additional document appended to the original patient record at the request of the patient. Section 164.526 of the HIPAA privacy rule outlines an appeal process that must be made available to the patient if their request for amendment is denied, and the patient wishes to appeal that denial.

Authentication and Authorship Issues

One aspect of protecting the integrity of health information that has become increasingly controversial is the issue of **authentication.** In other words, how can facilities identify the author of a particular record or computer entry into a health information system? In a paper record system, this is done through the original signature or through the use of a personal signature stamp (under written agreement with the facility not to delegate the use of the stamp to another person). Authentication not only serves to identify the author of an entry but also indicates that the author has reviewed the entry or report for accuracy and attests to it. In electronic health record systems, authentication of documentation is often achieved through a unique identification code and password entered by the person making the note or report. As is true with the use of signature stamps, it is important to ensure that the user's identification code and password are not shared with others; if they are to be reliable indication of authorship, they must be used only by the person to whom they belong.

HIPAA's regulations include a section proposing electronic signature standards. These proposed standards would require that any electronic signature systems for health care information provide a reliable way of identifying the signer, ensure the message's integrity, and provide for non-repudiation (to prevent a signer from later denying having signed the message).

The proposed standards noted that the only current electronic signature system that meets all these requirements is cryptographically based digital signature technology.* Any system used would have to guarantee the identity of the signer and prevent changes to the document in question after it is signed. As of late 2005, we are still awaiting the final rule on electronic signature standards.

Validity of Health Information as Evidence

One of the reasons it is important to protect the integrity of health information is so that the information or record may be used as evidence in court proceedings as an exception to the hearsay rules, which generally bar out-of-court unsworn statements from being used in court as proof. State laws governing the admissibility of health information as evidence vary.

In some states, health information can be admitted as an exception to the hearsay rule. The **hearsay rule** bars the legal admissibility of **evidence** that is not the personal knowledge of the witness. For example, a defendant physician may want to use the patient record to defend a malpractice claim, but the record contains information beyond the physician's personal knowledge—statements of nurses, descriptions of treatments given by respiratory therapists, recording of laboratory results prepared by medical technologists, and so on. In some states, however, medical records and health information may be admitted either as a business record or as an explicit exception to the hearsay rule in the state's rules of evidence. Business records are presumed to be reliable because they are routinely prepared in the course of business and are created as business is transacted, not specially prepared months later for use in court. In any event, it is up to the judge to decide whether any record is admissible in court proceedings according to the applicable rules of evidence.

When submitting the record for use in court as a business record, the HIM professional must attest that the record was made in the normal course of business. If anything has happened to that record or information that departs from the normal course of business, such as an alteration of original documentation, the information no longer has that presumption of reliability and may no longer be admissible. As discussed earlier, this action can cripple a malpractice defense and destroy the information's value as evidence in other types of proceedings, such as personal injury cases.

What if a record has been microfilmed or put onto other storage media, such as an optical disk or a computer tape, and the original destroyed? Can the information still be used as evidence? Rules of evidence require that when originals are still available, they must be produced. This is called the **best evidence rule.** When it becomes necessary to prove the contents of a document, the original must be produced or its absence accounted for. The best evidence rule was adopted to prevent fraud or mistake as to the contents of a document or record. If the original has been destroyed pursuant to a facility's records retention program and only copies of that information remain, that secondary evidence (e.g., the microfilm or optical disk) is probably admissible if the court is satisfied that the secondary record accurately reflects the original and that destruction of the original was done in good faith (e.g., as part of a facility-sponsored record retention program and not specifically to prevent the information's use in court). The testimony of the HIM professional is important in explaining the retention

---

*For a good overview of digital signatures, see Ballam H: HIPAA, security, and electronic signature: a closer look, *J Am Health Inform Manage Assoc* 70:26-30, 1999.

program and the secondary information or record system. Because of the length of time microfilming has been used, most courts admit microfilm copies without much question, but more recent technologies often must be explained by the HIM professional before the information can be used. This is one of the reasons that careful thought must go into the selection of new technology for information storage and retrieval. Obtaining the opinion of legal counsel about the admissibility of information stored in new ways and forms is a wise step to take before adopting new technology.

Retention of Other Records and Information

Patient records and information are not the only important documents to retain. Medical staff credential files, incident reports, surgical videos that identify patients, peer review data and minutes, radiographs, surgery schedules, and emergency department logs are just a few of the items for which a retention schedule must be established.[14] (See Chapter 8 for a full discussion of record retention.)

Duty to Maintain Confidentiality

Think about a past visit to a physician. What information was shared? If a patient discovered that his or her physician repeated that information to another patient, a neighbor, or the local newspaper, wouldn't that patient be angry? Might that not deter patients from sharing all relevant health and history information with their care providers, thus threatening the quality of care they receive? Today's society considers communications between patients and their health care providers to be confidential communications. For the sake of discussion, this chapter defines a confidential communication as one that transmits information to a health care provider as part of the relationship between the provider and the patient under circumstances that imply that the information shall remain private. Patients rely on that promise of confidentiality in disclosing intimate details to health care providers.

Health care providers are bound by various laws and ethical standards to maintain the confidentiality of private health information. Physicians, for example, are required by their Hippocratic Oath to maintain confidentiality: "What I may see or hear in the course of the treatment, or even outside of the treatment in regard to the life of men, which on no account one must spread abroad, I will keep to myself."

The AHA's patient rights statement, called *Patient Care Partnership: Understanding Expectations, Rights and Responsibilities* addresses the health facility's obligation. One of the key elements in that statement addresses the protection of the patient's privacy by the health care organization. AHIMA's own Code of Ethics sets the standard for HIM professionals to "advocate, uphold and defend the individual's right to privacy and the doctrine of confidentiality in the use and disclosure of information." Protecting the confidentiality of **protected health information** is one of the primary aims of the HIPAA privacy rule. And as part of the rule, organizations covered by the rule must provide patients with a notice of privacy practices. This notice is intended to explain to patients how their protected health information is used—both with their permission and without their permission. The HIPAA privacy rule specifies certain issues that must be addressed in the notice. The actual privacy notice is most often developed by the organization's privacy officer, who often is an HIM professional. In addition, handling requests related to the use and disclosure of health information is most often a function of the HIM department. Also, numerous state laws address the subject, as do Medicare's *Conditions of Participation*, The Joint Commission standards, and a growing body of court decisions.

To understand fully their obligation to keep patient health information confidential, health care providers need to understand what information is and is not confidential, or in the language of HIPAA, "protected." Some of the information that may appear in patient records is not "protected" health information.

Determining what information is confidential is not always as straightforward as it might seem. For example, for substance abuse treatment facilities, the very fact of a patient's admission for treatment is confidential, according to federal law, and may not be disclosed without patient **authorization** except under limited circumstances.[15] Under the HIPAA privacy rule, however, the fact of admission could be shared without completing an authorization, as long as the patient has agreed to inclusion in the facility's directory and as long as applicable state laws are not more restrictive. The HIPAA privacy rule does not **pre-empt** (or override) more protective privacy laws and regulations—either federal or state, unless they are in conflict with HIPAA's provisions. So, if HIPAA were to permit the release of directory information, but the applicable state law required patient authorization before release of directory information, that state law would be followed and not be pre-empted by the HIPAA privacy rule.

HIPAA's provisions protect a broad range of health information. The HIPAA privacy rule defines "protected" health information (PHI) as "individually identifiable health information that is transmitted by electronic media; maintained in any medium described in the definition of *electronic media* at § 162.103 of the rule; or transmitted or maintained in any other form or medium."

Thus, the decision as to whether an item is considered protected depends largely on the definition of individually identifiable health information (IIHI). The rule defines IIHI as information that is a subset of health information, including demographic information collected from an individual, and the following:

- Is created or received by a health care provider, health plan, employer, or health care clearinghouse and
- Relates to the past, present, or future physical or mental health or condition of an individual; the provision of

health care to an individual; or the past, present, or future payment for the provision of health care to an individual
• That identifies the individual or
• With respect to which there is a reasonable basis to believe the information can be used to identify the individual

It is important to note that the HIPAA privacy rule's provisions only apply to "**covered entities**," as defined by the rule. The definition of covered entities includes any entity as follows:

   • A health care provider that conducts certain transactions in electronic form
   • A health care clearinghouse
   • A health plan

So, although that covers the majority of health care organizations (because electronic transactions are the most common methods of billing for services), that definition does not cover all organizations that may have access to protected health information, such as personal health record sites on the Internet, companies that provide services related to health information storage and processing, and so on. Covered entities using outside agents or organizations (not part of the facility's own workforce) to handle or process PHI on their behalf must use a special agreement with that agency to ensure that the agency follows rules set by the covered entity for handling PHI. This agreement is called a "**business associate agreement**," and the HIPAA privacy rule outlines what must be addressed in these agreements, at a minimum.

Still, there are many recipients of health information that are not covered entities and are therefore not governed by the HIPAA privacy rule. In addition, many of those recipients are not "business associates" of the covered entity and are therefore not even covered by business associate agreements. This issue has been of great concern to many privacy advocates, who argue that the legal protection should follow the protected health information, regardless of who possesses that information.

Beyond health information, there are other documents in the health care facility that must be kept confidential if they are to serve their purpose adequately. Incident reports in which adverse occurrences are reported and investigated must be kept confidential to the extent permitted by state law so that staff members feel free to report such occurrences. Peer review records, such as committee minutes and credentialing files, also must be kept confidential to encourage candor in monitoring, managing, and improving the quality of clinical care.[16] HIM professionals are often involved in developing facility policies to protect the confidentiality of this information and in teaching staff to follow those policies.

In developing facility policies to protect the confidentiality of health information, HIM professionals must ensure that those policies adhere to federal and state laws and regulations on the subject. Many state HIM associations publish excellent legal guides to cover the basic tenets of individual states' laws. Plan to become familiar with these resources. Additional federal laws and regulations are described next.

Privacy Act of 1974

The Privacy Act was designed to give citizens some control over the information collected about them by the federal government and its agencies. It grants people the following rights:

   • To find out what information about them has been collected
   • To see and have a copy of that information
   • To correct or amend the information
   • To exercise limited control of the disclosure of that information to other parties[17]

Health care organizations operated by the federal government (e.g., military hospitals, Veterans Administration health facilities, Indian Health Service facilities) are bound by the act's provisions. The act also applies to record systems that are operated pursuant to a contract with a federal government agency—for example, a disease registry operated under a grant from the DHHS.

Freedom of Information Act

The Freedom of Information Act (FOIA) became law in 1966. It requires that records pertaining to the executive branch of the federal government be available to the public except for matters that fall within nine explicitly exempted areas. Under certain circumstances, medical records may be exempt from the act's requirements. One of the nine exempt categories includes "personnel and medical files and similar files, the disclosure of which would constitute a clearly unwarranted invasion of personal privacy."[17] To meet the test of being an "unwarranted invasion of personal privacy," the following conditions must exist:

   • The information must be contained in a personnel, medical, or similar file
   • Disclosure of the information must constitute an invasion of personal privacy
   • The severity of the invasion must outweigh the public's interest in disclosure
   • Interpreting this three-part test has been the subject of a number of court cases[18-20]

Regulations on Confidentiality of Alcohol and Drug Abuse Patient Records

These regulations, restricting disclosures of patient health information without patient authorization, apply to facilities that provide alcohol or drug abuse diagnosis, treatment, or referral for treatment—a substance abuse program in the language of the regulations. For a health care facility to be considered such a program, it must offer either an identified unit that provides alcohol or drug abuse diagnosis, treatment, or referral for treatment or medical personnel or other staff whose primary function is the provision of alcohol or drug abuse diagnosis, treatment, or referral for treatment and who are identified as such providers.[21] General hospitals and clinics are not considered to be such programs unless they have either an identified unit for this type of diagnosis or treatment or providers whose primary function is the provision of those types of services.

The regulations apply only to health information obtained by federally assisted programs, but because the definition of this is quite broad (e.g., all Medicare-certified facilities or those that receive funds from any federal department or agency, among other things), it applies to virtually all programs that meet the other requirements of the definition.

The regulations are important for several reasons. They prohibit the disclosure of substance abuse patient records unless permitted by the regulations or authorized by the patient. The regulations require specific content in an authorization to release health information; those issues are discussed later in this chapter.

These regulations are lengthy and detailed. HIM professionals who work in health care facilities that qualify as a "program" under these regulations must become very familiar with the key provisions.

Internal Uses and External Disclosures of Health Information

When one is sorting through the maze of parties who request health information, it is sometimes useful to categorize the requests as internal uses or external disclosures. Why? Because in a few, but by no means all circumstances, internal uses may not need patient authorization for access to that information, whereas external disclosures usually (but not always) do. Under the HIPAA privacy rule, internal uses for treatment, payment, or **health care operations** do not require patient authorization, unless other applicable laws or regulations require their use. For example, sharing patient information with employees on the facility's quality improvement staff would be an internal use for health care operations. Those staff members would be entitled to review the records of patients in the course of their duties. Staff physicians, nurses, and therapists caring for the patient would have access to the patient's information as an internal use for treatment. The health care organization's in-house counsel who is coordinating the defense of a malpractice claim would be an example of an internal use for health care operations, whereas a lawyer who represents a patient, a physician, or an employee of the health care organization would be considered an external disclosure and would require patient authorization.

Do not fall into the trap of thinking that just because a person works for the facility, he or she has carte blanche access to all patient information. Although it is true that health care personnel involved in the treatment of a patient should have access to the information they need to know, it does not follow that nurses should know the medical details of patients for whom they are not caring. This can be a serious problem in health care facilities and has taken on special significance with the growing number of patients who test positive for the human immunodeficiency virus (HIV). Is there any reason for a dietary aide who delivers food trays to each nursing unit to know whether a patient on that unit is HIV positive? Certainly, it can be argued that key staff involved in the patient's treatment should know. But often this knowledge goes far beyond the boundaries of those who need to know. The issue goes well beyond HIV status, however. HIM professionals should provide leadership and training to their coworkers on the appropriate and inappropriate uses of health information.

In addition, the HIPAA privacy rule recognizes and incorporates the principle of "**minimum necessary**." (See section 164.514(d) of the privacy rule.) Generally, only the minimum necessary amount of information necessary to fulfill the purpose of the request should be shared with internal users and external requestors. There are only a few situations in which the minimum necessary standard does not apply (e.g., uses or disclosures for treatment purposes, or where the patient has specifically authorized the release of more information, and in a few other circumstances).

General Principles Regarding Access and Disclosure Policies

Health Information Ownership

As a prerequisite for discussing specific access requests, it is important to have a basic understanding of health information ownership. Who owns the record and information? It is generally accepted that the health facility owns the record itself, but the exercise of those ownership rights is subject to the patient's ownership interest in the information within that record. Health information is, after all, a legal record of what was done for the patient and proof that billable services were rendered and that standards of care were (or were not!) met. On the other hand, patients have a right to control, to the extent possible given state and federal laws and regulations, the flow of their private health information. This is one of the reasons why every health care facility needs policies and procedures to guide employees in handling health information access and disclosure requests. Those who violate the patient's right to control the flow of his or her health information may be liable to that patient.

Resources on Releasing Patient Information

Various sources are available for setting policies and writing procedures to guide staff in handling health information and in responding to requests for information. As mentioned before, many state HIM associations have published excellent legal manuals. Peers in other local facilities are usually willing to share samples. AHIMA publishes various guidelines and practice standards, updating them and addressing new issues through position statements and practice guidelines. HIPAA's privacy rule required almost all health care organizations to update their practices on release of information. Because laws can change and case law evolves over time, it is important to use the most up-to-date sources available when establishing policies and procedures and to revisit those policies periodically to ensure that they reflect current legal and regulatory standards. Many health care facilities use in-house or outside legal counsel to review such policies.

Authorizations for Disclosure of Patient Information

As mentioned earlier in this chapter, both the HIPAA Privacy Rule and the regulations on Confidentiality of Alcohol and Drug Abuse Patient Records contain standards for what must be present in an authorization form for the authorization to be considered valid. (See Figure 15-2 for the privacy standards.) In addition, many state laws also have requirements for authorization content and timeliness of presentation. The HIM professional must ensure that the forms and processes for handling authorizations meet all applicable standards. Authorizations that do not contain all required elements are considered invalid authorizations, and releasing information on the basis of an invalid authorization is a violation of the HIPAA privacy rule and can result in penalties.

Each disclosure from records covered by the federal regulations on confidentiality of alcohol and drug abuse patient records must be accompanied by a notice specified in the regulations. That notice is a prohibition against redisclosure. In other words, recipients of the original disclosure are put on notice that they may not redisclose the information to anyone else or use the information for anything but its intended purpose because the records are protected by federal confidentiality rules in 42 Code of Federal Regulations (CFR) Part 2. The notice states the following:

> This information has been disclosed to you from records whose confidentiality is protected by Federal regulations (42 C.F.R. Part 2) which prohibit you from making any further disclosure of it without the specific written consent of the person to whom it pertains, or as otherwise permitted by such regulations. A general authorization for the release of medical or other information is not sufficient for this purpose.

There are some exceptions to the general prohibition against disclosure from alcohol and drug abuse patient records. In a medical emergency, for example, the regulations permit disclosure to medical personnel to treat a condition that "poses an immediate threat to the health of the patient."[22] Records of these disclosures must be maintained, including the following:

- Patient's name or case number
- Date and time of disclosure
- Description of circumstances that require emergency disclosure

- Description of information disclosed
- Identity of the party receiving the information
- Identity of the party disclosing the information

There are also some provisions for interagency disclosures (e.g., to the Food and Drug Administration), research, and Medicare or Medicaid audits.[23]

This list of required elements for authorization is similar, but not completely identical, to the requirements for a valid authorization under the HIPAA privacy rule. This means that HIM practitioners who work in facilities considered covered entities under the HIPAA Privacy Rule, which are also covered by the regulations on the confidentiality of alcohol and drug abuse patient records, must take care to ensure that their authorization forms meet the requirements of both sets of regulations (Figure 15-3).

Who should sign the authorization depends on the patient and his or her status. See Figure 15-4 for some general guidelines.

Disclosure for Direct Patient Care

When patients come to a health care facility or provider for treatment, it is reasonable to assume that they authorize their care providers to have information about their conditions and treatments. The HIPAA privacy rule supports this and allows internal uses of protected health information for treatment purposes without specific patient authorization. What is *not* reasonable to assume is that patients are granting access to anyone in the facility who may be curious to know that information as well. Internal uses for patient care purposes should be on a need-to-know basis. This means that those who really need to know the patient's health information to diagnose or treat that patient should have access.

Sometimes requests for disclosure of health information for patient care purposes come from outside the health facility where the information was originally collected. For example, if the patient chooses to begin seeing a new physician or is treated at another health facility, it may be important for that new health care provider to obtain a copy of the patient's health history, a test result, or the entire record. In fact, certain regulations (such as Medicare's *Conditions of Participation*) anticipate and require the transfer of relevant patient information on direct transfer of a patient from a hospital to a nursing facility. HIPAA's privacy rule permits disclosures of protected health information for treatment purposes without authorization. (However, some state laws continue to require authorization for external disclosures for treatment.) Some HIM professionals cite arguments in favor of obtaining written authorization for any disclosure under this category, which involves releasing information outside the original facility, unless there is an emergency situation in which patient authorization *cannot* be obtained (e.g., the patient is unconscious and the care providers cannot wait for the information until the patient recovers enough to authorize release). But in facilities that take that conservative view,

(c) *Implementation specifications: Core elements and requirements*

(1) *Core elements.*
A valid authorization under this section must contain at least the following elements:
(i) A description of the information to be used or disclosed that identifies the information in a specific and meaningful fashion.
(ii) The name or other specific identification of the person(s), or class of persons, authorized to make the requested use or disclosure.
(iii) The name or other specific identification of the person(s), or class of persons, to whom the covered entity may make the requested use or disclosure.
(iv) A description of each purpose of the requested use or disclosure. The statement "at the request of the individual" is a sufficient description of the purpose when an individual initiates the authorization and does not, or elects not to, provide a statement of the purpose.
(v) An expiration date or an expiration event that relates to the individual or the purpose of the use or disclosure. The statement "end of the research study," "none," or similar language is sufficient if the authorization is for a use or disclosure of protected health information for research, including for the creation and maintenance of a research database or research repository.
(vi) Signature of the individual and date. If the authorization is signed by a personal representative of the individual, a description of such representative's authority to act for the individual must also be provided.

(2) *Required* statements. In addition to the core elements, the authorization must contain statements adequate to place the individual on notice of all of the following:
(i) The individual's right to revoke the authorization in writing, and either:
(A) The exceptions to the right to revoke and a description of how the individual may revoke the authorization; or
(B) To the extent that the information in paragraph (c)(2)(i)(A) of this section is included in the notice required by §164.520, a reference to the covered entity's notice.
(ii) The ability or inability to condition treatment, payment, enrollment or eligibility for benefits on the authorization, by stating either:
(A) The covered entity may not condition treatment, payment, enrollment or eligibility for benefits on whether the in dividual signs the authorization when the prohibition on conditioning of authorizations in paragraph (b)(4) of this section applies; or
(B) The consequences to the individual of a refusal to sign the authorization when, in accordance with paragraph (b)(4) of this section, the covered entity can condition treatment, enrollment in the health plan, or eligibility for benefits on failure to obtain such authorization.
(iii) The potential for information disclosed pursuant to the authorization to be subject to redisclosure by the recipient and no longer be protected by this subpart.

(3) *Plain* language *requirement.* The authorization must be written in plain language.

(4) *Copy to the individual.* If a covered entity seeks an authorization from an individual for a use or disclosure of protected health information, the covered entity must provide the individual with a copy of the signed authorization.

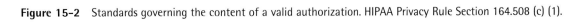

Figure 15-2 Standards governing the content of a valid authorization. HIPAA Privacy Rule Section 164.508 (c) (1).

According to the regulations on Confidentiality of Alcohol and Drug Abuse Patient Records, all authorizations must include the following:

- Specific name or general designation of the program or person permitted to make the disclosure
- Name or title of the person or name of the organization to which disclosure is to be made
- Name of the patient
- Purpose of the disclosure
- How much and what kind of information is to be disclosed
- Signature of the patient and, when required for a patient who is a minor, the signature of a person authorized to give consent under §2.14 of the regulations or, when required for a patient who is incompetent or deceased, the signature of a person authorized to sign under §2.15 in lieu of the patient. For minors, state law matters. If state law permits minors to obtain substance abuse treatment without parental or legal guardian consent, then only the minor can authorize the release of that information. If, however, the state does not allow minors to obtain substance abuse treatment without parental or legal guardian consent, both the minor and legal guardian's signatures are required to release this information.
- Date on which the consent (authorization) is signed
- Statement that the consent is subject to revocation at any time, except to the extent that the program or person that is to make the disclosure has already acted in reliance on it. Acting in reliance includes the provision of treatment services in reliance on a valid consent to disclose information to a third-party payer.
- Date, event, or condition on which the consent will expire if not revoked before. This date, event, or condition must ensure that the consent will last no longer than reasonably necessary to serve the purpose for which it is given.

Figure 15-3 Requirements for a valid authorization from the Confidentiality of Alcohol and Drug Abuse Regulations.

SITUATION	AUTHORIZING INDIVIDUAL
The patient is:	
An adult of sound mind, (age of majority defined in state statutes)	Patient
A minor	Parent or legal guardian
Deceased	Legal representative Executor of estate
Legally judged incompetent	Legally appointed guardian
Emancipated minor	Patient
Married Pregnant, or treated for pregnancy Treated for: (varies for each state) • Venereal disease • Birth control • Drug or alcohol abuse	
Minor and his parent is also a minor	Parent

Figure 15-4 The individual who can sign the form to authorize release of confidential information depends on the patient's situation.

steps must be taken to ensure that emergency patient care is not delayed by withholding information that is needed, pending the receipt of an authorization.

Disclosure for Performance Management and Patient Safety

Health information can be used to evaluate the quality of care and services provided to patients. The information provides evidence of exactly what was done, when it was done, why it was done, and how things turned out. For that reason, it is a valuable tool in quality management activities. Using the information in quality management is an impersonal use. In other words, committee members are interested not in who the patient is but in the quality of services provided. Specific patients are referred to by record or identification numbers when individual cases must be mentioned in peer review or quality management minutes and records. Members of the medical and professional staff may have access to patient health information, without patient authorization, in this context. The HIPAA privacy rule classifies this use as part of "health care operations"— and uses for health care operations do not require patient authorization. Even so, it is unwise to hand over records to someone just because that person happens to be on a peer review committee. Do not assume that quality management is the purpose for which all requests are made. A simple inquiry as to why the record or information is needed can help to ensure that the request is indeed related to the requester's quality management responsibilities.

One other caveat on this point: it is not unheard of for health professionals to use health records to gather unflattering evidence of a competitor's professional skill. Although records may be released without patient authorization for bona fide quality management activities, these informal "research" requests may not be sanctioned, official quality management activities. HIM professionals who are approached by a physician or other health professional with a request for records pertaining to other physicians or health professionals should ask the purpose of the request. If the answer does not indicate that the activity is official quality management business, then the requester should be asked to seek the approval of an appropriate committee or department chairperson. This protects the interests of all concerned.

Disclosure for Educational Purposes

Health information is a valuable teaching tool, both for student health professionals who are involved in formal training programs and for staff who must continue their education. Because some student health professionals may not be employed by the facility or otherwise bound to abide by the facility policies on confidentiality, it is important to ensure that any students with access to patient-identifiable health information agree to follow facility policies on confidentiality. Some facilities write such an agreement into the contract or in a separate agreement between the facility and the educational program or school; others require

students to sign individual confidentiality agreements, or to do both. The HIPAA privacy rule permits outside students to be considered as part of the organization's **workforce** and treated as an employee for the purposes for information access. But if the organization chooses to classify the students as part of the workforce, they must then be responsible for training those students in the privacy-related policies and procedures relevant to the student's role.

The educational use of the record is, like quality management, an impersonal use. It matters little who the patient is; what matters is what can be learned from the case. Teaching tools, such as case summaries, test results, photographs, surgical videos, and the like, should not identify the patient. Photographs and videos should be made in such a way that the patient cannot be identified, unless authorization to do so is obtained. Valid educational uses of health information are considered health care operations under HIPAA privacy rule and do not require patient authorization.

Again, care must be exercised in responding to these requests. Facility procedures should provide for some way to verify the validity of a student's request for information access. Sometimes this is done by having the student's preceptor or supervisor sign off on all student record requests. If no such controls are in place, students may be tempted to review health information about friends, relatives, and other people in whom they have no valid interest.

Disclosure for Research

Research, like educational purposes, usually involves an impersonal use of health information. The researchers are not interested in the identity of the patient, just that the patient falls within some predefined research population or control group. Even so, facility policies should define the circumstances under which researchers may have access to health information without patient authorization. Under the HIPAA privacy rule, those circumstances are fairly limited. Ordinarily, authorizations would not be required only if an institutional review board (described below) has waived the requirement, if the request involves a review that is preparatory to research (e.g., the use is simply to help a researcher prepare a research proposal and they will not use the information in any other way), or if the research involves decedent's information.

In many facilities, researchers must have their projects approved by an **institutional review board** (IRB), an advisory board that reviews the proposed research project for its objectives and proposed methods. If the researchers will have access to patient-identifiable data, it may be important to specify expected data security provisions in a written research agreement between the facility and the researcher. For example, the facility may want to require researchers to do all data collection on site in the HIM department and not remove original records or copies of records from the health facility. The HIM professional may expect to review proposed data collection forms to ensure that patient-identifiable data are not being collected. Be aware that the HIPAA privacy contains a number of provisions to guide the decision-making process of IRBs in deciding whether to waive the requirement for patient authorization.

Research projects in which the researchers want to contact patients directly pose a special problem because the simple act of verifying whether a patient is part of a specified group may, in many circumstances, be a breach of confidentiality. For those research projects believed to have sufficient merit to warrant cooperation, some facilities agree to act as intermediaries, notifying selected patients of the planned research and giving them the opportunity to determine whether they want to be contacted by the researchers. Only the addresses of patients opting to participate are then provided to the researchers.

Uses for Administrative Purposes

Uses for administrative purposes refers to the many internal activities that support the day-to-day functioning of the health care facility other than direct patient care, billing, and quality management. For example, a department manager or administrator may need access to certain limited patient information if he or she is responsible for responding to a complaint about the services provided to that patient by an employee of that department. Or a security manager may need access to a patient record to review an inventory of patient valuables to determine the validity of a patient's claims of lost property. A health care organization's professional liability insurer may want to review a sample of records to evaluate documentation practices and then use its assessments in determining the organization's insurability, although in this case, because the insurer is not part of the facility's own workforce, a business associate agreement would also be required. The health care organization's attorney, in preparation for expected litigation, may need to review the record of a patient who was involved in a serious incident. These activities generally qualify as health care operations under the HIPAA privacy rule and may use patient information without authorization (and are subject to the minimally necessary provision), but facility policies should define the situations in which patient authorization is required. In addition, all such requests should be funneled through the HIM department to facilitate consistency in handling them.

One of the more potentially problematic administrative uses of health information involves marketing activities. Ordinarily, the use of the patient information for marketing requires authorization. But there are certain exceptions under the HIPAA privacy rule. In some marketing strategies, specific health care services are marketed to patients who are most likely to have a need for those services. For example, brochures that describe a facility's new cardiac catheterization laboratory are mailed to patients who have been treated for cardiac-related problems or who are known to be at risk for such problems.

Marketing strategies make economic sense, but unless they are handled carefully, they run the risk of breaching confidentiality by publicly identifying patients as belonging to certain disease categories.[24] The HIPAA privacy rule has a very complex set of rules surrounding what activities qualify as marketing, the need to provide "opt-outs" so that patients can remove themselves from certain marketing lists, and when authorizations are required. HIM professionals should be involved in defining policies about the use of health information for marketing purposes and educating potential users about the risks. HIM professionals should also be evaluating proposed marketing uses of patient information to guard against abuses.

Disclosure for Payment Purposes

One of the most frequent disclosures of health information involves billing insurers for services provided to patients. Through clinical codes on the bill, and through claims attachments, information about the patient's diagnoses and procedures is relayed to the insurer, who then pays for the services provided. Under the HIPAA privacy rule, disclosures taking place for payment purposes do not require patient authorization, but some state laws may still require authorization. Disclosure for payment purposes is a controversial subject because quite frequently the patient who receives the services is not the same person who authorized disclosure as part of the application for insurance coverage. Therefore, the person whose information is being disclosed may not have given written authorization for disclosure. Many facilities try to handle this situation by making authorization for disclosure of health information part of the general consent to treatment signed by all patients on admission for treatment. HIM professionals should always exercise caution in disclosing information on the basis of a release that was signed before the information was collected. Probably the most practical way to exercise such caution is to make it clear to all patients before treatment that information will be released to their health insurer. If a patient does not want information to go to the health insurer for this treatment episode, he or she can make other arrangements for payment of the bill. The form suggested in the form in Figure 15-5 offers the patient the option of either authorizing disclosure to the health insurer or assuming financial responsibility for the services provided.

Disclosure to Attorneys

Written authorization from the patient or the patient's legal representative or a valid subpoena that meets HIPAA's special requirements is required for release of health information to an attorney, unless that attorney represents the health care provider that owns the record. In other words, the hospital's legal counsel does not require patient authorization to obtain access to a specific record, but the attorney for the respiratory therapist employed by the hospital and involved in the case does. If the records sought are from a physician's office, that physician's attorney does not require authorization, but the attorney of a codefendant hospital does require patient authorization.

SELECT ONE OPTION BELOW

1. _____ I authorize the forwarding of my name, address, birthdate, the name of the test(s) and charges to my insurance company.

2. _____ I consent to allow the disclosure of my name, address, birthdate, name of the test(s), and the charge to Medicaid or other medical assistance programs.

Patient's Full Name:_____ Birthdate:_____

Address: _____

City, State, Zipcode: _____

Medicaid Number: _____

3. _____ I do not give my consent to release the name of the test(s) to my insurance company, or medical assistance program. I will pay the bill myself.

Signature: _____

I also authorize the following persons or agencies access to my HIV antibody test results:

_____   _____   to _____
Name of Person/Agency   Date valid

_____   _____   to _____
Name of Person/Agency   Date valid

Figure 15–5 Patient's billing consent form. (Courtesy of the American Health Information Management Association.)

HIM professionals should take care in reviewing authorizations submitted by attorneys. Some attorneys use blanket authorizations with their clients, general statements that permit just about anyone to give an attorney just about any document related to the client. As with all other authorizations, the content of the authorization should be reviewed to make sure it complies with the health care facility's and applicable laws' requirements as to form and content.

Disclosure to Law Enforcement Personnel and Agencies

Occasionally, law enforcement representatives, including the medical examiner, are interested in gaining access to health information. For example, a police officer who accompanies an unconscious injured patient to the emergency department may need access to the patient's past records to contact family members. Federal Bureau of Investigation and Internal Revenue Service investigators have also been known to request access to health information. The HIPAA privacy rule, in section 164.501, defines law enforcement officials quite broadly: an officer or employee of any agency or authority of the United States, a state, a territory, a political subdivision of a state or territory, or an American Indian tribe, who is empowered by law to investigate or conduct an official inquiry into a potential violation of law or prosecute or otherwise conduct a criminal, civil, or administrative proceeding arising from an alleged violation of law.

Ordinarily, patient authorization is required for disclosures to law enforcement officials, but there are numerous exceptions (e.g., reporting of certain abuse, neglect, or domestic violence situations; compliance with mandatory state reporting statutes for conditions such as gunshot wounds and communicable diseases [see Chapter 7 on reporting requirements]; limited information for identification and location purposes; and information sought in response to law enforcement inquiries where **deidentified** [in other words, data that have been stripped of certain patient identifiers specified in the HIPAA privacy rule at 164.514(b)] data could not be used and the official makes those representations in writing). In addition, there are exceptions for certain situations involving the reporting of crimes on the health care facility's premises, crimes in emergency situations, and crimes where the patient is the victim. All these situations require certain conditions to be met, so the facility needs to have clear policies on release of information to law enforcement to guide the staff when they receive those requests. Many such requests come to staff other than the HIM department, such as the emergency department or nursing units, so it is very important for those policies to be well known throughout the organization. Involve the facility's legal counsel if health care facility policies do not address the particular situation that presents itself. And in any event, it is wise to verify the credentials of anyone representing themselves as a law enforcement officers by checking badge number or ID card or making a phone call to the agency involved, if there is a question as to identity.

In circumstances in which a suspicious death has resulted in the medical examiner or coroner being called in to conduct a postmortem examination, the medical examiner may have access to the patient's health information for use in conducting the autopsy, and no authorization for release of information is required from the next of kin or legal representative.

Disclosure to Family Members When the Patient Is a Minor

Generally, patients control access to their own health information. They may review the information themselves and choose either to share the information with family members or to withhold it. However, there are some exceptions, one of which is when the patient is a minor. Before a child reaches the age of majority, his or her parents or legal guardian generally makes authorization decisions on behalf of the child. In some limited circumstances, there are exceptions under various state and federal laws, such as when a minor child seeks treatment without parental involvement or consent (e.g., sexually transmitted disease, alcohol or substance abuse treatment) and when the minor is emancipated. Except in those circumstances, parents or guardians have access to the health information of their child or ward, and they may sign an authorization for disclosure on behalf of their unemancipated minor or ward. In cases of divorce and separation, disclosure decisions are typically made by the parent who has legal custody of the child. Unless one of the parent's parental rights has been terminated by the court, both parents retain the right to access and authorize the release of their child's information. In foster care situations, parental rights are generally terminated, albeit temporarily, and the foster parents assume those rights. The HIPAA privacy rule generally defers to state laws on matters involving parental rights.

Disclosure to Family Members When the Patient Is an Emancipated Minor or an Adult

State laws permit certain minors to make their own health care decisions without parental or guardian involvement. In other words, they are treated as adults, under the law, and have the right to consent to treatment and authorize disclosure of their own health information. Although the conditions vary, they generally involve minors who are married, living away from their parents and family, and responsible for their own support. In those circumstances, that person is considered to be an **emancipated minor** and can obtain proof of that emancipation. An emancipated minor can consent to treatment without parental involvement and may authorize disclosure of his or her health information. Because many state laws do not specifically state this, caution should be exercised in drafting facility procedures.

Disclosure to Family Members in Cases of Incompetence or Incapacity

A sad comment on the treatment of America's elderly population—especially those who are involved in residential treatment programs such as nursing facilities—is that sometimes health care providers assume that the patient is incompetent to make decisions so younger family members are consulted about all treatment and disclosure issues. This is a mistake. Patients typically control access to and disclosure of their protected health information. Confidential information should not indiscriminately be shared with family members without the patient's authorization. It should never be assumed that a patient is incompetent to make such decisions unless that patient has been legally declared incompetent. The patient should be capable of deciding what health information, if any, is to be shared with family members or others, subject to applicable laws or regulations.

The HIPAA privacy rule does permit health care providers to make certain assumptions about sharing information with family members who are involved in the care of the patient. For example, if a person comes to the pharmacy to pick up prescriptions for a patient, the pharmacy may assume that the patient wished the information about those prescriptions to be shared with that individual. The rule does, however, support the practice of asking the patient directly—when the patient is present—whether he or she wishes their information to be shared with others, including family members.

Incapacity is a different issue altogether. Competent patients may otherwise be unable to make access and disclosure decisions for various reasons. They may be unconscious, under anesthesia, comatose, and so on. In cases of temporary incapacity, health care providers should use common sense, good judgment, and some restraint in sharing appropriate health information with family members who are concerned for their relative. It may be appropriate to discuss the basic facts of the patient's condition and what the immediate plan is, but it may not be appropriate to disclose each and every detail. In cases of lengthy or permanent incapacity, a legal guardian for the patient may be appointed through court proceedings. When incapacity is anticipated, a person may grant **power of attorney** (the legally recognized authority to act and make decisions on behalf of another party) to another person, which authorizes the designee to act on behalf of the person who is now incapacitated. The person with power of attorney or the legally appointed guardian is then responsible for making decisions regarding the disclosure of health information to others. Be mindful, however, of the fact that there are different types of power of attorney. Some grant very broad powers to the holder; others are limited to specific issues, such as consenting to care. Reviewing the documents associated with the power or attorney will make it clear whether that person has the right to merely consent to treatment or to authorize the release of information as well.

Patient Access to Personal Health Information

Although the health care organization or provider owns the physical record of care, state statutes grant patients varying degrees of ownership interest in the health information in their records or data sets. Patients have no constitutional right to that information.[25] However, the HIPAA privacy rule does grant patients fairly broad rights to access their health information held by entities that are covered by the rule. In general, subject to any statutory prohibition or qualification such as those found in the HIPAA privacy rule, patients have a right to review and obtain copies of their health information.

Partly because of the variation in state requirements, health care organizations' practices with respect to granting patients access to their health information differ considerably. Even within states, some health care organizations take a consumer-oriented approach, whereas others try to discourage access requests by imposing additional hurdles for the patient to jump, such as inconvenient hours for accepting and handling such requests. The HIPAA privacy rule has helped to make these practices more uniform and patient friendly, but striking differences are still found. Some hospitals, for example, permit patients to review their health information during their hospitalization (with the attending physician present to answer questions), whereas others require that a brief waiting period take place before such access is granted. The HIPAA privacy rule requires that covered entities act on patients' request for access within 30 days of the request. HIM professionals must ensure that their facility policies comply with state and federal laws governing patient access. Within those limitations, the facility may have some latitude in the handling of patients' requests for information.

Whatever approach is taken, the HIM professional must establish reasonable safeguards for the security and confidentiality of the information. For example, before information is handed over in response to a patient request, there should be some reliable means of identifying the requester as the patient. It may be reasonable to obtain the patient's request in writing by way of a signature on an authorization for release of information form, although this is not required by the privacy rule, and lack of a signed authorization form should not serve as an arbitrary barrier for acting on the patient's request. This form may also be used to document that the review or release occurred. If the original hard copy record is being reviewed, that review should be closely supervised to guard against alterations or destruction of the record. If an electronic health record is being reviewed, similar security provisions are necessary to guard against alterations. Some facilities notify the attending physician or other health care practitioner that his or her patient has requested record access. Facilities may also choose to set certain reasonable hours for such on-site reviews. Again, any facility-imposed restrictions should not conflict with relevant laws.

Interesting questions can arise in the context of patients' requests for access to their health information. For example, what should the HIM professional do if the attending physician thinks that allowing patients to see their health information would be harmful to their recovery? Sometimes this question arises with respect to mental health therapy. Some state laws severely restrict access to mental health records. Some require attending physicians to document in the record that they believe that access to the information would harm their patients. Under the HIPAA privacy rule, if a licensed health care professional has determined, in the exercise of professional judgment, that the access requested is reasonably likely to endanger the life or physical safety of the individual or another person, the facility may then refuse such a request; however, this is a reviewable decision that affords the patient an appeal option.

Other Patient-Directed Disclosures

There are many other situations in which patients authorize other parties to receive their health information. For example, when patients apply for life insurance, disability insurance, or admission to certain schools or programs, they may authorize disclosure of health information. Provided the authorization meets the facility's valid requirements as to form and content, these requests should be promptly honored. Although HIM professionals do not encounter these requests every day, former patients occasionally want to examine their birth records to gain information about their natural parents if they were adopted. Problems may arise because of conflicts between some state laws that grant patients access to their records and adoption laws that may require sealed records to protect the privacy of the birth parents. The sealing of adoption-related records is common. Only a few states permit the adoptee to access these records, and a few provide for the disclosure of health information to the adoptee but strict confidentiality regarding the birth parents' identities. Disclosure of health information about the parents can be important to the adoptee when health conditions that may be genetically based arise later in life. Courts are often sympathetic to these "good cause" requests to open adoption-related records, but this is a decision to be made by a court, not by an individual facility. Keep in mind that not all requests for birth records necessarily require the identity of the parents to be revealed. If the former patient is interested only in time of birth, for example, the facility may be able to honor the request without jeopardizing the privacy rights of the birth parents.

Redisclosure Issues

Once a patient authorizes the disclosure of health information to other parties, such as insurers, control of the information is out of the facility's—and often the patient's—hands. For this reason, health care organizations often include a notice along with the information being disclosed that advises the party receiving the information that redisclosure of the information is prohibited. Through this notice, the third-party recipient is informed of its responsibility not to disclose the information further and to protect it from unauthorized use. Many health care facilities try to discourage redisclosure by stamping a redisclosure prohibition on all information sent out of the facility to alert the recipient that redisclosure issues must be referred to the facility's HIM department. However, except with respect to information covered under the Confidentiality of Alcohol and Drug Abuse Patient Records regulation, the receiving party is not generally bound by that prohibition on redisclosure. In fact, the HIPAA privacy rule anticipates redisclosure in many circumstances, such as in the case of a covered entity who receives another provider's records about a particular patient and then incorporates that information into his or her designated record set. If a valid request was received for release of that information, the second covered entity would be expected to release it.

Another interesting practice with respect to redisclosure involves the insurance industry and the Medical Information Bureau (MIB). The MIB has been described as a kind of medical "credit bureau."[26] Its data bank contains files on millions of people that are shared among hundreds of member insurance companies. The purpose of the MIB is to alert insurers to certain information about applicants for insurance within the past 7 years—information that could be used as the basis for denying insurance. Insurers cooperatively share health information they receive through the claims payment process, pooling it in the MIB for use by all members. How can they do this? The fine print on insurance contract applications generally gives the insurer both the right to use the MIB to access health information (if any information is on file there) and to redisclose information about any health claims into the MIB. The person signing the insurance application may not have been the patient. Thus, information about any given patient may end up being redisclosed into the MIB without the patient's knowledge or permission.

It is possible for patients to contact the MIB to see whether the bureau contains information about them. After contacting the MIB, patients are required to complete and sign a written request form.

Disclosure to Outsourcing Firms Handling Health Information Functions

External release-of-information vendor services are being used with increasing frequency in HIM departments, and outside contractors have been used over the years to microfilm records, digitally image records for storage, and perform medical transcription, coding, and other functions. Many departments use release-of-information vendors to handle routine release-of-information tasks. Some managers have found that these services can supply a staff person on site in the HIM department to do the job more economically and efficiently than the HIM department personnel can.

Regardless of whether these services make financial sense, their use raises some interesting disclosure issues. The function that these outside contractors perform, by its nature, involves access to confidential health information. HIM professionals who use these services must take steps to oversee the confidentiality, security, and appropriate handling of

health information. They must also ensure that the vendor executes an agreement with the covered entity, as required by the HIPAA privacy rule. The vendor should also be contractually bound to handle the confidential information appropriately. In situations in which confidential health information (e.g., dictated reports or hard copy records) must be physically removed from the facility, such as when data are manually delivered to an outside transcription firm or dictation is digitally transmitted over telephone lines to off-site locations, the HIM professional must ensure that adequate security measures are in place to prevent theft, loss, alteration, or destruction of the information. The HIM professional must also ensure that the removal of health information from the facility under this circumstance does not violate state laws. Check state laws to determine what restrictions apply to the removal of health information from the originating facility without patient authorization. Recently, several states have considered bans on sharing patient information with vendors outside the United States.

Disclosure to the News Media

A health care organization has no legal duty to disclose health information to the news media. In past years, hospitals often released basic information about admissions and births to the news media, but many facilities have discontinued this practice. Under the HIPAA privacy rule, no such routine disclosure to the news media of admissions and births should take place without patient authorization. A patient's right of privacy, however, does not bar the publication of information that is of public interest. Courts hold that with regard to a public figure, the celebrity's right to privacy must be weighed against the public's right to know and the freedom of the press. Therefore, if the patient is a public figure, health care organizations usually try, when releasing information to the media, to balance the public's need to know with the patient's need for privacy. For this reason, many health care facilities have adopted policies that permit a spokesperson merely to confirm admission and classify the patient's condition (e.g., critical, poor, fair, stable, good), except under extraordinary circumstances (e.g., treatment of the president or other key public figures, or where the patient requests that absolutely no information be shared or has opted out of the facility's directory). Disclosure of more detailed information should be avoided to minimize the risk of liability to the organization. At the same time, even confirming a patient's admission to a program for alcohol or drug abuse treatment would violate federal law if it were done without the patient's permission.

Some segments of the media have been known to use unusual measures to try to obtain health information on celebrity patients. Staff members may even be approached with bribes. Facility policies should address the measures to be used in handling celebrity records. Special security procedures for preserving the confidentiality of these patients' health information may be appropriate. Some facilities use special code names or an alias on printed reports, with the code known only to the HIM director, physician, and chief executive officer, but these procedures may conflict with the laws of some states with regard to identifying the patient. Some facilities remove such records from their regular filing or information systems and store hard copy reports in a locked file in the HIM department with limited access. The HIM professional should work with the organization's legal counsel or risk manager to devise an appropriate strategy for dealing with celebrity records.

Disclosure Pursuant to Legal Process

When health information must be used in court, the request for information comes in the form of a **subpoena duces tecum,** a **subpoena** (which may also be called a subpoena ad testificandum), a written court order, or simply a verbal order issued in court to the health care organization's attorney. A subpoena is a written order that requires someone to come before the court to testify. A subpoena duces tecum is a written order that requires someone to come before the court and to bring certain records or documents named in that order. When health information is needed in court or in pretrial discovery, such as a deposition, those orders are typically directed to the HIM department director.

State laws vary on who is empowered to issue subpoenas; judges, court clerks, and other officials may be authorized— even attorneys. The form and process that the subpoena must follow to be valid is also a matter of state law and is also addressed in the HIPAA privacy rule, but generally a subpoena must contain the following:

- A docket number (an identification number assigned by the court, generally referring to the year the lawsuit was filed and the numerical order in which the cases are filed; for example, the 318th case filed in that jurisdiction for 2001 might have a docket number of 01-318 with some other identifiers appended)
- The names of the parties (plaintiffs and defendants) involved in the case
- The name of the court or agency before which the proceeding is being held
- The details as to when and where the HIM director's appearance is being requested
- The documents that must be brought
- The signature and seal of the official issuing the subpoena

State laws vary with regard to the method by which and the time limits within which subpoenas can be properly served. Some court systems require service by sheriffs or other public officers. Other jurisdictions permit service by mail or messenger. In still other jurisdictions, service must be accomplished in person, by handing the subpoena to the HIM professional. There are also jurisdictions in which the service must be accompanied by a fee to reimburse the person subpoenaed for his or her time and expense. This nominal fee (called a witness fee) is usually set by statute or

court rules. HIM professionals must become familiar with the requirements applicable to their state and federal jurisdictions to ensure that they respond properly to the subpoenas received.

There are also some special rules associated with a subpoena of information from organizations covered by the Federal Regulations on Alcohol and Drug Abuse. Any subpoena of this specific information must also be accompanied by a court order before it can be released. And for a subpoena duces tecum for health information to be valid under the HIPAA privacy rule, it must be accompanied by court order, or the covered entity must receive "**satisfactory assurance**" from the party seeking the information that reasonable efforts have been made to ensure that the individual who is the subject of the protected health information that has been requested has been given notice of the request or that the party seeking the information has made reasonable efforts to secure a qualified protective order that meets the requirements of the HIPAA privacy rule. The HIPAA privacy rule outlines the qualifications for this "satisfactory assurance at section 164.512(e)(1)(iii)."

Responding to any subpoena that requires the production of health information usually involves the same basic steps (Figure 15-6). These steps, especially when electronic health records are is involved, vary somewhat depending on the design of the facility's information system. Most state HIM associations' legal manuals offer good step-by-step procedures for responding to subpoenas, based on the statutes and rules of that jurisdiction. Roach and the Aspen Health Law and Compliance Center recommend that the procedures include the following steps at a minimum:

1. Examine the information subject to subpoena to make certain that it is complete, that signatures and initials are legible, and that each page identifies the patient and the patient's identification number. (If the information is not yet complete, try to complete it. However, do not ignore a subpoena because the information is not yet complete.)
2. Examine the information to determine whether the case forms the basis for a possible negligence action against the health care organization; if so, notify the appropriate administrators, legal counsel, or risk manager.
3. Remove any material that may not properly be obtained in the jurisdiction by subpoena, such as, in some cases, notes referring to psychiatric care, copies of information from other facilities (unless they have been properly incorporated into the patient's information), and correspondence.*

---

*For a discussion of the issues involved in relying on other health care facilities' tests and records and incorporating them into the patient's record, see King PD: Inclusion of reports from other sources in hospital records, *Top Health Record Manage* 5:81-88, 1984.

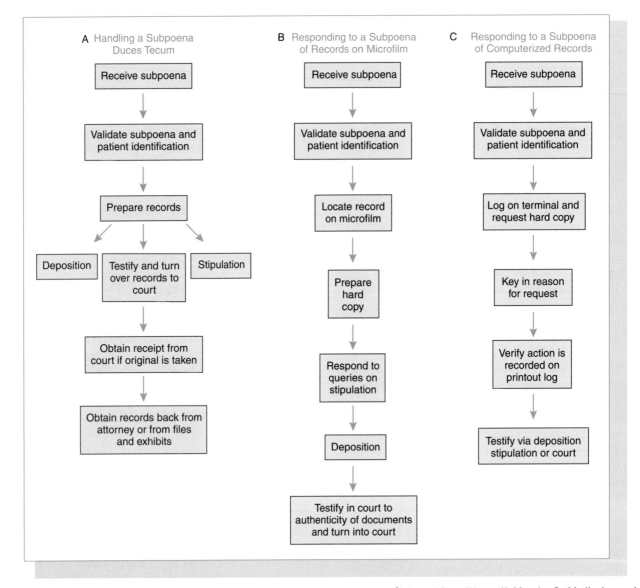

Figure 15-6 Flow charts outlining steps in responding to subpoena duces tecum. (Adapted from Waters K, Murphy G: *Medical records in health information,* Germantown, MD, 1979, Aspen Systems.)

4. Number each page of the patient record, and write the total number of pages on the record folder.
5. Prepare a list of the record contents to be used as a receipt for the information if it must be left with the court or an attorney. (Most facilities use a standard form for this purpose.)
6. Whenever possible, use a photocopy of the record rather than the original in responding (in person) to legal process. (A certificate of authentication can be helpful in convincing the court to accept the photocopy as a true and exact copy of the original.)[27]

The facility's procedures should describe these steps and the steps to follow if a subpoena is defective in some way (e.g., issued by the wrong party, conflicts with state or federal law, asks for records not in the facility's possession, or fails to provide satisfactory assurance where required). Ignoring a subpoena or court order creates trouble, possibly serious trouble. Involve the facility's legal counsel in drafting procedures for dealing with subpoenas and court orders, and do not hesitate to refer unusual problems to your facility's legal counsel. Legal counsel may decide to file a **motion to quash** the subpoena or order in which the court is asked to set aside the subpoena or order.

As mentioned earlier, court orders can be issued in writing or verbally in court to the facility's attorney. A health care organization should make every effort to comply with a court order as long as the order does not place the facility in the position of violating a statute or regulation. Again, as with the subpoena, if the court order is defective in some way (e.g., would force the facility to violate state or federal law), legal counsel must be involved immediately to work out a solution and to help the facility's leaders avoid being cited for contempt of court.

The fact that health information has been subpoenaed does not mean that it will be admissible as evidence. Here again, state laws vary concerning the admissibility of health information. As explained earlier, admissibility issues have become somewhat murky as new technologies for collecting, storing, and retrieving health information are put into use.

HIM professionals are occasionally called on not only to produce the subpoenaed health information but to testify as well. This process typically involves being sworn in and answering questions that lay the foundation for introduction of the patient's record into evidence. HIM professionals may be asked questions about whether the record or information was prepared in the normal course of daily business or according to established policies and procedures for documentation and recordkeeping. It is important for them to answer honestly and not speculate on matters that are beyond their knowledge. They should not guess at the "correct" answer to a question. When the answer to a question is not known, the proper response is simply to say, "I don't know" or "I am not qualified to answer that."

Health Information Management Department Security Measures to Prevent Unauthorized Access

Ensuring that all formal releases of information are appropriately handled is only one aspect of protecting the confidentiality and security of health information. Careful, thorough release-of-information policies are ineffective if internal security measures and systems are inadequate to protect health information from loss, theft, destruction, and alteration. One important aspect of protecting health information is preventing unauthorized access. In other words, how can facilities and HIM professionals keep health information out of the hands of unauthorized users?

Who might that "unauthorized user" be? It may be a curious employee or coworker who knows that his or her neighbor was recently admitted and wants to find out what is wrong with the person. It may be a private investigator who is trying to get information about someone on behalf of a client. It may be a computer hacker who breaks into the facility's health information system just for the challenge. It may even be a physician who is reviewing the records of a competitor's patients and trying to collect ammunition for a battle over delineation of privileges or medical staff membership. One of the most important responsibilities of HIM professionals is to keep confidential health information out of the hands of unauthorized users through appropriate policies and procedures, facility and space planning, information systems design and selection, staff education, security management, and other measures.

HIM policies and procedures should specify who has access to what—ideally, as specifically as possible. In an issue of the AHIMA's former confidentiality newsletter, *In Confidence,* information system security expert Dale Miller

recommended that information security policies define, by specific job function, information access. "An individual should have full and timely access to the information they need to perform their current tasks, but only for the purposes of fulfilling their responsibilities."[28] This advice is consistent with the approach taken by HIPAA's security regulations, which require access control decisions to be based on need, for example, by the role or function that person fulfills within the organization. When a facility employee asks to review a patient's health information, HIM professionals should not hesitate to inquire about the employee's purpose or need, if that need is not known from the circumstances of the request. Many times, legitimate information needs can be handled by less intrusive means than handing over a complete record. The question itself may discourage or defeat illegitimate or suspicious requests. Likewise, HIM professionals should not hesitate to verify the propriety of a request. Anyone can buy a laboratory coat and walk into a nursing station where health information is readily displayed. A person so attired may even be able to stroll unchallenged through an HIM department if staff are not adequately trained in security measures. Many health care organizations are so large that it is impossible for HIM department employees to know all the employees in other departments. Verification of employee identification is a legitimate security measure, as is checking with the employee's supervisor about the validity of certain requests. Locked access to information technology or server storage areas is a legitimate security measure, as is locked access to record storage areas. Sometimes even these basic security measures are not observed. Part of an HIM professional's job is to insist on adequate security measures for both manual and electronic health information systems.

See Chapter 8 for a more in-depth discussion of security issues.

Duty to Provide Care That Meets Professional Standards

In addition to a health care organization's or provider's duty to maintain the confidentiality of a patient's health information, there is a duty to provide care that meets professional standards. Simply put, health care providers must provide a reasonable quality of care to patients—care that meets professional standards. Liability can and does arise when providers fail to meet professionally accepted standards of quality, such as the practice guidelines and standards issued by various medical specialty societies, professional associations, and other consensus groups and those dictated by statute or regulation.

Before liability can be found, the claimant or plaintiff must meet certain requirements and overcome certain obstacles. First, the complaining party must file the claim within the statute of limitations. For this chapter's purposes, this means that once a plaintiff knows (or reasonably should have known) that he or she has a potential claim against a health care organization or provider, that claim must be filed within a certain period of time (e.g., within 2 years of discovering the malpractice). Otherwise, the claim will not be heard by a court. Statutes of limitations are designed to encourage the timely filing of claims, when evidence is fresh and witnesses are likely to be available. Through prompt filing of claims, the search for the truth is facilitated.

In some states, the plaintiff must also obtain a statement from a neutral health care provider (such as a physician) before filing a malpractice claim, certifying that the claim has some merit. Some states use this approach to discourage the filing of nuisance and groundless claims.

For any negligence or malpractice claim to succeed, the plaintiff must show that all the following elements of negligence or malpractice are present:

- *Duty.* The defendant must have had some duty to the plaintiff to use care. A physician, for example, owes a duty to his or her patients to use care that meets professional standards but owes no professional duty to the letter carrier who delivers the office mail.
- *Breach.* The defendant must be shown to have breached that duty (by action or inaction). In other words, the defendant's conduct must have failed to conform to the applicable **standard of care.**
- *Proximate cause.* The breach must be the "proximate" cause of the harm that befell the plaintiff.[29]
- *Harm or damages.* The plaintiff must show that he or she was harmed in some way (e.g., physical pain, suffering, emotional distress, monetary losses).

How does a judge or jury decide whether a defendant acted unreasonably—breaching his or her "duty" to the plaintiff? If the claim involves simple (not professional) negligence such as in a personal injury suit, the judge or jury uses the **"reasonable man" standard.** In other words, the jury is told to evaluate the defendant parties' conduct in light of the jury's own general experience and background. In professional negligence (malpractice) cases, the jury has no experience and training to draw from in evaluating the parties' actions. Therefore, the standard used to judge a professional's actions is the generally accepted standard of care for that profession. For example, orthopedic surgeons' actions are judged against the current standard of care in orthopedics. Pediatricians' actions are judged against pediatric standards of care and so on. These guidelines can be established by expert testimony, professional literature, or published standards. The applicable standard of care is often determined by referring to current standards published by the relevant specialty society and the professional literature. Sometimes referring to accreditation and licensing standards determines it. By pointing to deficiencies in meeting those standards, plaintiffs' attorneys hope to bolster their allegations of negligence.

When a plaintiff brings a civil suit against a defendant, the plaintiff has the **burden of proof.** In other words, unless the plaintiff can convince the judge or jury by a **preponderance of evidence** (making it more likely than not) that the claims against the defendant are valid, the defendant will prevail. The preponderance of evidence standard is not a particularly high one—unlike the "beyond a reasonable doubt" standard found in criminal cases. In a case in which the standard of proof is a preponderance of evidence, it may be helpful to think of it as a "51%" requirement. In other words, in weighing whether something is true or not true, if it is just 51% or more likely to be true (versus 49% or less likely that it is false), then the standard is met.

In a malpractice case against health care providers or organizations, the burden of proof often shifts to the defendant under a concept called **res ipsa loquitur** ("the thing speaks for itself"). An inference of negligence or malpractice is permitted simply because an injury to the plaintiff occurred under the following circumstances:

- The event would not normally have occurred in the absence of negligence.
- The defendant had exclusive control over the instrumentality (e.g., instrument, equipment, procedures) that caused the injury.
- The plaintiff did not contribute to the injury.[30]

For example, if postoperative abdominal adhesions developed in a patient after a surgical sponge was inadvertently left in the abdomen during surgery, the burden of proof would shift to the defendants (probably the surgeon and facility) for the following reasons:

- Surgical sponges are not supposed to be left in the operative site and sewn up inside a patient.
- The sponge, surgical technique, and sponge-counting procedures were within the exclusive control of the defendants.
- The patient did nothing to contribute to the injury.

All three elements must be present to shift the burden of proof in a negligence or malpractice case to the defendant. Otherwise, the plaintiff retains the burden of proving the defendant's negligence by a preponderance of the evidence.

Health information is extremely important in cases that revolve around the health care providers' and organizations' duty to provide care that meets professional standards. In many cases, the documentation of the care provided is the most important evidence available to the trier of fact (the jury, or the judge in cases without a jury). As health care providers soon come to realize, their documentation practices can either help them or hurt them in defending against malpractice claims. Care taken in thorough documentation can make all the difference in the outcome of malpractice litigation.

Incident, or **occurrence, reports** can be important pieces of documentation in investigating, pursuing, and defending against claims against health care organizations and providers. These reports, which should not be treated as part of the patient's health information, are factual summaries of unexpected events that have resulted (or could have resulted) in injury or harm to patients, staff, or visitors. They are used by health care organizations' risk managers or attorneys to investigate incidents that have the potential to become claims against the organization or individual provider and to identify areas where improvements are needed. In many facilities, these reports serve as an important data source for the performance measurement or patient safety program by identifying shortcomings and suggesting possible solutions.

State laws vary considerably with respect to protecting the incident report from discovery by plaintiffs and their attorneys. In some states, the reports are protected as part of the attorney-client privilege as long as the incident report is handled as a document prepared in anticipation of possible litigation and not used for other purposes (e.g., performance measurement or patient safety). In other states, the incident report may be protected from discovery as part of the facility's peer review and quality improvement efforts. In still other states, the incident report is not protected, and therefore users must be extremely careful about what is documented in the report. Facility legal counsel should be actively involved in defining incident report preparation and handling procedures so that the maximum protection possible can be obtained for these reports.

Duty to Obtain Informed Consent to Treatment

One important duty to patients that HIM professionals must be aware of is the physician's duty to obtain the patient's **informed consent** to treatment. Many times, when health professionals refer to obtaining **consent,** they mean getting a permit signed by a patient. Actually, obtaining consent refers to a communication process between the health professional and the patient. Unless that communication successfully informs the patient about the anticipated treatments and meets certain basic requirements, it cannot be considered a valid informed consent.

For practical purposes, the duty to obtain informed consent splits into the following two parts:

- The duty to obtain a general consent for treatment (a largely administrative process that consists of obtaining the patient's signature on a form, often preprinted on the back of the facility's "face" sheet or emergency department record)
- The attending physician's or surgeon's duty to obtain a separate informed consent before the performance of surgery or other invasive procedures

Because the patient has presented at the facility for treatment and that implies (to a certain extent) his or her consent to at least basic care, obtaining a signature on the general consent to treatment is typically a simple process. Obtaining an informed consent before the performance of surgery or

other invasive procedures is often much more complex. How, for example, does the care provider know that the patient is truly making an informed decision?

For a consent obtained by a health care provider to be valid, the health care provider must meet certain requirements. These requirements may be specified in state law and commonly include the following:

- The informed consent should be obtained by the person who will carry out the procedure. In other words, the process of communicating the planned procedure or treatment and its risks, benefits, and alternatives should be handled by the person who will do or supervise the procedure. In the case of surgery, it would be the surgeon. Keep in mind that some states and case law permit the physical act of obtaining a signature on the consent form to be delegated to others, provided the process of informing the patient has already taken place.

- The patient must be capable of giving an informed consent. In other words, the patient must be legally and mentally capable of understanding what is being proposed and making a decision. If the patient has been judged legally incompetent or because of certain emergency circumstances (such as unconsciousness accompanied by a life-threatening injury) cannot give an informed consent, the guardian or next of kin (designated by state law to act in the patient's stead) must receive the information and sign the consent.

Are minors capable of giving informed consent? In some circumstances and for some treatments they are. But how young is too young? This criterion varies from state to state. Barring any state law that prohibits this action, minors may indeed be capable of giving informed consent. Yet another aspect of this question is whether the otherwise competent patient can understand what is being said because of language barriers, hearing impairment, literacy problems, or other issues. Care providers must ensure that a patient can understand the risks, benefits, and alternatives to the proposed procedure before they obtain the patient's signature. Many facilities maintain a list of employees who can speak a foreign language and who can use sign language. In locations where there are large populations of patients for whom English is not their native language, it may be important to prepare patient educational materials and consent forms in the most common non-English languages.

The patient must be free from coercion or undue influence when giving consent. The consent of a patient who agrees to an incidental tubal ligation during gynecological surgery because her husband threatens not to pay the hospital bill unless she does so is considered invalid.

The consent should be granted for a specific procedure or treatment. In other words, if the physician asks for permission to do "abdominal surgery," it would be difficult to argue that the patient is giving a truly informed consent. If the diagnosis is uncertain, however, and exploratory surgery is required, the patient may indeed grant valid consent for the physician to do exploratory surgery and to proceed with more extensive surgery if, in the surgeon's opinion, it is warranted (e.g., when frozen-section results indicate cancer). The key issue is whether the patient has been adequately informed of this possibility and agrees to proceed.

The patient must indeed be adequately informed. State laws provide some guidance on the standard to be used in judging questions as to whether the patient was given enough information. In some states, it is within the caregiver's discretion to decide whether enough information has been given. In other states, a "reasonable man" standard is used. Generally, the standards require that the patient receive information about the nature and purpose of the proposed procedure, the risks and benefits of the proposed treatment, any reasonable alternatives to this procedure, and the risks of refusing the proposed procedure or treatment.[31]

The patient is given an opportunity to ask and receive answers to questions. This is a fairly common problem faced by health care facility staff when trying to obtain the patient's signature on the consent form after the physician has discussed the procedure with the patient and left. The patient may have been reluctant to pose certain questions to the physician or may not have had time to think through all his or her questions, and the facility staff are faced with a dilemma. Does the fact that the patient still has questions mean that he or she has not been adequately informed? Facility policies should define how far staff should go, if they should be involved at all in answering questions, or whether they should immediately notify the physician so that the patient might speak with the physician directly. Most facilities take an intermediate approach: if the question is not really related to the decision-making process (e.g., the patient wants to know about how long the procedure will take), staff may attempt to answer without questioning the validity of the consent. In cases of doubt, however, the physician should be involved. Otherwise, staff may find themselves involved in a postprocedure suit alleging a lack of informed consent.

There are a few circumstances in which informed consent is not required. In life-threatening situations in which the patient is incapable of expressing consent, consent is implied by law. In addition, there are situations in which although consent is required, it need not be accompanied by the normal disclosure of risks, benefits, alternatives, and so on. For example, if there is not time for full discussion of all relevant facts because treatment must begin immediately, some care providers have been excused for giving only a brief summary of the facts as long as the patient agrees to the treatment itself. And in limited circumstances, some care providers have been excused from providing all relevant facts when the provider believes that full disclosure would be harmful. "Therapeutic privilege" could apply when a patient is clearly beyond his or her ability to cope with the details of needed treatment, but this would have to be clearly documented to withstand court scrutiny. Patients may also waive the right to be informed. For example, if the physician attempts to inform the patient but the patient says that he or she would rather not know, just go ahead, the physician should clearly document the patient's waiver and all attempts to inform the patient. In addition, some patients may have had similar procedures or treatments before and may already be familiar with the relevant facts. Again, this situation should be documented.

Along with the right to grant consent is the right to refuse any treatment. Public attitudes toward death with dignity and outcries over heroic attempts to keep patients alive at all costs (both financial and human) have led to the enactment of the Patient Self-Determination Act.[32] This legislation requires health care facilities to query patients about whether they have already documented their life support– and treatment-related wishes (called advance directives) on admission. These wishes are documented as **advance directives** to health care providers in the event they become necessary. An advance directive can be either a **living will,** a written document that allows a competent adult to indicate his or her wishes regarding life-prolonging medical treatment should they be unable to consent, or a **durable power of attorney for health care,** in which a competent adult names in writing another adult to make any medical decisions on his or her behalf in the event he or she becomes incapacitated (although the extent of the decision-making power varies according to state law). The documentation requirements for these advance directives vary by state. The directives, if they exist, are then maintained with the patient's health information.

In some locales, HIM professionals have been faced with patients wanting to put their advance directives on file, although the patient has not been treated at that facility and does not have a health record. Although the facility is not legally obligated to file materials and create records for people who are not yet patients, it does seem prudent to develop a simple filing system (perhaps an alphabetical file separate from the health record) so that those directives can be retained and retrieved if the individual subsequently becomes a patient. This is a service to the community and may speed the location of the advance directives if or when that person is seen in the facility for treatment in the future.

Duty to Provide a Safe Environment for Patients and Visitors

A common duty of health care facilities and providers is to provide a safe environment for patients and visitors. If a patient is dropped and injured while being moved from an emergency department stretcher to an x-ray table, the facility (as employer of the people involved) is likely to be held liable for any damages. If a visitor stumbles in the facility's parking lot because the lot lights were not functioning and lawn care equipment was carelessly left in the lot's walkways by the facility's maintenance employees, the facility is liable for damages. If an infant is abducted from the neonatal nursery because the nursery was short staffed and the babies were momentarily left unsupervised, the facility is likely to be held liable for damages.

When health care facilities open themselves up to the public and to patients for "business," they assume a duty to provide a reasonably safe environment. That is not to say that any injury is compensable. For example, if a visitor who is not watching where she is going stumbles over a clearly marked step and crashes through a plate glass window, the facility may not be responsible. Likewise, if a distraught person enters the facility's emergency department with a gun and begins firing, killing patients and employees, the facility might not be liable.

The key issue in determining whether the facility breached its duty to provide a safe environment is whether the facility's actions (or lack of actions) were reasonable under the circumstances. What is reasonable? How much is enough? That determination is often difficult to make in advance. Certainly, at a minimum, the public expects health care facilities to meet the following criteria:

- To comply with life safety and building codes and other recognized standards
- To provide certain training to employees
- To make sure that the equipment and materials used on patients are clean and functioning properly

Duty to Supervise the Actions of Employees and the Professional Staff

Just as health care organizations must take reasonable steps to provide a safe environment for patients and visitors, they must also supervise the actions of employees and the professional staff (including medical staff). As discussed earlier in the chapter, a health care organization can be held liable for damages when its employees fail to perform their duties adequately, under the doctrine of **respondeat superior** ("let the master answer").

This does not apply just to patient care duties. A health care organization can be liable for an employee's failure to perform other duties as well. For example, if an employee of a large physician group practice inappropriately releases confidential information to an unauthorized party, the group practice could be held liable in a breach of confidentiality suit filed by the patient. Employers are responsible for training their staff to exercise their duties properly. Using this example, a health care organization should certainly ensure that staff members understand proper release-of-information practices and follow them. In fact, training in privacy and security-related issues germane to the employee's job is required by HIPAA. Many facilities go even further and insist that employees with access to confidential information sign an agreement to keep that information confidential and to follow facility policies on confidentiality. Figure 15-7 is a sample nondisclosure agreement by AHIMA that is designed for use with employees, volunteers, and students in the HIM department.

EMPLOYEE/STUDENT/VOLUNTEER

Non-Disclosure Agreement

[Name of health care facility] has the legal and ethical responsibility to safeguard the privacy of all patients and protect the confidentiality of their health information. In the course of my employment/assignment at [*name of health care facility*], I may come into possession of confidential patient information, even though I may not be directly involved in providing patient services.

I understand that such information must be maintained in the strictest confidence. I hereby agree that, unless directed by my supervisor, I will not at any time during or after my employment/assignment with [*name of health care facility*] disclose any patient information to any person whatsoever or permit any person whatsoever to examine or make copies of any patient reports or other documents prepared by me, coming into my possession, or under my control.

When patient information must be discussed with other health care practitioners in the course of my work, I will use discretion to assure that such conversations cannot be overheard by others who are not involved in the patient's care.

I understand that violation of this agreement may result in corrective action, up to and including discharge.

_____

Signature of Employee/Student/Volunteer   Date

Figure 15-7 Sample employee/student/volunteer nondisclosure agreement. (From Brandt M: *Release and disclosure: guidelines regarding maintenance and disclosure of health information,* Chicago, 1997, American Health Information Management Association. Used by permission.)

Medical Staff Credentialing Process

Under the doctrine of corporate negligence, a health care organization can also be held liable for the acts of its non-employee staff, such as the medical staff. In one of the most important cases on the doctrine of corporate negligence, *Elam v. College Park Hospital,* the court held that a hospital is liable to a patient for the negligent conduct of independent physicians and surgeons who are neither employees nor agents of the hospital.[33] A hospital owes patients a duty to ensure the competence of its medical staff and to evaluate the quality of medical care rendered on its premises. This is one of the main reasons behind medical staff credentialing programs, in which prospective members of the medical staff apply for membership and request that certain privileges to practice medicine at that facility be granted. Likewise, current members of the medical staff periodically (usually every 2 years) renew or request new or changed privileges to render certain types of care and services at the facility.

The purpose of the medical staff credentialing process is to ensure that only qualified physicians and other credentialed health professionals practice within the facility. During the appointment and reappointment process, the applicant's background is reviewed, licenses and certifications are checked, proof of current liability insurance is verified, and practice patterns and quality review data are evaluated to determine whether the applicant should be granted the privileges he or she seeks to gain or renew. If the evaluation is done poorly, medical staff credentialing decisions can result in liability for the health care organization. In *Rule v. Lutheran Hospitals and Homes Society of America,* a hospital was liable for birth injuries that occurred during an infant's breech delivery.[34] The jury found that the hospital had failed to investigate adequately the background and qualifications of the attending physician before granting him delivery privileges. The hospital had, in fact, failed to check with other hospitals in which the physician had practiced. If that check had been made, the hospital would have discovered that the physician's privileges to perform breech deliveries at one of those other hospitals had been substantially curtailed. This probably would have led to similar restrictions on the physician at the defendant hospital and perhaps would have made the physician ineligible for that privilege altogether.

The actual investigative and documentation procedure that is followed in acting on initial appointment and reappointment applications is outlined in the facility's medical staff bylaws and medical staff rules and regulations. Some state statutes address credentialing requirements, and The Joint Commission standards impose certain criteria that should be met. The Health Care Quality Improvement Act of 1986 also imposes some credentialing-related requirements on health care organizations. These requirements are discussed in Chapter 13, "Performance Measurement and Patient Safety."

Payers also have similar systems to verify the credentials of the physicians and other providers that they admit to their panels of "preferred" providers (in the case of preferred provider organizations), or the providers who participate in their health maintenance organization.

There is another body of federal and state laws that can affect the credentialing process. These laws are related to antitrust liability. Antitrust laws were developed to protect and encourage competition. Antitrust liability can arise in this context when the medical or professional staff credentialing process interferes with a physician's or health professional's ability to pursue his or her profession. This interference may be alleged to be a **restraint of trade.** This claim could arise, for example, when the only hospital for miles around enters into an exclusive employment agreement for certain specialty care consulting services and declares that any inpatients who need this specialty care may use only the employed specialist. The following laws protect against restraint of trade:

- The Sherman Act, which prohibits monopolies created by agreements among competitors[35]
- The Clayton Act, which prohibits certain arrangements that tend to lessen competition, such as certain "tying arrangements" that deny freedom of choice in selecting services and products[36]
- The Federal Trade Commission Act, which prohibits unfair methods of competition that affect commerce

Sometimes physicians try to use these acts to support their claims that their denial of staff privileges has the effect of reducing competition. Probably the best defense to actions that arise out of the denial of staff membership to an individual is for the health care organization to show a valid basis for the denial of privileges (e.g., quality-of-care problems). The defense strategy is different when the complaint involves the denial of privileges to a whole class of plaintiffs, such as podiatrists, but that is beyond the scope of this chapter. Be aware, however, that physicians and other health professionals are increasingly sensitive to antitrust problems and that the avoidance of antitrust liability should be considered when developing credentialing-related policies and procedures.

The credentialing process has its own set of confidential information: the credentials file and the practitioner's quality profile. The credentials file is basically a dossier on each medical or professional staff member. It typically contains at least the following:

- Completed medical staff application for appointment or reappointment
- Copies of the practitioner's license, diplomas, board certifications, controlled substances permit (for prescribing certain drugs), proof of current professional liability insurance, response to the facility's query of the National Practitioner Data Bank (NPDB) (established by the Health Care Quality Improvement Act of 1986) and perhaps other organizations (e.g., the Federation of State Medical Boards and American

Medical Association Physician Masterfile), and other documents required by the bylaws (e.g., results of any proctoring or observation of the practitioner that is done during the initial "provisional" appointment to the staff)

- Completed references from various sources (e.g., program directors for residencies, department chairpersons at other facilities where the practitioner works)
- Specific listing of the privileges requested by the physician and approved by the medical staff

This background information is supplemented with a quality profile for the practitioner, which is usually kept apart from the credentials file. The profile typically contains statistical information on the volume and type of cases treated in the past by the practitioner at that health care organization. It also contains information on the number and type of cases that have been subjected to quality reviews and the results of those reviews. Department chairpersons and credentials committee members use this information in evaluating the practitioner's competence. This helps them to decide whether to grant the requested privileges. The practitioner may treat only the kinds of cases and perform only the kinds of procedures for which he or she possesses clinical privileges in that facility. For this reason, credentialing and privileging decisions often involve sensitive issues and may be the subject of debate, disagreement, and even litigation (if requested privileges are denied).

Accessibility of Credentials Files and Quality Profiles

Because of their sensitive contents, the credentials file and quality profile are treated as confidential information. As a result, health care organizations need to establish clear policies on who may have access to the files and information, how the files and information are kept secure, and how long the information must be retained. HIM professionals are often involved in developing such policies.

To develop appropriate access policies that govern credentialing-related information, the HIM professional needs to understand who plays a role in the credentialing and privilege delineation process. Although the scenario may vary with individual organizations' medical staff bylaws, the following key players are commonly involved:

Applicant or practitioner. This refers to the person who is applying for either initial appointment or reappointment and is requesting certain clinical privileges. The practitioner has the right to review the contents of his or her own credentials file and quality profile.

Department chairperson. This is the clinical chairperson of the medical or professional staff department to which the applicant or practitioner belongs or wants to belong. The department chairperson must meet with the applicant or practitioner, review the contents of his or her credentials file and quality profile, and make a recommendation to the credentials committee or medical executive committee with respect to the application or request for privileges.

Credentials committee. Members of this medical staff committee are charged with responsibility for reviewing the contents of the credentials file and quality profile and recommending action to the medical executive committee or governing body. Credentials committees are usually made up of a cross-section of the medical and professional staff and provide a sort of check and balance on the appointment and privilege delineation process. For example, if the department chairperson of pediatrics does not want a new pediatrician added to the staff because that would mean more competition for patients, the chairperson might recommend against appointment of an otherwise qualified pediatrician. A cross-sectional credentials committee would probably not have the same biases and therefore could help prevent claims of unfairness.

Medical executive committee. This committee, commonly made up of the officers of the medical staff and clinical department chairperson, is often involved in reviewing the recommendations of the individual department chairperson and credentials committee and then passing that information along to the facility's governing body with its own recommendation. Access policies should define whether executive committee members should have direct access to credential files and quality profiles in their capacity as committee members or whether their review and recommendations should be limited to the information presented by the credentials committee and department chairperson. Because the executive committee often has major responsibilities for supervising the quality of clinical practice in the facility, members often have direct access to related files and information.

Governing body or Board of Directors. As the group ultimately responsible for ensuring the quality of services provided by the facility and its professional staff, the governing body makes the final decision on requests for appointment or reappointment and clinical privileges. This group often relies heavily on the recommendations made by the medical executive committee, department chairperson, and credentials committee but need not be bound by those recommendations. Facility access policies should define whether board members have direct access to credential files and quality profiles.

Medical staff coordinator. This person is responsible for collecting, organizing, filing, and controlling access to information within the credentials file and, often, the quality profile. By the nature of his or her responsibilities, this person must have access to the files and information. Some facilities choose to separate the handling of the quality profile, delegating that responsibility to the staff who coordinate all quality management and improvement activities. In those cases, the person responsible for the credentials file might not have access to quality profile data.

To the extent that HIM professionals are involved in credentialing-related activities, they have some access to credential and quality profile information. In some facilities, HIM professionals serve as medical staff coordinators. In other facilities, those responsibilities are separate from the HIM function, and HIM staff do not have access to this information.

Legal Risks

As mentioned earlier, the tasks of professional staff appointment, reappointment, and delineation of clinical privileges are fraught with potential problems. Physicians who are dissatisfied with the decisions made by a facility may choose to sue the facility, using a wide variety of legal theories. The elements essential to a successful defense vary with the legal theories involved, but generally, in defending these attacks, it is important to be able to show the following:

- That the facility's bylaws, rules, and regulations related to credentialing and privilege delineation were carefully followed and that those provisions meet relevant state and federal requirements
- That the complaining party was not singled out for special treatment but was treated in the same way as other similarly situated people were treated
- That the adverse decision was clinically justified (e.g., supported by something more than just the hunches of the decision makers) and that the justification for the decision was documented in the credentials file, quality profile, or related papers

The procedures for granting medical and professional staff membership and delineating clinical privileges are closely tied to the facility's performance management and improvement activities. Health care organizations use quality management and improvement monitors and indicators not only to improve the systems that support the provision of patient care but also to gather data about the clinical performance of staff members. In this way, the governing body can fulfill its responsibilities to supervise the actions of both employees and the professional staff.

Contract Liability Issues and the Health Information Management Department

Contracts (actual and implied) are another common source of liability for health care facilities and providers—even HIM professionals. Some courts have begun to enforce ethical and statutory obligations regarding the confidentiality of patients' health information as part of the contractual relationship between health care providers and their patients. In the *Hammonds* case cited earlier, the court found that the physician breached an implied condition of his physician-patient

contract when he disclosed patient information to an insurer without the patient's authorization.[9] Thus, breach of contract is another theory under which a patient may seek relief for breach of confidentiality.

Contract liability typically arises in response to more traditional scenarios. For example, one party to a contract fails to abide by the terms of the agreement and the other party sues for damages or specific performance (basically, a court order that requires the losing party to do what it contractually agreed to do). Health care organizations enter into written contracts every day. They may contract for certain professional services, such as emergency medicine or anesthesia services. They may sign contracts for the purchase or lease of equipment or supplies. Sometimes breach of contract problems arise because a contract has been entered into without careful, advance review by legal counsel or risk manager, and, as a result, the health care organization has agreed to unfavorable terms that may be difficult or impossible to meet.

How can this apply to a manager of an HIM department? Think of the potential contracts with which a typical HIM professional may be involved. There may be a contract with a transcription service. There may be a contract with a consulting company. There may be a contract with a release-of-information service or an imaging service. There may be contracts with local schools and educational programs in which liability issues regarding student-trainees are discussed. There may be managed care contracts in which the facility agrees to share certain health information with the managed care company. There may be a contract for purchase of hardware or software to support the facility's information system—the list goes on. If the HIM professional signs an agreement without benefit of legal or risk management review, he or she may be agreeing to terms that will later come back to haunt the facility.

The following are some of the typical things attorneys and risk managers look for in contracts:

- *Independent contractor clauses.* In signing a contract for professional services, the facility may want to clarify that the professional is not an employee but an independent contractor who is responsible for his or her own actions.
- *Hold harmless or indemnification clauses.* In these clauses, the health care facility generally wants the other party to accept financial and legal responsibility for its own actions and to agree to indemnify or compensate the health care facility for any claims against the facility that are the result of the other party's actions or inaction.
- *Termination or notification clauses.* Health care facilities typically want the process for terminating the contract to be clearly specified, including responsibility for advance notification of the other party of plans to terminate. The wording of such a clause is extremely important, and the health care facility will want as much latitude and flexibility as can be negotiated.

- *Confidentiality obligations.* Particularly with respect to contractors who will have access to confidential health information, the facility and HIM professional will want to specify the contractor's obligations to safeguard the confidentiality and security of that information. In fact, the HIPAA privacy and security rules require that these issues be addressed in a business associate agreement between the covered entity and all contractors who qualify as business associates under the rules. Although certain clauses are required in the rules, the actual language of the agreement is up to the covered entity to develop. The HIM professional may even want to specify the exact procedures that must be followed in handling the information.

In determining the safeguards and clauses that should be included in any contract, the HIM professional should use a variety of resources. Literature searches can locate articles specifically devoted to negotiating certain types of agreements, such as transcription contracts. The health care organization's risk manager and in-house counsel, if they exist, can also be of great assistance. The HIPAA privacy rule and security regulations should also be referenced. Because of the expense involved in obtaining legal review of a contract, many facilities establish a policy describing the characteristics of contracts that must be reviewed by counsel versus those that can be entered into with just a departmental review or risk management review (Figure 15-8).

Legal Resources for Health Information Management Professionals

No one expects HIM professionals to be lawyers. They are, however, expected to understand basic legal concepts, such as those described here. They are also expected to know how to find the information needed to help avoid legal problems for the HIM department, the health care organization, and, to a certain extent, the facility's professional staff. In larger facilities, HIM professionals may have access to a risk manager, in-house counsel, and outside attorneys to assist them in finding answers and developing appropriate policies, procedures, and system safeguards. Smaller facilities probably have fewer internal resources, and HIM professionals may need to work more closely with outside counsel on the most important questions, recognizing that there are often very limited budgets for outside legal services.

Regardless of the setting, HIM professionals should use important external resources that are available, such as the following:

- The *Journal of the American Health Information Management Association* and other professional journals and newsletters
- AHIMA's FORE (Foundation of Research and Education) Resource Center, where professional staff are available

to assist in literature searches and to loan library materials to members
- AHIMA's on-line body of knowledge, where articles and other AHIMA publications are available to members, including practice briefs
- The state's HIM association and any legal manuals it may have compiled
- Law firms' client newsletters and client advisories. Some firms with health law departments are glad to put HIM professionals and other health care providers on their free distribution list.
- State hospital associations or other health care industry groups, which keep members up to date on medicolegal issues
- The loss-control staff of any professional liability carriers that insure the health care organization
- Reference librarians at the public library or at law libraries, who can assist in locating and obtaining copies of legislation and regulations
- The *Federal Register,* a daily government publication that keeps the public apprised of proposed federal rules and regulations so that all interested parties have an opportunity to comment or prepare
- State government Web sites
- The HIPAA Web site of the DHHS, where copies of the regulations and the answers to frequently asked questions about privacy can be reviewed
- HIM peers in local health care facilities, who are usually more than glad to share information

With all the information that is available, there is no excuse for ignorance. HIM professionals have important responsibilities in today's health care organizations. Patients, health care organizations, and colleagues rely on HIM professionals to protect their confidential information and to assist them in successfully navigating a maze of standards, rules, regulations, laws, and guidelines related to health information, confidentiality, and patient care issues. In so doing, HIM professionals earn their professional credentials, achieve professional success, and improve the quality of health care.

Key Concepts

- HIM professionals must make decisions every day regarding who may have access to confidential health information. These decisions must protect the patient's privacy and be based on the many state and federal laws that govern access to health information.
- There are four main sources of law: (1) federal and state constitutions, (2) federal and state statutes, (3) rules and regulations of administrative agencies, and (4) court decisions.

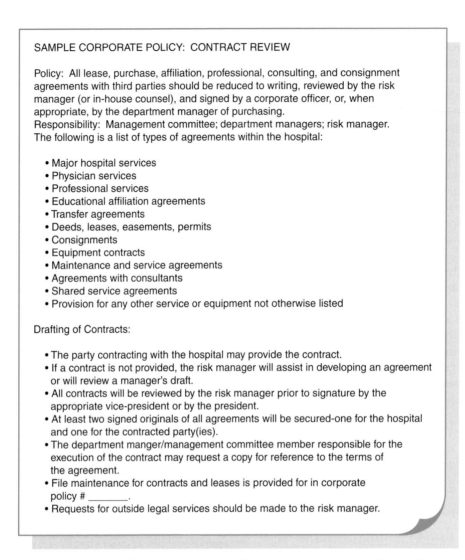

SAMPLE CORPORATE POLICY: CONTRACT REVIEW

Policy: All lease, purchase, affiliation, professional, consulting, and consignment agreements with third parties should be reduced to writing, reviewed by the risk manager (or in-house counsel), and signed by a corporate officer, or, when appropriate, by the department manager of purchasing.
Responsibility: Management committee; department managers; risk manager.
The following is a list of types of agreements within the hospital:

- Major hospital services
- Physician services
- Professional services
- Educational affiliation agreements
- Transfer agreements
- Deeds, leases, easements, permits
- Consignments
- Equipment contracts
- Maintenance and service agreements
- Agreements with consultants
- Shared service agreements
- Provision for any other service or equipment not otherwise listed

Drafting of Contracts:

- The party contracting with the hospital may provide the contract.
- If a contract is not provided, the risk manager will assist in developing an agreement or will review a manager's draft.
- All contracts will be reviewed by the risk manager prior to signature by the appropriate vice-president or by the president.
- At least two signed originals of all agreements will be secured-one for the hospital and one for the contracted party(ies).
- The department manger/management committee member responsible for the execution of the contract may request a copy for reference to the terms of the agreement.
- File maintenance for contracts and leases is provided for in corporate policy # _____.
- Requests for outside legal services should be made to the risk manager.

Figure 15-8 Sample contract review policy. (From Carroll R, editor: *Risk management handbook for health care organizations,* Chicago, 1997, American Hospital Publishing. Used by permission.)

- The right to privacy is the right to be left alone, to make decisions about one's own body, and to control one's own information.
- The federal court system and many state systems have three levels of courts: (1) trial courts, (2) intermediate courts of appeals, and (3) a supreme court.
- One of the most fundamental duties of HIM professionals and their health care facility employers is the duty to maintain health information about their patients. This duty is imposed explicitly by state and federal statutes and regulations and by accreditation standards.
- It is essential that patient health information that is transmitted to health care providers remain confidential. Health care providers are bound by various laws and ethical standards to maintain this confidentiality.
- It is generally accepted that the health care facility owns the record or information itself but that the exercise of those ownership rights is subject to the *patient's* ownership interest in the information within that record or information.
- When health information is needed for use in court, the request for information comes in the form of a subpoena duces tecum, a subpoena (which may also be called a subpoena ad testificandum), a written court order, or simply a verbal order issued in court to the health care organization's attorney.
- One of the most important responsibilities HIM professionals have is keeping confidential health information out of the hands of unauthorized users through appropriate policies and procedures, facility and space planning, information systems design and selection, staff education, security management, and other measures.
- Health care organizations owe patients a duty to provide care that meets professional standards. Health care providers must provide a reasonable quality of care to patients—care that meets professional standards.

- For a negligence or malpractice claim to succeed, the plaintiff must show that all the following elements of negligence or malpractice are met: duty, breach, proximate cause, and harm or damages.
- Physicians owe patients a duty to obtain the patient's informed consent to treatment. This duty is not just having a patient sign a consent form. Obtaining an "informed consent" refers to a communication process between the health professional and the patient. The patient must be informed about the anticipated treatment and its risks and alternatives.
- Health care organizations must take reasonable steps to supervise the actions of their employees and professional staff (including medical staff) under the doctrine of respondeat superior ("let the master answer"). They can be held liable for damages when their employees fail to perform their duties adequately.

REFERENCES

1. *Griswold v. Connecticut,* 381 U.S. 479 (1965).
2. 42 U.S.C. 12101-12213.
3. Sec. 51(a), (b) of the Federal Food, Drug and Cosmetic Act, as amended, 21 U.S.C. 360i.
4. *Darling v. Charleston Community Memorial Hospital,* 33 Ill. 2d 326, 211 N.E. 2d 253 (1965), *cert. denied,* 383 U.S. 946 (1966).
5. Keeton: Medical negligence—the standard of care, *Specialty Law Digest Health Care* 3, 1980.
6. *Peete v. Blackwell,* 504 So. 2d 22 (Ala. 1986).
7. *Johnson v. Women's Hospital,* 527 S.W. 2d 133 (Tenn. Ct. App. 1975).
8. *Greer v. Medders,* 336 S.E. 2d 329 (1985).
9. *Hammonds v. Aetna Casualty and Surety Co.,* 237 F. Supp. 96 (N.D. Ohio 1965) and 243 F. Supp. 793 (N.D. Ohio 1965).
10. 42 U.S.C. 1395x(e)(2) (1974); 42 C.F.R. 482.24(c) (1994).
11. *Minnesota v. Andring,* 342 N.W. 2d 128 (Minn. 1984).
12. *Fox v. Cohen,* 84 Ill. App. 3d 744, 406 N.E. 2d 178 (1980).
13. *Pisel v. Stamford Hospital,* 180 Conn. 314, 340, 430 A.2d 1, 15 (1980).
14. Tomes J: *Healthcare records: a practical legal guide,* Westchester, IL, 1990, Healthcare Financial Management Association.
15. 42 C.F.R., Chapter 1, Part 2, Section 2.13, Revised (1983).
16. McCann R: Protecting the confidentiality of peer review information, *J AHIMA* 64:52, 1993.
17. 5 U.S.C. 552a(b) (1977).
18. *Plain Dealer Publishing Co. v. U.S. Dept. of Labor,* 471 F. Supp. 1023 (D.D.C. 1979)
19. *Florida Medical Ass'n, Inc. v. U.S. Dept. of Health, Education and Welfare,* 479 F. Supp. 1291 (M.D. Fla. 1979)
20. *Washington Post Co. v. U.S. Dept. of Health and Human Services,* 690 F. 2d 252 (D.D.C. 1982).
21. 42 C.F.R. Part 2, Subpart B, 2.51.
22. 42 C.F.R. Part 2.51, Subpart B, 2.12.
23. 42 C.F.R. Part 2, Subpart B, 2.51.
24. Dennis JC: Profits and patient information: does database marketing breach confidentiality? *In Confidence* 1:4-6, 1993.
25. *Gotkin v. Miller,* 379 F. Supp. 859 (E.D.N.Y. 1974).
26. Are you "on file" in the Medical Information Bureau? *In Confidence* 1:11-12, 1993.
27. Roach WH Jr, Aspen Health Law and Compliance Center: *Medical records and the law,* ed 3, Gaithersburg, MD, 1998, Aspen Publishers.
28. Miller D: Glad you asked: Answers on information security and confidentiality, *In Confidence* 1:2, 1993.
29. *Palsqraf v. Long Island R.R. Co.,* 248 N.Y. 339, 162 N.E. 99, *rehearing denied,* 249 N.Y. 511, 164 N.E. 564 (1928).
30. Pozgar GD: *Legal aspects of health care administration,* ed 7, Gaithersburg, MD, 1999, Aspen Publishers.
31. Carroll R, editor: *Risk management handbook for health care organizations,* Chicago, 1997, American Hospital Publishing.
32. Public Law 101-508, 4206 (Medicare) and 4751 (Medicaid), 104 Stat. 1388.
33. *Elam v. College Park Hospital,* 183 Cal. Rptr. 156 (Ct. App. 1982).
34. *Rule v. Lutheran Hospitals and Home Society of America,* 835 F. 2d 1250 (8th Cir. 1987).
35. *Patrick v. Burget,* 108 S. Ct. 1658 (1988).
36. *Jefferson Parish Hospital District No. 2 v. Hyde,* 466 U.S. 2, 104 S. Ct. 1551 (1984).

Management

Human Resource Management

Wesley M. Rohrer III

Additional content,
http://evolve.elsevier.com/Abdelhak/

Review exercises can be found
in the Study Guide

Human Resource Management
　Navigating Through Turbulent Times
　Broad Environmental Forces
　　New Challenges in the Twenty-First Century
　　The Federal Regulatory Context
　　The Demographic Imperative
　Forces Transforming Health Care
　Challenges for Health Information Management
　　Professionals
　　Leadership and Human Resources Management
　　Overview of Leadership Theory
　　Relationships and Leadership Style
　　Transformational Leadership
　　Leadership Development
　　The Ethics of Leadership
　　Other Core Values in Health Care Management
　　Ethics of the Ordinary
　　Power and Ethical Decision Making
　　Values Clarification
　　Servant Leadership
　　Applications to Human Resources Management
　　Codes of Ethics
　Systems Perspective on Human Resource Management
　Systems Approach Applied to Health Information Services
　Systems Perspective Applied to Human Resources
　　Management
　Environmental Influences and Human Resources
　　Management
　　Women's Participation in the Workforce
　　Technological Change
　　Health Policy and Industry Developments
　　Economy Forces and Trends
　　Demographic Changes in the Workforce
　Legal and Regulatory Requirements Affecting Human
　　Resources Management
　　Institutional Accreditation
　　Civil Rights and Equal Employment Opportunity Legislation
　　Gender Discrimination and Sexual Harassment

Key Words

Affirmative action programs	Graphic rating scales	Power
Behaviorally anchored rating scales	Grievance procedure	Preventive discipline
Cafeteria benefit plan	Halo effect	Progressive discipline
Career counseling	Human resource audit	Protected group
Career planning	Job analysis	Reasonable accommodation
Compensation management	Job description	Recruitment pool
Counseling and referral	Job evaluation	Replacement charts
Critical incident method	Job grading	Selection process
Disparate impact	Job performance standards	Self-appraisal
Disparate treatment	Job ranking	Sexual harassment
Employee assistance program	Job sharing	Staffing table
Employee handbook	Key indicators of demand	Strategic human resource planning
Employment at will	Layoffs	Transactional leadership
Equal employment opportunity	Management by objectives	Transformational leadership
Factor comparison	Performance appraisal	Undue hardship
Flex time	Point system	Values clarification

This chapter contains revised information from a previous edition authored by Peter M. Ginter and W. Jack Duncan.

    Protecting the Rights of Persons with Disabilities
    Age Discrimination
    Immigration Control and Employment
    Employee Health and Workplace Safety
    Privacy of Information
    Employee Compensation
    Labor Union Legislation
    Managing Human Resources Within the Unionized
      Environment
Internal Environment of the Health Care Organization
    Organizational Culture
    Information Systems
    Role of Human Resources Management System in Health
      Care Organization
    The Employee as Client of the Human Resources
      Management System
    Employee Assistance Programs
    System Inputs
    Performance Appraisal Systems
    Adverse Outcomes of Employee Performance
    Employee Counseling and Discipline
    Grievance Process
    Compensation Management
    Training and Development
    Employee Health, Safety, and Well-Being
Future Issues

Abbreviations

ADA—Americans with Disabilities Act

ADEA—Age Discrimination in Employment Act

AFL-CIO— American Federation of Labor-Congress of Industrial Organizations

AHIMA—American Health Information Management Association

BARS—behaviorally anchored rating scales

BFOQ—bona fide occupational qualification

BLS—Bureau of Labor Statistics

CEO—chief executive officer

CQI—continuous quality improvement

EAP—employee assistance program

EEO—equal employment opportunity

EEOC—Equal Employment Opportunity Commission

ERISA—Employee Retirement Income Security Act

FLSA—Fair Labor Standards Act

FMCS—Federal Mediation and Conciliation Service

FMLA—Family and Medical Leave Act

FTE—full-time equivalent

HIM—health information management

HIPAA—Health Insurance Portability and Accountability Act

HIS—health information services

HMO—health maintenance organization

HRM—human resource management

IRCA—Immigration Reform and Control Act

ISO—International Standards Organization

JCAHO—Joint Commission on Accreditation of Healthcare Organizations (now The Joint Commission)

LAN—local area network

MBO—management by objectives

NLRA—National Labor Relations Act

NLRB—National Labor Relations Board

OFCCP—Office of Federal Contract Compliance Program

OSHA—Occupational Safety and Health Administration/Act

PHI—personal health information

POS—point of service

PPO—preferred provider organization

QWL—quality of work life

SEIU—Service Employees International Union

SQC—statistical quality control

TQM—total quality management

WAN—wide area network

Objectives

- Define key words.
- List and explain the human resource management responsibilities of all managers.
- Discuss the external and internal environmental challenges that face a health information services department manager in the twenty-first century.
- Apply the legislative and regulatory agency requirements for managing employees in a health care organization.
- Describe the societal, organizational, functional, and personal objectives and activities of human resource management in health care organizations.
- Understand the systems model of human resource management as it applies to health information services.
- Develop methods of recruiting, selection, retaining, and terminating employees who staff a health information services department.
- Describe various performance evaluation and compensation management programs used in health care organizations.
- Implement effective strategies for building a health information management team.
- Describe orientation and training needs for health information services departments.
- Define and explain career planning programs for health information management personnel.

HUMAN RESOURCE MANAGEMENT

Navigating Through Turbulent Times

As we plunge into the uncharted waters of organizational life of the twenty-first century, it seems wise to reflect on the dramatic changes in organization structure, technology, incentive structure, and strategies that have occurred in health care during the past two decades. Many of these changes can be seen as organizational responses to broad environmental influences that have had a pervasive impact across virtually all industries and enterprises, including those in health care, rehabilitation, and long-term care. We have witnessed the emergence of the "informated" organization,[1] the learning organization, the horizontal organization,[2] the virtual organization, and the consumer-driven health care organization. Every manager, worker, and professional has been considerably affected by the explosion of access to information from links to local area networks (LANs) to wide area networks (WANs), data warehousing, and the virtually unlimited resources of the Internet. Both the benefits and the excesses of re-engineering have been chronicled (as either a boon or a curse) and directly felt by both the victims and survivors of corporate "downsizing" and outsourcing work to off-shore sites. A bewildering array of alternative philosophies, methods, and buzzwords—continuous quality improvement [CQI], statistical quality control [SQC], total quality management [TQM], quality of work life [QWL], employee participation teams, empowerment, benchmarking, the Toyota manufacturing quality program, Baldridge awards, International Standards Organization (ISO) 9000, and Six Sigma certification among others associated with stimulating, monitoring, and sustaining quality of performance, products, and services—have competed for managerial and scholarly attention during this period of the transformation of the health care industry.

Broad Environmental Forces

New Challenges in the Twenty-First Century

The new century had barely begun before life as we knew it, at least in the privileged nations of the Western World, changed forever on September 11, 2001. Not only did these devastating acts of terrorism on U.S. soil result in thousands of personal tragedies, the event and its aftermath eroded the assumptions of safety and security of the homeland for many U.S. citizens. Beyond that it had profound geopolitical, economic, religious, and cultural repercussions across the globe. A whole new industry focused on emergency preparedness, and homeland security was created. Public health and health care leaders joined with community leaders and public officials to plan to respond to acts of bioterrorism and other potential catastrophic assaults. Airline transportation routines were radically affected and internal governmental surveillance increased dramatically, but in most cases invisibly. Although it is impossible to predict the future in detail, it is likely that the new level of heightened awareness, sense of insecurity, and vulnerability throughout the West will have long-lasting consequences in the workplace as well as across society.

Adding to the complexity and risk that all organizations face in the twenty-first century is the increasing threat of pandemics (e.g., avian influenza A [bird flu]). Not only could such an epidemic have devastating effects on the health of populations—according to the World Health Organization, 30% of the world's population might be affected in the first year, resulting in two million deaths[3]—but also would likely have severe if temporary effects on the economic, social, and political infrastructure. That a current issue of the *Harvard Business Review* (May 2006) devoted a lengthy Special Report to alerting the business community to the importance of monitoring and planning for a pandemic is a telling indicator of the breadth and severity of the likely impact of such a public health assault on the individual organization and the corporate community. Clearly, because the health care services organization will be on the front lines of addressing the consequences of a pandemic along with its public health partners, the organizational effects of such an event would almost certainly be immediate and profound.

The Federal Regulatory Context

Although the pace of regulatory growth affecting human resource management (HRM) slowed somewhat after the explosion of legislative initiatives and regulatory mechanisms of the 1960s and 1970s, subsequent federal legislation continues to have a significant impact on the workplace. Most notable of these federal policies are the Americans with Disabilities Act (ADA) of 1990, the Civil Rights Act of 1991, and the Family and Medical Leave Act (FMLA) of 1993. The continuing, although far from complete, elimination of legal and attitudinal barriers to women and minority group participation in the workplace has led to formal recognition of diversity management programs at the same time that the philosophical justification for equal employment opportunity (EEO) and especially affirmative action programs is being challenged. One could argue with some confidence that during the past two decades the single greatest force affecting organizational dynamics generally and HRM specifically has been the assertion by women of their rights to participate fully in the workplace in all professions and at all levels of decision making.

The Demographic Imperative

The phenomenon of an aging population is beginning to acutely affect the workplace both in the United States and the highly developed societies worldwide. This demographic trend, coupled with the legislative constraints on employer discretion embodied in the Age Discrimination in Employment Act (ADEA) (1967, as amended), has led to a "graying" of the workforce, at least in some regions of the United States. Also, the cultural and ethnic mix of workplaces in the United States and abroad are feeling the effects of sustained growth and migration. The U.S. Hispanic population reached

41.3 million on July 1, 2004, demonstrating a growth rate of 3.6% over the previous year. This was more than three times the growth rate of the total population.[4] The steady erosion of union representation within the U.S. workforce (from 25% of the private sector workforce in 1973 to just below 8% in 2004)[5] was the major theme of labor relations through the end of the twentieth century and into the twenty-first century. Although no major legislative developments have affected collective bargaining significantly during the past decade, recent political events portend significant changes in the near future. There have continually been skirmishes over management's right to hire replacement workers and the ramifications of team participation in quality management efforts for traditional labor relations. However, the separation in 2005 of roughly four million members of three major collective bargaining structures, including the Service Employees International Union (SEIU), from the American Federation of Labor–Congress of Industrial Organizations (AFL-CIO)[6] posits a strong challenge for the future or organized labor. The long-term decline in union membership as a proportion of the workforce and the decline in political power of organized labor at least at the national level begs the question of whether traditional collective bargaining structures and processes will be able to adapt to and survive the environmental and workplace changes discussed.

Forces Transforming Health Care

Beyond these broad influences affecting all organizations are the constellation of forces that have reshaped traditional health care and rehabilitation. The traditional model of health services delivery that focused on acute-care (hospital) services and that was orchestrated by independent physicians has been radically transformed into an environment of competing managed care networks coordinating an array of linked services and settings across the continuum of care. "Managed care" includes an increasingly diverse set of institutional structures and affiliations, including the established health maintenance organizations (HMOs), physician provider organizations (PPOs), point-of-service (POS) agreements, integrated delivery systems, and other types of health plans and networks. A common element for managed care across these variations of organization design is the commitment to accept the financial and other risks of providing cost-effective services of high quality to enhance the health and well-being of a defined population. This commitment has resulted in priority given to aggressive cost control, organizational consolidation, system integration, market concentration, and image marketing on the basis of perceived differences in quality.

These rather profound changes in health care organization, provider incentives, and relationships among providers, consumers, and purchasers have had a considerable impact on HRM within health care and rehabilitation service organizations. As provider organizations have reduced staff to lower personnel costs, thereby increasing labor productivity

in the short term, the potential for work-related stress, conflict, erosion of employee commitment and loyalty, and professional "burnout" has increased accordingly. Concomitantly, the implementation of new technologies, especially information technology, entails greater demands on employees to develop and continuously upgrade their skills and knowledge base to adapt to the plethora of information management tools and resources. Managers especially are faced with the pressures of maintaining their own professional and clinical competence while accommodating the new developments in information technology and information systems and adapting their leadership style and philosophy to the realities of changing employee values and expectations and to innovative structures (i.e., the horizontal, loosely linked, team-based organization).

The inevitability of change, if not of its specific forms or trajectory, is perhaps the only safe prediction about health care organization and delivery in the long term. Consequently, it can be argued that the most critical competencies of the health care manager and professional of the twenty-first century are the capacity to do the following:

- Exercise flexibility in response to continuous environmental change
- Communicate effectively with various stakeholders representing multiple and often conflicting priorities
- Direct the efforts of an increasingly diverse and mobile workforce resistant to traditional forms of control

Challenges for Health Information Management Professionals

Managing health information in the twenty-first century places special demands on health information management (HIM) professionals to obtain, train, retain, use, fully develop, and direct the efforts of the human resources required to achieve the goals of health care organizations. Several serious studies have concluded that the health care labor force of the future will demand multiskilled workers who have the flexibility of working in interdisciplinary teams in various provider settings within integrated health care systems and networks. As early as 15 years ago, the Pew Commission had concluded that "the evolving nature of our health care system will require health professionals with different skills, attitudes and values … creating a growing demand for the skills of collaboration, effective communication and teamwork."[7] Health information managers, professionals, and technologists will be required to serve health care delivery systems that emphasize preventive, rehabilitative, and long-term care and will increasingly coordinate services across providers, disciplines, levels, and loci of care. As community-based and home health services expand, there will be increased demands for integration of clinical and financial data and capturing information relevant to various outcome measures at the individual patient or client level, that is, the health record, and aggregated at the service population or community level. In the presence of considerable uncertainty about exactly how health care will be organized and delivered in the next generation, it can be predicted with confidence that health information managers must be prepared to respond to accelerating changes in technology, public policy, competitive markets, population distribution, employee diversity, and organizational structures.

Leadership and Human Resources Management

Leadership and management are closely related terms that convey different but complementary aspects of the behavior associated with ensuring effective organizational performance. Bennis and Nanus make the distinction in this way: "Managers are people who do things right and leaders are people who do the right things" (p. 221).[8] One implicit difference suggested by this characterization is that managers focus on efficiency and control, whereas leaders focus on the "big picture" (i.e., communicating a vision of the organization and inspiring and influencing people to invest in achieving it). Both perspectives and the associated activities of working managers and leaders at all levels are necessary to sustain effective, high-performance organizations. Although this applies to all complex organizations, it might be argued that in no sector of society is the need for visionary leadership and effective management of organizational resources more important than in health care in the twenty-first century.

One of the most obvious but surprisingly complex questions is "What is leadership, actually?" A massive volume of literature in leadership theory and practice has attempted to address this question during the past century, including controlled social science research studies and more descriptive, intuitive narratives from practicing leaders and executive managers. Some researchers have concluded, on the basis of a lack of reliable findings about the nature of leadership in thousands of studies, that its usefulness as a research variable may no longer be warranted. Nonetheless, common wisdom would suggest that leaders do make a difference in influencing the satisfaction, motivation, and achievements of their followers and in effecting organizational outcomes—even if these outcomes are difficult to measure reliably. Most working professionals would agree that, even if they are not absolutely certain about what makes leaders effective, they know that we need effective leaders, especially when we face difficult challenges, rapid change, and crises.

Overview of Leadership Theory

Even a summary of the basic themes and models of leadership developed during the past 50 years would go beyond the limits of this chapter. However, an overview of the key themes and approaches to leadership should be useful in demonstrating the direct relevance of HRM to leadership. One basic difference in the evolving models of management has been the distinction between those that focus on the characteristics of leaders independent of other factors affecting leadership and those that emphasize leadership as a set of relationships. The former is the "trait" approach, which is based on the assumption that leadership could be fully explained by identifying a cluster of personality and character traits that are necessary and sufficient for the leader to be effective. Stogdill's[9] meta-analysis of many such studies found that there was little correlation among the various sets of traits identified, although some characteristics (e.g., intelligence, initiative, and self-confidence) were frequently identified.

Beyond the lack of agreement about a common and sufficient core of traits was the recognition that different situations seemed to call for different kinds of leadership. For example, the ideal leader for handling a true crisis (i.e., effective decision making under fire) may not necessarily have the best qualities for gaining commitment to a pervasive and long-term process of organization change. This contingency approach to leadership recognizes that other variables in the leadership situation or context are likely to influence the leader's behavior and effectiveness. Among the variables identified in research studies using this model are the nature of the task, the expectations and maturity of followers, and the stability of the environment.[10] One implication of a contingency approach to leadership is recognizing that what it takes to be an effective leader all depends on the situation the leader faces.

Relationships and Leadership Style

The fact that the nature of followers is recognized by the contingency approach as being an important variable suggests the importance of considering the relational nature of leadership. On one level it is obvious that the concept of leadership entails that some others are being led as followers. A credentialed health information manager might be an exceptionally competent and knowledgeable professional. But unless he or she has responsibility for directing the efforts of others, he or she is not a leader. So the aspect of relationship is inherent to a full understanding of leadership. This is also suggested by the leadership style approaches to leadership exemplified by the University of Michigan[11] and Ohio State studies[9] of leadership style or behavior. In both these classic studies researchers attempted to determine which leadership styles were associated with effective group and organization performance. In these studies, two dimensions of leadership behavior were identified as characterizing different leadership styles: the Ohio State study identified these behavioral aspects as "initiating structure" and "consideration," whereas in the Michigan State studies the comparable dimensions were called "production orientation" and "employee orientation." The first dimension focused on task behaviors and structuring and organizing work, whereas the second emphasized maintaining supportive relationships, especially between the leader (supervisor) and the followers (subordinates). These same dimensions are also the basis for the popular Managerial Grid, developed by Blake and McCanse,[12] which describes five contrasting leadership styles (Figure 16-1).

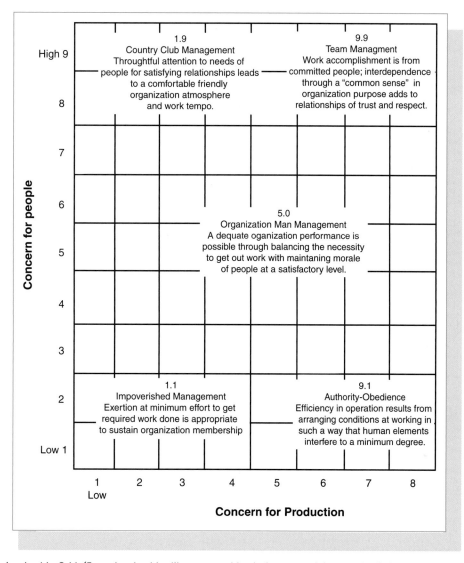

Figure 16-1 The Leadership Grid. (From *Leadership dilemmas—grid solutions,* copyright 1991 by Robert R. Blake and the estate of Jane S. Mouton, Austin, TX. Gulf Publishing Co.)

A more sophisticated and dynamic approach to leadership is the situational leadership model developed by Hersey and Blanchard,[13] which builds on the task behavior and relationship behavior vectors. However, this model also incorporates a situational variable, the maturity of followers, to suggest which leadership style might be most appropriate in a given situation. The quadrants on the charts (see Leadership roles matrix) correspond to four distinctive leadership roles: controller, coach, partner/colleague, and delegator. The effectiveness of these roles, in terms of individual and team satisfaction and productivity, will depend on the degree of team development and maturity achieved (Figure 16-2).

Although by no means conclusive, the leadership style studies collectively suggested that effective leaders generally are those who exhibit both a high concern for productivity and for people. Fiedler's[10] research linking leadership behavior to similar dimensions suggested that a structuring style was more appropriate when the leadership situation was either very favorable or very unfavorable to the leader, whereas a more people-oriented behavior was more appropriate when the leader faced ambiguous circumstances. What seems clear is that over the long term the leader must attend to both production and people concerns to continue to be effective.

Human resource management can and should provide support to the operating manager to enhance his or her efforts in both domains. For example, effective employee recruitment and selection and job analysis processes can be useful tools in task structuring, whereas diversity

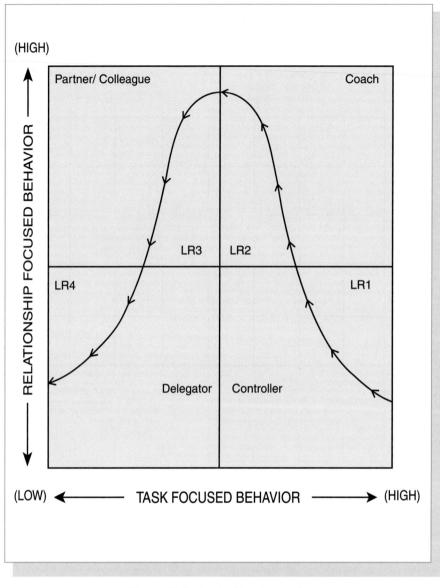

Figure 16-2 Leadership roles matrix.

management training can enhance the manager's relational skills. Even a significant investment in the HRM function cannot guarantee effective leadership in the specific case, but without effective HRM processes, the manager may be at a distinct disadvantage. It could be argued that the more effective and efficient are the HRM technical functions, the more time and energy the manager will have to invest in his relationship-building activities with his employees and peers.

Transformational Leadership

Another useful perspective on leadership is that provided by Burns in his historical and psychological analysis of leadership.[14] Burns contrasts two aspects or types of leadership: transactional and transformational. **Transactional**

leadership refers to those behaviors associated with the more routine and continuing exchanges of effort and commitment between managers and employees in carrying out the business of the organization and sustaining effective working relationships. The **transformational** role of the leader refers to the visionary, motivational, and charismatic aspects of leadership. The transformational leader is able to articulate a vision of the organization's future, to convince followers that they have a stake in the achievement of that vision, and to achieve commitment to change (personal and organizational) as not only inevitable but also beneficial both to the organization and to the employee's self-interest. Schein[15] focuses on the role of the leader as a change agent transforming organizational cultures by destroying dysfunctional ones and stimulating cultures supportive of growth and innovation. Hunt and Conger[16] cite Tosi's insistence that these aspects of leadership are complementary and necessary: "Supporting most successful charismatic/transforming leaders is their ability to effectively manage (transact with subordinates) the day-to-day mundane events that clog most leaders' agendas. Without transactional leadership skills, even the most awe-inspiring transformational leader may fail to accomplish his or her intended mission." Rohrer[17] has proposed a third dimension, **translational** leadership, that allows for the effective communication of the charismatic vision into practice at the operating level—and that this aspect of leadership is an especially important responsibility of the middle manager as the key liaison between executive management and the first-line supervisory and operating staff. From this perspective the HRM director can be viewed as playing a "translational" role in establishing, communicating, and helping to implement HRM policies and procedures that support the strategic direction and goals of the health care organization.

Leadership Development

Another aspect of leadership that has direct implications for HRM is that of emerging leadership and leadership development. If leadership is viewed primarily as being most characteristic of executive level management, then leadership identification and development efforts are very narrowly focused. However, if leadership is viewed as a capacity that is more widely distributed throughout the organization, the issues of emerging leadership and leadership development become more challenging and complex. Although a useful distinction has been made between management as a set of technical and control activities focused on maintaining day-to-day operations and the status quo in the short term and leadership as entailing a proactive, visionary, strategic, and empowering perspective, it could be argued that both are required at all managerial levels in the organization. Health care organizations present additional challenges in this respect because of the professional specializations that go with the territory so that each health professional is subject to the claims and influences of both clinical and administrative leaders. Both training and development and performance appraisal functions within HRM should play a critical role in leadership development at the lower and middle management levels, including the early identification of potential executive managers from lower in the ranks.

The Ethics of Leadership

Although not necessarily recognized as an HRM responsibility, the development of ethically responsible managers and leaders has profound implications for HRM. A justification for serious consideration of the ethical dimension of leadership, specifically in health care is expressed by Darr[18]: "For the health services manager, a personal ethic is a moral framework for relationships with employees, patients, organization, and community. In these relationships, the manager is not, and cannot be, a morally neutral technocrat. The manager is a moral agent ... (p. 1)." What follows from Darr's claim is that all managerial behavior—at least all activity that is relational rather than purely technical—must be considered from an ethical or moral perspective. This also suggests that ethical decision making is complicated by the fact that the manager must consider his or her decisions in terms of the interests of various constituency groups. Burns's[14] theory of transformational leadership also places the ethical dimension at the core of leadership in that it is rooted in individual, organizational, and societal values. He contends that "transforming leaders 'raise' their followers up through levels of morality (p. 426)." He notes that transformational leaders are more concerned about "end values" such as justice and equality, whereas transactional leaders focus more on modal (means) values such as honesty and fairness. Characteristic of both types of leadership is the leader's role in serving a common purpose that transcends individual needs and interests (of the leader and the followers).

Normative ethics may be defined as the science or art of determining principles, rules, and guidelines for right conduct (i.e., how one should behave responsibly in the community). For example, the preamble to the American Health Information Management Association (AHIMA) Code of Ethics (2004) states[24]:

> The ethical obligations of the health information management (HIM) professional include the protection of patient privacy and confidential information; disclosure of information; development, use and maintenance of health information systems and health records; and the quality of information. Both handwritten and computerized medical records contain many sacred stories—stories that must be protected on behalf of the individual and the aggregate community of persons served in the healthcare system. Healthcare consumers are increasingly concerned about the loss of privacy and the inability to control the dissemination of their protected information. Core health information issues include what information should be collected; how the information should be handled, who should have access to the information and under what conditions the information should be disclosed.

Ethical obligations are central to the professional's responsibility, regardless of the employment site or the method of collection, storage, and security of health information. Sensitive information (genetic, adoption, drug, alcohol, sexual, and behavioral information) requires special attention to prevent misuse. Entrepreneurial roles require expertise in the protection of the information in the world of business and interactions with consumers.

It would be difficult to argue with this statement of ethical accountability—and these standards—for HIM professionals could be applied to all health care professionals and managers through the health care system. Yet what specifically are the exemplary values that are to ground and guide ethical behavior in health care? Although numerous lists of values have been presented as core or fundamental to ethically responsive behavior in health care, the following values have achieved a broad consensus as *prima facie* ethical duties:

Respect for Person. Regarding each person (patient, subordinate, boss, peer, neighbor) as an end in himself or herself rather than as a means to some end or as an impersonal stereotype. This value entails granting the other person the maximum freedom that the nature of the relationship allows without impairing the freedom or welfare of others.

Beneficence (Service). Represents a commitment to doing good for, or providing service to, the other person, community, or broader society. A disposition toward competent, caring service to specific individuals (e.g., clients) or the broader community seems to be intrinsic in the health care professions. Although the focus of the direct care provider, physician, or therapist is usually on the health and well-being of the individual patient, the health care manager must also consider the effects of his or her decisions on the organization, the population or community it serves, and the broader society, including the global impact, if any. That the interests of the individual and the community may differ and conflict is a challenge faced often by the ethically responsive public health professional.

Nonmaleficence. This value forbids the ethically responsive person from doing harm or injury to the person or welfare of another. In one sense this represents the other side of the coin of the duty to do good. This is represented by the Hippocratic oath, which indicates that the physician's primary responsibility is to "do no harm." Like beneficence, this value challenges the ethical manager to consider and balance the needs and interests of all his or her key constituencies in making decisions with ethical consequences.

Justice. Often regarded as synonymous with fairness, acting justly in practice almost always is more complex than it appears. One more elaborate definition of justice is ensuring that equals are treated equally while "unequals" may be treated differentially. For example, all patients presenting with diabetes symptoms at the same stage of the disease should be given equivalent (if not strictly identical) treatment by the physician. However, if two patients present in an emergency department at the same time, the one with massive head trauma from an automobile accident should be given priority attention over the patient with a broken toe. The grounds for making these distinctions are addressed in discussion of the concept of distributive justice. For example, if the manager is allocating the end-of-year salary increases, which factors should be given most weight—past performance, recent acquisition of new skills, seniority, or some other consideration?

Other Core Values in Health Care Management

Northouse[19] adds two other values critical to leadership that generally are certainly worth consideration: honesty and building community. A compelling argument could be made that honesty or truth telling is a bedrock value on which all others are founded. Certainly our entire social fabric and the stability and integrity of our organizational culture depends on the assumption that most people, most of the time, are telling the truth as they see it. Without this ethical foundation, we could not make any reliable assumptions about the link between intentions, speech, and behavior of ourselves or of those with whom we interact. Honesty is not only the best policy ethically; it is the only reasonable basis for group behavior, organizational effectiveness, and managerial decision making in the long run.

If honesty is seen as a necessary precondition for ethical behavior, community building may be viewed as an outcome of ethical leadership. Northouse[22] argues that ethical leadership requires a community-oriented perspective. "Transformational leaders and followers begin to reach out to wider social collectivities and seek to establish higher and broader moral purposes …. An ethical leader is concerned with the common good—in the broadest sense (p. 316)." Implicit in this statement is that ethical leaders will attempt to align their actions to the extent possible with the good of the community and broader society. For example, the Board of Directors and executive management team of a hospital should consider the impact of a potential relocation of the facility from the urban core to a growing suburb on both communities affected.

Ethics of the Ordinary

Students of HIM often assume that the really important ethical issues in health care are those "life, death, and well-being" decisions made primarily by physicians and other hands-on practitioners and that most health care managers and support professionals would have little or no direct involvement in such ethical decisions. Historically the focus of ethics as applied to health care has been on the problems of biomedical and clinical ethics faced by the practitioner or researcher. Although these issues are of considerable concern to society as a whole and to ensuring ethical practices in medicine and research involving human subjects, this perspective is too narrow because it ignores the ethical implications of managerial practice in health care. Worthley[20] emphasizes the need for greater attention to the "ethics of the ordinary" in health care and for developing ethically responsive health care providers and managers at the level of the "routine and humdrum in which many less visible [ethical] challenges surface on a daily basis (p. 2)." Worthley focuses instead at the "microlevel" of ethical behavior: on the innumerable ethical decisions faced in the midst of the daily routine of the health care manager and HIM professional. He argues for the importance of this largely ignored realm of behavior on the basis that "the life of the individual healthcare provider—doctor, nurse, technician, administrator—is largely one of routine and humdrum in which many less visible challenges surface on a daily basis, and in which many ordinary, indirect, and subtle actions must be and are taken" (p. 2).[20] It is within this domain of "the ordinary" that health information professionals will be making most of their ethical decisions, including ones of real consequence to the welfare of the patients, their coworkers, their bosses and their own families. Even in the midst of their routine work, the HIM professional and the health care manager are moral agents—and this responsibility goes with their professional territory.

Power and Ethical Decision Making

In this context the concepts of power and values clarification on the decision-making process are fundamental. **Power** has famously been defined as the ability of person A to influence person B to do something he or she would otherwise not decide to do.[21] Understanding the effects of power, especially differences in the power held or sought by key players in the decision-making situation, is necessary in sorting out the ethical implications of alternative decisions. For example, the ethical health information manager should consider as a criterion in her decision making about a coding strategy the implications for the most vulnerable groups affected (i.e., the self-paying, uninsured). Those decision makers who are relatively powerful on the basis of their positions in the organization or their expertise have special responsibility for considering the ethical consequences of their behavior as it affects those with less power and influence, including their staff and clients within and outside the organization.

Values Clarification

Values clarification is also an essential process as a precondition for ethically responsive decision making and leadership. Rokeach[22] has characterized values as "standards that guide ongoing activities" and value systems as "general plans employed to resolve conflicts and to make decisions (p. 21)." He goes on to identify two sets of values, the instrumental, which identifies behavioral attributes such as "ambitious" and "responsible," and terminal or end-state values, such as "wisdom" and "a world at peace" with the former set of values seen as means to achieving the latter. Rokeach's instrumental approach to ethics suggests the practical nature of values and the real advantage, if not absolute necessity, of reflecting on and being clear about our own value commitments and priorities. For example, if we are forced to make a decision that seems to sacrifice "respect for persons" or individual autonomy for societal justice, are we willing to make that tradeoff? What, in fact, are our own ethical "nonnegotiables"? We are likely to be more confident, dependable, and balanced decision makers (and perceived to be fair and trustworthy leaders) to the extent that we continue to engage in thoughtful values clarification internally and with our employees.

Servant Leadership

Servant leadership was a paradoxical approach to leadership behavior developed by Greenleaf[23] that had a clear ethical foundation and spiritual undertones. Greenleaf argued that the essence of leadership was rooted in effectively serving, nurturing, and empowering one's followers. By taking on the role of servant, the emerging leader would gain the trust, respect, and loyalty of his or her followers. Also by serving to empower his or her followers, the leader should increase the productive capabilities of those to whom he or she is accountable. In this way ethical responsiveness is linked directly to performance improvement. Greenleaf also extends the scope of the leader's servant role to encompass social responsibility, equity, and justice. Ideally, the leader also serves by championing those outside the organization who are marginalized, powerless, and disadvantaged.

Greenleaf's primary contribution was to give serious attention to the ethical and good citizenship dimensions of leadership and to provide a foundation for a "business case" for altruistic and ethically responsive leadership. The core concept is certainly not new as it draws on early Christian sources (e.g., "Rather let the greatest among you become as the youngest, and the leader as one who serves." [Luke 22:26]). This perspective which was consistent with the countercultural ethos of the 1970s may seem somewhat anachronistic today. Nonetheless, given the leadership failures and financial crises in the last decades of the twentieth and the early twenty-first centuries both in corporate board rooms and in health care (e.g., AHERF, Columbia/Hospital Corporation of America [HCA], and HealthSouth), a re-examination of the servant leader model is timely.

Applications to Human Resources Management

The preceding discussion of ethics highlights the pervasiveness of the ethical aspects of decision making in health care both for the hands-on provider, other support professionals, the health care manager, and the HIM professional. It could be argued that, in spite of its absence in many discussions of the field, ethics is critical to effective HRM. For example, ethical responsibility or maturity should be included as a criterion in managerial recruitment and selection processes if we indeed give priority to the ethical conduct of our managers and intend to inculcate or reinforce a set of core ethical values in our organization's culture. Certainly the training and development function is an appropriate venue for addressing managerial ethics in formal supervisory training. HRM can also play a role in communicating and monitoring policies and procedures with ethical implications (e.g., ensuring due process in the disciplinary function, fair and justifiable allocation of employee compensation, etc.). Perhaps just as important, HRM leaders should serve as advocates for and models of ethical responsiveness in decision making by emphasizing the organization's core values in the implementation of top management's vision, the organizational mission, and strategic direction.

Although the role modeling of ethical behavior must flow from the top of the organization, as being an explicit and high priority endorsed and sanctioned by the Board of

Directors and the chief executive officer (CEO), it must be evident in practice at the supervisory level if employees are to regard this commitment seriously. One way to ensure that ethical behavior is given priority by management is to include it as a behavioral dimension within the formal performance appraisal process. This presents a challenge in developing clear criteria and objective measures that allow for valid and reliable assessment of the employee on this dimension. Nonetheless, if management is genuinely committed to fostering ethical behavior and ethical sensitivity in decision making, these goals must be given more than token endorsement. Managers, clinicians, and other health professionals must be held accountable for ethical behavior in practice.

Codes of Ethics

Methods to encourage ethical practice in an administrative environment include specific organizational policies and procedures to ensure compliance, formal expressions of core values, and organizational and professional codes of ethics. For example, Mercy Hospital of Pittsburgh, a member hospital of the Catholic Health East system, operated by the Sisters of Mercy, makes its value commitments explicit as a set of core values directly related to its mission statement. These core values (i.e., reverence for each person, community, justice, commitment to the poor, stewardship, courage, and integrity) reflect the values of the Roman Catholic faith and the religious community that sponsors and supports the hospital. However, these values as understood by the organization can also be used as standards to develop criteria and measures for evaluation of organizational and individual performance.

The following excerpt from the AHIMA Code of Ethics suggests the tenor and scope of professional codes of ethics and the profound implications for managerial behavior and decision making:

> The mission of the HIM profession is based on core professional values developed since the inception of the Association in 1928. These values and the inherent ethical responsibilities for AHIMA members and credentialed HIM professionals include providing service, protecting medical, social, and financial information, promoting confidentiality; and preserving and securing health information. Values to the healthcare team include promoting the quality and advancement of collaboration. Professional values in relationship to the employer include protecting committee deliberations and complying with laws, regulations, and policies. Professional values related to the public include advocating change, refusing to participate or conceal unethical practices, and reporting violations of practice standards to the proper authorities. Professional values to individual and professional associations include obligations to be honest, bringing honor to self, peers and profession, committing to continuing education and lifelong learning, performing Association duties honorably, strengthening professional membership, representing the profession to the public, and promoting and participating in research.[24]

Although specifically addressed to HIM professionals, this statement could be applied to virtually all health care managers at any level and functional specialization. The purpose, limits, and utility of professional codes of ethics are presented explicitly in the following AHIMA statement:

> A code of ethics cannot guarantee ethical behavior. Moreover, a code of ethics cannot resolve all ethical issues or disputes or capture the richness and complexity involved in striving to make responsible choices within a moral community. Rather, a code of ethics sets forth values and ethical principles, and offers ethical guidelines to which professionals aspire and by which their actions can be judged. Ethical behaviors result from a personal commitment to engage in ethical practice. Professional responsibilities often require an individual to move beyond personal values. For example, an individual might demonstrate behaviors that are based on the values of honesty, providing service to others, or demonstrating loyalty. In addition to these, professional values might require promoting confidentiality, facilitating interdisciplinary collaboration, and refusing to participate or conceal unethical practices. Professional values could require a more comprehensive set of values than what an individual needs to be an ethical agent in their personal lives.[24]

The most notable aspects of this section of the AHIMA code is the pervasiveness of the ethical accountability suggested (i.e., that the ethical HIM professional lives an ethical life in every respect and venue as opposed to making ethical pronouncements). Also, this statement explicitly grounds the ethical imperative to the employer, the public, and the individual—the primary constituencies of the health care system (i.e., the patient, resident, and client of services). This standard then serves not only as the ultimate criterion of quality, it also serves to ground all ethical decision making in health care.

Systems Perspective on Human Resource Management

This treatment of HRM will adopt the image or metaphor of the organization as an open system, that is, the organization as a living organism that attempts to achieve and maintain an equilibrium with its ever-changing environment.[25] Within this conceptual framework, HRM is viewed as a subsystem linked to and interdependent with other subsystems, such as financial management, within the internal environment of the organization. Each subsystem and the organization as a whole are subject to continuing influences from the external environment. To survive and thrive, the organization must respond and adapt effectively to these environmental forces. The latter can be distinguished as an unstable array or irregular flow of resources, constraints, threats, and opportunities. To maintain equilibrium with its environment, the organization must ensure an adequate flow of resources to sustain energy for continuing activities

CASE ANALYSIS: ETHICAL ASPECTS OF ADMINISTRATIVE DECISION MAKING

Donna Veritas, Assistant Director of HIM at St. Andrew's MetroCare Hospital, was asked to attend a department chair's meeting in place of her boss, Sam Murky. In response to her asking how she should prepare for the meeting, Murky warned her that she might be asked about the late budget requests from their department. He advised Donna that, if questioned about this, she should suggest that a chronic software problem compounded by excessive absence on the part of a senior member of the staff led to a medical record processing backlog that had further delayed the completion of their budget package. Donna was unaware of any software problem but was quite aware that one of her recently hired coding staff was on short-term leave for the past 2 weeks for hospitalization for an acute illness. The medical record processing backlog, however, had been a chronic problem for the past 2 years in part because of higher-than-anticipated turnover among coders and clerks in the department.

As the first agenda item, the Vice President for Fiscal and Support Services, Rhonda Requisite, announced that, as indicated in an earlier e-mail to all department heads, each manager would be expected to make a short presentation on his or her unit's budget proposal. The head of radiology, who was asked to begin the process, made a polished presentation with the use of PowerPoint slides. After some tough questions about his budget assumptions, Rhonda turned to Donna and asked her to make the presentation for the HIM department.

Questions for Analysis

How should Donna respond in this situation? What, if any, ethical issues are relevant to her decision? What actions should Donna take after the department head meeting? Who is affected ethically by her response to this situation? Who has primary responsibility for ensuring that ethical considerations are given due consideration within the department—and who within the St. Andrew's Hospital as a whole?

WORDS FROM THE SOURCE: THE LEADER REFLECTS ON LEADERSHIP

The following interview* with an experienced and especially thoughtful executive manager and leader in the field of rehabilitation and disability services addresses many of the aspects of leadership discussed above.

Would you briefly describe your organization, its mission, structure, and history?

Condeluci: UCP of Pittsburgh, Inc. is a multipurpose, nonprofit organization that provides services and supports to more than 1800 individuals with all types of disabilities and their families in Allegheny County, Pittsburgh, Pennsylvania. With a budget of more than $20 million dollars and a staff complement of 500 folks, UCP is working toward a community where each belongs. The agency was founded in 1951 and serves as United Cerebral Palsy affiliate, part of a national alliance of more than 120 disability-oriented agencies.

How would you characterize your leadership role in UCP?

Condeluci: In nonprofit organizations, as in most other organizations, the CEO is responsible for the overall operation of services and accomplishment of the agency mission. Of course, to do this requires the development of a culture and community of people dedicated to the vision and mission. To this end, I believe my most important role is to articulate the mission in a clear and compelling way so as to have the community and all key stakeholders invest in the cause. This means to communicate, nurture, empower, and validate all the stakeholders in their efforts to achieve our vision and mission. Given the goal of full participation of all the people with disabilities that we serve, the culture and community we create must accommodate to all types of physical and cognitive needs. To this extent, we must be fully accessible in architecture as well as attitude. This includes slowing down the pace, minimizing jargon, and removing other barriers to communication to ensure that everyone can participate effectively.

What traits or behaviors do you believe are important for effective leadership?

Condeluci: In thinking about the traits and behaviors associated with leadership, five words came to me fast. The leaders need to be **flexible** (nimble and able to adjust), **focused** (to keep your eyes on the tasks and challenges in front of you), **fair** (to create a culture where people feel valued, listened to, and treated fairly), **firm** (to hold your principles and values firmly in hand when making decisions), and **fun loving** (to create an environment where people can find happiness). In discussing the mental habits of leaders, John Kotter (1996) identifies risk taking, humble self-reflection, solicitation of opinions, careful listening, and openness to new ideas as key habits that successful leaders show. Regardless of the organizational context, effective leadership requires that all these things be balanced.

Do you believe that leaders are born or made? In other words, is leadership genetic or can it be developed?

Condeluci: Are leaders born or made? Probably both. There are some people who are destined to be leaders, though I would assume that this is a small group. Their destiny, however, was clear from the time they were children. Yet, most people, when given the challenge and using key principles and strategies, can emerge as leaders. Most of leadership strategies are ones that can be developed and practiced. One can clearly get better as a leader if he or she works at it. I study, think, and have written (Condeluci, 2002) about leadership actions and strategies every day. On this same point, Donald Krause (1997) says that "The power to lead is a function of character, not an accident of birth or a prerogative of position." This suggests that character traits can be developed and leaders can be shaped.

Continued

*Reflections on leadership I: An interview with Al Condeluci, PhD, Chief Executive Officer, UCP of Pittsburgh, Inc., July 6, 2005.

Do you consider leadership to be primarily the responsibility of top executives in the organization, or is it more widely distributed?

Condeluci: Leadership is definitely about orchestration. I have a dear friend who is Professor of Jazz and Orchestration at Rowan University's School of Music in New Jersey who constantly talks about musical success in terms of orchestration. Certainly you need good musicians, a variety of instruments, and well-written musical scores, but a truly great orchestra is more than the sum of these parts. The conductor is the key to bringing out the best in all three elements. The same is true for the successful leader in any organization. No one person can do it alone—the leader needs to hire the right talent with a broad range of skills, and the ability to motivate these talented individuals to rally around a clear and compelling vision and then to guide them, as a well coordinated and committed team all playing together in harmony.

How would you characterize your own decision making style as a leader?

Condeluci: Successful leadership is the ability to make clear and focused decisions. To this end, decision making is one of those strategies that leaders can develop. When any of us are confronted with a challenge, there is usually an intuitive alternative you are leaning toward. Current research suggests that intuitive decisions on average are as good as long, drawn out decision making (Gladwell, 2005). For me, timing is critical. If I have the luxury of time, I will put my intuitive decision through the classic decision making steps. If time is short, however, intuition will play a greater role. Always, information from my staff and other reliable sources is welcomed and considered.

Is team development important in your agency? If so, what is the process for developing effective teams?

Condeluci: Team development is critical at UCP. When I became the CEO in 1991, we put together a management team that essentially makes key agency decisions. Each person on the management team, which represented all our major units, had their unique perspective, and when time permits, I attempt to attain a consensus that we all can accept. However, if we are pressed for time, we try to get consensus from at least three of the seven members. *Developing teams is about developing social capital*. The more people get to know each other and find similarities, the easier it is to bond and to bend with each other (Putnam, 2000). Our management team tries to foster both social integration and personal growth, along with achieving our task-oriented goals.

What are your views about the concept of emotional intelligence presented by Goleman (1998) as a dimension of effective leadership?

Condeluci: I am a strong proponent of emotional intelligence. There is no question that people who can relate well and respond to each other on an emotional level will create a deeper bond. The more bonded people are, the more tolerant and flexible they will become. Emotional intelligence is usually associated with "right brain" thinking and it is important to note that, although this type of thinker is considered to be strong in emotional intelligence, he or she can be weak in other important aspects. "Left brained" thinkers often have critical leadership skills such as data analysis, focus, precision and objectivity as strong attributes. As stated earlier, leadership is more about balance, but I'm convinced that emotional intelligence is one of the more important facets of leadership.

Considering the recent examples of leadership failure in the corporate board room, including health care, what is the role of the leader in maintaining ethical behavior within the organization and in relationships to its environment?

Condeluci: Ethical behavior is a must in leadership. If a leader endorses or even passively accepts a position that is unethical, the foundation of trust and respect will be eroded if not lost completely. Leaders who stay focused on the organization's mission and vision and apply honest, forthright principles in their decision making will never go astray. This is not to suggest that every decision will be effective, or that ripples and fallout might not occur. However, the integrity and coherence of the culture that leaders create will be maintained as an organizational strength as long as the leader stays principled. This is consistent with Covey's (1900, 2004) discussions about the importance of principle-centered leadership.

What is your take on the importance of "transformational" and visionary leadership that has been given so much attention in the management literature?

Condeluci: Organizations must always try to be current and responsive to new thinking; but to change or adjust, just to appear "transformational," is wasted energy. Certainly, visionary leadership is a key component for a forward thinking CEO. Sashkin (1992) writes about visionary leadership, but his basic framework revolves around the vision itself. If the vision is not compelling and focused, the organization will flounder. What is more important is for the leader to keep the mission and vision fresh in the eyes of the key stakeholders.

What do you expect will be the greatest challenge facing leaders in health care and social services within the next 10 to 20 years? And how can leaders be better prepared to deal with such challenges?

Condeluci: The biggest challenge for leaders in the future will relate to building and maintaining a strong organizational culture and community. Changing demographics will result in a generation of newly emerging workers who will likely have quite different perspectives on work than those of our generation. What will remain constant, I believe, is that people will continue to value and seek out community, connections, and social capital. If the organization culture offers a strong sense of community to all members and if the leader strives to empower workers at all levels and creates supportive work environments, the more likely the employees will be committed to and invest in their organization.

Do you have any other wisdom or guidance you want to share with entry-level health information managers and professionals about leadership on the basis of your own experience as an executive and your own academic work in this area?

Condeluci: Leadership is one of those topics, like communication, that people often think is automatic and simple. Yet the concept of leadership is more akin to the Asian concept of *shibumi*. The notion of *shibumi* is applied when a situation or idea is both simple yet complex. A good example of *shibumi* would be found in the concept of a bridge. Often bridges are built simply to connect two otherwise separated places. Yet, as any engineer will tell you, designing a bridge is a very complex process. To safely connect two places requires a detailed and well-thought-out plan. I think this same notion of *shibumi* applies to leadership. Many of us will have the opportunity to lead some group, team, or organization unit in the course of our lives. Those who are in this position must make key decisions that may affect the organization as a whole and certainly the working lives of their followers. Although some of the issues discussed in this interview may seem simple, leadership is actually very complex and the process is filled with contingencies, nuances, and feelings. In many ways leadership is an art and you can bet that the successful leader has thought very deeply about his or her role, actions, and the consequences.

Bibliography

Condeluci, A: Cultural shifting: Community leadership and change, Ste. Augustine, 2002, TRN.

Covey S: 7 Habits of highly effective people, New York, 1990, Simon & Schuster.

Covey S: The 8th habit, New York, 2004, Free Press.

Gladwell M: Blink, New York, 2004, Little, Brown.

Kotter J: Leading change, Boston, 1996, Harvard Press.

Krause D: The way of the leader, New York, 1997, Parigee.

Putnam R: Bowling alone, New York, 2000, Simon & Schuster.

Sashkin M: Strategic leadership competencies. In Phillips RL, Hunt JG, editors: Leadership: A multiorganizational-level perspective, New York, 1992, Quorum.

and growth. It must adapt to constraints on its access to resources, its decision making, and its actions. The organization must maintain environmental sensing and intelligence functions to answer the questions "what is out there?" and "how is it going to affect us?"

Technology (or throughput) can be defined as the hardware and software (means) by which the organization transforms inputs into outputs (products, services, and benefits to the community). Technology, however, can also be regarded as an environmental factor that affects the organization as resource, threat, constraint, or opportunity. During the past quarter century the impact of technology on health care and rehabilitation in general and HIM especially has been dramatic and pervasive. The almost incredible developments in information technology not only have changed the way that we access, process, distribute, store, and manage data but also have transformed the fundamental structures and processes of organizations in virtually every industry, including health care. The impact of technology, especially information technology, is recognized, if not always made explicit, as a most important factor affecting HRM practice within health information services.

From a systems perspective, then, we can identify inputs, technology, outputs, and environmental influences as system variables that must be addressed in the organization's strategic management and planning processes. The human resources of a health care organization must be considered to be a key, arguably the most critical, strategic variable. Consequently, this systems perspective should be useful in our examination of HRM with applications relevant to the health care environment and especially to the health information manager.

Systems Approach Applied to Health Information Services

A systems approach to HRM is useful in understanding the organization and dynamics of any human collective enterprise including health information services because this perspective enables our recognition of the complex interrelationships of individual parts to the whole organization (Figure 16-3). It also encourages viewing the organization as being nested within one or more larger, more comprehensive systems, for example, a health information services (HIS) department within an acute care hospital within a comprehensive medical center affiliated with a managed care network as part of a regional health care system. When this systems framework is applied, the interdependence of subsystems within the organization and the important boundary relationships with relevant sectors of the environment must be considered. For example, applying a systems perspective, the HIS manager must deal not only with the relationships between HIS and financial management (internal) but also with a state-level regulatory agency (external).

As information technology becomes increasingly complex, pervasive, and central to the mission of the health care system, the typical HIM department might be more appropriately conceived as a "service center" for the whole enterprise rather than being limited within the confines of a traditional department. This makes a systems view especially useful in understanding how health information services fit within the organization and might be linked to both internal and external constituencies, including patients, providers, insurers, legal offices, regulatory staff, and other clients.

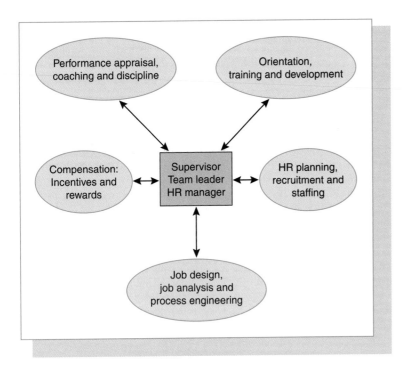

Figure 16-3 Activities and objectives of human resource management.

Systems Perspective Applied to Human Resources Management

Although there are various bases for distinguishing subsystems within any system, the following clusters of human resource functions represent a reasonable and familiar approach:

- Recruitment and employee selection
- Job analysis, job design, and process engineering
- Training and career development
- Performance appraisal and employee development
- Quality management and team building
- Employee and labor relations
- Compensation management
- Employee health and safety
- Regulatory compliance and reporting (e.g., EEO, Occupational Safety and Health Administration [OSHA])

All these subsystems have distinct territories based on historical practice, regulatory scope, and professional or specialist role identification, training, and, in some areas, certification. However, all are interrelated processes, each one addressing some aspect of maintenance and development of the human resources of the system. The health information professional must understand the purpose of these interdependent functions and his or her role in supporting and using these processes. As discussed earlier, these human resource subsystems can be associated with the dynamics of the open systems model: obtaining inputs (employee skills, knowledge, and energy) and transforming these inputs through HRM processes and technologies into outputs (desired results, outcomes, or impact).

Applying a systems view to HIM assists in defining the key variables that affect production within the department (Figure 16-4). Processing the relevant information for a discharged hospital inpatient provides a good example of the interdependence inherent in the systems model. After the patient is discharged, the data must be collected, scanned, or otherwise abstracted and collated in a prescribed order and format. The next step is an analysis of missing data elements before forwarding the records to the physician for completion, if necessary. Completed records are routed to the clinical coding staff to assign diagnosis and procedure codes for billing and indexing. When complete, the records are committed to a permanent storage medium. Unless the volume of records and transactions is very small, one person cannot perform all these functions. Employees with different skills and roles are needed to perform the various functions in the required sequence at appropriate times. If the information is not collected and available in one place when needed, the record cannot be effectively coded or analyzed; and, if data elements are missing, the record cannot be committed to permanent storage. At the least this will result in inefficiencies in processing and decreased productivity. At the worst it could interfere with timely and appropriate patient care.

Human resource activities may be considered by using the same logic. Job analysis, including the creation or revision of a valid and useful job description, should provide the foundation for setting and communicating performance standards and expectations to the employee. Using the job description as a blueprint, the supervisor can prepare for an effective performance review and appraisal with the employee. The performance appraisal process should be completed and

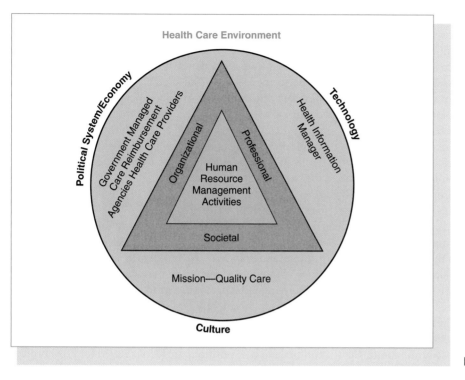

Figure 16-4 Systems model diagram.

documented before sound decisions can be made concerning compensation adjustments and promotions, transfers, or (when circumstances warrant it) disciplinary actions. Effective planning for employee orientation and training programs depends on information generated by the recruiting, selection, and performance appraisal processes and, in some organizations, the quality management subsystem. Environmental challenges from regulatory and legislative changes, economic conditions, and employee lifestyle and cultural influences continually affect all of the subsystems that constitute HRM in health care.

A systems model facilitates a comprehensive and integrated approach for HRM. To provide highly skilled and high-achieving workers, it is critical for the health information manager to match qualified employees with the positions that best fit their knowledge, skills, and job-related personal characteristics. The manager must take responsibility for maintaining staff competence and motivation through continuing education and staff development activities. In addition, it is important to facilitate career ladders and professional or career growth pathways. These programs should be planned, implemented, and evaluated continually to promote qualified and productive HIM professionals and support staff who will facilitate the delivery of high-quality health care and represent their employers and their profession effectively. By applying a systems perspective, managers, consultants, and students in training to be professionals can better appreciate how these processes and roles are linked and interdependent and the implications for addressing organizational problems and challenges strategically.

Environmental Influences and Human Resources Management

The structure and function of health care organizations and providers are continually changing to adapt to the external environment. The organization is limited in its capacity to control these outside forces, so it must develop appropriate HRM solutions in response to external challenges. These responses are more likely to be successful and persist to the extent that they (1) address the problem, (2) are efficient and cost-effective, and (3) are perceived as compatible with the core beliefs and values of the organization culture. The number of potentially relevant influences on the health care organization in general and the health information manager in particular is great, ever changing, and uncertain because what is "relevant" depends on the individual's and the organization's local context and circumstances. Consequently, we must be selective in which environmental influences to address. The following factors are given special attention: women's participation in the workforce, technological change, health policy and industry developments, economic forces and trends, demographic change and diversity, health policy and competition in health care, and the legal and regulatory constraints on HRM.

Women's Participation in the Workforce

Over the past three decades, there has been a rapid increase in the participation of women in the workforce. This trend has had profound consequences for the family, including reallocation of responsibilities for child care and other aspects of parental gender roles, as well as for the economy and the workforce. The increasing level of women seeking work outside the home not only has increased the labor pool for the traditionally "female" jobs including the health care and related jobs of nurses, housekeepers, food service workers, and clerical staff but also has led to pressures for expanding employment and career opportunities for women.

As more women with children assumed full-time jobs and careers outside the home, demand for different types of employee benefit programs and more flexible work schedules grew apace. The increasing presence of women in highly professional, managerial, and executive roles has resulted in a raised level of expectations for equal opportunity, equal compensation (for work of comparable value), and the elimination of irrelevant barriers based on gender rather than on ability to perform the job. During the period from 1975 to 2004, the number of women in the workforce with children at home increased from 14.6 million to 25.9 million, a 77% growth.[26] These changes in women's participation in the workforce and in the prevailing societal attitudes about women's (and men's) roles are reflected in the passage of the FMLA in 1993. This legislation forced many employers to examine and revise policies and procedures about the granting of appropriate leave time and ensuring job security for the employee facing new child care responsibilities or serious illness of a family member.

The increasing number of women in the workforce accompanied by the greater number of single working mothers and of families with both parents working outside the home has affected employee benefits and work schedules. **Cafeteria benefit plans,** in which employees can choose from an array of benefits to fit their needs or lifestyles, are common. For example, working parents may choose a subsidy for on-site child care, whereas a childless worker may choose additional dental insurance. Family leaves for both mother and father and increased number of personal days (which might be used to care for sick children) are other examples of how employers have responded to this profound sociocultural trend.

Job sharing and **flex time** have been offered by employers to accommodate the needs and preferences of working women. Job sharing is a staffing option in which a full-time position is shared by two or more persons. This can provide advantages for both the employer and the employee. The employer has gained some staffing flexibility, for example, reliable coverage for vacations, illness, jury duty, and family emergencies. If additional work hours are required for the short term, two job-sharing employees could be scheduled to perform the job without incurring overtime pay. Advantages for the employee include work schedules that may be arranged to accommodate child care or other lifestyle situations.

Flex time allows employees to control their work schedule within parameters established by management. The employer usually defines a core structure of hours of the day and days of the week in which the employee must work to provide needed services and coverage. The employee's preferred schedule can be arranged flexibly around these core hours and days of the week. Other employers allow flexible scheduling but require employees to submit their schedules in advance, such as 2 weeks to 1 month ahead. The use of flex time often depends on the nature of the work to be performed, that is, the predictability of work flow and how flex scheduling for one job affects overall department operations. If, for example, a project must be completed by a given deadline regardless of the hours expended, the employee or project team may be allowed to schedule work hours at will, provided that the project is completed within the required time period.

Technological Change

Technology continues to be a significant influence on HRM, especially within health information services. Increasingly, routine and standardized tasks, such as most clerical and filing functions, previously performed by lower skilled employees are being converted to computer-based processing. Because this evolving information technology facilitates more time-efficient and cost-effective methods of collecting and displaying data for analysis, new expanded opportunities and new positions are being created for HIM professionals to manage and use information generated by these decision support tools.

New medical equipment and procedures are changing the way medicine is practiced. Increasingly, clinical practice is becoming evidence or outcome based. These trends have had considerable effects on the type of data and methods of data collection that are required for medical practice and rehabilitation. Health care providers continue to explore ways to free clinicians' time to provide patient care and education rather than spending unnecessary time and effort in documentation and administrative procedures. Event-capturing information systems, such as videotape or handheld data entry devices, can provide more accurate and timely information capture with less effort and can provide a greater benefit to patient care than retrospective, narrative documentation can. Digitized documentation can be transmitted over fiberoptic networks, which will allow facilities to manage incoming and outgoing data from other organizations as well as internally generated information. Such information management tools and methods have begun to change the job titles, **job descriptions** (narrative presentations of the key responsibilities, activities, and working conditions associated with a designated job), and allocation of responsibilities within health information services units. Human resource managers must recognize, understand, and accommodate these changing approaches to information capture, transfer, and retrieval.

Health Policy and Industry Developments

As noted earlier, the health policy environment will continue to affect the organization of health care delivery, the dynamics of the health care market, and the incentive structure and priorities of health care providers and managers. These broad and pervasive effects will have direct implications, immediate and long term, for health information managers and HRM. Health care reform measures at federal and state levels, both proposed and enacted, have stimulated the development of managed care organizations to further the policy goals of controlling costs and improving efficiency while enhancing the access to and quality of health care services. In concert with earlier legislative efforts to stimulate competition among health care providers, health care managers have focused on cost-efficiency and productivity enhancement. A common strategy has been to decrease staff, outsource services, and, whenever possible, shift to lower-cost providers in response to changes in Medicare and Medicaid reimbursement, increased competition, and managed care. Continuing trends in federal policy compounded by state legislatures' attempting to trim their human services budgets will force many organizations to make even deeper cuts in staffing and substitute investments in technology for human resources. Unless increased access to care and associated revenues improve health care systems' operating and profit margins, health care reform will probably result in greater consolidation and a net reduction of new jobs and career opportunities in the health care sector.

The philosophy of managed care covering a continuum of health care, rehabilitation, and related support services has already altered the health care landscape by reconfiguring the organizational structure and practice patterns of health care delivery and the risk and incentive structure of key stakeholders. The organizational designs associated with managed care—health management organizations, PPOs, integrated delivery systems, POS, and health networks—will probably persist in some form for the foreseeable future. Unless some version of a nationalized and universal health plan were to become law, the logic that has driven piecemeal and incremental health reform during the past two decades is unlikely to be replaced. One implication of these policy changes and their structural and strategic implications for providers and payers is the critical need for real-time access to health information to support clinical, financial, and other managerial decision making. These developments have opened up a whole new industry centered on electronically based clinical information processing, including data collection, distribution, and storage, perhaps using patient-carried cards or accessing clinical data repositories by way of fiberoptic networks. Along with the increased demand for an integrated, electronic patient record is the need for co-ordinating clinical data with associated financial data both for the individual patient and across a covered population. These and other health information technology and system requirements will provide challenges and opportunities for health information managers, information technologists, and human resource managers in this environment.

Economy Forces and Trends

The state of the economy and the values of key economic variables, such as inflation, unemployment, business growth,

and interest rates, have a profound if somewhat indirect effect on HRM. These and other relevant economic variables shape the size and fluidity of the labor markets for health care workers, stimulate or inhibit the health care organization's capital expansion and enterprise development, and influence the organization's staffing plans and management's ability to use compensation to recruit and retain skilled employees. Normal economic cycles and periodic perturbations in the local, national, and increasingly the global economy will continue to affect the management of human resources.

It is critical for managers continually to anticipate economic trends in relation to the organization's strategic plans, technological developments, and health policy and regulatory changes. Organizations that monitor economic trends can avoid being blindsided by sudden crises that directly affect their HRM goals and activities. If, for example, the regional economy enters a recession because of the contraction or relocation of a dominant business or industry, the multiplier effects could be experienced as lower patient volumes, reduced revenue streams, changes in case mix, and less favorable credit and lending terms of local vendors. Longer-term or chronic economic downturns could result in the health care organization's contracting its business objectives and reducing employment levels. The health care organization might increase its use of contracted services, including temporary staffing, to lower its personnel costs and avoid long-term commitments. However, this approach also threatens the development of relationships of trust and long-term commitment. In certain areas of health care, including imaging and information technology services, contracts are being extended overseas and services outsourced that were once kept in house. The multitude of cost-saving measures can reduce the stress and anxiety associated with uncertainty and instability of the organization's continued economic presence but can increase anxiety among staff for fear of replacement.

As we saw in the 1990s, downsizing of organizations' workforces was a common if not always justifiable component of a more comprehensive corporate re-engineering. These often extensive and hurriedly implemented reductions in force were typically justified on the basis of process rationality, enhanced productivity, and gains in operating and financial performance. In too many cases, however, these draconian measures were an attempt to provide a "quick fix" to "bottom lines," stock market values, and shareholders' impatience. In all too many cases, management discovered in the following business cycle that these drastic cuts in staffing led to understaffing, employee burnout, and threatened lower quality of service.

Reduction in total hours worked, increased overtime, conversion of full-time to part-time or job-shared positions, and net loss of jobs through attrition are alternative methods of cost reduction that address the human costs and dislocation experienced by laid-off workers. Severance pay and outplacement assistance may be offered to smooth the terminated employee's transition to another job, career retraining, or period of unemployment. To preserve the values of trust, mutual respect, and commitment within the organization—all of which have been severely eroded by "downsizing," outsourcing, and layoffs—executive management and leadership at all levels must demonstrate respect for each employee as a valued person and recognize the contributions of all employees, including those exiting the organization. HRM must assume responsibility for ensuring that the appropriate number and type of staff with necessary skills and knowledge are obtained and retained to carry out the mission of the organization effectively and efficiently while sustaining the core values of the organization's culture.

Demographic Changes in the Workforce

Multicultural Workforce. A number of demographic changes evident in U.S. society present challenges in HRM. The population continues to become more diversified in most if not all areas of the country because some minority groups have higher birth rates than the majority. Accordingly, we are experiencing a greater representation of minority group persons in the workforce. The U.S. Department of Labor Statistics predicts a continuing influx of Asians, Hispanics, blacks, and women into the workforce, along with a decline in the proportion of white males. Among current workers scheduled to retire, the majority will be male and almost half will be white. The Bureau of the Census predicts that by the year 2050 non-Hispanic whites will represent only 53% of the population, a decline from 72% in 2000.[27] It can be reasonably predicted that in the twenty-first century the white male of working age will indeed be in a minority position in the U.S. workforce.

Gender Roles. The growing prominence of women in the workforce, not only in numbers but also (at least in some industries) by attainment of managerial and executive leadership roles, is a cultural phenomenon that has had a profound impact on power and interpersonal relationships in most organizations, including health care. As the roles of men and women in our society have become less narrowly defined and more fluid and ambiguous, we have experienced considerable tension and potential for conflict in the workplace. An obvious example in health care is the changing perception of gender roles and power relationships between physicians and nurses. At midcentury, the majority of physicians were men and almost all nurses were women. Subsequently, increasing numbers of women have become physicians and men have become nurses. Furthermore, nurses, regardless of sex, are asserting their claims to professional recognition and autonomy. At the same time, many physicians are feeling frustration from threats to their economic well-being and constraints on their decision-making authority and independence imposed by managed care and other regulatory mechanisms.

In health information services historically, most positions—managerial, technical, and clerical—have been filled by women. Almost certainly this gender segregation has suppressed salary levels and career mobility for health information managers and professionals. As our societal distinctions between male and female roles, capabilities, and career expectations continue to blur, we can anticipate more opportunities for women in health information services and greater upward mobility into executive management and less gender "ghettoization" within HIM.

Age Distribution. As more and more individuals work beyond the typical retirement age of 65 years and the children born in the latter years of the twentieth century begin entering the workforce, the workplace will see a continually lengthened age distribution. Many senior workers of the World War II era have entered retirement, but a significant number are continuing to work beyond the traditional retirement age of 65 years. In health care, it is not uncommon to see physicians either practicing or serving on advisory boards well into their 80s. This cohort models a traditional work ethic and values of loyalty, responsibility, and dedication to coworkers, employers, and patients.

Baby boomers, born between 1946 and 1963, are well advanced in their careers. Some have already assumed executive management and professional leadership roles, whereas others have experienced midcareer dislocations as victims of downsizing. This group tends to be goal oriented but more skeptical about and less motivated by allegiance to an organization or industry than their predecessor generation.

The next major age cohort was born and reared after the societal turmoil of the 1960s. They have experienced general economic affluence, the information revolution, and a backlash against the countercultural values of the 1960s. This generation tends to be politically more conservative than their parents' generation, motivated by personal development, self-actualization, and consumption. As employees, this generation responds to workplace autonomy, "loose" structure and controls, participatory supervision, and non-work-related goals and priorities. In contrast to the World War II generation, the post-1960s employees are less likely to define themselves by their jobs and more likely to engage in multiple careers in the course of their working lives.

Children born in the last two decades of the twentieth century, who are now becoming a formidable presence in the workplace, have grown up in an era dominated by information technology, telecommunications, and the entertainment culture. Many have been perceived as being antagonistic to or apathetic about formal authority, bureaucratic routine, and deep or long-term commitment to a job, organization, or cause. A more accurate appraisal may be that this generation is accustomed to frequent and dynamic changes in their environment and expects unrestricted and real-time access to unlimited sources of information and instant gratification of personal needs and wants. This attitude is reflected in the health care setting as more health information is accessed on-line and a consumer-driven approach to health care is adopted across society.

Each age group shares some characteristics and values based on the impact of societal, cultural, and economic factors that have affected its generation uniquely, and each suffers to some degree from the stereotypes imposed by other generations. These differences in beliefs, attitudes, and expectations, especially about the relationship among work, career, and personal lives, affect how they approach their jobs, coworkers, and managers. The members of the 50- and 60-year-old preretirement generation have a work ethic and value commitments related to careers not necessarily shared by subsequent generations. Intergeneration tensions and conflicts can be anticipated, especially at points of transition, as younger managers assume authority over older employees. The potential for conflict between generations is likely to be exacerbated by the shifts in, and confusion about, the gender roles discussed earlier.

Diversity in the Workplace. Diversity issues and diversity management are receiving more and more attention from businesses and the health care sector. Many believe that the term "diversity" translates only to the term "multicultural" or "multiethnic." Although each workplace will pinpoint a unique definition, the concept encompasses just as much variation as the term implies: differentiation by sex, gender, race, ethnicity, age, sexual orientation, or physical ability.

Until recently, encouraging diversity in the workplace was more or less a "feel-good" tactic. Many organizational leaders will agree that increasing or supporting diversity is strong ideologically and possibly beneficial economically. Supporting diversity allows workers to feel respected and valued for the qualities each can individually bring the organization. Economically, a more diverse workforce should provide more flexibility and adaptability toward the changing needs of the consumer population.

However, while giving the idea lip service, very few organizations have been able to go beyond this point. Hiring managers have indeed been well versed in employment law surrounding affirmative action, gender discrimination, age discrimination, and Americans with disabilities. But, most do little to examine the characteristics of the current environment and do not attempt to recruit individuals that would fill a void in representation of race, ethnicity, age, or sex.

Over the past decade, diversity management has emerged as a new HRM paradigm.[28] While many organizations struggle to realize any economic benefits of their transformation, St. Luke's Health System of Kansas City, Missouri, has emerged as a diversity leader in the health care arena.

Legal and Regulatory Requirements Affecting Human Resources Management

The primary mission of the health care organization is to address the health needs of a given community or defined population. Because it is a very labor-intensive industry, health care is especially dependent on the full and cost-effective use of its human resources in fulfilling this mission. Society's values and priorities are expressed in a formal way through legislation, policies, and regulations. Compliance

CASE STUDY: DIVERSITY MANAGEMENT IN ST. LUKE'S HEALTH SYSTEM

A market survey done by St. Luke's Health System (SLHS) revealed that the populations served by the system would be dramatically changing. Over a 5-year span, certain facilities would face a 23% increase in the Hispanic population and a 17% increase in the African-American population compared with an 8% increase in the white population. The population over age 65 years would increase by 19% and those aged 45 to 64 years would increase by 22%.

The first step taken by SLHS was to create a diversity council to provide direction to the senior management on diversity policy issues. The president and CEO sit on the diversity council and appoint new members from within the system. SLHS then created and recruited a system vice president for diversity to spearhead change throughout the organization.

The SLHS diversity council identified six functional areas in which to target diversity efforts: communications, education, patient relations, employee recruitment and retention, medical staff recruitment and retention, and supplier diversity. A diversity council committee was created within each functional area, cochaired by a director-level staff person and a council member. Successes of the diversity council committees include regular publications on diversity topics in both Web-based and paper forms, production of an exceptional new hire orientation video,

development of a new diversity training curriculum, design of cultural tool kits for nurses' stations, and partnerships with local career building organizations and health care professional institutions such as "Welfare to Work" or the Women's Employment Network.

Cultural tool kits contain a quick reference for nurses and other health care providers to make patients feel comfortable. The correct contacts for interpreter services within the hospital are listed, as well as contacts for appropriate community or religious organizations. A basic "Do and Don't" list will also be included with room for nurses to add notes about their personal experiences. For example, for new Hispanic prenatal patients, DO involve the father and other members of the family in the decision-making process involving care of the mother or new baby.[28a] Many American Indian populations have a more holistic view of health care and often use herbal remedies that are not considered "medicine" but would still have implications regarding drug interactions that clinicians should take care to note.[28b]

Overall success of the diversity initiative within SLHS can already be quantified by the increased number of women in various positions and lower staff turnover throughout the system. These short-term gains speak well of future achievements.

with these statutory and regulatory requirements, such as the *Conditions of Participation* for Medicare and Medicaid, is an important example of the organization's need to be responsive to relevant forces and constraints in its environment.

Another societal expectation that health care and other organizations must address is the right of employees to experience a safe and healthy work environment. Safety is not limited to the corporal environment alone; private information used for identification and benefit information also requires a number of safeguards. Furthermore, during the past half century we have established as public policy that all employees have equal opportunity to satisfy their economic and psychological needs by participation in the workforce generally and through specific jobs and professions of their choosing without facing barriers of discrimination and exclusion. Most human resource activities either directly support or are affected by compliance with legislation and regulatory mechanisms furthering the societal objectives of equal opportunity and fair employment, employee health and safety, and effective union-management relations.

A complex, evolving array of legal and regulatory requirements mandated as public policy through federal, state, and local legislation has pervasive effects on HRM in health care organizations (Table 16-1). These laws, judicial determinations, regulatory agency actions, and administrative guidelines influence and constrain HRM in all its functions, from recruitment and hiring through employee evaluation, promotion, and compensation to the termination process. These legal and regulatory factors impose a considerable administrative burden on line managers, who depend on support from human resource professionals to avoid preventable exposure to legal and financial risk and to provide efficient and cost-effective systems for resolving human resource problems. It could be argued that HRM has become the most regulated set of functions and activities in the workplace. Some of the most pertinent legislation, regulatory processes, and agencies with greatest impact on HRM in health care and rehabilitation are discussed in the following section.

Institutional Accreditation

The Joint Commission. Many health care organizations submit themselves to voluntary accreditation by agencies such as The Joint Commission. The Joint Commission publishes standards, rationale, and elements of performance to measure the effectiveness of leadership, HRM, and organizational performance in health care organizations. The *2006 Comprehensive Accreditation Manual for Hospitals* addresses standards and performance elements that relate specifically to the organization's HRM functions. The Joint Commission calls for hospital leadership to plan, initiate, and oversee the implementation of the following human resource functions:

- *Planning* to ensure "an adequate number and mix of staff that are consistent with the hospital's staffing plan" (HR.1.10).
- *Orientation, training, and education* of competent staff so that they "can describe or demonstrate their roles and responsibilities, based on specific job duties or responsibilities, relative to safety" (HR.2.20).
- Continuing *competence assessment* to ensure that "competence to perform job responsibilities is assessed, demonstrated and maintained" by regular administration of performance evaluations (HR.3.10-3.20).[29]

These standards and performance elements are then used as the basis for the organization's self-assessment and scoring to determine compliance with The Joint Commission's quality standards.

Civil Rights and Equal Employment Opportunity Legislation

Civil Rights Act of 1964, Title VII (as Amended). Title VII of the Civil Rights Act of 1964, which prohibits discrimination in employment on the basis of race, color, religion, sex, or national origin, was the legislative culmination of a growing societal consensus that the vestiges of racial, gender, and other forms of discrimination and segregation had to be eliminated in the workplace as well as in housing and public accommodations. The *Equal Employment Opportunity Act* of 1972 expanded the scope of Title VII and increased the powers of the *Equal Employment Opportunity Commission* (EEOC), the federal agency created to monitor and enforce compliance with Title VII. **Equal employment opportunity** requirements were mandated during the 1960s and 1970s through federal, state, and local legislation and through *Executive Orders* of the President of the United States, which, although not requiring Congressional approval, have the force of law. An example of the latter is EO 11246, which prohibits job discrimination on the basis of race, color, religion, sex, or national origin by contractors and their subcontractors doing business with the federal government and requires that they take certain affirmative action. The Office of Federal Contract Compliance Program (OFCCP) has responsibility to monitor and ensure compliance among enterprises covered under the order.

Affirmative action programs are written, systematic human resource planning tools that outline goals for hiring, training, promoting, and compensating minority groups and women who are protected by EEO laws. Although critics have argued that affirmative action goes beyond the legislative intent and language of Title VII, affirmative action plans are specifically mandated in EO 11246 for businesses under federal contract to address past discrimination and to achieve a workforce that reflects the diversity of the population. In the 1990s, affirmative action plans and other forms of preferential treatment, especially those that set quotas for hiring or selection, were under increasing assault

Table 16-1 FEDERAL REGULATIONS AND AGENCIES THAT AFFECT HUMAN RESOURCES IN HEALTH CARE

Legislation or Agency	Effective Date	People Affected and Key Points
The Joint Commission	Continuing	Voluntary accreditation Leadership and organizational performance
Occupational Safety and Health Act	1970	Safe and healthy environment for all workers
Fair Labor Standards Act	1938; amended 1963	Sets minimum wage, overtime pay, equal pay, child labor, and recordkeeping requirements for employers; 1963 Equal Pay Amendment forbids sex discrimination in pay practices.
National Labor Relations Act (Wagner Act)	1935	Gives employees the right to collective actions and outlaws unfair labor practices by management
Labor Management Relations Act (Taft-Hartley Act)	1947	Outlaws unfair labor practices by unions
Labor Management Reporting and Disclosure Act	1959	Forces unions to represent properly their members' interest
Civil Rights Act of 1964 (Title VII)	1964, amended 1972, 1991	Prohibits discrimination on the basis of race, color, religion, sex, or national origin and ensures equal employment opportunity
Health Care Amendents to the National Labor Relations Act	1974	Extends the coverage and protection of the act to employees of nonprofit hospitals and other health care organizations.
Vietnam Era Veterans' Readjustment Assistance Act	1974	Affirmative efforts to provide employment for qualified disabled veterans and veterans of the Vietnam era
Age Discrimination in Employment Act	1967	Protects employees between the ages of 40 and 70
Americans with Disabilities Act	1990	Outlaws discrimination against disabled people and assures reasonable accommodation for them in the workplace
Family and Medical Leave Act	1993	Grants unpaid leave and provides job security to employees who must take time off for medical reasons for themselves or family members

as representing reverse discrimination. The overturning of affirmative action programs based on racial or ethnic identification for admission to public higher education in California, Texas, and other states reflected unresolved tensions in society about EEO. The conflict can be regarded as one between advocates of providing an even playing field for all citizens (nothing more, nothing less) and those attempting to ensure specific socioeconomic outcomes for one or more preferred groups.

In response to some decisions of the Supreme Court that shifted the burden of proof in alleged discrimination cases to the plaintiff, Congress passed the *Civil Rights Act of 1991*. This legislation, which represents the current phase in the evolution of the statutory foundation for EEO, requires the employer charged with discrimination to demonstrate that the alleged discriminatory employment practices are job related and justified on the basis of business necessity. Furthermore, the act holds the employer liable for discrimination in "mixed motive" cases in situations in which the employer uses the defense that

an employment decision would have been the same (against the interests of the employee) even absent the discriminatory practice. On the other hand, the law also prohibits "race norming," in which the employer uses different cutoff scores as employment criteria for the Title VII–protected classes, for example, holding Hispanics to lower cutoff scores than whites on a standardized cognitive test.

In summary, the thrust of the civil rights movement in the workplace as embodied in EEO legislation was to remove artificial, irrelevant, and unfair barriers to full employment opportunity not relevant to performance in the job. It is recognized that employers may and should discriminate among workers on the basis of effort, skills, productivity, merit, and other job-related criteria. The law is not intended to discourage employers from rewarding excellence or penalizing employees for unacceptable performance. The law requires, however, that employment actions be related to work-related criteria rather than gender, race, religion, or any other prohibited factors.

Two types of discrimination have been acknowledged in case law under Title VII claims: direct discrimination (disparate treatment) and indirect discrimination (disparate impact or effect). **Disparate treatment** occurs when members of a **protected group**, such as women or minorities, receive unequal treatment in an employment action. For example, if a health care provider regularly hires female applicants as file clerks but rarely or never as executive managers, this practice would be liable to claims of disparate treatment. **Disparate impact** occurs when an otherwise neutral employment practice has a differential and adverse impact or effect on one or more of the protected groups. Requiring at least a 2-year college degree for all jobs in an HIM department may have a discriminatory effect on minority workers, who historically have a greater percentage of high school dropouts and lower proportion of college participation than whites or Asian Americans. Any test, standard, or criterion applied must (if challenged) be shown to be necessary for performance of the job and not result in screening out any protected classes.

Gender Discrimination and Sexual Harassment

Pregnancy Discrimination Act of 1978. The *Pregnancy Discrimination Act of 1978* extended Title VII prohibitions against discrimination on the basis of gender by broadening the definition of this form of discrimination to include pregnancy status, childbirth, and related medical conditions. Essentially, the act prohibits the employer from providing the covered employee less favorable benefits than other employees eligible for short-term sick leave or extended disability benefits.

Sexual Harassment. Sexual harassment is not a new problem in the workplace but has been given greater legal scrutiny and media attention as women's participation in the workforce has grown, especially in professional, managerial, and executive positions. According to the Supreme Court's interpretation, sexual harassment falls under the prohibitions against gender discrimination of Title VII of the Civil Rights Act. The EEOC guidelines define sexual harassment as "unwelcome sexual advances, requests for sexual favors, and other verbal or physical conduct of a sexual nature" when such conduct "is made either explicitly or implicitly a term or condition of an individual's employment," when submitting to or rejecting such behavior becomes the basis for an employment decision(s) affecting that person; or when such behavior creates "an intimidating, hostile or offensive working environment" (pp. 4-32).[30]

The ground-breaking legal decision in this area was the Supreme Court's decision in *Meritor Savings v. Vinson* (1986), in which the Court held that the plaintiff did not need to demonstrate a quid pro quo relationship between accepting or rejecting sexual advances and employment decisions (e.g., promotion or termination). Rather, the Court determined that the plaintiff had the burden only of

showing that the harassment resulted in an unfavorable or hostile working environment for the victim.

Sexual harassment as one form of gender discrimination can produce a number of negative effects in the workplace, including decreased productivity, increased worker stress and illness, higher turnover and absenteeism, lower morale, interference with team building, additional recruitment and training costs, and potential legal liabilities. Although it is generally viewed as a "women's issue," both men and women can claim protection against sexual harassment under Title VII, and the victim and alleged harasser may be of the same sex.

Given the Court's interpretation of the prohibitions of sexual harassment law extending to "hostile environment" cases, management's potential liability to such complaints is significant. Indeed, the employer may be held liable for sexual harassment on the basis of employee, supervisory, or managerial behavior even when specific complaints were not brought before management. Consequently, from both a risk management and an ethical perspective, it is clearly in management's interest to take assertive action to prevent such behavior and to take quick action to address any complaints that are reported.

To prevent problems with sexual harassment in the workplace, specific policies should be developed and communicated to all employees prohibiting such behavior and explaining the procedures for reporting, reviewing, and resolving complaints. All supervisors and managers should have training in these policies and procedures and in how to respond effectively to both complaints and observed incidents of sexually offensive behavior. Management must ensure that all complaints of sexual harassment are fully and fairly investigated. The employer's legal liability will be influenced by whether management knew or should have known about the harassment and by what actions, if any, were taken to prevent or stop it. As in most other areas of HRM with consequences for employees' rights and welfare, complete documentation of the relevant facts of the situation and management's actions to respond to the complaint is essential.

Protecting the Rights of Persons with Disabilities

The Individuals with Disabilities Education Act (1970), the Rehabilitation Act of 1973, and the Americans with Disabilities Act (1990) form the legislative foundation for equal opportunity for individuals with disabilities in the workplace, in school, for transportation services, and for other public accommodations. The Rehabilitation Act, comprehensive legislation that prohibits discrimination against "the handicapped" and encourages equal access in employment, education, and medical and rehabilitation services for those with disabilities, is limited in its scope to institutions receiving federal funds and federal agencies. Note that the term "handicapped" is generally avoided by HRM professionals because it is regarded within the disability community as being insensitive and potentially offensive. Section 504 prohibits discrimination by any organization or program receiving federal funds against otherwise qualified individuals on the basis of their disability. Section 501 protects federal employees from discrimination on the basis of disability. Section 502 provides that people with disabilities have barrier-free access to federal and federally financed buildings constructed after 1968. Section 503 mandates that employers with federal contracts in excess of $2500 must avoid employment discrimination against people with disabilities and develop affirmative action plans to employ and promote these individuals. Because Medicare Part A and Medicaid are considered to be federal financial assistance, most health care organizations are covered by this act.

The *Americans with Disabilities Act* extended and expanded the protections of the Rehabilitation Act and has been viewed by advocates of those with disabilities as the culmination of decades of effort and as a crowning achievement of public policy in this area. The National Council on Disability affirms that "the ADA is about enabling people with disabilities to take charge of their lives and join the American mainstream. It seeks to do so by fostering employment opportunities, facilitating access to public transportation and public accommodations, and ensuring the use of our nation's communication systems."[31] Title I of the ADA makes it illegal for organizations with 15 or more employees to discriminate against an *otherwise qualified person* with disabilities if that person can perform the significant job duties with or without **reasonable accommodation.** Recruitment, hiring, promotion, compensation, termination, leaves, layoffs, job assignments, and benefits are all covered under this act.

The definition of disability is broad, stating that a disabled person is one who has a physical or mental impairment that substantially limits one or more of his or her major life activities, has a record of substantially limiting impairment, or is regarded as having a substantially limiting impairment. The courts have tended to interpret disability narrowly within the breadth suggested by the legislative language, although several test cases heard by the Supreme Court in April 1999 would significantly widen its coverage to those with correctable conditions, including visual impairment and hypertension.[32] Recent Supreme Court decisions have tended to narrow the scope of application of those covered by the act, however.

Although the ADA could be regarded as the most sweeping civil rights legislation since Title VII of the Civil Rights Act of 1964, the language of the act does not require the employer to commit to affirmative action initiatives for those in the workforce with disabilities. The applicant with a disability must be qualified by meeting all the job requirements with or without accommodation. The act requires that qualified employees with disabilities receive reasonable accommodation in the workplace to perform the essential job functions without causing undue hardship to the employer. If a job description has marginal functions included,

---

Box 16-1 EXAMPLES OF REASONABLE ACCOMMODATION

- Modifying existing facilities to be readily accessible to and usable by a person with a disability (e.g., widening a cubicle for wheelchair access)
- Restructuring a job to facilitate the employee's disability (e.g., minimizing travel by use of conference calls and e-mail conferencing)
- Modifying work schedules (e.g., providing flex time to accommodate outpatient therapy)
- Acquiring or modifying equipment (e.g., adapted computer keyboards)
- Providing qualified readers or interpreters
- Appropriately modifying examinations, training, or other programs (e.g., on-line versus paper-and-pencil responses)
- Reassigning a current employee to a vacant position

---

the person with a disability cannot be screened out because of inability to perform the nonessential duties if they could reasonably be assigned to someone else (Box 16-1).

What constitutes **undue hardship?** Any action that would require significant difficulty or expense when considered in light of the nature and cost of the accommodation in relation to the size, resources, technology, and structures of the employer's operation is viewed as undue hardship. The courts have tended to place a narrow interpretation on this condition because most accommodations have proved to be easily implemented and neither disruptive nor costly.

The health information manager can comply with the intent of this law by taking the following actions:

- Determine and *document* the essential functions of each job.
- Review job applications to eliminate questions or statements regarding people with disabilities that would make the employer legally liable.
- Inform and train anyone doing employment interviews about the ADA regulations.
- Review the justification for physical examinations as a requirement for employee selection. If medical or physical examinations are necessary, they can be required only after a conditional job offer is extended and must be required of all applicants in this situation as a condition of employment.
- Increase supervisory awareness about the ADA and issues affecting employees with disabilities; for example, post an appropriate ADA poster in a location and format accessible to applicants, employees, and visitors.

Age Discrimination

The *Age Discrimination in Employment Act* of 1967 (as amended) protects employees and applicants 40 years old and older from discrimination on the basis of age. From a public policy perspective, the ADEA can be regarded as a regulatory response to the negative and largely false cultural stereotypes about the aging process generally and about older workers specifically. These stereotypes portray an employee who is transformed into a low-energy, apathetic, cynical, injury-prone, and disengaged hanger-on with nothing left of value to contribute to his or her organization or profession. From this perspective, the best course for management is to encourage and rigidly enforce retirement at an arbitrary age. Not only has this been a needless waste of human resources and proven talent (i.e., losing the skills, knowledge, wisdom, and work ethic of older workers), but also forcing retirement or otherwise marginalizing the older employee generates other social and personal costs.

Several exceptions are recognized in the act to the prohibitions against age discrimination. The employer may be able to demonstrate that age is a *bona fide occupational qualification* (BFOQ), an otherwise prohibited factor construed to be reasonably necessary to the operation of the enterprise. Also, the ADEA makes allowances for forced retirement at age 65 years for "bona fide executives" or those in "high policy-making positions."

The ADEA applies to private employers with 20 or more workers, labor unions, employment agencies, and federal, state, and local government employers. The EEOC, the agency that administers this law, requires employers to demonstrate that "reasonable" factors other than age were considered in making an adverse employment decision once a prima facie case for age discrimination is established. With the graying of the U.S. population and Congressional discussion about increasing the age for Social Security benefit eligibility, a higher proportion of older employees could be anticipated in the workforce. This could lead to more intergenerational conflict over jobs and economic security and consequently to increases in litigation under the ADEA.

Immigration Control and Employment

The *Immigration Reform and Control Act* (IRCA) of 1986 was primarily designed in response to growing public concern in certain regions of the United States about the influx of illegal aliens, including those from Mexico, Central America, and the Far East. Concerns were raised about the impact of these illegal immigrants on employment opportunities for U.S. citizens and legal aliens and on the social service network. The IRCA prohibits employers from hiring or retaining unauthorized and undocumented workers after the effective date of the legislation. However, the act also prohibits discrimination in employment against noncitizens who can document their legal right to work in the United States. The impact of this legislation has been somewhat localized, affecting California, Texas, other southwestern states, and Florida more than other areas. However, political debate has intensified about the impact of illegal and undocumented aliens in the context of homeland security and economic concerns, making this a major public policy issue with direct implications for human resource management.

Employee Health and Workplace Safety

Occupational Safety and Health Act. Growing concern about worker health and safety in the workplace, especially in manufacturing and the extractive industries, with strong backing by organized labor led to Congressional passage of the *Occupational Safety and Health Act* in 1970. In passing OSHA, Congress intended that "certain [occupational and health] standards would define the conduct expected from employers covered by the OSHA, and that adherence to these standards would bring about a safe and healthy workplace."[33]

OSHA covers all workers except those who are self-employed or protected under other federal agencies and those who work on family-owned and -operated farms. It has jurisdiction over every chemical substance, piece of equipment, and work environment that poses even a potential threat to worker health and safety. The extremely detailed OSHA standards are administered by the Occupational Safety and Health Administration, the regulatory agency that issues work and safety standards and schedules inspections to ensure employer compliance.

Health care organizations are also subject to OSHA's regulatory oversight. They are required to communicate to their employees information on the known risks associated with any hazardous materials encountered on the job and label all hazardous materials. A written orientation and training program must be developed and used to educate all employees. Examples of hazards that may affect HIM are electronic equipment operation and exposure to hazardous materials, such as alkaline batteries. Efforts to guarantee protection from exposure to communicable disease may also be required by OSHA for employees who have patient contact. Recordkeeping requirements are extensive but justified on the basis that such documentation constitutes the only effective method of tracking, identifying, and correcting safety and health hazards. Detailed reports must be filed for all occupation-related injuries, illnesses, and deaths.

Through OSHA, the U.S. government has tried to preserve worker health, safety and well-being by requiring employers to provide a safe and hygienic workplace. Severe penalties are imposed on organizations that violate this law because violations could lead to serious injuries or occupational diseases. In its early years of implementation, OSHA was much criticized by the employer community as an example of heavy-handed overregulation. Although business associations and smaller business enterprises might be especially likely to complain about the administrative burden imposed, the general consensus among both management and organized labor is that OSHA has increased the overall awareness of safety and occupational health issues in the workplace.

Privacy of Information

The Health Insurance Portability and Accountability Act of 1996 (HIPAA) has affected employees in the health care sector in two distinct ways. First, HIPAA has mandated the ways in which patients' medical information should be stored and transmitted electronically to ensure that it remains private and is only used for appropriate means. During new-hire orientation, employees learn about the safeguards that must be followed and then take a quiz to ensure comprehension. For example, conversations by nurses and physicians about patient-specific medical concerns should not take place in a busy hallway where details could be easily overheard. HIM specialists working in cubicles or in other areas where multiple pairs of eyes may be present must safeguard any personal health information (PHI). PHI should not be left in plain view of any passersby—this includes the computer monitor, for which a privacy screen may be required. Adherence to HIPAA guidelines is of utmost importance; violations can come with a punishment up to and including immediate termination depending on the severity of the breach.

Second, HIPAA affects the employees of the health care entity. The HRM functions of benefits enrollment and management, Employee Assistance Programs (EAP), and even OSHA compliance will require that employee PHI is handled in some way. The same caution that employees of the health care entity use to protect their patients and consumers must be used by the internal HRM team.

Employee Compensation

The *Fair Labor Standards Act* (FLSA) of 1938 was passed at the end of the Depression era to address a number of employer abuses involving the compensation of employees in various industries. This act (sometimes referred to as the Wage and Hour Law) establishes minimum wage, overtime pay, child labor restrictions, and recordkeeping requirements for employers. For every "covered" job, overtime compensation must be paid at one-and-a-half times the employee's regular rate of pay for every hour over 40 worked in a week or over 80 hours for some health care organizations that use a 14-day pay period, that is, the 8/80 plan. Several categories of employees—executive, administrative, and professional—are exempt from the overtime provisions of the act.

The *Equal Pay Act* of 1963 amended the Fair Labor Standards Act to eliminate gender-based discrimination in pay practices. It requires employers to pay men and women equal wages when the jobs that they perform are equal in skill, effort, and responsibility and are performed under equivalent working conditions. Exceptions are allowed for valid merit or seniority award systems and when individual productivity determines compensation, such as in sales commissions or piece rate work. Some advocates of gender equity have promoted the *comparable worth* doctrine, which calls for equivalence of wages for jobs that, although not identical in content, require comparable skills, knowledge, training, and responsibility. However, the federal courts have not been sympathetic to this expansion of the equal pay logic.

Congressional passage of the *Family and Medical Leave Act* of 1993 reflects the increasing role of women, especially working mothers, in the workforce and the implications for child care arrangements. The FMLA grants up to 12 weeks of unpaid leave annually and affords job security to employees of either sex to address family health care needs and childbirth. Specifically, the FMLA authorizes either parent who is eligible under the act to take leave associated with the birth or adoption of a child. The act also covers leave for care for a spouse, child, or parent as well as for the employee's own extended illness. The FMLA is administered by the U.S. Department of Labor, which enforces compliance with the FMLA for all private, state, and some federal employees.

On return from FMLA leave, employees must be restored to their original jobs or equivalent positions with equivalent pay, benefits, and other terms and conditions of employment. Advance notice of leave of at least 30 days is required from the employee for "foreseeable" circumstances. An employer may require medical certification to support all medical leave requests, including second or third opinions and a fitness-for-duty report to return to work.

The *Employee Retirement Income Security Act* (ERISA) of 1974 is a comprehensive and exceedingly complex federal law governing the administration of employee pension and welfare benefit plans. ERISA evolved in response to increasingly widespread and cynical corporate abuses of employees' pension rights and funds. Although the original version of ERISA passed in 1974 was derided as "lawyer's dream" legislation and as being so complex that employers would not be able to comply even with good intention, the law has furthered the goal of reducing the more notorious examples of pension fund abuse. Among the major objectives of this legislation are to ensure that (1) retirement funds are adequately safeguarded, (2) future benefit obligations are ensured through prudent financing, and (3) benefits are provided to all employees, not just the highly placed and highly paid.

ERISA establishes the fiduciary responsibilities of pension plan administrators and specifies conditions of employee participation, eligibility, vesting, funding, and reporting. The law stipulates management's obligation to communicate clearly to all employees about their pension and welfare benefit rights and options.

Labor Union Legislation

The *National Labor Relations Act* (NLRA), also known as the Wagner Act, has served as the foundation for U.S. labor law and collective bargaining since it became law in 1935. The major legislative intent was to establish as national policy the need to "eliminate the causes of certain substantial obstructions to the free flow of commerce and to mitigate and eliminate those obstructions … by encouraging the practice and procedure of collective bargaining and by protecting the exercise by workers of full freedom of association, self-organization, and designation of representation of their own choosing, for the purpose of negotiating the terms and conditions of employment or other mutual aid or protection" (pp. 4-5).[34]

Several factors led to the passage of this legislation at the end of the Great Depression, including growing public concern about the disruptive effects of labor-management conflict and violence and the recognition that workers had legitimate rights to organize to better represent their interests. In striking contrast to the English common law principle, which considered unions to be a criminal conspiracy against property rights of owners, the NLRA established a formal justification of and mechanisms to implement collective bargaining. The latter was established as an effective and preferred means of formalizing labor-management relations and resolving conflict between these two forces in the workplace.

Specifically, the NLRA gives employees the right to collective action free of employer interference or repercussion. It gives employees the right to form labor unions and bargain with management about wages, hours, and other terms and conditions of employment with the goal of achieving written agreement. When ratified by both sides, the written agreement or contract becomes the basis for managerial actions, employee behavior, and mutual expectations for the life of the agreement.

The NLRA originally prohibited the following unfair labor practices directed toward management (Box 16-2).

To monitor and enforce the NLRA, the act established the National Labor Relations Board (NLRB). The role of the NLRB is to determine an *appropriate bargaining unit* for elections and negotiation, to conduct secret ballot elections that determine whether a union will be recognized, and to investigate and adjudicate any *unfair labor practices* claimed by the employer or the union.

The *Labor Management Relations Act* (1947), commonly referred to as the "Taft-Hartley Act," is a set of amendments to the NLRA passed in response to public concerns about renewed labor conflict threatening the post–World War II economic prosperity and perceptions in the business community that "big labor" had gained unfair advantage under the NLRA. The Taft-Hartley Act addressed these concerns by specifying unfair labor practices committed by unions (Box 16-3).

The *Labor Management Reporting and Disclosure Act* was passed in 1959 as additional amendments to the NLRA in

---

Box 16-2 UNFAIR LABOR PRACTICES

- To interfere, restrain, or coerce employees from engaging in or refraining from collective action covered in the law
- To dominate or interfere with the formation or administration of any labor organization by contributing money or other support to it
- To discriminate against anyone in hiring, retention, or any other condition of employment because of their union activity or noninvolvement
- To discharge, discipline, or otherwise discriminate against employees who have exercised their rights under this act
- To refuse to bargain in good faith with employee representatives

---

Box 16-3 ILLEGAL UNION CONDUCT

- To restrain or coerce employees or employers in the exercise of their legal rights under the NLRA
- To force an employer to discriminate against an employee because of the employee's membership or nonmembership in the union
- To refuse to bargain with an employer in good faith
- To engage in certain kinds of picketing and strikes, such as recognition picketing to force the employer to recognize or bargain with an alternative union than the one already certified
- To engage in "featherbedding," in which management agrees to pay for work not actually performed
- To demand excessive or discriminatory initiation fees
- To engage in secondary boycotts and "hot cargo" agreements

---

response to reported corruption and abuse of power of some influential union leaders. Its major provisions include the following:

- An employee bill of rights
- Financial reporting requirements
- Fair election practices for union offices
- Other measures to curtail and correct abuses of power of union leaders.

The *Health Care Amendments of 1974* represent the most recent revisions of the NLRA and those of special interest to health care organizations. In passing this legislation, Congress attempted to balance its desire to bring most health care workers under the protection of the NLRA with the need to protect health care from the potential conflict and instability associated with some aspects of collective bargaining. In fact, it is estimated that the 1974 amendments covered about 1.5 million health care workers who had not been afforded NLRA protection by extending the act to all voluntary, nonprofit, nongovernmental health care institutions.

The health care amendments include several constraints on collective bargaining unique to health care in recognition of Congressional concern and that of the broader public about preserving stability and reducing conflict within health care organizations and ensuring continuity of service delivery. The most notable of these amendments is the 10-day strike notice, which requires the union to provide written notice to the employer and the *Federal Mediation and Conciliation Service* (FMCS) 10 days in advance of a strike, picketing, or other collective action disrupting work. The 1974 amendments also contain an extended notice period for resolving disputes before contract expiration. Another mechanism is provided to facilitate contract dispute resolution through establishing a *Board of Inquiry* when negotiations reach an impasse and a strike or other disruptive action is threatened. The Board of Inquiry is selected by the director of the FMCS to investigate the facts in dispute, allow a cooling off period, and make a written report of findings of fact and recommendations to resolve the dispute. Although the recommendations are nonbinding, they can be instrumental in highlighting and narrowing differences between the two parties and pointing toward resolution. Finally, this legislation recognizes the historical roots of health care in religious tradition by exempting individuals with faith-based, conscientious objection from showing allegiance to labor or other secular organizations by permitting a waiver of paying union dues.

Built on these foundation blocks of labor legislation are innumerable judicial decisions and administrative law rulings and guidelines that collectively have shaped the process and boundaries of collective bargaining both across industries and within health care. One example is the Supreme Court's decision in 1991 to uphold the NLRB regulations issued in 1988 that reversed the Board's former logic concerning the appropriate composition of bargaining units in health care organizations. This court decision resolved a long-standing conflict between the federal courts and the NLRB over the impact of bargaining unit determination on health care delivery and resulted in establishing clear rules that specified eight narrowly defined bargaining units following the logic applied in the manufacturing sector. Although dealing with an apparently narrow and technical issue, this judicial decision has had significant effects on the direction of collective bargaining in health care with implications for human resource managers.

Managing Human Resources Within the Unionized Environment

The primary objective of labor unions is to become a counterbalancing power to management by presenting a unified and assertive voice calling for improved wages, benefits, job security, or working conditions for the employees represented. Unions justify their claims on workers' support and loyalty by promising to achieve economic and well-being objectives (Box 16-4).

Management almost always opposes vigorously any new attempt at union organization affecting its enterprise or facility. At one level it could be argued that no individual or group holding power would choose rationally to dilute or give up that power except by force or subterfuge. Consequently, executive management collectively (and probably most managers individually) operates so as to preserve and if possible expand its sources of power and degree of control. Consequently, management's response to a unionization drive is predictably assertive opposition.

However determined management is to defeat a union effort, its capacity to mount an aggressive campaign is constrained by the NLRA and the union's right to file unfair labor practice charges with the NLRB. Furthermore, management (more so than union leadership) must consider the long-term effects of its actions on employee satisfaction, morale, and productivity; workforce stability; and quality of service. Accordingly, the employer's wisest campaign strategy is to provide complete, objective information in presenting management's arguments against unionization within the organization. Management has the right under the law to counteract the union's claims but should do so with facts rather than appeals to emotion or unsubstantiated claims. Probably the most important factor is the attitude management demonstrates toward all its employees, those favoring the union and those opposed. Management is best served if it maintains a genuine attitude of respect, trust, and commitment to the welfare of all its employees. If the employer cannot make these value claims authentically, it probably deserves the constraints and costs associated with dealing with a union at the bargaining table. It could be argued that weak, ineffective, and unresponsive management is a good predictor of successful unionization.

Management can provide facts that place its past efforts for the employees in a favorable light and, conversely, that show the adverse effects of unionization in general or the union seeking representation in particular. For example, management can communicate information about union dues; history of picketing, strikes, and election "win rates"; salaries of union officers; and any other relevant facts about the union and its likely behavior and effects on the organization (Box 16-5). However, the ultimate outcome will be influenced by local circumstances and cannot, of course, be guaranteed.

Internal Environment of the Health Care Organization

Organizational Culture

Every organization has its own unique culture that maintains and symbolically represents the meaning and value of organizational roles and functions and managerial and employee activities. Organizational culture is shaped primarily by the organization's leadership, historical factors, core technology, the organization's mission, and key environmental forces. Schein[35] has argued that the leader's key function is to transform organizational culture by destroying confining and dysfunctional aspects of culture that no longer fit its mission and environment and creating

---

Box 16-4 EXAMPLES OF UNION BENEFITS

- Protect jobs within the bargaining unit
- Negotiate the best possible total compensation package for the life of the contract, that is, wages and benefits
- Preserve against the erosion of economic benefits in the future
- Defend workers' rights, including the right to engage in political activity
- Ensure a safe and healthy working environment for all workers

Box 16–5 GUIDELINES FOR MANAGERS AND SUPERVISORS DURING A UNION ORGANIZING CAMPAIGN

Management has both the right and the obligation to

- Tell employees that the organization does not believe that union representation is in their best interest and therefore encourage them to vote "no" on the ballot.
- Answer employees' questions honestly about organizational policy, strategy, and goals in relation to the union's campaign issues.
- Explain the costs of unionization to the employees personally, for example, the necessity of paying union dues and fees.
- Assure employees that with or without the union, management is committed to providing high-quality health care and a desirable working environment and culture for all employees.
- Explain that if the employees choose to recognize the union, any improvements in wages, benefits, and working conditions will thereafter be subject to negotiation and not guaranteed, as the union might suggest.
- Administer appropriate disciplinary action against any employee who threatens or coerces other employees, whether for or against the union.
- Enforce the organization's policy against solicitation and distribution of union literature in compliance with prevailing NLRB rules.

Management should not risk unfair labor practice charges or the erosion of mutual trust and respect of the majority of the employees by engaging in any of the following:

- Surveillance of employees or other kinds of espionage to determine the level of union sentiment or to "finger" employees as union activists
- Interrogating individual employees about their union sympathies or union activity
- Threatening, coercing, or intimidating any employees because of their union support or activities
- Making any specific promises contingent on the outcome of the election
- Offering unilateral improvements in wages, benefits, or working conditions during the election campaign

Data from Werther WB Jr, Davis K: *Human resources and personnel management,* ed 3, New York, 1989, McGraw-Hill, pp. 500-519.

Box 16–6 MAJOR COMPONENTS OF AN ORGANIZATION'S CULTURE

- Foundation assumptions about the person and his or her world
- Basic ideology about the organization's role within society and the economy
- Core values and beliefs that define membership in or affiliation with the organization
- Visible symbols that reflect organization membership and allegiance
- Norms, customs, rituals, and taboos that reflect core values and beliefs

inevitable change, while remembering and appreciating the traditions and legacy of the past, is essential for effective management of organizational culture.

Another challenge is based on the existence of multiple subcultures in all complex organizations. The existence of subcultures with associated differences in values, beliefs, norms, language, dress code, and so forth creates potential misunderstanding, tension, and conflict. For example, accountants in the financial management division are likely to have different values, priorities, jargon, and behavioral expectations than software design engineers. Managers above the unit level, especially human resource managers, must be able to recognize, understand, and respond to this source of potential conflict. Organization leadership must try to channel the potential energy and creativity associated with cultural diversity in productive efforts to further the broader goals of the organization.

Information Systems

Information systems continue to improve in power, efficiency, accessibility, and ease of use. For efficient management of human resource functions, appropriate use of information systems and technology is necessary. Because managing people requires an increasingly large base of relevant information, an adequate information system should be developed to facilitate decision making and to accomplish more work of higher quality with less effort. In many health care organizations, electronic processing has replaced the manual paperwork formerly used for most HRM functions. Increased use of electronic, on-line processing of information should result in better services to employees (as internal clients), more powerful planning tools for the manager, and more cost-effective and accessible information processing for all users in the organization.

Managers and supervisors have an important, continuing responsibility in maintaining complete and accurate information concerning their human resources. The amount of information that must be maintained for each employee has grown exponentially along with the dramatic growth in regulatory oversight and demands for compliance affecting HRM. For example, the FLSA requires that accurate records

new cultural forms and symbols that provide a better fit (Box 16-6).

The challenge for management in the twenty-first century is to create a culture of receptivity to change because this will be necessary for survival given the likelihood of accelerated developments in science, technology, and the global economy. At the same time, leadership must preserve the cultural linkages to its past heroes and achievements and to a clear sense of mission, ties that provide and maintain a sense of greater purpose and commitment among the members of the culture. Preparing the organization for be maintained on all employees to include the employee's identifying information, hourly rate of pay, total hours worked, total earnings, and other data relevant to administering the compensation system.

In addition to this compensation system data, other types of information relevant to HRM are required for each employee. Hire dates and anniversary dates of promotions are needed for **performance appraisal** and ERISA administration. The employee's pay rate and range, job grade classification, current job title, and position number must be recorded. Copies of performance appraisals, job descriptions, disciplinary actions, commendations, and other performance-related documents should be maintained consistent with management policy and (if applicable) terms of the prevailing written agreement. Documentation of participation in orientation, training, or management development programs is important in maintaining a workforce skills inventory and in making decisions about promotions, transfers, and job sharing. These records are essential to provide a justification of and legal defense for various staffing decisions and actions affecting individual employee's compensation and terms and conditions of employment.

Role of Human Resources Management System in Health Care Organization

Human resource activities in the HIM department mirror the activities found in enterprises in other industries (Figure 16-5). A common set of HRM functions, processes, and activities are required to obtain, maintain, and sustain a competent, motivated workforce that through individual and team efforts accomplishes tasks to achieve the goals associated with satisfying the needs of the internal and external consumers of health information services.

HRM systems are also used to assist an organization in fulfilling its specific mission, strategic goals, and business plans. Human resource planning, recruitment and selection, job analysis, training and development, performance appraisal and productivity measurement, quality management and empowerment, compensation management, employee assistance and counseling, discipline, and occupational health and safety are essential human resource processes maintained to further the organization's objectives while addressing broader public policy goals.

The Employee as Client of the Human Resources Management System

Human resource functions can also be seen from the perspective of the individual employee with unique needs, goals, concerns, and priorities. The employee typically attempts to satisfy various needs through participation at work. In Abraham Maslow's model of human motivation, the individual responds to a hierarchy of needs ranging from lower-order physiological and safety needs to higher-order ego and spiritual (peak experience) needs.[36] At least to the degree that the employee's individualized needs and objectives are congruent with the goals of the organization, which must be given priority, HRM systems can be expected to address the individual's needs also. Indeed, not only is it ethically well founded for management to consider the employee's welfare in its decision making, it is essential in the long term for attracting, retaining, and motivating knowledgeable and skilled workers in today's dynamic health care market. Certainly, those employed or seeking employment in HIM with computer science or information technology and systems expertise have many alternative career options within and outside health care.

If the organization routinely fails to satisfy the individual's needs, employee satisfaction is eroded, performance and

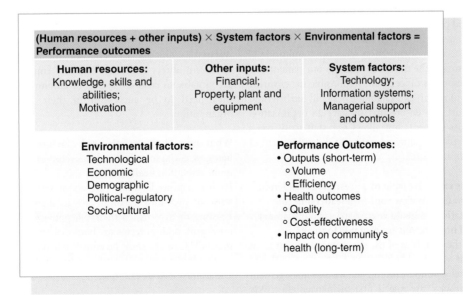

Figure 16-5 Application of the systems model to productivity.

productivity decline, and turnover rates increase. These adverse trends are likely to result in increased costs to the organization both in the direct costs of recruitment, selection, and training and in indirect costs of lost productivity and, ultimately, lower quality patient care. High turnover rates and low employee morale may result in lower levels of customer satisfaction, adverse public relations, loss of market share, and decline in financial viability.

The personal goals and objectives of employees may be addressed through the following human resource activities:

- Supervisory coaching
- Training and development programs
- Career ladders and job rotations
- Performance appraisal and feedback
- Team development and empowerment
- Compensation management
- Employee discipline (linked to a progressive improvement plan)
- Employee assistance services (matched to individual needs)

Clearly, the importance of competent and responsive first-line supervision is paramount because the supervisor often serves as either the facilitator of the employee's growth and well-being in the workplace or as an obstacle to the individual's development.

Employee Assistance Programs

Employees experiencing personal problems may obtain support and referral services through an **employee assist-ance program** (EAP) in most health care organizations. EAPs have emerged as specialized in-house service centers, staffed by professionals such as social workers, counselors, and health educators. Increasingly, the health care organization provides the employee seeking assistance referral to an external provider under contract to ensure professionally competent and confidential services. The purpose of these programs is to help employees who have significant personal, family, or community-based problems that interfere with job satisfaction and performance. Some common employee problems that might lead to EAP services are substance abuse, financial problems, family conflicts, difficulty coping with stress, and chronic physical and mental health conditions.

Employees may seek these confidential services on their own initiative or be referred by a supervisor. Whichever route is pursued, maintaining strict confidentiality is a key element in achieving effective EAP services. The primary goal of the EAP approach is to help employees help themselves. In addition to the personal rewards and problem solving facilitated by this assistance, these programs can be justified as cost-effective investments for the organization to the extent that they lower the costs of excessive absenteeism, lost productivity, interpersonal conflict, and turnover. An EAP referral may result in retention of an employee who would otherwise leave the organization perhaps with diminished capacity or it might eliminate or lower barriers to optimal performance of the employee.

REFLECTIONS ON LEADERSHIP II: AN INTERVIEW WITH GREGORY PEASLEE, SENIOR VICE PRESIDENT, HUMAN RESOURCES, UNIVERSITY OF PITTSBURGH MEDICAL CENTER, PITTSBURGH, PENNSYLVANIA

Briefly describe your role as Senior Vice President/Human Resources, University of Pittsburgh Medical Center as it contributes to furthering the mission, strategic direction, and goals of the medical center.

Peaslee: The University of Pittsburgh Medical Center (UPMC) as primarily a health services organization relies on a multitude of different staff to provide the needed services to our patients. As the chief human resources officer I am responsible for ensuring that UPMC is able to recruit and retain the best and the brightest in all areas. We must also ensure that we have an organization culture that not just supports but allows our staff to thrive, a culture that supports continuing education and development of each individual within UPMC.

As a member of the executive team of a prestigious academic medical center, how do you view your own leadership role within the organization? Who do you regard as your primary constituencies and how are you accountable to them?

Peaslee: As one of the members of the senior management team (one of four senior vice presidents reporting to the CEO) and who has a broad background including finance and management of our physician groups, my role is first to manage effectively those direct areas that report to me (human resources, construction, property management, and security) but also to assist in the overall management of UPMC. In other words, I view my role as ensuring the success of UPMC in all areas. My leadership style is one of a *servant leader;* I am there to serve the rest of the senior management team, the management of the areas under my direct authority, and our employees at large. I am accountable to ensure that all our employees are receiving what they need to be successful in their various roles in the organization.

What traits, characteristics, or behaviors do you regard as being essential for effective leadership in human resource management in health care?

Peaslee: The leader must care about serving others, not in the sense of providing medical care to them but in the sense of assisting them to reach their full potential. He or she must be intelligent, both in terms of "book smarts" but also with "people smarts." He or she must be empathetic but at the same time able to require exceptional performance from staff. The effective leader must lead by example.

Do you view leadership as being primarily associated with key positions in the organization's hierarchy or should it be developed at all levels of the organization? If the latter, how can it be developed most effectively?

Peaslee: Leadership must be developed at all levels of the organization. Most services are provided at the front-line staff level and the management of those functions must be on-site to lead effectively. Development of front-line leadership is a multifaceted approach. First it must start with effective selection of candidates for these positions. Most organizations have a habit of "promoting the best doer" of a function to be the front-line leader. Although he or she indeed may be a good leader as well, leadership is generally different than [functional] "doing." Organizations must first examine their process of identification of this group of leaders. Once an emerging leader has been identified, organizations must provide the new leader the appropriate tools and training for him or her to be effective in the leadership role.

To what extent is team development an important component of HRM in your organization? What is required for the organization to develop and manage teams effectively?

Peaslee: Currently, this process is not a distinct part of the HRM function except as it is addressed in our leadership training initiative.

What is the greatest or most difficult challenge to the effective and efficient use of human resources at UPMC (or in health care generally) during the next decade? What strategies might be developed to respond to this challenge?

Peaslee: The greatest challenge in HRM in health care during the next decade will be ensuring that the organization has the supply of professional clinical staff needed for the organization to thrive and meet its mission. Among the strategies that need to be enhanced or developed is more effective recruiting of talented people to enter into health care clinical training programs to reduce the shortages of such trained workers. Development of programs to break down the barriers to the education of these needed workers, including tuition costs and employment during training/education, are critical as is presenting the professions in a proper manner to showcase the many attractive health care careers.

Please identify and discuss a situation representing a significant human resources problem or challenge that you or your organization has addressed effectively.

Peaslee: Related to the challenge noted in the last question, we have expanded our own schools (nursing and radiology techs) to be able to train more workers and to offer free tuition for these programs. Also we have worked with various other providers of training and educational programs in these areas to foster and support the quality and relevance of their programs as related to UPMC's staffing needs.

Considering the recent examples of leadership failure within the corporate board room, including health care, what do you see as the role of the human resources executive in maintaining ethical behavior within the organization and in its relationships with its external environment?

Peaslee: I think the role of the human resources executive is a key one in this area. For example, I serve on our board/staff ethics committee, which is responsible for providing education and guidance on UPMC ethics philosophy. The human resources department also plays a significant role in developing and monitoring policies that promote the ethical behavior of our staff. It is also incumbent upon the human resources leader to be on the look out for questionable behavior within the management ranks.

Do you believe that traditional labor relations processes (e.g., collective bargaining) and priorities are relevant (effective) in health care systems in the twenty-first century? What are the benefits and costs of these processes from the perspective of executive management?

Peaslee: I have the pleasure of working in a largely "bargaining unit–free" environment with only 1500 unionized members out of 40,000 employees. I do not believe that collective bargaining is helpful for the organization or for our employees' welfare. I am convinced that unionization places a needless barrier between the employees and management.

What do you see as the greatest challenge(s) affecting leaders in health care within the next several decades? How can leaders be better prepared to deal with these challenges?

Peaslee: The greatest challenge I see being faced by health care leaders in the future is the continuing demand to provide more and better services to the population while also being responsive to societal demands that payers (i.e., employers, insurers, and individuals) pay less for health care, overall.

System Inputs

Human Resource Planning and Forecasting. One of the most important roles that the HIM professional can assume is that associated with **strategic human resource planning**. This should be a proactive rather than a reactive HRM activity in which managers must continually forecast and coordinate the supply of qualified human resources with the predicted demand on the basis of workflow cycles in health information services. This strategic approach to planning anticipates and prepares for future staffing needs on the basis of **key indicators of demand,** which are measures of program operations (i.e., volume, activity, or output) that can be reliably linked to staffing levels. The greater the number of workers employed by health information services and the greater the degree of complexity in the relationships between jobs and functions both within and external to the unit, the more important is systematic human resource planning in providing health information services effectively and efficiently.

Planning improves use of resources by providing a systematic and reliable method of matching personnel requirements with organizational and departmental goals and priorities. A human resource (staffing) plan can achieve efficiency in hiring new workers because similar position vacancies can be filled at the same time, saving advertising and referral source costs. By having newly hired workers oriented and trained together, the organization can also reduce administrative and training costs. As health information services become more distributed with organization-wide rather than department-level accountability, astute and reliable planning becomes an essential role for the HIM professional.

Human resource planning can provide useful tools for the HIM professional in developing and justifying staffing supply and demand projections. These include trend (demand) analysis, replacement charts, flow (Markov) analysis, and staffing (census) tables. These and other techniques support strategic HRM and encourage contingency thinking in which the decision maker can pose and respond to a number of "what if" questions related to future HR supply and demand. For example, if a digitized patient record is to be implemented within the year, the need for manual record filing positions will decline and proactive human resource actions can be taken. If a credible human resource plan is prepared 6 months to 1 year in advance and periodically reviewed and updated, the affected employees can be reassigned other duties, retrained, or transferred to another unit so that terminations and layoffs are minimized. On the other hand, more data imaging and analysis staff will be required, so necessary recruitment and training can be initiated early to meet this need. Continuous human resource planning ensures that external environmental challenges and opportunities can be addressed by effective use of available human resources and support systems.

The management of staffing always requires timely and thorough planning to support short-term operations and long-term strategies. Thoughtful human resource planning to maintain the desired level of service is essential in a competitive environment, especially when facing significant resource constraints, for example, after a drastic "downsizing" or an especially tight labor market for critical skills. As expense budgets tighten to meet anticipated shortfalls in revenue, departments are likely to be required to do as much or more work with a smaller staff. This not only reduces the available "hands and minds" but also places greater demands on line managers, supervisors, and human resource specialists (Box 16-7).

Effective staffing is dependent on useful and reliable forecasting. Forecasting or prediction ranges in sophistication from a manager's intuitive "guesstimates" to the scenarios generated by computer simulations of complex systems using multivariable algorithms. The most appropriate forecasting method depends on the nature of the problem, for example, as being well defined and routine or ambiguous and complex, and the level of resources available. In real-world situations, the forecasting method used and the priority given to it are often driven by time and resource constraints.

Box 16–7 HUMAN RESOURCE PLANNING PROCESS

- Forecasting (predicting or estimating) key staffing variables:
  - Volume of activity or output for the period projected
  - Application of productivity measures or targets
  - Level of staffing required for that volume, that is, *demand estimate*
  - Staff available to satisfy demand for labor, that is, *supply estimate*
- *Reconciliation* of supply and demand estimates (a process of validating the net shortfall or excess of available staff)
- Developing or revising external recruitment plan
- Projection of training needs and schedules
- Identifying or reviewing promotion, transfer, and retirement opportunities
- Continuous evaluation of planning activities

This situation entails estimates based on information easiest to access, considering only a limited set of relevant variables and making conservative projections. The most common approach is to extrapolate from past trends and current values of key variables into the short-term future. In other words, we base our forecasts on the implicit assumption that the future will most likely resemble the recent past.

Staffing projections and plans are needed to ensure that a supply of educated workers is available to meet the demand for information services at the time and place required. Cross-training technical staff through a regular rotation of job duties and assignments accomplishes several objectives. It not only ensures a pool of potential substitutes for employees on leave or for position vacancies but also alleviates the boredom, frustration, and declining motivation that have been associated with turnover in positions with highly structured and routine activities.

A human resource strategic plan for staffing the coding function, for example, should be based ultimately on the projected volume of patients and the associated workload for coding staff. This can be translated into demand estimates for coding staff based on employee or unit productivity standards. A comparable supply estimate can be determined by adjusting the current census for projected flows into and out of these jobs and by considering the size of the recruitment pool for these positions from traditional sources, such as local colleges and technical institutes. Once the demand and supply estimates are verified and reconciled, specific recruitment, training, and internal promotion and transfer plans and schedules can be developed or revised (Figure 16-6). An unexpected gap in projected supply of trained coders or analysts could result in more aggressive campus recruitment or increased in-service and external training activities. Another response might be increased reliance on temporary staffing agencies to address peak workload needs for transcriptionists (for example) on a

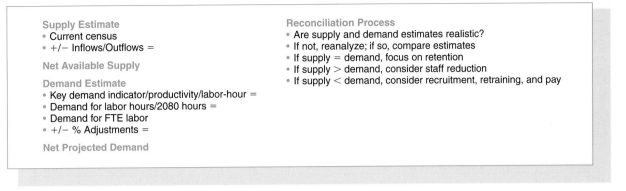

Figure 16-6 Reconciliation of supply and demand estimates.

short-term or as-needed basis. Such solutions can lower the overall costs of staffing in the long term while addressing fluctuations in the workload, both those that are cyclic and those that are less predictable. With the development of such plans, staffing levels can be managed cost-effectively by minimizing lost productivity and any compromising of essential services.

Tools for Human Resource Planning. Some of the methods and tools useful in developing a human resource or staffing plan are described next:

Replacement Charts
Replacement charts present a visual representation of who is available to fill projected vacant positions. Typically, these

charts are reserved for key managerial or highly professional positions. The replacement chart usually identifies individual incumbents, the most likely (or all potential) replacements, and summary measures of performance and promotion potential. The information in the chart should include that obtained from supervisory performance appraisals, assessment centers, training and career development activities, skill inventories, performance audits, and other sources relevant to the employee's career mobility. For example, the replacement chart in Figure 16-7 shows that if there is a vacancy at the manager level (M. Jones leaves), J. White is more likely to be promoted than B. Benson. If J. White moves to manager, then B. Benson succeeds White as assistant manager and presumably both F. Brown and S. Green would be considered for an upcoming vacancy.

Date Compiled: _____

Possible HIS Position Vacancies	Name of Employee	Attributes
Manager, Health Information Services	M. Jones	A, 1
C. Smith, Incumbent	B. Benson	B, 2
	J. White	B, 1
Assistant Manager, HIS	J. White	A, 1
M. Jones, Incumbent	B. Benson	B, 2
Supervisor, Clinical Data	F. Brown	A, 1
J. White, Incumbent	J. Jones	B, 2
Supervisor, Medical Language Division	S. Green	A, 1
B. Benson, Incumbent	C. Black	B, 1

Key to Attributes:
A 5 Ready for Promotion
B 5 Needs More Experience Before Promoting
C 5 Not Suitable for Promotion At Present
1 5 Performance Appraisal Rating Excellent
2 5 Performance Appraisal Rating Acceptable
3 5 Performance Appraisal Rating Unacceptable

Figure 16-7 Replacement chart.

Job Title	J 1	F 2	M 3	A 4	M 5	J 6	J 7	A 8	S 9	O 10	N 11	D* 12	Total FTE's
HI Analysts		2							1		1		4
Data Entry Specialists	3				1					2			6
Optical Imaging Specialists								1					1
Release of Information Coordinators					1				1				2
Director of HIS													
												Total	13

*Months of the year.

Figure 16-8 Staffing table. Anticipated openings for this budget year by month of the year.

Staffing Table

A **staffing table** also provides a graphic representation of job titles and anticipated position vacancies (Figure 16-8). Because of increased computerization of health records processing, management predicts that additional data entry clerks must be hired in February, May, and October. A total of six full-time equivalent (FTE) clerks will be needed in the current budget year.

Human Resources Audit

A **human resources audit** is conducted to assess which openings can be filled with internal candidates already employed within the organization. An audit results in the integration of relevant information about the skills, knowledge, abilities, and leadership potential of all employees in the workforce into one document. This report should be useful in developing and coordinating effective recruitment, selection, orientation, training, and career planning activities.

Skill Inventories

These profiles of employee skills, knowledge, and capabilities can be developed for both nonmanagerial and supervisory-management employees. Demographic information, such as job title, job experience, and length of service with the organization, is typically provided. The most essential data presented in the inventory characterize the employee's performance history, current assessment of the employee's performance, and managerial judgment about the employee's potential for promotion. This tool should provide a coherent and comprehensive summary profile of the employee's credentials, including specific skills, areas of expertise, capabilities, and potential for professional growth.

Job Analysis and Design. Job analysis is a key human resource function that is undervalued and misunderstood by many managers and employees. Although job analysis is generally viewed as a technical function performed by HRM specialists, it cannot be implemented effectively without the active involvement of supervisors and the employees whose jobs are subject to analysis. Because first-line supervisors and the employees themselves are in the best position to understand what is required to perform the job, how it can be performed most efficiently, and what outcomes are expected from doing the job right, these individuals must be recognized as primary sources of information. Consequently, every supervisor and line manager must understand the purpose, processes, and outcomes associated with job analysis and his or her responsibilities in ensuring that it is done effectively for all jobs within that area of accountability. Ultimately, **job analysis** should result in the design of jobs and work processes that maximize the cost-effective use of human resources to support the mission and goals of the organization while addressing the individual employee's needs, concerns, and goals.

Improvements in employee performance, productivity, quality, and cost control are founded on systematic analysis of job functions, activities, and responsibilities. The manager must have a clear understanding of each job and how it relates to other jobs within the system to organize, coordinate, and use effectively the resources available, especially the people resources. Specific outcomes of job analysis include but are not limited to the following:

- Job requirements necessary for performing the job
- *Essential functions* of the job for ADA compliance
- Job specifications or qualifications (required of the employee)

- Selection criteria (based on the job specifications)
- Formal job description
- Performance standards (established or reviewed)
- Productivity measures (established or reviewed)
- Training needs and priorities
- Data to inform job evaluation or "pricing"

This representative list of outcomes of job analysis suggests the importance of this function to the organization. Indeed, it can be argued that job analysis, if done well, serves as the foundation and "glue" for the HRM system as a whole. Consequently, managers must be held accountable for fulfilling their responsibilities to support this process. The supervisor or manager should also directly benefit from this process by gaining tools, such as current and accurate job descriptions, useful in managing individual and team performance and coaching. It should be noted, however, that the focus for job analysis is not the employee holding the job but the job itself as a component of the total structuring and coordination of effort within the whole organization.

The following tools are some of those more commonly used to conduct formal job analysis:

- Job analysis forms (Figure 16-9)
- Questionnaires
- Interviews (individual and group)
- Checklists (supervisor or employee)
- Employee logs or diaries

- Work process, activity, and output records
- Direct observation (by supervisor or consultant)
- Video recording or taping (infrequent, special circumstances)

Any one or a combination of these methods may be used, but some form of survey or checklist is typically used as the basic data collection instrument. When teamwork is inherent in the work process, observation of the team process or group interviewing is very appropriate. Direct observation of a complex work process may be useful but is also time intensive, costly, and subject to perceptual bias of the observer. Self-reported activity or incident logs can be useful for analyzing managerial and professional positions characterized by a high degree of flexibility, exercise of discretion, and complex behavior. However, this method can be disruptive and also prone to bias and subjective reporting.

Job analysis should be an established human resource activity scheduled so that all jobs in the organization are subject to review and analysis on a predictable cycle. With the rapid changes in technology, regulation, and other environmental factors, it can be argued that the job analysis cycle should be no longer than 3 to 5 years, although organizational and industry factors will determine the appropriate frequency of formal job analyses. Certainly the job description should be reviewed at least once a year, preferably as part of the performance appraisal process, by both the employee and the supervisor.

Position Title: Health Information Secretary

Department: Health Information Services

Supervisor: Manager, Health Information Services

Current Supervisor's Name: Kathy Castlerock

General Job Objectives:
- Acts as department receptionist and first telephone contact.
- Processes daily work schedules.
- Demonstrates effective relationships with co-workers, patients, public, physicians, administration, and outside agencies.

Essential Job Duties:
(List all tasks required to perform the routine functions required for the position.)
Example:
- Greets visitors to the department.
- Routes incoming phone calls and takes messages when intended party is unavailable.

Meets Standards of Performance By: (Example)
(For Greeting Visitors) Receiving no complaints in the performance period concerning discourteous service.

Exceeds Standards of Performance By: (Example)
(For Greeting Visitors) Receiving compliments by visitors, coworkers, or physicians on helpfulness and courteous service.

Figure 16-9 Sample job analysis form.

In addition to the organization-wide rationale for conducting regular job analysis, individual managers might want to perform job analysis to do the following:

- Evaluate the effects of external challenges, such as a change in Medicare reimbursement regulations, on a specific job (e.g., billing clerk).
- Identify and eliminate irrelevant or potentially discriminatory job requirements and specifications.
- Identify job elements and working conditions that can be addressed to enhance the quality of work life.
- Develop an effective staffing plan to respond to changes in departmental mission, technology, or workload.
- Ensure better match of applicants with projected job vacancies and new positions.
- Develop a unit-wide training and career development plan and schedule for in-services.
- Develop untapped potential in a specific position. For example, a review of the position of insurance clerk at a neighborhood health clinic reveals that basic knowledge of ICD-9-CM (*International Classification of Diseases*, Ninth Revision, *Clinical Modification*) coding is required. The clinic often faces a backlog in coding of outpatient service records. By identifying this untapped resource, the clinic director can obtain training for the insurance clerk to prepare the clerk to help with backlog coding. This job redesign not only enhances the facility's capacity to provide more efficient service but also may improve the job satisfaction and career opportunities of the employee.
- Rotate an employee to another position in the unit in which he or she will learn new skills and use already developed skills more fully.
- Determine whether the salary difference between two employees with different jobs but similar responsibilities and performance records is fair and reasonable.
- Initiate a unit-wide study to establish realistic productivity standards.

Job Descriptions. A job description is the most tangible output of the job analysis process. The job description is a written document of the essential requirements, responsibilities, reporting relationships, qualifications, working conditions, and other significant aspects of the job. Within the organization, normally all job descriptions should follow the same format for ease of comparison and analysis. Form and content of job descriptions among health care organizations vary, however. Some job descriptions also include **job performance standards** that are used as the primary criteria for performance evaluation. For the job description to be a useful supervisory tool, the performance factors applied in practice must be consistent with the job description, even if these standards are not included in the text of the job description.

The job description can be a relatively brief summary or profile of the job requirements or a more comprehensive

Table 16–2   STRUCTURE AND KEY ELEMENTS OF THE JOB DESCRIPTION

Element Required	Purpose
Date	Date it was created and most recently revised
Author/responsible manager	Establishes accountability and source to refer any questions
Organization level/ unit (department, division, office, etc.)	Places the job within the organizational structure
Job grade or classification	Ranks the job's level and importance for compensation purposes
Supervisory relationships	Identifies immediate supervisor and employees supervised (if any)
Job status	Exempt or nonexempt from overtime and other FLSA requirements
Job summary	Concise description of the basic purpose and functions of the job
Essential functions, duties, and activities	Major tasks and responsibilities of this position; estimated time and effort distribution; "essential functions" must be identified for ADA compliance
Job specifications	Qualifications in terms of education, experience, skills, knowledge, certification, etc., needed to perform the essential job responsibilities
Working conditions	Physical and psychological demands of the work environment. Any unusually challenging aspects should be addressed, such as handling hazardous materials, need to maintain strict confidentiality

and detailed report. All job descriptions should contain, at a minimum, a set of key elements to serve the many purposes discussed earlier (Table 16-2).

Employee Handbooks. The **employee handbook** provides a written reference manual of organizational policies and procedures covering employee rights, benefits, obligations, norms and standards of conduct, and other expectations of and constraints on employee behavior. With increasing challenges to the employment-at-will doctrine, the content and language of employee handbooks have come under considerable scrutiny by employers, unions, their respective legal counsel, and individual employees. For example, in some state courts employee terminations have been challenged on the basis that language in the employee handbook implied a contractual obligation to offer continuing employment to the employee unless specific grounds for due cause of termination were proved. Subsequently, most employers have screened and revised such language to reduce the likelihood of a successful legal challenge on the basis of the handbook. The following guidelines pertain to their appropriate content and use. Employee handbooks must be as follows:

- Presented to communicate precisely and clearly the relevant policies and procedures established by management
- Reviewed periodically by legal counsel to minimize legal risk
- Updated continually to reflect changes in policy and procedures
- Distributed to all employees at orientation and on any significant revisions
- Covered as an essential component of supervisory training

All employees, at the time of orientation or release of revisions to the handbook, should be required to sign a statement to be maintained in the employee's file indicating that they have received a handbook and reviewed its contents within a definite time period. Management must assume the burden of ensuring that employees have access to the handbook and understand its scope and purpose. Also, employees must be informed that it is their responsibility to inquire of their managers or supervisors if they need clarification about any material in the handbook.

Job analysis should yield accurate and useful job descriptions that describe the essential functions of the job, how these are to be performed, and what qualifications the employee must present to perform the position effectively. Management policies and procedures governing employee conduct and working conditions should be clearly communicated through employee handbooks, personnel manuals, and supervisory coaching. These human resource processes and tools should provide the foundation for recruiting and selecting qualified individuals to fill the target positions consistent with human resource staffing plans and current needs.

Recruitment. Recruitment is the process and set of activities performed to identify and maintain a **recruitment pool** of potential applicants presumably qualified and willing to perform one or more target positions in the organization. The recruitment function includes setting specific targets and schedules for filling vacant positions, selecting appropriate media for communicating the staffing needs, notifying external recruitment sources, announcing specific position vacancies, and identifying a group of potentially eligible applicants.

Key Activities in the Recruitment Process
The following key activities involved in employee recruitment must be performed whether recruitment is provided under contract with external agencies or is conducted by in-house staff:

- Identify a position vacancy or need
- Review and (if needed) revise the job description
- Develop a recruitment plan, including appropriate internal and external communications about the position
- Create and maintain a recruitment pool of eligible applicants

The job opening has been identified either in the human resource plan or by request of a manager facing an immediate or foreseeable future need. The recruiter becomes familiar with the job requirements by reviewing the current job description, job specifications, and related information developed during the job analysis process. This review enables the recruiter to achieve a better match between the job requirements and the applicant's qualifications. The recruiter (staff or contractor) should discuss this job with the immediate supervisor or other responsible managers to ensure that they have a common understanding of the organization's expectations for filling this position. If necessary, the job description should be revised to reflect any changes in requirements or other aspects of the job before the position is advertised.

Once a common understanding of the essential requirements and expectations of the job has been achieved, recruiting specialists must consider and select appropriate recruitment sources and media for communicating the position opening. Cost-benefit considerations should be applied on the basis of systematic and continuous evaluation of the recruitment effort. A pool of potentially qualified applicants should be identified among those who respond to the position announcements and those referred by employees or external agents.

Sources of Applicants.
Entry-level positions are usually filled by newspaper and trade journal advertisements, walk-in and on-line inquiries, or employee referrals. Health care organizations also use professional recruiters, such as executive search agencies, for managerial and highly skilled professional positions. If a professional recruiter is used, the employer must be vigilant in discovering any intentional or unintentional biases of the recruiting agency, such as referring only applicants younger than 40 years, that might unnecessarily limit the applicant pool and expose the employer to legal risk. Executive search and other professional recruiting agencies typically charge fees for their services to the hiring organization, and the employer must understand its obligations and include such expenses in any cost-benefit analysis of its recruitment program.

Recruitment channels that are both available to most health care organizations and relatively low in cost include walk-in, write-in, and on-line, self-initiated application, and employee referrals. The latter process might be especially useful and even encouraged by management if it proves to be a reliable source of appropriate applicants. Not only are current employees likely to be effective recruiters for desirable positions but also management can signal its respect for the employees by welcoming such referrals.

Targeted advertising is the most common channel of recruitment and can be cost-effective. Local daily newspapers, professional journals, and trade periodicals are the most likely places to advertise. Many organizations post or publish new positions on bulletin boards and in in-house newsletters often in advance of externally focused efforts to encourage internal applicants. Increasingly, organizations announce position openings on-line. Increasingly, employers and job seekers rely on on-line recruitment and application processes to accomplish the initial screening.

Local and regional educational institutions, including community colleges, are usually excellent sources of recruitment for HIM positions at all levels. Medical assistant, medical transcriptionist or secretary, physician office management, nursing administration, HIM, information sciences, and business administration programs are likely sources of potential employees, depending on the nature of the position and level of training and certification required. Often, graduates from entry-level health profession and technologist programs have been required to complete relevant clinical education in health care, rehabilitation, or health administrative settings. These applicants should have an easier transition to the health care environment and a shorter learning curve than others who lack this experience.

Constraints on Effective Recruitment

Constraints arise from the organization's strategic plans and objectives, current financial position, compensation policies, environmental conditions, job requirements, and departmental or unit budgets and from federal and state regulation and legislation, especially EEO requirements.

Management's human resource policies in support of their long-term strategic plans and short-term operational objectives can constrain line managers and the recruitment staff by limiting the recruitment pool or by increasing the cost of maintaining an adequate pool of qualified applicants. For example, a promotion-from-within policy that mandates that qualified employees in place be given preferential consideration for promotion before external applicants are considered will probably be justified on the basis of effective employee relations and lower recruitment and training costs. However, this policy might also make the filling of any one position more difficult. A hire-from-within policy also might work against some organizational and public policy objectives, such as achieving a more diverse workforce, while supporting other values and policy objectives, such as extending the working life of older employees before retirement. Awarding preference to military veterans for civil service positions—for example, municipal, state, or federal agencies—is another constraint affecting the discretion of the recruiting staff or manager.

Certainly, compensation policies may constrain recruiting and influence the performance levels and productivity within the organization. For example, if the pay range for coders is significantly below the prevailing market rate or that of a key competitor, the recruiting effort for these jobs could be adversely affected. However, if the pay rate cannot be improved at least in the short term because of organizational constraints, the job might be made more attractive to applicants in other ways, such as flex time scheduling, on-site child care, or subsidized parking.

Health care organizations may have employment status policies that can act as an impediment to effective recruitment. For example, an organizational policy against hiring part-time workers (or hiring only part-time workers) would probably limit the applicant pool, although the effects on the quality of applicants are uncertain. The health information manager might be able to take advantage of, or argue for initiating, a job-sharing option to respond to such a policy constraint.

Employee Selection. Once an adequate pool of applicants has been recruited, the **selection process** begins. As a practical matter, the line between recruitment and selection processes is a fuzzy one. The selection process involves a sequence of activities that should result in the hiring of a well-qualified employee to fill the target position. The number of available and qualified applicants for the position is an important consideration. For example, if there is a surplus of trained medical transcriptionists in the region given the number of competing health care providers and total number of position vacancies, the hiring health information services unit is likely to identify and hire a qualified candidate without great difficulty. However, if the local or regional labor market is tight, the hiring unit may need to take very aggressive measures to fill open positions, for example, by making recruitment trips to colleges and job fairs outside the region to identify and recruit health information managers and technical staff. In the latter situation, recruiting methods should be reviewed to determine which recruitment sources, communication channels, and strategies for widening the recruitment pool are most effective. Consideration must be given to increased use of on-line recruitment methods, especially for positions related to information services.

Each health care organization must implement a set of activities essential to effective employee selection within regulatory and budgetary constraints. The process is sufficiently flexible that each organization can develop a recruitment and selection plan appropriate for its own needs and constraints. For example, some employers take aggressive steps to increase staff diversity by targeting recruitment and selection efforts to attract minority group applicants to fill key positions, such as by sending mailings to African American church leaders or social fraternities and sororities.

Components of the Employee Selection Process

Initial Contact

The screening process actually begins during the first interaction, usually face to face or by telephone, between the employer (as represented by a receptionist or interviewer) and applicant in which the applicant and employer's representative each form initial impressions of the other in terms of a potential match. These initial perceptions may be quite robust, especially in influencing the applicant's decision to continue pursuing the open position. Although the HRM staff person should avoid making judgments based primarily on initial impressions, the first encounter is likely to influence subsequent interactions between the applicant and the organization. It is indicative of the dramatic changes brought about by the "information revolution" and the development of the Internet that the applicant's initial encounter with the organization is increasingly likely to be through its Web presentation.

Application Review

Research has shown that the standard application form may be the single most valid and reliable selection tool commonly used, especially if used in conjunction with personal contact reference checks.[37] If the application form has been developed to meet the needs of the organization, it should be essential to the completion of the initial screening phase of the selection process. The application could be developed to produce weighted scores based on specific selection criteria identified during job analysis. A rating cutoff score could be established to screen out applicants who do not meet the basic criteria of eligibility for the position. Structuring the selection process as a set of increasingly rigorous screens should increase the efficiency of the process and validity of the final selection decisions.

Although some organizations consider career resumes to be a substitute for the application form, this approach is not advisable. Because all applicants should be evaluated fairly and objectively *against the same set of criteria*, it is essential that the same information is collected and considered for each applicant. Failing to do so could subject the employer to legal liability under Title VII or other EEO legislation and lead to an inconsistent and unreliable selection process; that is, poor decisions might be made about both well-qualified and less-qualified applicants. Consequently, the HRM specialist must make an additional effort to convert the resume data that are not standardized into the desired data set of the application.

Furthermore, there is some evidence that applicants distort, exaggerate, or otherwise misrepresent their academic attainments, work experience, or other credentials in the prepared resumes. Some notorious cases have been documented of individuals creating separate and fraudulent identities through their resumes and paper record. Of course, applicants can also embellish or present false information on the application. Consequently, the use of reference checks should be considered an essential component of the selection process. In the case of verifying credentials of HIM professionals, the validity of the certification or registration should be confirmed with AHIMA.

Reference Checks

References are checked to accomplish two objectives: (1) to obtain new information about the applicant's performance history and likely future performance and (2) to verify information already obtained from other sources. For various reasons, including concerns of employers about exposure to legal liability, it is difficult although not impossible to obtain useful and accurate information about performance history and personal characteristics of an applicant from previous supervisors or coworkers. Many organizations have adopted a policy that requires the supervisor or other manager asked to provide a reference by another employer to refer that request to an HRM specialist. Typically, the HRM staff verifies dates of employment with that organization, the last position held, and perhaps whether the person left the job voluntarily or was terminated. The organization is reluctant or unwilling to provide relevant and useful performance-related information and subject itself or its managers to the risk of being sued by the applicant if that information could be regarded as prejudicial or defamatory. Consequently, it is more likely that the HRM staff specialist or manager will at best be willing to verify the accuracy of the work history reported by the applicant.

If the person conducting the reference check is able to reach the previous supervisor directly, he or she might obtain more candid feedback about performance strengths and deficiencies, disciplinary or interpersonal problems, and the circumstances of the applicant's separation from the previous position. However, it is increasingly unlikely that such important information can be obtained. It is notable that employers are also being challenged from the opposite position, that is, being held legally liable for failing to obtain information relevant to job performance or behavioral problems of an applicant who is hired during or subsequent to the selection process. These competing legal principles place the hiring official between the proverbial "rock and a hard place" and certainly impede the organization's ability to base its selection decisions on what is usually considered the most effective predictor of future performance, that is, past performance.

Testing

All selection tools normally used to make assessments about the applicant can be considered "tests" of some aspect of the applicant's abilities, knowledge, or personal characteristics. In effect, the entire selection process can be seen as an elaborate process of prediction of future performance: which applicants are likely to perform the job successfully and which ones not likely to do so? The various selection tools in this respect serve as tests or predictors of some aspect of future job performance. From this perspective, even the application form and personal interview should be regarded as tests.

However, in common usage, "tests" refer to evaluative devices—written, oral, and electronic—that specifically measure some skill, knowledge capability, interest, or psychological trait. In the HIM environment such tests would include but not be limited to instruments or methods measuring knowledge of coding and medical terminology, quantitative analysis ability, keyboarding and transcription skills, and understanding of effective supervisory or management principles.

All employee selection tests must be reviewed and validated so that they can be defended against a Title VII charge of being discriminatory. The acid test legally is whether any challenged test can be demonstrated to be job related as established in the Supreme Court's decision in the landmark EEO case of *Griggs v. Duke Power* (1971). In this case, the Supreme Court held that a test not demonstrated to be job related could be considered illegal under Title VII if it had adverse (discriminatory) effects on members of a protected class, in this case African Americans, even if the test was not intended to do so. Management has the burden of proving that all selection tests used are valid and reliable indicators of some aspect of future job performance and that all applicants for the position are administered the test(s) under the same testing conditions. In the language of the Supreme Court, "Congress has forbidden giving [testing or measuring procedures] controlling force unless they are demonstrably a reasonable measure of job performance."[38] For example, requiring applicants to achieve some target score in a mathematics proficiency test would probably not be considered appropriate if the position does not require numerical calculations or use of statistical methods.

Although once commonly used as screening tools, aptitude, intelligence, personality type, and other psychometric measures are not considered performance tests and, except in special situations, would be quite difficult to justify as job related. Aptitude tests and interest inventories presumably predict the probability of a person's being successful in some activity independent of his or her training or experience. Psychometric tests provide measures of a range of psychological, personality, and cognitive characteristics and predispositions, some of which might be linked to job-related behavior. Such tests should be administered and results interpreted only by testing experts if the test(s) has been validated in terms of measuring specific job or performance requirements. In no case should a line manager apply a test "locally" to an applicant or employee without review and approval by the appropriate human resources professional.

Selection Interview

The personal interview is widely regarded within management circles as the most important of all selection tools or predictors, and many managers have great confidence in their ability to use this technique effectively. Unfortunately, the interview is considered by many HRM professionals and scholars to be often quite unreliable and prone to bias and errors of judgment. Why is there this mismatch between expectations and actual experience?

The justification for using the personal interview as an essential selection tool is that it gives the supervisor or other interviewer the opportunity to get a "good look" at the applicant, to determine whether the applicant will "fit in" with others in the unit, and to confirm whether the applicant can really get the job done. The problem with the personal interview as a tool for achieving these objectives is its susceptibility to various distortions and bias. The face-to-face nature of the personal interview suggests that the applicant's physical appearance and ability to communicate orally dominate the interviewer's impressions. This can easily result in **halo effect** bias in which the observer's perception of one characteristic of an individual dominates other perceptions to result in an undifferentiated overall impression, positive or negative. For example, the applicant appears to be physically attractive and well dressed. This perception leads the interviewer to make the judgment on the basis of this perception alone that the applicant is intelligent, well educated, and has leadership ability, none of which can be reliably assessed from only these visual cues. This, of course, is not to suggest that physical presence and good grooming are irrelevant to effective performance in a given position.

The problem is that such first impressions based primarily on visual and oral cues encourage quick and all-encompassing judgments that tend to be resistant to subsequent data that are contrary to that overall positive or negative halo. Some research has shown that dominant impressions are formed within the first several minutes of the interview. If the interview process is regarded as a data collection tool as well as a test, it will be inefficient and invalid to the degree that data that are available after the formation of the initial impression are discounted or ignored. Consequently, the validity and reliability of the interview as a test of future job performance could be severely compromised by halo effect bias.

Many managers believe that they are intuitively good interviewers, that they know how to make accurate and reliable judgments of the person's fit with the organization, intelligence, integrity, dependability, leadership potential, and like characteristics on the basis of one relatively brief interaction. The manager may in fact be able to assess fit with the organization's culture, the applicant's ability to "think on his or her feet," and other characteristics relevant to the job on the basis of the interviewer's wisdom and years of experience. However, without specific training in interviewing, effective listening, and other human relations skills, as well as knowledge of the implications of Title VII, the ADA, and other legal constraints on the selection interview, the manager may misperceive and inflate his or her abilities in this role.

In spite of these real concerns about the personal interview as a selection tool, virtually no organization would make a decision to hire for a position vacancy without the interview. Clearly, the interview process can be a useful tool for obtaining job- and performance-related data. For example, the interview could test the applicant's problem-solving abilities if this activity is planned as part of the process. As another example, the interviewer could assess the applicant's conflict resolution skills by using a role-playing exercise during the interview. Finally, it is important to ask the same questions under similar interview conditions of all applicants to permit fair comparisons of all applicants and to avoid grounds for charges of discriminatory treatment under Title VII. In summary, then, the reliability and validity of the interview process can be enhanced by training the interviewer, structuring the interview to address important selection factors, and standardizing the process to ensure fair treatment for all applicants.

Finally, we should recognize the value of the interview as an opportunity for the applicant to evaluate the organization and his or her fit within the job and the organizational culture. Furthermore, the employer has an opportunity not only to evaluate the applicant but also to market the position to a well-qualified applicant. If this two-way communication process is implemented effectively, it can assist both parties in their decision making about the employment match.

Typically, a series of interviews are conducted by individuals with different perspectives on the selection process. An HRM specialist usually conducts an initial screening interview to determine the applicant's eligibility on the basis of essential selection factors. If the applicant meets these criteria, subsequent interviews are scheduled with the immediate supervisor, the unit or division manager, and other managers with a relevant perspective on this position. In some organizations, peers or employees to be supervised by the applicant (if selected) are included in the interview process. For example, in selection of a quality improvement director or tumor registrar, a higher level administrator or physician may want to participate in the interview process. When there are multiple interviews, the person who retains final hiring authority must be clearly designated. It is critical that the immediate supervisor be given a significant role in the selection process even if not given final decision-making authority. Certainly, this manager has the greatest stake in achieving a good employment match and is usually the person in the best position to predict the applicant's fit within the job and the unit.

The job description and specifications should be reviewed with the applicant during the interview and a copy given to the applicant for consideration. The applicant should be encouraged to ask any questions about the job requirements, working conditions, compensation level, work schedule, and so forth, and the applicant should be given a tour of the work environment. Professional, courteous, and informed interviewing can only benefit the employer regardless of the outcome of an individual selection decision.

Medical Examination

The medical examination is provided to evaluate or certify that the applicant is sufficiently healthy and physically fit to carry out the duties and activities of the target position. This step is critical in health care organizations, especially when the employee is likely to have frequent contact with patients.

Management and the general public have acknowledged concern about the potentially destructive effects of substance abuse in the workplace. However, a study of human resource managers' attitudes about drug abuse and mandatory testing in hospitals disclosed that only 9% of the employers in the survey had mandatory drug testing as part of their employee selection processes and only 7% required drug testing of current employees.[39]

It should be noted that the ADA has directly affected the use of this selection tool, which had previously been routinely required in many organizations. Under ADA guidelines, the organization may impose a medical examination only after a bona fide job offer has been extended and only if required of all applicants extended job offers for this position.

Probationary Employment

Although not usually considered part of the selection process itself, the period of probationary or provisional employment covering the first phase of the selected applicant's employment in the target position is closely linked to it. This period, typically lasting 3 months for nonprofessional and technical positions and 6 months or longer for professional and managerial positions, gives the applicant an opportunity to become oriented to the job and organization under lower performance expectations than when the employee achieves regular employment status. For the employer, the probationary period provides an opportunity to set expectations and closely monitor the new employee's performance and conduct with his or her supervisor and coworkers. Furthermore, it allows either the employer or the employee to terminate the relationship voluntarily during the probationary period in the case of an unsuccessful match without adverse effects on either party.

Employee Retention. Retention of staff, although not considered to be a separate and distinct specialization or function within HRM, is in fact one of management's most important responsibilities. Not only must a system obtain inputs (resources) to transform into outputs (products and services), but also the system itself must be maintained through the application of these resources. This requires the steady availability or flow of resources for the system to sustain its endeavors and to survive. In practice, the organization must give priority to retention of its employees (or at least those who provide net benefit to the organization) because employee turnover is so costly to the organization. The costs associated with placing a new employee in a target position ready to perform the job are considerable. These include the costs of reviewing and updating job descriptions, developing recruitment plans, media advertisements and recruiter's travel expenses, employee relocation, separation compensation, interviewing, reference checks, test administration and analysis, and employee orientation and supervisory training. Implicit costs are also incurred, such as decreased productivity associated with position vacancies and the learning curve for employees in training. Various estimates have been made of the total costs of employee turnover. Cascio[40] reported a study of this issue within the pharmaceutical firm Merck & Company that showed turnover costs ranging from 1.5 to 2.5 times the annual salary paid for the affected job. By applying his turnover cost model to hypothetic hospital cost data, Cascio[40] estimated an average turnover cost of almost $8000 per employee.

Supervisory Coaching

All of remaining HRM functions and activities discussed in this chapter can be considered to have direct or indirect effects on employee retention. Although supervisory coaching is inherent in the supervisor's role and not an HRM staff function, it could be argued that this process has the greatest long-term impact on employee satisfaction, morale, level of performance, and, ultimately, retention.

Providing regular feedback on performance to employees is perhaps the most critical aspect of the supervisor's coaching role in encouraging, developing, and retaining employees. Employees typically want to have constructive and useful feedback about aspects of their performance that require improvement and would benefit from additional guidance, practice, or formal training. Without clear and candid feedback, employees quite naturally assume that their performance is at least satisfactory and that it fulfills the supervisor's expectations.

Orientation. Human resource management involves more than identifying, evaluating, and hiring qualified individuals for positions within the organization. Unless the employer ensures that the new employee has an appropriate and supportive transition into the job and the broader organization, the efforts and cost associated with recruitment and selection may be wasted. When the employee reports for the first day of work, processes must be in place to facilitate the new employee's transition. The process of becoming a productive employee effectively socialized into the culture of the organization is critical to the organization and to the employee. This process includes both orientation to the environment, such as locating the restrooms, obtaining an identification card, meeting coworkers, and orientation to the job itself in terms of performance expectations and standards, work process, and cultural norms. Various methods are used in the orientation process, including formal group presentations, self-guided instructional media, supervisory "walk-throughs," review of orientation manuals and employee handbooks, and the shadowing of veteran employees and supervisors.

Formal orientation programs may be provided for all new employees within a health care organization through scheduled group or individual sessions conducted by the human resources department. This orientation *never* substitutes for the job-specific departmental orientation and the personal interchange between the new employee, the supervisor, and the peer group.

Orientation programs are a key ingredient of employee satisfaction in an organization. The central objectives of orientation are to reduce a new employee's anxieties about fitting in and to make sure that the employee is sufficiently familiar with the job requirements and expectations to begin to make a positive contribution in the position. Effective orientation can reduce down time, error rates, and the new employee's stress and accelerate the learning process. Furthermore, an effective program should address all aspects of the work environment including the social, technological, cultural, and political dimensions relevant to performance in the position.

One of the major benefits to the employer of a formal, integrated orientation program is to provide accurate, relevant, and consistent information to all new employees in contrast to their obtaining information and misinformation piecemeal from new coworkers and acquaintances. An effectively designed orientation program utilizes HRM staff, supervisors, and well-respected coworkers to provide a comprehensive and participatory learning experience.

The Changing Work Environment and Employee Expectations. In today's environment of geographical, career, and social mobility, it is rare for an employee to hold the same job in one organization for longer than several years. The erosion of organizational loyalty and identification has been aggravated by the aggressive downsizing efforts associated with the corporate re-engineering movement of the early 1990s. Furthermore, we have witnessed increasing "externalization" of the workforce in the form of part-time and casual employees, off-site work, and contracting for temporary workers, which has further eroded the expectations of the traditional employment relationship.[41] It is notable that by the early 1990s, the largest private employer in the United States was Manpower, Inc., a temporary help agency.[42]

College graduates are cautioned to maintain a high level of current and transferable skills, to "travel light" without making or expecting long-term commitments, and to anticipate a career of continuing transitions from one project to another with an ever-changing set of team members and rotating leaders. Organizational identities blur as mergers, buyouts, and restructuring leave the outsider (and perhaps even the employees and other stakeholders most affected) confused and frustrated. As traditional organizational structures seem to "morph" rapidly into new, less-familiar ones, defining accountability, maintaining controls, and sustaining vision over the long term (i.e., beyond the end of the quarter) seem increasingly elusive goals. In health care it is especially important that managers, health care professionals, technologists, and support staff all stay focused on the mission of providing high-quality health care and related services continuously while doing so cost-effectively.

Performance Appraisal Systems

Performance appraisal is one of the most critical and most problematic of all the human resource subsystems. Most employees and many supervisors approach the performance appraisal process with suspicion, cynicism, frustration, and anxiety. Typically, neither employees nor supervisors expect any positive or lasting outcomes, at least for most employees. It is not uncommon for supervisors to regard the process as something to get out of the way so that more productive and less unpleasant work might be accomplished. All too frequently, performance appraisal has been done carelessly, unreliably, and even destructively in terms of the employee's motivation, productivity, and relationship with the supervisor. Indeed, sometimes performance appraisal as a systematic method for observing, evaluating, documenting, and giving feedback to employees about their performance is not done at all.

Given the importance of performance appraisal and its potential benefits to both the employee and the organization, its negative characterization is especially unfortunate. When the process is understood by supervisors and employees and the evaluators and the evaluated, has been well designed, and is effectively managed, it should further the goals of individual employees, managers, and other stakeholders of the organization. For the health care organization, the benefits of effective appraisal should ultimately enhance the quality of health care provided to the community.

Performance appraisal entails three interrelated processes: measurement, judgment, and communication. Although each of these processes must be done competently to achieve the objectives of appraisal, it can be argued that the last is the most critical because it has the most pervasive impact on the supervisory relationship. The measurement dimension is addressed by the determination of the assessment method, for instance, quantitative rating of performance factors, and the design of the appraisal instrument(s). **Graphic rating scales,** one of the most common rating techniques in practice, calls for the rater to assess performance according to numerical scales often anchored by brief descriptors of performance. This measurement aspect of appraisal is a technical specialization performed by HRM staff or under contract. The judgment aspect is a special (and especially challenging) case of the supervisory coaching function. The effectively trained supervisor, who understands the supervisory role, has gained the respect of his or her team, and typically exercises good sense in day-to-day decision making, is likely to demonstrate good judgment in the performance appraisal process.

Communication is a fundamental supervisory-management process and organizational dynamic. Effective multiway and reciprocal communication is a requirement for any open system to sustain itself and maintain internal coordination. Communication as a critical aspect of performance appraisal entails the presentation of clear performance expectations, attempts to validate the employee's understanding and "buy in" to enhancing performance, and the supervisor's feedback on performance, such as encouragement, identifying deficiencies, and praising extra effort.

Unless the supervisor provides the employee with specific, action-oriented, candid, but supportive feedback, investment in other aspects of the process is likely to be wasted and the primary objective, shaping employee behavior in achieving individual, unit, and organizational goals, frustrated.

Structured and comprehensive evaluation of employee performance should provide valuable information to management to support various organizational systems. Compensation decisions, such as merit-based increases, and promotions are often linked to performance appraisal results. These results can identify training and development needs to plan for individual, team, and unit-wide training. Alternatively, the appraisal process might be used to justify a disciplinary response to a "problem" employee or referral to an EAP for counseling and referral. Managers can monitor output from performance appraisal reviews to identify patterns or trends that reflect strengths and deficiencies in recruitment, selection, or training programs.

A performance appraisal system should produce an accurate and comprehensive profile of the employee's job performance. One approach calls for a *360-degree evaluation*[43] that identifies, observes, and assesses the totality of the employee's responsibilities and contributions. For this to be done effectively, job performance factors, standards, weights, and criteria must be established, defined, communicated, and accepted by both managers and employees. The performance appraisal system then uses this information as the foundation for the evaluation process.

Ideally, performance factors, standards, and criteria should be developed through a rigorous consensus process that includes input from a representative group with relevant perspectives on the job(s) subject to job analysis. Typically this would include job incumbents, supervisors, peers in jobs linked to those being analyzed, and, when feasible, clients. The 360-degree approach is built on the assumption that diverse perspectives that "wrap around" the entire job can be obtained. For example, one performance factor for a database management specialist might be "quality of client services." The related performance standard might be "providing database design solutions that are responsive to the client's expressed need within resource and time constraints" and the criterion establishes one or more specific conditions that define success, such as some measure of efficient design or productivity target.

Although some performance factors and standards might be common to many jobs within an organization, such as quality of patient care, no two units or supervisors are likely to apply precisely the same criteria for evaluation in practice. For performance appraisal to be valid for any one position or unit, the factors, standards, and criteria must be established with the target jobs in mind. Poor fit between the performance appraisal process and the reality of the jobs subject to this process works against valid, reliable, and useful appraisal outcomes.

Methods of Performance Appraisal

Employee Ranking

Although no longer commonly used as the primary appraisal method, employee ranking has been used in the military for leadership assessment and promotional review and in higher education for faculty recruitment and appointment processes. Two types of ranking have been used most often: simple ranking and forced distribution. In *simple ranking,* all employees (or candidates) are ranked from 1 to *n* on one or more summary or global measures of performance, such as overall contribution to the department's goals. The supervisor should consider and rank all employees under his or her authority, often in descending order from "best" to "least" (or "worst") contributor. This approach has the benefit of simplicity and efficiency, assuming that the number of employees supervised is not too large, that is, 15 or fewer. The major disadvantages are that one global performance factor is usually too broad to be a useful measure for employee feedback and performance improvement and that a ranked list of employees does not facilitate effective feedback.

Forced distribution ranking requires the supervisor to place the employees into a set of ordered groups, for example, "top 10%," "above average 20%," "middle 40%," on the basis of a global measure. In effect, this forces the employees into a more or less normal distribution along this performance factor. Because it does not require the supervisor to rank within these categories, it eases the ranking burden and may make the ranking more useful as a feedback measure of "where the employee stands." However, it shares the other deficiencies of simple ranking.

If used as the sole or primary method of employee evaluation, ranking is too limited and subjective to be a useful measure of performance in most situations. However, ranking could be applied as a supplement to another method that is considered generally more valid and reliable.

Graphic Rating Scales

Various approaches and tools (instruments) have been used to rate employee performance. A set of graphic rating scales is probably the earliest and most common method in practice (Figure 16-10). A graphic rating scale is a linear, continuous scale representing performance for a predetermined performance factor, dimension, component, or some personal characteristic. Typically, the scale displays a discrete but arbitrary range of numerical increments, with four-, five-, and seven-point scales the most common. Often the scales are labeled by using verbal "anchors," such as "fails to meet standards," "meets standards," and "far exceeds

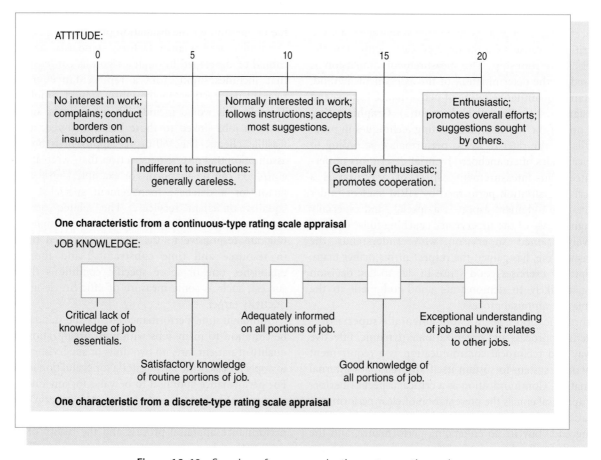

Figure 16-10 Sample performance evaluation system—rating scale.

standards," to enhance the reliability of the rating. Some scales are anchored only at the end points, and raters are asked to check the appropriate location on the continuum corresponding to their intuitive rating. To be useful and valid measures of job performance, the scales must be clearly understood, designed to be reliable indicators of performance, and based on the critical behaviors and skills that determine job performance.

Critical Incident Method

The **critical incident method** of employee performance evaluation requires the supervisor to document exceptional job-related behavior, that is, extremely effective or ineffective performance, actually observed or reported. Such statements, identified as critical incidents, collectively represent the range of behavior typical for that employee. Documented positive critical incidents may be used as the basis for merit pay decisions and negative ones used as the basis for performance correction plans or disciplinary action. Although this method is a potentially powerful source of job-specific feedback, it is very prone to various biases and subjectivity in observation and reporting. Nonetheless, documenting exceptional incidents of performance is on balance likely to be worth the supervisor's effort.

Behaviorally Anchored Rating Scales

Behaviorally anchored rating scales (BARS) were developed in part to address concerns about the reliability of traditional graphical rating scales. The BARS method anchors the numerical scales with brief narrative descriptions of a range of behavior from highest to lowest level of performance on that dimension. These narrative descriptions may be drawn from critical incidents documented in real-world supervisory situations. For example, on a scale of "interpersonal effectiveness with clients" as an aspect of the performance of physical therapists, a brief scenario representing especially cordial, responsive, and client-centered behavior could be used to anchor the highest level of performance on this dimension. Other realistic scenarios would be developed and matched to the range of discrete points on the scale. This method offers several advantages over the traditional rating scales in addition to the objective of improving the reliability of the rating itself. When the numerical ratings are anchored in "slices of life" familiar to both supervisor and employee, the employee has a clearer, more concrete understanding of how the supervisor views his or her performance. Although this method does not guarantee that the supervisor will rate the employee fairly or "objectively" or that the employee will agree with the supervisor's rating, both parties should have a common ground for discussion on the basis of specific job behavior. It should be noted that research has not demonstrated that the BARS method results in more reliable ratings statistically (Figure 16-11).

Goal Setting and Performance Improvement Plans

During the 1970s and 1980s, **management by objectives** (MBO) dominated corporate thinking as *the* model paradigm or system to integrate business planning, productivity

Behavioral Anchors	Rating	Score
Manager consistently models the highest standards of ethical behavior as demonstrated in her/his leadership in organizational, professional and community roles.	Outstanding	4
Manager holds her/himself and her/his staff to high standards of ethical performance by addressing this dimension explicitly in the performance appraisal review with her/his employees.	Excellent	3
Manager periodically acknowledges the core values of the health system and the HIM profession in staff/team meetings and other modes of communication, emails, bulletin board postings, etc.	Good	2
Manager's behavior complies overall with organizational policies and AHIMA Code of Ethics.	Satisfactory	1
Manager has one or more documented incidents of violations of organizational conduct and/or professional ethical standards.	Unacceptable	1

Figure 16-11 Behaviorally anchored rating performance appraisal system.

management and control, employee performance evaluation, and supervisory coaching. MBO, developed as an integrated planning process by George Odiorne and popularized by the management guru Peter Drucker, became so pervasive and its advocates so committed that it might be regarded as a total philosophy of management. Although MBO has largely been replaced by waves of alternative approaches, such as strategic management, total quality management, and re-engineering, one of its core principles, the systematic setting and periodic review of performance goals, has survived the passing waves of management fads.

In fact, there would be considerable consensus among scholars and managers that goal setting should be an essential part of any performance appraisal process. When any evaluation method reveals a significant performance or skill deficiency, behavioral problem, or other obstacle to peak performance, the supervisor has a responsibility to address this concern. One effective approach is to set specific, actionable goals within a coherent performance plan. The goals should be clearly understood by both supervisor and employee, as concrete and quantifiable as possible, and their attainment measurable or observable. A specific target date for completion of the goal or a sequence of projected progress points must be established for the goal to be effective. Although some flexibility should be built into the performance plan to recognize the effects of factors beyond the employee's control, agreement about projected dates of key milestones is critical. A goal without a time frame for implementation is at best an expression of good intention but not a genuine performance goal statement. The employee should be encouraged to participate actively in the goal-setting process, but at the very least the employee must "buy into" whatever goals are established for the employee.

Self-appraisal can be a useful complement to traditional rating schemes and goal setting. The employee is encouraged to reflect on his or her performance for the period, identify strengths and weaknesses, and identify accomplishments and obstacles to progress before the formal performance appraisal review. The employee and supervisor, using the same evaluation tool, can then compare one another's perceptions of the same performance history. Although this process does not guarantee agreement about ratings or the value added by the employee's contribution, it certainly encourages the exploration of common ground, a more objective approach to analysis of performance problems and mutual goal setting.

An example of a performance improvement plan is shown in Figure 16-12.

Checklists

Standardized checklists may be used to select statements or words that most clearly describe an employee's performance (Figure 16-13). They may also be associated with weights when scored so that the more critical job duties have greater impact than less important ones. A forced-choice method requires the supervisor to choose the one statement in each

For professional development and growth, the following goals will be established to improve personal productivity and enhance contributions to department objectives and the hospital mission.

Within each goal, selected objectives are outlined to serve as benchmarks and measure towards that goal.

Area of Accountablilty—Clinical Data Coordination

I. Reduce unbilled accounts due to coding to 0 days with minimum oversight.

   A. Report status every Monday to department head using the Health Information Services weekly statistics form.

   B. Outline reasons for variance from the standard.

   C. Perform timely follow-up to assure that all records are released for billing within the time parameters established.

II. Improve productivity in coding and abstracting. Industry standards for coding hospital inpatients are 8 minutes per record and Outpatient Services, 2.5 minutes per record.

   A. Document obstacles that prohibit this level of performance at this hospital.

   B. Increase coding expertise through continuing education from a variety of resources.

   C. Code all patient types to enhance skills.

III. Use Continuous Quality Improvement (CQI) principles to improve work efficiency in your responsibility area.

   A. Organize work area to exhibit neatness and efficiency.

   B. Prioritize daily work to optimize adherence to department CQI standards. Report when not attainable to reasons beyond your control.

Figure 16-12 Sample performance development goal plan.

pair of statements that is more descriptive of some relevant aspect of the employee's performance being evaluated. Examples of paired statements follow:

1a. The employee is a quick learner.
1b. The employee is often late in completing assigned work.
2a. The employee is a diligent worker.
2b. The employee takes longer than the typical employee to learn new procedures.

Forced-choice methods often use a standardized instrument, so that the process is not likely to include job-specific performance factors and criteria. Another disadvantage is that the supervisor may find this method unfamiliar and difficult to complete by choosing between statements that appear to be unrelated or abstract. Furthermore, it is not obvious that the output of this process lends itself to useful feedback to the employee.

Weights	Performance Appraisal Criteria	Check
6.5	Employee is accountable to essential job duties.	
4.0	Employee keeps work area well organized.	
3.9	Employee works cooperatively with others as a team.	
4.3	Employee considers consequences before taking action.	
0.2	Employee adheres to dress code.	
etc.		
Total 100		
	Total of All Weights Checked	

Employee Name_____ Department_____
Position_____ Date_____
Supervisor_____

Figure 16-13 Representation of a sample weighted performance checklist.

Each of the methods just presented and variations of them have relative strengths and deficiencies as performance evaluation tools. The human resource manager has responsibility to ensure that a reliable, useful, and credible process is tested, implemented, and monitored for effectiveness. It is critical that all employees are educated about the process and that supervisors are trained to understand their role in the process and how to conduct performance appraisal effectively.

Rater Biases That Affect Appraisal. A major problem associated with the measurement aspect of performance appraisal is the potential for rater bias. The following are common biases that can invalidate any evaluation method if not recognized and addressed:

- **Halo effect**—When one performance factor or personal characteristic dominates the evaluator's perceptions and judgments. This is one of the most common and difficult to remedy sources of bias.
- **Central tendency error**—When the evaluator rates all employees similarly as "average" on most performance factors. This predisposition to "play it safe" distorts the process by failing to make valid distinctions among employees in level of performance and between factors of performance for the same employee that are demonstrated in practice.
- **Leniency or strictness bias**—The tendency to be consistently too lenient or too strict in evaluation relative to the actual level of performance.
- **Recency effect**—The phenomenon in which the most recent incidents or trends in employee's performance have disproportionate influence on the overall per-

ceptions of and judgments about the employee's performance. Ideally, the entire range of employee behaviors across all job duties and activities for a specified time period should be reviewed and assessed based on reliable documentation.

- **Stereotyping**—Founding evaluative perceptions and judgment on stereotypes on the basis of racial, ethnic, gender, age, disability, or other personal or cultural characteristics. Bias based on these deep-seated stereotypes and attitudes independent of an individual's competence and level of performance has proved to be very resistant to change.
- **Personal prejudice or favoritism**—The supervisor's personal likes and dislikes of employees independent of their performance and conduct should not affect performance evaluation. Assessments should be based as firmly as possible on applying clearly communicated performance factors and criteria to observed and documented performance.

Implementation of the Performance Appraisal System. Effective implementation of the employee performance appraisal system is one of the most critical and challenging of management's responsibilities because it is so central to the organization's strategic planning and control functions. The system must be demonstrated to be useful and valid both to justify the resources committed to it on a cost-benefit basis and to withstand any legal challenges. An effective system should make a measurable difference in terms of improved performance, whereas an ineffective system can actually result in deterioration of performance, job satisfaction, and supervisory and employee motivation. The risks of ineffective performance appraisal are great indeed.

The key element in the process resides in the fabric of the supervisory relationship itself. If the supervisor applies effective coaching and interpersonal skills, understands team process, and has earned respect among the employees as a fair, competent, and ethical leader, that will provide a solid foundation for the performance appraisal system. Without this foundation of consistently effective supervision, even a technically sound method backed by strong top management endorsement is likely to fail.

Adverse Outcomes of Employee Performance

Although the goals of the HRM system are focused on the effective use and full development of all the individuals participating in the organization, it is a fact of our organizational experience that too often these objectives are not fulfilled for some employees. Employees fail to live up to supervisory expectations and probably their own as well. Individuals with an excellent work history suddenly demonstrate declining performance or erratic behavior. After a generally positive but somewhat critical supervisory evaluation, employees become less enthusiastic about the job, distance themselves from coworkers, and begin to miss work frequently without clear justification. On failing to obtain an expected promotion, a manager "retreats" into the technical aspects of work and becomes increasingly absorbed in Internet stock investment. A single parent has an interruption of child care coverage and begins to leave before the shift ends, spends excessive time on the phone, and periodically displays fits of temper with coworkers. Such signs of performance failure, career frustration, or personal and family problems interfering with on-the-job performance can point to adverse consequences to follow for the employee and for the organization. Instead of promotions, career mobility, compensation increases, and job satisfaction, many employees experience the anger, frustration, and erosion of self-confidence and credibility among their peers associated with career plateaus or performance decline.

Adverse organizational responses to real or perceived deterioration of performance and problematic behavior— for example, inappropriate sexual references or abusive conduct—can lead to invoking of the employee discipline process, referral to an EAP, demotions, or job transfers. In the extreme case, the employee may be terminated for cause on the basis of performance deficiencies, unacceptable conduct, or failing to provide net benefit to the organization. Because of a disruptive personality, poor work ethic, refusal to accommodate to the organizational culture, or some other factor, management has determined that the employee's behavior incurs higher costs to the organization than whatever benefits might result.

Most organizations have termination-for-cause events that require immediate dismissal. These situations are usually clearly defined and, although unpleasant, not usually as troublesome for the manager as subtler and more chronic problems (Box 16-8).

Box 16-8   EXAMPLES OF EMPLOYEE BEHAVIOR THAT MIGHT JUSTIFY FOR-CAUSE TERMINATION

- Prolonged absence from work without notification
- Chronic history of irregular attendance and failing to report
- Threatening behavior directed toward patients, coworkers, or managers
- Reporting for work under the influence of drugs or alcohol
- Being caught in the act of theft, embezzlement, or fraud against the employer or clients
- Extremely offensive or chronic acts of sexual harassment
- Significant use of the organization's resources for private business or gain without prior approval

---

Wrongful Discharge. The employer almost always justifies an employee termination on the basis of "just cause," on the basis of the employee's outrageous, dangerous, negligent, or insubordinate behavior or chronically deficient performance. In spite of the legal tradition of "at-will" employment discussed next, employees increasingly (and in some state courts, successfully) have challenged presumed just-cause terminations. Because this legal doctrine is evolving and differs among states, this remains an ambiguous and therefore risky area for HRM professionals and the employer.

An attempt to negotiate a resolution with the problem employee is recommended if an employee is likely to take court action to pursue a wrongful discharge. A negotiated severance payment, outplacement assistance, and transfer to another, more suitable position in the organization are some alternatives to termination that may be mutually acceptable. Whatever the facts of a specific situation, the health information manager must be aware of the legal constraints and consequences imposed on employers to protect employees from wrongful discharge.

At-Will Employment. Historically, employers and employees have operated under the English common law doctrine of **employment at will.** Under this doctrine, an employment contract without a specified length of term could be terminated by either party with or without cause. Recently, this doctrine has been eroded in the courts at least in some states as a reflection of the expanding scope of employee rights initiated by the EEO revolution.[44] Such claims of unjust termination are generally based on one of these legal foundations:

Tort law. The termination is based on the premise that the employee has economic injury or damages from the action of the employer. This application of civil law principles does not entail breach of contract.

Implied contract. Courts in many states have recognized claims based on statements made in employee manuals and handbooks or oral statements made by managers. The managers' statements or the handbooks are interpreted with the implication that an employee would be retained for a certain length of time or indefinitely as long as the employee meets standards of satisfactory performance.

Implied covenant of good faith and fair dealing. This approach challenges the termination on the basis that the employee was discharged for reasons other than just cause, violating an implicit covenant. The good faith and fair dealing principle would most likely be recognized on the basis of an employee's seniority, record of satisfactory performance, and positive representations of the employee's performance by supervisory management. Relatively few states recognize such an implied covenant in the employment context.

Public policy exception. This covers a situation in which a termination for any cause conflicts with the intent of another public policy. For example, an employee demonstrating irregular performance is discharged for filing a Workers' Compensation claim or for threatening to report abuse of hospital patients to state authorities.

It must be emphasized that differences in legal precedent and interpretation among state courts make this area uncertain and difficult. In general, management is in the best position by treating terminations as a last resort, being prepared to prove just cause, and by applying this remedy equitably to all employees under similar circumstances.

Wrongful Discharge Defense. Before taking steps to terminate a problem employee, managers should review the following considerations to protect themselves and their organizations against wrongful discharge allegations and further conflict:

- Were any promises about terms of employment made to the employee at the time of hiring or subsequently that were not fulfilled?
- Is there a good cause for the termination in terms of documented violation of organizational policies, codes of employee behavior, or a pattern of behavior that in the aggregate could be considered as justification for termination?
- Has this employee filed any claim, charge, or complaint with any government agency or engaged in any "protected" activity, for example, in unionization efforts?
- Will the decision to terminate appear to the reasonable person to be fair, deliberate, and reasonable?
- Do other managers aware of the situation support the decision?
- Is there complete documentation of the events leading to the decision to take action?
- Was this employee in a particularly vulnerable position at the time of termination?

For additional safeguards for management contemplating disciplinary action, please refer to Figure 16-14.

Layoffs. Involuntary separation occurs whenever the employer terminates the employment relationship for whatever reason, sometimes as a result of low patient volume, restructuring, or adverse economic conditions. As previously discussed, **layoffs** should be avoided when possible if the same result can be achieved by reduction of the employee's hours, early retirement, or job sharing. Involuntary separation usually provides the employees affected with no direct benefits other than eligibility for unemployment compensation benefits administered by a state agency. If layoffs affecting a significant number of employees can be

Prior to taking disciplinary action, a manager may complete this checklist. If one or more "no's" are checked, it is a good idea to discuss the action with the Director of Human Resources or someone from Administration to assure the disciplinary action planned is appropriate under the circumstances.

	Yes	No
1. Has the work rule or the policy that was violated been published or otherwise clearly communicated to this employee?		
2. Did this employee ever receive a written copy of this rule or policy?		
3. Is the rule posted on bulletin boards or similar areas?		
4. Is the infraction reasonably related to the orderly, efficient, and safe operation of the unit, department, or organization?		
5. If others have similar infractions, did they receive the same disciplinary action as is being contemplated for this employee?		
6. Are there factual records available on all employees covering violation of the rule or policy in question?		
7. Does this employee have the worst record of all employees on violation of this rule or policy?		
8. Have there been any previous warnings for violation of this rule or policy given to this employee?		
9. Does the documentation surrounding the infractions include dates, times, places, witnesses, and pertinent facts on all past violations?		
10. Is there a factual written record showing the steps taken by the manager to correct the improper conduct of all employees?		
11. Is the degree of discipline to be imposed related to the seriousness of the offense, the degree of fault, and any mitigating factors?		
12. Has this employee had an opportunity to tell his or her side of the story?		

Figure 16-14 Disciplinary checklist.

anticipated, it is sound management policy and ethically responsive to notify the affected employees as early as possible to give them the opportunity to plan for the economic dislocation involved.

Retirement. Retirement is another type of separation, which may be voluntary or involuntary. The number of involuntary retirements is likely to decrease in large part because of amendments to the ADEA, which eliminated forced retirement at an arbitrary age for most employees, with the exception of some highly paid executives. With the increasing affluence of older individuals due in part to the extended "bull market" in equities and the corresponding growth in retirement assets, however, we might anticipate an increase in voluntary retirements at an earlier mean age. It will be the responsibility of HRM staff to track retirement patterns and identify key individuals facing retirement so that recruitment and replacement plans and targets may be developed. In some environments, including health care, some older professionals may choose to negotiate contacts on a part-time or per-project consulting basis. This could provide advantages to the employer by reducing employee benefit costs while retaining access to the considerable knowledge, skills, and experience that the preretiree has to offer the organization. At the same time, this arrangement could ease the older employee's transition into his or her later career.

Employee Counseling and Discipline

Employee **counseling and referral** and **progressive discipline** are problem-solving processes to halt the decline in a troubled employee's performance and to prevent excessive employee turnover through termination or supervisor-initiated transfers. Whatever managers can do to prevent unnecessary terminations is likely to provide net benefit to the organization. Employees do not resign voluntarily, except under exceptional circumstances, if they enjoy a satisfying work environment, a challenging job, communication with their supervisors, and personal opportunities for growth.

All organizations have policies, procedures, and standards for employee conduct that serve as guidelines to expected employee behavior. These policies and procedures are usually documented in organizational and departmental policy manuals and in employee handbooks. These personnel policies should include a description of a progressive disciplinary process and the **grievance procedure.** The disciplinary process should be invoked when neither performance appraisal nor assertive supervisory coaching has been an effective remedy for problem behavior. The grievance process, on the other hand, provides a communication and problem-solving mechanism for employees to express a complaint that management has violated one of its own policies (or the union contract) with adverse consequences for the employee. The proactive health information manager communicates these policies and procedures

to current staff and to new employees in orientation, staff in-services, and periodic performance reviews. Critical incidents of problem behavior and specific violations of management policies must be documented for follow-up actions, such as initiating the disciplinary process. When employees fail to follow these policies and rules of acceptable conduct, it is the manager's responsibility to assist the employee in taking corrective action and achieving an effective level of performance.

Counseling and Referral. Employee counseling is provided to assist the employee in addressing personal and other problems that might originate outside the workplace but affect job performance and behavior in the workplace. Referral is the process of linking the employee with an array of resources to address the specific problem(s) identified. Informal counseling and referral on a very limited basis has traditionally been regarded as a supervisory role. However, within the past two decades most large organizations, including those in health care, have recognized the need to provide counseling and referral services on a more professional and consistent basis by establishing Employee Assistance Programs (EAPs). EAP services may be provided in-house through a centralized staff of trained counselors who provide counseling and referral to address an array of problems and issues including financial concerns, family and community conflicts, depression, eating disorders, alcohol and substance abuse, and other behavioral problems. Alternatively, EAP services may be provided under contract with one or more external agencies. This arrangement might reduce the total costs of providing these services and should mitigate concerns about maintaining strict confidentiality for employees who seek these services.

In either approach, the supervisor has a key role in providing a link between the troubled employee and appropriate resources to address the employee's problems. One of the most critical aspects of this role is that the supervisor recognizes employee verbal and nonverbal behavior that indicates more serious problems and responds to any employee's suggestions that he or she requires assistance and resources in handling problems interfering with work performance and overall well-being. The other obligation is to ensure that the supervisor and all others involved in any referral to the EAP maintain complete confidentiality to preserve the integrity and credibility of the program.

Employee Discipline. Although it is not a comfortable issue for most managers of the "baby boomer" generation, maintaining employee discipline is a prerequisite for organizational effectiveness and even viability in a competitive, uncertain environment. Every system must maintain internal order to survive and grow. An employee disciplinary process must be invoked in cases in which that basic order is threatened or disrupted by challenges to authority, insubordination, dangerous or abusive behavior to coworkers or clients, chronic violation of management policies, criminal activity, or other behavior that brings discredit or legal liability to the organization.

Progressive Discipline. There is a consensus among practitioners that a progressive discipline process is most effective, one in which there is a planned sequence of managerial responses of increasing severity to correct continuing violations of policy regarding acceptable employee conduct and performance standards. Its purpose is to give the employee subject to the disciplinary process several opportunities to correct the offensive behavior before the final irrevocable step of termination is invoked. It is in the best interests of both management and the employee to have the problem(s) resolved satisfactorily at one of the earlier stages in the process. When the infraction is of a less disruptive nature, such as chronic tardiness or absenteeism, employees may be motivated to take corrective action without additional incentives, having realized the risks entailed by continuing the challenged behavior. In other situations, progressive discipline may not be as effective or even appropriate, for example, in response to outrageous behavior endangering the lives of others.

The progressive disciplinary process usually includes at least the following stages after the supervisor has identified a chronic or emerging behavior problem:

1. Oral warning (with a note to the employee's file)
2. Written warning and reprimand
3. Suspension with final warning
4. Termination

It should be noted that depending on the severity of the infraction, the employee's history of conduct, and his or her response to the disciplinary warning, steps in the process may be adjusted or omitted. However, management should ensure consistency of disciplinary response in like situations to avoid charges of favoritism or discriminatory treatment.

Oral Warning

Progressive discipline is initiated by an oral warning from the supervisor to the employee about the offending behavior. The warning should include a candid description of the problem, what measures are required to correct it, and the specific deadlines or target dates to accomplish the behavior change. A summary of this conversation should be documented in the manager's records but not placed in the employee's permanent personnel file.

Written Warning and Reprimand

If the behavior is not corrected within the expected time frame, the next step is a written warning and reprimand. The written warning must clearly indicate the following information:

- Nature of the problem behavior
- Reference to the specific policy, guidelines, or standards violated

- Record of the date of the verbal warning
- Documentation of any critical incidents of the employee's behavior subsequent to the initial warning
- Restatement of the corrective action required
- Explanation of the consequences of failure to correct the sanctioned behavior

A separate statement reprimanding the employee for engaging in the offending behavior might be provided as well. The purpose of this stage is to put the employee clearly on notice that pursuing the unacceptable behavior or failing to take the corrective action specified will result in clear and certain disciplinary consequences, including termination if circumstances warrant it.

Suspension or Final Written Warning

Suspension from work without pay may be an appropriate "last resort" disciplinary action before termination. This step might be especially appropriate in situations involving the threat of violence or especially disruptive behavior as it provides a "cooling off" period for all parties involved. Suspension (usually for a 3- to 5-day period) also gives management an opportunity to do a thorough investigation of the facts of the situation when the employee's presence might interfere with that process. This should facilitate management's making a more informed decision about whether to proceed to termination or alternative disciplinary actions. It should be noted that suspension per se should not be invoked as a punishment of the employee. In fact, the employee facing further disciplinary action would probably be feeling considerable stress and might welcome a temporary separation from the workplace.

Termination or Discharge

Termination should be reserved as a last resort when other good faith efforts have failed. It is only partly in jest that this step is referred to as the workplace "death penalty" because of the adverse personal, economic, and career consequences. Although in some extreme cases it might be appropriate to skip other stages in the disciplinary process and proceed to termination, this should be done only with caution and strong justification because it appears to conflict with the "progressive" aspect of the process. Termination in one sense represents a system failure, a waste of organizational resources, even when the employee is given full and fair opportunity to correct the problem. Furthermore, termination decisions are subject to employee grievances and the risk of legal action. Consequently, this disciplinary action should never be taken without the most serious deliberation and after all other options have been explored.

Progressive discipline works well with violations of policy and rules of acceptable conduct but may not be appropriate or effective in problems involving skill deficiency or quality of work performance. In fact, invoking the disciplinary process may produce a negative reaction that would complicate efforts to help the employee develop a performance improvement plan. In-service education or focused counseling is likely to be more effective in these situations. It should be recognized that in some "gray area" situations the determination of whether to treat a performance problem as a disciplinary one may be difficult. In these cases, the supervisor should seek advice from his or her manager or the designated HRM professional to make a fully informed decision. It should be emphasized that the objective of the disciplinary process is *not punishment but correction* and compliance.

Preventive discipline is another approach consistent with the purposes of the disciplinary process already discussed. A preventive approach encourages understanding of the rationale for and compliance with policies, standards, and rules so that significant violations of policy are avoided. These efforts might be most effectively incorporated within continuing team development activities, such as quality team leadership training. However, it is reasonable for the employer to expect self-discipline and that all employees will make reasonable efforts to comply with organizational policies, rules of conduct, and expected standards of performance.

Grievance Process

Management must ensure that employees have full access to an effective mechanism for expressing their concerns and the opportunity to obtain satisfaction when they believe that management has violated organization policy in taking some adverse action against them. The grievance process then is provided to facilitate communication and problem solving when management or the supervisor specifically is in conflict with the employee. A grievance is a formal charge that management has violated a specific management policy or provision of the written agreement (labor contract) that results in denial of some benefit to the employee or an infringement of some alleged right or privilege of employment. Not infrequently, a grievance is filed in response to a disciplinary action taken against the employee, especially in a unionized environment.

Employee grievance or complaint procedures are established because no matter how clearly defined or well communicated an organization's policies and procedures might be, they are always subject to misunderstanding, being applied inappropriately, overlooked, or, less frequently, intentionally disregarded. Questions of interpretation and application of policies or contract language often arise that require a systematic investigation and structure for problem resolution and redress.

Critical to an effective process for handling complaints and disagreements that arise over policies and rules governing the workplace is that prompt and fair action be taken on the basis of informed and balanced judgment. The employee must perceive that a fair hearing will be given and that the final judgment will be equitable and impartial. Ideally, employees who believe that they have been unfairly treated should be able to discuss their concerns with their supervisors. However, the employee's grievance is often directed against the behavior of the immediate supervisor. In these circumstances, it may be difficult to resolve the problem at this level in one-to-one negotiation. When this occurs, a progressive grievance process ensures that the employee will have a fair hearing, that the issue will be thoroughly and fairly investigated, and that a good faith effort will be made to resolve the grievance reasonably and efficiently at the lowest level possible.

The progressive grievance process gives an employee the opportunity to present his or her case to increasingly higher levels of management, recognizing that the problem may not be resolved at the supervisory level. The grievance is presented first to the immediate supervisor for resolution. Failing that, the case may proceed through a sequence of higher levels of authority in the hierarchy for subsequent review and decision. In the nonunion environment, the final decision is typically made at the top executive level, by (for example) the vice president for HRM/labor relations or ultimately the CEO.

In a unionized environment, the grievance process is negotiated as part of the labor contract and usually parallels the process for nonunion employees. The presentation of a grievance by an employee or a group of employees is a protected activity under the NLRA. This entails that the employer cannot fire, penalize, or otherwise discriminate against an employee because the employee has filed a grievance. If the employer takes such an action, the employee has the right to file a complaint with the NLRB.

The primary difference between the nonunion and the unionized environment is that the grievance procedure achieved through collective bargaining almost always includes external arbitration as the final stage. This entails vesting authority for final disposition of the grievance in an impartial third party from outside the organization. The arbitrator, who is typically quite knowledgeable about the industry and experienced in the role, makes a judgment (award) that is "final and binding" on both sides. Because final arbitration places the decision beyond the control of either party and the costs are split equally between management and the union, there is some incentive to settle the grievance at a lower level in the process. Indeed, the logic of the process at least from management's perspective calls for resolution of the issues at the lowest possible level to avoid unnecessary costs and emotional escalation of the dispute.

Developing an Effective Grievance Policy. When communicating a grievance procedure through a policy statement, management must ensure that the following issues are clearly addressed:

- State the purpose and goals of the process.
- Identify which complaints may be handled through the grievance process and which may not, for example, terminations for active drug abuse.

- Describe each stage of the process and the respective time frames for review and decision.
- Specify who is to participate in the presentation of and response to the grievance.
- Describe the mediation and final arbitration process, if applicable.
- Communicate critical time limits for grievance handling to encourage prompt action, investigation, and resolution.
- Clarify the responsibilities of management at each level for documentation, notification, and subsequent action.

A representative (and condensed) model of an effective grievance process for nonunionized employees that is appropriate for most health care organizations is provided next.

Sample Health Information Management Complaint Procedure

Goal of the Complaint Procedure

This procedure was established to create an avenue for problem resolution so that questions or conflicts could be investigated and resolved quickly, thoroughly, and within the appropriate organizational structure.

Valid Complaints

- Questions about or concerns with policies and procedures
- Disagreement with performance appraisal
- Concerns about the physical work environment
- Questions about or concerns with compensation and benefits management

Invalid Complaints

Appeal of termination for cause as specified in the policies and procedures manual is an invalid complaint.

Procedure

1. Complaints should be presented orally to the immediate supervisor.
2. The employee may present the complaint personally or organize a group to present the complaint.
3. The supervisor hears the complaint and makes every effort to resolve the problem at this step. The supervisor shall write out the complaint, whether it is resolved or not, sign it, and then ask the employee or the employee group representative to sign, so that the complaint is documented and clearly defined.
4. If the outlined plan or the resolution proposed by the supervisor is unsatisfactory to the employee or group, a copy of this report is sent to the division chief with the "Request for Review" box checked.
5. The division chief conducts a review and responds to the employee or employee group representative within 3 working days with a plan for problem resolution.

6. If, after this step, the employee or group still believes that the problem is not resolved, the last step is to present the issue to the personnel action committee for consideration. This committee convenes in special session within 10 working days. The decision of this interdisciplinary committee is binding, and no other appeals will be heard.

Compensation Management

Definition. Compensation management entails understanding of wage and salary administration, payroll systems, employee benefits, knowledge of applicable federal and state legislation and regulation, and effective communication strategies. It can be argued that the most critical aspect of compensation management is to communicate effectively the goals, procedures, and constraints associated with the organization's compensation policies and to maintain the credibility of the system as being managed fairly and with integrity. Employees at the least expect to see some stable relationship between their training and experience, level of effort, productivity, and quality of performance (as their contribution) and their total compensation (as their return). Unfortunately, various constraints on the organization often make it difficult if not impossible for management to achieve, sustain, and demonstrate this relationship.

Compensation Management and Other Human Resource Management Functions. Compensation management is interdependent with all the other HRM functions, but especially with recruitment and performance appraisal. If the health care organization is not able to offer competitive salaries and benefit packages to the qualified applicants for health information services, nursing, physical therapy, occupational therapy, dietetics and food service, business office, and other positions, its recruitment efforts are significantly constrained. This affects not only recruitment but also the capacity of the organization to retain its high-performing employees. Inability to maintain competitive compensation almost inevitably has adverse effects on the quality of care provided. If employees have no faith in the fairness of the merit pay or pay-for-performance program and believe instead that favoritism dominates annual pay decisions, this perception can stimulate or reinforce cynicism, frustration, and declining motivation and performance. When the department manager is committed to rewarding superior performers, to acknowledging performance improvement in underachievers, and to correcting historical salary inequities but is given no significant increase in the department's personnel budget, what are the likely effects on the manager's morale and credibility with the staff?

By fairly rewarding meritorious performance, productivity gains, extraordinary effort, notable commitment to customer (patient) service, and other desired outcomes, the organization is more likely to attain employee behaviors over the long term that are consistent with the organization's goals and strategic plans. Human resources planning, recruiting, selection, placement, career planning and development, and performance appraisal also contribute to furthering the organization's mission. However, compensation management programs are somewhat unique in the immediacy of their effects, positive and negative, on individual employees' perceptions of their value to the organization, motivation to perform, and sense of economic security and well-being.

Objectives of Compensation Management. The following objectives are anticipated as a consequence of effective compensation management:

- Attracting well-qualified applicants for positions when needed
- Retaining and motivating employees who are making positive contributions to the organization's mission
- Ensuring that high-quality health care services are continually provided
- Rewarding desirable work behaviors and attitudes
- Controlling costs by managing human and financial resources effectively
- Complying with laws and regulations governing wage and salary administration and employee benefits
- Communicating the goals and policies supporting compensation management programs to sustain employees' understanding and acceptance
- Achieving a system that is perceived by the employees to be fairly and prudently managed

Job Evaluation. Job evaluation, a technical function at the foundation of the compensation management system, provides a formal procedure to determine the relative worth of each position in the organization. In other words, job evaluation results in the fair "pricing" of all jobs in the organization. To be effective, the job evaluation process must be based on a current and useful job description. In fact, job evaluation can be regarded as a process parallel to job analysis that translates a hierarchy of jobs into a pay structure for the organization. Because job evaluation requires special expertise and training, it is usually performed by human resource staff or contracted out to a consultant specializing in compensation systems.

Understanding the process used by the organization to determine the worth of a job to the organization is important for the HIM manager. The manager has a responsibility to ensure that the pay established for health information services positions is equitable with that for comparable positions in the organization and competitive in the relevant labor market. If health information services managers and staff are paid significantly less than staff in similar positions within or external to their organization, the health information manager faces a major constraint in attracting and retaining well-qualified and highly motivated employees. This results in higher costs for recruitment, orientation, and training and the lost productivity because of excessive turnover and supervisory stress and burnout.

Job ranking, job grading or classification, **factor comparison,** and the **point system** are alternative methods used to evaluate jobs. Figure 16-15 compares these methods along two matrices: whether they consider the job as a whole or divide the job into factors for comparison and whether jobs are compared against one another or against some relevant standard.

Job Ranking

The simplest method, but also the least precise, is the ranking method. In this approach, whole jobs are ranked by comparing them with other positions within the organi-

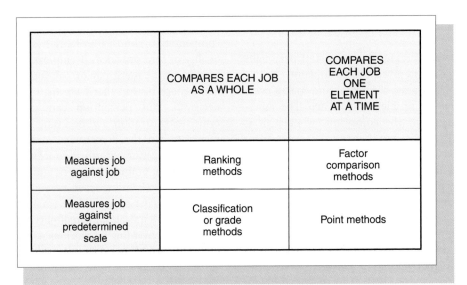

	COMPARES EACH JOB AS A WHOLE	COMPARES EACH JOB ONE ELEMENT AT A TIME
Measures job against job	Ranking methods	Factor comparison methods
Measures job against predetermined scale	Classification or grade methods	Point methods

Figure 16-15 Job evaluation systems chart.

zation on the basis of one or more key characteristics. A file clerk in the health information services department may be ranked near the bottom, whereas the diagnosis-related group coordinator is closer to the top. This ranking is based on the relative levels of responsibility of these positions and their impact on revenue generation. The ranking method is best used in organizations with a small number of positions.

Job Grading

Job grading is more sophisticated than ranking but not necessarily any more precise. This process classifies each job by assigning it to the narrative description of a grade that it most closely resembles. A common example of this method is the traditional civil service classification. This method is not precise because the jobs are compared and categorized on the basis of broad descriptions and judgments about overall similarity. This intuitive assignment process is likely to be least reliable when classifying new jobs that are unlike any of those already classified. The health information manager in an organization using this system must be knowledgeable about the distinctions between job grades to ensure that the jobs within the department are fairly classified and valued.

Factor Comparison

The factor comparison method requires identification of essential factors or elements common to all jobs and comparison of jobs on the basis of rating those elements, not the job as a whole. Factors typically applied in this method are as follow:

- Level of responsibility, including supervision
- Essential skills and knowledge
- Mental effort (demands)
- Physical effort
- Working conditions, including hazardous situations and confidentiality

When these factors have been determined, a set of key or benchmark jobs are identified on the basis that they reflect the array of jobs in the organization. Generally, the pay level of these jobs should reflect market wages for similar positions. The key jobs are then ranked by applying a rating scale to each of the common factors. By using a current average salary or prevailing market rate for each job, weighting the common elements, and distributing this wage rate among the job factors, a pay level or range is established for each job. Finally, all other jobs are evaluated and priced using the key jobs as benchmarks.

Point System

A point system evaluates jobs by analyzing key elements of the job and assigning point values to these factors on the basis of predetermined descriptive standards or criteria. The latter define each factor and specify the levels or degrees within the factor. For example, if education were one of the evaluation factors, degrees within this factor might be as follows:

- Level of education:
  - Master's degree or beyond
  - Bachelor's degree
  - Associate's degree or technical training beyond high school
  - High school diploma or equivalent

Points are then assigned to each degree within the factor for each job. Job grades or levels are established by specifying a range of evaluation scores for each grade. Pay ranges are then associated with each job grade by establishing arbitrary but reasonable bands around some average or target wage, which might be based on a prevailing market rate for such jobs. Actual jobs in the unit are then matched to the pay grades and priced. By applying the linear regression technique, a statistical relationship between the point scores and target prices (wages) can be established. Current pay levels for all jobs or those being given priority attention can be plotted against their point scores to identify any "outliers," those significantly above or below the established pay range for that grade. This analysis could support managerial action to address any jobs whose pay levels seem inappropriate.

To manage effectively under the constraints associated with this method, the health information manager needs to be familiar with the logic of the pricing procedure, the factors and degrees identified, and the relationship between points assigned and pay ranges for the job grades. The appropriate compensation specialist within the HRM department should be a useful resource to the line manager who needs more information about the point system or other method of pricing jobs in the organization.

Many variations of these methods are tailored to meet the strategic goals, financial health, and environmental and market challenges faced by the organization. The Hay plan is a popular proprietary method commonly used in health care organizations. This job evaluation method is a variation of the point and factor approach that uses a committee process for evaluating critical job factors to determine each job's relative worth.

Why Job Evaluations Are Used

Regardless of the specific method used, all job evaluation approaches seek to determine a position's relative worth to maintain pay equity within an organization and competitive compensation for target jobs within the relevant labor markets. No matter which method of job evaluation is in place, the responsible manager should review all wage rates for employees under the manager's authority and advocate adjustments for any pay levels that do not appear reasonable and fair compared with the job requirements. For example, health record analysts review the patient record after discharge and identify missing documents or data. The supervisor of the health record analysts might determine that workers doing comparable jobs in the outpatient surgery center were ranked two job grades above the health record analysts. Investigation reveals that the inpatient health record analyst position had been ranked lower because the current job description fails to reflect the medical terminology skills, data entry experience, and frequency of interaction between this position and the medical staff. After the job descriptions have been revised to better reflect the actual skills, knowledge, and responsibilities of this position, the job is re-evaluated. The newly determined "price" might result in a pay adjustment for the health record analysts to correct this inequity.

Wage and Salary Surveys

Some organizations use data from wage and salary surveys to determine the market value of a given position. These surveys are often conducted by industry or professional associations, such as state hospital associations. In using this information in managing compensation, management determines how it wants to be positioned competitively relative to its labor markets. For example, if the director of health information services has had difficulty retaining coding analysts, she may argue, on the basis of regional wage and salary data, that her organization needs to bring the average salary for these positions above the regional mean salary.

The organization typically uses such data when overhauling its compensation program through a comprehensive job evaluation program. Management must be cautious in using survey data to ensure that the jobs included in the survey data are comparable to the target positions within the organization. A position of "data analyst" can represent quite different responsibilities, tasks, and skill requirements from one organization to another. Also, if the study was based on very small samples of jobs or otherwise not representative of the relevant labor market, the survey pay ranges might provide misleading and unreliable benchmarks.

Another concern is that survey data should not necessarily be imposed as standards, overriding the organization's unique circumstances and compensation experience. For example, if the average salary data for clinical coders reflects a shortfall in supply of qualified applicants statewide, then this standard may be inappropriate (too high or too low) given their relative worth in the organization. When any unit within the workforce has been unionized, the negotiated wages in the contract covering that bargaining unit could have an escalator effect on comparable positions outside the bargaining unit. Negotiated wages that exceed their value relative to other nonunionized positions in the organization could cause an imbalance in the organization's wage and salary program that eventually should be identified and addressed through job evaluation.

Training and Development

Training and development is a critical function for maintaining the health care organization as a productive system in a competitive environment. The importance of training and development has grown with the explosion of information technology, telecommunications, and health-related technologies during the past several decades. The focus of training and development has traditionally been on individual skill building and growth of knowledge to facilitate upward mobility along some career track or pay scale. With the growth of quality management programs, employee empowerment, and innovative, "looser" forms of organizational design, such as the horizontal organization, the emphasis today is more on team development. In his model of the learning organization, Senge[45] defines the learning organization as one that "is continually expanding its capacity to create its future" (p. 14) and this requires commitment to five disciplines including team learning. Senge[45] claims that "team learning is vital because teams, not individuals, are the fundamental learning unit in modern organizations" (p. 10).

Rationale for In-Service Training and Development. Credible and cost-effective training programs must be linked to the mission and strategic goals of the organization, leadership priorities, environmental challenges, and needs for training and development identified at the operating level. Clearly, employee development is not only desirable but also a necessary investment for the long-term survival and growth of the organization. However, as aggressive competition and changes in federal health care policy constrain traditional revenue streams for many health care providers, management increasingly focuses on areas to control costs. Unfortunately, some organizations have cut back or eliminated some educational and training programs on the basis that they are expendable "frills." This view is short sighted and likely to prove unwise in the long term. The failure to make sound investments in full development and use of its human resources threatens the organization's ability to retain well-qualified employees, respond effectively to environmental change and market pressures, and benefit from technological developments.

Historically, hospitals have emphasized skill building and maintenance and keeping staff current with the latest clinical, technological, and regulatory developments affecting the health care professions through regular in-service, targeted, on-site training. Although training and development programs can entail a significant operating expense, failure to provide continuing investment in training can result in an even higher cost in the long term. For example, if the coding staff has not kept up to date with diagnosis-related group coding and reimbursement changes, a hospital could have huge revenue losses as a result of inappropriate code assignment or denied claims because of incorrect coding. Failure to keep abreast of changing regulatory and accreditation requirements may place an organization in danger of unfavorable accreditation decisions or sanctions. At the same time, management must practice systematic assessment to determine its most important training needs and match these needs with appropriate training and development opportunities, in-service and externally based.

Furthermore, each training and development program and activity should be subject to cost-benefit consideration to maximize the net benefits from the total investment in this area.

Designing a Training Program

Needs Assessment

A needs assessment provides the foundation for a well-designed training program and should precede curricular development and scheduling. Programs already in place should be evaluated periodically to ensure that they continue to be relevant to identified training needs. Teaching and instructional methods should be reviewed to ensure that content is effectively presented and learning reinforced consistent with established principles and practices for the adult learner. Special attention should be given to incorporating new on-line technologies into the training programs to ensure an active learning experience for the employees. As discussed earlier, the importance of team building and team learning to new organization designs, relationships among coworkers, and work processes is likely to require the development of new training models and materials appropriate for team approaches (Box 16-9).

Staff Development

After the formal orientation of the new or promoted employee as the employer's initial training investment, managers must be responsive to any training need that is identified for the employee to remain competent, knowledgeable, and responsive to changes in clinical practice, technology, and regulatory requirements. During the departmental or unit orientation, the manager should review the job description in detail and emphasize the expectations of performance for every significant job responsibility. The employee cannot be expected to perform at or above standards if those expectations and standards are not clearly communicated and reinforced. Many employees become frustrated, dissatisfied, and demotivated because they were reprimanded by a supervisor for performance deficiencies and failed expectations that were never adequately communicated. The supervisor must never assume that employees can "read the manager's mind" or intuitively understand the organizational priorities. Job responsibilities, work procedures, productivity standards, performance criteria, and management's goals and priorities must be communicated clearly, explicitly, and often. The supervisor has the responsibility to take the guesswork out of performance.

Training and development programs may be provided by in-house staff, under contract with external consultants, by funding employees' participation in external educational programs, or by a combination of these approaches. Instructional methods and designs include but are not limited to the following:

- Traditional lecture and discussion
- Group role playing and problem solving
- In-service demonstrations by supervisors and experienced clinicians
- Professional mentoring and partnering
- Programmed instruction
- On-line interactive learning (LAN or Internet based)
- Participation in part-time external degree or certificate programs
- Accredited continuing education, such as workshops and conferences

Career Planning

Career planning enables employees to be promoted from one job in a career path or ladder to another within an organization. It also provides an incentive for motivating and retaining effective performers and identifying potential managers and leaders for appropriate training and placement. It should support and encourage a learning culture in which all employees have the opportunity for challenging work, responsibilities, and social interaction that sustain job satisfaction, motivation to achieve, commitment to quality service, and desire for career-long learning and skill development. Effective career planning activities benefit the organization by ensuring a continuous supply of qualified workers to accomplish the objectives of the organization (Box 16-10).

The health information manager can assist in career planning within the organization and within the profession. Executives from the organization can be asked to give presentations on developments in health information technology and systems and career and leadership opportunities within and outside the organization. **Career counseling** may be offered formally by the human resources staff, through an EAP, or less formally by the mentoring of veteran professionals and managers.

Box 16-9 POTENTIAL TRAINING NEEDS FOR THE HEALTH INFORMATION SERVICES ORGANIZATION

- Monitor professional journals and other relevant information sources to identify changing requirements in the collection, analysis, dissemination, and regulation of health information.
- Survey employees to assess their need for new skills or knowledge.
- Identify skill, knowledge, and interpersonal strengths and deficiencies within the performance appraisal and disciplinary processes.
- Access and analyze training need indicators from other sources including quality assessments, management and peer feedback, grievance reports, claims denial reports, productivity monitoring systems, and accreditation reviews.
- Observe and review employee participation in quality management activities and other team-based processes, presentations, and project reports.

Box 16-10 EXAMPLE OF CAREER PLANNING ACTIVITIES

Sally is a health information specialist whose main responsibility is inserting late reports in discharge records. As a result of this job, Sally knows the document filing system well and is familiar with the various parts of the record and the sequence required by various users. She could be easily trained to assist with release-of-information requests several times a week. The release-of-information coordinator position has a higher pay rate and requires more skills than Sally's position. When Sally has had time to learn the extra skills, she will be an excellent choice for promotion to release-of-information coordinator.

An in-service resource center with current materials relevant to professional advancement and educational programs should be provided to supplement the employee's access to the wealth of resources and linkages available through the Internet. Another means of promoting career planning is to post job descriptions within the department so that job requirements and specifications for position openings are communicated and accessible to all employees. Trainee or transitional positions can be created for people who want to advance but lack the job experience to apply for a desirable, higher-level position.

Training and development programs are especially helpful in preventing obsolescence and career plateaus. Obsolescence threatens when employees no longer have the skills required to perform successfully in an ever-changing workplace, for example, medical transcriptionists who have not kept current with medical terminology or financial analysts who have not mastered the latest generation of electronic spreadsheets.

Career plateaus represent stages in an employee's career when a decline in performance or failure to achieve a newly imposed, higher standard of performance or level of commitment might place the employee at risk for demotion, termination, or career stagnation. The employee may be labeled fairly or not as a burnout, an individual who has peaked and will no longer be considered for promotional, professional development, or other career-building opportunities. Key signs of career plateaus are reluctance or refusal to adapt to new technology and insistence that "this is the way we've always done it here." These employees may lose interest in volunteering for professional growth activities and may require assertive supervision, including mandatory training in conjunction with realistic goal setting and career planning.

Employees at this stage who have a proven record of good performance and continuing value to the organization should be identified and given consideration for developmental opportunities as an investment in career prolongation. The costs of career rejuvenation are likely to be far less than the "hidden" costs of losing the benefits of work experience,

expertise, professional relationships, and role modeling associated with the older employee at a plateau stage. On the other hand, supervisory management should candidly but humanely discuss future prospects within or outside the organization with employees who are not perceived by their managers to have much potential for career renewal and performance improvement. EAP counseling or outplacement services might be appropriate resources in these situations.

Employee Health, Safety, and Well-Being

The work environment consists of the physical, psychological, sociocultural, and political factors associated with a community of diverse individuals participating together more or less voluntarily to perform work to achieve their own personal and career objectives, consistent with furthering the mission and goals of the organization. These individuals are motivated by physiological, social, and psychological needs as well as by their economic objectives. Today's workforce expects the employer to provide a working environment that addresses this array of needs, one that is at least comfortable, safe, hygienic, and accessible.

The influence of social and psychological factors in the workplace on employees' job satisfaction, sense of well-being, and motivation has been a recurring focus of research and managerial concern.

Hertzberg demonstrated that some groups of professional employees regarded working conditions, including the physical and psychological factors of the work environment, as factors that, if not perceived to be adequate or sufficient, would act as "dissatisfiers" and erode employee motivation and performance. On the other hand, the presence of a positive working environment would serve as a foundation necessary for management to address factors associated with job performance itself, which could enhance employee motivation, that is, the "satisfiers."[46] This accords with our common work experience: when the work environment is perceived to be comfortable, pleasant, and safe, we are more likely to be satisfied with our job and organization and less likely to have our working conditions interfere with our performance and productivity.

Legal Requirements and Recommendations. Some of the laws and regulations previously discussed in this chapter affect the design, safety, and accessibility of the workplace. OSHA (1970) requires that employers furnish a workplace that is free from health and safety hazards that are likely to cause injury, harm, or death. The Vocational Rehabilitation Act of 1973 requires that federal buildings and buildings that were constructed with more than $2500 in federal funds be accessible to people with handicaps. The ADA expands the scope of organizations covered by such accessibility requirements to include most types of service establishments, including hospitals; rehabilitation facilities; physician's, dental, and other health providers' offices; pharmacies; insurance offices; banks; and virtually all others that provide "public accommodation." The employer is required under

ADA to make reasonable accommodations in the workplace to the individual's ADA-relevant disability, including physical disability, mental health, and other medical conditions. Adjustments to the workplace to accommodate the employee's disability are usually simple and inexpensive to implement without being disruptive to the normal work processes. Of course, if more elaborate facilities' renovation is required, for example, making restrooms ADA accessible for wheelchair users, the initial investment will benefit all future applicants, employees, clients, and visitors with disabilities using these facilities.

"Green Building" Design in Health Care. A relatively recent development related to employee health and satisfaction is the use of "green building" design and construction for health care facilities. "Green" or "high performance" architectural design and construction approaches and standards have been applied for decades in commercial facilities but have only recently been implemented in health care. The argument for green buildings in industry has been based largely on cost efficiencies and environmental protection concerns. However, there is some evidence that green facilities also are associated with employee (and customer) satisfaction, improved health, and enhanced performance and productivity. An architect's perspective on these relationships follows: "The most compelling argument for improving building efficiency and performance may be found in the relationship between occupant comfort and worker productivity [given] … that worker salaries comprise the major cost of operating a commercial building.…"[47]

There have been few hard data beyond testimonials to support the link between green buildings and employee satisfaction and outcomes in health care. However, the Center for Health Design, a research and advocacy organization, whose mission is to "transform health care settings … into healing environments that contribute to health outcomes through the creative use of evidence-based design"[48] has funded research and advocacy efforts to encourage best practice in facilities design that will enhance employee satisfaction and performance and health care outcomes. This is an area that seems very promising for health care system managers as they face the challenge of controlling costs, retaining productive and well-motivated employees, and increasing patient satisfaction and other desired performance measures.

FUTURE ISSUES

Managing human resources within a health information services environment through the twenty-first century will be an especially challenging endeavor. This chapter has provided only a selective overview of the dynamic and complex field of HRM. The accelerating rate of technological

development in both information services and clinical knowledge in health care delivery, uncertainties about the direction of national health care policy, continuing pressures for accountability on all health care providers to maintain quality improvement in health care delivery while doing so cost-effectively—all these forces and probably others not foreseeable will increase the complexity of managing human resources effectively while addressing the priorities of various key constituencies. The health information manager of the twenty-first century must be prepared to face this challenge along with the opportunities for life-long learning, career growth, professional recognition, and personal satisfaction associated with this career commitment.

Key Concepts

- Human resource management is among the most regulated of all organizational systems and processes. This characteristic compounds the challenges management faces in understanding and responding effectively to individual and group needs and concerns in the workplace while fulfilling the organization's mission and objectives.
- The thrust of equal employment opportunity and related legislation since the 1960s has been to remove artificial impediments to full opportunity for all persons to participate in the workplace, to fully develop and use their skills and knowledge, and to receive fair compensation for their contributions. Legislatively, this has taken the form of prohibiting employers from discriminating on the basis of race, color, religion, national origin, gender, age, and disability status.
- Advocates of the modern approach to human resources management argue that eliminating these discriminatory barriers will enhance the broader goals, that is, obtaining, developing, fully using, and retaining the organization's best human resources.
- The human resources management system depends on effective coordination among its various subsystems to ensure effective individual and group performance directed toward achieving organizational goals. For example, job analysis, training and development, performance appraisal, and compensation subsystems and processes are interdependent and must be effectively integrated. Intelligent, responsive, consistent, and creative supervisory coaching is the critical component of human resources management in practice.
- In spite of effectively designed systems and processes, competent management and supervision, and appropriate technology, ineffective performance, inappropriate employee behavior, and violation of important policies, norms, and values will almost certainly occur. Mechanisms must be provided to address these performance problems that are

cost-effective, reliable, and responsive to the individual's legal rights and ethical standards. These include a progressive disciplinary process and a reliable employee assistance program.

• Management must address factors inherent in job performance and those in the working environment, for example, health and safety, management policies, and procedures, to eliminate barriers to individual motivation and performance while enhancing opportunities for job satisfaction, a sense of achievement, and appropriate recognition.

• Managers can no longer rely exclusively on traditional organizational structures, procedures, and incentives to respond effectively to environmental change or to attain optimal performance from employees. Flexibility and innovation in organization design, the structuring of work, and strategies for facilitating peak performance from individuals will be increasingly necessary.

• The team will probably retain its importance as the key organizational unit in health care; therefore, team management and facilitation skills are essential for the health information services manager.

• Finally, for the first-line supervisor in health information services to attain and retain competence as a supervisory manager, he or she must balance technical expertise, general knowledge of organization and management principles, and some understanding of current human resources management "best practice" with effective communication and interpersonal and team-building skills.

Acknowledgments

The author thanks Ms. Heather Barr, MHA, for her creative contributions to and editorial assistance with the preparation of revisions to this text.

REFERENCES

1. Zuboff S: *In the age of the smart machine: the future of work and power,* New York, 1988, Basic Books.
2. Ostroff F: *The horizontal organization,* Oxford, 1999, Oxford University Press.
3. Staples J: A new type of threat, *Harv Bus Rev* 84:20-22, 2006.
4. U.S. Census Bureau: Hispanic population passes 40 million, USCB 05-77. 9, June 2005.
5. U.S. Department of Labor: Union members in 2004, USDL 05-112. 27, January 2005.
6. Matthews RG, Maher K: Labor's PR problem: As more workers find unions weak and irrelevant, leaders seek to restore positive image, *Wall Street J* Aug 15, 2005, p. B1.
7. Health Professions Education for the Future Schools in Service to the Nation: *Report of the Pew Health Professions Commission,* San Francisco, February 1993, Pew Health Professions Commission, p. 7.
8. Bennis WG, Nanus B: *Leaders: The strategies for taking charge,* New York, 1985, Harper & Row.
9. Stogdill RM: *Handbook of leadership: a survey of theory and research,* New York, 1974, Free Press.
10. Fiedler FE: *A theory of leadership effectiveness,* New York, 1967, McGraw-Hill.
11. Cartwright D, Zander A: *Group dynamics research and theory,* Evanston, IL, 1960, Row, Peterson.
12. Blake R, McCanse A: *Leadership dilemmas—grid solutions,* Houston, TX, 1991, Gulf Publishing.
13. Hersey P, Blanchard K: *Management of organization behavior: utilizing human resources,* ed 6, Englewood Cliffs, NJ, 1993, Prentice Hall.
14. Burns JM: *Leadership,* New York, 1978, Harper & Row.
15. Schein E: *Organizational culture and leadership,* San Francisco, 1985, Jossey-Bass.
16. Hunt JG, Conger TA: From where we sit: an assessment of transformational and charismatic leadership research, *Leadership Q* 10:335-343, 1988.
17. Rohrer W: The three T's of leadership: leadership theory revisited, *Top Health Record Pract* 914-25, 1989.
18. Darr K: *Ethics in health services management,* ed 4, Baltimore, MD, 2005, Health Professions Press.
19. Northouse PG: *Leadership: theory and practice,* ed 3, Thousand Oaks, CA, 2004, SAGE Publications.
20. Worthley JA: *The ethics of the ordinary in healthcare: concepts and cases,* Chicago, 1997, Health Administration Press.
21. Robbins SP: *Essentials of organizational behavior,* ed 8, Upper Saddle River, NJ, 2005, Pearson/Prentice Hall.
22. Rokeach M: *The nature of human values,* New York, 1973, Free Press.
23. Greenleaf RK: *Servant leadership: a journey into the nature of legitimate power and greatness,* New York, 1977, Paulist Press.
24. American Health Information Management Association: *Code of ethics,* Chicago, 2004, American Health Information Management Association. Revised and approved by AHIMA House of Delegates on July 1, 2004.
25. Morgan G: *Images of organization,* Thousand Oaks, CA, 1998, SAGE Publications.
26. U.S. Department of Labor, Bureau of Labor Statistics: Women in the labor force: a datebook, report No. 985, Washington, DC, 2005, U.S. Department of Labor.
27. Day JC: *Population projections of the United States by age, sex, race, and Hispanic origin: 1995 to 2050,* U.S. Bureau of the Census, Current Population Reports, P25-1130, Washington, DC, 1996, U.S. Government Printing Office.
28. Gilbert JA, Stead BA, Ivancevich JM: Diversity management: a new organizational paradigm, *Journal of Business Ethics* 21:61-76, 1999.
28a. Kaiser Family Foundation: South Florida Sun-Sentinel examines prenatal program hoping to improve care for women by targeting, educating men. *Kaiser Daily Women's Health Policy Report:* http://www.kaisernetwork.org. Accessed November 16, 2004.
28b. Sanchez TR, Plawecki JA, Plawecki HM: The delivery of culturally sensitive health care to Native Americans, *J Holist Nurs* 14: 295-307, 1996.
29. Joint Commission on Accreditation of Healthcare Organizations: *2006 hospital accreditation standards,* Washington, DC, 2006, Joint Commission on Accreditation of Healthcare Organizations.
30. Kahn S, Brown B, Zepke B et al: *Legal guide to human resources,* Boston, 1996, Warren, Gorham & Lamont.
31. Young J: *Equality of opportunity: the making of the Americans with Disabilities Act,* Washington, DC, 1997, National Council on Disability.
32. Kaufman L: Adjusting the legal bar for disability, *New York Times,* April 18, 1999.
33. Kahn S, Brown B, Zepke B et al: *Legal guide to human resources,* Boston, 1996, Warren, Gorham & Lamont.
34. Leslie D: *Labor law in a nutshell,* St. Paul, MN, 1986, West Publishing.
35. Schein E: *Organizational culture and leadership,* San Francisco, 1985, Jossey-Bass.
36. Maslow A: A theory of human motivation, *Psychol Rev* 50:370-396, 1943.
37. Cascio W: *Applied psychology in personnel management,* Reston, VA, 1982, Reston Publishing.

38. Douglas J, Feld D, Asquith N: *Employment testing manual,* Boston, 1989, Warren, Gorham & Lamont, 1989.

39. Tanner J, Kinard J, Cappel S et al: Substance abuse and mandatory drug testing in health care institutions, *Health Care Manage Rev* 13:33-42, 1988.

40. Cascio W: *Costing human resources: the financial impact of behavior in organizations,* Boston, 1991, PWS-KENT Publishing.

41. Pfeffer J: *New directions for organization theory: problems and prospects,* New York, 1997, Oxford University Press.

42. Castro J: Disposable workers, *Time* March 29, 1993, pp 43-47.

43. Bernardin H, Russell J: *Human resource management: an experimental approach,* Boston, 1998, Irwin/McGraw-Hill.

44. Employment at will: Alive and well in Pennsylvania? *Penn Employment Law Lett* 5:1, 1995.

45. Senge P: *The fifth discipline,* New York, 1990, Doubleday/Currency.

46. Pugh D, Hickson D: *Frederick Hertzberg in writers on organization,* Thousand Oaks, CA, 1997, SAGE Publications.

47. Lehrer D: Building a case for building performance, *AIA SF Newsletter* (August 2001) http//techstrategy.com/lineonline/aug01. Accessed June 3, 2005.

48. Center for Health Design: Fact sheet (2006): *www.healthdesign.org.* Accessed November 16, 2006.

chapter 17

Operational Management

Carol Venable
Anita Hazelwood

Additional content,
http://evolve.elsevier.com/Abdelhak/

Review exercises can be found
in the Study Guide

Chapter Contents

Introduction

Individual Work Processes (Micro Level)

Organizing Work
    Serial Work Division
    Parallel Work Division
    Unit Assembly Work Division

Work Distribution Chart

Productivity
    Productivity Standards

Work Simplification or Methods Improvement
    Identifying a Problem Area or Selecting a Work Process or
        Function to Improve
    Gathering Data About the Problem
    Organizing and Analyzing Data Gathered on the Problem
    Formulating Alternative Solutions and Improvements
    Selecting the Improved Method
    Implementing the Improved Method and Evaluating the
        Effectiveness of the Improvement

Systems and Organizational Level (Midlevel)

Systems Analysis and Design
    Systems Model Concept
    Input-Output Cycle
    Goals of Systems Analysis and Design Process
    Components of Systems Analysis and Design
    Designing the System
    Evaluating the Proposed System
    Implementing the System

Organizational Structure
    Formal Organizational Infrastructure
    Informal Organization

Organization–Wide Level

Change Management

Strategic Management

Situational Analysis
    External Environmental Analysis

Key Words

Accent lighting
Adaptive strategies
Ambient lighting
American plan of office design
Benchmarking
Carpal tunnel syndrome
Critical path
Decision grid
Decision matrix
Decision table
Decision tree
Directional strategies
Ergonomics
External environmental analysis
Flowchart
Flow process chart
Functional strategies
Gantt chart
Informal or unwritten organization
Internal environmental analysis
Linkage strategies

Market entry strategy
Methods improvement
Mission
Movement diagram
Office landscaping
Open office design plan
Operation flowchart
Operational strategies
Organization chart
PERT network
Policies
Population
Procedures
Process
Productive unit of work
Productivity
Productivity standards
Project management
Proximity chart
Random selection
Re-engineering

Relative humidity
Sample
Staff hour
Stopwatch study
Strategic control
Strategic implementation
System
Systems analysis and design
Systems flowchart
Task-ambient lighting
Task lighting
Time-and-motion study
Trip frequency chart
Values
Vision
Work breakdown structures
Work distribution chart
Work sampling
Work simplification
Work station

This chapter contains revised information from a previous edition authored by Peter M. Ginter and W. Jack Duncan.

     Internal Environmental Analysis
     Mission, Vision, and Values
Strategy Formulation
Strategic Implementation
Strategic Control
Project Management
     Characteristics of a Project
     Characteristics of Project Management
     Project Planning
Information Technology Applications
Re-Engineering
     Objectives
     Use of Policies and Procedures in the Re-Engineering Process
     Relationship to Quality Improvement
     Applications to Health Information Management

Design and Management of Space in Health Information Services
Work Space Design
     Work Flow
     Traffic Patterns
     Functions Performed in the Work Space
     Need for Confidentiality of Work Performed
     Shift Workers-Sharing Work Space
     Flexibility for Future Needs
     Employees' Personal Needs
Design of the Workstation
     Ergonomics
     Components of the Workstation
     Environmental Considerations

Abbreviations

ADA–Americans with Disabilities Act

BLS–Bureau of Labor Statistics

CMS–Centers for Medicare and Medicaid Services

CTD–cumulative trauma disorder

CTS–carpal tunnel syndrome

DRG–diagnosis related group

EPA–Environmental Protection Agency

HIM–health information management

HVAC–heating, ventilation, and air conditioning

JCAHO–Joint Commission on Accreditation of Healthcare Organizations

NIOSH–National Institute for Occupational Safety and Health

OSHA–Occupational Safety and Health Act

RSI–repetitive stress (or strain) injury

Objectives

- Define key words in operational management.
- Describe various methods of organizing work.
- Define productivity, productivity standards, and a productive unit of work.
- Describe the various methods of measuring output to establish productivity standards.
- Apply the work simplification process to improve a system.
- Explain the concepts applied to the systems model.
- Utilize the systems analysis and design process to analyze and improve a system.
- Differentiate between the formal and the informal organization.
- Introduce the concept of strategic management and how it concerns the achievement of a fit between the organization and its environment.
- Examine the characteristics of projects and project management.
- Utilize the project management process to achieve an organizational goal.
- Define re-engineering.
- Outline the considerations that must be examined in designing work space for health information services.
- Apply the employee's individual needs to the design of the work space.
- Describe the components of a workstation.

INTRODUCTION

Health information is not limited to one department or even to one organization. It is developed, disseminated, and used throughout organizations and communities. The effective use of health information depends on the systems that can create, analyze, disseminate, and use it. To be effective, the systems must effectively use the resources of people, processes, and equipment.

An important skill for the health information manager is the ability to analyze the processes that create and handle health information to be sure that they are functioning in the most efficient and effective manner. These processes could involve paper, computer systems, or both. There are numerous software programs available to assist with the various operational functions.

This chapter describes the tools that can help to analyze and improve the methods used in health information systems. The discussion begins at the micro level of individual jobs and procedures and moves through a midlevel look at systems analysis and design and organizational concepts to a larger macro or organization-wide level with the concepts of project management, re-engineering, and design.

INDIVIDUAL WORK PROCESSES (MICRO LEVEL)

Organizing Work

The method of organizing, or allocating, the work among the employees depends somewhat on the type of organization and the nature of the work to be accomplished. Work division can be accomplished by any of the following methods:

Function—Similar tasks are performed by one unit within a department or an organization.
Project—A work unit performs all steps for a particular project (an example is a task force).
Product—In a manufacturing company, one unit performs all the work to produce a single product.
Territory—Sales forces are divided in this manner, with each representative responsible for a certain geographical area. Another example may be the organization of the hospital nursing service by patient care units.
Customer—This concept can be applied in a health information management (HIM) department when teams are organized to work on patient records of particular physicians.
Process—Similar work processes or procedures are grouped together and performed by a particular unit or group of employees.

Work processing can be further subdivided to the individual employee level. This subdivision can be classified into serial, parallel, and unit assembly (Figure 17-1).

Serial Work Division

The serial work division is one of consecutive handling of tasks. A series of small tasks is grouped together. Each task in the series is performed by a specialist in that type of work. The work passes from one employee to another until all tasks have been performed and the work is complete. An example of the serial arrangement is an assembly line in a factory, where each step in the process is performed by a different person.

Parallel Work Division

Parallel work division demonstrates a concurrent method of handling work. One person performs a series of tasks. The tasks may be, but are not necessarily, related. Several employees may be performing the series of tasks at the same time. An example of this method in an HIM department is one in which four persons are employed to assemble and analyze patient records. Each employee assembles and analyzes records.

Unit Assembly Work Division

In unit assembly work division, each employee specializes in a particular task, as in serial work division, but the sequence of tasks on each unit is not identical. For example, in Figure 17-1, Poly Ester specializes in tasks 1 and 2. She may perform these tasks before anyone else works on a particular item, after tasks 3 and 4 are done, after tasks 5 and 6 are complete, or even after all steps—3, 4, 5, and 6—are done. A great deal of coordination is necessary in the unit assembly method because the amounts of time needed to perform individual tasks differ. The advantages and disadvantages of the three methods of organizing work are delineated in Table 17-1.

Work Distribution Chart

The **work distribution chart** is a useful tool that provides data to analyze the processes performed by a work group and the individual employee within the work group. Examination of the data assists in identifying problems but not solutions. The work distribution chart is a matrix that displays the tasks being performed in a work group, the employees who perform them, and the amount of time spent on each task by each employee and the work unit as a whole.

Preparation of the work distribution chart requires the following steps:

1. *Each employee prepares a task list* (Figure 17-2). The employee should be instructed that the task list should reflect what the employee actually does, not what he or she should be doing. To gain cooperation from the employees, the supervisor should explain the purpose of gathering these data. The purpose is not punitive

Table 17-1 ADVANTAGES AND DISADVANTAGES OF WORK DIVISION METHODS

Serial	Parallel	Unit Assembly
Advantages		
Employees are skilled in their own tasks.	Because employees know all functions, absences and volume fluctuations are managed.	Saves time; employees can work on the item without waiting for others to finish their tasks.
Causes of delays are easily identified.	Work is more interesting to the staff because they see it through to completion and it encompasses a wider variety of functions.	Employees are skilled at their own tasks
If one step in the process requires a specialized skill or use of specialized equipment, fewer skilled staff or pieces of equipment are needed.		
Disadvantages		
Employee absences can cause backlogs.	If one or more of the steps require specialized skills or equipment, more skilled staff or pieces of equipment are needed, making the process more expensive.	Work can become boring because employees' work has limited variety and scope.
Slow employees can delay the final product.	Recruiting and training of staff to complete multiple functions may be difficult.	Difficult to use unless work can be easily divided into tasks that do not depend on the results of other tasks.
Work can become boring because employees' work has limited variety and scope.		Coordination of work flow and scheduling of completion of individual items would be difficult.
The work items are handled numerous times because each step is performed by different employees. This may increase the total processing time for all steps.		

Serial Work Division

Employee	Poly Ester	Justin Case	Cindy Rella
Processes	Tasks 1 & 2 on all records	Tasks 3 & 4 on all records	Tasks 5 & 6 on all records
Sequence	Before tasks 3, 4, 5, & 6	After tasks 1 & 2 and before tasks 5 & 6	After tasks 1, 2, 3, & 4

Parallel Work Division

Employee	Poly Ester	Justin Case	Cindy Rella
Processes	Tasks 1, 2, 3, & 4 on 1/3 of the records	Tasks 1, 2, 3, & 4 on 1/3 of the records	Tasks 1, 2, 3, & 4 on 1/3 of the records
Sequence	First to work on this group of records	First to work on this group of records	First to work on this group of records

Unit Assembly Work Division

Employee	Poly Ester	Justin Case	Cindy Rella
Processes	Tasks 1 & 2 on all records	Tasks 3 & 4 on all records	Tasks 5 & 6 on all records
Sequence	First to work on record, or after tasks 3 & 4, or after tasks 5 & 6, or after tasks 3, 4, 5, & 6.	First to work on record, or after tasks 1 & 2, or after tasks 5 & 6, or after tasks 1, 2, 5, & 6.	First to work on record, or after tasks 1 & 2, or after tasks 3 & 4, or after tasks 1, 2, 3, & 4.

Figure 17-1 Methods of organizing work.

TASK LIST

Name of employee: Doc Tors Helper
Job title: Incomplete charts clerk
Department/area: Incomplete charts area
Date compiled: 02/01/07-02/05/07

Task number	Activities	Hours per week	Posted to activity #
1.	Pulling records for physicians to complete	10	
2.	Checking physicians' completed records	6	
3.	Inputting changes into computer system	4	
4	Corrections or changing of deficiency stamp on front of folder	2	
5.	Preparation of delinquent list	4	
6.	Copying transcribed discharge summaries and operative reports	5	
7.	Distributing copies of discharge summaries and operative reports to designated physicians	3	
8.	Miscellaneous (lunch, breaks, other assigned tasks)	6	

Figure 17-2 Task list.

but to analyze how time is spent in the work group to improve the jobs. Over a 1-week period, each employee lists the tasks he or she performs and the amount of time spent on each. The task statements should be brief and specific and include no more than 15 statements. The duties should be listed in order of importance. Every minute need not be accounted for. Hours should be entered to the nearest 15 minutes, and breaks and other nonproductive time should be included in a miscellaneous category.

2. *Supervisor prepares a list of the major activities of the work group* (Figure 17-3). This is a list of general categories into which all activities of the employees can be classified. As a rule, no more than 10 activities should be listed. They should be listed in order of importance with the most important listed first. When the activity list is completed, each task shown on the individual employee's task lists should be classified under one of the major activities. It may be necessary

to add a miscellaneous category to accommodate all the tasks that may not fall under one of the major activities of the section.

3. *Supervisor combines the employee task list and the activity list into the work distribution chart* (Figure 17-4). The work distribution chart is complete when the following entries are made:

- The major activities are listed in the left-hand column.
- The employees are listed across the top of the chart; the columns should be assigned in the order of responsibility starting with the department head or supervisor at the left.
- The tasks performed by each employee and the amount of time required for the performance of each task are listed in the column under the employee's name.
- The total time spent on each major activity by all employees is recorded in the right-hand column.

Analysis of the work distribution chart can answer the following questions:

ACTIVITY LIST

Department: Health information management
Area: Incomplete chart area
Number of employees: 4

Task number	Activities	Hours per week
1.	Pulling records for physicians to complete	21
2.	Analysis of completed records and updating of computer system/folder	26
3.	Preparation of delinquent list	5
4.	Copying and distributing transcribed discharge summaries and operative reports	21
5.	Filing transcribed summaries and operative reports on medical records	13
6.	Supervision	20
7.	Audit of the incomplete files	7
8.	Checking in charts that have been returned from the OB-GYN unit	9
9.	Answering the telephone	12
10.	Miscellaneous incomplete area activites and nonproductive time	26
	Total Hours	160

Figure 17-3 Activity list.

What tasks are employees performing? Are these tasks important to achieving organizational goals? Question the total time of the group on a particular activity and then that of individual employees. Are the activities that take the most time really the most important ones? Is a lot of time spent redoing work that had errors? Handling complaints?

How are tasks distributed among employees of the work group? Does each employee do a little bit of one task? Does any one employee do the bulk of one task while the others are not using their time effectively?

Are employees' qualifications being used? Are highly skilled, highly paid employees using those qualifications? For example, are medical transcriptionists filing the reports that they type? On the other hand, are employees doing tasks that they are not qualified to do—for example, does a person with only knowledge of medical terminology assign codes to Medicare patients' diagnoses and procedures?

How are individual jobs constructed? Are employees performing too many unrelated tasks, or are they doing one thing all day long? Performing too many

WORK DISTRIBUTION CHART

TASKS	SUPERVISOR	HR	DOCTOR'S HELPER	HR	CLERK 3	HR	CLERK 4	HR	TOTAL HOURS
Supervise	Supervisory duties	20							20
Prints delinquent list and checks for accuracy; makes copies			Pulls records for physicians	10	Pulls records for physicians	5	Pulls records for physicians	6	21
Analysis of completed records			Check each completed chart; put on shelf for filing; make changes in computer	12	Check each completed chart; put on shelf for filing; make changes in computer	8	Check each completed chart; put on shelf for filing; make changes in computer	6	26
Prep of delinquent list			Prints delinquent list; checks for accuracy; makes copies	4	Distributes delinquent lists	1			5
Copy and distribute reports	Receives transcribed reports; make copies and distribute to originating physician	4	Receives transcribed reports; make copies and distribute to originating physician	8			Receives transcribed reports; make copies and distribute to originating physician	9	21
Filing					Files transcribed reports	10	Files transcribed reports	3	13
Audit of files	Audit of charts for quality	4			Physical audit of files	3			7
Check-in charts					Check charts from OB-GYN	6	Check charts from OB-GYN	3	9
Answer phone	Handles complaints from physicians	4					Receives physicians' requests to pull records	8	12
Miscellaneous	Orders supplies; meetings; breaks	8	Assists supervisor; breaks	6	Pulls for medical staff committee; breaks	7	Messenger duties; breaks	5	26
Total		40		40		40		40	160

Figure 17–4 Work distribution chart.

unrelated tasks wastes effort and is costly. Changing from one task to another decreases productivity because of the time spent setting up and ending each task. The monotony of performing one or a few tasks for most of the work time causes boredom and, possibly, dissatisfaction with the job.

Analysis of the work distribution chart may also aid the manager in choosing one of the above types of work division (serial, parallel, or unit assembly). By including the number of units produced in the work distribution chart, managers can use the chart to establish **productivity standards** in an organization.

Productivity

Productivity is the process of converting an organization's resources (labor, capital, materials, and technology) into products and services that meet the organization's goals. Productivity is also defined as the number of items produced per staff hour that meet established levels of quality.[1] A productive organization is one that produces quality products or services with the least expenditure of resources.

Productivity is often expressed as a ratio:

$$\frac{\text{Output (services or products)}}{\text{Input (resources consumed)}}$$

or

$$\frac{\text{Quantity and quality}}{\text{Staff hours}}$$

Some related definitions are important to the understanding of productivity. A **staff hour** is defined as 60 minutes of time during which an employee is working on a task or a particular function and being paid for that work. A **productive unit of work** is an item produced that meets established levels of quality. The quality (or accuracy) level is an important aspect of this definition. When a product does not meet the quality level, it often has to be redone. Therefore, if products that do not meet the quality level were counted as output, the number of products would be inflated because of counting the rework and the original work as outputs. Quantity, in the preceding ratio, generally refers to the number of work units that are produced by an employee who is trained and who is working at a normal pace. Examples of outputs in an HIM department are coded patient data, completed response to a request for information, and a transcribed report.

Productivity Standards

Productivity (also known as performance or work) standards are the tools that are used to specify the expected performance and to measure actual performance. Productivity standards have many uses in managing an HIM department. They can assist in determining the number of personnel, equipment, and supplies needed to accomplish the projected workload; in scheduling completion and distribution of tasks; in evaluating proposed changes in processes or systems to see whether a savings in personnel time would occur; in setting goals for a work group or individual employee; and in evaluating the performance of a work group or individual employee. Productivity standards can also be used to determine the actual cost of producing a given product or service.

Setting Productivity Standards

Getting Started

When a productivity program is designed, the work requirements and resources of the department must be clearly understood and the following should be addressed:

- All departmental activities should be identified and defined.
- An area of productivity focus should be selected.
- For the specific functions that are studied, quantity and quality must be defined.
- Current performance as well as past performances should be reviewed.
- Staff members should be involved in the establishment of the expectations of the program.
- Reporting mechanisms should be developed; then performance should be monitored.
- As a final step, the improvements identified should be implemented.

Measuring Input

To set productivity standards, certain determinations must be made. First, the methods of quantifying inputs must be determined. This is usually in terms of employee time expressed in paid staff hours worked. Second, the unit of work for measuring output must be established. For given processes, this can take various forms. For example, for the coding function, should the number of codes be counted or the number of records? Should the output be classified by level of difficulty (e.g., outpatient versus inpatient, Medicare versus non-Medicare)?

Measuring Output

Actual Performance. Various methods are used to measure output. They range from using past performance data to using time studies and work sampling. Using data from actual performance is the most common method of measuring output and is the easiest, quickest, and least expensive method. Data can be collected by the organization's own staff; therefore, specialists are not needed. Methods used to collect this information include employee-reported logs in the form of time ladders or diaries, as shown in Figure 17-5. Equipment can also be used to count items of work; for example, dictation equipment can record the number of minutes transcribed or characters entered.

Work Sampling. **Work sampling** is another method of collecting actual performance data. This method is based on the statistical laws of probability. The research concepts of population, random selection, and sample must be comprehended to understand the work sampling method.

TIME LADDER			
Employee's name: Mary Knowall		Date: July 1, 2000	
Employee's job: Chart analyst			
Time	Task	Time	Task
8:00	Receive charts from floor	3:20	
8:05	Place discharged charts (40) in alphabetical order	3:25	
8:10		3:30	Input deficiencies into computer system
8:15	Assign service assignment on each chart	3:35	
8:20		3:40	
8:25		3:45	
8:30	Place each chart in chart order	3:50	
		3:55	
10:30	Analyze charts for deficiencies	4:00	Place charts in doctors' incomplete chart area
10:35		4:05	
10:40		4:10	
		4:15	
11:00	Coffee break	4:20	Clean up work area
11:05		4:25	
11:10		4:30	Head for home
11:15	Continue chart analysis		
12:30	Lunch break		
1:30	Continue chart analysis		
3:00	Coffee break		
3:05			
3:10			
3:15	File loose reports in charts		

Figure 17-5 Time ladder.

Population. All items or members of the group to be studied.

Sample. The group of items chosen to represent the whole population. The size of the sample is important because it must be large enough to represent all members of the group but small enough to be manageable and cost effective.

Random selection. The method of choosing the sample that gives each item in the population an equal chance of being chosen.

In work sampling, the supervisor observes employees at times randomly selected, as opposed to continuous, all-day observations, and records the task the employee is doing at the time of the observation. The observations are tallied to determine the percentage of all work time (the population) spent on each task. Combining these percentages with the number of items produced determines the productivity standards for these tasks. Advantages of the sampling method as opposed to the use of continuous observations are as follows:

1. Detailed information can be gathered that might otherwise be difficult to obtain by using continuous observations.
2. Data can be obtained in less time and with less expense by using the sampling method.
3. Personnel who are being studied complain less often than individuals being observed continuously.
4. Data can be easily obtained without any interruption of the normal work routine by using the sampling method.
5. The sampling method is likely to produce more accurate results than continuous observations.

Using actual performance data has several problems. These productivity standards are based on existing procedures, processes, employee performance, and qualifications, all of which might not be the most effective for this process. Therefore, expected results would be based on poor performance and ineffective processes.

Benchmarking. **Benchmarking,** another method of setting standards, is the comparison of one organization's performance with that of another organization that is known to be excellent in that area. Benchmarking is beneficial because it is more than comparing productivity. It involves discovering how the benchmark organization achieves its goals and then incorporating these methods into the other organization. The aim of benchmarking is the improvement of the organization's processes. More information on benchmarking is in Chapter 13.

Stopwatch or *time-and-motion.* **Stopwatch** or **time-and-motion studies** are the most expensive techniques for setting productivity standards. Stopwatch studies require a skilled analyst to observe the employee performing the task and to record stop and start times for each portion of the task. The selection of the employee to be observed is an important element of this technique. The employee should be one who performs the task at an average speed, not the fastest or the slowest. This method is a poor public relations tool. Having to watch every move an individual makes can be quite unsettling and puts the individual on edge.

Whichever method is used to collect data and set productivity standards, the concept of quality cannot be overlooked. Techniques for ensuring the expected quality level of the output must be built into the methods for measuring the quantity. See Chapter 13 for more information about quality measurements.

Efficiency is as important in setting work standards as it is elsewhere in the organization. If it becomes too expensive to set standards and measure work, the goal of productivity monitoring is defeated.

Productivity standards must be understandable, realistic, reliable, and attainable under normal working conditions. Clear communication between employers and employees is important for the program to be a success. An effective productivity management program is based on accurate, reliable standards that have earned credibility with the employee.

Increasing Productivity

Productivity can be increased by the following methods:

- Increasing output while holding input constant
- Decreasing input (resources) while maintaining the same level of output
- Increasing output while decreasing resources
- Increasing resources and output but with a proportionately greater increase in output
- Decreasing output and resources with a proportionately greater decrease in resources

Research findings on productivity improvement show the following[2]:

- Productivity goes up when it is measured.
- Productivity improves as it becomes a primary goal of management.
- Productivity increases as managers and staff are held accountable for its measurement and evaluation.
- Productivity increases as its benefits are shared with the employees responsible for the increase.
- Productivity increases as employees are rewarded for extra output.
- Productivity increases as the resources allocated are in direct proportion to the productivity improvement potential.

Implementing a Productivity Program

For the program to be useful, an organization needs a focused approach to improving productivity. A productivity improvement program needs well-defined goals. To be effective, as many employees as possible should be involved in the development of the program. Organizational goals should be integrated with employee goals. All employees should be part of the program and should be accountable for productivity improvement in their own work areas. Employees should share in the benefits of improved productivity and should be rewarded and reinforced for their contributions. Implementing a productivity improvement program is a six-step process.

1. Identify an area in the organization for improvement.
2. Establish a unit of measurement (productivity ratio) and measure current performance in that area.
3. Develop a *measurable* productivity objective.
4. Identify a strategy for meeting the objective.
5. Establish time frames and identify checkpoints.
6. Analyze results and provide feedback.

An example of a productivity improvement program in an HIM department is shown in Figure 17-6.

Monitoring and Improving Performance

The department head or supervisor should develop a mechanism for analyzing the productivity of each employee and a means for summarizing overall section or departmental productivity. Depending on the specific management needs, reporting may be done on a daily, weekly, or monthly basis.

Once overall productivity is established, management should review the areas that are in need of improvement. This improvement may be in the form of additional staff or training, improvement of work methods or individual work performance, or a change in the structure of the section or department. Time management and motivational techniques for employees may also prove to be beneficial in many cases.

Motivation

Managers in the workplace today often forget how important a role motivation plays with their employees. To be effective, managers need to understand what motivates an employee in the context of the job they perform in the department/facility. Greater productivity and increased employee morale is a natural result of a properly motivated employee. In general, motivation for better job performance depends on job satisfaction, individual recognition, personal achievement, and professional growth.

According to Kovach,[3] managers should ask themselves the following 10 questions when attempting to provide a more positive motivational climate for employees:

1. Do you personally thank staff for a job well done?
2. Is feedback timely and specific?
3. Do you make time to meet with—and listen to—staff on a regular basis?
4. Is your workplace open, trusting, and fun?
5. Do you encourage and reward initiative and new ideas?
6. Do you share information about your organization with staff on a regular basis?
7. Do you involve staff in decisions, especially those that will affect them?
8. Do you provide staff with a sense of ownership of their jobs and the unit as a whole?
9. Do you give associates the chance to succeed?
10. Do you reward staff on the basis of their performance?[3]

Aside from motivational theories and information published by notable authors such as Douglas McGregor, Frederick Herzberg, and Abraham Maslow, managers must understand that they are dealing with human beings and that very basically motivation involves getting people to do something simply because they want to do it. The manager's reward is productive employees.

Work Simplification or Methods Improvement

An organizational goal is to provide the best service or make the best product with the least expenditure of resources while maintaining a healthy and contented workforce. The effectiveness of the individual employee depends on the effectiveness of the processes used. **Work simplification,** sometimes called **methods improvement,** is an organized approach to determine how to accomplish a task with less effort in less time or at a lower cost while maintaining or improving the quality of the outcome. It uses commonsense concepts to eliminate waste of time, energy, material, equip-

Productivity Improvement Area:	Coding
Productivity Ratio:	Number of records coded per man hour
Current Level of Productivity:	6 correctly coded patient records per man hour
Productivity Objective:	10 correctly coded patient records per man hour
Improvement Strategy:	Weekly educational programs on coding. Each coder will attend a coding seminar each year.
Time Frame:	Six months
Checkpoints:	Monthly
Evaluation and Feedback:	Measure productivity; if level meets goal, praise and congratulate. Establish incentive pay program.

Figure 17-6 Productivity improvement program for coding.

ment, and space when performing work processes. Sometimes work simplification is misunderstood to mean work speed up. When work simplification tools are correctly used, the rate of production is enhanced by performing only the essential steps in the best way possible at a standard pace.

The fundamental objectives of work simplification are as follows:

- Simplify
- Eliminate
- Combine
- Improve

The simplest means of performing the work is usually the easiest and most practical.

Questioning is fundamental to improving work processes. The first question that must be asked is, "Does this process assist in achieving the organization's goals?" When the answer is no, the process should be eliminated. Remember to question the statement "That's the way it has always been done." The questions of who, what, when, where, and how must be answered.

The philosophy of work simplification is that there is always a better way to perform every task. The statement that the process has always been done this way is a red flag that the process could use change and that the employee does not understand why the procedures are done in this way. The goal of a work simplification program is to increase efficiency through the elimination of unnecessary work and through the optimal structure of necessary work.

The individual who performs the tasks must be given significant attention when individual jobs are dissected. Employees need to be involved in the process because they are the experts in their own work processes. If they are involved in change, they are more likely to accept the change. However, care must be taken so that the content of the job does not become oversimplified and boring.

The steps in the work simplification method are similar to those in the scientific method:

1. Identify a problem area or select a work process or function to improve.
2. Gather data on the problem.
3. Organize, analyze, and challenge the data gathered on the problem.
4. Formulate alternative solutions or improvements.
5. Select or develop the improved method.
6. Implement the improved method and evaluate the effectiveness of the improvement through follow-up.

Identifying a Problem Area or Selecting a Work Process or Function to Improve

Identification of a problem is not an easy task. A competent manager must be able to differentiate between a symptom and its cause or problem. What appears to be the problem may only be a symptom. This step is essential because if the symptom's cause is not correctly identified, the problem will not be solved and the symptom may be only temporarily eliminated.

In health care, distinguishing between symptoms and diagnoses (problems) is a familiar process. The patient comes to the emergency department with the symptom of abdominal pain. On testing and evaluation, the patient is diagnosed with acute appendicitis. When the cause of the abdominal pain is identified, treatment can be initiated to remedy the symptom.

By use of the same approach of symptom versus diagnosis, common work symptoms can be examined to find the diagnosis or problem. For example, the symptom of poor productivity may be traced to the problem of inefficient work flow. High employee turnover may be a symptom of low morale caused by poor workload distribution.

The following list indicates potential problems that should be investigated:

- Duplication of work processes
- Overlapping of responsibilities
- Frequent backtracking
- Inconsistencies
- Frequent delays and interruptions
- Poor workload distribution (congestion and clutter)
- Inaccuracies and errors
- Lack of controls
- Lack of instructions or procedures
- Low employee morale
- High absenteeism or turnover
- Complaints from customers and employees
- Apparent waste of materials, effort, personnel, time, and space
- Obvious fatigue
- Poor safety record
- Excessive time required to carry out an activity in comparison with results achieved
- Chronic backlog
- Regular overtime

Managers need to be sensitive to cues from their employees and their surroundings. When managers are not responsive to these cues, a potential problem may develop into a crisis situation. Once a sign is recognized as a potential problem, the manager must proceed to investigate and move to resolution of the problem. Nothing is more discouraging to employees than to raise a concern and have no response from management. After a while, employees complain among themselves and fail to make management aware of problem areas.

Another approach to selecting an area of work to be simplified is to review areas with high labor requirements and a large number of diverse work activities and those in which excessive time is needed to perform the work, the costs are high, or the end product is inadequate.

Gathering Data About the Problem

Data collection methods vary with the type of problem and the work performed. Data-gathering methods include the collection of blank forms used in the process, completed forms, office or work layout, organizational charts, job descriptions, work logs, manuals/standards/procedures, interviews with employees, and observation. Additional facts may be obtained from supervisory staff.

The key to gathering data is to ask the right questions to find out how the work is being performed. The following are key questions to ask:

- Why is this process performed? How does it move the organization toward achievement of its goals?
- Who does the work? Why this particular individual? What are the individual's qualifications for performing these processes?
- What work is currently being done and why is it being done?
- When (in what sequence) is the work being performed and why in this manner?
- Where is the work being performed and why there?
- How is the work being done? Why is it being done this way? Is there a better way to achieve the same result?
- At what rate does the work flow to the employee? Is the rate consistent?

A flow process chart can be used to analyze procedures and to determine opportunities for improvement through eliminating, combining, or resequencing any part of the process.

Flow Process Chart. A **flow process chart** is a tool used to collect information on the steps of a work process and to analyze and improve the process. It is especially helpful in analyzing manual operations. The flow process chart is used to show the steps or actions involved with respect to a single person (job), a single material, or a single form.

There are several basic steps in constructing a flow process chart:

- Accurately describe the job or activity that is being studied, for example, "Processing a request for copies of medical records." Flow process charts may be constructed for current or proposed jobs.
- Select the employee, material, or form to be followed.
- Determine the beginning and ending points of the process to be studied.
- List each step in the procedure or job. A separate line should be used for each step, no matter how insignificant it may seem.
- Select the symbol that best describes the activity. The symbols used to represent each step in the process are shown in Figure 17-7. The symbols that represent each step are connected with a line to facilitate analysis.
- Indicate distance traveled if the transportation symbol is selected. The amount of time should be indicated when there is a delay in the process or whenever indicating the time would be of some use in analyzing the process.
- Each of the operations should be counted and entered in the summary box. The distance traveled and the minutes delayed should also be entered.

Each step in the process should be subjected to the following questions:

- Is that particular step necessary or of value?
- Can the step be eliminated?
- Can the step be streamlined or combined with another step?
- Is the step properly sequenced within the process?

SYMBOL	PROCESS	END RESULT	EXAMPLE
○	Operation Make-ready	Get-ready to do	Sorting
●	Operation Do	Produces or accomplishes	Coding, data entry
⇨	Transportation	Moves	Walking
▽	Storage	Keeps	Object placed in permanent storage
□	Inspection	Verifies	Proofreading
D	Delay	Interfaces	Object is in temporary storage or waiting

Figure 17-7 Flow process chart symbols.

This analysis of the flow process chart can identify problems such as duplication of effort, too much travel time from one workstation to another, and delays in transferring work.

Figure 17-8 shows a completed flow process chart for a current and a proposed release-of-information function.

Flowcharts. Additional types of **flowcharts** are used to verify and obtain information about how a procedure is being performed. Flowcharts are essentially road maps that show the logical steps and the sequence involved in a procedure. Flowcharts are used to depict all levels of operations

	Present	Proposed	Difference
○ No. of Operations	8	7	1
⇨ No. of Transportations	4	1	3
☐ No. of Inspections	3	2	1
No. of Delays	1	1	0
D No. of Storages	1	1	0
▽ Distance Traveled	65	20	45
Minutes Delayed	60	30	30

Job: Processing a request for copies of medical records
Charted by: S. Smith
Department: HIM
Date: 4/4/07

Present Method

Present Method	Marked Symbol (Operation / Transportation / Inspection / Delay / Storage)	Distance in Feet	Time in Minutes
written request opened by receptionist	Operation		
request forms alphabetized	Operation		
receptionist transports to release of info	Transportation	15 Ft	
ROI clerk checks for completeness	Inspection		
ROI clerk makes outguides for charts	Operation		
ROI waits for clerk to pull charts	Delay		60 MIN
clerk pulls charts	Operation		
charts transported to ROI	Transportation	20 Ft	
ROI reviews medical record	Inspection		
ROI tags pages to copy	Operation		
ROI copies charts	Operation		
chart and copies transported to supervisor	Transportation	15 Ft	
supervisor inspects request and copies	Inspection		
chart and copies transported back to ROI	Transportation	15 Ft	
ROI documents copies sent	Operation		
chart to file	Storage		
copies mailed	Operation		

Proposed Method

Proposed Method	Marked Symbol (Operation / Transportation / Inspection / Delay / Storage)	Distance in Feet	Time in Minutes
written request opened by ROI	Operation		
ROI clerk checks for completeness	Inspection		
ROI alphabetizes request forms	Operation		
ROI reviews chart locator system	Operation		
ROI prints list for clerk	Operation		
ROI waits for clerk to pull charts	Delay		30 MIN
clerk pulls charts	Operation		
charts transported to ROI	Transportation	20 Ft	
ROI reviews charts	Inspection		
ROI copies charts	Operation		
chart to file	Storage		
copies mailed	Operation		

Figure 17-8 Flow process chart for release of information *(ROI).*

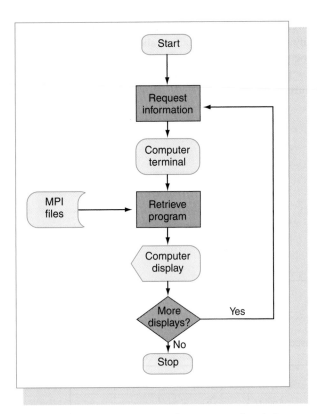

Figure 17-9 Systems flowchart for master patient index.

from whole systems that involve many departments and people, as in a systems flowchart, to the work of one person or procedure, as in an operations or procedure flowchart. The **systems flowchart** depicts the flow of data through all or part of the system, the various operations that take place within the system, and the files that are used to produce various reports or documents. Figure 17-9 shows an example of a systems flowchart for the master patient index.

Operation or Procedure Flowchart. The **operation flowchart** is a graphical representation of the logical sequence of activities in a procedure. In addition, it points out the decision points encountered in carrying out that function. The operation flowchart should specify how a function is performed, not the methods used. This type of flowchart is a superb communication tool between employees and management (Figure 17-10).

Flowchart Symbols and Guidelines. The standard symbols shown in Figure 17-11 are used to construct flowcharts. When unique symbols are used, their meaning should be identified in a key or legend on the flowchart (Box 17-1).

The flowchart can be used for both planning and controlling activities. As a planning tool, the flowchart may be used to help develop a new procedure. The chart will show the linkage points among the various aspects of the task and will show areas that need to be changed. It can also

be used to compare current and proposed procedures. As a control tool, the flowchart can be used to compare the actual work flow with the original procedure and also as a means of constant evaluation of processes.

Movement Diagrams. The **movement diagram,** sometimes called a layout flowchart, represents graphically the physical environment in which the processes are performed. The purpose of a movement diagram is to depict the flow of work activities through the desks and equipment. A movement diagram can show movement of paper or an employee. This type of chart can be beneficial in identifying the problem of backtracking or bottlenecks in procedures. With a graphical display of the physical layout, a more efficient route for accomplishment of the task can be achieved.

Movement diagrams or layout flowcharts are especially useful in the analysis of manual systems (Figure 17-12).

Organizing and Analyzing Data Gathered on the Problem

The third step of the process entails organizing and analyzing the facts or data obtained from step 2. As with all steps in work simplification, the employees who perform the work need to be included in this process.

Data can be organized in many ways. One is by chronological sequence of the work under study. Another is by problems or source of problems, such as the department or function in which they originate.

Formulating Alternative Solutions and Improvements

By use of the fundamental belief of methods improvement that there is always a better way along with the information

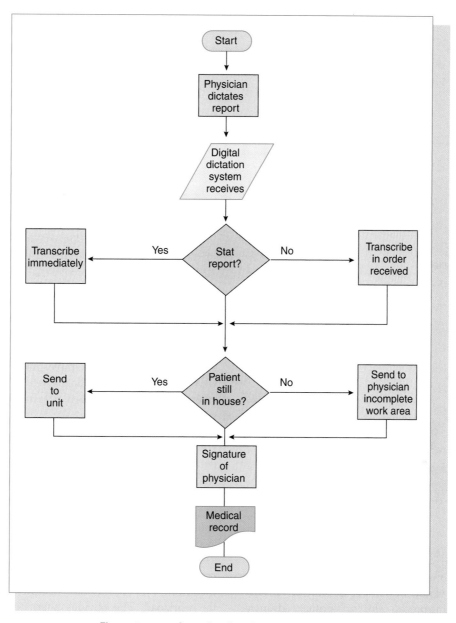

Figure 17-10 Operation flowchart for transcription.

gathered, questioned, organized, and analyzed from the prior steps, several alternatives should come to mind. Employees who are close to the situation might not see the value of making changes, but their input must be acquired. Journal articles and conferences with colleagues within and outside the organization may stimulate some new and different thinking.

Selecting the Improved Method
To identify the best alternative for rectifying the problem, several decision-making tools are available.

Decision Grid or Matrix. The **decision grid** or **matrix** (Figure 17-13) is the most basic of the decision support tools. The alternatives are compared with one another by various criteria. The alternatives are listed down the left side. The elements or criteria are listed across the top. Examples of criteria frequently considered in selecting alternatives are cost, feasibility, desirability, acceptance, effect on productivity, and effect on quality.

This grid may be used to arrive at a decision concerning any type of problem once the alternatives are defined and the criteria selected. Another option is to weigh the criteria.

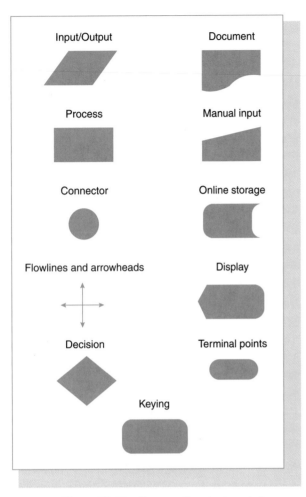

Figure 17-11 Common flowchart symbols.

The element of cost may be weighted three times that of any other element. This would mean that cost is the first priority in this decision-making process. The grid's primary advantage is that all relevant information can be displayed and viewed at the same time. This is useful when a committee or group is attempting to arrive at a consensus.

Decision Table. A **decision table** is an analytical tool that provides a means of communication of the logical sequence of a particular operation. This type of decision support tool can be used in situations where the logic and sequential flow of data cannot be clearly shown on a flowchart. The decision table was originally designed to explain the logic found in computerizing a manual process.

A basic decision table is divided into four segments:

Conditions segment. These are usually questions that form the conditions that may exist in a system. Condition statements or questions are assigned row numbers and entered in the left-hand column. A heavy line separates the condition statements or questions from the action statements.

Condition-entry segment. This is the set of rules (or scenarios) that provide yes or no answers to the questions in the conditions segment. The rules should be numbered. The rule numbers are then assigned horizontally across the top of the form. The condition entries are entered opposite the applicable condition questions.

Action segment. This lists the action to be taken for fulfilling each condition. Action statements are assigned row numbers and are entered below the condition statements below the heavy line.

Action-entry segment. This section uses an "X" to indicate the suitable action concluded from the answers entered in the condition-entry segment.

A decision table may be simple and characterize only a few conditions. It can, however, be complex and contain dozens of conditions and actions. Examples of the usage of decision tables in the HIM department may involve a complex process within the department or may assist in employee decisions. For example, in Figure 17-14, employees who are employed less than 1 year will receive no raises whereas individuals who have been employed for 1 to 3 years will receive 3% raises.

Decision Tree. Decisions are often linked to other decisions. In effect, sometimes one decision necessitates future decisions. A **decision tree** is used to chart alternative courses of action for solving a problem. It also depicts some of the probable consequences or risks resulting from each course of action. Decision trees are a valuable tool for evaluating decisions that are linked together over time with assorted potential outcomes. As an example, the transcription supervisor has an unanticipated heavy load of dictation. He or she has insufficient staff to handle the workload. The obvious alternatives in this situation include (1) hiring more transcriptionists, (2) paying overtime to current transcriptionists, (3) contracting work out to a transcription service, and (4) hiring temporary help (Figure 17-15).

When this decision tool is used, the decision centers on the objective of making the wisest expenditure of money. This decision tool is effective when probabilities can be determined for the various outcomes. In this example, it would be helpful for the transcription supervisor to determine the probability of an increased demand for transcription services or the probability of continuation of the heavy load of dictation. After evaluating additional services rendered and considering previous year figures, the supervisor may estimate that there is a 70% probability that the workload will increase next year and a 30% probability that the workload will decrease. Monetary values have to come into play in evaluating the risks compared with the alternatives.

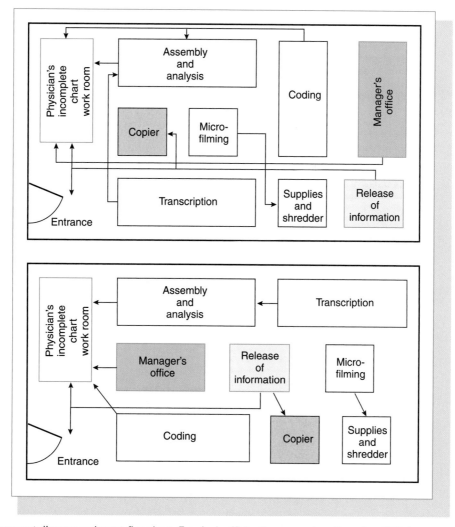

Figure 17-12 Movement diagram or layout flowchart. *Top,* An inefficiently arranged section of an HIM department. The release-of-information employees are not located near the photocopier, and the manager and coding staff are far removed from physician access. *Bottom,* Improved physical layout, making movement and work flow more efficient.

	Alternative	Cost	Feasibility	Desirability & Acceptance	Decision
1	Hire new coding supervisor	$28,000 position	Requires recruitment; few qualified applicants; usually new grad	Coding staff will resist new graduate	3rd priority
2	Promote lead coder to coding supervisor	$8,000 raise ($28,000) $20,000 savings	Places heavy burden on work load	Coding staff may resist	2nd priority
3	Promote operations supervisor to Assist. Director supervising both operations and coding	$12,000 raise ($28,000) $16,000 savings	Excellent; supervisor has previous coding experience	Poses minor acceptance problem with coders; very desirable to operations supervisor	1st priority

Figure 17-13 Decision matrix or grid showing the elements considered by the director of the HIM department in the hiring decision for a coding supervisor.

Employee Raises	Rule 1	Rule 2	Rule 3	Rule 4
Employed less than 1 year	Y	N	N	N
Employed 1–3 years	—	Y	N	N
Employed 3–5 years	—	—	Y	N
Employed 5 or more years	—	—	—	Y
No Raise	X			
3% Raise		X		
5% Raise			X	
7% Raise				X

Conditions / *Condition Entry*
Actions / *Action Entry*

Figure 17-14 Decision table used to determine employee raises.

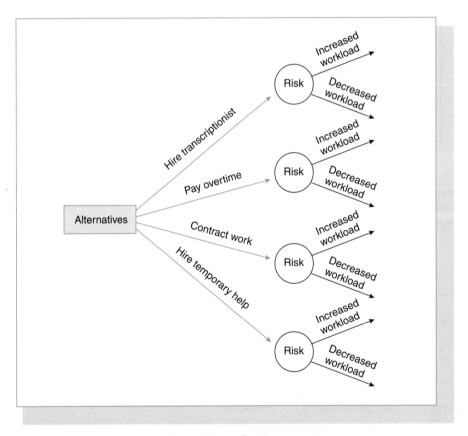

Figure 17-15 Decision tree.

Implementing the Improved Method and Evaluating the Effectiveness of the Improvement

Provided that the employees have participated in the entire process, this step should be easy and simple to apply. The improved method should result in a more simplified, better, faster, more convenient, and less costly method of performing the task. The purpose of the work simplification and the reasons for its importance should be made clear to every employee affected by it.

To ensure success with the improved process, the new procedures should be documented and reviewed with all employees involved. People, by nature, tend to resist change. However, if employees realize that this change is part of their own efforts, resistance should be minimal. Sometimes it is helpful to demonstrate work simplification examples from other departments. If the employees can see results in reducing waste and accomplishing the work effectively, they will work together to meet the challenge that work simplification offers (Box 17-2).

Box 17-2 GUIDELINES FOR WORK SIMPLIFICATION

- Encourage employee participation in planning for work simplification. Promote employee knowledge of work simplification objectives, process, and results. In-service training may be necessary.
- The series of work activities needs to be simple and productive. Each adopted activity must be justified for its necessity. All unnecessary or duplicative activities should be eliminated. The activities that contribute directly to the goal should be maximized.
- Whenever reasonable, combine work activities. Duplication of effort is frequently found in evaluating a procedure. In various activities, certain data are copied over and over. If feasible, these writing activities should be combined into a single method or operation.
- As much as possible, reduce the distances traveled. Sometimes the movements of people and paper are costly and may be wasteful. Closely examine such movements and attempt to reduce them to the shortest distance possible. However, when movement is essential, it is typically a more efficient process to move the paper than to move the person. Some specific guidelines are as follows:
  1. Equipment, materials, and supplies often used should be located within an individual's normal grasp area.
  2. The quickest way to move small objects is usually by sliding rather than carrying.
  3. Hand motions should begin simultaneously and be completed at the same time, motions should be as simple as possible, and individuals should work to achieve rhythm.
  4. Continuous curved motions are more desirable than straightline motions requiring sudden changes in direction.

Strive to arrange activities to provide a smooth work flow. When more than one clerical step is included in the process or activity, a pattern of steady, constant flow of work is ordinarily desirable. The employee may feel overwhelmed by workloads that are too heavy. On the other hand, the employee may become frustrated and bored if workloads that are too light appear frequently. Hesitations and delays in the flow of work should be minimized.

SYSTEMS AND ORGANIZATIONAL LEVEL (MIDLEVEL)

Systems Analysis and Design

Systems analysis and design is a method used to evaluate and study all types of systems. This process is usually used at an organizational level involving several departments and functions. The main benefit of using this process is that it is a defined and accepted method for gathering and "analyzing a great quantity of data in a logical, documented format" (p. 118).[4] Like work simplification, it follows the scientific method of problem solving, using tools of description, investigation, research, creativity, and judgment. The analysis portion involves examining the way things are currently done and defining the users' requirements for the system. The design segment determines the best way to meet the users' specified requirements for the system.

The systems analysis and design process can be used for various types of systems, ranging from paper-and-pencil systems to paperless computer-based systems. Its use with computer information systems is detailed in Chapter 5. The process can be lengthy and time consuming and it requires dedication of staff and financial resources. It is usually used when an existing system no longer meets the organization's needs or when new needs are identified.

The health information manager can be involved in this process in a variety of ways, including being a user of a system, defining its requirements with a systems analyst, or even assuming the systems analyst role.

The use of the systems analysis and design method does not guarantee success. The choice of solutions (designs) is still a human one and fraught with possibilities of human bias and error.

Systems Model Concept

The process of systems analysis and design is based on the systems model concept. A **system** is an assemblage of things that form a connected whole, a complex but ordered whole, a plan or scheme, or a method. A system refers to various elements that are interrelated according to a plan for achieving a well-defined goal. In an organization, the elements are employees or human resources, equipment and supplies, and raw material. These elements are linked together by processes or procedures to achieve the organization's goals or desired outcomes (Figure 17-16).

Hierarchical Structure. The systems model concept also recognizes the hierarchical structure of systems. Large systems are composed of subsystems, which in turn are composed of subsystems. For example, the human body is a system composed of subsystems of the digestive, respiratory, and cardiovascular systems. The digestive system is composed of the stomach system, the small intestine system, the large intestine system, and so on.

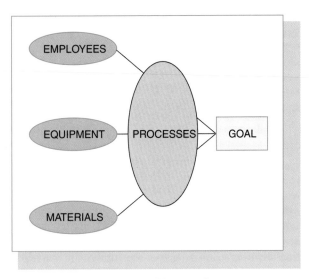

Figure 17-16 Diagram of a system.

- Sorting
- Filing
- Calculating
- Retrieving data and information

Processing refers to the procedures and methods involved in the system. Procedures are an established series of work steps used to accomplish a goal and commonly include the efforts of several people. Procedures handle recurring transactions consistently and uniformly. In viewing procedures microscopically, we see that they consist of a progression of methods. Procedures consist of related methods that are essential to complete various work processes. Methods apply to the tasks of an individual employee and may represent a manual, mechanical, or automated way of performing a procedure. An example of a method is alphabetizing the names of the physicians on the medical staff by their last names.

Output. The ultimate goal of a system is output. Output is a result of transforming input into a desired form. For example, the transcriptionist transforms the physician's dictation into a typed report. Other output examples are release-of-information correspondence, coded diagnoses and procedures, and productivity reports. Output is usually in paper or computer screen format and is needed as the input for another process or system.

Feedback. Feedback is crucial for the success of the entire system. It compares the output with expected standards of performance. In other words, feedback contrasts what was produced with what should have been produced. An example of feedback would be the physician's evaluation of the typed report or the quality improvement plan. If the feedback shows that the quality standards were not met, a modification is sent back to the input phase for improvement of the system.

Feedback can also occur concurrently with the input-processing-output cycle. The input and processing are evaluated and improved before the preparation of the output.

Controls and Constraints. Systems do not operate in a vacuum; they are controlled and constrained by internal and external factors. These factors dictate what can and cannot be done in every phase of the system. An internal dimension of controlling encompasses the organizational policies, procedures, and standards that affect the system. An example of an internal control for a health information process is the policies and procedures that govern the release of health information. This policy stipulates the type of information that may or may not be released without the patient's written authorization. Additional internal controls may be those required for profit as a profit margin or for quality of service and those required by the customer.

The external controls include the local, state, and federal rules and regulations and social, economic, and ethical

Unity of Purpose and Boundary Concepts. Embedded in the systems model concept are the principles of unity of purpose and boundary or integrity of the system. These concepts are important for effective application of the systems analysis and design process. A system has unity of purpose when the system and its subsystems all focus on achieving a single purpose. The boundary concept refers to separating the system from other systems. It identifies what is included and what is excluded in the system being studied. The boundaries define the scope of the study and the possible limits of the system. For example, the process under study may involve several departments, but the study may be limited to the part of the process that occurs only within one department. Determination of the system's boundaries is often an administrative or management decision.

Input-Output Cycle

Systems are composed of input, processing, output, feedback, and control.

Input. The flow of work through a system begins with some type of input. Examples of input include labor, energy, money, and attitudes. In a health information system, the types of input are commonly data, information, or materials. Examples of materials include the mail, demographic data on the health care facility's patients, and telephone calls received by the receptionist. Incorporated in this input are employees' skills and knowledge and the equipment and supplies needed to perform the task.

Processing. The processing element transforms the input into a desired output. Sometimes this phase is called the transformation process. The following are traditional processing activities:

- Classifying
- Storing

values. External controls that affect the HIM department are the federal regulations on the confidentiality of drug and alcohol patient records, the information management standards of the Joint Commission on Accreditation of Healthcare Organizations (JCAHO), and the diagnosis related group (DRG) weights published in the *Federal Register*.

Goals of Systems Analysis and Design Process

The goal of the systems analysis and design process is to produce a well-designed system that can be described as follows:

Effective. The system accomplishes its purpose and achieves its established goals.
Efficient. The system accomplishes its purpose while remaining cost-effective.
Dependable. The system meets established time frames.
Flexible. The system can accommodate unusual circumstances.
Adaptable. The system can absorb changes, if necessary.
Systematic and logical.
Functional. The system serves its intended purpose.
Simple.
Resourceful. The system is useful within the organization.
Accepted. The system is accepted by those who work with it.

Components of Systems Analysis and Design

The major components of systems design are as follows:

- Determination of the need and objectives of the system
- Systems analysis
- Design of the system
- Evaluation of the proposed system
- Implementation of the system

Determining the Need for the System. Before the analysis process is begun, the users must determine the need for the system. The needs, which are often determined by management, are in the form of objectives. They should provide answers to the following questions:

- What information is needed?
- Who needs the information?
- When do they need it?
- In what format do they need it?

Systems Analysis. The analysis of the system has three components: accumulation of facts, organization of facts, and evaluation of facts.

Accumulating the Facts

Gathering of data is made possible by envisioning the course that a piece of paper follows in a process and then tracking each step in that particular process. The tracking can begin at any point and work backward or forward from there.

Sources that may be used in the accumulation or gathering of facts include the following:

- Organization charts
- Procedure manuals
- Job descriptions
- Flowcharts
- Financial data

Investigation methods include group discussions and interviews with managers and operations employees and questionnaires to all affected personnel and users of the system. Before the investigation is begun, the existing manuals and charts should be reviewed. The interview should focus on obtaining facts pertinent to the system analysis. At this point in the process, solutions should not be suggested. Strategic questions should be devised to verify facts from previous sources.

Organizing the Facts

The facts obtained in the previous step must be organized or classified in some way. Conventional ways to organize facts are in the following categories:

- Interrelated objectives
- Organizational structure
- Input and output
- Processing modes
- Major complaints or problems disclosed

Organizing facts by organizational structure can be advantageous because it shows not only who has authority to make decisions but also the flow of data among organizational units. Organizing facts by major complaints or problems is also beneficial because only valid problems and significant complaints should be included. The organization of facts is helpful in proceeding with their evaluation. The means of organization should also show meaningful relationships.

Evaluating the Facts

As much as possible, the facts should be ranked, rated, measured, weighed, and evaluated. The assignment of quantitative values to facts should be accomplished in as many areas as possible. In reality, some evaluation may be subjective and based on opinion. Information tends to include some nonquantifiable components. Again, try to adhere to the facts, not to feelings or beliefs. At this point in the process, possible solutions to the problems may be examined.

Designing the System

After the facts have been gathered, organized, evaluated, and analyzed, a design of a new system or a proposed revision to an existing system is explored. People must be committed to this process. The design of a system should be a team effort that includes management, operations personnel, and users of the system. Often, numerous systems could fit the requirements. However, they can differ in many aspects, especially cost.

The following factors should be considered when designing the new system:

- Effects on employees (retraining, layoffs, transfers, schedules)
- Profits and costs (salaries, space, materials, and supplies)
- Customer service

System design should not be performed in a rush. Various possibilities must be considered with their strengths and weaknesses. The term "trade-off" is routinely used in this part of the process. In other words, sometimes one need must be sacrificed for another.

Evaluating the Proposed System

In this step of systems design, the proposed system should be evaluated to determine whether it is satisfactory. A review of the overall arrangement and a specific check of the design's critical areas are crucial. The proposed system must meet the needs of the employees and managers as well as the organizational needs.

Implementing the System

The last step in systems design is the implementation phase. This phase may be time consuming. To implement a new system smoothly, it is imperative that the employees have a stake in the new system. Again, the employees and management should have been actively involved in the entire system design process. The new system may be implemented on a trial basis by a few employees. Employee acceptance should be taken into consideration. Some retraining may need to take place at this time. Modifications to the new system may occur during this trial period. If the new system involves a large operation, parallel operations may be conducted. This procedure allows the old system to continue to function while the new system "bugs" have been worked through and removed or modified. After the trial period, the old system can be phased out.

Organizational Structure

Organizational structure can be either formal or informal.

Formal Organizational Infrastructure

The formal organizational infrastructure is designed to plan work, assign responsibility, supervise work, and measure results. The formal relationships between various people and the organizational structure are identified on an **organization chart**. This chart clearly identifies hierarchical relationships, the lines of authority, responsibilities, and span of control. In an organization chart, the primary functions of the organization and the subfunctions within each primary function are identified. It should also aid in the identification of any areas of overlap in responsibility. The major disadvantage of the formal organization chart is its inability to show the informal interaction between employees as they carry out their everyday activities.

Informal Organization

The **informal or unwritten organization** refers to the many interpersonal relationships that occur in an organization that do not appear on the formal organization chart. A typical informal organization is composed of two or more persons who develop mutually satisfying interactions pertaining to personal or job-related matters. An informal organization develops over time.

Positive Aspects of Informal Organization. The most positive aspect of an informal organization is its blend with the formal organization to produce an operable system for the accomplishment of the work. If management can motivate the informal leaders to accept a new procedure, these leaders may be able to convince others to accept it. The informal organization provides the necessary social values and stability to work groups.

A well-known benefit of informal organization is that it provides an additional channel of communication. It is capable of efficiently sending and receiving communications. This informal channel is called the "grapevine." The grapevine can be described as the informal oral communication network that aids employees in learning more about what is happening in the organization and how it might affect them. Often it is more effective than the formal line of communication in distributing information, obtaining feedback, solving problems, and revising procedures.

Negative Aspects of Informal Organization. Informal organizations can also be a hindrance to management. In some organizations, the disadvantages far outweigh the benefits. A common example of abuse of the informal organization is one in which the employees find opportunities to work together even when no such work assignments have been made.

When an informal group loses confidence in a manager, they may combine forces to make life miserable for the manager. On occasion, informal groups may develop cross-purposes with the goals and objectives of the formal organization.

Potentially negative impacts or conflicts resulting from informal organization must be weighed against its constructive and practical function in nurturing creativity and innovation. A relatively conflict-free organization tends to be rigid, static, and inflexible.

Acceptance and Balance

Managers must accept three additional facts about the formal and informal organizations:

1. Informal organization is inevitable. Management creates the formal organization and can alter it as it so desires. The informal organization is not created by management. As long as organizations are composed of people, informal organizations will exist.

2. Small groups are the central component of the informal organization. Group membership in the informal organization strongly influences the overall behavior and performance of its members. Many sociologists agree that the group, not the individual, is the basic component of the human organization.[5]

3. Informal organization always coexists within the formal structure. This is a fact of organizational life. The formal and informal organizations must be balanced to achieve optimal performance and attain organizational objectives. Management trying to suppress the informal organization creates a destructive situation that results in reduced effectiveness. On the other hand, if the formal organization is too weak to accomplish its objectives, the informal organization can grow in strength, resulting in abuse of power, insubordination, and disloyalty.

The ideal situation is one in which the formal organization is strong enough to achieve its objectives and at the same time permit a well-developed informal organization to maintain group cohesiveness and teamwork. The informal relationships that exist in an organization deserve attention from employees and managers concerned with the organization's effectiveness.

ORGANIZATION-WIDE LEVEL

Change Management

Simply put, change management can be defined as the task of managing change. One meaning of managing change refers to "the making of changes in a planned and managed or systematic fashion."[6] This is a proactive approach where an organization plans to implement new systems or processes to grow and thrive. Managing change may also refer to a reactive response "to changes over which the organization exercises little or no control."[6] This may include implementing new systems or policies in response to new JCAHO standards or Centers for Medicare and Medicaid Services (CMS) directives. There are various methods for managing change, including strategic management, project management, and re-engineering.

STRATEGIC MANAGEMENT

One useful model of the strategic management process is illustrated in Figure 17-17.

Strategic management involves four primary stages. These stages are situational analysis, strategy formulation, strategic implementation, and strategic control.

Situational Analysis

Analyzing and understanding the situation is accomplished by three separate processes: (1) **external environmental analysis**, (2) **internal environmental analysis**, and (3) the development of the organization's **directional strategies** or its **mission**, **vision**, and **values**. The interaction and results of these processes form the basis for the development of strategy.

Issues in the external environment directly and simultaneously affect all three situational analysis processes. Issues in the external environment affect the process of environmental analysis, provide the context for internal analysis, and influence the mission, vision, and values. For example, a regulatory change may very well affect independently the analysis of the external environment, the determination of factors to be considered strengths or weaknesses of the organization, and the way managers view the mission, vision, and values.

External Environmental Analysis

To operate in today's changing environment, health care managers need a method for obtaining and assessing external information that will affect the organization. This process is referred to as external environmental analysis. As information is accumulated and classified, managers must determine the environmental issues that are significant to the organization. In addition, they must monitor these issues, collect additional information, evaluate their impact, and incorporate them in a strategy.

External environmental analysis is the process by which an organization crosses the boundary between itself and the external environment to identify and understand changes (issues) that are taking place outside the organization. These changes represent both opportunities and threats. Health care managers need to understand the nature of these opportunities and threats before they affect the organization. These external opportunities and threats represent the fundamental issues that will spell success or failure for the organization. Opportunities and threats should influence the strategy adopted by the organization, that is, what the organization *should* do.

Internal Environmental Analysis

The organization itself has an internal environment that represents the resources, competencies, and capabilities of the organization (what the organization *can* do). An understanding of these factors requires an extensive, in-depth analysis of the internal functions, operations, structure, resources, and skills.[7]

An internal environmental analysis should reveal the strengths and weaknesses of the organization. An understanding of the strengths and weaknesses provides a foundation for strategy formulation and is essential if a strategy is to be developed that optimizes strengths and de-emphasizes and overcomes weaknesses.

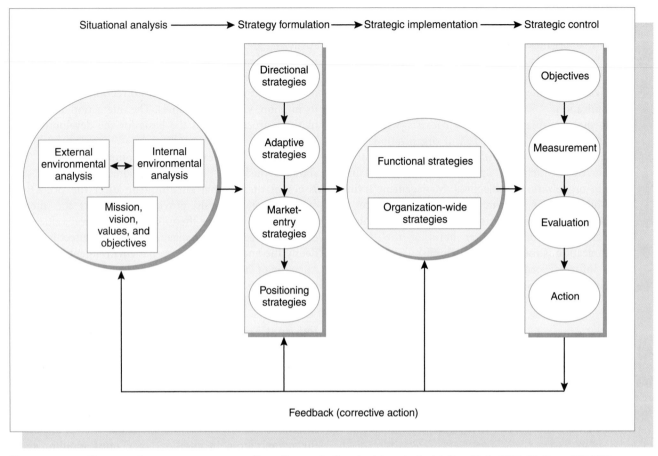

Figure 17-17 The strategic management process. (From Swayne L: *The physician strategist,* New York, 1996, McGraw-Hill. With permission of the McGraw-Hill Companies.)

Mission, Vision, and Values

The mission, vision, and values of an organization greatly affect the strategy it ultimately adopts. The organization's *mission* represents the consensus and articulation of the organization's understanding of the external opportunities and threats and the internal strengths and weaknesses.[8] It is a general statement of what distinguishes the organization from all others of its type and answers the questions "Who are we?" and "What do we do?" *Vision,* on the other hand, is the view of the future that management believes is optimal for the organization (ideally, it is based on an understanding of the external opportunities and threats and internal strengths and weaknesses) and is communicated throughout the organization. Vision profiles the future and constitutes what the organization *wants* to do.

The *values* of an organization are the fundamental beliefs or "truths" that the organization holds dear. Values are the best indicator of the philosophy of the organization and specify what is important (honesty, integrity, customers, and so on) in the organization. Values are sometimes referred to as guiding principles. These become the *directional strategies* of the organization and the basis for setting organizational objectives.

Mission, vision, and values are considered part of the situational analysis because they rely on and influence external environmental analysis and internal environmental analysis. Taken together, these directional strategies express an understanding of the situation, what the organization is now, and what it wants to be. They are also a part of strategy formulation because they provide a definition of the broadest direction for the organization.

Strategy Formulation

Situational analysis involves gathering, classifying, and understanding information. Strategy formulation involves making decisions using that information. These decisions result in a strategy for the organization.[9] As noted earlier, the first set of decisions concerns the mission, vision, and values and provides the general direction for the organization. Next, more specific strategic decisions must be made. These decisions include determination of the adaptive strategies, market entry strategies, and the positioning strategies.

The **adaptive strategies** are more specific than the directional strategies and indicate the method for carrying out the directional strategies. The adaptive strategies specify how the organization will expand (diversification, vertical integration, market development, product development, or penetration), contract (divestiture, liquidation, harvesting, or retrenchment), or stabilize (enhancement or status quo) operations.

Market entry strategies indicate whether the adaptive strategy will be accomplished through buying into the market (i.e., acquisitions), cooperating with other organizations in the market (i.e., mergers and alliances), or internal development. Positioning strategies delineate how the organization's products and services will be positioned vis-à-vis competitors' products and services in a given market and might include strategies such as cost leadership or product differentiation.

Decisions concerning these strategies are sequential. Directional strategies are developed first; then adaptive strategies are formulated. Next, market entry strategies are selected. Finally, positioning strategies are formulated. These strategic decisions explicitly answer the following questions: What business(es) are we in? What business(es) should we be in? How are we going to compete? At this point, the broad organizational strategies have been selected.

Strategic Implementation

Once the directional, adaptive, market entry, and positioning strategies have been formulated, **operational strategies** that support these organizational strategies are developed and the process of **strategic implementation** is initiated. Operational strategies are made up of strategies developed within the functional areas of the organization and strategies that link the functional areas and develop the capabilities of the organization. **Functional strategies** and supporting programs and budgets must be developed for the key areas in the organization, such as marketing, information systems, finance, and human resources. These functional areas are directly and independently affected by the strategy formulation process, yet functional strategies must be integrated to move the organization toward realizing its mission. In addition to the functional strategies, organizations often develop **linkage strategies** that enhance the general capabilities and link organizational processes. These operational strategies include initiatives such as changing the organization's culture, reorganization, upgrade of facilities and equipment, and social and ethical strategies. These strategies generally affect the entire organization and cut across all functional areas.

Strategic Control

The final stage of strategic management is strategic control. Strategic control is similar to the general management control process discussed later in this chapter. **Strategic control** is a process that includes (1) establishment of standards (objectives), (2) measurement of performance, (3) evaluation of organizational performance against the standards, and (4) taking corrective action, if necessary.

However, strategic control is much broader and, in turn, affects the operational strategies, the organization's general strategy, and situational analysis processes. As managers monitor these various organizational processes, they learn what is effective and take corrective action as necessary.

Sometimes it is difficult for managers to plan or envision the long-term future of an organization in a dynamic environment. Managers often need to react to unanticipated developments and very new competitive pressures. Strategy becomes an intuitive, entrepreneurial, political, culture-based, or learning process. In these cases, previous experience is of limited value. Managers must create and discover an unfolding future, using their ability to learn together in groups and to interact politically in a spontaneous, self-organizing manner. When there are provocative atmospheres conducive to complex learning, organizations may change and develop new strategic directions. In such atmospheres, the destination and the route may turn out to be unexpected and unintended. As a result, strategy emerges spontaneously from the chaos of challenge and contradiction through a process of real-time learning and politics.[10] At the center of this process is the manager, who must carefully craft the decisions that will contribute much to the success or failure of the organization. Therefore, we must understand the manager if we are to understand management.

Project Management

Project management as defined by some experts is management plus planning.[11] It uses the basic management principles of planning, organizing, directing, and controlling (with an emphasis on planning) to bring a project to a successful conclusion. Because projects are unique and demand that people do things differently from before, the team is following an unknown path and must plan ahead.

Project management techniques are used by many varied professions—engineers, construction contractors, and military and government agencies. Today's health care managers also find project management techniques helpful in confronting the conflicting responsibilities of completing continuous and routine work while exploring and implementing new health care delivery models and technologies with less resources, greater time constraints, and continuous communication links across organizational units.

Characteristics of a Project

To understand the concepts of project management, the characteristics of a project must be defined.

Unique. This process has never been done before. It is a one-time event or one-of-a-kind activity. It will never be repeated in precisely the same way again. There is no practice or rehearsal. Experience can be gained from previous projects. However, this particular combination of time, place, people, and project is unique.

Product or Result. The outcome of the project is a single, definable product, such as a bridge that is built, a rocket that is launched, or a hospital that is constructed. Projects are goal oriented and work through the process to achieve that goal. The product is different for each project.

Finite. The project is usually on a fixed time scale with start and finish dates. It can be viewed as a temporary activity. The project is undertaken to accomplish a goal within a set period of time. Once the goal is achieved, the project ceases to exist.

Complex, Numerous, and Sequenced Activities. Projects involve a variety of complex and sequenced activities used to achieve the goal or objective.

Team. Projects are completed by a team of people from diverse professions and organizational units. Projects may be task interdependent and may use advanced technology. However, projects are human endeavors and cannot be performed by technology alone.

Cross-Functional. Often projects cross several functional areas in an organization, involving multiple skills and talents of many people. The actual work may be performed by many functional areas. Because of this, the project does not neatly fit into the organizational structure.

Limited Resources. Projects usually have a set limit of resources and budget. The end result is specified in terms of cost, schedule, and performance requirements.

Change. Projects have the characteristic of being somewhat unfamiliar. Projects may comprise innovative technology and possess pivotal elements of uncertainty and risk. However, the essence of project management is to create change. When the project is completed, the world (i.e., organization, department) is a little different.

Characteristics of Project Management

The following are some characteristics of project management[12]:

- A single person, the project manager, administers the project and operates independently of the normal organization chart or the chain of command. The project manager has the authority to plan, direct, organize, and control the entire project from start to finish.
- Decision making, accountability, results, and rewards are shared among the members of the project team.
- Although the project activities are temporary, the functional areas performing the work are usually a permanent part of the organization. After the completion of the project, the individual workers are returned to their original assignments or reassigned to a new project.

- The project focuses on delivering an end product or end result at a certain time, with certain resource allotments, and to the satisfaction of performance or technical requirements.
- Project management can set into motion other support functions, including personnel evaluation, accounting, and information systems.

Project Planning

Planning is essentially thinking ahead. In project management, planning involves two phases: defining the project and planning the project.

Defining the Project. Defining the project is often called project overview. Four areas are detailed in the definition phase.

1. The *problem statement* answers the following questions:
   - What is the problem?
   - What is the opportunity?
   - What is to be done?
   - Who is responsible for the project?
   - When must it be completed?
2. The *goal statement* is the final outcome of the project. It serves as a point of focus and reference that keeps all activities on track. A goal statement tells precisely what the outcome will be and when it will be done. It needs to be action oriented, short, simple, and straightforward. An example of a project goal is to implement a computer-based patient record by the year 2006.
3. To achieve the stated goal, several steps have to take place. These steps represent milestones in the project and are considered *objectives*. They define major components that must be accomplished to achieve the overall goal. Objectives are more precise and measurable than the goal statement. A project objective for the goal of implementation of a computer-based patient record is an on-line connection between the hospital computer system and the medical staff offices within 6 months.
4. *Resources* include people (human resources), materials, space, and money that are needed to achieve the goal.

Plan. A project is initiated with the preparation of a written plan. The purpose of the plan is to direct and guide the project manager and the project team members through the project. Basically, planning is thinking ahead, communicating the plan, and using the plan as a yardstick to measure the progress toward achievement of the goal. The five areas detailed in the planning phase are as follows:

1. *Project activities.* Every objective of the project should encompass separate activities. These activities define the work to be accomplished to attain the objective. The method of **work breakdown structures** is often used in projects. It divides the project into major objectives, partitions each objective into activities,

further divides the activities into subactivities, and creates work packages that must be done to complete the project.

2. *Time and cost.* The time and cost for completion of each activity are estimated. Variations in time may be due to the skill level of the people performing the activity, material availability, technology or machine variations, and unexpected events, such as illness and employee turnover. Estimates of time may contain the most optimistic completion time, the most pessimistic completion time, and the most likely completion time. Cost estimates are typically categorized into labor, materials, other direct (e.g., telephone, postage) costs, and indirect costs or overhead.

3. *Activity sequence.* Once the activities have been identified along with their time and cost estimates, they need to be sequenced. Some activities are dependent on others; that is, one activity cannot be started until another is completed. They must be done sequentially. Other activities may be done simultaneously.

4. *Critical activities.* Management tools such as the **Gantt chart** and **PERT network** can be used to determine the sequence and the amount of time needed to complete the project. The sequence of activities that makes up the longest path to complete the project is called the **critical path.** When activities are completed on schedule, the whole project will be completed on time. However, sometimes activities take longer than anticipated or materials cannot be obtained, and then the project completion time is extended.

5. *Project proposal.* The purpose of a project proposal is to provide a complete description of the project activities, time lines, and resource requirements. It is a statement of the general approach being taken and the results expected. It is a decision-making tool, a key to management control, a training aid for new project team members, and a reporting document. The project proposal portrays the transition from project management planning to project management implementation.

Project Implementation. Once the project has been approved, the work begins. The implementation process contains three phases: organize, control, and termination.

Organize. Organizing includes the assembly of the required resources (materials, personnel, and money) to accomplish the work defined in the plan. Organizing also includes the development of the structure needed to administer the plan. The following three areas are detailed in the organization phase:

1. *Project manager.* The most important element of project management is the project manager. This person has the responsibility to integrate work efforts and plays a major role in planning and executing a project. The project manager is accountable for the project and dedicated to achieving its goals. The criteria for selection of a project manager vary according to organizations. The usual characteristics include the following:
   - Background and experience
   - Leadership
   - Strategic expertise
   - Technical expertise
   - Interpersonal skills
   - Managerial capability

   Selecting the most qualified project manager can be the key to the project's success or failure.

2. *Project team.* Project management entails bringing individuals and groups together to form a single, cohesive team working toward a common goal. Project work is teamwork accomplished by a group of people. Once the project manager is selected, he or she can assist in the selection of the project team members. The size and composition of the project team depend on the resources allocated to the project. The following characteristics are desirable in a member of a project team:
   - Commitment to the project goal
   - Communication skills
   - Flexibility
   - Technical competence
   - Task orientation
   - Ability to be a team player
   - Experience with project management tools
   - Dependability, history of meeting deadlines

3. *Work activities.* Now that the planning and organizing have been done, work on the project gets started. The project manager assigns responsibilities for completing activities to members of the project team. As discussed previously, activities can be subdivided into subactivities and work packages. A work package as one continuous activity is assigned to a project team member who has the authority, expertise, and access to the appropriate resources necessary to complete the assignment. A work package has beginning and ending tasks with a definitive description of each task. The project manager schedules the start dates of each work package. Because many activities are interrelated, work packages must be clearly documented so that their completion can be tracked.

Control. Controlling is the monitoring and maintenance of the structure of the project. Part of control is the reporting at specified points throughout the project. The reports should indicate potential problems. The following two areas are detailed in the control phase:

1. *Effective project leadership.* The project manager and the project team must work together to reach the project goal. Group cohesiveness, open communication, team development, and empowerment of members are top priorities for the project manager (Box 17-3).

2. *Control tools.* Controls focus on performance levels, cost, and time schedules. Controls also track progress, detect variance from the plan, and allow the project manager to take corrective action.

The project manager reports the status of every activity in the project at least monthly. This report summarizes the progress for that month and for the length of the entire project. The project manager should also report the variances from the plan. These variances may be related to budget, labor, time, or materials. Positive variance examples are being ahead of schedule or under budget. Negative variances may include an extended time schedule or a greater budgetary item than anticipated. Negative cost variances may not be under the project manager's control, such as unexpected equipment failure or increased cost of supplies.

When each milestone of the project is completed, the project manager should review the project. Despite all the extensive planning, things will not automatically happen according to the plan. To get back on schedule, the project manager may have to reallocate resources, consider alternatives, and re-evaluate activities. This is where good project managers prove their worth by getting the project back on schedule.

Termination. There are three types of project termination.

1. *Termination by extinction.* The project work as scheduled is either successfully or unsuccessfully done and the decision to terminate is agreed on.
2. *Termination by inclusion.* The successful project is institutionalized or transformed into the organization as a unit.
3. *Termination by integration.* A common way of closing successful projects occurs when equipment, material, and personnel are distributed back into the organization.

Termination Process

The four phases in the termination process are as follows:

1. *Approval.* Obtain the client's or administration's approval of the project. The termination or closing down of the project depends on their satisfaction and the quality of service the project provided.
2. *Logistics.* Assign a termination manager and team to assist in the termination phase, conduct a termination meeting, prepare personnel reports, and terminate work orders and contracts.
3. *Document.* Document the entire project. Document the completion and performance of all team members and the performance of vendors, consultants, and contractors.
4. *Final report and audit.* The final project report is a history of the project. Items included in the final project report are the overall success and performance of the project, techniques used, strengths and weaknesses, organization, and recommendations from the project manager and project team. An audit of the project should be conducted after implementation. The essential questions that need to be asked in evaluating the success of the project are the following:
   - Was the goal achieved?
   - Was the work done on time? Within budget? Within specifications?
   - Was the client or administration satisfied with the results?

Project Tools. Project tools may be used in the planning or controlling phase of project management. The two most common tools are the PERT network and the Gantt chart.

PERT Network

PERT is the acronym for Program Evaluation Review Technique. It is a scheduling device that was originally developed early in the space age as a tool for missile development programs. It is a system of diagramming the steps or component parts of a large, complex project that is usually nonrepetitive in nature. The various components of a PERT network and the estimated completion time for each component must be identified. All events in the network and all subsequent activities that are performed flow from and are aimed toward the completion of a specific goal. The basic components of a network (goal, events, and activities) are discussed further as follows:

1. *Goal:* The acknowledgment and statement of the goal is the most basic concept of the PERT network and all major events and activities flow toward this goal. The network is essentially a diagram representing the overall plan for achieving the final goal. An example of a goal statement in the construction of a PERT network is the following: Conversion of the computer system in the HIM department is fully operational.

2. *Events:* Events in the network are discrete control points in time and reflect either the starting or ending points for one activity or a group of activities. Events are usually represented on the network by circles, rectangles, or ovals and usually contain the descriptive wording of an element. For ease of reference, events are usually numbered, but letters can also be used if there is a limited number of events. Examples of the wording of an event are as follows: Computerized coding system selected and Renovation of department begun.

3. *Activities:* In the network, activities must be performed to move from one event to the next and finally to the actual goal. Activities generally require time, money, and resources for completion and usually represent the work or action required to move from one event to another. Activities may also involve staff members. Remember that activities connect events in the network and along with events constitute the diagram reflecting the starting point through the accomplishment of the actual goal. Activities in a PERT network are generally depicted by a solid line (or a solid line with an arrow on one end) between the events to which they are related. Because activities reflect work being done, examples of the wording of activities would be as follows: Developing job procedures and Training file clerks.

Included in the preparation of a PERT network is the determination of a critical path. The critical path is the longest route and estimated completion time in the PERT network for a given project. This route would consist of the events and activities that must be completed, the order in which they must be completed, and the time frame in which they must be completed for the project to be accomplished (Figure 17-18). The critical path therefore controls the time required to complete the project.

In Figure 17-18, the circled letters represent events and the solid line with the arrow at one end represents an activity or a group of activities that leads to the next major event. The goal is represented by the letter N in this network. The critical path is the A-B-D-G-J-M-N path, and the time needed to complete this project is 66 days.

The following steps are suggested for constructing a PERT network:

1. The final goal should be stated in detail and then worked forward from the beginning to the end.
2. All possible events should be listed, followed by a description of all activities for each of the events in the network.
3. All events should be analyzed and should be placed in the proper sequence. At this point, relationships between events, logical flow of events, and dependences should be considered.
4. Remember that the length of the line representing an activity or a group of activities does not represent time. There may be burst events (events that stem from one event) or merge events (events that merge together into another event). For example, in Figure 17-18 events C and E would be burst events and events J and I would be merge events.
5. The flow of events and activities is always forward because there can be no backward loops or backtracking in a PERT diagram.

Advantages of a PERT Network and the Critical Path

A PERT diagram is a valuable tool for the systems analyst because it can be used to plan an individual, detailed project or to plan an entire department's workload. The advantages of such a diagram are as follows:

1. The analyst is forced to determine and define all the individual events that must take place from the start of the project through its completion.

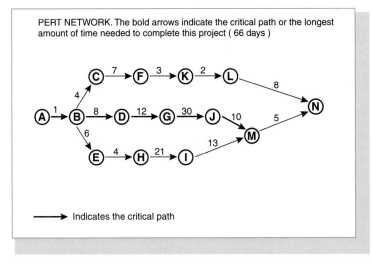

Figure 17-18 PERT network.

2. The analyst is also required to predict time estimates for the completion of each activity in the network.

3. Once the diagram is drawn, the analyst can determine the critical path or the longest time needed to complete the project.

4. Because estimated times are listed on the diagram for completion of each event, the analyst can determine whether the project is moving along according to schedule. If more time is needed than indicated on the diagram, then that extra time taken must be made up during some other event for the project to remain on schedule. (See Example of Setting Up a PERT Schedule.)

Example of Setting Up a PERT Schedule

The director of an HIM department in XYZ Hospital is responsible for supervising the enlargement and renovation of the reimbursement section of the HIM department. The director must determine the length of time needed to complete the project. The following events must be accomplished to complete the project:

START (A): A meeting is called to discuss thoroughly the plans for the departmental renovation.

STEP B: During the meeting, a committee is established to oversee the renovation of the reimbursement section.

STEP C: One duty of the committee is the recruitment of additional employees for this section. Recruitment ads must be written and approved before advertising in professional journals, newspapers, and so forth.

STEP D: A second duty of committee members is to finalize the departmental layout for this section.

STEP E: Finally, the committee must make decisions regarding the additional equipment needs of the reimbursement section.

STEP F: Prospective applicants for the reimbursement section are interviewed by committee members and the director of the HIM department.

STEP G: After the approval of the layout, construction on the new renovation begins.

STEP H: Additional office equipment and furniture must be ordered for the renovated section.

STEP I: When all equipment is received, it must be thoroughly checked and installation must be scheduled.

STEP J: This step involves the completion of all construction on the new section.

STEP K: After the applicant interviewing phase, a decision is made to hire four new employees.

STEP L: Orientation and training sessions are scheduled for the four newly hired employees.

STEP M: All equipment is installed in the renovated section of the department.

FINISH (N): The reimbursement section of the HIM department begins operation.

As shown in Figure 17-18, some activities may occur at the same time. Other activities must wait for an activity to be completed before they can begin.

Gantt Chart

Named after the famous management consultant Henry Gantt, a Gantt chart is a common project scheduling tool. Gantt charts are appropriate for complex projects with multiple steps. The chart consists of a horizontal scale divided into time units (days, weeks, months) and a vertical scale depicting project work elements (tasks, activities, work packages). The length of the horizontal bar corresponds to the expected length of time to complete the activity. As time progresses, the bar is filled in with symbols related to projected completion, actual progress, and actual completion (Figure 17-19). When the chart is used as a visual control tool, shading or color coding could be used.

The Gantt chart can also be used for personnel planning, resource allocation, and budgeting, and it is often used to track the progress of computer-based projects. It provides an excellent view of project status and it is a useful tool for monitoring progress. As with the PERT network, the Gantt chart plays an important role in the planning and controlling of projects.

Information Technology Applications

According to Wayne Niemi, "Project management software is designed to improve communications between the project manager and project team members, transfer information about project deadlines, assign tasks and track the status of multiple projects. One of the many benefits of these programs is that they allow users to manage more projects and accounts with fewer staff members. With a more organized approach to project management, job tasks are simplified with improved communication."[13] Some programs allow the manager to break out each participant's tasks, goals, and deadlines so that they have their own project program. Software programs also give managers the ability to help keep track of action items from several projects at once.

There are various types of software packages available that will assist with project management. Charting software provides tools for drawing flowcharts, organizational charts, and other types of diagrams. Specifically, these tools can help a supervisor see whether the steps of a project have problems or miscommunications, defines the boundaries of a process, and develops a common base of knowledge. They will often bring to light redundancies, delays, dead ends, and indirect

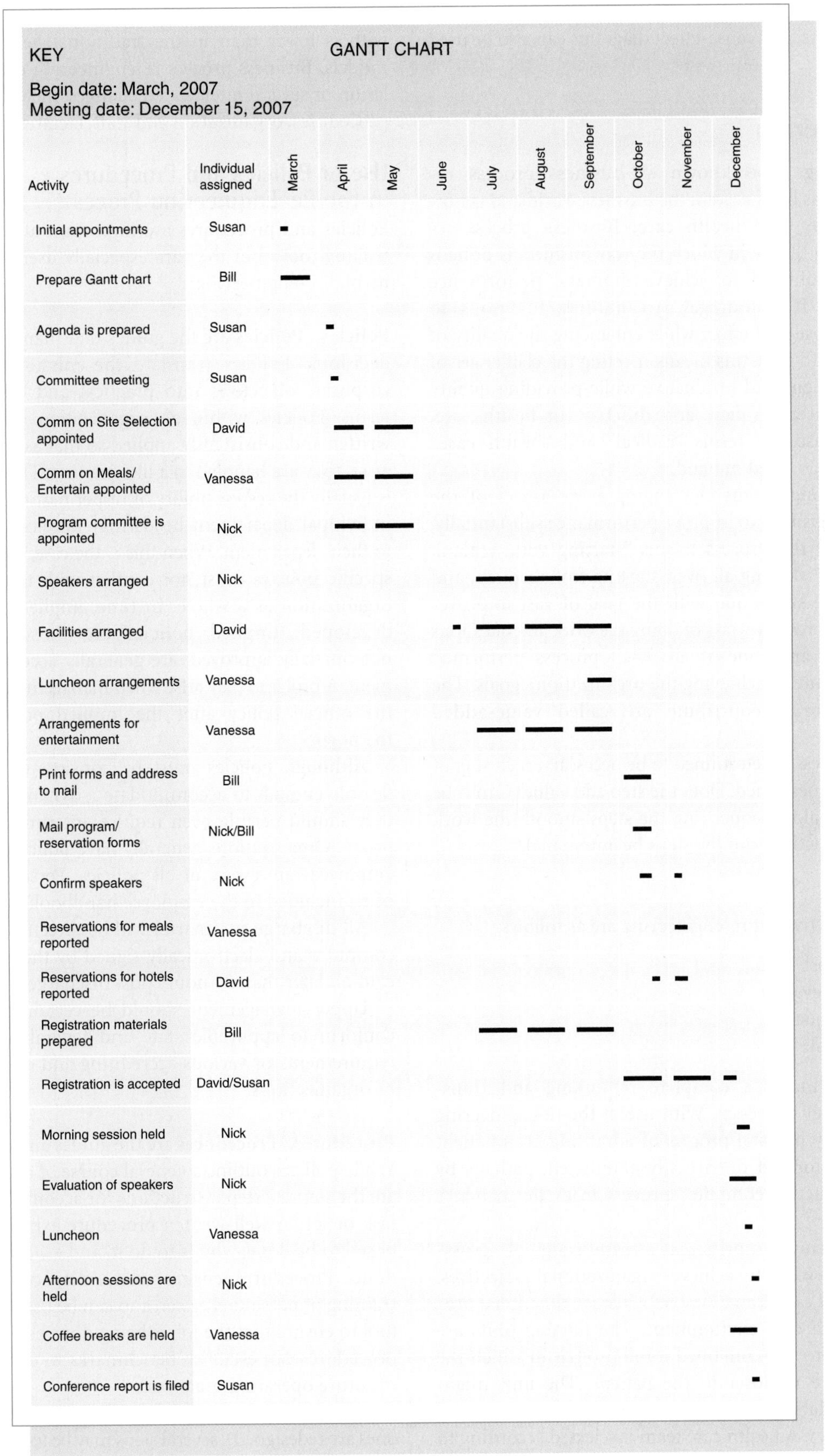

GANTT CHART

KEY

Begin date: March, 2007
Meeting date: December 15, 2007

Activity	Individual assigned	March	April	May	June	July	August	September	October	November	December
Initial appointments	Susan	■									
Prepare Gantt chart	Bill	■									
Agenda is prepared	Susan		■								
Committee meeting	Susan		■								
Comm on Site Selection appointed	David		■	■							
Comm on Meals/Entertain appointed	Vanessa		■	■							
Program committee is appointed	Nick		■	■							
Speakers arranged	Nick					■	■	■			
Facilities arranged	David				■	■	■	■			
Luncheon arrangements	Vanessa							■			
Arrangements for entertainment	Vanessa					■	■	■			
Print forms and address to mail	Bill								■		
Mail program/reservation forms	Nick/Bill								■		
Confirm speakers	Nick								■	■	
Reservations for meals reported	Vanessa									■	
Reservations for hotels reported	David								■	■	
Registration materials prepared	Bill					■	■	■			
Registration is accepted	David/Susan								■	■	■
Morning session held	Nick										■
Evaluation of speakers	Nick										■
Luncheon	Vanessa										■
Afternoon sessions are held	Nick										■
Coffee breaks are held	Vanessa										■
Conference report is filed	Susan										■

Figure 17-19 Gantt chart.

paths that can go unnoticed or ignored. Time lines, PERT and Gantt charts, and cause-effect diagrams can also be used in this process.

Re-Engineering

Re-engineering (also known as business process re-engineering) has been used in the business world and is now finding its way into health care. Business process re-engineering is a theory in which the way business is done is radically re-evaluated to achieve dramatic performance improvement. It encourages streamlining functions to reduce time, cost, and effort while enhancing the quality of service. In health care, this means meeting the challenges of becoming efficient and productive while providing quality care. This concept is new and different in health care, possibly because the terms "radical" and "health care" usually do not go hand in hand.

Re-engineering means challenging every aspect of the way of doing business to improve performance substantially. Re-engineering the process means "starting with a blank sheet of paper," starting all over, starting from scratch, and challenging the status quo with the goal of vast improvements.[14] It explores new ways of doing the work and questions why processes are done at all. Each process performed should contribute to achieving the organization's goals. The processes that do contribute are called value-added activities.

Once a process is determined to be necessary, each step of the process is questioned. Does the step add value? Can it be simplified? Would resequencing the steps smooth the work flow? When practical, can the steps be automated?

Objectives

The main objectives of re-engineering are as follows:

- Reduce cost
- Increase revenue
- Improve quality
- Reduce risk

Re-engineering is a complete rethinking and transformation of key processes. With use of the re-engineering approach, a key hospital process of admitting an inpatient could be transformed or virtually eliminated, perhaps by using an interactive computer process from the patient's home.

Re-engineering emphasizes streamlining of cross-functional processes to achieve organizational objectives. Patient-focused care is an example of a cross-functional process in a health care environment. The nursing units are transformed into self-contained minihospitals in which the delivery of care is closer to the patient. The unit might contain a mini laboratory, a mini radiology department, and a mini pharmacy. A health care team is selected according to the patient's diagnosis, procedure, or severity of illness. That health care team delivers all the care to the patient. The actual number of health care workers the patient has contact with is fewer than in the traditional health care delivery models. Business process re-engineering entails the assimilation of several interrelated changes, including policies and procedures, organization and staff, facilities, and technology.

Use of Policies and Procedures in the Re-Engineering Process

Policies and procedures are important at all times as controlling tools, but they are especially useful during departmental re-engineering.

Policies. **Policies** are the guides that managers use to make decisions. Policies translate the mission statement and corporate objectives into practical and easily understood terms. Policies within an organization should be clearly written and consistently applied so that as similar situations arise, they are handled in a like manner. Thus, policymaking is usually the responsibility of upper management, although individual department heads may develop policies specific to their department. When this is the case, these department-specific policies must not conflict with the policies of the organization as a whole. In time, implied policies may be developed. Implied policies are those that, although not officially approved, are generally accepted by management. A problem may arise when management tries to enforce the official policy after the implied policy has become the norm.

Although policies must be consistent, they should be flexible enough to accommodate a dynamic workplace and they should permit, even require, interpretation, as appropriate. Organizations generally have policy manuals so that employees are aware of all policies. Personnel policies are often included in the employee handbook.

All discharge summaries will be directly entered into the computer and electronically signed by the attending physician no later than 24 hours post discharge.

Upper management should be certain that all policies conform to applicable state and federal laws and to the requirements of various accrediting and certifying agencies or organizations.

Procedures. **Procedures** are the guides and plans for action. While policies outline a general course of action, procedures are the step-by-step instructions for accomplishing a specific task or job. A well-written procedure explains what is supposed to be done, who is to do it, and exactly how it is to be done. Procedures ensure uniformity of practice, make training of personnel easier, and can be used as a controlling tool to ensure that the job is being done as planned. Written procedures can establish benchmarks to compare with past or future operating practices.

When procedures are written or evaluated (or existing ones are redesigned), several steps may be followed (Box 17-4).

Procedures are generally written in either narrative, step-by-step outline, or playscript style. In narrative style, the

Box 17-4 STEPS IN WRITING PROCEDURES

- List each step in the procedure.
- Determine a logical sequence for the steps.
- Can any steps be eliminated?
- Are the steps too difficult for the employees' skills?
- Are there any potential bottlenecks or obstacles to completion?
- Determine the impact of this procedure on other procedures.
- Will this procedure create potential problems in related areas?
- Will changes need to be made in other procedures?
- Test the procedure for several weeks and ask for employee input.
- Evaluate the effectiveness of the procedure.
- Make changes as necessary.
- Implement the new procedure.

procedure is written in story or paragraph format and includes all of the parts of the procedure. It is usually the hardest style to write because there must be transition statements between all of the parts of the process.

The step-by-step procedure is written in outline format and takes the employee through each individual task in the procedure. It is generally the easiest style for the employee to follow.

The playscript format is often used when several employees are involved in a particular task. In this method a number is assigned to each step in the procedure and action verbs are used to describe the key steps in the task. It also identifies which employee or "actor" completes each step. (See Example of a Statement Written in Playscript Style.)

Example of a Statement Written in Playscript Style

Actor	Step Sequence	Action Word	Action Sentence
Receptionist	1	Greets	Greets visitors as they enter the health information department

After all procedures are written, they should be organized into a procedure manual. Effective communication and writing skills should be used in creating this manual. Clarity and brevity are essential elements of the procedure manual, as is the use of action verbs to convey the steps in the procedure. The purpose of the manual and the intended audience are factors in deciding on the writing style used, the level of detail, and the kinds of examples used.

How the procedure manual is to be arranged and disseminated must also be considered. The procedure manual should be accessible, easy to read, and arranged so that infor-

mation is easily found. It should be updated frequently. It is often distributed in a binder for ease in updating.

Relationship to Quality Improvement

Because re-engineering advocates radical change that might be too risky for health care organizations, the more cautious and acceptable approach of quality improvement is often used in conjunction with re-engineering. Sometimes total quality management is used in conjunction with re-engineering to restructure a process to create the most efficient operation model for delivering an outcome. Total quality management starts with minor successes and builds.

Applications to Health Information Management

HIM professionals need to become involved in the organization-wide re-engineering process. They need to look at processes and procedures in a whole new light. Looking forward to the computer-based patient record, HIM professionals need to view how it will radically change the delivery of patient care and management of information. For its full potential to be realized, HIM professionals have to be willing to let go of old ways and change things dramatically.[15] The same forms that are used in paper records cannot simply be computerized and expected to meet the information needs of the future. Given the HIM role in the health care field and the dramatic changes in health care delivery systems, HIM professionals need an understanding of and commitment to the re-engineering process.[16]

DESIGN AND MANAGEMENT OF SPACE IN HEALTH INFORMATION SERVICES

This section focuses on the arrangement of the physical components of furniture, equipment, and environment with the goal of providing maximum effectiveness and coordinating these physical components into a comfortable work area, thus contributing to maximum efficiency of the department/organization.

Work Space Design

When the work space is designed, the following aspects should be considered.

Work Flow

Considering the purpose of the organization, the primary objective in work space design is efficient and effective work flow. Is the work moving to the next person with a minimum of backtracking and bottlenecks? Work flow is a greater concern in an environment where paper is used than in a totally computerized system. As discussed earlier in the chapter, several tools are available to use in analyzing and improving work flow, including flowcharts.

Traffic Patterns

Along with work flow, the traffic patterns of employees and visitors to the area are important considerations. To determine these patterns, the location of entrances to the area, the employees who work together, and the employees who frequently receive visitors or leave the area need to be identified. A **trip frequency chart** shows which employees frequently interact with one another (Figure 17-20). The various employees and locations are listed along the horizontal and vertical axes. The number indicates how many times one employee visits the work space of another employee. Low numbers indicate which employees do not interact frequently and, therefore, do not need to be close to one another, whereas high numbers indicate a need for closeness.

Work groups or teams are commonly found in today's workplace. Space design must facilitate the work of these teams, not prohibit it. The supervisor or team leaders also need to be located in proximity to their staff to provide more effective supervision and to facilitate communication.

The work space allotted to a particular departmental function or work group should conform to the number of employees performing that function. Equipment, references,

and other materials needed to perform the job can then be located in one central area so that they are easily accessible to all employees performing similar tasks.

Functions Performed in the Work Space

When the work space is designed, an obvious consideration is the type of function performed in the space. Some specific functions beyond those of the data entry–clerical type must be considered. The reception area has a public relations aspect. Because visitors see this area first, it should be neat, well organized, and functional. It should be located so that visitors do not interrupt the work flow. Serving as a buffer zone between the outside and the place of work, the reception area provides privacy for the staff. This area should be monitored constantly to assist and screen visitors, letting only those people enter who have legitimate business.

Another special-purpose area is a conference room. This area is needed for meetings that are too large to take place in a private office, that might disturb others in the office, or that need special equipment (e.g., an overhead projector). This area can also be used for training.

In the overall design of a department, it is often desirable to place certain areas next to each other and other areas far away from each other. A restaurant designer would not place the patron waiting area near the garbage dump. This would be undesirable. A **proximity chart** shows the need to place

FROM \ TO	Director	Secretary	Health Information Analyst	Release of Information Specialist	Clinical Coder	Optical Image Specialist
Director		14	5	3	7	8
Secretary	30		4	9	2	10
Health Information Analyst	8	3		4	12	20
Release of Information Specialist	16	9	5		5	14
Clinical Coder	12	4	10	6		9
Optical Image Specialist	25	19	9	11	7	

Figure 17-20 Trip frequency chart.

some areas close to or far from each other (Figure 17-21). It can also show why the proximity is important.

Need for Confidentiality of Work Performed

If the work being performed is of a confidential nature, access to the work area may need to be controlled. If the confidential information is audible—for example, physicians dictating reports for the patient record or employee conferences—then the space design must provide for this speech privacy. If the work is performed on a computer, the use of screens or panels around work areas may be advisable to prevent others from reading information displayed on the computer screen. The location of a fax machine also involves security concerns. In a health care organization, confidential information is often transmitted by way of fax machine. Fax machines should be located in areas that are secure from access by unauthorized employees.

Shift Workers–Sharing Work Space

Sometimes it is necessary to divide a particular job function into shifts. This is true if space is restricted or if equipment to perform the job is costly and limited in supply. Shift work may mean that employees must share their work space. Under these circumstances, each employee should have some private space in the work area that is his or her own for displaying photographs and for storage of personal items. Employees sharing work space need to respect one another's privacy. Adjustability of chairs and other work equipment is important so that the needs of all may be met.

Flexibility for Future Needs

Work space design should be as flexible as possible to accommodate the future needs of the organization. These needs might include downsizing, expansion, or further computerization. The use of partitions instead of solid-

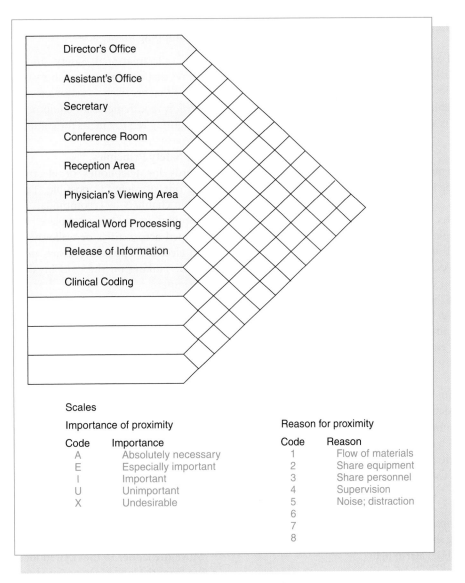

Figure 17-21 Proximity chart.

walled offices is recommended for organizations that anticipate change, either in size or in the work functions being performed. Workstations whose components may be added or subtracted as necessary (i.e., modular furniture) increase the capability of organizations to implement change without loss of efficiency.

Expanding technology demands increase the need for power capabilities of the work space. Regular electrical power and "clean" power for computers and telecommunications systems are located beneath access floors so that necessary power is available at any given location. This system allows for flush-to-floor outlets and flexible placement of furniture and equipment.

Employees' Personal Needs

The work environment is composed of people gathered together to perform work that will accomplish the objectives of an organization. These people have physical, safety, social, and psychological needs that must be met as well as the need to collect a paycheck. Today's workforce wants a comfortable, safe, and user-friendly environment.

Physical Size and Structure. Because employees vary in physical characteristics such as height, weight, and length of torso and extremities, workstation components should be as flexible and adjustable as possible. More information on the workstation and its components is presented later in the chapter.

Age. Older people may require special considerations in the workplace regarding lighting, sound, and temperature.

Medical Conditions. In addition to the special considerations of age, workplace requirements for physical handicaps or other medical conditions of the worker must be addressed. The Vocational Rehabilitation Act of 1972 requires that federal buildings and buildings that were built with more than $2500 in federal funds be accessible to handicapped people. These requirements include wide aisle space for wheelchairs, 28-inch height for desks, 32-inch-wide doors, ramp entrances to buildings, and appropriate (time-delayed) entry doors.

The Americans with Disabilities Act (ADA), which became effective in 1992, provides that if a facility is a "public accommodation," it must take "barrier removal" steps. Public accommodations include many types of service establishments, such as professional offices of health care providers, pharmacies, insurance offices, banks, and hospitals. Barriers that affect work space access can be modified in the following ways:

- Installing ramps where steps are located
- Repositioning shelves
- Installing flashing alarm lights
- Widening doors
- Installing offset hinges to widen doorways
- Installing accessible door hardware
- Removing high-pile, low-density carpeting[17]

Adjustments to the work space to accommodate special equipment or handicaps without causing the employer undue hardships are required by the ADA.

Safety Needs. A safe work environment is important to management and to workers. It reduces the number of work-related accidents, which are costly to the organization in terms of lost work time and Workers' Compensation claims.

Management is responsible for providing a safe work environment for employees. These responsibilities include the following:

- Maintaining a favorable climate for safety
- Ensuring that the equipment and furniture are in the best working condition
- Being a good example
- Teaching principles of safety (see Basic Safety Principles)
- Stressing an orderly work environment
- Stopping unsafe acts

The Occupational Safety and Health Act (OSHA) requires that employers furnish a workplace that is free from hazards that are likely to cause serious harm or death. OSHA has safety requirements for equipment, noise level standards, and lighting requirements for computer users.

Basic Safety Principles.
- Cords for telephones or electrical equipment should be out of sight, if possible. Furniture often contains cable channels to accommodate the multitude of cords required in today's workplace. Cords should never be draped across aisles or walkways. Whenever unplugging an electrical appliance, always pull on the plug, not the cord. Yanking on the cord breaks insulation or loosens terminals.
- File and desk drawers should not be left open for people to trip over or walk into. They should not be used as a step-stool because they will not hold a person's weight.
- Office tools such as scissors, staples, razor blades, and pencils should be used only for their intended purpose. Pencils are not to be used as hole punchers. Letter openers are not to be used for prying open stuck drawers.
- Paper cuts are an annoying type of injury that can be avoided by proper handling: using rubber finger guards, picking up individual sheets of paper at the corner instead of the side, and encouraging the use of hand lotion for dry skin, which is more susceptible to paper cuts.
- Drawer files can tip over if more than one drawer at a time is opened or if heavy objects are placed in top drawers or far in the front of a drawer.
- Stepladders should be fully open and locked before use. Move the ladder to the desired location instead of reaching from the ladder. Do not use boxes, chairs on rollers, or tables in place of ladders.

- Open-shelf files should be bolted to a wall or to the back of another file. Trying to remove records from files that are too tightly packed can cause the files to sway or topple if they are not bolted to some other support.

Social Needs. The atmosphere in the office affects employees' happiness and feelings of well-being. A positive environment can motivate employees to improve productivity and decrease use of sick days.

Employees, especially those engaged in similar activities, like to work in proximity to one another, where they can easily ask questions or otherwise confer on the work at hand. Workstations in clusters are effective in encouraging the team approach concept.

Personal Space. Personal space is the private area that surrounds an employee and is felt to belong to him or her. Personal space requirements vary among cultures, with those from Middle Eastern countries, for example, typically requiring less personal space than Americans do.

Territoriality is another concept that should be considered in office space planning. Territoriality refers to the physical area that is under the control of the employee or is specifically for his or her use. It may be the employee's workstation or a private office.

Employees take pride in their physical surroundings. The workstation becomes a reflection of employees' personalities. They like the freedom to decorate or personalize it to suit themselves.

Reflection of Status in the Organization (Is the Corner Office Dead?). The status of an employee within an organization, especially the managerial staff, used to be reflected by whether the employee had a private office, the size of that office, and whether the office had windows. The large corner office in a building or suite was seen as the most desirable space in terms of status within the organization.

Private offices are not as common or as widely used as they were in past years. The trend is toward a more open type of **office landscaping**. The private office still denotes prestige, however, and most managers prefer to have some degree of privacy in their work setting. The work may be of a personal or confidential nature that requires a location in which business matters cannot be overheard by other employees. The work may also require a high degree of concentration. Such a case would require locating the workstation in an area free from distractions and interruptions.

The disadvantages of private offices are interferences with heat and air conditioning systems, a decrease in supervisory effectiveness, and increased construction costs.

Managers can enjoy almost as much privacy with an open plan as with a private office by using high divider panels to surround the office furnishings. Panels with doors are available in a wide variety of fabrics and materials, including glass.

Evaluation of individual needs is necessary to decide whether a private office is needed. Combining the conventional office plan with private offices with the open plan maintains the status and privacy needs of the executive. Such a combination is referred to as the **American plan of office design**.

Design of the Workstation

Ergonomics

Ergonomics is the science concerned with the relationship of people to their working environment and more particularly to the study of how to design a work environment that promotes comfortable, safe, and injury-free work. The science of ergonomics includes the analysis of psychological and physiological influences.

Background. Repetitive strain (or stress) injuries (RSIs), also called cumulative trauma disorder (CTD), are the fastest growing workplace injuries in the United States today. The most common RSIs are **carpal tunnel syndrome** (CTS) and tendinitis. CTS often occurs in workers who spend long hours using computers or workers who perform repetitive tasks. According to the Bureau of Labor Statistics (BLS), the median of days missed from work was highest for carpal tunnel syndrome.

Employers are becoming increasingly interested in workplace design as the absenteeism rate related to CTD increases and Worker's Compensation claims soar.

OSHA is committed to achieving safer workplaces and is in the process of developing industry- and task-specific guidelines that assist employers and employees in recognizing and controlling potential ergonomic hazards. A guideline is a voluntary tool and is designed to be flexible so that employers can adopt innovative programs to suit their workplaces. OSHA is developing these guidelines for a select number of industries taking into account injury and illness incidence rates.

The National Institute for Occupational Safety and Health (NIOSH) sets standards in office design, construction, and use of equipment, especially in the use of computers. The results of an NIOSH study showed that computer users have various types of health complaints. Among them are optical problems (thought to be brought on by stress), painful or stiff muscles and joints, and loss of strength in arms, hands, wrists, and fingers. After the study, NIOSH stressed ergonomic solutions to these problems. In other words, they recommended that managers provide employees with furniture and equipment that can be adjusted to the physical traits of each worker to eliminate strain. NIOSH sets standards for lighting as well.

Successful Ergonomics Programs. Organizations that have implemented ergonomic programs report decreases in work-related injuries and subsequent health care costs and increases in productivity and worker morale. A successful ergonomics program requires a strong commitment from management. Education and training are important parts of any such program. Workers and supervisors should have an understanding of the potential risks of injuries, symptoms to be aware of, and prevention and treatment. Managers should attend training sessions with the employees. Sharing the responsibility for a comfortable and productive work area increases the success of the ergonomics program.

Identifying ergonomic risk factors (situations in which extra demands are placed on the employee) is essential for preventing ergonomics-related injuries and illnesses.

There are several ways to identify risk factors:

- Use employee interviews or questionnaires. Employees are asked to identify what they consider risk factors present in their jobs. Anonymous written questionnaires may elicit more honest responses than one-on-one interviews.
- Use an ergonomics checklist to survey the workplace. Many commercial checklists are available for purchase. The types of questions asked include:
  1. Does the work area allow a full range of motion?
  2. Is the height of the work surface adjustable to accommodate varying heights of employees?
  3. Is the employee able to vary posture?
  4. Are objects within easy reach?
  5. Is the chair adjustable to assist in maintaining good posture?
  6. Does the chair have an adjustable backrest?
  7. Is there sufficient leg and knee room?
  8. Is the lighting sufficient for comfort?
  9. Are employees trained in handling and lifting heavy objects?
  10. Are materials and forms moved over minimal distances?
- Examine the absenteeism rate.
- Review employee grievance logs.
- Look for signs of stress among workers.

Components of the Workstation

The **workstation** is a collection of desks or work surfaces, equipment, storage facilities, and chairs shaped by technology, the tasks to be performed, and various human needs.

Desk or Work Surface. The office desk serves as a work space, storage space, filing area, and place where office and communications equipment rests. Efficiently organized, the desk can enhance productivity. Made-to-order drawer arrangements facilitate storage and make supplies accessible.

The height of the work surface should be adjustable, if possible, to accommodate the height of the user and the task to be performed. Work surface height should be about 28 inches for tasks other than keyboarding. Keyboard or typing tasks require a lower work surface than other tasks. Keyboards should be at least 2 to 3 inches lower than the regular work surface so that the users' arms do not have to be raised to type. Keyboards may be attached under the desk in a pull-out arrangement, or a special lower work surface may be built into the workstation to accommodate the keyboard.

There should be adequate knee clearance to accommodate a full range of movement, and feet should lie flat on the floor or on a footrest so that the knees are parallel at a 90- to 110-degree angle.

The size of the desk often depends on employees' organizational levels and the tasks assigned. The work surface should be at least 30 inches wide. When possible, the desktop should not be crowded with equipment. Managers who do many types of desk work may require a larger work area.

Guidelines for Work Surface of Desktop Arrangements. The positioning of key workstation components is extremely important in an organization concerned with efficiency and ergonomics. Employees should be able to reach all work surfaces and equipment with a minimum of movement. Frequent stretching to reach key workstation components causes fatigue and other musculoskeletal problems related to the arms, neck, and back. Short, frequent breaks and rest pauses assist in reducing these problems. Employees should incorporate exercises, stretches, and movement into these short breaks or rest pauses. Software programs are available to remind workers to take a break. Some flash instructions on the screen for simple neck, shoulder, wrist, and arm exercises. For example, medical transcriptionists commonly sit at word processing stations for many hours without changing position or routine. Breaks do not always have to be rest breaks. Interspersing different functions into the transcriptionist's day can also alleviate the strain and muscle fatigue that come from sitting for long hours in the same position. Transcriptionists should break their routine occasionally by doing other tasks to relieve the boredom and fatigue. Changing the routine may not work well if an incentive or other type of productivity program is in place.

The positioning of the components on the work surface depends on the frequency, sequence, and duration of the task. The more frequent and longer-duration tasks are done in the primary zone; the materials that are used to support the more frequent tasks are stored in the secondary zone.

Writing, keying, and reading use the primary zone or front area of the work space. This is the area of the work surface that is within bent arm's reach. Computers may be located in the primary space in the workstation for full-time computer operators and in the secondary space for managers and others who operate computers only part of the time.

Supporting materials and equipment only occasionally used or waiting to be used are placed in the secondary area or the area of extended arm's reach.

Space that does not fall into the primary or secondary zone categories should be used for storage.

The Chair. The office chair is probably the single most important component of the workstation because of its ergonomic impact. Ergonomic chairs have positive effects on posture and circulation and minimize stress placed on the back. Chairs should be adjustable to support the body. Chairs should have the following adjustments:

- Seat pan tilts forward and backward
- Pneumatic height adjustment
- Independent back adjustment
- Individualized lumbar support in both height and firmness

Chairs should be adjusted so that the forearms are parallel to the floor with both feet flat on the floor or on a foot rest with thighs parallel to the floor. When the chair is too high, the feet lack the proper support and the chair places pressure on the blood vessels in the thighs, leading to pain and poor circulation. A seat that is too low increases back fatigue.

Backrests support and distribute the upper body weight. The back support should follow the natural curve of the back. A towel or lumbar pad can be used if the chair does not provide adequate support.

Computer and Peripherals. As with the chair, flexibility and adjustability are prime factors in monitor selection and placement. Monitors should swivel and tilt and, if possible, be adjustable in height. The top of the monitor screen should be just slightly below eye level when the employee is sitting. Employees who wear bifocals or trifocals may need to have the monitor at a lower position. The center of the screen should be about 20 degrees below eye level. Maintaining a distance of 18 to 28 inches between the eyes and the monitor allows easy focusing and reduces eyestrain and fatigue. The employee should refocus the eyes periodically by looking away from the monitor. Blinking, yawning, and moving the eyes up and down and right and left also help. Source documents should be positioned to be at the same height as the screen to reduce neck and eye movements, thus reducing neck discomfort and eyestrain. Hanging document holders may be provided with the monitors or purchased separately. Finally, filter screens reduce glare and relieve eyestrain.

Printers should be located so that the user does not have to get up from the chair to retrieve printed pages.

The design of the keyboard should allow the hand to be in a neutral position while keying. A neutral position is similar to a handshake position. Traditional keyboard design forces the palm downward and the wrist outward, called an ulnar deviation. New designs for keyboards attempt to alleviate these problems. Newer detachable keyboards can be positioned for ergonomically correct keyboarding. Wrist rests or supports help to keep the wrists in a straight position while allowing freedom of movement.

Ergonomic software that monitors how much the computer is used and prompts the employee to take a rest break at appropriate intervals and even suggests simple exercises is available.

Partitions. Partitions surrounding the workstation are usually less than ceiling height and designed to house shelves or closed-in storage space, bulletin boards, and other components that may be useful to the employee. Such panels or partitions provide privacy and diminish distractions from the surroundings.

Shelving, Filing, and Storage Space. The efficiently designed workstation contains filing and storage space located conveniently for the seated worker. Shelves may be located above the workstation within easy reach of the worker, and drawers for supplies can be attached to the work surface for easy accessibility.

Telephone. The telephone and any accessory equipment should be positioned so that they are convenient to the user but do not interfere with the primary work space. Telephone cords should be long enough to permit the employee to reach the phone from any position in the workstation. Cordless telephones and headsets are useful for various applications.

Shared or Multifunction Workstations. Workstation furniture or components must accommodate a number of functional tasks. Many workstations used by general or technical employees are shared, either on the same shift or between shifts. This means that it is even more important to purchase furniture with as many adjustable features as possible.

Space Standards and Guidelines for the Office. One of the first steps that should be done is to secure a drawing or blueprint of the available area. Blueprints are generally drawn to scale; for example, $\frac{1}{4}$ inch on the blueprint is equal to 1 actual foot of space. Many variables must be considered when allocating space in an office, but there are some guidelines to assist the supervisor in making decisions (Box 17-5).

Environmental Considerations

Ergonomics encompasses many aspects of the workplace, including lighting, sound, air temperature, air quality, and color. Workers who participated in the Steelcase Study II on office comfort stated that, if they could change physical conditions in their offices, they would most often make improvements in the heat and air conditioning, regulate temperature, reduce noise, obtain more space and privacy, and acquire more comfortable chairs.

Given a choice between getting a raise with no improvements in the office environment and getting a smaller increase with improvements, more than half the employees in the Steelcase Study selected the larger raise. A substantial number, however, stated that they would select a smaller raise if they could control heat and air conditioning (30%) and general office comfort (27%), had a chair with back support (26%), had a private office with a door (21%), and had a quieter place in which to work (20%). It is interesting to note that heat and air conditioning ranked highest as the item employees most wanted to control; it ranked eleventh as the item that executives believed that their company

Box 17-5 GUIDELINES FOR ALLOCATING OFFICE SPACE

- Generally, each clerical employee should be allocated at least 60 square feet for his or her work area (this includes the desk, aisle space, and storage space). The amount of space allocated depends on the job assignment, total space available, need for privacy, and number of pieces of equipment used. When space permits, 75 to 85 square feet per clerical worker is allocated.
- Space standards for aisles:
  - Main aisles: 4 to 5 feet wide
  - Secondary aisles: 3 to 4 feet wide
  - Aisle space between desks: not less than 36 inches
- Spacing of filing cabinets depends on the frequency of use and the type of cabinet.
- Equipment used should be placed near the user.
- A supervisor should be placed at the back of the group of workers whom he or she supervises.
- The file area should be placed in a location that is inaccessible to unauthorized personnel.
- Do not have employees working too near a heat source, in an air conditioning draft, or facing a window.
- Provide sufficient floor electrical outlets for office machines.
- Paper or forms should move to the employee rather than having the employee move to the paper.
- Movable files are the most space-efficient type of filing units.

would consider a motivator or reward for high employee performance. Employers greatly underestimated the need of employees to control their own environment.

Air Quality. Heating, ventilating, and air conditioning (HVAC) systems are an integral part of office design. Heating and air conditioning systems are easier to operate in the **open office design plan** of most modern offices than in the traditional or closed plan.

Good air quality improves productivity. Air pollution (stale, dusty air), on the other hand, produces undesirable effects, such as headache and fatigue. Air circulation is important in the work environment. Fifteen cubic meters of fresh (outside) air per hour per person is desirable in a non-smoking environment. Air conditioning not only cools the air but also removes undesirable pollutants such as smoke, asbestos, soot, dust, and chemicals. Clean air is important for equipment operation as well as for its effects on employees. Mechanical air filters are helpful, as are frequent cleaning, sweeping, and vacuuming.

OSHA has set indoor air quality standards and can take action against employers who fail to comply. The Environmental Protection Agency (EPA) lists indoor air pollution as one of its top five environmental issues, causing a wide range of problems such as bronchitis, asthma, emphysema, cancer, and heart disease. The EPA states that a common problem in

businesses is that the HVAC system operates only on weekdays and not when the building is unoccupied. It suggests starting the system several hours before workers arrive and continuing it for several hours after they leave for maximum effectiveness. The EPA also promotes restricted areas for smokers. The agency recommends regular inspections of the building and the HVAC system. Data on symptoms suffered by building occupants and likely contamination sources should be collected and analyzed periodically.

Temperature. Temperature means the hotness or coolness of the air. A comfortable office temperature is about 70° F or lower, with older employees requiring a slightly warmer environment. Thermostats are often set at 65° F during the heating season to conserve energy. Human bodies in large numbers generate heat, especially when they are performing physical tasks such as walking and typing. A computer also generates heat equal to that generated by one person.

Humidity. The percentage of moisture in the air is called **relative humidity.** The most comfortable standard for office workers is 30% to 60% with a temperature ranging between 65° F and 70° F. Automated equipment requires a relative humidity range between 20% and 80%. Too much humidity causes short circuiting in equipment, and too little humidity produces static electricity.

Lighting. Proper lighting is more important today than ever before with so many people using computers. Lighting affects not only productivity but also employee health.

In planning a good lighting system, the following factors should be considered:

- Flexibility and adjustability
- Ease of installation
- Low energy use
- Low initial cost
- Efficiency of the system
- Safety
- Effect on employees (comfort level)
- Integration of sunlight into lighting systems

Amount and Type of Light. The amount and type of light should be evenly diffused over the work area. Moving from areas of greater light intensity to areas of lesser intensity causes eyestrain, fatigue, and headache because of pupil expansion and contraction.

The amount and type of light used depend on the color scheme of the office decor, the type of work being performed, and the age of the worker. Less light is needed in areas that are decorated with light colors because light colors reflect light, whereas darker colors absorb light.

High levels of illuminance are needed for many tasks that involve paper documents, whereas lower levels are needed in computer-user environments, reception areas, storerooms, and stairways. In areas where work is both paper based and done on computers, appropriate lighting is difficult to achieve because of the different lighting needs.

Also, older workers require more light for performing the same tasks as younger workers. After age 50 years, light requirements may be 50% higher and after age 60 years 100% higher than for younger workers.

Light Source Design. Light sources are designed as direct lighting, indirect or reflective lighting, or combinations of the two. Direct lighting reflects directly on the work surface. Semidirect lighting reflects some light off the ceiling but most shines directly on the work surface. Indirect lighting reflects all light off the ceiling. Lights may be suspended from the ceiling, recessed in the ceiling and enclosed, placed in troughs near the top of the wall, suspended from partitions, or attached directly to modular furniture.

Task Lighting. The number one priority for lighting is to achieve the best task visibility possible. A second priority should be to create the most comfortable visual environment possible. **Task lighting,** also referred to as **accent lighting,** often involves building the light fixtures into the furniture or workstations to illuminate specific work areas. Task lighting is especially important in an open office design.

Sometimes variable-intensity task lighting is used in work areas. Variable-intensity lighting achieves adjustability by using a plastic cylinder with a network of dark lines enclosing a fluorescent lamp. By turning the cylinder, employees can adjust the illumination to suit themselves or the tasks.

Ambient Lighting. Indirect lighting fixtures provide **ambient lighting.** Light is directed upward so that it is reflected off the ceiling onto the work area. It provides light for a large area, but the light is insufficient to work by. Ambient lighting is often combined with task lighting to provide a lighting system that is flexible, lower in energy costs, and easier to install than direct overhead lighting. **Task-ambient lighting** can be used with reduced overhead lighting, or it can supply light by means of fixtures that emit light both upward and downward. It is an attractive and economical means of providing adequate light for an open office design.

Lighting and Computers. The lighting at computer workstations should be lower than for areas in which concentrated work on paper documents is performed. Glare on the monitor from lights and windows can be avoided by using antiglare filters with proper placement and by having the capability of adjusting the computer screen. Computers should be placed at right angles to outside windows. The user should not directly face the window when working at the computer. Window coverings such as louvered blinds can be used to adjust the amount and glare of sunlight.

Sound and Acoustics. Sound control is important for a healthy and productive work environment. Without a sound

control program, employees experience physiological and psychological problems such as increased blood pressure, accelerated heart rate, increased muscle tension, mental stress, and irritability.

Sound is measured in decibels. One decibel equals the smallest degree of difference or change in loudness that is detectable by the human ear. Maximum sound levels for various types of office environments are as follows:

- General offices—60 dB
- Private offices—40 dB
- Data centers (with computers, printers, copiers, telephones, and other equipment)—70 dB

The sound control system has two main goals: speech privacy and controlling noise generated inside and outside the work area.

Levels of Speech Privacy. Various levels of speech privacy can be attained through the use of construction materials, acoustic decorations, and sound-masking devices. Levels of speech privacy are as follows:

- *Absolute:* Nothing can be heard, not even mumbling. It is the most difficult and expensive level to achieve.
- *Confidential:* Cannot understand what is said but mumbling can be heard.
- *Normal:* Sound of incoming conversation is loud enough to distract people from their work; a fair amount of conversation could be heard if one concentrated on listening; recommended where the confidential level is not needed.
- *None:* Most common level; incoming speech is distracting and easy to understand.

Guidelines for Controlling Sound. Controlling sound can be done by confining the source of the noise within a separate room, muffling the sound source with acoustic materials, or submerging it in the background hum of a white noise system. Some additional guidelines for controlling sound should be considered in work space design (Box 17-6).

Box 17-6 GUIDELINES FOR CONTROLLING SOUND

- Use barriers to block sound.
- Locate desks so that employees do not face traffic.
- Use sound-absorbent materials.
- Position overhead lights so that sound reflection is minimized.
- Angle windows outward if possible.
- Use acoustic covers on printers and other equipment to reduce noise levels.
- Use felt or rubber cushions under equipment.
- Carpet the work area where equipment is being used.

Pleasant background noise such as music is often used in the workplace. Music has a calming effect, reduces fatigue, and lessens monotony. Music appropriate for the office environment and the type of work being performed should be selected.

An effective sound control system results in increased efficiency, decreased errors, a higher level of concentration, increased physical comfort, and elimination of distractions.

Color. Using color appropriately not only adds to the attractiveness of the office but also contributes to the efficiency and productivity of the workers. Certain colors cause employees to have positive feelings, whereas other colors have the opposite effect.

One popular approach to selecting colors is the monochromatic approach, which uses various shades of one color for floors, walls, and draperies with one bright accent color for furniture, pictures, or lamps. Color choices vary depending on the task of the employees and the function of the area.

Light colors are appropriate in offices where close paperwork is done. White is a neutral color and is non-threatening as long as it is not too bright a shade of white. Earth tones evoke a feeling of safety in the environment. Blue is a good color for a break area because it is relaxing and reduces blood pressure, pulse, and respiration. Violet is the most restful color but should not be used as a solid color for walls. It is a good accessory color that helps people to relax. The color red is rarely used in offices because it has such a strong stimulating effect that it can cause headaches and increased blood pressure.

An ergonomically designed health information department contributes to the overall efficiency of the organization. Considering all the factors mentioned here in the design of the department will accomplish this goal.

Key Concepts

- Work division can be accomplished by function, project, product, territory, customer, or process. The three methods of dividing work are serial, parallel, and unit assembly.
- The work distribution chart can be used to answer the following questions:
- What tasks are employees performing? Are these tasks important to achieving organizational goals?
- How are tasks distributed among employees of the work group?
- How are employees' qualifications being used?
- How are individual jobs constructed?
- Productivity standards are used to accomplish the following:
- Determine the number of personnel, pieces of equipment, and amount of supplies needed to handle the projected workload.

- Schedule completion and distribution of tasks.
- Evaluate proposed changes in processes or systems to see whether a savings in personnel time would occur.
- Set goals for a work group or individual employee.
- Determine actual cost of producing a given product or service.
- Managers should provide a positive motivational climate for employees.
- The fundamental objectives of work simplification are to simplify, to eliminate, to combine, or to improve the work processes. The simplest means of performing work is usually the easiest and most practical. The philosophy behind work simplification is that there is always a better way to perform every task.
- The steps in the work simplification process are as follows:
- Identify a problem area or select a work process or function to improve.
- Gather data about a problem.
- Organize and analyze the data gathered on the problem.
- Formulate alternative solutions or improvements.
- Select the improved method.
- Implement the improved method and evaluate the effectiveness of the improvement.
- Systems are hierarchically structured in that a system is composed of subsystems. Subsystems can be further broken down.
- Identifying the boundaries of the system—what is included and what is excluded—identifies the scope of the study.
- Systems design consists of five major components:
  1. Determination of the need for and objectives of the system
  2. Systems analysis
  3. Design of the system
  4. Evaluation of the proposed system
  5. Implementation of the proposed system
- In systems analysis, the sequence of steps is the accumulation of facts, the organization of facts, and the evaluation of facts.
- The formal organizational infrastructure is designed to plan work, assign responsibility, supervise work, and measure results.
- Facts about the informal organization are as follows:
  - Informal organizations are inevitable as long as there are people in the organization.
  - Small groups are the central component of the informal organization. Group membership in the informal organization strongly influences the overall behavior and performance of its members.
  - The informal organization always coexists with the formal structure.
  - Informal relationships deserve attention from employees and managers concerned with the organization's effectiveness.
- Strategic management: situational analysis, strategy formulation, strategic implementation, and strategic control.

- Project management focuses on completion of a project with the following attributes:
  - Unique; never having been done in precisely the same way before
  - Focused on producing a single definable product
  - Has defined deadlines
  - Involves a variety of complex and sequenced activities
  - Completed by a team of people with diverse qualifications and skills
  - Does not fit neatly into the formal organizational structure
  - Has a set amount of financial resources
  - Creates change
- The major objectives of re-engineering are to reduce costs, increase revenue, improve quality, and reduce risk.
- A goal is designing a work place that integrates the needs of the organization with the needs of the employees in a healthy and productive environment.

Acknowledgments

Special credit is given to Karen Youmans and Carol Barr for contributing information from the first edition.

REFERENCES

1. Amatayakul MK, Schraffenberger LA: Productivity: A handbook for health record *departments,* Chicago, 1988, American Medical Record Association.
2. John Sheridan Associates: Management for productivity. Presented at the Southeastern Medical Record Conference, Miami, May 13, 1981.
3. Kovach K: *Employee motivation: Addressing a crucial factor in your organization's performance,* Ann Arbor, MI, 1999, University of Michigan Press.
4. Waters K, Murphy GF: Systems analysis and computer applications. In *Health information management and systems analysis,* Rockville, MD, 1983, Aspen Systems.
5. Longest B Jr: *Management practices for the health professional,* ed 3, Reston, VA, 1984, Reston Publishing Co., p. 122.
6. Nickols F: Change management 101: A primer (Sept 12, 2004): http://home.att.net/~nickols/change.htm. Accessed. February 1, 2004.
7. Duncan WJ, Ginter PM, Swayne LE: Competitive advantage and internal organizational assessment, *Acad Manage Exec* 12:6-16, 1998.
8. Duncan WJ, Ginter PM, Kreidel WK: A sense of direction in public organizations: an analysis of mission statements in state health departments, *Admin Soc* 26:11-27, 1994.
9. Duncan WJ, Ginter PM, Reeves T et al: Consensus building about the future in a local public health organization: from strategic thinking to strategy formulation, *J Public Health Manage Pract* 4:13-25, 1998.
10. Senge PM: *The fifth discipline,* New York, 1990, Currency Doubleday.
11. Reiss G: *Project management demystified,* London, 1992, E&FN SPON.
12. Cleland D, Kin W: *Systems analysis and project management,* New York, 1983, McGraw-Hill.
13. Niemi W: Project management software keeps track of multiple tasks and improves communication, *Foodservice Equipment Supplies Specialist* 50:82, 1997.
14. Hammer M, Champy J: *Re-engineering the corporation: a manifest for business revolution,* New York, 1993, Harper Business.
15. Brandt M: Re-engineering—starting with a clean slate, *J Am Health Inform Manage Assoc* 65:61-63, 1994.
16. Fox L: Organizational change: re-engineering the work flow, *J Am Health Inform Manage Assoc* 65:35-36, 1994.
17. *American jurisprudence,* ed 2, New York, 1992, Lawyers Cooperative Publishing.

BIBLIOGRAPHY

Bessell I, Dicks B, Wysocki A et al: Understanding motivation: an effective tool for managers, Department of Food and Resource Economics, Florida Cooperative Extension Service, Institute of Food and Agricultural Sciences, University of Florida, Gainesville, FL (July 2002): http://edis.ifas.ufl.edu.

Brandt MD: Measuring and improving performance: A practical approach to implementing a productivity program, *J Am Health Inform Manage Assoc* 65:46-51, 1994.

Brodnik M, editor: Reengineering in health information management, *Top Health Inform Manage* 14, 1994.

FitzGerald J, FitzGerald A, Stallings W: *Fundamentals of systems analysis,* New York, 1981, John Wiley.

Kallaus N, Keeling BL: *Administrative office management,* ed 10, Cincinnati, 1991, South-Western Publishing.

Kish J Jr: *Office management problem solver,* Radnor, PA, 1983, Chilton.

Liebler J: *Managing health records: administrative principles,* Germantown, MD, 1980, Aspen Systems.

Littlefield CL, Rachel F, Caruth D: *Office and administrative management,* ed 3, Englewood Cliffs, NJ, 1970, Prentice-Hall.

Longest B Jr: *Management practices for the health professional,* ed 3, Reston, VA, 1984, Reston.

Nicholas JM: *Managing business and engineering projects,* Englewood Cliffs, NJ, 1990, Prentice-Hall.

Quible Z: *Administrative office management: an introduction,* ed 5, Englewood Cliffs, NJ, 1992, Prentice-Hall.

Stallard J, Terry G: *Office systems management,* ed 9, Homewood, IL, 1984, Richard D. Irwin.

Weiss J, Wysocki R: *5-Phase project management,* Reading, MA, 1992, Addison-Wesley.

Wulf P: Performance improvement: a case study. Presented by Patrick Wulf from Ernst & Young, FHIMA Mid-Year Symposium, Orlando, FL, February 4, 1994.

chapter 18

Revenue Cycle and Financial Management

Bryon D. Pickard

Additional content,
http://evolve.elsevier.com/Abdelhak/

Review exercises can be found
in the Study Guide

Chapter Contents

Historical Perspective
   Payment for Health Care Services
Managing the Revenue Cycle
   Front-end Activities
      Contracting
      Licensure and Provider Enrollment
      Charge Master—Fee Schedule
      Registration and Admitting—Access Management
      Utilization Management—Case Management
      Patient Encounter
      Coding—Charge Capture
   Back-end Activities
      Patient Accounting
      Claims Processing
      Collection Follow-up and Claim Denial Management
      Payment Processing
      Reimbursement Analysis
      Case Mix Analysis
Financial Aspects of Fraud and Abuse Compliance
Setting Priorities for Financial Decisions
   Management Accounting
   Mission
   Goals
   Objectives
The Budget and Business Plan
   Budgets

Key Words

Accounting rate of return	Discounting	Operating budget
Accounts receivable	Double-distribution method	Operating margin ratio
Accounts receivable turnover ratio	Entity	Opportunity costs
Accrual basis accounting	Equity	Participating provider
Action steps	Fee schedule	Payback method
Activity ratio	Financial accountant	Per case
Assets	Financial accounting	Per diem
Balance sheet	Financial analysis	Performance ratio
Budgets	Flexible budget	Productive time
Business plan	Fund balance	Profit
Capital expenditure	Goals	Prospective payment system
Capital expenditure committee	Liabilities	Ratio analysis
Capitalization ratios	Liquidity ratios	Revenue
Capitation	Long-term debt/total assets ratio	Rolling budget method
Cash basis accounting	Managerial accountant	Simultaneous-equations method
Certificate of need	Managerial finance officer	Stable monetary unit
Charge description master	Master budget	Statement of cash flow
Charge master	Master charge list	Statement of revenues and expenses
Chart of accounts	Matching concept	Statistics budget
Compounding effect	Medicare	Step-down method
Controlling	Mission	Third-party payer
Current ratio	Net	Time value of money
Days of revenue in patient accounts receivable ratio	Net operating revenue	Turnover ratio
Depreciation	Net present value	Variance report
Disclosure	Objectives	Whole service
	Objectivity	Zero-based budget

This is a revision of the chapter in the previous edition authored by Mary Alice Hanken.

    Statistics Budget
    Operating Budgets
    Master Budget
  Who Participates in Budget Development?
  Budget Periods and Types
    Flexible Budget
    Zero-Based Budget
  Budgeting for Staff
  Using the Budget as a Control
    Variance Reports
Preparing a Business Plan
  Identifying Trends
  Staffing Information
  Program and Automation Assessments
  The Four M's
  Developing the Business Plan and Budget
Cost Allocations
  Why Does Allocation Occur?
  Allocation Methods
    Step-Down Method
    Double-Distribution Method
    Simultaneous-Equations Method
  Why Is Cost Allocation Methodology Important for the
  HIM Professional?
Financial Accounting
  Fundamental Accounting Principles and Concepts
  Financial Management Duties
  Cash and Accrual Systems
  Fiscal Periods
Using Financial Reports to Provide Management
Information
Using Ratios to Evaluate Financial Data
  Liquidity Ratio
  Turnover Ratio or Activity Ratio
  Performance Ratio
  Capitalization Ratio
Capital Expense and Investment Decisions
  Capital Expenditures
  Capital Request Evaluation Process
  Time Value of Money
  Compounding
  Discounting
  Net Present Value
  Accounting Rate of Return
  Payback Method
  Arguments Pro and Con for Evaluation Methods
Other Phases of Financial Management
  Implementing
  Seeking Alternatives
  Role of the HIM Professional in Financial Management

Abbreviations

AHA—American Hospital Association
AICPA—American Institute of Certified Public Accountants
ANSI—American National Standards Institute

CDM—Charge description master
CFO—Chief financial officer
CLIA—Clinical Laboratory Improvement Amendment
CMS—Centers for Medicare and Medicaid Services
COB—Coordination of benefits
DRG—Diagnosis related group
EDI—Electronic data interchange
EFT—Electronic Funds Transfer
EOB—Explanation of Benefits
ERA—Electronic remittance advice
FASB—Financial Standards Accounting Board
GAAP—Generally Accepted Accounting Principles
GASB—Government Accounting Standards Board
HCPCS—Health Care Procedure Coding System
HCFA—Health Care Finance Administration
HIM—Health information manager
HIPAA—Health Insurance Portability and Accountability Act
HMO—Health maintenance organization
IRS—Internal Revenue Service
NCQA—National Committee for Quality Assurance
NPI—National Provider Identifier
PCAOB—Public Company Accounting Oversight Board
PHI—Personal health information
PPO—Preferred provider organization
PPS—Prospective payment system
RBRVS—Resource-based relative value scale
RVU—Relative value unit
UB-04—Uniform Billing Code of 2004

Objectives

- Define key words.
- Use fiscal terms with understanding
- Describe the various stages of the revenue cycle
- List different reimbursement methodologies.
- Explain the differences between financial and managerial accounting
- Calculate key financial ratios.
- Understand the difference between cash and revenue.
- Explain the role of the health information professional in the budgeting process.
- Recognize that organizational planning drives financial management activities.
- Prepare a business plan and a budget.
- Explain the purpose of each budget type.
- Use capital evaluation methods.
- Describe various cost allocation methods.
- Assist in charge master updates.
- Review and analyze variance reports.
- Define general principles of accounting
- Review and apply ratios to financial reports.
- Understand the potential financial implication of noncompliance with Medicare fraud and abuse regulations

Health information professionals have long been considered experts and industry leaders when it comes to understanding health care information regulations, statutes, data standards, and clinical vocabularies and terminologies. It is the assurance of reliable standards, data integrity, and ethical principles and guidelines that makes health care information of use for clinical decision making and ultimately most valuable toward improving the quality of patient care. In the same manner, financial management and accounting principles exist to ensure the quality, integrity, and reliability of financial data and information. Generally accepted accounting principles (GAAP) provide a common set of rules and procedures recognized as the accepted standard for financial management and reporting.

This chapter highlights the many different roles and responsibilities health information managers may find themselves engaged in pertaining to the management and stewardship of an organization's financial resources. Financial management principles apply not only to finance department staff and accountants, but also to an organization's entire management team. The precise scope and nature of the health information manager's (HIM's) role in regard to financial management responsibilities will vary from one organization to another; however, a common theme prevails. First, the information found in health care records is at the very core of patient care, clinical decision making, and ultimately delivering quality outcomes. And at the same time, the economic aspects of providing health care and being able to effectively communicate financial and monetary matters covering every facet of health care delivery are essential. Health information managers have always contributed to the organization's fiscal viability through productive and proficient data collection and information processing for patient care and reimbursement and research and by management of the resources under their control. In today's health care environment it becomes increasingly clear that clinical and financial health care information go hand in hand, and being able to effectively analyze, communicate, and use this strategic resource offers even greater opportunities for health information professionals to flourish.

HISTORICAL PERSPECTIVE

Financial management in health care has become increasingly complex over the past 20 years. Concurrently, the roles held by the HIM professional and health information services have become pivotal positions in the fiscal success of any health care organization. The dependence on the health record's content to define accurately and completely the services provided and conditions treated for reimbursement purposes contributed to this escalation in

status. Skilled HIM professionals have the expertise to analyze the health record for pertinent data and information to maximize reimbursement without compromising the integrity of data quality.

During this dynamically changing period, the financial aspects of health care organizations have become much more important. Health care managers not only must know how to adjust their operations to respond to the dynamics of the economy and regulatory changes, but also must understand the concepts and principles of financial management.

Payment for Health Care Services

In the 1930s, the customary method of paying for health care was direct, out-of-pocket remuneration. Some payments were monetary, others were in goods. When hospitals started being used more often than physician offices or house calls, both hospitals and industry explored ways to insure for the cost of health care. This exploration resulted in the establishment of insuring agents that served as the forerunner for what became Blue Cross and led into multiple private insurance companies, both nonprofit and for profit. These companies provided a new service to the public: coverage for health care expense.

As more people paid health care insurance premiums, they began exercising their "right" to make use of services paid for by their premiums. The increasing use of health care services contributed to rising premiums and greater than anticipated demands on health care providers and organizations. The demand was but one factor leading to building more hospitals and more people seeking training in health care as physicians. Insurance provided an avenue that not only insured the individual but also assured the hospital that it could receive payment for the care provided. Such assurances were atypical before the 1930s. Those insured had no incentive to limit or judiciously seek health care services. Access to full or nearly full payments for services did not encourage hospitals to limit the realm of services provided or control duplication of services within the same community.

By the mid-1960s, social reform required the establishment of a government-subsidized health care program. This program became known as **Medicare.** The Medicare program further encouraged hospitals to provide services without regard to cost because most costs were reimbursed under the Medicare reimbursement program. Over the past 40 years, the government's perspective has become one that embodies the philosophy that all citizens have a right to health care. This trend began with the passage of Titles 18 and 19 to the Social Security Act in 1965.

As health care expenditures continued to increase (Figure 18-1), the federal government found it necessary to impose controls on its insurance costs. It was not until the

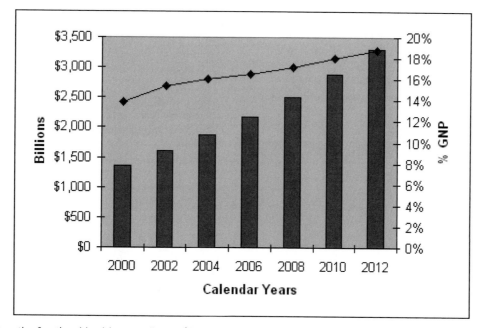

Figure 18-1 Growth of national health expenditures. (From the National Health Expenditures and Selected Economic Indicators, Levels and Annual Percent Change: Selected Calendar Years 1999–2015. http://www.cms.hhs.gov/NationalHealthExpendData/downloads/proj2005pdf.)[1]

1980s that the reimbursement formula was modified to restrict reimbursement and control the government's expenditures for health care. In 1982, the Health Care Finance Administration (HCFA) (since restructured to become the Centers for Medicare and Medicaid Services [CMS]) implemented the Tax Equity and Fiscal Responsibility Act. The law mandated a **prospective payment system** (PPS) for most hospital inpatient services. The PPS became effective in 1983. This program attempted to balance the payments made for the same services rendered by different providers and pay the providers on the basis of the diagnosis at a fixed rate. Diagnosis related groups (DRGs) were established in the United States and case mix groups in Canada.

Reimbursement modifications occurred in the private insurance industry as well. Some contracts established between insurance companies and hospitals paid the hospital a specific rate for care provided to its subscribers (covered insureds). Different reimbursement methods now exist, including prenegotiated amounts, reimbursement based on a discount off billed charges, **per diem** payments, reimbursement based on audited costs, DRGs, ambulatory care groups, resource utilization groups, and payment for services at billed or full charges. Reimbursement at billed or full charges seldom occurs anymore. Some insurance organizations provide payments directly to the insureds or subscribers, who then must pay the health care provider.

The sequence of events that have occurred over the past 40 years has created the third-party payer concept. A **third-party payer** (the insurance company) pays for services provided by health care organizations or practitioners to the "insured." In addition, the "payer" often receives premium payments from the insured's employer. Health insurance has become entwined with employee benefits rather than insurance purchased by the individual as is the case for automobile or homeowner insurance. The employers have gained considerable purchasing power in regard to health insurance and, at the same time, have a significant interest in the cost of health care services. The federal government and state governments also cover or insure nonemployees in significant programs such as Medicare and Medicaid.

Reimbursement modifications have extended beyond hospital providers to home health agencies (converted from **whole service** cost based to discipline cost based), skilled nursing facilities (resource utilization groups), outpatient departments (ambulatory patient classifications), ambulatory surgery centers, and rehabilitation facilities (case-mix function-related groups).

The philosophical change in reimbursement to control costs affected physicians and other independent practitioners as well. The resource-based relative value scale (RBRVS) was implemented in 1992. The intent of the RBRVS was to ensure equity in payment for like services. The scale assigns a certain number of units (or partial units) to each procedure of service. In effect, payments were based on current procedural terminology (CPT)–4 codes, regardless of the practitioner's specialty.

Example of Work–Based Relative Value Unit (RVU)

Description of Service	CPT Code	Associated Work RVU
1. Evaluation and management, new patient, comprehensive office/outpatient visit—approximately 30 minutes	99203	1.34
2. Arthroscopically aided anterior cruciate ligament repair/augmentation or reconstruction	29888	13.88

Source for work RVU: CMS National Physician Fee Schedule Relative Value File.

Other attempts at controlling costs included reducing the options available to a person to obtain health care services. In the 1980s, the growth of managed care programs (e.g., health maintenance organizations [HMOs], preferred provider organizations [PPOs], and prepaid group practice plans) was significant. Growth continued through the 1990s. Some communities had as much as 60% of their insured population enrolled in a managed care program. The programs require the insured person to comply with specified rules of access, obtain approval for routine care, seek services from a preselected directory of providers, and fulfill other utilization requirements. Substantial financial disincentives are imposed on those who choose to receive services outside the predefined network of providers or without obtaining the necessary approvals.

In truth, health care costs increased uncontrollably when health care was paid for "in full." Controls using a variety of methods, fee structures, prospective rates, access mandates, and so on have slowed the rate of increase in expenditures to some degree. Provider dropout through hospital closure and state-mandated authorization processes such as **certificate of need** programs to set up new services or purchase expensive equipment has reduced some duplication of services. However, even with the advancements and efforts that have been made in an attempt to control and maintain health care expenditures, most experts agree that the U.S. health care system is still considered to be one of the most costly and inefficient (Box 18-1). It is projected that health care expenditures will continue to outpace the rest of the economy and by the year 2010 will exceed 18% of gross national product (see Figure 18-1).

In 2005 there were more than 46 million people with no health insurance coverage, representing 15.9% of the U.S. population.[3] One of the principle drivers for the increased numbers of uninsured is the high cost to employers offering

---

Box 18–1 FACTORS DRIVING HEALTH CARE COSTS[2]

General inflation
Consumer demand
Drugs, medical devices, other medical advances
Rising health care expenses
Government mandates and regulation
Litigation
Fraud and abuse

Source: PricewaterhouseCoopers analysis.

---

health care benefits to employees. In 2005 much of health care insurance continued to be employment based, and businesses found it necessary to share the burden through increased employee premiums, deductibles, and co-payments. Simply put, employers have limited financial resources and seemingly endless competing needs for these same resources. In many cases employers have even discontinued offering health benefits completely. This is particularly seen in small businesses or companies that are able to use greater numbers of part-time workers—employees who may not qualify for health care benefits.

The debate over a solution on how best to provide access to high-quality, affordable health care is sure to be a major campaign theme for future political agendas. One thing becoming increasing clear is that information technology and the ability to deliver health information where and when needed seem to be right at the heart of the answer to controlling health care costs. If past attempts to control costs are any predictor for the future, health care providers should prepare for decreased reimbursements for services rendered. It is essential for health care managers to provide services *efficiently and effectively*, at a cost lower than or equal to the payment that will be received. The health information manager's role now includes much more than effective and efficient management practices.

MANAGING THE REVENUE CYCLE

Because of the high cost of health care and corresponding financial pressures faced by most health care provider organizations and individual practitioners alike, significant emphasis is placed on both generating revenue and maximizing potential sources revenues. In accounting terms, an organization's revenues can be classified as either operating revenue or nonoperating revenue. When we speak of accounting terms, we are referring to generally accepted accounting principles (GAAP) mentioned earlier. For the purposes of our discussion of managing the revenue cycle, we focus on operating revenues, which include those revenue sources generated from the actual delivery of clinical patient care activities and services; that is, charges for the services that are provided. Nonoperating revenues can also be important in contributing to the bottom line of health care providers and may include such items as gifts and donations, income from endowment funds, research grants, interest from investments, and other miscellaneous income.

Health information professionals have learned as part of their biomedical education that human beings are complex organisms comprised of multiple interrelated systems and that without the nourishment of constant blood flow the human body would stop working. Much in the same manner as red blood cells and white blood cells make up the lifeblood contributing to the growth and overall health of the human body, organizations cannot survive without sufficient streams of revenue. Applying a similar analogy to financial management and specifically to the revenue cycle, without a constant flow of revenues and subsequent cash flow, health care organizations would cease to exist. For most health care organizations or providers, revenues result from performing the services and equate to the charges for services provided. Cash results from the collection of payments for services provided. You can think of revenue as what is earned and cash as what has been collected. A health care organization's revenue stream and subsequent cash flow enable its ability to acquire and retain sufficient operational and capital resources for providing ongoing patient care services.

It is well documented that the revenue cycle and the management of an organization's revenue streams can be a rather complicated process, particularly when striving to keep up with constantly changing regulatory requirements, technology enhancements, and specific detailed reimbursement contracts. The scope and breadth of interrelated functions making up the revenue cycle comprise many essential HIM competencies, making HIM professionals well positioned to step in at almost any point in the revenue cycle. In many cases HIM professionals may oversee the entire revenue cycle process for an organization.

Front-end Activities

Most health care is not cash and carry that is paid for at the time of service, but rather a complex network or group of operations and systems interwoven with multiple participants and administrative processes. When revenues are generated, the outstanding accounts receivables (dollar amount owed) that result are often an organization's largest asset following its physical plant and facilities. The actual makeup of the revenue cycle can vary greatly from organization to organization and often is best described by breaking down into component front-end and back-end activities. The revenue cycle consists of all previsit and postcare activities and systems associated with a patient entering the health care system, the patient receiving services, and eventually the provider being paid for the service (Figure 18-2).

Contracting

Because the major source of revenue for most health care organizations comes not from patients, but rather from third-party insurance companies, it is important for providers to understand and negotiate the best reimbursement contract terms up front. Of course, the effectiveness in negotiating payer contracts is often dictated by the power of the major health care players in the local market. Individual physicians in private practice may find it more difficult bargaining with a payer dominating the market. On the other hand, if the payer needs a certain hospital, medical specialty, or provider group in their network, the tables may be turned as far as negotiating. In addition to actual negotiated payment rates, it is important that specified reimbursement rules and such items as technical coding and billing requirements be identified beforehand and agreed to by both parties. Payer contracts are legally binding documents describing the obligations for both providers and payers in providing health care services to patients (e.g., insurance plan members or beneficiaries in the case of government payers). Contract language will typically include essentials for submission and payment of claims, including reimbursement specifics for modifiers, HCFA Common Procedure Coding System (HCPCS), medical necessity determination, services to be carved out (e.g., Behavioral Health, Vision, or Dental), and any contract exclusions. Language provisions will also be included describing provider requirements for granting payer access to confidential patient records and other personal health information (PHI). There are numerous opportunities for health information professionals to lend their expertise as part of the contracting process. Common contracted methods of reimbursement might include the following:

- Percent of billed charges
- Percent of Medicare
- Per diem arrangement
- DRG or case rate
- Per unit
- Predefined fee schedule
- Capitation

Once a provider has come to terms with a payer and is under an approved contractual agreement, the provider is considered a **participating provider** and agrees to provide services to covered plan members, or Medicare beneficiaries, and must abide by established payment rates. A nonparticipating (noncontracted) provider is considered out-of-network by the payer, which most frequently results in a reduced payment or nonpayment. Most payers offer out-of-network benefits, enabling the patient to receive care from a nonparticipating provider at a higher rate of coinsurance, which must be collected directly from the patient. In the case of Medicare, if an individual provider is considered nonparticipating, government regulations specify a limit on how much the patient can be charged.

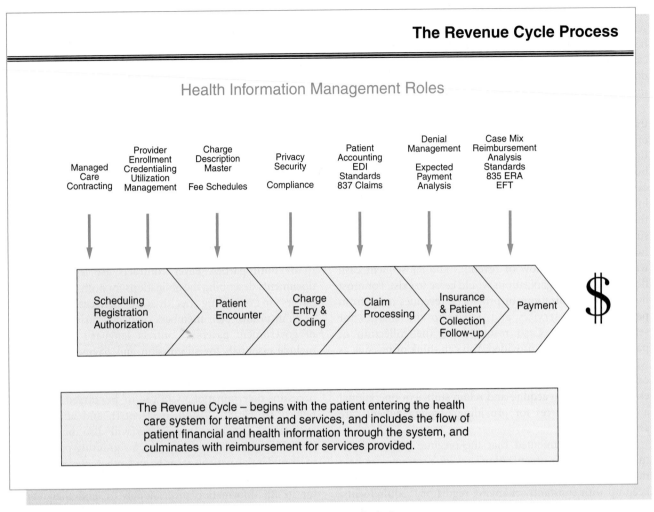

Figure 18-2 The Revenue Cycle Process.

Licensure and Provider Enrollment

Apart from actual payer contracts, government and non-governmental commercial payers alike, require providers rendering health services to patients to be fully licensed and fulfill rigid credentialing requirements. The credentialing process enables both payers and providers to document a certain standard of quality of care. Provider enrollment documentation must be completed prior to a payer granting billing privileges to individual providers. The National Committee for Quality Assurance (NCQA) establishes accreditation standards that payers and providers use to oversee the credentialing process. The credentialing process essentially provides a screening mechanism for verifying provider education, credentials, licenses, board certifications, clinical experience and practice history, and malpractice coverage and professional claims history. In the case of clinical laboratories, the Clinical Laboratory Improvement Amendment (CLIA) of 1988 mandates completion of a certification process before obtaining billing

privileges. Payers also require that a specific tax identification number be included as part of their enrollment information. The Internal Revenue Service (IRS) requires health care business organizations and individual provider or group entities conducting business to file an application for obtaining a federal tax identification number. Depending on the terms of payer contracts, delays in completing and submitting provider enrollment licensing and credentialing information to a payer can delay or possibly prevent reimbursement all together. The Health Insurance Portability and Accountability Act (HIPAA) requires health care providers to obtain and use a National Provider Identifier (NPI) for health care transactions by 2007. HIM professionals already engaged in handling medical staff credentialing responsibilities will note that many of the same licensing and credentialing source documents already used in the medical staff office are needed for this integral front-end revenue cycle function.

Charge Master–Fee Schedule

Because health care services rendered generate revenues, it is imperative that services be priced (charged for) effectively and that the price be consistent with the cost to provide the service and at a level above contracted rates for each given service. This requires regular analysis of contracted reimbursement rates and expenses associated with services or product costing. HIM professionals have access to all data associated with various clinical treatment and procedures to resolve health conditions because they have access to the health record. The HIM professional can be key to collecting and classifying tests and procedures performed for the various conditions treated. Likewise, HIM professionals can assess the various expenses (costs) associated with a service. Charges must be assigned so that costs are covered for the various supplies and services used. Each health care organization has a **master charge list**, sometimes called the **charge master**, **charge description master (CDM)**, or **fee schedule**. This list reflects the charge for each item that may be used in the treatment of a patient and the charge for most services; that is, respiratory therapy treatments, physical therapy services, laboratory tests, and so on. The charge description master is most always automated and linked with the billing system. In some organizations, it is also linked with the clinical data system maintained by HIM services and can be used to perform fiscal-clinical analyses (Table 18-1). In many organizations information system logic may be established to automatically generate both technical and professional charges.

Associated with each service is a charge and either a CPT-4 code, or a HCPCS code from the CMS Common Procedural Coding System. CPT-4 codes are an industry standard, updated annually by the American Medical Association. HCPCS codes are updated periodically by the CMS. Also, individual charge amounts can be impacted by the addition of clinical modifiers. Modifiers are specific numerical or alpha codes that when appended to a given charge can affect the level of reimbursement. The HIM professional's knowledge of classification systems can be beneficial in ensuring that the master list is up to date at all times. Organizations may also maintain an expanded list of activities and services that are performed but not billable. This expanded list may assist in measuring activity and service volumes or account for resources used.

Registration and Admitting–Access Management

The health care delivery system requires that numerous front-end activities take place before a patient ever receives treatment or health care services. For a patient to be effectively scheduled and registered for admission to a hospital or other health care facility or for the patient to be seen by an individual medical provider, numerous previsit verification processes are used to capture necessary information for billing purposes. In addition to appropriately handling all the clinical aspects of a patient registration leading up to the actual encounter, the registration function requires the collection of complete and accurate demographic, financial, and insurance information. The actual process of obtaining this information can be cumbersome and may include accessing a multitude of varying sources and systems to effectively gather. Not only must providers verify whether a patient is covered under a given health plan, but they must also determine what specific benefits are available. This task becomes even more complex when considering the increasing variations of copayments and deductibles and other complexities coinciding with the growth of consumer-driven health plans. Failure to accurately register a patient and obtain all necessary demographic,

Table 18-1 EXAMPLE FROM PINE BEHAVIORAL HEALTH CHARGE MASTER
Charge Master–Pine Behavioral Health
(Providers are all employees of Pine Behavioral Health)

UB Code	CPT Code	Description	Provider	Facility Charge	Provider Charge	Comments
915	90801	Diagnostic psychological assessment	MD/clinical psychologist	20.75	198.25	Split bill for Medicare
915	90853	Group Tx	CSW	15.75	45.00	Split bill for Medicare
915	90853	Group Tx	MD/clinical psychologist	15.75	55.00	Split bill for Medicare
915	90853	Group Tx	Other clinician	50.00		
510	90862	Medication management	MD	15.75	72.25	Split bill for Medicare

CSW, Clinical social worker; *MD*, medical doctor; *Tx*, therapy.

financial, and insurance information on the front-end can lead to costly claim errors, claim denials, and subsequent reimbursement delays later on in the revenue cycle.

Health care payer policies set administrative standards that necessitate that some treatments and services require a referral (formal request) from a physician before the patient can be seen by another specialist provider. Other policies mandate that hospital or physician services be precertified (preapproved) by the payer before the patient receives services. This is particularly true for hospital admissions and surgical procedures and enables the payer to monitor and control potential costs (expenditures) prior to services being performed.

Utilization Management— Case Management

Because health care is expensive, payers and providers alike expend significant resources and efforts toward determining the medical necessity and appropriateness of patient care. A patient's insurance and coverage requirements can change quickly, making it essential that services be constantly evaluated and authorized in advance. A payer may deny services or refuse to reimburse providers if a patient's care or course of treatment does not meet certain clinical protocols and established benchmarks. Services that are not authorized result in lost patient revenues. Using the documentation found in the patient's health record, utilization management staff can evaluate the appropriateness and necessity of medical services based on established guidelines and clinical criteria. Utilization staff members perform up front prospective reviews and concurrent and retrospective reviews to evaluate the medical necessity of procedures, admissions, treatment plans, length of stays, and discharge plans.

Patient Encounter

Whether it is an admission to the hospital, skilled nursing facility, a surgical procedure, clinical lab test, x-ray examination, physician office visit, home health visit, or any other mode of patient treatment, it is the actual service and corresponding documentation that provide the ability to generate revenue. Not only is documentation of the patient encounter necessary for continuity of care purposes, but it also serves as a source document for billing purposes. Source documents may be in the form of electronic health records and automated information systems or traditional paper health records and encounter forms. The adage that "if it is not documented it is not done" holds true. Billable services must be appropriately documented, and failure to do so can result in nonpayment.

Coding—Charge Capture

In many health care organizations there can be one distinct information system, or on the other hand there may be several different order entry and ancillary clinical systems interfacing with the core billing system. Many of these information systems may include system logic established to automatically generate both technical facility charges and professional charges. In some organizations, charges may be manually entered from encounter forms decentralized in provider offices or input centrally in data control. In yet other cases, complex manual coding or computer-assisted coding may be required prior to a charge being released to the billing information system and for a bill to be generated. In these cases, a reasonably complete clinical health record must be accessible to coding staff to meet the goal of timely and accurate coding and submission of data for billing. Physicians and other clinicians support this activity by timely, accurate, and complete documentation. Coding staff may also confer with physicians and other practitioners to obtain information needed to clarify a code assignment.

As we mentioned earlier, cash flow is the lifeblood of any organization. The HIM manager holds an important key to expediting the time lapse between the recording of revenue and the receipt of cash. This key is in the coding and classification function. The health information manager must implement procedures and practices to monitor work flow to ensure the timeliness of work flow through the coding and classification section of the department and identify causes for any delays (Box 18-2).

Because codes are required for proper billing and complete accurate codes are required for optimum reimbursement, the health information manager must ensure that the coding and classification staff members are up to date in their work and in the application of coding rules and principles. This holds true whether manually assigning codes from paper or electronic record documentation or functioning to validate and edit codes generated from computer-assisted coding tools.

Back-end Activities

Keeping in mind that the revenue cycle is composed of an interwoven system with multiple participants and systems, the actual distinction between front-end and back-end revenue cycle activities will vary depending on such reasons as organizational structures, staffing patterns, historical performance, or information systems within the organization.

Box 18-2 CAUSES FOR DELAYS IN CODING AND BILLING

- Untimely receipt of health records after care or service
- Incomplete health records
- Lost records or misplaced records
- Inadequate coding staff or scheduling
- Untimely transcription or key reports

Patient Accounting

The patient accounting department or business office typically has primary responsibility for the back-end billing, collection, and cash processing associated with patient accounts. Many patient accounting departments also have responsibility for the front-end registration or patient access function. With the advent of DRGs, a cooperative relationship has evolved between the HIM department and patient accounting. The need to keep each other informed of accounts receivable status requires that each area's manager and staff work closely and respect the other's constraints. Each area has expertise that should be shared with the other. The HIM department has a good working relationship with medical staff members. Patient accounting has extensive experience working with patients and insurance companies to collect balances due on the accounts. Sharing techniques with each other on how best to get results from people benefits both departments. Each department receives newsletters, regulatory notices, and other information that can be shared with the other to allow both departments to be more knowledgeable.

Each area works with medical terminology. The staff members in patient accounting are often trained from within. HIM professionals can teach medical terminology to the patient accounting staff and educate them in medicolegal aspects, such as patient confidentiality and proper release rules concerning personal health information (PHI).

Patient accounting is expected to effectively manage billing and collection of revenue earned by the organization, otherwise known as managing the accounts receivable. The HIM department can also support increased reimbursement by ensuring that the organization's CDM (master listing of services) is kept up to date with current CPT-4 codes.

Claims Processing

Generating clean and accurate claims has become complex with the number of payers and the variety of administrative and technical reimbursement rules associated with obtaining payment for health care services. Health care providers use in-house billing systems and external clearinghouse vendors to define specific claim billing formats and edit checks unique to particular clinical services and individual payers. Example claim edits might include the following:

- Correct patient or subscriber information
- Valid subscriber number formats
- Correct Coding Initiative (CCI) edits
- Local Medical Review Policy (LMRP) edits
- Confirmation of accident date when diagnosis code indicates an accident
- Confirmation that age- or sex-related procedure codes match
- Valid authorization number present.

Claims for health care services are most often billed to insurance companies with a standardized health insurance claim form and are submitted electronically or by the traditional paper format. For years, hospital technical charges have been submitted with a UB-92 (Uniform Billing Code of 1992) claim form, and physician professional charges have been submitted with the CMS 1500 claim form. In the current electronic data interchange (EDI) environment driven by HIPAA, the recommended standard transaction set to define claim formats and data content is the American National Standards Institute (ANSI) 837 health care claim. Providers will be required to use a new UB-04 health insurance claim form and new CMS 1500 health claim form version beginning in 2007. See examples of UB-04 and CMS 1500 in Figure 18-3.

Patients covered by multiple insurance plans may necessitate the submission of both primary and secondary health care claims. Primary insurance coverage provides reimbursement to providers regardless of other insurance coverage. Secondary coverage reimburses providers after considering benefits paid by the primary insurance plan. Specific coordination of benefit (COB) rules deter-mine which payer is responsible for paying full benefits and which becomes the secondary payer for a given claim.

Collection Follow-up and Claim Denial Management

Submission of clean health care claims and collecting the proper reimbursement of what is owed are common and essential goals amongst all health care providers. With that stated, defining what constitutes a clean claim and being paid accurately and timely can be allusive goals for providers and payers alike. A novice might come to expect that accurate and timely payment would follow the submission of clean claims. Although advances have indeed been made in standardizing electronic systems and workflows to verify eligibility, provide coding edit checks, adjudicate third-party claims, and remit payments, health care reimbursement is still fraught with potential pitfalls. There are a number of reasons why payers may delay or deny a claim, resulting in the provider having to file an appeal or resubmit the claim to receive payment. Common denial reasons might include lack of coverage, bundled services, coordination of benefits, missing referral or authorization, or additional information needed to process a claim. Patient accounting collection staff must frequently coordinate with the HIM department to obtain requested clinical documentation to support a claim. In addition to delayed reimbursement, the added cost of reworking denied claims makes it essential that denial trends be scrutinized for corrective action. Denial reasons can also evolve from internal systems, from payer systems, or within the systems of an external clearinghouse. HIM professionals can be exceptionally helpful in formulating appeal letters to address medical necessity and coding related denials.

The collection of self-pay balances after insurance pays or for those patients without insurance coverage can be a

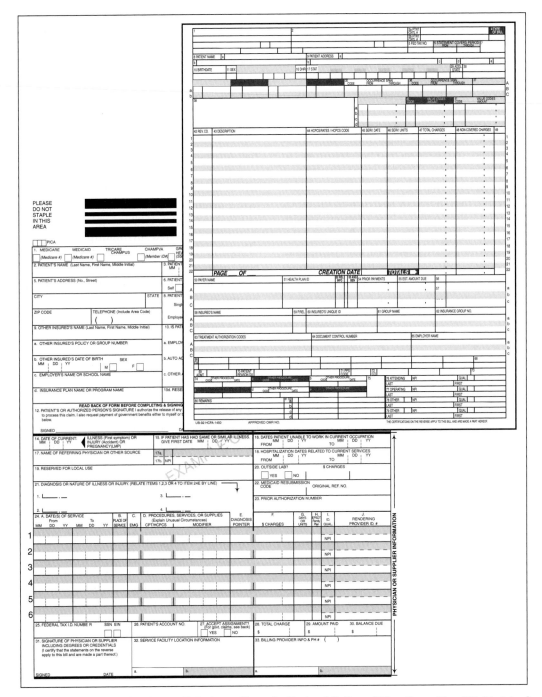

Figure 18-3 UB-04 Claim Form and CMS 1500 Claim Form. (From the National Uniform Billing Committee: UB-04 claim form: www.nubc.org and the National Uniform Claim Committee: CMS 1500 form: www.nucc.org.)

resource intensive and elaborate task. For accounts not paid in a timely basis, providers may have to file liens, handle probate matters, and assist with the collection of delinquent accounts. This may include giving depositions to stipulate that charges are reasonable and customary and that charges coincide with documented clinical services. In the case of delinquent patient accounts, sometimes the remaining accounts receivable balance will be referred (outsourced) for professional collection. When a patient balance is referred to collection and written off as a bad debt, it is no longer an active accounts receivable. An unpaid patient balance may also be written off as a charity allowance should the patient be eligible for a health care organization's financial assistance program.

Payment Processing

The patient accounting office is also responsible for handling daily deposits, bank reconciliations, and cashiering duties, as well as accurately recording insurance and patient payments. Because of the volume of transactions, providers may use a bank lockbox service to receive individual insurance and patient payments. Insurance payments are accompanied by a remittance advice (RA) or explanation of benefits (EOB), defining the amount adjudicated (paid) by the payer. The remittance advice may vary from payer to payer, although it will typically include the following:

- Charges billed amount
- Amount allowed by insurance
- Payment amount
- Patient liability (balance)
- Amount disallowed by insurance

The HIPAA ANSI-835 electronic remittance advice (ERA) standardizes claim payment formats enabling health care payment transactions to be electronically transmitted and posted to provider billing systems. Actual payments are deposited either by hardcopy check or wired through electronic funds transfer (EFT). The patient accounting office may also be responsible for issuing insurance and patient refunds for accounts with overpayment credit balances, providing cashier services, and maintaining patient valuables.

Reimbursement Analysis

Decision support systems provide comprehensive reporting tools to help health care managers track and report on all aspects of reimbursement and financial performance. These are the systems that unite both clinical and financial information, which is useful to measure, for example, revenue cycle performance, case mix, budgeting, cost accounting, clinical protocols and pathways, and outcomes. Many of these performance measurements can occur annually, monthly, weekly, or daily (Table 18-2) and may be trended over time to compare with historical performance and available benchmark information.

It is essential that accounts be reviewed to ensure that correct payment was made according to the terms of each individual payer contract. Configuring information systems to coincide with the language found in each individual reimbursement contract can be difficult for payers and providers alike, making it necessary to closely monitor payment trends. As mentioned earlier in the chapter, insurers pay for services in one of several ways, including the following:

- Percent of billed charges
- Percent of Medicare
- Per diem arrangements
- DRG or case rate
- Per unit
- Predefined fee schedule
- Capitation arrangement

Routinely analyzing paid claims to determine how much was paid by the insurer for a service, test, procedure, and so on and comparing the payments with the charge master are important also. If the insurer pays full charges, no variances are noted, but for other arrangements, the payments may be less than or more than the amount charged by the health care provider. Frequently, charges must be compared with health record documentation to ensure accuracy.

DRGs are an example of a **per case** or fixed payment system. Care provided for a given condition classified into a DRG may cost more than the approved payment for the given DRG. If payment rates are less than the amount charged, a revenue deduction or adjustment occurs. If adjustments are significant, expenses may not be fully covered. If expenses are not covered, management must consider alternatives to providing the care, such as modifying the supplies and services included in the treatment of a condition. Coding professionals who recognize the effectiveness of different tests in treating a condition can identify the more effective tests for utilization management professionals and physicians to consider in establishing treatment guidelines for other physicians to follow. It is important to consider possible outlier payments in addition to the contracted DRG payment. A day outlier can occur when a patient's length of stay extends beyond what is considered normal (standard) for a particular DRG.

Table 18-2 COMMON REVENUE CYCLE PERFORMANCE MEASURES

Measure	Description	Example
A/R days	Average time to receive payment	Accounts receivable/average daily revenue
A/R aging	Distribution of accounts receivable by aging days	1-30 days, 31-60 days, 61-90 days, >90 days
Collection rate	Effectiveness of collecting	Cash collections/revenue
Payer mix	Distribution of revenue by payers	Commercial, Medicare, Medicaid, private-pay
Denial rate	Number or dollars of denied claims	Denied charges/total revenue
Bad debt rate	Write-offs due to bad debt	Bad debt write-offs/total revenue
Charity rate	Write-offs due to charity	Charity write-offs/total revenue

A/R, Accounts receivable.

If payment rates are higher than the amount charged by the health care provider, the provider should assess its charges. Typically, health insurance companies set their rates on the basis of community averages. If the amount paid by the insurance company is higher than the provider's charges, then the provider's charges are lower than the community average. Insurers also pay based on a practice of paying the lower of the insurance company's fee schedule or the provider's charges. Whenever charges are paid, the same analysis of the provider's charges should occur. This type of periodic review of payments and charges helps the provider maximize reimbursement for the organization.

In some areas of the country where managed care is a dominant method of insurance, another payment arrangement known as **capitation** may apply. Capitation payments are used in health maintenance organizations (HMOs). Insured members enroll with an HMO. For each month an insured remains with the HMO, the HMO's providers are paid a fixed amount (capitated payment), usually at the beginning of the month. The providers (physicians, therapists, and sometimes facilities such as hospitals and ambulatory surgery centers) are required to provide any care needed by the insured during this period, regardless of whether the capitation amount is sufficient to cover the cost to do so.

Case Mix Analysis

When the DRG system for payment was introduced, hospitals began looking not only at the number of services provided (e.g., the number of days of care) but also at the "case mix" or types of care classified by estimated resource use.

A case mix value is assigned to each DRG. The values may vary by payer. Medicare values are published each year in the *Federal Register*. For example, if a DRG has a case mix value or weight of 1.4 and the hospital's payment for 1.0 value of service is $4000, then the hospital will receive $5600 as payment for the entire hospital stay. The system allows some flexibility for unusual cases that are "outliers," which consume more than the normal amount of resources.

Aggregating the case mix data for a group of patients allows the hospital to compute a case mix average or "index."

Example of Case Mix

DRG	Case Mix Value	Number of Cases in Period	Total Value of Service
DRG XX1	1.2	45	54.00
DRG XX2	0.95	15	14.25
DRG XX3	1.4	60	84.00
DRG XX4	2.1	10	14.25
Case mix index	1.3	130	173.25

Case mix index for the period = total value of service/total number of cases. Total value of service = case mix value × number of cases in the period.

Analyzing the case mix for all inpatients for a given period of time is useful for tracking trends. Is the overall case mix increasing (or decreasing)? Is the hospital treating sicker patients? Are patients consuming more resources? Does the case mix vary by payer? Does the case mix vary by type of service? When you compare case mix with other data (length of stay, age groups of patients, charges for services, actual reimbursement for services), what do you find?

FINANCIAL ASPECTS OF FRAUD AND ABUSE COMPLIANCE

Because of improprieties among the ranks of some publicly traded companies, the Sarbanes-Oxley Act of 2002 was created to provide greater and much needed financial accountability. Now an organization's management must attest annually to the effectiveness of internal controls and undergo an external audit, attesting to the effectiveness of internal controls. This legislation is of particular interest to nonprofit organizations as well because they evaluate their own internal controls and financial reporting. The Public Company Accounting Oversight Board (PCAOB) was created as a result of Sarbanes-Oxley to oversee the audit of public companies and guard the public interest.

The federal government, through the Centers for Medicare and Medicaid Services (CMS), is focusing on eliminating fraud and abuse in its health care program. With annual health care costs topping $1.7 trillion in 2003, national health care fraud estimates place annual losses at 3% ($51 billion) and as high as 10% ($170 billion).[5] Major efforts have been put in place to recover these losses from health care providers. As identified in a few publicly traded companies, some of the losses experienced in health care have been due to dishonest providers and outright calculated efforts to defraud. Other health care providers have inadvertently not met one or more complex Medicare requirements. The federal government has won judgments against health care providers and settled cases with others without any admission of guilt. For some health care providers it was a better decision to settle a potential case for an agreed upon dollar amount, that is, pay a fine, than to engage in detailed and prolonged scrutiny. Some of these cases involve tens and hundreds of millions of dollars.

The Office of the Inspector General publishes an annual work plan that details its focus for Medicare fraud and abuse. The work plan gives health care providers an indication of general and specific areas that are targets for review (Box 18-3).

Box 18-3 DEFINITIONS AND EXAMPLES OF FRAUD AND ABUSE

Medicare fraud is defined as "making false statement or representations of material facts to obtain a benefit or payment for which no entitlement would otherwise exist." Fraud is committed knowingly.[6]

Medicare abuse is defined as using "practices that are inconsistent with accepted medical practice and directly or indirectly result in unnecessary costs to the Medicare program."[4] It is not required that the acts were committed knowingly.

Examples of fraud:

1. Claim submitted for services not rendered.
2. Bill submitted for more costly procedures than those actually rendered.

Examples of abuse:

1. Providing services that are not medically necessary.
2. Billing Medicare on a higher fee schedule than used for non-Medicare patients.

Providers have set up compliance programs within their organizations to implement necessary programs that meet the complex Medicare requirements. The American Health Information Management Association (AHIMA) has information and resources designed to help organizations set up and administer compliance programs. Health information managers often manage or actively participate in their organization's compliance program.

Medicare laws and regulations are promulgated by the federal government. The federal government contracts with organizations that help process and adjudicate bills for services (fiscal intermediaries). These intermediaries also have administrative rules and guidelines. Health care providers must become familiar with and use the laws, rules, regulations, and guidelines from both federal and local levels in designing their workflow processes and information systems.

Health care providers that participate in the Medicare program are expected to have systems for coding diagnoses and procedures and for submitting claims that meet Medicare requirements. The documentation in the clinical record must accurately describe the service provided and justify the need for the service. The diagnoses, and any services or procedures, must be coded correctly with national guidelines. The bill for services must be submitted with sufficient information in the correct format. As stated, interpretation of these complex and changing rules can be a complicated process, and reconciling the appropriate action to take may not always be clear for every practice-related decision faced.

One of the ways for HIM professionals, or any profession for that matter, to stay focused in carrying out day-to-day responsibilities without sacrificing ethical principles, is to rely on their core values. Professionals have an ethical obligation to do what is right and, by their nature, recognize a standard code of ethics. HIM professionals have an obligation to follow a specific code of ethics as put forth by AHIMA. One key ethical principle, included in the code of ethics clearly articulates the HIM professional's responsibility to "refuse to participate in or conceal unethical practices or procedures".[7] These ethical principles hold true regardless of whether handling clinical or financial health information. The American Institute of Certified Public Accountants (AICPA) adheres to a similar code of professional conduct for certified public accountants.

Unfortunately, not everyone involved in health care adheres to a professional code of ethics, and the potential for fraud is a growing concern. The Office of the National Coordinator for Health Information Technology (ONCHIT) recognizes that the transition to electronic health records and a national health information network will go a long way toward minimizing health care fraud. And at the same time, there is an awareness of new challenges this may bring as well. Health information technology is being looked on to accelerate efforts to hardwire necessary internal controls and for combating health care fraud.

SETTING PRIORITIES FOR FINANCIAL DECISIONS

Up until this point in our discussion we have concentrated on effectively and appropriately managing an organization's revenue cycle. We have examined how the revenue cycle bridges the gap between clinical practice and the attainment of necessary economic resources. Managing the revenue cycle is just one component of overseeing an organization's financial resources, and ir does not happen in a vacuum. Health care leaders are also responsible for planning future activities and must learn to use and interpret many different types of financial accounting information.

Management Accounting

Managerial accounting provides economic information and an internal framework to enable health care leaders to make effective decisions concerning the activities and overall performance within an organization. Information in the form of internal accounting reports, budgets, business plans, cost analysis and other reports measuring an organization's performance make up management accounting. In establishing priorities, planning and controlling are essential management functions. Health care organizations and individuals engage in planning to provide a framework for their actions. The strategic and operational plans set the targets for performance. Budgets are plans for the financial resources associated with these performance plans. Most organizations have a mission, goals, and objectives that departmental managers use as an umbrella for developing and linking departmental objectives and budgets to organizational goals.

Mission

The **mission** is a statement of the organization's purpose in broad terms. It defines the geographic environment and population that the organization serves—for example, "The Mission of Citywide Surgi-Centers, Inc. is to provide convenient, state-of-the-art, surgical services for all residents of the City of Citywide and its surrounding neighborhoods."

Goals

To implement the mission, organizational leaders define **goals** to support the mission. A goal is a statement of what the organization wants to do. One of Citywide's goals may be "to increase the number of nontraditional surgeries performed at the center by supporting research into safe surgery techniques." The goals established by senior leaders or administration serve as a foundation, offering the direction management needs to determine the organization's intent.

Objectives

Once the intent is known, management can formulate **objectives.** Objectives are more specific statements that define the expectations or outcomes given the goal direction. One of Citywide's objectives may be "to begin performing eye surgery as a new service next year." Objectives provide clear guidelines for management and supervisors to define the **action steps** to achieve the objective. The action steps define the dates when certain activities are to be completed, how much labor or funding will be required, how resources will be used, and the expected outcomes or results. During action step formulation, budgets are developed.

THE BUDGET AND BUSINESS PLAN

Budgets

Budgets are detailed numerical documents that translate the goals, objectives, and action steps into forecasts of volume and monetary resources needed. The managerial accounting process includes the activities of planning and preparing budgets consistent with the strategic plan. Just as we have an accounting component responsible for recording transactions as they occur (financial accounting), there are other people who work with administration and management to assign the anticipated fiscal resources of the organization. These people may work in the budget or controller's office. Their primary responsibilities include helping management to prepare budgets, conducting cost-finding studies to set rates, and determining productivity. The reports they produce include the budget, the budget variance reports, cost reports, and third-party reimbursement reports. The types of budgets that result from the planning process include the statistics budget, the operating budgets, and the master budget.

Statistics Budget

The first of several budgets developed from the planning process is the **statistics budget.** Future volumes are often predicted from historical data. The HIM department is the primary source of historical data, such as discharges by clinical service, payer type, DRG, and physician; operations by type and surgeon; length of stay by DRG, diagnosis, clinical service, and physician; number and type of ambulatory visits; number and type of home health visits; number and type of ambulatory surgery cases; number and type of emergency department visits; and many other volume indicators. Unless significant changes have occurred in the regulatory and external and internal environments, relying on historical data to predict the future is appropriate. But history should not be the only source of volume predictions.

Key medical and other clinical staff members should be interviewed for their prediction of future demands for services. The medical staff is a valuable source of information and may be aware of plans for service changes and expansions of competing organizations. The staff members also have access to literature that describes technological advances in patient care. Such advances could drastically reduce volumes experienced in the past. In the 1990s, it was not uncommon for patients who had coronary artery bypass surgery to be hospitalized for 6 or more days. Today, cardiac stents can be implanted to open a blocked artery as an outpatient procedure.

The statistical analysts in the HIM department can also predict declining volumes by comparing data from month to month and identifying trends in utilization of the facility by different physicians or by the community. Sometimes physician utilization declines as a physician ages and cuts back his or her practice or when a physician brings patients to a health care facility that is more convenient to his or her office.

When new services are contemplated, the staff involved in providing the service should be involved in predicting the utilization of the services or the volumes anticipated. Staff optimism should be tempered by management querying staff and the anticipated users of the service. Sometimes health care leaders use marketing research firms to predict volumes on the basis of the demographics of the community. If a hospital is anticipating opening a long-term care facility or skilled nursing facility, an analysis of the age demographics of the community should be done to ascertain the number of elderly people residing in the community today and the number expected to be residing in the community in the next 5 to 10 years. Furthermore, an assessment of the competition would be completed.

If a departmental activity is directly tied to the volume of activity of the organization, then statistical projections can form the base for a departmental budget. For example, if the organization projects a 15% increase in the volume of home health encounters because of a new service market, what HIM activities are related to this statistic? How will the HIM budget reflect these data in budget planning?

Operating Budgets

Once patient, physician, and procedure volumes are determined, managers can begin building their **operating budgets**. These budgets predict the labor, supply, and other expenses required to support the work volume predicted.

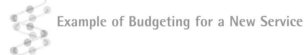 **Example of Budgeting for a New Service**

If Citywide implements an outpatient service with a volume of 3600 eye surgeries annually, what does Citywide's HIM department need to do to support this new service? The supervisor may predict the following:

- An average of 12 operations will occur per working day.
- The department will be responsible for gathering preservice information by telephone or other means.
- A coder will need to be trained to code eye surgery services.
- Four additional personal computers will need to be purchased to access the organization's electronic health record (EHR) and other information systems.
- A scanner will be necessary to scan hardcopy records into the EHR.
- If some of the eye surgeries involve implants, the HIM department may need to set up and maintain a registry component in the organization's patient information system.

The supervisor must now assign costs to each of these items and budget them in the correct categories as they apply: labor, file supplies, training and education, hardware, and software.

When budgeting for supplies and services it is helpful "to segregate expenses into at least two categories, (1) fixed expenses (those that are not related to the volume of business) and (2) variable expenses (those that fluctuate as a result of changes in volume)."[1] If managers must adjust their budgets because of a reduction or an increase in volume, it will be easier to identify the supplies and services that are volume dependent.

The departments that provide direct patient care prepare both the expense portion and the revenue portion of their operating budgets. To determine their revenue budget, the patient care departments assign estimated charges and estimated payment to the services they will be delivering on the basis of the statistics budget.

Master Budget

After all departments develop their operating budgets, the same categories of expenses (e.g., labor, supplies, training and education) and revenues (patient care, nonpatient care [e.g., cafeteria, gift shop]) are consolidated into one **master budget** with each of the operating account's combined balances.

When the organization has aggregated this information, organizational leaders determine whether the budget will go forward as constructed or whether it needs rework in certain areas.

Additional information on budgeting for capital expenditures is covered later in this chapter.

Who Participates in Budget Development?

Many people participate in the budgeting process. Organizations find it advantageous to include supervisory and frontline staff members in the development of budgets because they are closer to the consumption of resources. This is known as the participatory approach to budgeting. But management is ultimately responsible for the budget and its compliance with organizational objectives, goals, and mission. Because the budget is a prediction of expenses, revenues, services, and volumes to come some time in the future, it cannot be exact but should be used as a guide to measuring and improving management's predictive capability.

Budget Periods and Types

The budget period may differ from organization to organization. Budgets may be prepared for 1 year or several years. Typically, budgets are prepared for 12 months, running parallel to an organization's fiscal year. Some organizations use a **rolling budget method.** This method requires management to prepare a budget for a period of time and add to the end of that period another month when a month is consumed. For example, a budget may be prepared for 6 months (January through June), and when the first of the 6 months (January) ends, the manager would prepare the budget for the new sixth month (July).

Flexible Budget

Another type of budget is the **flexible budget.** This budget is predicated on volume. All supplies, labor, and other variable expenses are budgeted in proportion to the anticipated volume. If the volume anticipated is not reached, labor and other expenses are expected to decrease accordingly, and vice versa if the volume exceeds expectations.

Zero-Based Budget

Because many facilities are experiencing reduced reimbursement for their services, modified approaches to budgeting are being considered. One such approach is the **zero-based budget.** In the zero-based budgeting approach, management must complete a program assessment and define consequences if specific programs are terminated or reduced. Cleverley et al[9] defined the seven steps of zero-based budgeting:

1. Define the outputs or services provided by the program or department (statistical reports, coding, quality assurance study preparations, responses to requests for information, transcription, filing, and so on).
2. Determine the costs of these services or outputs.
3. Identify options for reducing the costs through changes in outputs or services (modify current procedure, eliminate an activity).
4. Identify options for producing the services and outputs more efficiently (use of a contracted service, voice recognition, optical imaging, and so on).
5. Determine the cost savings associated with options identified in steps 3 and 4.
6. Assess the risks, both qualitative and quantitative, associated with the identified options of steps 3 and 4.
7. Select and implement the options with an acceptable cost-risk relation.

Budgeting for Staff

Because staffing expenses usually consume a major portion of any health care organization's budget, careful attention is given to preparing the supporting detail for this component of the budget. A detailed staffing plan is useful for comparison during the year with staffing utilization and other reports. Calculating staffing needs "involves the merging of productivity data with volume data."[8] Many HIM departments have a number of functions that have associated productivity data that can be gathered and used in budgeting.

Example of Merging Productivity Data and Volume Data

A department has an annual volume of 9500 requests for information per year. A staff person can usually complete about 15 request responses per day. Each staff person uses an average of 11 holidays, 8 sick days, and 12 days of vacation per year. How many full-time equivalents (FTEs) should be included in the budget?

15 requests per day × 5 days × 52 weeks = 3900
9500 requests/3900 = 2.4 FTEs (without productivity adjustment)

Nonproductive time =

11	holidays
8	sick days
12	vacation days
31	days off
× 8	hours a day
248	hours/year

Productive time 2080 hours per year − 248 nonproductive time = 1832 hours
Productivity rate 1832/2080 = 0.88 or 88%
FTEs needed 2.4 FTEs/88% = 2.7 FTEs
Also see Table 18-3.

Using the Budget as a Control

The activity of **controlling** is one of several management duties. In this chapter, it refers to the activities that management typically pursues when what was planned does not occur financially. The chapter on human resources management (see Chapter 16) identifies the budget as a feedback tool. Once established, the budget is a "non–self-correcting feedback control" that managers can use to make decisions.

Variance Reports

One tool that most organizations have is a **variance report.** This document reflects the budget that was prepared and approved and shows the actual results on at least a monthly basis. "Given the manager's responsibility to control the use of resources, variance analysis is one of the most important tools a manager can use."[8]

Variances may occur for a variety of reasons. Reviewing the reports and identifying areas where the variance is significant in either a positive or negative fashion is appropriate. Significance can be determined by a dollar amount and/or a percentage. Commonly, variances are due to volume and rate differences from what was planned. It is helpful to be able to determine how much of the variance is due to volume and how much is due to rate or cost. Some variances are due to a combination of factors. Various approaches are used—some more basic, others more complex.

If the real cause of the variance is understood, then the management action taken, if any, is more likely to be informed and appropriate (Tables 18-4, 18-5, and 18-6).

PREPARING A BUSINESS PLAN

As mentioned earlier, the organizational planning process links departmental objectives and budgets to the over-

Table 18-3 EXAMPLE OF SALARY BUDGET FOR DEPARTMENTAL STAFFING (PARTIAL WORKSHEET WITH ESTIMATED TOTALS)

Lealand Clinic

Salary Budget Worksheet for Health Information Department

Classification of Position	Staff Name	FTE	Hourly Pay Rate	Current Year Base Salary	Increase Planned Next Year	Date of Increase	Amount of Increase	Total Next Year
Manager	Hansen	1.0	42.00	87,360	7%	3/1	6,115	92,460
Supervisor	Holden	1.0	25.00	52,000	7%	5/1	3,640	54,426
Data Specialist	Hillier	0.8	25.00	52,000	7%	1/1	3,640	44,512
Tech I	Hardy	1.0	20.00	41,600	7%	7/1	2,912	43,056
Totals		32.5		954,000			66,800	1,006,000

Example of calculations: $87,360 \times 0.07 = 6115/12 = 510 \times 10$ months $= 5100 + 87,360 = 92,460$.

FTE, Full time.

Table 18-4 BASIC VARIANCE ANALYSIS–SUNSHINE HOSPITAL

Service	Actual	Budget	Variance
Inpatient revenue	190,000	180,000	10,000
Sunshine Hospital volume and rate data			
Inpatients	Actual	Budget	Variance
Patient days	950	900	50
Average rate per day	200	200	0

This reflects a positive variance because of an increase in volume.

arching goals. In some cases organizations may require their managers to prepare business plans in addition to compiling a budget. A **business plan** is a formal written document that evolves from the input of others, listing objectives that support the organizational goals. The plan includes the following:

- Specific actions steps
- Quantifying resource requirements and cash flow benefits
- Prediction of expected outcomes
- Programmatic outline that may span a fiscal year or a longer time frame

All budgets and business plans rely on data. Collected data must be in a format that conveys information to the manager. There are many sources for data useful in the development of budgets and business plans (Box 18-4).

Identifying Trends

For the business plan data gathering to be completed, the statistics gathered should be compared with those of prior periods to identify trends that imply a need to change operations or staffing. For example, in the health information department if the statistics showed that the number

Table 18-5 VARIANCE ANALYSIS WITH AN ADJUSTMENT FOR VOLUME–MELROSE OUTPATIENT

Initial Report

Outpatients	Actual	Budget	Variance
Visits	16,500	13,500	3,000
Salaries (variable item)	460,000	360,000	(100,000)
Supplies (variable item)	75,000	55,000	(20,000)

Outpatient is over budget; however there is an increase in service and there should be a corresponding increase in revenue unless this is a capitated or managed care contract environment. If the report is adjusted for volume, it presents a different picture.

3000 visits/13,500 visits = 22% higher volume than budget plan

Melrose Outpatient Clinic

Budget with a 22% increase in the variable cost items

Adjusted Report

	Budget	Actual	Adjustment	Adjusted Budget
Salaries	360,000	460,000	79,200	439,200
Supplies	55,000	75,000	12,100	67,100
Total	415,000	535,000	91,300	506,300

When the adjusted report is compared with the actual expenses, the salary variance is $20,800 instead of $100,000 and the supply variance is $7,900 instead of $20,000. The clinic is exceeding anticipated expenses given the 22% increase in volume; however, the variance is significantly less when adjusted for volume. The unexplained variance is now $20,888 + $7900 = $28,700 instead of $100,000 + $20,000 = $120,000.

of minutes of dictation was increasing by 10% per month, it could be anticipated that additional transcriptionists would be required or external assistance would be needed to transcribe the dictation.

Table 18-6 PRODUCT LINE VARIANCE REPORT USING DRGS
AS A PRODUCT LINE

	Actual			Budget		
DRG	Net Revenue	Cost	Profit	Net Revenue	Cost	Profit
XX1	75,500	63,400	12,100	81,200	61,000	20,200
XX2	61,400	44,500	16,900	59,300	38,800	20,500
XX3	82,800	84,700	(1900)	63,600	61,200	2,400
Totals	219,700	192,600	27,100	204,100	161,100	43,100

Staffing Information

Staffing information is a necessary component of business planning and budgeting. Staffing information maintained by the HIM manager should include the following:

- Current organizational chart by function and by name
- Productivity standards
- Skills assessment inventory for each staff member
- Training obtained or needed
- Average time off by categories of staff (nonproductive time)
- Salary or hourly wage for each position or staff member
- Hire dates or planned raise dates and amounts
- Accrued vacation and sick leave (if accrual is allowed)
- Staffing utilization reports

Maintaining these data allows management to know which staff members are prepared to assume new duties,

Box 18-4 COMMON DATA SOURCES FOR THE HIM DEPARTMENT

- Monthly discharge, operations, and visit statistics by payer type (e.g., Medicare, public aid, commercial, managed care)
- Monthly discharge, operations, and visit statistics by service type (e.g., medical, surgical, obstetric)
- Length of stay by clinical service and payer type
- Incomplete medical records, per week or month, per physician, per clinical service, and so on
- Requests for records from insurers, patients, other health care providers
- Average pages per records, number of pages generated by automated sources, number of pages handwritten
- Lines, minutes, or words of diction per month, per physician, per report type
- Records requested and pulled
- Discharges by DRG
- Cases by physician (encounters, discharges, operations).
- Records and loose sheets filed
- Research studies (e.g., organized, searches)
- Quality improvement studies (e.g., organized, supported)
- Records, encounters scanned, and quality reviewed

what training must be planned or budgeted for to allow other staff members to take over activities, what amounts of staff resources were actually used during a period, how much vacation time and sick time are accrued for this department, and the true productive time of staff members. **Productive time** is the time a worker is present and working. A full-time position is typically 2080 hours annually (40 hours per week × 52 weeks). Yet a full-time position does not equate to 2080 productive hours. Some hours are not worked because of vacation, holidays, sick time, and so on, and thus would be considered nonproductive time. Productive hours are further reduced by training and meeting hours. Monitoring time off and nonproductive time allows management to estimate more closely the productive hours available to meet workload demands.

Program and Automation Assessments

Two assessments may be completed before proceeding with a business plan and budget: automation assessment and program assessment. These assessments are similar to doing an internal environment assessment of the HIM department. When the assessments are completed, the health information manager knows whether the tools are available to achieve the outcomes necessary. If administration has determined that no additional staff can be added this year, then a manager's dependence on automation may increase. Automation may be less expensive to add than staff and increase productivity as well. The assessment of programs requires the staff to consider seriously the adequacy of each service it offers and decide whether the services meet the users' or customers' needs and how critical the service is to the organization.

The Four M'S

All managers have the responsibility to manage the four M's:

- Manpower
- Machinery
- Materials
- Money

When preparing the business plan and, ultimately, the budget, all proposed expenditures must balance the M's; that is, an increase in one should attempt to offset the cost of another. If we request a computer to help us do our work, we should be able to do the work with fewer persons. This is a trade-off between machinery and personnel. Sometimes, however, machinery is needed to offset the need for more personnel to meet volume increases.

Developing the Business Plan and Budget

Now that we have gathered and assessed the data, we have identified the needs we want to address. The first step is to figure out whether the needs we identified are consistent with the organization's mission and goals.

If your proposal is consistent with the organization's mission and goals, then you must decide what you want to do and how you want to do it. Several questions can be answered during the process (Figure 18-4).

Example of Departmental Objectives for Budget Planning

- Develop an implementation, training, and evaluation plan for a clinician electronic signature program for transcribed reports and other electronic components of the electronic health record. (new objective)
- Meet or exceed the state-regulated time frame for response to release-of-information requests. (ongoing)
- Continue to receive, prepare, image, index, and do a quality review of all outpatient documentation within 24 hours of receipt, 7 days a week. (ongoing)

As each objective is developed and linked to organizational goals, the action steps must be prepared in detail to ensure that the objective is attained. Costs to do each step of the planned objective must be determined and associated with the timing of the steps. Some expenses may be evenly distributed throughout the year. Other expenses may be "one time" expenses planned for a particular month. Some objectives will be new objectives and others will be ongoing objectives.

The organization's goals include increasing cash flow. Your proposal is to establish a courier service to deliver incomplete records to physicians' offices to decrease the number of incomplete records.

Objective
To decrease the number of incomplete records by 25%.

When do you plan to do it?
By second quarter of next year

What will be achieved?
- Reduction in accounts receivable days by 2 or $140,000 by delivering records to physicians' offices. This will reduce the time for the physician because he/she does not have to come to the HIM department to do his/her records.
- Reduction in physician complaints or increase in compliments.
- Avoidance of purchase of additional file shelving units to store incomplete records.

What is needed to achieve the objective?

Resources:	Capital:	Small Car*:	$10,000
	Operating Expenses:		
	Labor:	0.5 FTE	$ 7,200
	Auto Costs:		4,000

Collaboration Required: Security, Personnel and Purchasing Departments

*Car to be used by courier. Courier must be licensed driver.

How does the hospital benefit from this objective?
Cashflow impact: The reduction in incomplete records will result in 2 fewer days in accounts receivable or the equivalent of $140,000. Invested annually at 10%, the $140,000 will yield at least $14,000 interest income.

Figure 18-4 Questions to ask when preparing a business plan.

COST ALLOCATIONS

Another important tool in management accounting is cost analysis and being able to measure the impact on various subunits within an organization. To determine the approximate costs to provide services, an organization must develop and maintain a cost allocation system. The cost management system allocates direct and indirect costs. Costs are classified by department or responsibility center. Non–revenue-generating departments are considered indirect cost departments, whereas revenue-generating departments are considered direct cost departments. Cost allocation allocates the costs of indirect, non–revenue-generating departments to direct, revenue-generating departments.

Why Does Allocation Occur?

Some payers reimburse on the basis of the full costs of direct departments and permit the allocation of indirect departments to the direct departments only to the extent that the indirect departments contribute to the direct departments' provision of care or generation of revenue. Many indirect departments support the provision of care through the assistance provided to the direct departments. For example, telecommunications is an indirect department. If no one answers the organization's phone during an emergency, services are not provided. The HIM department supports the efforts of the nursing service, the therapy departments, and the ancillaries by serving as the central controller of all records and reports. The HIM department is considered a non–patient revenue-generating department. The total costs of the department are therefore considered indirect and must be allocated to patient revenue-generating departments such as nursing, therapy, and laboratory.

The HIM department does have revenue-generating opportunities. Some departments charge for copies of health records provided to insurance companies and lawyers. Other departments provide transcription services for their physicians and charge accordingly. These services are revenue generating; however, they are not directly related to the primary mission of the organization–patient care.

Allocation Methods
Step-Down Method
The **step-down method** is a common method that is supported by Medicare in its cost-reporting requirements. In this method, the indirect department that receives the least amount of service from other indirect departments and provides the most service to other departments has its costs allocated first.

The chaplain service is an indirect department that may offer less service to other departments than the HIM department offers to direct departments. Both provide services to nursing, but seldom does the chaplain provide services to the therapy departments or the laboratory. So the HIM department costs would be allocated before those of the chaplain service.

The allocation is made on the basis of the ratio of services provided to each department or some other basis, such as square footage, employees, or worked hours.

Example of Step-Down Cost Allocation

Housekeeping serves more indirect departments than laundry/linen or health information services. Housekeeping's services are used 20% of the time by laundry/linen, 5% of the time by health information services, 5% by radiology, and 70% by nursing. Laundry/linen's services are used 3% by health information services, 5% by radiology, and 92% by nursing. This results in allocation of the costs of the indirect departments to the direct departments of nursing and radiology.

The step-down approach is most common in health care institutions. The steps in the allocation table's appearance show how the approach was named.

Double-Distribution Method
The **double-distribution method** is similar to the step-down method. This method assumes that the allocation of costs cannot be linear and that some indirect departments need to be allocated to less commonly dispersed departments before the costs of these departments are fully allocated. In the example discussed earlier, housekeeping was fully allocated to the remaining departments of laundry/linen, health information services, radiology, and nursing. Then laundry/linen's costs were fully allocated. In the double-distribution method, we would now have the opportunity to distribute some of laundry/linen's costs back to housekeeping. In the step-down method, that option is not available.

Simultaneous-Equations Method
The **simultaneous-equations method** (also known as the algebraic or multiple apportionment method) permits multiple allocations to occur through sophisticated mathematical software and the use of simultaneous mathematical equations. This method may require 10 to 12 different distributions of costs.

Why Is Cost Allocation Methodology Important for the HIM Professional?

Some forward-thinking organizations provide comprehensive budgeting reports to their department managers.

Example of Cost Allocation Method

Department	Total Costs	Housekeeping	Laundry/Linen	HIS	Total
Housekeeping	$ 30,000	$30,000			
Laundry/linen	$ 15,000	$ 6,000 (.20)	$32,000*		
Health information services	$100,000	$ 1,500 (.05)	$ 630 (.03)	$102,130	
Radiology	$135,000	$ 1,500 (.05)	$ 1,050 (.05)	$ 10,213 (.10)	$147,760
Nursing	$270,000	$21,000 (.70)	$19,320 (.92)	$ 91,917 (.90)	$402,240
Total	$550,000	$30,000	$21,000	$102,130	$550,000

*The laundry/linen department costs were $15,000, and the allocated housekeeping costs were an additional $6000.
HIS, Health information systems.

The managers see not only the direct costs incurred by the department-that is, the supplies they order and pay for, the labor they paid for, and so on-but also the allocations of costs from other departments. The HIM department may find it unusual to see costs for the laundry department allocated to the HIM department. If the HIM department uses no laundry services, then the allocation should be removed and reallocated to the departments that use this service. The health information manager must fully investigate the services of laundry before removing the allocation because the laundry department may assist housekeeping in removing stains that may appear on the carpet in the HIM department.

Furthermore, the HIM department should assess whether costs are being properly allocated to its user departments. This may require HIM department management to monitor the user demand for several months, perhaps by counting the number of records, reports, or statistics requested and then determining what percentage of all requests should be allocated to each user department. For example, the HIM director may decide that the simplest method for allocating the HIM department costs is by record requests (Figure 18-5).

Given this information, the HIM professional can now approach the cost accountant and review current allocations to the new data and then may make adjustments as indicated on the basis of the factual data provided.

Some organizations allocate costs in a less scientific manner for simplicity. Some methods include allocating costs of other departments to user departments based on the total square feet occupied by all user departments. In our example, if the HIM department represented 5% of the total square feet served by housekeeping, then 5% of housekeeping's costs would be allocated to the HIM department. Clearly, one could argue that the HIM department area requires less cleaning than perhaps the operating room, but the allocation method is simple to apply and keep up to date.

FINANCIAL ACCOUNTING

The role of managerial accounting was explained previously in our discussion of how budgets, business plans, and cost allocations are linked to organizational goals and provide financial information to internal decision makers. **Financial accounting,** on the other hand, refers to recording and reporting the financial transactions of the organization for both internal management and users outside of the organization. External users might include loan officers, creditors, investors, and payers. For the purposes of financial accounting, organizations must adhere to generally accepted accounting principles promulgated by the Financial Standards Accounting Board (FASB). FASB is a rule-making body of the American Institute of Certified Public Accountants (AICPA), which establishes general accounting principles for all types of financial accounting transactions and reporting. A separate Government Accounting Standards Board (GASB) provides financial accounting and reporting standards for state and local governments.

Fundamental Accounting Principles and Concepts

It is these basic underlying concepts and principles that help ensure the quality of financial accounting information made available to users. Generally accepted accounting principles and assumptions provide a common framework for both recording individual accounting transactions and communicating financial information. An understanding of these important concepts will provide a foundation for understanding how financial accounting information develops and is communicated. Some of the more important accounting principles and concepts follow.

Entity: General accounting principles define an **entity** as the business unit or activity for which accounting

RECORDS REQUESTED FOR FIRST NINE MONTHS OF YEAR

Requestor	Number Requested	% of All
Administration	5	.004
Fiscal Services	210	.16
Quality Management	400	.30
Risk Management	17	.01
Nursing Service	323	.24
Respiratory Therapy	105	.08
Physical Therapy	90	.07
Anesthesiology	47	.04
Surgery	143	.11
Medicine	180	.13
Social Work	12	.01
Total	1340	1.01 (due to rounding)

Figure 18-5 Example of record request.

records are maintained. Separate financial statements must be prepared for each individual business entity. Just as a physician in private practice should not combine funds with his or her own personal household finances, an individual hospital as part of a large publicly traded health care corporation should not combine accounts with the parent corporation. Each entity must keep its own unique set of books and prepare separate and distinct financial statements.

Going Concern: According to generally accepted accounting principles, an assumption is made that an entity will continue for the foreseeable future. The **going concern** concept assumes that the owners of a business entity will continue operating indefinitely to fulfill the business plans of the organization.

Stable Monetary Unit: Accounting entities use a **stable monetary unit** of measure to record and report financial transactions. In the United States this stable monetary unit is represented by the U.S. dollar. It is understood that inflation could affect the reporting of financial information; however, for the purposes of accounting standards it is assumed that this would not be significant enough to cause alarm.

Matching Concept: The importance of recognizing revenues and expenses in the same accounting period is represented by the **matching concept**. Earlier in the chapter during our discussion of the revenue cycle we mentioned that revenue is accounted for when the actual charge is posted to a patient account. The matching concept recognizes that any associated expenses such as labor, supplies, and travel would be recorded in the same accounting period and matched with the revenue for that accounting period.

Objectivity: Because of inflation and market dynamics, there can be considerable differences between the current value of an asset and its original cost. For this reason, accounting principles recognize the historical cost of an asset as the most objective measure for financial reporting. As an example, a physician office building currently valued at $1.5 million that was purchased 5 years ago for $500,000 would be recorded on the balance sheet at $500,000. Even though the market value of the office building is $1.5 million, the **objectivity** concept states that historical cost is a more objective measure than current value.

Disclosure: An entity's financial statements provide a mechanism to communicate the economic activities of an organization. In the event supplemental data are available to better clarify or offer additional information for decision makers, this should be disclosed on pertinent financial statements. **Disclosure** of additional information through the use of footnotes on an organization's financial statements is a commonly accepted accounting practice.

Financial Management Duties

When the HIM professional interacts with the financial accounting staff of the organization, it might be to request a payment to a publisher for a departmental reference book. The payment is recorded as an expense to the HIM department and classified by the type of expense, for example, books and subscriptions. Besides recording the expense, financial accounting professionals must reduce the cash balance to allow for the payment to be issued to the publisher. The people employed in the financial accounting section of fiscal services capture the data necessary to build the foundation for reports used in understanding the financial management of the organization. Just as there are numerous diverse job roles within the HIM profession, the duties of the **financial accountant, managerial accountant,** and **managerial finance officer** cover different aspects of financial management (Table 18-7).

Cash and Accrual Systems

The financial transaction processing associated with financial accounting can be accomplished in one of two manners: **cash basis accounting** or **accrual basis accounting.** In a cash basis environment, each transaction is recorded when cash is exchanged, as with one's personal finances. Revenues are recognized when money is received for services provided, and expenses are recognized when money is paid out for the resources used to provide those services. The cash basis accounting method may have worked in health care providers in years past, but it does not work today because services rendered today are seldom paid for today. Instead, health care providers often must wait 30 or more days to receive payment from a third party, typically an insurance company.

Accrual basis accounting uses the matching concept, enabling revenues to be matched with the actual expenses incurred to produce the revenue. The accrual method records the revenues expected as "revenues," although the "cash" has not yet been received. The revenues are matched as closely with the expenses as possible. For example, if an operation occurred today, the expenses associated with performing the operation are operating room staff, anesthesia, medications, disposable medical-surgical supplies, and so on. The charges associated with each of these items are recorded as revenue, and the actual cost or expense of these items is recorded as expenses of the operation.

Profit represents the amount of money (cash) actually received from the payer (patient or insurance company) less the actual cost to do the service, assuming that the cost is less than the cash received.

Each financial transaction must be recorded during the financial accounting process. Transactions are assigned to designated accounts. Several health care associations, such as the American Hospital Association (AHA), have developed a standard **chart of accounts**, although there may be slight variations from one health care organization to another. Typically, the largest expense items are in the lower number account categories, whereas the expense categories that have limited expenses appear in the higher number account groups. Labor expenses may be classified in the 100 series, and dues expenses may be classified in the 900 series. A chart similar to the standard chart of accounts for expenses exists for revenues.

Financial accounting using the accrual basis requires the accountant to comply with the double-entry method of transaction recording. This means that when revenues and expenses are matched and recorded, another set (double) of entries must occur simultaneously. These entries typically record an amount equivalent to the revenue in a category called **accounts receivable**; the expense amounts reduce categories of assets, such as medical-surgical supply inventory and pharmaceutical inventory, or increase liability categories, such as wages payable. The statement of revenues and expenses and balance sheet results from the double-entry activities.

Table 18-7 FINANCIAL MANAGEMENT DUTIES

Financial Accounting	Managerial Accounting	Managerial Finance
Record financial transactions (e.g., payments, orders, expenses, revenues, accruals)	Prepare reports such as budgets, cost reports, productivity and volume schedule; set rates or charges; monitor variances	Financing and funding activities; planning for future expenditures; investment decisions and planning
When Past and current activities	*When* Current and future activities	*When* Future activities
Titles Staff accountant, accountant, bookkeeper	*Titles* Cost accountant, budget coordinator	*Titles* Chief financial officer, treasurer

Fiscal Periods

Organizations can choose a calendar year as a fiscal year; that is, it begins January 1 and ends December 31. Or a fiscal year may not coincide with a calendar year. It may be July 1 through June 30. Fiscal periods are selected by organizations because they more consistently conform to activity cycles of the organization. A teaching institution may choose the fiscal period of July 1 through June 30 because students finish one level of training in June and are ready to start the next level in July. Budgets often correspond to fiscal periods. Specific IRS rules require that a health care organization's fiscal year must coincide with the tax year for tax accounting reporting purposes.

USING FINANCIAL REPORTS TO PROVIDE MANAGEMENT INFORMATION

The **balance sheet** displays the organization's **assets, liabilities,** and **fund balance** or **equity** at a fixed point in time, for example, December 31 of a given year (Figure 18-6). The balance sheet may be computed at any time. It is a snapshot at that time and may vary considerably during a time period. The balance sheet lists assets and liabilities and the difference between assets and liabilities. This financial

report is best represented by the following basic accounting equation:

$$\text{Assets - Liabilities} = \text{Fund Balance (Equity)}$$

Assets are cash or cashlike items or other resources that can be converted to cash. Assets may be considered as short-term assets (those easily converted to cash) or long-term assets (items more difficult to convert to cash quickly or items needed to operate the business). Liabilities are the debts or obligations the organization owes. They may include wages accruing between paydays and mortgage payments owed to the bank. The fund balance category is the residual category that collects the profits and losses that result from the differences between revenues and expenses.

The **statement of revenues and expenses** reports the expected or earned income and the associated expenses for an accounting period (Figure 18-7). This financial report may also be referred to as the income statement and is best described by the basic equation:

$$\text{Revenue} - \text{Expense} = \text{Net Income}$$

The **statement of cash flow** is an important financial report that provides additional detailed information about the source and use of funds (Figure 18-8). This report documents the change in cash balance for a given accounting period and is useful in evaluating an organization's ability to pay its bills. The statement of cash flow looks at sources and

RKK Memorial Hospital Balance Sheets for years ending December 31 (thousands of dollars)	Year 2	Year 1
Cash and securities	7,250	5,850
Accounts receivable (estimated net)	22,760	20,850
Inventories	4,780	3,440
Total current assets	34,790	30,140
Gross plant and equipment	152,420	145,780
Accumulated depreciation	26,930	21,550
Net plant and equipment	179,350	167,330
Total assets	214,140	197,470
Accounts payable	5,680	5,250
Accrued expenses	5,790	5,420
Notes payable	945	2,870
Current portion of long term debt	2,670	2,200
Total current liabilities	15,085	15,740
Long-term debt	29,420	30,800
Capital lease obligations	1,720	2,140
Total long term liabilities	31,140	32,940
Fund balance	167,915	148,790
Total liabilities and funds	214,140	197,470

Figure 18-6 Balance sheet.

RKK Memorial Hospital- Income Statements for years ending December 31
(Revenues and Expenses) (thousands of dollars)

	Year 1	Year 2
Net patient services revenue	110,500	98,500
Other operating revenue	7,300	8,800
Total operating revenue	117,800	107,300
Operating Expenses		
Nursing services	54,300	50,200
Dietary services	5,200	4,640
General services	12,680	11,450
Administrative services	11,290	10,360
Employee health and welfare	9,560	9,240
Provision for uncollectibles	4,220	3,980
Provision for malpractice	1,450	1,220
Depreciation	4,200	4,050
Interest expense	1,890	2,300
Total operating expense	104,790	97,480
Income from operations	13,010	9,860
Contributions and grants	3,290	890
Investment income	540	345
Nonoperating gain or loss	3,830	1,235
Excess of revenues over expenses	16,840	11,095

Figure 18-7 Statement of revenues and expenses.

RKK Memorial Hospital Statement of Cash Flow for Year 2 (thousands of dollars)

Cash Flow from Operations

Total operating revenue	117,800
Total cash operating expenses	(100,590)
Change in acounts receivable	(1,910)
Change in inventories	(1,340)
Change in accounts payable	(430)
Change in accruals	370
Net Cash Flow from Operations	13,900

Cash Flow for Investing Activities

Investment in plant and equipment	(6,640)

Cash Flow from Financing Activities

Repayment of long term debt	(1,380)
Repayment of notes payable	(1,925)
Capital lease principal repayment	(420)
Change in current portion of long-term debt	470
Net cash flow from financing	3,255

Nonoperating Cash Flow

Contributions and grants	3,290
Investment income	540
Nonoperating cash flow	3,830
Net increase (decrease) in cash	7,835
Beginning cash and securities	5,430
Ending cash and securities	14,285

Figure 18-8 Statement of cash flow.

uses of cash based on the organization's operating, investing, and financing activities.

USING RATIOS TO EVALUATE FINANCIAL DATA

The statement of revenues and expenses, the balance sheet, the statement of cash flow, and other reports allow management to compare the success of providing services cost effectively. **Financial analysis** or **ratio analysis** is the management process of formulating judgments and decisions from the relation between the numbers represented on two reports: the balance sheet and the statement of revenues and expenses.

A ratio expresses the relation between two numbers, such as one asset category, cash, to all assets. Professional associations, such as the Healthcare Financial Management Association, the Medical Group Management Association, and the AHA and health care systems collect data from their member organizations and members and publish average or benchmark ratios. Sometimes the data are reported by region, facility size, and facility type. The publication of average ratios permits organizations to compare their individual ratios with the average to determine how well they compare with others. Benchmarking performance against peer data provides a good yardstick for measuring performance.

When conducting ratio analysis, it is important to be consistent in defining the ratio components. When HIM professionals calculate the average length of stay of adult patients, they must be careful not to include infant discharges or infant days. This means that the definition for adult length of stay demands that the composition of the denominator and numerator be consistently determined. In addition, one should not assume that published average ratios are developed in the same way by all who submitted data to the collecting organization.

There are four commonly recognized ratio categories:

- Liquidity
- Turnover
- Performance
- Capitalization

Liquidity and capitalization ratios focus on balance sheet numbers (assets, liabilities, and equity/fund balance accounts). They measure the ability of the health care organization to meet its short- and long-term financial obligations. Performance ratios use data from the statement of revenues and expenses. Ratios in this category evaluate the effectiveness of resource use to deliver services and products. Turnover or activity ratios use data from the balance sheet and the statement of revenues and expenses. These ratios measure the organization's ability to generate net operating revenue in relation to its various assets.

Liquidity Ratio

One of the most common **liquidity ratios** is the **current ratio.** This ratio compares current assets with current liabilities. Both categories appear on the balance sheet. What the current ratio tells a manager is whether there are sufficient cash and cashlike assets to cover the immediate liabilities (bills) that will come due in the short term (1 year).

Example of Liquidity Ratio

The Citywide Surgi-Center has cash, marketable securities, and accounts receivable of $300,000. Citywide has payroll liabilities, payables due to their suppliers, and the mortgage on the surgery equipment and building due this year in the amount of $150,000.

Current assets = $300,000
Current liabilities = $150,000
Current ratio = 2:1 or 2.0

The ratio says that Citywide can meet its current obligations twice. It has twice as much cash and other liquid assets as it needs to meet its bills.

Turnover Ratio or Activity Ratio

One ratio that is affected by the activities of the health information services department is the **days of revenue in patient accounts receivable ratio.**

This **turnover ratio,** or **activity ratio,** divides patient accounts receivable by the average daily patient revenues. Patient revenues are found on the statement of revenues and expenses and patient accounts receivable are found on the balance sheet because accounts receivable are considered an asset to an organization. Accounts receivable are eventually paid and converted to cash. Patient revenues can be expressed as either net or gross. Gross patient revenues, sometimes referred to as patient services revenues, refer to the value of services provided at full billed charges. Net patient revenues, sometimes referred to as net patient services revenues, refer to the amount the health care provider expects to receive as payment for the services. Therefore net revenue is gross revenue less any contractual discounts or adjustments agreed to between the insurance company and the provider or the difference between full charges and fixed fees established by the government (e.g., DRG) or insurer. The 1990 American Institute of Certified Public Accountants' audit and accounting guide, *Audits of Providers of Health Care Services,* requires that reports prepared for public use reflect net patient revenues, not gross patient revenues.

When using net patient revenues in the **accounts receivable turnover ratio** (AR days ratio), one must be certain to use net accounts receivable. For consistency, if gross patient revenues are used, then the divisor must be gross accounts receivable. Most reports are now expressed in terms of net patient revenues and receivables.

Net days of revenue in
patient accounts receivable

$$= \frac{\text{Net patient accounts receivable}}{\text{Average daily net patient service revenue}}$$

Average net daily patient service revenue

$$= \frac{\text{Net patient service revenue for the period}}{\text{Days in the period}}$$

The days of revenue in the patient accounts receivable ratio provide a measure of the average time that receivables are outstanding or the period for which a health care organization extends credit to its debtors. High values for this ratio imply longer collection periods and may signal a need for the health care organization to seek cash or financial resources from other sources to pay its ongoing day-to-day expenses until the receivables are collected.

Example of the Average Number of Days of Revenue in Accounts Receivable

Compare Citywide Surgi-Center's days of revenue in patient accounts receivable (also known as AR days) with the hypothetical average published by U.S. Surgi-Centers:

	Citywide Surgi-Center's AR Days					U.S. Surgi-Centers Average
	May	*June*	*July*	*August*	*Sept*	
AR Days	37.6	37.9	38.4	39.1	39.7	45.8

Conclusion: Citywide is collecting their receivables effectively, yet the collection period is increasing. Management should assess the causes for this trend.

Performance Ratio

The **performance ratio** evaluates the use of resources to achieve a goal. A common performance ratio is the **operating margin ratio.** This ratio displays the relation between the net revenues received and the expenses required to supply the revenues. **Net operating revenue** is the amount of revenue *expected* to be received or total charges less the deductions expected by third party payers resulting in revenues **net** of deductions or net operating revenue. If Citywide had net operating revenue this month of $100,000 and expenses of $96,000, the revenues in excess of expenses would be $4000 ($100,000-$96,000). Citywide's operating margin ratio would be 0.04 or 4%.

Capitalization Ratio

There are several **capitalization ratios.** One that may be experienced by anyone who works in an organization that has an anticipated building project is the **long-term debt/ total assets ratio.** This ratio compares the amount of long-term debt the organization has (bills that will come due in a period more than 1 year from now [e.g., mortgages]) with the amount of assets (things the organization can convert to cash [e.g., furniture, land, inventories, marketable securities]) it has to pay those debts. The banks will consider the organization's ability to pay back the estimated additional debt it will incur.

CAPITAL EXPENSE AND INVESTMENT DECISIONS

You may ask who has the overall responsibility for capital decisions. This responsibility is another component of the fiscal services area. The overall capital planning function is part of the managerial finance role. Some institutions assign this duty to a chief financial officer (CFO); others, a treasurer. The role of the managerial finance officer is one of planning for the future. We have discussed the role of the financial accountant. It is one of recording what has happened today or in the past, such as paying staff for work performed. We have also discussed the role of the managerial accountant during the budget review. This person helps record what is happening currently or previously (variance analyses) against what was anticipated and what is still anticipated to happen (the budget).

The managerial finance officer, CFO, or treasurer works with financial organizations (e.g., banks, investors) to obtain funding and financing for an organization's plans. If an organization wants to build a new building, financing support is required. This person may also make investment decisions to maximize the income on idle money the organization may have at any given time. The thrust is to ensure that the organization is effective in delivering the services suggested by the mission statement while doing so efficiently so that funds are not being spent on inappropriate items. The following reports result from these activities:

- Balance sheet
- Statement of changes in financial position
- Investment reports
- Financing reports

Capital Expenditures

Some facilities establish a **capital expenditure committee** to evaluate all capital requests so that cash resources are used to purchase the high-cost items that will yield the most benefit to the organization. When the final list is approved, proposed acquisition dates are assigned. The proposed acquisition date does not guarantee that a manager will be able to purchase the item on that date. The CFO or controller must assess the condition of the cash budget to determine whether sufficient cash will be available to meet not only the upcoming expenses to support the upcoming service levels but also the one-time expense associated with the piece of capital.

Because capital requests are typically considered by a committee, it is important for department managers to know how to prepare a well-developed and justified request for the equipment needed for their departments. To do so requires an analysis of the opportunity cost of funds.

The capital expenditure committee considers all requests received. A capital investment should be evaluated in terms of the following:

- From the perspective of its contribution to the mission and from a financial perspective relative to the cost of the capital acquisition
- Revenues it may generate for the organization
- Period of time the acquisition will contribute to the organization (economic life)
- Cost to the organization to borrow the funds or loss of interest on the funds
- Regulatory hurdles, such as requirements to obtain approval from planning or rate-setting agencies and any reimbursement opportunities through Medicare or taxation

Any organization has limited funds to invest in new capital. Each decision to use funds for one acquisition means that another must be foregone. Financial managers describe this process as weighing opportunity costs. **Opportunity costs** are benefits that would be received from the next best alternative use of the investment funds. Some providers use as a measure of opportunity cost the interest rate received on invested funds.[10] Cleverley et al[9] define opportunity costs as "values foregone by using a resource in a particular way instead of in its next best alternative way."

The health information manager is obligated to contribute to conserving the facility's cash and adjusting the department's operations to meet the actual levels of service.

Capital Request Evaluation Process

In most organizations, there is a formalized process for obtaining approval of a capital expenditure. The process is usually initiated by a department manager preparing a written request on a capital expenditure approval form (Figure 18-9).

Some forms are elaborate, requiring the manager to calculate various financial analyses. Others are more verbiage oriented, requiring the manager to define the need, alternatives considered, volume of business related to the item being requested, analysis of various vendors or suppliers considered or bids obtained to determine the item's cost, and an economic feasibility study.

Each facility defines its capitalization value. For the sake of this example, any expenditure in excess of $500 for equipment or furniture is considered a **capital expenditure.** Capital items usually have a high initial cost and a "life" of more than 1 year.

Time Value of Money

No discussion of capital expenditures would be complete without including the concept of the **time value of money.** This concept includes several premises. The first is that a person who invests money should be entitled to a return or interest. The return is based on at least two conditions: the length of time the money is invested and the degree of risk associated with the investment. If the investment carries great risk, the rate of return should be higher and vice versa.

The time value of money says to the layperson that it is more beneficial to receive a dollar today than to receive it 1 year from now. The reason is that a dollar received today can be invested and gain interest for 1 year longer than a dollar received 1 year from now. That is, a dollar received today and placed in a savings account at 5% interest accrues a minimum of $0.05 in interest. At the end of the year, the savings account closes at $1.05. If the dollar is not received until the end of the year, there would be $1.00, not $1.05.

Compounding

The value of the investment is determined by the length of time the investment is in place because of the **compounding effect.** In the example previously discussed, we started with $1, but at the end of the year we had $1.05, simply by selecting a safe bank in which to deposit this dollar. If that dollar was left in the bank for 3 years at the 5% interest rate, we do not end up with $1.15, but rather $1.16. An extra $0.01 is earned because of the compounding effect. By the fourth year, $0.22 is gained. Although the gain may not seem significant in this example, consider the effect if $10,000 is invested. Compounding can mean significant gains for the investor.

Discounting

The concept of **discounting** is the opposite of compounding. The question we ask ourselves when we are considering discounting is, How much must one invest today at a compound interest rate of x to receive a given amount at the end of N years? What we know is how much we want to have at the end of the period—say, our retirement age. What we do not know is the *present value* of the money we need to invest today at today's interest rate to accumulate the sum we want by retirement age. For example, if you were to retire next year and today's interest rate is 5% and you want $105,000 next year, what is the present value you would need to invest today? ($100,000).

Description ______________________ Budget Year ______________
Budget Cost $ ______________
Manufacturer ______________________ Unity Cost ______________
Quantity ______________
Model # ______________________ Total ______________
Freight ______________
Vendor ______________________ Installation ______________
Quorum Discount ______________
Materials Manager Signature ______________________ TOTAL COST $ ______________

1. Type of expenditure: Replacement ________ New ________

2. Briefly define function of capital expenditure ______________________

3. Estimate # of procedures to be done ________ **4.** Average Charge per procedure ______________

5. Will the number of FTE's increase or decrease ________ **6.** By how many ______________

7. Briefly describe why item is needed ______________________

8. Financial Analysis		Annual	**REQUESTED BY:**	
a.	Gross revenue	$ ______	______________	
b.	Less: Salaries	______	Department Director	Date
c.	Supplies	______		
d.	Depreciation	______		
e.	Professional Fees	______		
f.	Other (itemize) ______	______	**APPROVED BY:**	
g.	______	______		
h.	______	______	______________	
i.	(Total sum b-h)	______	Dept. Asst. Administrator	Date
j.	Gross profit (a-i)	______		
k.	Less: Contractual adjustments	______	______________	
l.	Bad debts	______	Maintenance Director	Date
m.	Policy discounts	______		
n.	Total (sum k-m)	______	______________	
o.	Gross margin (j-n)	$ ______	Asst. Admin.–Finance	Date
p.	Asset cost	______		
q.	Return of individual asset O/P	______ %	______________	
r.	Payback—years (P/O)	______	Administrator	Date

Figure 18-9 Capital expenditure approval form. (From Huron Regional Medical Center.)

Continued

When the capital expenditure committee evaluates capital requests, they are evaluating the opportunities available to the organization. Should the organization leave its funds in the bank at a certain interest rate, or should it invest in a new program that predicts it may yield yet another level of revenue and do so for several years? Decisions such as these are confronted by managers every day. The managers must weigh the risk associated with the new program against the considerably lower risk of leaving the money in the bank. Unfortunately, it is not this simple because each year many capital requests are submitted and must be compared with one another.

Helping the capital expenditure committee is the fiscal management staff. Financial managers assess or weigh the value of an investment in equipment or other capital request against the interest that would be received on the funds if left

Capital Expenditure Request Instructions

Description	Please list the exact item you are requesting.
Manufacturer	If known, please list the manufacturer of the product you are requesting.
Model #	This is important to ensure you are ordering the item you really want.
Vendor	If known, please list who the vendor is from which this item can be ordered.
Budget Year	This should always be our fiscal year that ends on June 30 each year. e.g., October 4, 1993 is budget year 1994.
Budget Cost	This is the amount you list on your Capital Equipment Budget. If the item wasn't budgeted please insert "NONE."
Quantity	How many do you want to order?
Total	Multiply the number in Unit Cost by the number in Quantity.
Freight	Please include this total if known. You may ask the Materials Manager for this total. If the Unit cost included freight, insert "NONE".
Installation	Please have our Maintenance Department give you a figure to include here.
Quorum Discount	This must always be completed. If there is no discount, please insert "NONE".
Total Cost	This is the total you receive when adding together the freight and installation with the Cost.

The financial analysis, section 8, must be completed prior to approval by the Assistant Administrator–Finance and Administrator. Should you need any help in completing this section, please contact the Controller or the Assistant Administrator–Finance.

Figure 18-9, cont'd Capital expenditure approval form. (From Huron Regional Medical Center.)

in the bank by using one or more of the following capital evaluation methods:

- Accounting rate of return
- Payback method
- Net present value

Net Present Value

In its simplest format, a new piece of equipment or new program will have cash outflows and cash inflows. For example, St. Elsewhere Medical Center has two capital requests. One is from the HIM department for a new dictation system. The other is from the business office for a new charge auditing program.

We know that capital requests will require some cash outflows. The dictation system vendor will expect to be paid a certain sum at the time of installation. The charge auditing program will require additional staff and training costs before it is fully productive. Both proposals will have cash inflows. The HIM manager predicts that she will be able to eliminate the contract typing service expense and do all work in house, thus eliminating payments to the outside contract service. The business office manager says he will find items that have been used in the patient care process and not been charged. When they are found, his staff can

add these charges to the bill and obtain third-party reimbursement for them.

Both proposals have an expected life of 5 years. That is, the equipment will operate optimally for 5 years before the technology is outdated. Each will be depreciated over 5 years as well. Straight-line **depreciation** is calculated by dividing the capital cost by the years of life (in this example, the life is 5 years). The resulting amount is considered the annual depreciation expense.

The charge auditing program includes a training program for the departments that provide services. It is proposed that the program will use a continuous quality improvement approach to identify where charges are lost and assist these areas in reducing errors. Over a period of 5 years, all departments will have improved their charge-entering procedures to ensure that no charges are overlooked or lost.

The proposals will subtract cash outflows from cash inflows to result in a new cash inflow or outflow at the end of each year for the full 5 years. Depreciation expense is considered an outflow. The proposed annual nets for each project must be evaluated against the rate of interest the moneys would have earned if left in the bank. Because the net amounts are the remaining amounts received at the end of each year, we must use a discounting factor to determine the present value of each net amount or **net present value**.

Table 18-8 INTERNALIZING THE COPY SERVICE PROPOSAL

Year	New Cash Flows	Present Value 13%	Value of Cash Flows Today
1	1,000	0.88496	885.00
2	3,000	0.78318	2,349.54
3	7,000	0.69305	4,851.35
4	12,000	0.61332	7,359.84
5	15,000	0.54276	8,141.40
Total	38,000		23,587.13

To find this factor, use a table that can be found in most finance textbooks. Table 18-8 represents a portion of such a table.

Example Comparing Competing Projects-Net Present Value

	HIM	Patient Accounts
The project	Dictation system	Auditing program
Net cash flows	$25,000/year	$15,000/year
Project life	5 years	5 years
Initial capital	$75,000	$60,000
Annual depreciation	$15,000	$12,000
Return required	10%	10%
Net present value (NPV)	$94,775	$56,865
NPV—initial capital	$19,775	($3,135)

Decision: The health record project meets the criteria to have a 10% return and exceed the initial capital outlay.

Example of Net Present Value Evaluation—Copy Service

You want to bring the copy service in house. Because you know the volumes intimately, you can accurately forecast the service's growth. Your current contracted copy service pays your organization a retrieval fee, but your staff does all the logging, pulls all the records, and answers all the calls about the records requested. On the basis of the volumes you have experienced in the past and anticipate in the future, you can estimate the revenues from the copies and the related expenses. The revenues less the expenses are the net cash flows.

1. Prepare your pro forma (expected revenues and expenses) to provide this service internally.
2. Meet with your CFO and ask what interest rate he expects on investments or what return he expects from new programs. Review the table in a finance book labeled

"Present Value of One Dollar Due at the End of N Years" and the interest column that corresponds to the CFO's expectations. He expects 13%.

From the copy service example, one can see that even though the program is projected to generate $38,000 in net cash flows, the real value of those flows in today's dollars is $23,587.13. In other terms, if we had $23,587.13 today and invested it at 13% interest, at the end of 5 years it would yield $30,000. If we need $25,000 in capital to start this program, the investment ($25,000) would not be recovered in the 5 years and may be turned down. If we need only $19,000, perhaps to buy a personal computer and a big copy machine to support the logging effort, then the project may be approved because the investment is less than the net present value of the cash flows ($23,587).

Accounting Rate of Return

This evaluation method uses averages. The annual net inflows or outflows are averaged over the project's life for each project. The asset value or investment value is averaged over the life of the project as well. The asset value is depreciated on a straight-line basis for the life of the program.

Example of Accounting Rate of Return—Copy Service

If we use our same copy service example's facts, we can use the following **accounting rate of return** formula:

Average net income $38,000/5
Initial investment = $19,000

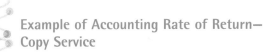

$$\frac{\$38,000 \; 5 \; years}{\$19,000} = 40\%$$

Accounting rate of return: 40%

Before proceeding further, we need to revisit the CFO and determine whether an accounting rate of return of 40% is acceptable.

Example Comparing Competing Projects—Accounting Rate of Return

	HIM	Patient Accounts
Net cash flows	$25,000/year	$15,000/year
Depreciation	-15,000/year	-12,000/year
Average net income	$10,000/year	$3,000/year
Average investment	$75,000/year	$60,000/year
Accounting rate of return	13%	5%

Decision: The HIM project has a higher accounting rate of return.

Payback Method

The **payback method** is probably the simplest of all methods. The payback period determines the number of years it will take for the cash inflows from each project to pay back the initial investment (cash outflow).

Example of Payback Method—Copy Service

Year	Net Cash Flows	Initial Investment	Remaining
0		$19,000	
1	$ 1,000	-1,000	$18,000
2	$ 3,000	-3,000	15,000
3	$ 7,000	-7,000	$48,000
4	$12,000	-12,000	
5	$15,000		
Total	$38,000		

We can see that by year 4, our initial investment will be paid back. To calculate the portion of year 4 that it consumes, we divide the remaining amount ($8000) by the net cash flow ($12,000). Therefore this investment will be paid back in 3.67 years.

Example of Payback Method—Comparing Competing Projects

The HIM project's initial investment is $75,000. Annual cash flows of $25,000 will result in a payback period of 3 years ($75,000/$25,000).

The patient accounts project's initial investment is $60,000. Annual cash flows of $15,000 will result in a payback period of 4 years ($60,000/$15,000).

Arguments Pro and Con for Evaluation Methods

Each of the evaluation methods has advantages and disadvantages. No one method is more effective than the others, and occasionally financial managers use more than one method to weigh the opportunities. The payback method is the simplest to use. No special tables are required, but it ignores the basic concept of money management—the time value of money.

The accounting rate of return is simple to use. No special tables are required, but it ignores the time value of money and does not take into consideration when inflows are received. The same average could result if the heavier inflows are received later in the project's life or earlier. If the time value of money was considered, a money manager would want to receive the larger inflows earlier rather than later.

The net present value approach requires calculations of the discounted amounts or the use of special discounting tables. It assumes, however, that net inflows are reinvested at the same rate as the cost of capital or the interest rate the investment would have received had the money been left in the bank. It also requires the evaluators to assume a rate of return.

OTHER PHASES OF FINANCIAL MANAGEMENT

Implementing

The implementation process is probably the most rewarding activity of management because it confirms whether your ideas were correct, your plans were accurate, and your achievements are worth reaching. It requires support from your entire staff and from administration and organizational leaders.

Because of the high cost of health care and the continuing impact on the overall economy, reimbursement pressures are certain to increase. Even in an economy operating under ideal conditions and in an environment of health care regulation and reform, the need to monitor closely all activities to ensure that services are delivered as cost effectively as possible is management's greatest challenge.

Seeking Alternatives

No manager can identify *all* alternatives to doing a task. Just as the composition of the business plan requires the involvement of all staff, during times of high growth and increasing volumes, all staff members need to be involved to find new and better methods to achieve the same outcome. This holds true for periods of economic downturns and lower volumes as well. Management should meet with staff (in teams if the staff size is large or as a whole if the staff size is small) at regular intervals to brainstorm alternatives to performing tasks. Ideally, this process should occur before the budgeting process so that management can fully investigate the options that surface and prepare any justification materials at budget time. This participative management approach is becoming more common in health care with the increased awareness of continuous quality improvement processes and need to hardwire excellence.

Role of the HIM Professional in Financial Management

The need for HIM professionals to be more adept in fiscal activities is apparent. The ability to understand, use, and communicate both financial and clinical information continues to take on a new level of importance in health care organizations. This chapter cannot review all aspects of financial management. To be truly successful, HIM professionals of tomorrow must be able to communicate as easily with the CFO as they are able to deal with the medical staff. If the HIM professional is to gain this level of expertise, additional training must be sought beyond the contents of this chapter.

REFERENCES

1. Centers for Medicare & Medicaid Services: National health expenditures and selected economic indicators, levels and average annual percent change: selected calendar years 1990-2013: www.cms.hhs.gov.
2. PricewaterhouseCoopers analysis: The factors fueling rising healthcare costs: www.pwchealth.com.
3. U.S. Census Bureau: Income, poverty and health insurance coverage in the United States: 2004: www.census.gov.
4. National Uniform Billing Committee: UB-04 claim form: www.nubc.org and National Uniform Claim Committee: CMS 1500 claim form: www.nucc.org.
5. National Health Care Anti-Fraud Association: A serious and costly reality for all Americans: www.nhcaa.org.
6. *St. Anthony's medical billing and compliance guide,* Reston, VA, 1998, St. Anthony Publishing.
7. American Health Information Management Association: *Code of ethics,* Chicago, 2004, American Health Information Management Association. Revised and approved by AHIMA House of Delegates on July 1, 2004.
8. Ward WJ Jr: *Health care budgeting and financial management for non-financial managers,* Westport, CT, 1994, Auburn House.
9. Cleverley WO, William O, Cameron AE: *Essentials of health care finance,* ed 5, Sudbury, MA, 2003, Jones and Bartlett Publishers.
10. Neumann BR, Suver JD, Zelman WN: *Financial management—concepts and applications for health care providers,* ed 2, Baltimore, 1988, National Health Publishing.

Additional Resources

American Health Information Assoc., Foundation of Research and Education: Report on the use of health information technology to enhance and expand health care anti-fraud activities, 2005. Available online at www.ahima.org.

American Health Information Management Association: Fraud and abuse compliance programs (journal articles and seminars). Chicago, 1998, 1999, 2000.

Berger S: Fundamentals of healthcare financial management: a practical guide to fiscal issues and activities Healthcare Financial Management Association, New York, 1999, McGraw-Hill.

Development of automated coding software: development and use to enhance anti-fraud activities, 2005. Available online at www.ahima.org.

Kovner AR, Jonas S, editors: *Health care delivery in the United States,* ed 6, New York, 1999, Springer.

Nowicki M: The financial management of hospitals and healthcare organizations, Chicago, 1999, Health Administration Press and Washington, DC, 1999, AUPHA Press.

Robinson-Crowley C: *Understanding patient financial services,* Gaithersburg, MD, 1997, Aspen Publishers.

chapter 19

Viewpoints

Linda L. Kloss
Don E. Detmer
Jeffrey J. Williamson
Marion J. Ball
Jean S. Clark
Bryant T. Karras
Mary Alice Hanken
Michael D. Gray
Bill G. Felkey

 Additional content,
http://evolve.elsevier.com/Abdelhak/

Chapter Contents

Transforming Health Information Management
The Case for a Wired Health Care System
A Compelling Vision
A Health Information Management Profession in Transition
Milestones for Change

Health Professionals for Translational, Clinical, and Public Health/Population Informatics
Biomedical/Health Informatics
Workforce Needs
AMIA's 10 × 10 Program
Other Educational Initiatives

Collaborating for Change
Technology and Change
Two Case Studies
Lessons Learned
Collaboration
Nursing
Health Information Management
Technology as Enabler

International Health Information Management
International Federation of Health Records Organizations
The Electronic Health Record
Clinical Data Management
Privacy, Security, and Confidentiality of Personal Health Information
Education
Needs of Developing Countries
The Joint Commission
International Opportunities

Public Health Information: A Strategic Resource
Public Health and Medical Care
Population-Based Data
Information Needs and Core Public Health Functions
Public Health Programs
Health Problems and Costs
Improving Health
Integrating the Information System
Legal Context
Cooperation

A Vision of Digital Information Convergence: "How Connected Do You Want to Be?"
Closed-Loop Solutions (On-Line and Real Time)
Telecommuting Oversight
Self-Care Management
Integration for Patient Safety
Digital Dashboards
Multidisciplinary Collaboration
Therapeutic Outcomes Monitoring
Digital Information Convergence
Priorities and Trends

Abbreviations

AIDS—acquired immunodeficiency syndrome
AHIMA—American Health Information Management Association
AMIA—American Medical Informatics Association
ATM—automated teller machine
CCR—continuity of care record
CDC—Centers for Disease Control and Prevention
CIO—chief information officer
CPOE—computerized physician order entry
EHR—electronic health record
EMS—emergency medical services
FORE—Foundation for Research and Education
GPS—global positioning system
HEDIS—Health Plan Employer Data and Information Set
HIM—health information management
HIPAA—Health Insurance Portability and Accountability Act

HIT—health information technology
HL7—Health Level 7
ICU—intensive care unit
IFHRO—International Federation of Health Records Organizations
IOM—Institute of Medicine
IP—Internet protocol
IT—information technology
JCAHO—Joint Commission on Accreditation of Healthcare Organizations (now The Joint Commission)
NHIN—National Health Information Network
PDA—personal digital assistant
RFID—radiofrequency identification
SARS—severe acute respiratory syndrome
TIGER— Technology Informatics Guiding Educational Reform
WHO—World Health Organization

The purpose of this chapter is to stimulate thinking and provide food for discussion. Industry leaders representing different health professions present their views regarding issues that will affect the future of health care. We hope that you will enjoy reading this chapter and find that the seeds planted by these contributors will stimulate health information management (HIM) professionals to meet the challenges of the next century. Transforming health care to meet the demands of the next decade requires collaborating and developing alliances with other professionals, committing ourselves to new roles, and being open to new ideas.

TRANSFORMING HEALTH INFORMATION MANAGEMENT

Linda L. Kloss

The scope of the national effort to bring up a fully interoperable information technology (IT) network for health care has been described as equivalent to converting one seventh of the U.S. economy from paper to computer. The case for this massive undertaking has become so compelling that the dialog has changed over the past 5 years from "if" to "how" and "how fast." The vision of what success will look like is coming into sharper focus and leadership for change is emerging in the public and private sector.

The Case for a Wired Health Care System

According to the Institute of Medicine (IOM) and others, the U.S. health care delivery system is one of the most complex systems in the world.[1] It is inefficient, highly fragmented, and very expensive. In 2004, the United States spent $1.79 trillion on its health system, or 15.5% of our gross national product. This is a substantially higher rate of spending than any other country, and at the current rate of growth the United States will be spending $3.58 trillion in 10 years.[2] Despite this level of spending, health care is simply not affordable or available for many of our country's citizens. Nearly 50 million citizens do not have health insurance and the gap between those who have access to world-class care and those who do not is increasing rapidly.

The problems of patient safety and variability in quality are also well documented. In its landmark 1999 study, researchers at the IOM documented that between 44,000 and 98,000 people die in hospitals in the United States each year as a result of medical errors.[3] It is projected that nearly one third of the $1.6 trillion the United States spent in 2003 went to care that is duplicative, fails to improve patient health, or may even make it worse. In addition to cost, access, and safety, the aging of our population also supports the case for a wired health care system because chronic disease cannot be effectively managed without access to information.

No one expects that an interoperable health information system is a panacea. But there is growing consensus in Washington, DC, in state capitals across the land, and in the private sector that the other problems of our health care system cannot be solved without an information infrastructure. Stated another way, it will not be possible to transform any aspect of health care delivery in the United States without better information and better information tools. Research has begun to document real cost and quality improvements achievable with advanced electronic health records (EHRs). For example, it is estimated that adoption of advanced computer systems for drug ordering in the outatient setting could eliminate more than two million adverse drug events and 190,000 hospitalizations per year. This would save $44 billion per year. Standardized exchange of health care information between providers would deliver national savings of $86.8 billion annually.[4]

A Compelling Vision

On April 27, 2004, President George W. Bush called for widespread adoption of interoperable EHRs within 10 years. He established the position of National Coordinator for Health Information Technology, and in July 2004 the National Coordinator released a report entitled "The Decade of Health Information Technology: Delivering Consumer-Centric and Information-Rich Health Care," which outlined a framework for strategic action consisting of four broad goals, each with three key strategies.[5] The general framework for action includes the following:

Informing clinical practice—This goal encompasses efforts to bring EHRs directly into clinical practice. The rate of adoption of EHRs is accelerating, but strategies and incentives are needed to scale the rate, particularly in solo or small practices.

Interconnect clinicians—A wired health care system must be capable of exchanging information among its components. This requires protocols, standards, and a common set of intercommunication tools such as authentication tools, Web services architecture, and security technologies. It also requires privacy practices that will hold up to public scrutiny.

Personalize care—People must learn to use information to better manage their own wellness and assist with their personal care decisions. This goal aims to encourage the use of personal health records and provide access to meaningful information to enable people to select clinicians and institutions on the basis of meaningful measures of their performance.

Improve population health—Goal 4 pertains to the need to use information to continually improve the quality of clinical care, health delivery, and the public health systems.

Taken together, these four goals form a powerful agenda for change to be carried out over the next decade through many national and local projects by the public and private sectors. Federal leadership from the Secretary of Health and

Human Services, the Office of the National Coordinator, federal health programs such as the Veteran's Health Administration and the Department of Defense are essential to advancing this vision. Public-private collaboration has been an effective way of securing commitment to the vision from multiple stakeholder health care organizations across the country that heretofore has worked in isolation.

As we move into 2006, the focus will be on deploying standards so that EHR systems can exchange information. The focus will also be on advancing our learning about how to implement and use systems for the greatest benefit realization. This calls into question the critical issue of having a knowledgeable workforce of HIM and informatics experts capable of supporting the transformation. And, of course, financing the transformation is a continuing challenge. Although payback is certainly anticipated, the up-front end cost is prohibitive for many health care organizations and for the federal and state governments.

In 5 short years, we have reached an important juncture in transforming health care through modern IT. There is a vision and a short-term set of action plans. There is leadership and a growing consensus on the criticality of this agenda to health care. The framework will undoubtedly be refined with experience. Some strategies will prove sound, whereas others will be adapted or abandoned. Although it will surely take the United States at least the next decade to accomplish change of this scale, the challenges today are about how to ensure that change happens, not whether change is needed. In itself, this is a very big step forward.

A Health Information Management Profession in Transition

HIM professionals have essential skills and competencies needed to build and operate an interoperable health information system. With the national agenda coming into sharper focus, the pressure is on the HIM field to be ready to lead.

In 2003, the American Health Information Management Association (AHIMA) appointed a task force of experts in HIM practice, medical informatics, academia, and IT from both the private sector and the government to help AHIMA develop a plan to help the field move more expeditiously by the following[6]:

- Promoting migration from paper medical records to electronic health information
- Reinventing and redesign how health information and records are managed
- Delivering measurable cost and quality results from improved information management

This is not a new focus for the field or AHIMA, but the initiative reflects the need for greater focus and acceleration of the pace of transformational change so that all HIM practitioners are contributing to the transition to an electronic practice environment. The initiative is a way of convening strategic conversations across the field about the need for proactive change leadership.

At the same time, AHIMA's Foundation for Research and Education (FORE) conducted extensive research on the health information workforce in the United States for the following reasons[7]:

- To assess the current workforce, its characteristics, and its roles
- To understand how IT will affect roles
- To understand new competencies that will be needed to manage electronic records and information

This included research about current characteristics, roles and functions of practitioners, and perspectives of students and educators. It also included examination of how HIM roles were changing at organizations that have more advanced IT in place. Regarding the field today, we learned that HIM professionals work in 40 different work settings in 125 different job titles. The emphasis of HIM has shifted in recent years from processing, safeguarding, and retrieving records to helping people access information to support clinical decision making, administrative oversight, financial management, medical research, and personal health management. HIM professionals, along with nurses, physicians, IT experts, and others are involved in projects to implement EHRs and to connect the health care system.

Our research confirmed the importance of the HIM domain of practice going forward, but it also confirmed the need for new and deeper skills necessary for electronic HIM. This will demand advanced degrees, additional specialty training, and a strong commitment to life-long learning. For example, areas of specialization include clinical terminologies and classification systems, management of EHR systems, managing information security and privacy, and data analytics. EHRs, personal health records, interconnected clinicians, and IT-enabled research, and public health will require an HIM workforce, but one that has a different set of skills and competencies than in the past.

Milestones for Change

It took the United States just 11 years from the time the National Aeronautical and Space Administration was set up to put a man on the moon. It took 18 years from idea to a completed map of the human genome. The United States and other countries have embarked on national projects not unlike space travel or genomics in complexity and the impact on the way we live. We are pursuing fundamental change in health and health care through a national health information vision and strategy.

Perhaps the most important milestones ahead will be feedback from those at the front line, the physicians who must incorporate technology into their day-to-day work and the patients they serve. Research is beginning to show that physicians and patients alike report a more satisfying relationship because of better information, more efficient and effective care, and improved access.

As we migrate from paper to electronic information, the nexus of the work of HIM professionals will be to design and manage systems and processes to ensure information integrity, real time access to the right information, sound privacy and security protections, and the effective use of information for a variety of purposes from quality improvement to clinical trials. The new work of HIM professionals will be critical to all health care stakeholders, most especially the patients served by our health care system.

AHIMA is now helping to educate consumers about personal health information—why it is important and how to access, manage, and protect it. No longer is medical record information for use by physicians, hospitals, payers, and researchers only. Personal health records and access to information about health and health care will transform health care delivery and will transform HIM. Helping people organize and use their personal health information may be a new job for HIM professionals, but it is not a new mission and value of the field. Helping people through quality information has been a sustaining value for nearly 80 years.

HEALTH PROFESSIONALS FOR TRANSLATIONAL, CLINICAL, AND PUBLIC HEALTH/POPULATION INFORMATICS

Don E. Detmer and Jeffrey J. Williamson

This chapter seeks to inform the reader of educational developments relating to the American Medical Informatics Association (AMIA) as it moves into the next 7 years (2014), by which time President Bush expects Americans to be using EHRs for their personal care. As such, the health professional workforce part of the national story is a compelling one, and one that continues to unfold. Most important, AMIA has focused itself on ensuring that, as these years pass, IT will be a central means for transforming American health care into a system that focuses on population health and personal health and not be simply having ICT be pursued as an end in itself. And, as the IOM Chasm report recommends, AMIA wishes to see Information and Communications Technology (ICT) help create a health care system that is equitable, safe, efficient, effective, and patient centered and one that offers timely care.[1]

Biomedical/Health Informatics

Over the past 20 to 30 years, a growing number of health professionals, especially physicians and nurses, have carved out a new profession generally known as **biomedical** and/or **health informatics.** This has occurred quite naturally in the complex adaptive systems manner of "self-organization" as ICT and computer science applied to health research,

education, and care has developed. AMIA considers informaticians to be health professionals with relevant expertise in health sciences, epidemiology, cognitive sciences, computer science, computational biology, and engineering, all tied together with the common theme of technology and information.[8] Behavioralists and communications specialists feel that informatics puts too much attention on the technology vis-à-vis communications. Certainly, if care is to be transformed, we need to ensure that the human behavioral, communication, and information technology, and computer and health sciences, come together in the proper mix.

Titles do matter in health care. Nursing and medicine appear to differ on what to call the graduates of their programs. Nursing appears to be converging around the title of **nursing informatics specialist,** whereas medicine typically describes graduates as being either biomedical or medical informaticians. Others use informaticists to describe a person who is an expert and engaged in the practice or research of informatics. In summary, it is clearly safe to say that not all in or related to the field are yet comfortable with the term *informatician*. As a founder (D. E. D.) of the discipline of administrative medicine in the mid 1970s, I can attest that it took 25 years for the term to gain general acceptance and that there are still detractors who favor executive medicine or other options. In any event, the next 5 years are certain to be pivotal for both the nation and its national health information infrastructure and for those professionals who cast their lot with this fascinating career choice.

In many respects, the 3500 or 4000 biomedical and health informaticians are essentially hybrid experts bridging a clinical discipline with knowledge and skills in ICT applied to health. AMIA and its honorific college, the American College of Medical Informatics, have been the principal organizations for this group of individuals whose interests and expertise are quite diverse. Sharing a keen interest in scholarship and also the practical applications of ICT, they have been key players in comprising the emerging disciplines we now refer to as translational bioinformatics, clinical informatics, and public health/population informatics. Each domain has fuzzy borders and there is ample opportunity for discussion and debate on what exactly constitutes each category and whether these categories do justice to all relevant areas of interest and concern. For example, visualization, imaging, and simulation are three other domains that intersect the field.

AMIA is measurably strengthened by those members who live in 52 nations around the world and as such, along with the International Medical Informatics Association, plays international and national roles. When it is considered that the first department of medical informatics was so named at the University of Utah in 1984, it can be realized how quickly the field has matured in the United States. Medical informatics in the United States is both theoretically and practically based in comparison with the field in Europe that has been more theoretically grounded historically.

In this country, the field of nursing informatics has led the health professions by developing both a formal process for program accreditation and graduate certification. It is now becoming evident that the house of medicine also needs to give full professional standing and stature to informatics as a discipline. The exact form certification will take in medicine is uncertain at the time, but a summit meeting will be held in 2007 for a number of interested national medical boards to discuss appropriate next steps. It is likely that a subcertificate within the current board structure, such as a subcertificate in emergency medicine, and a few other boards will develop.

The fact that AMIA was elected to membership in the Council of Medical Specialty Societies in November 2006 is clear evidence that medical informatics is here to stay and will only become more important in the years ahead. The growth in the knowledge base relevant to health and illness, the demands for evidence-based medicine, the move to computer-based record systems, and the growth of the Internet among other forces all point to a health care system with a robust ICT infrastructure needing experts to make it develop and function properly. Human memory unaided by access to knowledge bases and increasingly sophisticated decision support systems just will not get the right care delivered or support citizens wishing to manage their own health and its care.[8a]

Workforce Needs

How many informaticians are needed? As discussed previously, it is reasonable to state that AMIA considers informaticians to be health professionals who also have expertise in components of health sciences, epidemiology, cognitive sciences, computer science, computational biology, and engineering, all tied together with the common theme of technology and information.[8]

Using this definition or something quite akin to it, Charles Safran, MD, Chairman of the Board of AMIA in 2005, estimated that somewhere around 10,000 informaticians would be needed to help the nation meet the goal set by President Bush for computer-based health records. AHIMA and AMIA cohosted a summit in 2005 to examine the workforce needs for professionals who typically see these organizations as being their professional home base.[8b]

AMIA's 10 × 10 Program

In the summer of 2005 AMIA launched its 10 × 10 program[9] to address part of the workforce situation. The AMIA 10 × 10 program uses curricular content from existing informatics training programs and other AMIA educational initiatives with a special emphasis toward those programs with a proven track record in distance learning. The content provides a framework but also cover details, especially in areas such as electronic and personal health records, health information exchange, standards and terminology, and health care quality and error prevention. AMIA 10 × 10 programs mostly focus on applied clinical informatics but

others are developing in the three major domains in the field of informatics:

- Clinical or health care (including personal health management; electronic and personal health records, health information exchange, standards and terminology, and health care quality and error prevention)
- Public health and population informatics
- Translational bioinformatics principally bridging research findings from genomics, proteomics, and epigenetics.

We anticipate that there will continue to be many professionals who will pursue a doctor of philosophy degree, especially in translational bioinformatics. The 10 × 10 program is aimed generally at those who are clinicians seeking to build a research or practice career combining their clinical expertise with informatics. Corollary to this goal, the 10 × 10 program will bring recognition and awareness to the informatics expertise found in AMIA's member institutions and it will highlight the breadth of education opportunities that are available throughout the country and in some instances around the world as well. For example, the major 10 × 10 offering from Oregon Health Sciences University has been translated into Spanish and taught to over 200 clinicians in South America. The American College of Physicians and the California Health Care Foundation have also funded AMIA 10 × 10 programs for clinicians,

Other Education Initiatives

AMIA also wishes to support faculty in community colleges to gain the basic skills in informatics needed to prepare the broad spectrum of learners across the nation in basic ICT skills—both less intensively trained health workers and citizens. The International Computer Driving License Foundation is another model that the United States could support and of which AMIA is well aware because one of the authors (D. E. D.) has helped with others to build a health curriculum for Europe. The AMIA sees outreach to broader populations of ICT learners as being a relevant part of its "Got EHR?" initiative, an AMIA effort encouraging clinicians and citizens to adopt computer-based health records.[10]

Educators in the field of informatics have long desired a national framework by which managers in health care practice settings can define roles related to important informatics and health information technology (HIT) functions. In late 2001 the AMIA Education Committee discussed the need to identify such roles and began a process of developing comprehensive sets and subsets of "core health and biomedical informatics competencies." On November 13-14, 2002, a retreat of the Education Committee lead by Chairman John H. Holmes, PhD, was held in San Antonio, Texas, that resulted in a white paper presented to the AMIA Board of Directors. An updated version is nearing completion.

A clear application was seen for existing and emerging informatics training programs with value extending to other academic disciplines. The exercise of assigning a definition to each competency was determined to be best left to a broader constituency. The set of resulting information could be "viewed as the minimal knowledge, skill, values, experience, and judgment that a person needs to possess in order to function within a specific role in a particular craft or profession."

A consensus/delphi approach was used by the committee to gather educational outcome objectives of a broad range of informatics training programs, including informatics training programs, short courses, AMIA-sponsored education activities, and course documents such as syllabi and lecture notes. AMIA sees this work continuing in 2007 with the organization, analysis, and publication of these competencies. At its recent annual meeting, the AMIA expanded its tutorial sessions that have drawn on this work. Along the way, the notion of "core" competencies became unpopular in many circles and the trend in labeling this effort has moved toward "basic" or "informatics" competencies. Nonetheless, the informatics and broader HIT community must organize around a common set of education principles.

Another educational initiative that AMIA's strategic plan commits itself to develop is a common introductory curriculum in informatics for all entry-level health professional students. The goal is to identify a basic entry-level set of knowledge and skills that can be constructed in a modular fashion so that schools across the country can pick and choose from the various modules or simply adopt the full curriculum as their basic course in IT. The Macy Foundation has funded a basic curriculum in communications skills and this additional curriculum could be very useful. In the view of the authors, this course should examine basic understandings in organizational behavior and aspects of change management and more central dimensions of informatics. Obviously, the curriculum will be developed and will evolve as funding becomes available to pursue this objective. At least some major health professional associations have expressed interest in this initiative but a great deal of work will be needed before it becomes more than simply an attractive idea.

All the efforts presented here are viewed by the authors as vital to the field of biomedical/health informatics whose roots go back at least a few decades, and which seems now to be poised to play a pivotal role as an integrating force related to science and knowledge management in the transformation of the U.S. health care system. Collaboration and partnership with other disciplines will be crucial for future success in informatics because this field is intrinsically integrative in nature. It must remain flexible enough to incorporate new informations technologies and the explosive growth in the knowledge bases relating to health care.

COLLABORATING FOR CHANGE

Marion J. Ball

"A new technology does not add or subtract something. It changes everything. ... New technologies alter the structure of our interests: the things we think *about*. They alter the character of our symbols: the things we think *with*. And they alter the nature of community: the arena in which thoughts develop." So wrote communications theorist Neil Postman in 1992, early in the decade when the human factors movement achieved acceptance in the health informatics community.[11]

Technology and Change

As we work to create the EHR envisioned by President Bush and the National Health Information Network (NHIN) and what it requires for full functionality, we are banking on Postman's being right. Our plans to transform the health care system count on IT to enable the extent of change Postman described, change that includes everything—"interrelationships between humans, the tools they use, and the environment in which they live and work," what the IOM defines as human factors.[12]

Consider a "simple" tool, e-prescribing. According to one physician, it means "... you're not just digitizing a prescription pad, but rather, entering patients' recent history, recalls, interaction and allergy checks, perhaps other indications such as patient weight, co-morbid conditions and such. You're actually spending time and effort creating better input. So you're fundamentally changing what docs do."[13]

Any clinical system, including e-prescribing and computerized physician order entry (CPOE) among others, affects "nursing staff, ward assistants, pharmacists, and staff in the laboratory and radiology departments" as well as physicians.[14] Nurses especially are affected by changes in clinical workflow. When their roles "as an integrator (or coordinator) of care and as a reviewer (or checker/editor) of orders" were significantly reduced, nurses at one institution expressed dissatisfaction with their changed roles, despite having time freed up for direct patient care.[15]

An article in *Annals of Internal Medicine* concluded that, because CPOE "fundamentally changes the ordering process," its costs are "substantial both in terms of technology and organizational process analysis and redesign, system implementation, and user training and support."[14] Two very different experiences with CPOE are often reviewed for the lessons they offer on the importance of human factors in technology implementation. They are discussed briefly below.

Two Case Studies

Partners HealthCare and Brigham began development of their CPOE system in 1991. From the outset, the development team acknowledged that CPOE constituted "a radical cultural change." The team acted to lessen resistance by having a physician serve as chief designer for the system, soliciting clinician input through two pilot trials and phasing in implementation from 1993 to 1996. According to the chief technology officer at Partners, "... we smothered them with support. ... We had knowledgeable, pleasant people available to hold their hand and get them through implementation. After six months, things settled down." On the floors where clinicians worked, support was available 24 hours a day for what was regarded as "… a clinical initiative with an I.T. component."[16] Implementation at Massachusetts General Hospital and the Dana Farber Institute followed.

In January 2003, the $34 million CPOE developed in-house at Cedars-Sinai Medical Center in Los Angeles was turned off, 3 months after it had been turned on. Physicians protested mandatory certification (which had been approved by a physician-led executive committee) and the additional time it took to enter orders (despite using a clinical rules taxonomy expressly to facilitate physician acceptance and approval).[13] They complained about the system's inability to accommodate misspellings and its use of overly intrusive alerts. Human and organizational factors cited as contributing to its failure included involving only "a fraction" of doctors in system development, providing insufficient training, and not phasing in implementation but rather going for a "big bang" approach.[17]

Lessons Learned

Historically, physicians have been criticized for being slow to adopt institutional technologies such as CPOE. Perhaps, as one analyst suggested, "most of the information technology that has been put forward to doctors over the last 20 years has been designed to improve the rest of the health care system a little bit at the expense of the doctor," not to provide "clear business value" to physicians.[18] Recent survey data show that physicians are adopting technology at a "significantly higher rate" than the general public and are heavier users of computers at or for work and five times more likely to own personal digital assistants (PDAs).[19]

With almost a decade between them, the implementations at Cedars-Sinai and the Brigham are difficult to compare. Nonetheless, whatever technical issues were at play, it was physician resistance that brought down the system at Cedars-Sinai. As Lorenzi and Riley stated, "people who have low psychological ownership in a system and who vigorously resists its implementation can bring a 'technically best' systems to its knees." In their view, insufficient user ownership and communications deficiencies often cause implementation failure.[20,21]

In 2003, reports stated that many of the initial protesters at Cedars-Sinai were internists. This led to two theories: (1) they had not been included as a group in the planning and (2) as primary care physicians who treat a wider range of conditions than specialists, they may have needed more support when the system was introduced.[13] Certainly, the "big bang" approach allowed no time to fine tune the system or to grow constituencies of users among physicians and across physician groups.

Since 1997, a research team from Oregon Health and Science University has studied CPOE at successful sites. Their findings acknowledge the need to address different groups: "Context matters and it affects the way of doing things: The time and place, institutional context, professional and departmental context, and the individual's role cause perceptions to vary."[22]

One other theme sounded by the Oregon research team is particularly relevant: "multidisciplinary collaboration and trust." It is echoed in the phrase "professional and departmental context" and in the assertion that "it is a myth that only doctors give orders, since other clinicians like nurses and pharmacists are part of the process as well."[22]

Collaboration

Collaboration is an essentially human endeavor. As systems involve "larger, more heterogeneous groups of people and more organizational areas," human factors become more significant.[20] In initiatives of the scope we are now undertaking—to have an EHR for every American and the health information network to support it—technology does indeed change everything in health care. As the IOM explained, "When technology shifts workloads, it also shifts interactions between team members."[12] These are not trivial changes: they "change roles and the social order."[23]

Hence, collaboration is critical. In *To Err Is Human*, the IOM called on us to recognize technology "as a 'member' of the work team."[12] In like manner, the initiative known as TIGER, for Technology Informatics Guiding Educational Reform, calls on us to acknowledge the role of the nursing profession.

Nursing

In 2005, the TIGER initiative brought together nurses and nurse advocates from education, government, industry, and practice for a 1-day consensus building meeting. The participants expressed their determination to ensure the continued vitality of the nursing profession and to become key partners in the national efforts to transform the health care system. This, they agreed, required informatics competencies.

Although core competencies have been identified, they have yet to be incorporated into accreditation standards and performance appraisals to be disseminated to nursing organizations and others outside informatics. To meet this challenge and to give nursing the prominence it requires, the TIGER team explicated a vision for the nursing profession in the twenty-first century that focuses on integrating IT into nursing by bridging the gap between education and practice. To realize this vision, the team held a 2-day national invitational meeting October 31 through November 1, 2006, attended by nursing organizations, government agencies, and other key stakeholders (academic institutions, practice settings, the vendor community).

Outcomes of the meeting are to include action plans for specific institutions and a high-level report with exemplars and recommendations to guide the nursing profession as it works to transform health care and realize the goals of the IOM—care that is *safe, effective, patient centered, timely, efficient, and equitable.*[24]

Health Information Management

In 2003, AHIMA published a report setting forth its vision for 2010. The future state of health information, AHIMA concluded, is "electronic, patient-centered, comprehensive, longitudinal, accessible, and credible."[25] The same report acknowledged the impact of external forces on HIM, including workforce concerns and consumer awareness.

A number of the report's 10 recommendations echoed the precepts guiding the TIGER initiative. The first acknowledged the need for collaboration and recommended that AHIMA "lead a consortium of groups and organizations in influencing national efforts." The second called for expanding "the visibility of AHIMA and health information management." Other recommendations highlighted the need for changes in training, education, and curriculum and for recertification and continuing education.

Like the TIGER initiative, AHIMA has targeted nothing less than the transformation of an entire profession. They are actively advancing their vision through work with such groups as the EHR Collaborative, Connecting for Health, eHealth Initiative Foundation projects, the Alliance, and Health Level 7 (HL7). In addition, they have acted to address work force issues through such mechanisms as accreditation, recruitment, and faculty development.[19]

Technology as Enabler

As a tool, technology enables change, but it is humans who use those tools. To transform the health care system that serves us all, we must work to bring theory into practice. To succeed, we must acknowledge the importance of human factors and of the nursing profession as well.

INTERNATIONAL HEALTH INFORMATION MANAGEMENT

Jean S. Clark

HIM has changed tremendously over the years and no more so than over the last 5 years. Advances in technology, regulatory requirements, an increased attention to data quality, and the need to have a portable personal health record are factors contributing to the change. None is greater, however, than the public's demand for accurate, timely, and complete information about their health care and their care providers and the ability to easily transport their health information in a transient society. Furthermore, there is a consensus within the industry that we cannot address these issues without bringing a global perspective to our solutions.

No longer can we think of HIM as unique to the United States. Now and in the future, we should increase our global perspective and understanding of HIM and the professionals who work in that discipline throughout the world. My contribution to this chapter will explore HIM topics that are international in nature and the solutions applied to these issues that must be developed from an international perspective.

International Federation of Health Records Organizations

The International Federation of Health Records Organizations (IFHRO) was formed in 1968 by a group of "medical record" professionals who saw the need to bring together health records organizations across the world. Membership was composed of medical record associations and not individual members. For example, AHIMA was a founding member of IFHRO. Today, this organization has grown to include 22 countries' health information management associations and has expanded to include individual and corporate members. The goal of IFHRO is to promote health record practices and education throughout the world with a special emphasis on assisting developing countries in that regard. IFHRO identified the following five common issues facing the international community of HIM as the focus of its work[26]:

- The EHR
- Clinical data quality
- Privacy, security, and confidentiality of personal health information
- Education
- Needs of developing countries

It is clear that these issues are ones that transcend the global community and should be addressed from a broader perspective than just what is happening within an individual country. It is also imperative that the richer countries help with the developing countries to improve health information, which leads to better data and better health.

Over the next 10 years, continued changes in health care will require standardization in health information practice standards, educational requirements for HIM, and improved data quality and accessibility to data and information to improve health care around the world. It will also mean that the developed world must help the developing countries to develop and maintain at least an entry level of HIM practices to improve communication, understanding of disease, and ultimately patient care. It is a big job, indeed, but one that must be done and led by health information management professionals around the world.

The Electronic Health Record

The EHR is not unique to the United States. In fact, some countries are far ahead in this initiative. Many countries, such as the United Kingdom, Canada, and Ireland are promoting the EHR as a matter of public policy. It should be noted that beginning in 2005, the United States began to develop and implement a national health information network.

Standards development organizations are international in scope such as HL7 and International Organization for Standardization (ISO). Many EHR technology vendors are internationally based. Many countries are adopting Systematized Nomenclature of Human and Veterinary Medicine (SNOMED) and other terminologies and systems. Underlying these commonalities is the need to improve quality, control costs, manage chronic diseases, and improve public health surveillance.

Understanding how nations are approaching the EHR, identifying the skills and competencies needed by health information professionals who work in an electronic environment, identifying ways HIM associations can advance the EHR through collaboration, identifying resources and understanding ways organizations such as IFHRO can help support the work of national countries are global initiatives that will further the implementation of the EHR worldwide.

The EHR may never be implemented in every country of the world, but the need to improve the information and communications technology infrastructure from a global perspective supports the EHR as a key technology in this infrastructure.

Clinical Data Management

Accuracy, accessibility, comprehensiveness, consistency, currency, definition, granularity, precision, relevance, and timeliness are characteristics of data quality. The patient's health record serves as the means of communication among health care providers, it is the tool used to make decisions about the patient's care, it serves as a legal document, and it is used for planning, education, research, financial reimbursement, and quality and outcome measurement activities. Thus, the quality of the health record and the quality of its content are paramount to the delivery of quality health care.

How countries are approaching clinical data management and data quality and the skills and competencies identified as needed by health information professionals are issues that are important to ensuring consistencies and credibility of data and information around the world.

The World Health Organization (WHO) has recognized the need to promote better data quality through a collaborative effort with IFHRO to certify morbidity and mortality coders. Only through standardization of coding practices and education can clinical data and information become meaningful and useful to improve the quality of health care and ultimately the health of people around the world.

Privacy, Security, and Confidentiality of Personal Health Information

From a global perspective, this issue is probably the most sensitive. Because not all countries view the personal health record and health information as confidential, it is difficult to promote laws such as the United States' Health Insurance Portability and Accountability Act (HIPAA) as important or necessary. However, as the world becomes smaller and the commitment to improve the dignity and rights of human beings around the world increases, so will the need for laws (or processes) to ensure privacy, security, and confidentiality of personal health information.

It will behoove those in the global community who already recognize these needs to develop a broader understanding of how nations are, or are not, approaching the issue of privacy legislation, to also identify the skills and competencies needed by HIM professionals in this regard and to share best practice among HIM around the world to promote privacy, security, and confidentiality of personal health information.

Education

Of all the global issues facing HIM, education is most likely the biggest international opportunity. There are academic programs in this discipline in many countries, although degree status and curricular content varies. HIM is not widely recognized as a distinct body of knowledge. Changes in HIM are so rapid that advanced curricular content needs to be advanced quickly. In some countries, baccalaureate programs are at risk due to low enrollment, postgraduate programs are slow to develop, and some countries have no academic education at all but recognize the need.

Current issues that would benefit from an international educational standpoint include a shared professional definition; standardized competencies for HIM practice; curriculum models; faculty development; nurturing new programs at the technical, baccalaureate, and master's levels; sharing best practices in student recruitment; gaining recognition in the health informatics discipline; external program accreditation practices; and certification of individual practitioners.

Needs of Developing Countries

From a professional and ethical standpoint, it only seems appropriate that responding to the needs of developing countries cannot be left out of the international HIM equation. Many countries do not have health records at all but recognize the need for them. Communications among caregivers is by word of mouth in many cases. Formal academic programs do not exist and "on-the-job training" is limited. Although the world is getting smaller every day with the use of technology and communication, advanced HIM practice is not developing at the same pace.

It will be important to establish a broader understanding of the needs of developing countries as they relate to HIM and to identify how the developed world can help promote HIM practices in developing countries. By providing access to best practice, resources, and experts, the world of HIM in developing countries can improve.

The Joint Commission

So far, I have addressed issues facing HIM from a practice and professional standpoint. However, it would be an omission not to address another factor influencing the global community and that is accreditation. The Joint Commission has an international division and more and more countries' health care organizations are requesting The Joint Commission accreditation for their hospitals. HIM professionals in the United States have been traditionally involved in the success of their organizations' Joint Commission surveys. International accreditation can provide these same opportunities for involvement on the global level.

The Joint Commission has recently partnered with WHO to eliminate medical errors worldwide. WHO has designated The Joint Commission as the world's first WHO Collaborating Center dedicated solely to patient safety. In a press release issued in August 2005, Dr. Dennis S. O'Leary, President, The Joint Commission, said, "Together, we can measurably strengthen and improve patient safety worldwide by spreading proven practices without regard to borders or other barriers that frequently exist in the international arena. This partnership should truly make a difference in improving the safety and, the quality of health care for people throughout the world."[27]

HIM professionals around the world can be of assistance in this initiative by continuing to promote complete, accurate, and timely medical records and the quality of clinical data and information.

International Opportunities

As consultants, educators, and resources for best practice and collaboration, HIM professionals have a role in their own countries and in the international community. Understanding the issues and stepping out of the security of one's own country can provide opportunities and challenges that will have a far-reaching impact on health information practices around the world. The world will be a better place from HIM professionals' involvement. Think internationally; act nationally.

PUBLIC HEALTH INFORMATION: A STRATEGIC RESOURCE

Bryant T. Karras and Mary Alice Hanken

Public Health and Medical Care

As we take a more overall view of health, we recognize the value of lifestyles, safe and clean communities, and the myriad of things we can do to prevent injuries at home, at work, and in our communities. As organizations prepare to "manage" individuals' health care, they realize that the power and payoff are not in treating individuals for expensive diseases and conditions but in preventing disease and in educating consumers to take care of themselves. This shift is the impetus needed to bring the public health sector and the medical care sectors together. The long-range goals of both groups are similar, but to many observers it appears that the two sectors are not strongly connected.

Public health provides both direct clinical services and community services. It addresses both the individual and the population being served in a community or wider region. Public health goals for the year 2010 are expressed in terms of the entire population in the United States, for example, as follows:

- Environmental: Reduce pesticide exposures that result in visits to a health care facility. Target: 13,500 per year, (baseline: 27,156 visits to health care facilities were due to pesticides in 1997)[28]
- Respiratory: Reduce hospital emergency department visits for asthma per year. Target: Children under age 5 years: 80 per 10,000 population; age 5 to 64 years: 50 per 10,000 population; age 65 years and older: 15 per 10,000 population, (baseline: Children under age 5 years: 150.0 per 10,000 population; age 5 to 64 years: 71.1 per 10,000 population; over age 64 years: 29.5 per 10,000 population. 1995-1997 data).[28]

Population–Based Data

Managed care organizations that take on a group of enrollees are now asked to express their data in terms of the population they serve. The Health Plan Employer Data and Information Set (HEDIS) report card system looks at data much the same as the *Healthy People 2010* goals and has some similar goals in its quality of care measures. These are approximate measures of meeting a quality-of-care goal for a given population. Employers who purchase health care need some type of feedback regarding the quality of care purchased for the dollar spent. HEDIS includes a number of measures in a variety of categories. Although weighted toward measures based on data available on billing claims, data extracted from clinical records are also used to evaluate these measures, for example, use of appropriate medications for people with asthma. This measure estimates the percentage of enrolled members age 5 to 56 years with persistent asthma who received medications deemed acceptable by the National Heart, Lung, and Blood Institute for long-term asthma control. The rates are broken down by age group. Asthma was chosen because it is a costly and increasingly prevalent disease. It affects an estimated 20.3 million Americans, including 6.3 million children. Many health care visits, hospitalizations, missed work and school days could be avoided if individuals have appropriate medications and disease management.

Another HEDIS measure is adolescent immunization status. This is a measure of the percentage of enrolled adolescents who turn 13 years of age during the measurement year and who had a second dose of measles-mumps-rubella vaccine and three hepatitis B vaccinations by their thirteenth birthdays. The varicella (chickenpox) vaccination is also reported. The rationale notes that "of the estimated 125,000 new cases of hepatitis B each year, more than 70 percent affect adolescents and young adults. Hepatitis B is highly infectious and sometimes results in liver failure and death."[29]

As communities discuss and implement regional data systems, they expand the base of population data available. Although most care providers hope that these systems will also support individual direct care through coordinating and reduction of duplication, most policymakers and researchers see the benefit in gaining access to more population-based data. As HEDIS and regional and national systems demonstrate, data are valuable only if they are accurate and reliable. This requires appropriate definitions for data, standards for the content, collection, and quality of the data—all skills of the health information manager.

It has always been true that a hospital or health care system is not isolated from its surrounding community. For this reason, the health information professional must take seriously the role or partnership in protecting the health of his or her region. The activities are identified by the core functions, fundamental obligations, and essential services of public health. An important component of these functions that health information manager can assist in is in "assessment." The functions of assessment include monitoring, diagnosing, and investigating health problems and hazards. The other obligations and core functions of public health are outlined below.

Information Needs and Core Public Health Functions

The public health and managed care/medical care systems have similar information needs. The following discussion focuses primarily on public health. The goal of public health is prevention of disease, injury, disability, and premature death: public health is not simply medical care funded or provided through public means.[30] Sometimes the services of public health are less visible and may be more difficult to understand than medical services. We may not think of clean water as contributing to our health, but contamination of drinking water results in sickness. Even today, when floods or earthquakes hit areas of the United States, water supplies may be disrupted or contaminated. Leaching of chemicals from farmland fertilizers or pesticides or industrial plants is another source of contamination. Public health prevention measures are designed to protect entire communities or populations from such threats as communicable diseases, epidemics, and environmental contaminants (Box 19-1).

Box 19-1   PUBLIC HEALTH OBLIGATIONS

The fundamental obligation of agencies responsible for population-based health is as follows:

- To prevent epidemics and the spread of disease
- To protect against environmental hazards
- To prevent injuries
- To promote and encourage healthy behaviors and mental health
- To respond to disasters and assist communities in recovery
- To ensure the quality and accessibility of health services

Public health functions are organized around several core activities (Figure 19-1 and Box 19-2), which include the following[31]:

- Assessment—collecting, analyzing, and disseminating information on health status, personal health problems, population groups at greatest risk, availability and quality of services, resource availability, and concerns of individuals.
- Policy development—using the assessment data to consider alternatives and determine which actions and policies to pursue.

Box 19-2   ESSENTIAL SERVICES

Public health agencies accomplish these responsibilities by implementing the following 10 services[31]:

Assessment
1. **Monitor** health status to identify community health problems.
2. **Diagnose and investigate** health problems and health hazards in the community.

Policy Development
3. Inform, educate, and empower people about health issues.
4. Mobilize community partnerships to identify and solve health problems.
5. Develop policies and plans that support individual and community health efforts.

Assurance
6. **Enforce** laws and regulations that protect health and ensure safety.
7. **Link** people to needed personal health services and ensure the provision of health care when otherwise unavailable.
8. **Ensure** a competent public health and personal health care workforce.
9. **Evaluate** effectiveness, accessibility, and quality of personal and population-based health services.

Serving All Functions
10. **Research** for new insights and innovative solutions to health problems.

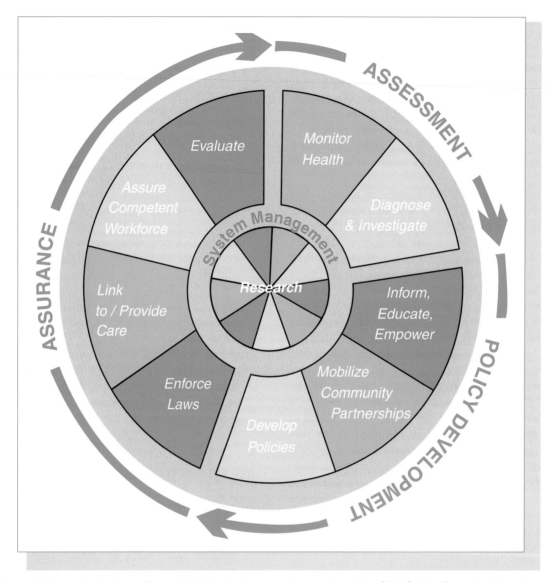

Figure 19-1 Public health functions. (From Public Health Functions Steering Committee [1994]: http://www.health.gov/phfunctions/images/pubh_wh2.gif.)

- Assurance—monitoring actions and policy decisions of public health and other community partners to attain the goals of public health.

Public Health Programs

Proven cost-effective public health measures include water fluoridation to prevent tooth decay, smoking cessation among pregnant women to prevent low birth weight, immunizations to prevent measles and mumps, and health education of consumers to reduce their need for medical services.[30] Many Americans take public health programs for granted. However, much like the health care system, there is a cadre of trained professionals with a system in place to prevent public health problems and to respond when an epidemic breaks out or a toxic chemical is spilled. When young children were being admitted to the hospital for treatment of *Escherichia coli* infection, it was the public health department that tracked down the source of the problem as contaminated hamburger meat and undercooking of the hamburger. All states have health departments with county and city coverage. Most public health departments work with the medical community on some aspects of care. For example, the *E. coli* outbreak was both a clinical treatment problem and a public health problem. Pediatricians and family practitioners usually work closely with the public health department in immunizing children against many childhood diseases. Both the medical care system and the public health system take an interest in prevention of injury, illness, and disease. The most intense development of those interests may be the catalyst that brings the community together.

For much of the last 40 years, public health has been defined by a series of categorical programs and problems such as acquired immunodeficiency syndrome (AIDS), tuberculosis, sewage treatment, immunizations, food-borne illnesses, and primary care for the underserved. When a problem was identified and brought into public view, legislators enacted laws and appropriated funds to address that specific problem. Public health agencies responded by organizing themselves to carry out disease-specific or problem-specific programs.[30]

The result of these disease- and program-specific efforts and their reporting requirements is often a disconnected, dysfunctional information system—the components are each intended to meet a specific program need. In many states this results in program-specific data systems. For this problem of having individual dedicated channels the term "*stove pipes*" is commonly used. To expand the analogy, it would be preferable to have one large smoke stack to clean and maintain rather than a dozen different stove pipes of various sizes and configurations. In analyzing its data collection forms for all programs, one state found that it was asking for the individual's address more than 300 times. A coordinated system that allows "registration" once would be a tremendous step forward in reducing the administrative paperwork burden. The next step in the transition would be to build a coordinated database and eliminate program-specific, free-standing information systems. The Washington State Public Health Improvement Plan for 2005-2007 contains several recommendations related to information technology, including developing a shared administrative structure, identifying areas where better use of technology could improve public health practice and evaluating standards for data collection.[30]

Health Problems and Costs

Public health takes a long look at the real causes of health problems in the United States. It is estimated that about half of all deaths are caused by tobacco use, improper diet, lack of physical activity, alcohol misuse, microbial and toxic agents, firearm use, unsafe sexual behavior, motor vehicle crashes, and illicit use of drugs. The element of personal and community responsibility in these causes of health problems is inescapable. With the possible exception of some microbes and toxic agents, all the causes listed are primarily a result of human behavior.

- In 2002, nearly 8000 Washingtonians died from tobacco-related illnesses. Tobacco-related illnesses are the leading cause of preventable death in Washington State. Direct medical costs associated with tobacco use in 2002 are estimated at $1.5 billion. One of Washington State's tobacco use goals is to reduce adult cigarette smoking to 16.5% or less by 2010 from a starting point of 22.4% in 2000. Since the launch of a smoking cessation program in 2000, there are about 115,000 fewer adult smokers.[32]
- Motor vehicle crashes were the leading cause of unintentional injury hospitalizations and deaths of children aged 0 to 17 years in Washington State in 1999 to 2001. Child safety seats lower a child's chance of death and injury by about 70%. About 45% of Washington State children who died as the result of a motor vehicle crash were unrestrained by a child safety seat or a seat belt at the time of the crash. During the time period of 1999-2001 there were approximately 355 hospitalizations and 10,600 emergency department visits annually as the result of motor vehicle injuries to children aged 0 to 17 years.[32]
- Wearing a bicycle helmet is estimated to reduce the risk of a head injury by 85%. Head injury is the most common cause of serious injury, disability, and death in bicycle accidents. In Washington State the leading cause of injury hospitalizations for children aged 5 to 14 years was a bicycle injury in 1999-2001.[32]
- Cardiovascular disease, including heart disease and stroke, is the leading cause of death in the United States and in Washington State, accounting for about 33% of all deaths.[30] Cardiovascular disease mortality and morbidity can be reduced by controlling four major modifiable risk factors: physical inactivity, tobacco use, high blood pressure, and high cholesterol levels.

The burning cigarette, the moving car, the raw hamburger, and the failed on-site sewage system are all carriers of health threats that are best dealt with early.

Improving Health

Public health can be a powerful tool. Its population-based focus helps to accomplish changes and evaluate the magnitude of the problem. Public health professionals also actively participate in public education efforts.

The connection between public health and better health is well established. Since 1900, the average life expectancy of United States citizens has gone up from 45 to 75 years. Public health improvement in sanitation, the control of diseases though immunizations, and other activities are responsible for 25 of the 30 additional years that Americans can now expect to live. In addition, population-based public health of the 1970s contributed greatly to recent improvement in reduced tobacco use, blood pressure control, diet, use of seat belts, and injury control, which in turn have contributed to declines of more than 50% in deaths caused by stroke, 40% in deaths from heart disease, and 25% in overall death rates for children.

Integrating the Information System

To achieve the goals and to demonstrate that goals are met, public health needs an integrated information system.

Although some basic systems are in place, improvements are still needed. Public health systems still need the following:

- Redesign of program-specific, free-standing data systems into integrated systems
- An integrated, centrally managed, electronic network that provides access to federal, state, and local information systems
- Data systems that facilitate the provision of services to consumers
- Data management systems that meet the local needs to systematically collect, analyze, and monitor standardized baseline data
- Data systems that contain decision support modules to help identify potential outbreaks of certain infectious diseases and alert communities to contamination of food or water or intentional introduction of harmful bacteria
- Linkage between local and statewide databases in both the private and public sectors
- Data use and dissemination standards
- Technical assistance to ensure a high standard of data analysis, dissemination, and risk communication
- A fully integrated, secure computer network
- Evaluation and dissemination of new health information technologies
- Tracking of clinical and environmental laboratory information

Public health professionals need good data systems to be able to provide accurate, understandable information for policymakers, community leaders, health plans, and health care providers. Outcome measures need to be tracked. Policy outcomes need data for evaluation. The main concern running through all of this data collection, analysis, and dissemination is the need for balancing the privacy and confidentiality of the individual with the protection of the public good. Most health care providers are aware of regulations that require reporting of communicable diseases. This reporting to the public health department allows the department to take further action, if necessary, to prevent spread of the illness. In most instances, the reporting does not endanger the privacy of the individual. The reports are not published as public information; however, some diseases do require follow-up with others who may have had contact with the infected individual. The granularity of the data depends on the authority of the agency and their need to act specifically on the information. For example, the state or local health department will need to know an individual's name and address to follow up for mandatory treatment, but the Centers for Disease Control and Prevention (CDC) only needs to know that a case occurred and was successfully treated; the patient's identity is not released to the federal agency.

Legal Context

All states have a set of diagnoses that are referred to as notifiable conditions. These are largely highly contagious

---

Box 19-3 IMMEDIATELY REPORTABLE COMMUNICABLE DISEASE CONDITIONS

- Animal bites
- Botulism
- Brucellosis
- Cholera
- Diphtheria
- Diseases of suspected bioterrorism, suspected food-borne or suspected water-borne origin
- Enterohemorrhagic *E. coli*
- *Haemophilus influenza,* invasive disease
- Hemolytic uremic syndrome
- Hepatitis A, acute hepatitis, unspecified, infectious
- Listeriosis
- Measles (rubeola)
- Meningococcal disease
- Paralytic shellfish poisoning
- Pertussis
- Poliomyelitis
- Rabies
- Relapsing fever
- Rubella, including congenital
- Salmonellosis
- Shigellosis
- Tuberculosis
- Typhus
- Unexplained critical illness or death
- Rare disease of public health significance

---

communicable diseases that require the health department to intervene to prevent the further spread of disease in the community. Box 19-3 has this set of diseases for Washington State.

At the time of this writing, several states, including New York and Washington, have laws that permit the reporting of clusters of cases that could be an indication of an epidemic from a unknown cause including bioterrorism (for example, covertly disseminated anthrax) or an emerging natural infection, such as SARS (severe acute respiratory syndrome). To enable this analysis, data including the chief complaints, preliminary diagnosis, and a limited demographic data set are permitted to be reported to public health. By aggregation of data from many different hospitals, the presence of an unnamed syndrome can be detected.[33]

Although the exact value of syndromic surveillance is not yet known, this method in one form or another represents the future of modern disease surveillance.

Cooperation

Despite all the media attention that public health has gotten in the wake of anthrax, monkeypox, and SARS outbreaks, the underlying budget to support the task of public health to monitor and detect disease is woefully underfunded. Hospitals have no direct financial gain to provide required information to their local health jurisdiction. However, the effect on the community could be devastating if these data are not shared with public health officials in a timely manner. As the sophistication of health departments increases, the methods for transmitting these reports securely will become commonplace.

Efforts to ensure access and quality of care require partnerships among many affected parties. The sharing of data and the tracking of measurements, programs, and changes over time are essential to obtain community and client perspectives on quality of care and services.

All states have plans and target goals for public health as well as a broad array of services. Tracking services and goals and assessing progress requires data (Box 19-4). If tracking is implemented appropriately, there is an opportunity to eliminate the individual "stove pipes" and instead use a standards-based unified approach that links the stakeholders of public health by common data channels (Figure 19-2). Electronic transmissions will ultimately save time and resources of hospital staff, who would otherwise have to prepare a paper report of these cases.

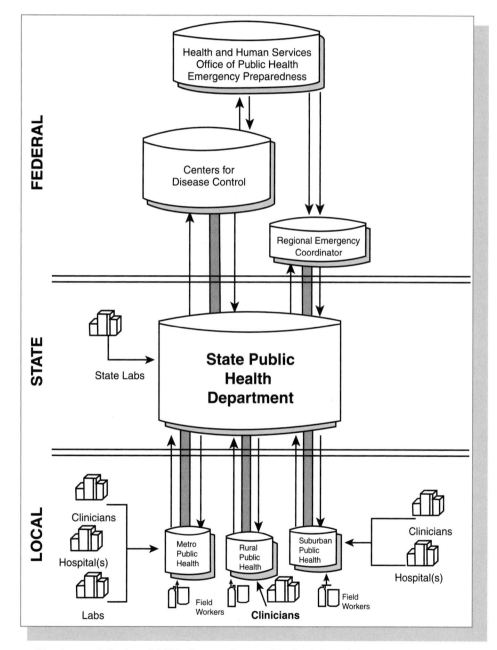

Figure 19-2 Diagram of local-state-federal model. This diagram shows an idealized view of the existing public health infrastructure. This describes the structure of the public health IT environment. Federal agencies include the CDC, the region X health director of the Department of Health and Human Services. State agencies include state department of health and local agencies include the county and local health agencies of various sizes. Single data channels rather than program specific "stove pipes" are shown and the flow of information is represented. (From University of Washington Center for Public Health Informatics.)

Box 19-4 LIST OF CORE PUBLIC HEALTH ACTIVITIES

Following are the core public health activities and services that a mid-size health jurisdiction would provide to meet 95% performance on the Standards for Public Health in Washington State.

Ensuring a Safe and Healthy Environment
- Food safety (inspections, education, permitting, data management including local responsibilities for shellfish monitoring)
- Water recreational facility safety (inspections, education, permitting, data management)
- Hazardous materials management (drug laboratory inspection, testing oversight, cleanup oversight)
- Solid waste management (permitting, inspection, enforcement, education)
- Water quality control: sewage (permitting, inspection, enforcement, education and operations and management), ground water, drinking water (permit, inspection, enforcement, education, drinking water data), surface water (drinking water permit, inspection, enforcement, education, and environmental monitoring)
- Vector/rodent control/zoonotic disease (inspection, enforcement, education, and sampling)
- Air quality monitoring (indoor investigations)
- Environmental laboratory services
- School safety (inspection, education, and consultation)
- Environmental health community involvement
- Environmental sampling
- Review of land use decisions

Protecting People From Disease
- Detection/case investigation: screening (specimen collection and analysis), testing, laboratory (identification and diagnosis), diagnosis (clinical and laboratory identification)
- Surveillance, reporting (transmission of information), data analysis (monitor and interpret), data gathering (collecting information and collection systems), epidemiological investigations, case finding (identifying cases and location), contact tracing (identifying potential exposure)
- Regional epidemiology
- Laboratory (identification and diagnosis)
- System intervention: immunizations (preventive preexposure or postexposure), treatment and prophylactic treatment (dispensing, shots, application, and observation), counseling (one-on-one education and therapy), tuberculosis program
- Public and provider education (informing general public and outbreak specific)
- Surveillance of chronic disease trends and behavioral changes, identifying clusters, special studies to identify risk factors and focus prevention efforts, prevention activities focused on behavioral and environmental/policy interventions, and evaluation
- Outreach and prevention with high-risk populations
- Plans and surge capacity for response to emergency situations that threaten the health of people

Understanding Health Issues
- Epidemiology (infectious and noninfectious disease trends monitoring, collection, and analysis of data on health risk behaviors, health status, and critical health services)

- Dissemination of assessment information in the community to support decision making
- Technical assistance, education, and leadership for community-level data use

Evaluation of Public Health Program Results
- Prevention is best: promoting healthy living
- Capacity for health education and systems work related to the following activities: engaging community agencies, organizations and constituencies to address and develop locally designed programs driven by locally identified health issues, strategic planning based on community needs, local data gathering and analysis, and coalition and stakeholder-building
- Resource assessments (develop assessment of resources based on specific needs), generate resources (design materials, find funding, write grants), designing and providing promotional materials or social marketing campaigns evaluating results of efforts, and collecting and disseminating research-based best practices
- Ensure and support healthy pregnancy, healthy birth outcomes, early brain development; includes maternal and child health programs, early intervention, health and safety promotion in child care centers, children with special health care needs, family planning, First Steps/Maternity Case Management/Maternity Support Services community outreach and Women, Infants, and Children (WIC) program
- Evaluating results of efforts, collecting and disseminating research-based, replicable best practices (including about chronic illnesses and health behaviors), provider and public education

Helping People Get the Services They Need
- System assurance role: bring people together and provide leadership and support, system infrastructure, support for local community SWOT (strengths, weaknesses, opportunities, and threats) assessment
- Provide information and education about critical public health services; create conditions that make action possible.
- Information and referral activities (maintain inventory of services, referral, resource broker)
- Create conditions that make action possible (standards, policy, quality assurance, materials and supplies, information, and education)
- Safety net services (direct services as identified through local assessment, Menu of Critical Health Services)

Administration
- Leadership, planning, policy development, and administration
- Financial and management services (accounting, budget, contracts, procurement, grants, and asset management)
- Leadership and governance (communication, public relations, relationship building, program planning, and fund raising)
- Legal authority (policies, procedures, and regulations)
- Human resources (personnel, employee development and recognition, compensation and benefits management, and employee policies)
- Information systems (hardware/software systems, networking, data sharing, policies)

From Public Health Improvement Plan 2004, Washington State Department of Health.[30]

Health information management professionals have the knowledge and skills to support the data and information systems of the public health system and can contribute to the overall health and well-being of the entire population.

A VISION OF DIGITAL INFORMATION CONVERGENCE: "HOW CONNECTED DO YOU WANT TO BE?"

Michael D. Gray and Bill G. Felkey

During the late 1970s we might have heard a child ask his father, "Daddy, what was it like to be alive before people were on the moon?" Today, we might reasonably expect that a child could ask her parents, "What was the world like before the Internet?" The current version of Internet protocol (IP) allows for 4.3 billion discrete machine addresses on the Internet. As of the date of this writing, two thirds of those addresses have been consumed. The next version of this protocol that is already being implemented will allow 3.4×10^{38} devices to be interconnected globally.

The number of potential machine addresses is so large in the expanded protocol that it is conceivable to connect virtually any electronic device with a network interface, whether wired or wireless, to any other network-enabled device. In other words, every car, every mobile phone, every watch, every appliance, and even every health care–related device on the planet could communicate with each other. Take a moment to ponder this phenomenon and interpolate how this level of ubiquitous connectivity will revolutionize health care. Then contemplate the magnitude of data that will be generated as more health-related devices are integrated into the existing health care IT infrastructure. As you read the following scenarios highlighting data-driving technologies, reflect on the level of innovation required to extract knowledge from the new data sources and deliver it to the decision maker on demand.

Closed-Loop Solutions (On-Line and Real Time)

Imagine the elderly patient whose heart condition can be monitored continually through a device that resembles a watch but is actually a continuous health status monitoring tool. The device uses a combination of cellular connectivity and global positioning system (GPS) technology. This patient is walking alone on a path in the woods near his home when his heart stops beating. His brain loses oxygen and he collapses. The instrument, which is available today, would alert a remote monitoring center of the patient's collapse and would transmit exactly how his heart had stopped beating. An implanted, wirelessly controlled defibrillator would be remotely activated to attempt to revive the patient. First responders would also be dispatched

to the exact location where he had collapsed and his current medical record would be downloaded and accessible on their mobile care information appliances. If an emergency medical services (EMS) unit servicing your hospital responded to this call, at what point would your organization be able to tap into and use this datastream? And more important how would these data converge with your current systems and processes to mobilize and manage critical resources that optimize this patient's chances for survival?

The hospital of tomorrow will be poised to receive these patient data at the onset of the incident. While the EMS unit is en route, the hospital's cardiac response team will be able to analyze and monitor the patient's heart rhythm, access the patient's complete electronic medical record, and construct a current prescription drug profile by extracting drug benefit utilization data from third-party payers. As the patient is received into the emergency department, the appropriate physical assets such as mobile diagnostic imaging devices are staged and ready and a team of critical care specialists will be fully prepped to take immediate action.

Furthermore, the hospital will have the option to push the patient's array of information to off-site consulting physicians who use sophisticated decision support systems based on clinical guidelines to distill the information and offer real-time clinical expertise. An off-site cardiac specialist will be virtually "in the room" with the patient and be able to confer with the on-site physicians by a high-definition, full-motion video and stereo-quality audio connection to a remote command center that serves multiple hospitals. This may sound futuristic, but a handful of progressive health care organizations that are moving toward digital convergence already have these resources at their disposal.

Telecommuting Oversight

Telemedicine, telepharmacy, and telenursing will help health care organizations manage critical shortages of medical disciplines and specialties. As you are reading this viewpoint, a pool of independent pharmacists, working part time from home, are verifying prescriptions for geographically dispersed pharmacies with the aid of a broadband data connection and streaming multimedia applications loaded on their computers. When staffing a 24-hour pharmacy operation within a hospital emergency department is no longer cost-effective, telepharmacy, as described, will be used in conjunction with robotic dispensing systems. This streamlined solution manages the end-to-end process, including medication selection, labeling, insurance adjudication, video-conferencing for counseling, and even collecting copayments by cash or credit card through dispensing kiosks located in the waiting area of the emergency department. Obviously, the initial focus of these alternative solutions will address service bottlenecks in high-demand markets, provide a standard level of care for underserved rural areas, and alleviate acute shortages of highly skilled medical specialists such as intensivists.

Virtual intensive care units (ICUs) and telemedicine are already operational in the United States. Currently, multiple hospital systems have access to a single off-site intensive care physician by transmitting real-time monitoring information from the hospitals' ICUs to the intensivist. Imagine this intensivist monitoring ICU patients at multiple hospital systems through a matrix of integrated digital displays. As one patient's vital signs become a point of concern, the intensivist can tap on the touch sensitive monitor and expand the view to access more detailed health information, including the patient's EHRs. At the same time, other screens in the nine screen array display real-time, full-motion video of the patient so that the intensivist can evaluate the patient's physical condition. With this command view, he or she can evaluate the multidimensional data and guide the attending physicians and nurses in the physical ICU with direct instructions for therapeutic intervention. Increasingly, telecommunication and the appropriate use of centralized or shared services will help fill the voids of our health care system nationally.

Self-Care Management

Patients, in most states, legally own the information contained in their medical records. However, patients do not feel that they actually own this information. The EHR will allow access to this information by patients and their designated caregivers. Currently, the electronic communication between health care providers and patients involving protected health information is transmitted by encrypted e-mail. As patients become more comfortable with electronic communication with respect to their health, health care providers will need to offer secured access to laboratory test results, current drug profiles, appointment scheduling software, and recommended links to health information libraries through a personalized Web portal.

Providing access to electronic medical records and those data they contain will require some form of patient consent. We believe that the banking industry's automated teller machine (ATM) card will be used as the model for controlling access to health information. Patients will potentially carry a health ATM card that will contain a radiofrequency identification (RFID) chip supplemented by a biometric fingerprint or iris scanned authentication. Thus, as patients approach the reception desk of the clinic, they will automatically be signed in, their medical case history will be electronically accessed, and insurance coverage verification will be completed. All that will be needed to complete the patient intake process will be for the patient to communicate their primary health concerns or medical reasons for the visit. Even this part of the process could be handled electronically by an integrated self-assessment kiosk located in the reception area.

Integration for Patient Safety

Existing implementations of bar code technology support the medication use process by helping to reduce medication administration errors associated with patient/drug identification and verification. But, as multiple technologies are combined, the ability to oversee the medication use process and the ability to monitor patient safety metrics will improve care precipitously. Bar codes, wireless connectivity, RFID product authentication, and real-time feedback at the point of administration will help reduce errors and provide additional evidence-based resources to analyze breakdowns in the process when they occur. From the moment a medication order is conceptualized in the mind of a prescriber to the pushing of the syringe into the intravenous port of the patient, rules engines will be integrated into each step of the process.

The benefits of integrating a suite of technologies such as bar codes, RFID, and other wireless technologies in the health care setting seem to be limited only by our imagination. For example, as a patient with a myocardial infarction is stabilized in the emergency department and is being prepared for transfer to the ICU, he or she is fitted with an identification wristband that integrates bar code and RFID technologies. The hospital is able to monitor patient flow throughout the organization with RFID sensors, analyze patient resource use, and measure all levels of process throughout against previously established benchmarks. If clinicians have RFID chips integrated into their identification badges, then clinician time associated with patient treatment could be tracked along the course of patients' hospital stays. Data gathered in each episode of care could be used to estimate the treatment time associated with a particular diagnosis. These data could also be used to assess clinicians' clinical performance or adherence to established care processes. In multigroup practice facilities, administrators will be able evaluate which physicians comply with quality, effectiveness, and efficiency requirements. Additionally, this use of technology would enable the automation of billable coding processes, which would establish the opportunity for near real-time claims processing.

Digital Dashboards

Creative use of wireless technologies can make physical assets such as beds, infusion pumps, computers on wheels, mobile medication dispensing cabinets, and so forth "network aware" for location tracking purposes. The locations of these network-enabled devices are graphically superimposed onto a digital floor plan located in the nurse's station. These "digital dashboards" display real-time feedback from operations on 42-inch plasma screens. These dashboard screens also illuminate patient location and current room/bed use data and incorporate clinician/staff tracking throughout the facility. So when a patient returns from radiology the nurse will notice a change on the digital dashboard corresponding to that patient's room and re-engage the patient's therapeutic process. Complementing this situationally aware environment are hands-free, wireless fidelity–connected, communication badges that make instantaneous communication and coordination a reality.

These tools are allowing hospitals to measure their performance against standard clinical targets such as a 20-minute delivery goal for the administration of "stat" medications.

Today, management of chronic diseases such as congestive heart failure, diabetes, hypertension, and cardiopulmonary obstructive disease consumes the majority of all health care spending.[34] As a result, medication regimen adherence for these chronic diseases will become a closed-loop process. In other words, systems that are matched appropriately for each patient's needs will tell patients what medications should be taken and indicate that medications have been taken to reduce doubling doses, regimen complexity will be reduced by appropriate prompting and organization, and refills for chronic medication will be staged for dispensing in a just-in-time manner.

Multidisciplinary Collaboration

An emerging form of medical record called the continuity of care record (CCR) will facilitate collaboration of multi-disciplinary teams by providing the clinicians with a view of the recent health status and treatment history of a patient. The CCR will enable the current physician providing treatment with an understanding of what the previous physician had diagnosed and the treatment that had been prescribed. With a standard format for transferable medical information, a more holistic approach to chronic care management is possible. As a result, significant therapeutic outcome and quality of life improvements can be realized for patients while costs are reduced.

It is conceivable that the CCR could also encourage coordination between the primary and supplemental insurers, health care organizations such as hospitals, home health care, emergency services, pharmacy, and non-health-related services. In essence, a comprehensive chronic disease management program supported through multiple channels could deliver the most appropriate and cost-effective care combinations to aid the patient's therapeutic process. For example, patients with diabetes can obtain specific treatment information and support through a customized Web portal connecting them to a multidimensional care team. Through this secure Web portal they get detailed information about their disease and the best preventative techniques to self-manage their care. If they have additional questions, they can initiate an on-line chat through their personalized Web portals by instant messaging a clinician such as a nurse who can promptly address their questions. Similarly, patients can dial a toll-free number to a diabetes management call center that could give immediate person-to-person response to questions relating to the management of their condition.

Therapeutic Outcomes Monitoring

By integrating network-enabled monitoring equipment such as blood glucose monitors, patients would be able to transmit real-time blood sugar data to their case management resource center. Clinical decision support systems would evaluate the blood glucose levels against individualized patient care plans and advise case managers to initiate phone calls to their patients or schedule a nursing visit to further evaluate patients' conditions. In the case where patient blood glucose levels are dangerously out of range, these data would trigger a number of events. One response might be a phone call from the care management center verifying that patients have begun to remedy the out of range blood glucose levels with appropriate insulin therapy.

We have already mentioned the use of implanted devices. However, it is important to emphasize that the use of implanted devices will proliferate and their specific applications will broaden. Currently, use of implanted devices assist in locating patients with Alzheimer's disease, regulate reproductive systems, aid neuromuscular strengthening, control hunger, control pain, and manage drug therapies. As next-generation nanotechnologies create implanted devices that function at the genomic level, the beneficial applications for human health will be virtually limitless. One thing is certain. There will be no slowing down of technology innovation in health care. Everything noted in this viewpoint is beyond the concept phase. Everything described is either available today or is being tested in human subjects. The future is closer than we think.

Digital Information Convergence

All of these enabling technologies provide health care organizations with massive amounts of clinical data that were never before available. With this new level of information, health care providers have the potential to dramatically improve the quality of patient care. However, the ultimate opportunity for health care organizations lies not in the discrete data that these systems generate in isolation, nor does it reside in relational data stores resulting from integrating multiple technologies. It is conceivable that these enabling technologies will generate more useful data then can be understood and analyzed through conventional query and reporting mechanisms. Therefore, we believe that a significant opportunity exists for health care organizations that can converge all these data-enabling technologies into an enterprise data architecture. By using data warehousing and data mining algorithms to push instantaneous, situationally relevant information to the point of need, care will be optimized. We call this optimal end state "digital information convergence." The clarity and enterprise intelligence that it delivers to the point where critical decisions are being made we call "total situational awareness."

Digital information convergence expands the health care organization's field of view and provides "total situational awareness" of its operational opportunities and process liabilities. Obtaining this degree of insight requires a change in how the organization architects its IT infrastructure, integrates systems into this environment, and distills knowledge from a veritable ocean of clinical and operational data.

We believe that the most fiscally prosperous health care organizations of the next decade will be those that internalize the strategic objective of digital convergence today and transform their current IT architecture by incorporating data warehousing methods with expanded decision support capabilities. The catalyst accelerating health care's interest in data warehousing and business intelligence is the massive amount of data generated from technologies and applications implemented over the last few years. In essence, health care firms are beginning to realize that their technology investments have continued to make them data rich but knowledge poor.

Priorities and Trends

A recent survey of hospital chief information officers (CIOs) supports our opinion. Given the implementation trends over the last 2 years, it is not surprising to see continued focus on wireless enabled technologies that use PDAs, bar code scanners, and speech recognition systems. Mobile care technologies are the conduits for new data acquisition and existing data dissemination. The survey also reveals that CIOs (last year more than previous years) recognized their need for data convergence and information analysis. In other words, they have a need to convert their data into knowledge. A year ago, 37% of CIOs participating in the survey planned to implement data-warehousing technologies. However, this year when they were asked this question, 51% of technologists forecast implementing a data warehouse within their health care organizations during the next 2 years.[35]

The integration of technology in and around the patient care process has given us more information than ever before. However, without a systematic approach to extracting and analyzing the data accumulating in real time from a host of integrated and stand-alone systems, the modern health care organization will not be able to fully leverage its IT investment and unlock the strategic insights stored within its existing data. If knowledge is power, then most health care organizations are currently generating mere watts from their current data instead of the megawatts that are available.

New technology adoption should not focus on how to simply automate what is currently being done. Rather it should be viewed as an opportunity to improve existing work processes. The path to digital convergence requires a mind shift by administrative, clinical, and technological leaders. These leaders need to embrace innovation within their organization that delivers the trifecta of process, clinical, and technology excellence.[36]

The advance of mobile computing capabilities on the health care system's horizon will continue to drive toward real-time information sharing and system ubiquity. Undoubtedly, these technologies have the potential to launch a health care enterprise to a level of care that has never before been possible. To make this a reality, health information professionals leading tomorrow's world-class health care organizations will embrace digital information convergence as the ultimate innovative achievement. They will evaluate technology with respect to its ability to broaden the situational awareness of decision makers throughout the continuum of patient care. Now is the time to invest in solutions that will put the organization on the path toward achieving this vision and securing a competitive advantage.

In the final analysis, systems that enable digital information convergence will continue to untether the mobile health care professional by intelligently delivering the right information, at the right time, to the right person, in the right format, on the right device. It is imperative that all the data-enabling systems and devices that can provide your organization with "situational awareness" about every clinical event be considered. Given the scenarios described above, organizations need to answer the questions, "How connected are you?" and "How connected do you want to be?" Ultimately, organizations need to determine at what point in the care continuum the process data, evidence-based information, and clinical protocols available will become aggregated for decision making. Also, these data will ultimately be used for process improvement at both the individual patient and population levels. All this will occur as a byproduct of every interaction and transaction across the health care enterprise. Most important, the information will need to be systematically applied at the point of care to achieve the best possible patient outcomes.

REFERENCES

1. Institute of Medicine: *Crossing the quality chasm: a new health system for the 21st century,* Washington, DC, 2001, Committee on Quality of Health Care in America, Institute of Medicine, National Academy Press.
2. Department of Health and Human Services, Centers for Medicare and Medicaid Services: *Data and projections to 2013 (2014 extrapolated),* Medicare Trustees Report, March 23, 2004.
3. Kohn L, Corrigan J, Donaldson M, editors: *To err Is human: building a safer health system,* Washington, DC, 2000, Committee on Quality of Health Care in America, Institute of Medicine, National Academy Press.
4. Walker J, Pan E, Johnston, Adler-Milstein D et al: The value of health care information exchange and interoperability, *Health Affairs (Millwood)* Jan-Jun:Suppl Web Exclusives: W5-10-W5-18, 2005.
5. Office of the National Coordinator for Health Information Technology: Framework: http://www.hhs.gov/news/press/2004pres/20040721.html. Accessed November 17, 2006.
6. AHIMA e-HIM resources: http://www.ahima.org/infocenter. Accessed October 4, 2005.
7. AHIMA Workforce Research Reports: http://www.ahima.org/fore/practice/workforce. Accessed October 4, 2005.
8. Chueh HC: Personal communication.
8a. AHIMA/AMIA: The value of personal health records: a joint position statement for consumers of health care. July 2006: http://www.amia.org/inside/releases/2006/ahima-amiaphrstatement.pdf.
8b. AHIMA/AMIA: Building the work force for health information transformation. February 2006: http:www.ahima.org/emerging_issues/workforce_web.pdf.

9. American Medical Informatics Association: 10 × 10 Program: http://www.amia.org/10x10/. Accessed December 4, 2005.

10. American Medical Informatics Association: http://www.amia.org/gotehr/. Accessed December 4, 2006.

11. Postman N: *Technopoly: the surrender of culture to technology,* New York, 1992, Alfred A. Knopf.

12. Institute of Medicine: *To err is human: building a safer health system,* Washington, DC, 2000, National Academy Press.

13. Hagland M: Reduced errors ahead, Healthcare Informatics (August 2003): www.healthcare-informatics.com. Accessed August 28, 2003.

14. Kuperman GJ, Gibson RF: Computer physician order entry: Benefits, costs, and issues, *Ann Intern Med* 139:31-40, 2003: at www.annals.org. Accessed October 2, 2003.

15. Horak B, Turner M: Involving health care professionals in technological change: comments on case 9.1: Williams Memorial Hospital—Nursing unit computerization. In Lorenzi M, Riley R, Ball M et al, editors: *Transforming health care through information,* pp. 233-246, New York, 1995, Springer-Verlag.

16. Briggs B: CPOE: Order from chaos. Health Data Management (February 2003): www.healthdatamanagement.com. Accessed August 23, 2003.

17. Connolly C: Cedars-Sinai doctors cling to pen and paper, *Washington Post,* page A012005 (March 21, 2003): www.washingtonpost.com/ac2/wp-dyn/A52384-2005Mar20? Accessed February 25, 2005.

18. Chin T: Doctors outpace consumers in embracing e-technologies, *AMNews2003* (October 6, 2003): www.ama-assn.org/sci-pubs/amnews. Accessed October 2, 2003.

19. Bloomrosen M: e-HIM: From vision to reality, *J AHIMA* 76:36-41, 2005 [expanded on-line version: http://library.ahima.org]. Accessed October 4, 2005.

20. Lorenzi NM, Riley RT: Managing change: An overview, *J Am Med Inform Assoc* 7:116-124, 2000.

21. Lorenzi NM, Riley RT: Organizational aspects of implementing informatics change. In Dewan NA, Lorenzi NM, Riley RT, et al: *Behavioral healthcare informatics,* pp. 156-170, New York, 2002 Springer-Verlag.

22. Ash JS, Sittig DF, Seshadri V et al: Adding insight: a qualitative cross-site study of physician order entry, *Int J Med Inform* 74:623-628, 2005.

23. Stead WW, Lorenzi NM: Health informatics: linking investment to value, *J Am Med Inform Assoc* 6:341-348, 1999.

24. Institute of Medicine: *Crossing the quality chasm: a new health system for the 21st century,* Washington, DC, 2001, National Academy Press.

25. American Health Information Management Association: A vision of the e-HIM future, *J AHIMA* (Suppl):2003: www.ahima.org. Accessed October 4, 2005.

26. International Federation of Health Records Organizations: General assembly, October, 2004, discussion papers on the five issues facing health information management.

27. Joint Commission on Accreditation of Healthcare Organizations: http://www.jcaho.org.

28. Centers for Disease Control and Prevention: *Healthy People 2010:* http://healthypeople.gov. Accessed March 7, 2006.

29. National Committee for Quality Assurance: HEDIS measures: http://www.ncqa.org. Accessed March 7, 2006.

30. Washington State Department of Health: Public health improvement plan 2004, p. 67-68: http://www.doh.wa.gov/PHIP/documents/PHIP2004phip.pdf. Accessed March 8, 2006. Tumwater, WA.

31. Harrell JA, Baker EL, Essential Services Workgroup: *Essential services of public health,* 1995, American Public Health Association: http://www.apha.org/ppp/science/10ES.htm. Accessed March 8, 2006.

32. Washington State Department of Health: Injury and violence prevention program (children), tobacco prevention and control, and public health action plan: http://www.doh.wa.gov. Accessed March 8, 2006.

33. Lober WB, Karras BT, Wagner MM et al. Roundtable on bioterrorism detection: Information system-based surveillance, *J Am Med Inform Assoc* 9:105-115, 2002.

34. U.S. Department of Health and Human Services: Prevention makes common "cents": http://aspe.hhs.gov/health/prevention/prevention.pdf. Accessed November 22, 2005.

35. Healthcare Information and Management Systems Society: 16th Annual HIMSS leadership survey (Feb 14, 2005), Healthcare CIO results: Key trends index: http://www.himss.org/2005survey/docs/Healthcare_CIO_key_trends.pdf. Accessed Nov 25, 2005.

36. Gray MD, Felkey BG: Computerized prescriber order entry (CPOE): Evaluation, selection, and implementation, *Am J Health System Pharmacy* 61:190-197, 2004.

Glossary

Abbreviation list An official list of approved abbreviations maintained by health care organizations, to avoid misunderstandings from either poor handwriting or the fact that many abbreviations have more than one meaning.

Abstracting (1) A process by which a set of predetermined data is obtained from the patient record and related sources; (2) the process of selecting specific data items from medical records for clinical and administrative decision making. Abstracting has a wide range of uses from billing and case-mix analysis, to selection of cases for quality review. Also known as statistical analysis.

Accent lighting (*See* Task lighting.)

Access time The time (in milliseconds) that it takes for the appropriate image to be located for display on the terminal screen once the disk is placed in the disk drive.

Accession of active case When patients are determined eligible and added to a registry.

Accounting rate of return An evaluation method that uses averages. The annual net inflows or outflows are averaged over the project's life for each project, and the asset value or investment value is averaged over the life of the project as well. The asset value is depreciated on a straight-line basis for the life of the program.

Accounts receivable The revenue (dollar amount) owed to an organization.

Accounts receivable turnover ratio A ratio that provides a measure of the average time that receivables are outstanding or the period for which a health care organization extends credit to its debtors.

Accreditation A voluntary process by which a private non-governmental organization or agency performs an external review and grants recognition to a program of study or institution that meets certain predetermined standards.

Accredited record technician A credential offered in the early 1950s after completion of a 9- to 12-month technical program and successful completion of a certification examination. This was eventually replaced by the RHIT (Registered Health Information Technician) credential.

Accrual basis accounting Financial transaction processing method that uses the matching concept, enabling revenues to be matched with the actual expenses incurred to produce the revenue. The accrual method records the revenues expected as "revenues," although the "cash" has not yet been received. The revenues are matched as closely with the expenses as possible.

Action steps Define the dates when certain activities are to be completed, how much labor or funding will be required, how resources will be used, and the expected outcomes or results.

Active record Active files that frequently need to be accessed on the basis of the health care activity of the patient.

Activity ratios Ratios that use data from the balance sheet and the statement of revenues and expenses to measure an organization's ability to generate net operating revenue in relation to its various assets. Also referred to as turnover ratios.

Acute care The treatment of common illnesses and injuries, such as nausea, vomiting, and abrasions.

Adaptive strategies More specific than directional strategies; indicate the method for carrying out the directional strategies.

Advance directive (1) A documented life support or treatment-related wish of a patient that is given to health care providers to follow in the event they become necessary; (2) a legal written document that specifies patient preferences regarding future health care or specifies another person to make medical decisions in the event the patient has an incurable or irreversible condition and is unable to communicate his or her wishes. The patient must be competent at the time the document is prepared and signed.

Adverse event Negative side effects or complications a patient may experience associated with health care.

Advocacy The support or promotion of something.

Affinity diagram A diagram often used after initial brain-storming sessions to organize and prioritize information into clusters or categories. Affinity diagrams are particularly useful when dealing with large amounts of complicated information because this technique reduces what may be considered an unmanageable amount of information into a smaller number of homogeneous groups.

Affirmative action programs Written, systematic human resource planning tools that outline goals for hiring, training, promoting, and compensating minority groups and women who are protected by EEO (Equal Employment Opportunity) laws. Affirmative action plans are specifically mandated in EO 11246 for businesses under federal contract to address past discrimination and to achieve a workforce that reflects the diversity of the population.

Aggregate data Data that have been collected or combined from many different sources.

Alphabetical identification When the record is identified by patient name. Alphabetical identification is the most basic identification system used in health care.

Alternative dispute resolution Rather than settling a dispute in court, a neutral party or panel hears both sides of a dispute and renders a decision, or by settling claims against them by negotiating a direct payment to the parties bringing the claim in exchange for the claimants' dropping the claim. Also referred to as arbitration or mediation.

Alternative hypothesis In a test of statistical significance, an alternative hypothesis states that there is a difference or relationship and that the observations are the result of the effect plus chance variation.

Alternative medicine Those practices that are used in lieu of conventional or what might be thought of as "Western Medicine."

Ambient lighting Light is directed upward so that it is reflected off the ceiling onto the work area. It provides light for a large area, but the light is insufficient to work by.

Ambulatory care A comprehensive term for all types of health care provided in an outpatient setting; the patient travels to and from the facility on the same day and is not hospitalized, institutionalized, or admitted as an inpatient.

Ambulatory payment classification system System of assigning groupings and weights to ambulatory care services. The groupings and weights are used by third-party payers such as Medicare to determine payment for services.

American plan of office design The combination of the conventional office plan with private offices and the open plan which allows the executive needed privacy.

Analytic study A type of epidemiologic research study design that includes case-control or retrospective, cohort or prospective, and historical-prospective. It examines diseases and health conditions to determine characteristics that may cause the disease or condition.

Ancillary services Departments that provide diagnostic and therapeutic services at the request of a physician to both inpatients and outpatients; the departments include radiology (medical imaging), clinical laboratory, physical therapy, occupational therapy, respiratory therapy, cardiographics, pharmacy, and so on. Ancillary services differ from other areas of the hospital because the hospital is able to charge patients or third parties directly and, therefore, generate revenue for the hospital. They are under the direction of physicians.

Anesthetic death rate A rate that indicates the number of deaths that are due to the administration of anesthetics for a specified period of time.

Antitrust Laws that prohibit anticompetitive behavior such as price discrimination, restraint of trade, and monopolies.

Applets Programs that are allowed by JAVA to run on top of HTML pages and are more efficient than CGI scripts. Applets, which run on the client side, are available through the user's Web browser. After the user clicks on the submit button, the JAVA applet is downloaded to the user's machine temporarily.

Application gateway A type of firewall solution that allows only certain applications to run from outside the network. This is applicable if an organization wants to prohibit outside entities from transferring files to its network.

Application software Sets of instructions used to accomplish various types of business processes. For example, software written to process laboratory orders.

Arbitration The settling of a dispute outside of court through a neutral party or panel. (*See* Alternative dispute resolution.)

ARDEN Syntax language for medical logic modules (MLMs) that allows encoding of medical knowledge (e.g., laboratory values, medication orders).

Ascension number A unique identifier.

Ascertainment Identification.

Assault A deliberate threat, coupled with the apparent ability, to do physical harm to another person without that person's consent. No contact is required.

Assets Cash or cashlike items or other resources that can be converted to cash. Assets may be considered as short-term assets (those easily converted to cash) or long-term assets (items more difficult to convert to cash quickly or items needed to operate the business).

Assisted living A type of long-term care facility that typically offers housing and board with a broad range of personal and supportive care services.

Authentication (1) The process of identifying the source of health record entries by attaching a handwritten signature, the author's initials or an electronic signature. (2) The process of verifying or confirming the identity of a user that is requesting access to the information.

Authorization In the context of patients authorizing disclosure of their protected health information, the term refers to the written permission that meets the requirements of the applicable law that is required to be able to disclose the information.

Autopsy rate A rate computed so that health care facilities can determine the proportion of deaths in which an autopsy was performed. This enables a facility to examine why a higher or lower autopsy rate may be seen from one month to another.

Average daily inpatient census The average number of inpatients in a facility for a given period of time.

Average length of stay The average length of stay of inpatients discharged during a specified period.

Bailiff Courtroom personnel who are present to assist in keeping order, administering oaths, guarding and the assisting the jury, and performing other duties at the direction of the judge.

Balance sheet A financial report that displays an organization's assets, liabilities, and fund balance or equity at a fixed point in time.

Bandwidth A measure of how much information can be transmitted simultaneously through a communication channel. Bandwidth is measured in bits per second (bps).

Bar chart (*See* Bar graph.)

Bar code A machine-readable representation of information in a visual format. Originally stored in the widths and spacings of parallel lines but now can be patterns of dots or circles and hidden images.

Bar code device Optical scanners, equipment that reads bar codes.

Bar code reader Equipment that reads bar codes.

Bar graph A type of graph used to illustrate nominal, ordinal, discrete, and continuous data. The discrete categories are shown on the horizontal, or x, axis and the frequency is shown on the vertical, or y, axis. The purpose of the bar graph is to show the frequency for each interval or category.

Basic interoperability One computer system can send data to another, but that does not necessarily mean that the receiving system can interpret those data.

Battery Nonconsensual, intentional touching of another person in a socially impermissible manner.

Bedside documentation systems Software and hardware located at the patient's bedside that encourages recording of information about patient care at or near the time of its delivery.

Bed size (bed count) The total number of inpatient beds with which the facility is equipped and staffed for patient admissions.

Bed turnover rate The number of times an inpatient hospital bed, on the average, changes occupants during a given period of time.

Behavioral health Services that include psychiatric, psychological, and social work services to the patient, often referred to as client, and characterized as including mental health, alcohol, drug abuse, foster care, case management, and developmentally disabled services.

Behaviorally anchored rating scales (BARS) A method used in employee evaluation that anchors the numerical scales with brief narrative descriptions of a range of behavior from highest to lowest level of performance on that dimension. These narrative descriptions may be drawn from critical incidents documented in real-world supervisory situations.

Benchmarking Comparing an organization's performance against organizations that have been identified as excellent. Benchmarking a commonly used tool for gathering data and identifying ways to improve processes and initiate change at all operational levels.

Beneficiary One who is eligible to receive or is receiving benefits from an insurance policy, a managed care program, or government program.

Benefit period Time frame in which the insurance benefits are covered; varies from insurance policy to policy.

Benefits realization A system evaluation method that determines if the system has delivered all the benefits that were anticipated.

Best evidence rule Rules of evidence require that when originals are still available, they must be produced. When it becomes necessary to prove the contents of a document, the original must be produced or its absence accounted for.

Bias Preference for a particular point of view, a flaw in the system or design caused by methods used in the selection of subjects, nonresponse of subjects, and interviewing techniques, to name a few.

Biomedical device A device (such as automated electrocardiogram systems and patient monitoring systems) that converts data from one form to another and transmits the data to a database.

Biometric A unique, measurable characteristic or trait of a human being that can be used for automatic recognition or identity verification.

Bioterrorism Terrorism using germ warfare, an intentional human release of naturally occurring or human-modified toxin or biological agent.

Brainstorming A structured but flexible process designed to maximize the number of ideas generated. Brainstorming requires a leader who serves primarily as a facilitator and recorder and a team of 6 to 10 persons brought together to generate ideas about a relevant issue. The issue is defined, a time limit for discussion is set, and ideas are recorded for all team members to discuss.

Breach of contract Occurs when one party to a contract fails to follow the terms agreed to in the contract.

Break glass Refers to a quick means for a person who does not have access privileges to certain information to gain access when necessary.

Break-even analysis A cost-benefit analysis (CBA) technique in which costs to operate the current system are compared with those to operate the proposed system. The point at which old system costs equal new system costs is the break-even point. After the break-even point, the proposed system should begin to generate a positive monetary return compared with the old system.

Budgets Detailed numerical documents that translate the goals, objectives, and action steps into forecasts of volume and monetary resources needed.

Burden of proof When a plaintiff brings a civil suit against a defendant, unless the plaintiff can convince the judge or jury by a **preponderance of evidence** (making it more likely than not) that the claims against the defendant are valid, the defendant will prevail.

Business associate agreement A special agreement required by HIPAA that covered entities must use when using outside agents or organizations (not part of the facility's own workforce) to handle or process protected health information on their behalf. This agreement ensures that the agency follows rules set by the covered entity for handling protected health information.

Business plan A formal written document that evolves from the input of others, listing objectives that support the organizational goals. The plan includes the following: specific action steps, quantifying resource requirements and cash flow benefits, prediction of expected outcomes, and a programmatic outline that may span a fiscal year or a longer time frame.

Business rules (1) As applied to an information systems environment, are the rules that determine the user interface and database services that may be required. The business rules reside on the application server; (2) as applied to an organization, describe the operations, definition, and constraints that apply to an organization in achieving its goals.

Cache memory Memory within the magnetic disk on the workstation.

Cafeteria benefit plan A common type of benefit plan that allows employees to choose from an array of benefits to fit their needs or lifestyles.

Capital expenditure Items that usually have a high initial cost and a "life" of more than 1 year. Each facility defines its own capitalization value.

Capital expenditure committee A committee that evaluates all capital requests so that cash resources are used to purchase the high-cost items that will yield the most benefit to the organization.

Capitalization ratios Ratios that focus on balance sheet numbers (assets, liabilities, and equity/fund balance accounts) to measure the ability of the health care organization to meet its short- and long-term financial obligations.

Capitation (1) A form of reimbursement in which a prepaid, fixed amount is paid to the provider for each person (per capita) served, regardless of how much or how often the patient receives health care services; (2) a type of fixed-payment arrangement used in health maintenance organizations (HMOs). For each month an insured member remains with the HMO, the HMO's providers are paid a fixed amount, usually at the beginning of the month. The providers are required to provide any care needed by the insured during this period, regardless of whether the capitation amount is sufficient to cover the cost to do so.

Care The management of, responsibility for, or attention to the safety and well-being of another person or other persons.

Career counseling A service that may be offered to employees formally by the human resources staff, through an employee assistance program, or less formally by the mentoring of veteran professionals and managers.

Career planning Enables employees to be promoted within an organization from one job in a career path or ladder to another. Career planning also provides an incentive for motivating and retaining effective performers and identifying potential managers and leaders for appropriate training and placement.

Carpal tunnel syndrome Swelling of the tendons through the carpal tunnel (located in the front part of the wrist), which puts pressure on the medican nerve, causing pain and weakness. The most common repetitive strain (or stress) injury that occurs in workers who spend long hours using computers or workers who perform repetitive tasks.

Cascading style sheets (CSS) A tool used to optimize the use and appearance of the Web page by allowing users to easily apply personalized formatting to Web documents. With CSS-styled pages, the user can transform Web content into a format that addresses the requirements for accessibility.

Case A person with a given disease or condition that is under study.

Case eligibility All of the organization's patients diagnosed (clinically or histologically) and/or treated for active diseases on or after the reference date or beginning of the registry are eligible for inclusion in the registry.

Case finding The method by which all of the eligible cases to be included in the registry are identified, accessioned into the registry, and abstracted.

Case law In deciding on cases when no statutes apply, judges refer to similar cases that have been decided in the past and by applying the same principles, courts generally arrive at the same ruling in the current case as in similar previous cases

Case management An aspect of health care that refers to all activities, including assessment, treatment planning, referral, and follow-up, that ensures the provision of comprehensive and continuous services and the coordination of payment and reimbursement of care.

Case studies Provide a richly detailed portrait of an individual, program, event, department, time period, culture, or community.

Case-control study A type of analytic study design where the researcher collects data on the cases (those who have the disease that is under study) and controls (those who are similar to the cases but do not have the disease that is under study) by looking back in time. The intent of the researcher is to establish some association between the disease and the exposure characteristic. Also referred to as a retrospective study.

Cash Money that results from the collection of payments for services provided.

Cash basis accounting Financial transaction processing method whereby each transaction is recorded when cash is exchanged. Revenues are recognized when money is received for services provided, and expenses are recognized when money is paid out for the resources used to provide those services.

Cash budget A forecast of estimated cash receipts and disbursements for a specified period of time.

Catchment area A defined geographical area that is served by a health care program, project, or facility such as a hospital or mental health center. Services provided are usually directed at population groups and range from immunizations, diagnostic testing, and screening to nutrition counseling and family planning.

Cause-and-effect diagram A diagram used for solving complicated problems by helping people consider many factors and the cause-and-effect relationships between those factors. Also referred to as fishbone diagrams.

Censored The subject in a research study is alive at the time of analysis or was alive when last seen.

Census statistics Ratios, percentages, and averages related to the length of stay, occupancy, bed turnover, and total number of patients present at a specified time within the institution.

Centralized filing A filing system that uses a single location for all records created throughout the facility. This centralized file location is staffed by specialized personnel who provide records that have been requested by authorized users.

Certificate of need A regulatory process that requires certain health care providers to obtain state approval before offering certain new or expanded services.

Certification Refers to the process by which government and nongovernment organizations evaluate educational programs, health care facilities, and individuals as having met predetermined standards.

Certified coding associate (CCA) An entry-level coding credential implemented by AHIMA in 2002. The recommended amount of experience for this credential is 6 months or completion of an AHIMA-approved coding certificate program or other formal training program.

Certified coding specialist An advanced coding credential implemented by AHIMA in 1992. To receive this credential, individuals must pass the CCS examination, which focuses on inpatient coding systems. The recommended amount of experience for this credential is 3 or more years.

Certified coding specialist–physician-based An advanced coding credential implemented by AHIMA in 1997. To receive this credential, individuals must pass the CCS-P examination, which focuses on ambulatory care coding. The recommended amount of experience for this credential is 3 or more years.

Certified in Healthcare Privacy and Security (CHPS) A credential offered by AHIMA that validates an individual's expertise in designing, implementing, and administering comprehensive privacy and security protection programs in all types of health care organizations.

Charge master (charge description master) A list used by health care organization that reflects the charge for each item that may be used in the treatment of a patient and the charge for most services (e.g, respiratory therapy treatments, physical therapy services, laboratory tests, and so on). The list is most always automated and linked with the billing system. (*See* Master charge list.)

Charitable immunity A doctrine that had, until the early to mid-1960s, protected nonprofit hospitals from liability for harm to patients. Courts now permit harmed patients to sue hospitals for their wrongful acts.

Chart of accounts Used by several health care organizations to assign transactions to designated accounts in the financial accounting process. The largest expense items are in the lower number account categories, whereas the expense categories that have limited expenses appear in the higher number account groups.

Chart order The reference that defines the facility's standard sequence of pages to be followed in each record.

Checksheet A form specially designed to collect data so that the results can be readily interpreted from the form itself.

Checksum A special character that is added to the bar code that tells the bar code reader that the bar code is correct. The checksum character is read by the bar code scanner, but it is not passed along as part of the data.

Claim—Request for payment by the insured or the provider for services covered.

Classification A scheme for grouping similar things in a logical way, based on common characteristics.

Classification system— A scheme for grouping similar things in a logical way, based on common characteristics. Classification systems vary in their level of detail; some offer very general groupings, whereas others allow more detailed groupings and subgroupings, enabling the user to capture a greater degree of specificity, or granularity, of data. (*See* Classification.)

Clerk of the court The administrative manager of the court who handles the paperwork associated with lawsuits. Complaints are filed with the clerk, as are other pleadings and documents.

Client A person who receives professional services; a patient in the behavioral health setting, adult day care, or home health care may be referred to as a client.

Client server technology Involves the splitting of an application into tasks that are performed on separate computers, one of which is a programmable workstation. Client server computing is a form of cooperative processing that distributes the processing tasks to different systems for optimal responsiveness.

Clinical case definition A list of signs and symptoms that establish a clinical diagnosis.

Clinical data repository Collects, organizes, and analyzes all institutional business and clinical data that have been summarized and aggregated for that purpose. Clinical data repositories are designed to deliver the individual patient's information to the care team through the clinical workstation.

Clinical decision support systems (CDSSs) Systems that provide diagnostic investigation tools and clinical guideline advice to patient care providers. Basic clinical decision support provides computerized advice regarding drug doses, routes, and frequencies, and more sophisticated CDSSs can perform drug allergy checks, drug-laboratory value checks, and drug-drug interaction checks and can provide reminders about corollary orders (e.g., prompting the user to order glucose checks after ordering insulin).

Clinical practice guidelines Specific procedures or protocols for medical professionals to follow for patients with a particular diagnosis or medical condition based on research.

Clinical privileges The permission granted by the appropriate authority (governing board) to practitioners to provide well-defined patient care services in the granting institution, based on licensure, education, training, experience, competence, health status, and judgment.

Clinical reference terminology Terminology that offers a consistent language for capturing, sharing, and aggregating health data across specialties and sites of care.

Clinical terminology Terminology used to represent the information in a medical record, whether that record is in paper form or electronic form.

Clinical trial A study consisting of two or more groups that have different exposures and that are followed forward to determine their outcomes. A certain medication or treatment is given to a group and the outcomes are compared with those of a control or comparison group (subjects who do not have the intervention). Also referred to as a community trial.

Close-ended questions Questions that provide a list of responses to choose from, similar to the multiple-choice type questions, dichotomous or yes/no questions, or questions based on level or measurement or ranking. Also referred to as structured format questions.

Code A unique identifier assigned to a specific term, description, or concept.

Code of ethics Guides the practice of people who choose a given profession and sets forth the values and principles defined by the profession as acceptable behavior within a practice setting.

Code set A list of codes and the terms or descriptions with which they are associated.

Coding The assignment of unique identifiers to the terms within a particular clinical terminology. In the field of health information management, coding commonly refers to the selection of alphanumerical codes to represent diseases, procedures, and supplies used in the delivery of health care. Also referred to as encoding.

Coding system A system primarily designed to support the administrative, financial, and regulatory functions associated with care. Coding systems serve as the primary communication tool between those providing services (e.g., physicians and hospitals) and those paying for services (e.g., insurance companies).

Coefficient of variation Used when two samples or groups have very different means. The coefficient of variation compares their standard deviations expressed as percentages of the mean.

Cohort study A study that begins in a community or an industrial setting or within a hospital. Subjects are separated into two groups on the basis of their exposures or health characteristic and then are followed forward to determine whether the disease develops. (*See* Prospective study.)

Coinsurance When the insured is partially responsible or liable for the debt (cost of their health care); usually expressed as a percentage of the cost (e.g., insured pays 20% and plan pays 80%).

Collaboration The combined labor of users and information systems staff in the pursuit of electronic health records.

Color coding A filing technique that uses colors to designate certain letters or digits helps to prevent misfiles and aids in rapid storage and retrieval. Color coding can also provide an easy way to distribute workload and make sorting of folders much easier.

Commission on Accreditation of Health Informatics and Information Management (CAHIM) The accrediting body established by AHIMA in 2004 that accredits undergraduate HIM programs that were previously accredited by CAAHEP (Council on Accreditation of Allied Health Educational Programs). The CAHIIM also offers an approval process for master's degree programs in HIM which will convert to an accreditation process in the future.

Common law The large body of principles that have evolved from prior court decisions. (*See* Case law.)

Communities of Practice (CoP) An on-line communication tool offered by AHIMA for connecting association members. The CoP provides up-to-date news and links to resources, helps keep members informed on the latest trends in HIM, helps members solve problems, network, and career build.

Community trial A study consisting of two or more groups that have different exposures and that are followed forward to determine their outcomes. A certain medication or treatment is given to a group and their outcomes are compared with those of a control or comparison group (subjects who do not have the intervention). (*See* Clinical trial.)

Community-acquired infection Infection that occurs in the community or less than 72 hours after admission as a hospital inpatient.

Comorbidity A condition that is in addition to a primary condition and affects course or treatment of a condition or length of stay.

Compensation management Entails understanding of wage and salary administration, payroll systems, employee benefits, knowledge of applicable federal and state legislation and regulation, and effective communication strategies. Compensation management should communicate effectively the goals, procedures, and constraints associated with the organization's compensation policies and to maintain the credibility of the system as being managed fairly and with integrity.

Complaint A written statement by the plaintiff that states his or her claims and commences the action in a lawsuit.

Complementary and alternative medicine Therapies (usually not included in Western medicine) that may or may not have been proven to be effective, including herbal remedies, massage therapy, natural food diets, acupuncture, and biofeedback. Complementary medicine includes those practices that could be used along with conventional therapies. Alternative medicine includes those practices that would be used in lieu of conventional medicine.

Compounding effect The result of applying an interest rate to the number of compounding periods in a year and the length of the term (i.e., number of years). The more frequent the interval of compounding the greater the effect—$100 invested at 8% after 5 years = $148.98.

Computer output microfiche (COM)   A process used in health care that allows large amounts of electronically stored data to be placed on microfilm quickly. In COM, the computer displays data on a special screen connected to a microfilm camera (recorder), which films the screen, reduces the image in size, and places the image directly onto a Mylar microfiche sheet. As more screens are filmed, they are added to the microfiche until it is full, and this process continues until the entire computer file has been copied to film.

Computer output to laser disk (COLD)   The automatic transfer of data to electronic document management. COLD is an important part of automating document images and index functions without the degree of manual labor required in scanning.

Computer-aided software engineering (CASE)   Computerized design tools that provide a mechanism for the electronic development of systems analysis aids such as structure charts, data flow diagrams, entity-relationship diagrams, and data dictionaries. Instead of developing charts and diagrams manually, the analyst can use a computer program with a graphical interface to assist in development.

Computer-based patient record   A term proposed by the Institute of Medicine (IOM) committee in 1991 to describe a patient record system that could be could be part of hospital information systems, medical information systems, or a type of clinical information system. This term has most recently been replaced by the terms electronic medical record or electronic health record.

Concept permanence   Once a concept has been created within a terminology, its meaning cannot change, and it cannot be deleted. The preferred name of the concept can change, or the concept may be deemed inactive, but its meaning must remain fixed as long as the terminology is in use.

Concurrent review   A review process that assesses the need for continued inpatient stay and the provision of care and services while the care is in process.

Conditions of Participation   Standards that are published by the Centers for Medicare and Medicaid (CMS) that establish the minimum that organizations must meet to be eligible to receive reimbursement for providing care to Medicare beneficiaries. The specifics of the regulations vary according to the provider setting.

Confidence interval   An estimated range of values with a high known probability of covering the true population value.

Confidential communication   Communication that transmits information to a health care provider as part of the relationship between the provider and the patient under circumstances that imply that the information shall remain private.

Confidentiality   An ethical and a legal concept endorsed by health professionals to meet the expectation of patients that their information, when provided to an authorized user, will not be redisclosed or misused.

Confounding variables   Variables that affect the dependent and independent variables.

Consent   Written permission from the patient allowing care or treatment.

Contemporaneous documentation   Documentation made while care is being provided, while the information is fresh in the care provider's mind.

Context representation   Formal, explicit information about how concepts are to be used. Context representation is essential to avoid the misinterpretation of health data.

Contingency table   A table that displays the joint frequencies of two qualitative variables used to compute Chi square statistic.

Continuous data   Data on quantitative variables that can assume an infinite number of possible values.

Continuum of care   The full range of health care services provided, moving from the least acute and least intensive to the most acute and most intensive or vice versa.

Contract   A formal and binding agreement (actual or implied).

Contracted amount   The amount of reimbursement that is negotiated between the provider and the third-party payer.

Control   A person who is similar to the case, but does not have the disease or condition that is under study.

Control chart   A data display tool used to monitor performance that can determine whether a process is statistically in control. Control charts have three important lines: the central line is the mean or median, and the upper and lower lines are termed control limits. Data points outside the control limits (or unusual data patterns) indicate a special cause that should be found and eliminated.

Controlling   The activities that management typically pursues when what was planned does not occur financially.

Cooperative processing   Distributes the processing tasks to different systems for optimal responsiveness. By separating shared data, it can provide more efficient computer functions. It seeks to achieve the best performance for low-volume and high-volume processing, optimal network traffic, and realistic security and control.

Copayment   A type of cost-sharing in which the insured (subscriber) pays out of pocket a fixed amount for health care service.

Core measure   A set of standardized metrics developed and used by The Joint Commission to assess the quality of health care organizations.

Corporate negligence   Under this theory, courts can hold health care organizations liable for their own independent acts of negligence. Organizations are responsible for monitoring the activities of the people who function within their facilities, whether those people are employees or independent contractors, such as physicians, and for complying with appropriate industry standards, such as accreditation (The Joint Commission) standards, licensing regulations, and *Conditions of Participation* issued by Medicare.

Correlation analysis   Determines the strength, direction, and statistical significance of a relationship between one or more performance variables.

Correlation coefficient   A statistic that shows the strength of a relationship between two variables.

Cost-benefit analysis (CBA)   A system evaluation method that attempts to measure benefits compared with system costs. Cost-benefit analysis is used to determine whether the information system decreases or increases benefits and whether it decreases or increases cost for the organization.

Cost-effectiveness analysis   A system evaluation technique that is used to evaluate certain beneficial consequences in nonmonetary terms. In cost-effectiveness analysis, desirable benefits are not valued in monetary terms but are measured in some other unit.

Council on Accreditation   This body is now the Commission on Accreditation for Health Informatics and Information Management Education. Its mission is to establish and enforce standards for educational preparation of health informatics and information management professionals by recognizing educational programs that meet their standards.

Council on Certification The certifying body of AHIMA that is responsible for developing and maintaining certification and recertification processes.

Counseling and referral Problem-solving processes used to halt the decline in a troubled employee's performance and to prevent excessive employee turnover through termination or supervisor-initiated transfers. Employee counseling is provided to assist the employee in addressing personal and other problems that might originate outside the workplace but that affect job performance and behavior in the workplace. Referral is the process of linking the employee with an array of resources to address the specific problem(s) identified.

Court order A written or verbal order issued by the court.

Court reporter The individual who is responsible for creating a verbatim transcript of court proceedings.

Covered entity Any entity that is a health plan, a health care clearinghouse, or a health care provider that conducts certain transactions in electronic form and must comply with the Privacy Rule of the HIPAA.

Credential Denotes that individuals have met specific standards and demonstrated a level of competence in their field of practice. Individuals who obtain credentials are required to maintain their credentials over time by meeting continuing education requirements as defined by the agency or organization that supports the credential.

Credentialing (1) Any process by which practitioners are evaluated with the intent to affect control over their professional practice. More specifically within health care organizations, credentialing refers to the policies and procedures used to determine the membership category and clinical privileges to be granted to each member of the professional staff. (2) The process of granting (or renewing) certain privileges to practice medicine to prospective or existing members of the medical staff at a facility. During the appointment and reappointment process, the applicant's background is reviewed, licenses and certifications are checked, proof of current liability insurance is verified, and practice patterns and quality review data are evaluated to determine whether the applicant should be granted the privileges he or she seeks to gain or renew.

Credentials registry Provides a document management service to individual professionals. The credentials registry maintains an individual's credentials verification documents and releases copies of the file or selected relevant documents to health care organizations at the individual's request when he or she seeks appointment or clinical privileges.

Credentials verification organization Makes the contacts necessary to verify an applicant's education, training, experience, and professional licenses and certifications through primary source agencies.

Critical path The sequence of activities on a PERT network that takes the greatest amount of time to complete.

Critical incident method A method of employee performance evaluation that requires the supervisor to document exceptional job-related behavior, either extremely effective or ineffective performance, actually observed or reported. These statements, or critical incidents, collectively represent the range of behavior typical for that employee. Documented positive critical incidents may be used as the basis for merit pay decisions and negative ones used as the basis for performance correction plans or disciplinary action.

Cross-reference Means of linking files or data.

Cross-sectional study A type of descriptive study that examines the distribution of disease or health characteristics in population at one point in time. This type of study is used to generate hypotheses and is also referred to as a prevalence study.

Current ratio This ratio compares current assets with current liabilities to determine whether there are sufficient cash and cash-like assets to cover the immediate liabilities (bills) that will come due in the short term (1 year). The current ratio is one of the most common liquidity ratios.

Data (1) A collection of elements on a given subject; the raw facts and figures expressed in text, numbers, symbols, and images; facts, ideas, or concepts that can be captured, communicated, and processed either manually or electronically. (2) Raw facts, characters, or symbols.

Data compression A mathematical technique that applies formulas to a file to produce a smaller file. Files are compressed by eliminating strings of redundant characters and replacing them with more compact symbols.

Data dictionary Serves as the central repository for all information about the database and functions as a catalog for identifying the nature of all the data in a system. The data dictionary provides the central resource for ensuring that standard definitions for data elements and data structures are used throughout the system.

Data flow diagram (DFD) A diagram used to track the flow of data through an entire system. Data flow diagrams identify the data flow within a system, providing a data map of what data go from an area, what data are received by an area, and what data are either temporarily or permanently stored in an area. In addition to tracking data flow, a DFD identifies transformations on data (processes) and data repositories (data stores).

Data interface standards Agreed on means of transmitting data and connecting data communications equipment. A formal standard is typically the product of a standards development organization and is recognized by the American National Standards Institute.

Data mapping The process of identifying and describing the link between two distinct data models or data bases. It is used to identify terms that have the same meaning in two different databases. It may be used in a classification system to identify specific terms that fit within a particular classification. It could be used to consolidate multiple databases into a single database identifying redundant data for consolidation or elimination. It could be used to identify data relationships as part of data lineage analysis.

Data mart A subset of data extracted from the larger database. It is a smaller application with a focus on a particular subject or department.

Data mining The process of searching large volumes of data for patterns using tools such as clustering, classification, association rule mining. The science of extracting useful information from large data sets or databases. An example is a retail company that can mine its data to identify which products are frequently purchased together. These products might then be placed in proximity to encourage other customers to do the same.

Data repository Brings together information from all or a few of the applications and databases for an organization. Useful when an organization has a number of different databases or systems from a variety of vendors that contain related pieces of information about an individual or a company function. The software can quickly organize the information that is needed and provide access to enable better decision making.

Data security The technical, physical, and procedural methods by which access to confidential information is controlled and managed.

Data set A group of data items or data elements and their definitions. Data sets frequently also have defined values for each data element. A data set that has defined values for each element is useful for systematic data collection and measurement.

Data sheet A form designed to collect data in a simple tabular or column format. Specific bits of data (e.g., numbers, words, or marks) are entered in spaces on the sheet.

Data standards Documented agreements on representations, formats, and definitions of common data.

Data warehouses Receive clinical data from a transactions system such as a pharmacy system or a radiology system and combine them with other organizational data from administrative and financial systems. Also referred to as information warehouses.

Database A collection of stored data, typically organized into fields, records, and files.

Database management system (DBMS) An integrated set of programs that manages access to the database.

Database model A collection of logical constructs used to represent the data structure and the relationships between the data. The four major database models are relational, hierarchical, network, and object oriented.

Data-driven rules Rules that are applied to data to trigger an outcome, for example, create an alert in an electronic health record.

Days of revenue in patient accounts receivable ratio Measure of the average time that receivables are outstanding or the period that a health care organization extends credit to its debtors.

Decentralized filing A filing system in which parts of the record are filed in different locations in the facility rather than a centralized location.

Decision grid Used to compare various alternatives in a decision with criteria that are the basis for making the decision. Also known as matrix chart.

Decision matrix (*See* Decision grid.)

Decision support systems Information systems designed to support planning functions of an organization by drawing from multiple databases to analyze the day-to-day business activities of the organization. Decision support systems range from simple analysis of cost per patient for specific departments or clinics to high-level strategic analysis, marketing, and policy development.

Decision table Analytical tool that provides a means of communication of the logical sequence of an operation.

Decision tree Used to chart alternative courses of action for solving a problem and subsequent consequences from each course of action.

Deductible The cost that must be incurred by the patient beneficiary before the insurer assumes liability for the remaining charges.

Deemed status Refers to facilities that are accredited by The Joint Commission and AOA and are in compliance with the Medicare Conditions of Participation (COP) for hospitals.

Defamation Oral (slander) or written (libel) communication to a person (other than the person defamed) that tends to damage the defamed person's reputation in the eyes of the community.

Defendant The party or parties in a lawsuit from whom relief or compensation is sought from the plaintiff.

Deidentified Refers to data that have been stripped of certain patient identifiers.

Demographics Personal data elements, sufficient to identify the patient, collected from the patient or patient representative and not related to health status or services provided.

Dependent variable A variable whose value is dependent on one or more other variables but which cannot itself affect the other variables.

Deposition A sworn verbal testimony.

Depreciation Systematic allocation of the cost of a capital asset over a predetermined time frame in a rational manner. Calculated by dividing the capital cost by the years of life.

Descriptive study A type of research design. In epidemiologic research it is used to describe the frequency and distribution of diseases in populations. Descriptive studies are usually the first study design chosen when little is known about the disease or health characteristics.

Designated Record Set (DRS) A term used in HIPAA to include the records that contain protected health information maintained by or for a covered entity. For a health care facility these records include medical records and billing records about an individual. For a health plan these records include the enrollment, payment, claims adjudication, and case or medical management records.

Destruction letter A letter that must be signed by two witnesses during the record destruction process and that contains (as an attachment) the complete manifest of all patient record numbers and patient names.

Diagnosis related group (DRG) A classification scheme to group cases into groups expected to use similar amounts of hospital resources. Developed for Medicare and used since 1983 as part of a prospective payment system for services.

Differentiation A term used for variation from normal tissue. (*See* Grading.)

Direct method of age adjustment An age adjustment method that uses a standard population and applies the age-specific rates available for each population. One then determines the expected number of deaths in the standard population. To use the direct method of age adjustment, age-specific rates must be available for both populations, and the number of deaths per age category should be at least 5.

Direct pay, self-pay, out-of-pocket Payment by the patient to the health care provider.

Directional strategies Basis for setting organizational objectives.

Disaster recovery An organization's plan detailing how it will restart operations after a natural or human-caused disaster. As part of the plan critical information stored by the organization in must be identified and a plan put in place to restore the records, data hardware and software needed for business operations. In health care the clinical and business records are critical resources.

Discharge days The duration of hospitalization for an inpatient. (*See* Length of stay.)

Discharge planning A utilization management (UM) function designed to assist patients in transitioning from one level of care to another. Often UM staff conduct an initial discharge assessment but will refer patients in need of intensive discharge planning to case management services.

Discounted payback period A cost-benefits analysis method in which an organization determines how much a system costs in future dollars. The basic concept underlying this approach is that today's dollars are worth more than future dollars. Future dollars that are anticipated to be made by installing an information system are discounted in calculations used to determine the discounted payback period.

Discounting The opposite of compounding. Discounting is used to determine how much one must invest today at a compound interest rate of x to receive a given amount at the end of N years.

Discovery A process whereby each party in a lawsuit seeks to discover important information about the case through a pretrial investigation. Discovery includes obtaining pertinent testimony (through depositions and through interrogatories) and documents that may be under the control of the opposing party. The purpose of the discovery phase is to encourage early out-of-court resolution of cases by acquainting all parties with all pertinent facts.

Discrete data Data on quantitative variables that can only take on a limited number of values, typically only whole numbers. Examples of discrete data include the number of medications a person is taking, the number of children in a family, or the number of records that are coded.

Disparate impact Indirect discrimination that occurs when an otherwise neutral employment practice has a differential and adverse impact or effect on one or more of the protected groups.

Disparate treatment Direct discrimination that occurs when members of a protected group, such as women or minorities, receive unequal treatment in an employment action.

Dispersion The extent to which scores within a set vary from each other.

Document A document contains information. A document may be something physical like one or more printed pages or a virtual document in electronic format.

Domiciliary (residential) A type of long-term care facility where supervision, room, and board are provided for people who are unable to live independently. Most residents need assistance with activities of daily living (e.g., bathing, eating, dressing).

Double-distribution method An allocation method that assumes that the allocation of costs cannot be linear and that some indirect departments need to be allocated to less commonly dispersed departments before the costs of these departments are fully allocated.

Downtime The length of time when the computer system is not available to the user community.

Due process The right to a full hearing.

Durable medical equipment Equipment such as wheelchairs, oxygen equipment, walkers, and other devices prescribed by the physician.

Durable power of attorney for health care An advance directive in which a competent adult names in writing another adult to make any medical decisions on his or her behalf in the event he or she becomes incapacitated (although the extent of the decision-making power varies according to state law).

E-health The use of emerging information and communication technology, especially the Internet, to improve or enable health and health care.

Electronic data interchange (EDI) The electronic (computer-to-computer) exchange of data.

Electronic-health (e-health) The use of emerging information and communication technology, especially the Internet, to improve or enable health and health care. The field of e-health includes a range of functions and capabilities such as specialized search engines focused on various kinds of health care, provider and payer Web sites, support groups, Web-based physician consultations, self-care or monitoring systems, telemedicine, and disease management, and so forth.

Electronic-health information management The use of emerging information and communications technology to manage health information systems.

Electronic health records (EHR) Patient records that are maintained electronically in a manner that is accessible to caregivers, the patient, and others who need access to specific information or to aggregate information to prevent illness and improve future treatment. (*See also* patient record.)

Electronic medical records (EMR) Electronic patient records that are developed by individual health care providers/ organizations. EMRs are composed of whole files as opposed to individual data elements. The data from the EMR are the source of data for the electronic health record (EHR). (*See also* patient record.)

Emancipated minors Minors who can make their own health care decisions without parental or guardian involvement. They are treated as adults, under the law, and have the right to consent to treatment and authorize disclosures of their own health information. Although the conditions vary, emancipated minors generally involve minors who are married, living away from their parents and family, and responsible for their own support.

Emergency care area (*See* Emergency department.)

Emergency department (ED) Facility that provides emergency services. Functional areas of an emergency department include a trauma area, a casting room, examination rooms, and observation beds. A patient in the ED can be managed in one of the following ways: treated and discharged to home, treated and admitted for observation, treated and admitted to an inpatient unit, assessed and sent to surgery, stabilized and transferred to another facility, or, in the event of death, transferred to the morgue.

Employee assistance programs (EAPs) Programs offered by most health care organizations, which provide support and referral services for employees experiencing significant personal, family, or community-based problems that interfere with job satisfaction and performance.

Employee handbook A written reference manual of organizational policies and procedures covering employee rights, benefits, obligations, norms and standards of conduct, and other expectations of and constraints on employee behavior.

Employment at will English common law doctrine under which an employment contract without a specified length of term could be terminated by either party with or without cause.

Encoding The assignment of unique identifiers to the terms within a particular clinical terminology. (*See* Coding.)

Encounter The professional contact between a patient and a provider during which services are delivered.

Encryption Protects transmitted information by changing readable text into a set of different characters and numbers on the basis of a mathematical algorithm. Computers on either end of the transmissions must have keys to encrypt the information being sent and then decrypt the text at the receiving end into the original text.

Entity-relationship diagram A diagram used principally to illustrate the logical design of information system databases by describing diagrammatically the relationship between entities and by identifying entity attributes. Entity-relationship diagrams are composed of three categories of items: entities, relationships, and attributes.

Epidemiologic case definition A definition set as a reportable condition by the Centers for Disease Control and Prevention. These are of diseases that must be reported to a public health agency.

Epidemiology The study of disease and the determinants of disease in populations. Also, the study of clinical and health care trends or patterns and the ability to recognize trends or patterns within large amounts of data.

Episodes of care Care for a specific condition during a period of relative continuous care.

Equal employment opportunity Requirements that were mandated during the 1960s and 1970s through federal, state, and local legislation that prohibit employers from discriminating on the basis of race, color, religion, national origin, sex, age, and disability status.

Equity The profits and losses that result from the differences between revenues and expenses. Also referred to as fund balance.

Ergonomics Study of the relationship of people to their working environment including the construction and adjustability of equipment and furniture, arrangement of workstation, and design of work processes.

Ethernet A standard defined by the Institute of Electrical and Electronics Engineers (IEEE) as having a data transmission speed across the LAN of either 10 million bits per second (Mbps) or 100 Mbps. The topology is designed with messages that are handled by all computers in the LAN until they reach their final destination. Ethernet is the most widely used LAN network topology in use today.

Etiology The study of the causes of disease.

Event engine A tool that tracks unexpected data and notifies the providers by e-mail and beepers that something unusual has occurred.

Evidence Refers to information legally presented at trial, which is offered to prove or disprove an issue under contention. If that information is allowed to be used at trial, it can be "admitted into evidence." Both the federal government and individual states have rules of evidence, which are interpreted and applied by the judge in deciding what information may fairly be admitted into evidence.

Evidence-based medicine Using guidelines developed through research in making clinical decisions.

Exchange time The time (number of seconds) that it takes the jukebox to locate the disk and retrieve it.

Ex officio A member of the governing board or committee who does not have voting privileges.

Experimental epidemiology Epidemiological research through two types of studies: clinical trial and community trial.

Expert system A program that symbolically encodes concepts derived from experts in a field and uses that knowledge to provide the kind of problem analysis and advice that the expert might provide.

Exposure characteristics Characteristics or risk factors that may cause (or increase the risk for development of) the specific disease.

External environmental analysis Process by which an organization crosses the boundary between itself and the external environment in order to identify and understand changes that are taking place outside the organization.

Extranet Allows users outside the network to gain access to the network through a password. Also known as a VPN.

Factor comparison A method for evaluating jobs that requires identification of essential factors or elements common to all jobs and comparison of jobs on the basis of rating those elements, not the job as a whole. Factors typically applied in this method are level of responsibility, including supervision; essential skills and knowledge; mental effort (demands); physical effort; and working conditions, including hazardous situations and confidentiality.

Failure mode and effects analysis (FMEA) A risk analysis technique now being used in health care organizations to analyze existing systems and to evaluate new processes before implementation. FMEA is a technique that promotes systematic thinking about the safety of a patient care process.

False imprisonment The unlawful restraint of a person's personal liberty or the unlawful restraining or confining of a person. Physical force is not required; all that is required is a reasonable fear that force will be used to detain or intimidate the person into following orders.

Federal Register A Monday-through-Friday publication of the National Archives and Records Administration that reports regulations and legal notices issued by federal agencies, presidential proclamations and executive orders, and other documents as directed by law or public interest.

Fee for service A reimbursement method in which the cost is based on the provider's charge for each service.

Fellowship of American Health Information Management Association (FAHIMA) A credential offered by AHIMA that is designed to recognize AHIMA members who have made significant and sustained contributions to the profession over time. Eligibility for fellowship requires that an individual have a minimum of 10 years of full-time professional experience in health information management or a related field, 10 years of continuous AHIMA membership, evidence of sustained and substantial professional achievement, and a minimum of a master's degree. An individual must complete an application that is reviewed for approval by the AHIMA Fellowship Committee.

Fetal death rate Computed to examine differences in the rates of early, intermediate, and late fetal deaths.

File guide (*Alphabetical*) A guide used to aid in the filing process that lists the letter of the alphabet and any vowel subdivisions within the main letter category (such as Da, De, Di, Do, Du, all within the main letter category of D). (*Numerical*) A guide used to aid the filing process that lists the primary and secondary numbers for the file sections (such as in terminal digit filing 25-30-80, the primary number is 80 and the secondary number is 30.)

File server A specialized PC, or larger host computer, that is used only to provide a common place to store all the data that the PC users may need.

Financial accountant Responsible for recording past and current financial transactions (payments, orders, expenses, revenues, accruals, etc.).

Financial analysis The management process of formulating judgments and decisions from the relationship between the numbers represented on two reports: the balance sheet and the statement of revenues and expenses. Also known as ratio analysis.

Firewall A system used to prevent access to a private network from the outside or to limit access to the outside from within the network. All data that enter or leave the organization's network must pass through the firewall, which acts as a filter, providing a single point of entry to a network.

Fiscal intermediary An organization that has contracted to manage the processing of claims and payments.

Fishbone diagram A diagram used for solving complicated problems by helping people consider many factors and the cause-and-effect relationships among those factors. (*See* Cause-and-effect diagram.)

Flex time Flex time allows employees to control their work schedules within parameters established by management. The employer usually defines a core structure of hours of the day and days of the week in which the employee must work to provide needed services and coverage. The employee's preferred schedule can be arranged flexibly around these core hours and days of the week.

Flexible budget A type of budget that is predicated on volume. All supplies, labor, and other variable expenses are budgeted in proportion to the anticipated volume. If the volume anticipated is not reached, labor and other expenses are expected to decrease accordingly and vice versa if the volume exceeds expectations.

Flow chart A graphical representation of a specific sequencing of steps in a process. A flow chart can be an outline or schematic drawing of the actual process that needs improving or a picture of the ideal process once improvement actions are taken. A flow chart consists of a series of connected symbols that represent actual or expected process steps.

Flow process chart Chart used to list each step in a work process; identifies the distance traveled and the time consumed by each delay. It is useful to collect information about a manual process, analyze it, and improve it.

Focus groups Interviews that include a small group of people (usually experts in the field or people whose opinion on the topic is being sought) that are brought together to answer and discuss specific questions. Participants can discuss issues, hear one another's viewpoint, and comment on those views. Focus groups enable a researcher to learn more about the topic because a group of experts is brainstorming.

Focused review A review conducted to determine the cause of less-than-desired performance.

Follow-up The processes used by cancer registries to determine the cancer patient's status. The primary purposes of follow-up are to ensure continued medical surveillance to determine outcomes of the treatment and to monitor the health status of the population under investigation. Follow-up information provides the documentation of residual disease or its spread, recurrences, or additional malignancies. Subsequent treatments should be included in the patient hospital database.

Force field analysis Analysis used to identify the variables that help and variables that hinder reaching the desired outcome or solution to a problem. In addition to identifying the causal order, force field analysis estimates the relative effect of each process variable (such as the number of available trained workers) on an outcome variable (such as increasing the number of outpatient visits).

Formal definitions Definitions that follow a formal structure and that are represented in a form that can be manipulated by a computer, as opposed to narrative text definitions intended for human readers.

Foundation of Research and Education (FORE) A separately incorporated affiliate organization (to AHIMA) that actively promotes education and research in the heath information management (HIM) field. The Foundation offers grants-in-aid to support research activities and professional self-development opportunities, scholarships, professional recognition awards, and more.

Frames Vertical and/or horizontal lines that structure the form on the screen. Frames divide the form into logical sections and to direct data entry length and location.

Fraud A willful and intentional misrepresentation that could cause harm or loss to a person or the person's property.

Frequency distribution The number of times that each category of a qualitative variable or value of a quantitative variable is observed within a sample.

Frequency polygon A method used to present a frequency distribution with continuous data. It is constructed by joining the midpoints of the tops of the bars of a histogram with a straight line. The total area under the polygon is equal to the sum of the areas of the bars in the histogram and therefore equal to total sample size multiplied by interval width.

Functional interoperability (syntactic interoperability) Specifies the syntax or format of the transmitted message so that it can be parsed and stored by the receiving system.

Functional model A description of the environment and what happens in that environment that is used to begin the process of developing a specific information system. (*See also* Use case.)

Functional strategies Developed in functional areas of the organization to support programs and budgets in key areas of the organization.

Fund balance The profits and losses that result from the differences between revenues and expenses. (*See* Equity.)

Gantt chart Scheduling and progress chart that emphasizes work time relations necessary to meet a defined goal; a common project scheduling tool.

Gatekeeper The primary care physician who participates in a comprehensive managed care plan and is responsible for coordinating all care provided to the managed care enrollee (patient). The focus of care is on prevention through regular physical examinations and other primary care services. If a patient needs to see a specialist, the gatekeeper must make the referral and thereby controls access to all other care.

General system life cycle A life cycle that can apply to all systems and includes a birth or development period, a period of growth and maturity, and a period of decline or deterioration.

Generalizability The ability to extrapolate or make inferences about a population on the basis of results of a study of a sample of the population.

Goals Statements of what the organization wants to do.

Governing body A group of individuals who have the ultimate legal authority and responsibility for the operation of the health care organization, including the quality and cost of care. Also called the board of trustees, board of governors, or board of directors.

Grading Variation from normal tissue. Also known as differentiation. Used in the description of tumors.

Granularity A term used to describe the level (degree) of detail in the data.

Graphic rating scales When employee performance is evaluated, graphic rating scales require the rater to assess performance by use of numerical scales often anchored by brief descriptors of performance. This is one of the most common rating techniques in practice.

Graphical user interface (GUI) A user-friendly screen application that is important for efficiency and user satisfaction for both the individuals involved with scanning and for clinicians.

Grievance procedure Provides a communication and problem-solving mechanism for employees to express a complaint that management has violated one of its own policies (or the union contract) with adverse consequences for the employee.

Gross death rate A crude measure that shows the number of hospitalizations that end in death out of all patients who were discharged or who died during the same period of time.

Group decision support software (GDSS)   Usually a network of workstations or portable personal computers that are all located in a conference or meeting room and used to facilitate the joint application design process. GDSS can be used to administer a survey or questionnaire electronically to a group of people at the same time and to facilitate brainstorming or a nominal group technique. GDSS allows anonymity of response, minimizes bias, and speeds up the deliberative process.

Halo effect   Bias in which an observer's perception of one characteristic of an individual dominates other perceptions to result in an undifferentiated overall impression, positive or negative.

Hardware   The physical equipment (both electronic and mechanical) that makes up computers and computer systems. It includes electric, electronic, mechanical, and other equipment.

Health   Defined by the World Health Organization as a state of complete physical, mental, and social well-being and not merely the absence of disease or infirmity.

Health care information   Information about wellness strategies, diseases, and conditions associated with treatment options. Information about how to use the health care system.

Health care operations   Under HIPAA's privacy rule, health care operations is a term used to describe activities such as conducting quality improvement activities, contacting patients with information about treatment alternatives, providing educational information, evaluating practitioner and provider performance, accreditation, licensing, and credentialing. These activities may need to use or reference protected health informationl however, when the use is related directly to the operation of the health care entity and is handled appropriately, no specific authorization is required on the part of the individual(s) whose information is being used.

Health care services   The processes that contribute to the health and well-being of the person. Services may be provided in a variety of health care settings, such as the hospital, ambulatory, or home setting and include nursing, medical, surgical, or other health-related services.

Health informatics   The intersection of information science, medicine, and health care. It deals with the resources, devices, and methods required to optimize the acquisition, storage, retrieval, and use of information in health and biomedicine. Health informatics tools include not only computers, but also clinical guidelines, formal medical terminologies, and information and communication systems.

Health Insurance Portability and Accountability Act of 1996 (HIPAA)   Legislation enacted in 1996 related to health insurance that also contained provisions for administrative simplification in the handling of health information. A primary focus was the adoption of standards that are required for electronic capture and transmission of billing and health insurance information. The legislation also recognized the need for privacy and security standards for health information. HIPAA regulations also invigorated the government's efforts to reduce health care fraud and ensure that health care organizations are complying with reimbursement regulations and coding guidelines associated with the submission of claims for services rendered to federally funded patients.

Healthy People 2010   A report generated by the U.S. Department of Health and Human Services (DHHS) that identifies national objectives for disease prevention and health promotion.

Hearsay rule   Bars the legal admissibility of evidence that is not the personal knowledge of the witness.

Hierarchical   A term used to describe a database model that supports a treelike structure that consists of parent (or root) and child segments. A parent can have more than one child segment, but each child segment can have only one parent. A user queries the database, and the search seeks the answer from parent to child. The answer to the query is found by matching the conditions by searching downward through the tree.

Hierarchy chart   A type of decomposition diagram that breaks down problems into smaller and smaller detail by identifying all the tasks in a process and grouping them into various hierarchical levels.

Histogram   A graphic representation of frequency distributions. Histograms are useful for identifying whether the variation that exists in the frequency distribution is normal or skewed.

Historical-prospective study   An epidemiologic research study design that uses past records to collect information regarding the exposure characteristic or risk factor under study. Then, over the next 10, 15, or 20 years, medical records, death certificates, and so on are monitored to determine the number of cases of a particular disease that have developed.

Home health care   The provision of medical and nonmedical care in the home or place of residence to promote, maintain, or restore health or to minimize the effect of disease or disability. Home health care services mainly provide care for rehabilitation therapies and after acute care.

Horizontal integration   A merging of health care organizations offering services at the same point on the continuum of care (e.g., a multihospital system).

Hospice   A multidisciplinary health care program that is responsible for the palliative and supportive care of terminally ill patients and their families, with consideration for their physical, spiritual, social, and economic needs.

Hospital   Defined by the American Hospital Association (AHA) as a health care facility that has an organized medical and professional staff, inpatient beds available 24 hours a day, and the primary function of providing inpatient medical, nursing, and other health-related services for surgical and nonsurgical conditions and usually providing some outpatient services, especially emergency care.

Hospital ambulatory care   "Hospital-directed" health care that is provided to patients who are not admitted as inpatients and for which the hospital is responsible, regardless of the location of the health care. Services include satellite clinics, observation units, outpatient departments, ancillary services, and other specialty clinics.

Hospital formulary   Provides information on drugs that are approved and maintained by the health care organization and contains information on drugs including, but not limited to, names, dosages and strengths, packaging, characteristics, and clinical usage.

Hospital inpatient   A patient who generally stays overnight and is provided room, board, and nursing service in a unit or area of the hospital.

Hospital patient   Person who is receiving or using health care services for which the hospital is liable or held accountable. Hospital patients include inpatients, observation patients, ambulatory care patients, emergency patients, and newborn inpatients.

Human resource audit   An audit conducted to assess which openings can be filled with internal candidates already employed within the organization.

Hypothesis An educated guess about the outcome of a study. A hypothesis is a claim or statement that poses an assertion to be supported and may predict a relationship between two or more variables.

Inactive record The record of a patient who has not received treatment or had other activity associated with the record for more than 5 years. Inactive records do not need to be as readily available as active records but do need to be accessible when needed.

Incidence The number of new cases of disease.

Incidence rate The number of newly reported cases of a disease in a specified time period divided by the population at that time. The quotient is then multiplied by a constant such as 1000 or 100,000. Incident rates are determined to examine the frequency of specific types of disease.

Incidence study (*See* Prospective study or Cohort study.)

Incident report A paper-based or electronic report completed by health care professionals when a variance occurs from the usual process of patient care or when a mishap or injury occurs involving a patient, staff member, or visitor. Incident reports are meant to be nonjudgmental, factual accounts of the event and its consequences, if any, and are prepared to assist the organizations in identifying and correcting problem-prone areas and in preparation for legal defense. Also referred to as occurrence reports.

Independent living facility A type of facility composed of apartments and condominiums that allow residents to live independently; assistance (e.g., dietary, health care, social services) is available as needed by residents.

Independent variable The variable that causes change in the other variables.

Indicator An indirect measure that describes events or patterns of events suggestive of a problematic process or behavior.

Indigent Someone who is without the means for subsistence—poor or impoverished.

Infant death rate A rate that is computed to examine deaths of the neonate and infant at different stages. An infant death is death of an infant at any time from the moment of birth through the first year of life.

Inference A generalization.

Informal or unwritten organization Composed of two or more persons who develop mutually satisfying interactions pertaining to personal and/or job-related matters. These relationships are not depicted on an organization chart.

Information Data that have been organized and processed into meaningful form, either manually or by computer, to make it valuable to the user. Information adds to a representation and tells the recipient something that was not known before.

Information system development life cycle See System Development Life Cycle.

Information system life cycle A life cycle that is similar to the general system life cycle. The information system life cycle consists of the following phases: design, implementation, operation and maintenance, and obsolescence.

Information warehouses Receive clinical data from a transactions system such as a pharmacy system or a radiology system and combine them with other organizational data from administrative and financial systems. (*See* Data warehouses.)

Informed consent A communication process between the health professional and the patient. The patient must be informed about the anticipated treatment and its risks and alternatives.

Infrastructure (technical) Technical infrastructure refers to the technology architecture required to maintain systems. Technology infrastructure includes the hardware, software, network, and communication resources required as underpinning to an electronic health record system.

Inpatient A patient who is receiving health care services and is provided room, board, and continuous nursing service in a unit or area of the hospital.

Inpatient bed occupancy rate The proportion of inpatient beds that are occupied (the percentage of occupancy).

Inpatient service days Unit of measure including services received by one inpatient in one 24-hour period. Synonyms: patient day, inpatient day, census day, bed occupancy day.

Institutional Review Board (IRB) A research and human rights advisory board that is part of most health care facilities and universities and that meets at least quarterly. The aim of an IRB is to protect human subjects or patients from research risks and invasion of privacy, by reviewing all research studies that involve subjects or patients, including experiments, interviews, and questionnaires, and any study that collects data from a patient's medical record.

Insurance A purchased contract (policy) in which the purchaser (insured) is protected from loss by the insurer's agreeing to reimburse for such loss.

Integrated delivery system (IDS) A network of health care organizations that provide or arrange to provide a continuum of services to a population; the network assumes the clinical and fiscal responsibility for the outcomes and health status of the population.

Intensity of service/severity of illness Criteria that measure a need for health care services that can be provided only in an inpatient facility or define a degree of acute physical impairment that requires inpatient medical intervention.

Intentional tort Claims pertaining to intentional harm. Legal claims that may be brought against health care facilities include assault and battery, false imprisonment, defamation of character, invasion of privacy, fraud or misrepresentation, and intentional infliction of emotional distress.

Interface engine A type of middleware (software and hardware that serve as a bridge between applications) that allows two applications to exchange information without having to build a customized interface for each application.

Internal environmental analysis Reveals the strengths and weaknesses of the organization.

Internet A telecommunications international computer network that serves as the gateway to a multitude of users.

Interobserver reliability Reproducibility or reliability between more than one research assistant or observer.

Interoperability The ability of different information systems to communicate. The ability of software programs to exchange data using a common set of business procedures and to read and write the same file formats and use the same protocols.

Interrogatory A form of testimony. Interrogatories are sworn written answers to questions.

Intranet Like an Internet that runs exclusively within a network. An Intranet is accessible only by users who can be authenticated as being within a specific network.

Intraobserver reliability Reliability within one research assistant or observer.

Invasion of privacy In health care, invasion of privacy is a negligent disregard for patients' privacy. For example, health care providers who divulge confidential information from a patient's record to an improper recipient without the patient's authorization have invaded the patient's privacy and breached their duty of confidentiality.

JAVA A programming language introduced in late 1995 by Sun Microsystems. JAVA is thought to be less complicated than the C programming language. The main objective of a JAVA program is to allow applications to be built as stand-alone ones that can be transferred across the Web and run independently on a client computer. JAVA is an object-oriented language that is compiled into a universal, non-machine-dependent format.

Job analysis Systematic collection, evaluation and organization of job performance; understanding of what is required to perform the job, how it can be performed most efficiently, and what outcomes are expected from doing the job right.

Job description A narrative presentation of the key responsibilities, activities, and working conditions associated with a designated job.

Job evaluation A formal procedure used in compensation management to determine the relative worth of each position in the organization. The process is usually performed by human resource staff or contracted out to a consultant specializing in compensation systems.

Job grading A job evaluation method that classifies each job by assigning it to the narrative description of a grade that it most closely resembles.

Job performance standards Included in some job descriptions and used as the primary criteria for performance evaluation.

Job ranking A job evaluation method that ranks whole jobs by comparing them with other positions within the organization on the basis of one or more key characteristics. This ranking is based on the relative levels of responsibility of these positions and their impact on revenue generation. The ranking method is best used in organizations with a small number of positions.

Job sharing A staffing option in which a full-time position is shared by two or more persons. This option is offered by some employers to accommodate the needs and preferences of working women.

Joint application design A data-gathering technique by which a group of people spend a concentrated time together in determining system requirements. The group is usually composed of end users, managers, analysts, and others who may have an impact on or be affected by the system under study. This method is also referred to as joint requirements planning (JRP).

Joint Commission on Accreditation of Healthcare Organizations (*See* The Joint Commission.)

Jukebox Holds and retrieves individual disks as they are requested (much like a musical jukebox does). Each box or cabinet holds multiple disks and is capable of high-speed retrieval.

Jurisdiction The power of a court (federal, state, etc.) to hear a dispute.

Key indicators of demand Measures of program operations (i.e., volume, activity, or output) that can be reliably linked to staffing levels.

Knowledge Derived from information once information is organized, analyzed, and synthesized by the user.

Knowledge base A collection of stored facts, heuristics, and models that can be used for problem solving.

Layoffs Involuntary separation that occurs whenever the employer terminates the employment relationship for whatever reason, sometimes as a result of low patient volume, restructuring, or adverse economic conditions.

Lean thinking A performance improvement model that is based on the principles of eliminating waste and retaining only value-added activities, concentrating on improving value-added activities, responding to the voice of the customer, and optimizing processes across the organization.

Leapfrog Group A collaboration of large employers that came together in 1998 to determine how purchasers could influence the quality and affordability of health care. The Leapfrog Group identified four hospital quality and safety practices that are the focus of its health care provider performance comparisons and hospital recognition and reward. The quality practices are computer physician order entry, evidence-based hospital referral, and intensive care unit (ICU) staffing by physicians experienced in critical care medicine.

Legal record analysis A review of the clinical records that focuses on the presence or absence or items that are required in clinical record based on state and federal regulations.

Length of stay The number of calendar days from admission to discharge for an inpatient. Also referred to as the duration of inpatient hospitalization or discharge days.

Level of significance The criterion or standard a researcher chooses when performing a test of significance usually 0.05 or 0.01.

Liabilities The debts or obligations an organization owes. Liabilities may include wages accruing between paydays, mortgage payments due to the bank, and so forth.

Libel Written defamation of character.

Licensed independent practitioner Defined by The Joint Commission as "any individual permitted by law and by the organization to provide care, treatment, and services without direction or supervision."

Licensure The legal approval for a facility to operate or for a person to practice within his or her profession. An individual must meet eligibility requirements defined by the state before the individual is granted a license to practice. Licensure occurs at the state level and is overseen by a state licensing board or agency.

Life care centers Centers that provide living accommodations and meals for a monthly fee. They offer a variety of services, including housekeeping, recreation, health care, laundry, and exercise programs. Also referred to as retirement communities.

Life-table analysis Examines survival times of individual subjects and is most appropriate for prospective studies or experimental studies when the researcher has a loss of subjects as a result of follow-up or the study ends before recurrence or death has occurred in some subjects.

Line graph A graph that provides a simple, yet highly graphic, visual method of monitoring trends over time.

Linkage strategies Initiatives such as changing the organization's culture, reorganization, upgrade of facilities and equipment, and social and ethical strategies.

Liquidity ratios Ratios that focus on balance sheet numbers (assets, liabilities, and equity/fund balance accounts) to measure the ability of the health care organization to meet its short- and long-term financial obligations.

Literature review A review of past research studies on the same subject. A literature review is the second step of a sound research study design (after the hypothesis or question is established).

Living will A written document that allows a competent adult to indicate his or her wishes regarding life-prolonging medical treatment should he or she be unable to consent.

Local area network (LAN) Connects multiple devices together by communications and is located within a small geographic area.

Logical system design Describes the functionality of the system and presents the vision of system performance and its features.

Longitudinal patient record A comprehensive record that provides the complete history of a patient, from birth to death. This record provides easy access to medical history, reduces repeated diagnostic testing and treatments, and promotes patient safety through medical alerts and information on allergies, drug reactions, and drug interactions.

Long-term care Health care that is provided over a long period of time (30 or more days) to patients who have chronic diseases or disabilities.

Long-term debt/total assets ratio A capitalization ratio that compares the amount of long-term debt the organization has with the amount of assets it has to pay those debts.

Lossless When data compression reproduces the original file exactly with no information loss.

Lossy When data compression causes some information to be lost in the translation.

Magnification ratio The inverse of the reduction ratio.

Mainframe Machines that are used for major applications, to maintain large databases, and for high-volume work.

Major birth defects Birth defects that affect survival, require substantial medical care, or result in marked physiological or psychological impairment.

Malpractice Professional negligence.

Malware Malicious software (can be any unauthorized software that is found in an information system).

Managed care A generic term for a health care reimbursement system that is designed to minimize utilization of services and contain costs while ensuring the quality of care. The term managed care encompasses a continuum of practice arrangements, including health maintenance organizations (HMOs), preferred provide organizations (PPOs), and other alternative delivery systems.

Management by objectives (MBO) A management planning process popular during the 1970s and 1980s, used to integrate business planning, productivity management and control, employee performance evaluation, and supervisory coaching. MBO has largely been replaced by alternative approaches, such as strategic management, total quality management, and re-engineering. One of its core principles, however, the systematic setting and periodic review of performance goals, is still used today.

Managerial accountant Helps record what is happening currently or previously (variance analyses) against what was anticipated and what is still anticipated to happen (the budget).

Managerial finance officer Plans for the future by working with financial organizations (banks, investors, and so on) to obtain funding and financing for an organization's plans. Also referred to as the chief financial officer (CFO) or treasurer.

Mapping Enables users to use data for multiple purposes without having to capture the data in multiple formats. Mapping is also valuable for retaining the value of historical data when migrating to newer database formats and terminology versions.

Market entry strategy Indicates whether the adaptive strategy will be accomplished by buying into the market, cooperating with other organization in the market, or internal development.

Master budget A consolidation of all department operating budgets with each of the operating account's combined balances.

Master charge list A list used by a health care organization that reflects the charge for each item that may be used in the treatment of a patient and the charge for most services (i.e., respiratory therapy treatments, physical therapy services, laboratory tests, and so on). The list is almost always automated and linked with the billing system. Also known as the charge master, charge description master (CDM), or fee schedule.

Master patient index (MPI) Index that identifies all patients who have been treated by the facility and lists the number associated with the name. The index can be maintained manually or as part of a computerized system.

Matching principle Recognizes the importance of recognizing revenues and expenses in the same accounting period. Any associated expenses such as labor, supplies, travel, and so forth would be recorded in the same accounting period and matched with the revenue for that accounting period.

Maternal death rate The rate is calculated by dividing the number of maternal deaths by the number of obstetric discharges. A maternal death results from causes associated with pregnancy or its management but not from accidental or incidental causes unrelated to the pregnancy.

Matrix A multidimensional tool that may be used to organize, categorize, and reduce information into a more usable form. The matrix may be used in the decision-making process by weighting information or in the evaluation of performance over an extended period.

Mean A measure of central tendency that summarizes an entire set of data by means of a single representative value. The mean or average is calculated by adding up the values of all the observations and dividing the total by the number of observations.

Median The middle value within a data set. When the values are arranged from lowest to highest, the number of values above the median is equal to the number of values below the median. For an odd number of observations, the median is the middle number in the ordered set of numbers; for an even number of observations, it is the mean of the middle two numbers.

Medicaid A joint program between the state and the federal governments to provide health care to welfare recipients in the different states.

Medical informatics The study of medical computing. (*See also* Health informatics.)

Medically indigent People whose incomes are above what would normally qualify for Medicaid but whose medical expenses are high enough to bring their adjusted income to the poverty level.

Medicare A government-subsidized health care program that provides health insurance for elderly people and certain other groups.

Messaging standard A consensus-based specification standard for exchange of data among electronic systems.

Methodology The way a research study is designed so that the hypothesis can be properly tested. Includes a step-by-step process of what is done in the research study and why this process is necessary to test the hypothesis properly.

Methods improvement (*See* Work simplification.)

Microcomputers Based on small microprocessing chips found in individual PCs. Microcomputers are used for desktop applications such as word processing and spreadsheets and, with the increase in computing power available on the PC, can serve as the hardware for a database management system.

Microfiche A copy of a microfilm jacket made on a special 4 × 6-inch sheet of polyester film (Mylar).

Microfilm jacket A 4 × 6-inch holder that has channels, or narrow sleeves, formed by fusing together two panels of transparent material. A strip of roll microfilm can be inserted into a channel. Each jacket can hold about 70 document pages, depending on the reduction ratio used when the documents were filmed.

Microfilm reader Used to read microfilm images. A reader, also called a viewer, is a projection box that magnifies the image, passes light through it, and displays it on a screen.

Microform A term used to describe any type of micrographics format.

Middleware Software and hardware that serve as a bridge between applications.

Minicomputers Often used in departmental systems such as laboratory or radiology systems. Minicomputers were popular in the 1980s and early 1990s because they were less expensive than mainframes and had some of the processing power of a mainframe and allowed devices and files to be shared.

Minimum necessary A principle of the HIPAA privacy rule, whereby only the minimum necessary amount of information necessary to fulfill the purpose of the request should be shared with internal users and external requestors. There are only a few situations in which the minimum necessary standard does not apply (e.g., uses or disclosures for treatment purposes or where the patient has specifically authorized the release of more information and in a few other circumstances).

Mirroring Records from one database are continuously sent from one server to another server. The originating database is the principal database and the receiving database (server) is the mirror. In the event of a failure of the principal database (server) the receiving database (server) can quickly take over the functions of the principal database.

Mishap A medical error made in the delivery of patient care.

Mission A broad-term statement of the organization's purpose. The mission statement defines the geographical environment and population that the organization serves.

Mode The value that occurs most frequently in a given set of values. The mode is the only measure of central tendency that can be used with nominal data.

Morbidity The extent of illness, injury, or disability in a given population.

Morbidity rates Complication rates, such as community-acquired, hospital-acquired or nosocomial, and postoperative infection rates. Morbidity rates can also include comorbidity rates and the prevalence and incidence rates of disease.

Morphology Cell structure and form.

Mortality The death rate in a given population.

Mortality rates Death rates, including gross death rate, net death rate, cause specific death rates, and neonatal and infant death rates. Death rates that are computed because they demonstrate an outcome that may be related to the quality of the health care provided.

Motion to quash A motion filed by legal counsel in which the court is asked to set aside the subpoena or order.

Movement diagram (layout flowchart) Graphically represents the movement of paper or people in the physical environment where the processes are performed.

Multifunctional device (MFD) A device that is able to serve as any combination of scanner, photocopier, fax, or printer output device.

Multimedia Information content and information processing using multiple formats (e.g., text graphics, video, audio).

Multiple consistent views Required to support the different views of the vocabulary depending on the utility.

National Practitioner Data Bank (NPDP) A database of practitioner-specific information that is used by hospital medical staffs considering applications for membership (either initial appointment or reappointment) or requests for clinical privileges to identify any available adverse quality of care information about the applicant.

Natural language processing The processing of data in natural language form. Natural language processing for cardiology, for example, would need to include all the terms and expressions used by cardiologists in their models of thinking. (*See* Text processing.)

Negligence Conduct that society considers unreasonably dangerous. Failure to provide a reasonable level of care.

Neonatal death rate A rate computed to examine deaths of the neonate and infant at different stages. A neonatal death is the death of an infant within the first 27 days, 23 hours, 59 minutes of life.

Net Income from revenue reduced by all relevant deductions.

Net death rate A rate that differs from the gross death rate in that it does not include deaths that occurred less than 48 hours after admission to the health care facility. The net death rate is useful because it provides a more realistic account of patient deaths related to patient care provided by a specific health care facility.

Net operating revenue The amount of revenue *expected* to be received or total charges less the deductions expected by third-party payers resulting in revenues net of deductions or net operating revenue.

Net present value Discounted or present value of all cash inflows and outflows of a project as a given discount rate.

Network A term used to describe a database model. A network model is similar to the hierarchical model except that a child can have more than one parent. In a network database, the parent is referred to as an owner and a child is referred to as a member. In other words, it supports the many-to-many relationship.

Niche vendors In health care a company that focuses on one particular market and may focus on particular software products.

Nomenclature A system of names that have been assigned according to pre-established rules.

Nominal data Data collected on variables where qualitative rather than quantitative differences exist between individuals. Nominal data are also called categorical, qualitative, or named data.

Nominal group technique (NGT) An idea-generating technique, similar to brainstorming, that uses silent generation of ideas and a sequential reporting approach to ensure participation by all group members.

Nonrepudiation In an electronic system, the electronic signature must ensure the signed document was not modified after the signature was affixed. Additionally, the electronic signature must ensure that only the signer could have created a signature.

Nonsemantic concept identifier An identifier that does not carry any meaning in itself and does not indicate the hierarchical position of the term it represents.

Nosocomial (infection) An infection that develops more than 72 hours after hospitalization.

"Not elsewhere classified" (NEC) Term used to collect concepts that are not covered elsewhere in a terminology.

Null hypothesis In a test of significance, a null hypothesis states that there is no difference or relationship in the population and the observations are the result of chance.

Numerical identification An alternative method of identification that uses a number to identify the patient record.

Nursing classification schemes Classification schemes used to classify the interventions that nurses perform and outcome evaluations based on those interventions. Two nursing classification systems include the Nursing Interventions Classification (NIC) and the Nursing Outcomes Classification (NOC). NIC and NOC are useful for clinical documentation, communication of care across settings, integration of data across systems and settings, effectiveness research, productivity measurement, competency evaluation, reimbursement, and curriculum design.

Nursing facility A comprehensive term for a long-term care facility that provides nursing care and related services for residents who require medical, nursing, or rehabilitative care.

Object In programming an object is an individual unit of run time data storage that is used as the basic building block of programs. In object-oriented programming a program works with a dynamic set of interacting objects. These objects include a very specific kind of typing that allows for data members to associate with the object and for methods that access the data members in predefined ways. An example of an object would be "my car," which is an instance of a type (class) called "car," which is a subclass of "motor vehicles."

Objectives Specific statements that define the expectations or outcomes given the goal direction. Objectives provide clear guidelines for management and supervisors to define the action steps to achieve the objective. Objectives are usually measurable.

Object-oriented A type of database model that embraces the concept of an object. An object-oriented database is a collection of objects. Objects support encapsulation and inheritance. Encapsulation is the technique by which an object such as a patient is defined with certain characteristics. The user does not need to know how the characteristics are stored, just that the object "patient" exists and has certain attributes.

Observation patient A patient who needs assessment, evaluation, or monitoring because of a significant degree of instability or disability that does not require admission to the hospital as an inpatient.

Occurrence report Factual summaries of unexpected events that have resulted (or could have resulted) in injury or harm to patients, staff, or visitors. Occurrence reports are used by health care organizations' risk managers or attorneys to investigate incidents that have the potential to become claims against the organization or individual provider and to identify areas where improvements are needed. (*See* Incident report.)

Odds ratio An estimate of the relative risk a person has if he or she is exposed to a certain characteristic.

Office landscaping The overall design of the office areas or spaces; the most common type is the open type.

Office of the National Coordinator for Health Information Technology In 2004 President Bush created the new position of National Health Information Technology Coordinator. This Office and role within Health and Human Services (HHS) is charged with providing national leadership in support of government and private efforts to develop the standards and infrastructure to more effectively use information technology to achieve quality health care and to reduce health care costs. The Coordinator reports to the Secretary of HHS.

Ongoing record review The review of a health care facility's clinical records on an ongoing basis, beginning at the point of care and based on organization-defined indicators that address the presence, timeliness, readability (whether handwritten or printed), quality, consistency clarity, accuracy, completeness, and authentication of data and information contained within the record.

Open architecture A system that uses different vendors to integrate the best possible products that provide the best speed and processing capabilities. Open architecture protects the facility's investment against possible vendor bankruptcy or complete closure and also allows individual pieces of equipment to be exchanged as rapidly as technology advances, not only as rapidly as one vendor makes upgrades.

Open office design plan Design for an office arrangement that features open space free of permanent walls. Workstations that are created with the use of partitions and furniture. The open plan focuses on work groups, traffic patterns, and work flow.

Open system A system in which the specifications are made public to encourage third-party vendors to develop add-on products for them. Open systems are designed to incorporate all kinds of devices, regardless of the manufacturer or model that can use the same communications facilities and protocols.

Open-ended questions Questions that do not provide a list of responses to choose from, similar to an essay type question, enabling the recipient to write out his or her thoughts in free form. Also referred to as unstructured format questions.

Operating budget A budget that predicts the labor, supply, and other expenses required to support the work volume predicted.

Operating margin ratio A common performance ratio that displays the relationship between the net revenues received and the expenses required to supply the revenues.

Operating system Directs the internal functions of the computer and serves as the bridge to application programs. Operating systems act as system managers that direct the execution of programs, allocate time to multiple users, and operate the input/output (I/O) devices and the network communication lines.

Operation flowchart A graphic representation of the logical sequence of activities in a procedure. It shows the decision points encountered in carrying out that function.

Operational strategies Made up of strategies developed within the functional areas of the organization and strategies that link the functional areas and develop the capabilities of the organization.

Opportunity costs The benefits that would be received from the next best alternative use of the investment funds.

Optical character readers A device used for optical character recognition.

Optical character recognition A data entry technique that uses a scanner to read typewritten or specifically formatted data such as bar codes into a computer at high rates of speed.

Order entry The on-line entry of orders for drugs, laboratory tests, and procedures, usually performed by nurses or unit clerks.

Ordinal data Data expressing rankings from lowest to highest according to some criterion.

Organization chart Illustrates the hierarchical relationships between various individuals, lines of authority, accountability, and responsibility; identifies the organization's primary functions and the subfunctions within each primary function.

Osteopathic medicine Based on the theory that all body systems are interconnected and therefore the focus of health care is directed at the whole person. Because two thirds of the body is composed of muscle and bone, osteopathic medicine places a great deal of emphasis on the musculoskeletal system.

Outcard A card that stays in a patient file permanently to tell the new location of the paper record or the new medium to which the file has been transferred. Outcards are usually cardboard to allow the patient name and record number to be written directly on them.

Outcome measures Performance measures that examine the end results or product of the patient's encounter with the system.

Outguide A plastic folder used in place of a record when the record has been removed from the files. An outguide serves as a placeholder and usually contains two separate see-through pockets, one to hold the requisition slip and one to hold any loose papers to be filed in the record that accumulate while the record is out of file.

Out-of-pocket A payment method in which the patient pays directly to the health care provider. (*See* Self-pay.)

Outpatient A patient who is receiving health care services at a hospital without being hospitalized, institutionalized, or admitted as an inpatient.

Outsourcing The use of contract services.

P value In a test of significance, the probability that the observed value of the test statistic could occur in the event that the null hypothesis is true. The P value can range from 0 to 1. The smaller the P value or closer it is to 0, the less likely the null hypothesis is true and the smaller the probability that the observed difference or relationship could be due to chance or sampling error alone.

Packet filter A type of firewall that examines data entering or leaving and accepts or rejects the data on the basis of system-defined criteria.

Palliative care Health care services that relieve or alleviate patient symptoms and discomforts, such as pain and nausea; it is not curative.

Pareto chart A chart that is similar in form to bar charts and histograms. However, unlike bar charts and histograms, occurrences plotted on a Pareto chart are ordered from the largest or most frequently occurring category (and presumably most important) to the smallest or least frequently occurring category. Pareto charts often are used in conjunction with brainstorming as a visual aid to demonstrate where attention to specific problems should be focused.

Participant observation A type of qualitative research in which the researcher is immersed into the subject's environment to learn what the subject experiences first hand. The researcher pays special attention to the physical, social, and human environment and formal and informal interactions and unplanned activities. The researcher can choose to be disguised or undisguised and is basically there to describe a problem to outsiders on the basis of the understanding of the insider's perspective.

Participating physicians A term that refers to physicians who participate in a preferred provider organization (PPO).

Passive case A term used to describe reporting systems that rely on reports submitted to the registry by hospitals, clinics, or other facilities, supplemented with data from vital statistics. In some states, staff submits reports voluntarily, but, in general, reporting requirements are established by state legislation.

Password aging The process whereby users must change their password at a specific frequency (e.g., 30 days, 90 days). This process enables the passwords to remain unique and identifies users who do not log in for a period of time.

Patient An individual, including one who is deceased, who is receiving or using or has received health care services.

Patient advocacy The promoting of health care quality and patient safety improvements. Patient advocacy is concerned with ensuring overall patient satisfaction with the process and outcomes of care episodes.

Patient assessment The process of obtaining appropriate and necessary information about each individual seeking entry into a health care setting or service.

Patient centered care Care that puts the patient in charge and gives him/her as much control as desired. It gives patients choices that allow them to express their cultural traditions, personal preferences and values, family situations, and lifestyles.

Patient health record The primary legal record (either paper or electronic) documenting the health care services provided to a person in any aspect of the health care system. The patient health record includes routine clinical or office records, records of care in any health-related setting, preventive care, lifestyle evaluation, research protocols, and various clinical databases. The principal repository for information concerning a patient's health care, uniquely representing patients and serving as a dynamic resource for the health care industry. (Synonymous with clinical record, medical record, health record, resident record, client record. In electronic format, synonymous with electronic health record, electronic medical record.)

Patient record system The set of components that comprise the system and mechanisms by which patient records, the data in the records, and the data about the records are created, used, stored and retrieved. The patient record contains administrative, legal, and clinical information about an individual. The individual and aggregate use of this information is essential to the delivery of health care. The patient record system also includes information about the system (e.g., policies and procedures, information on who may use the system, practice standards for clinical documentation). The system may use a paper-based patient record or a hybrid combination of paper and electronic patient record or use a fully electronic patient record. (Synonymous with medical record system, health record system, resident record system, electronic health record system.)

Patient safety improvement The actions undertaken by individuals and organizations to protect health care recipients from being harmed by the effects of health care services.

Patient safety indicators Indicators that screen for problems that patients experience as a result of exposure to the health care system and that are likely amenable to prevention by changes at the system or provider level.

Pay for Performance (P4P) A payment system initiated by some health plans that financially rewards providers who achieve specific quality or patient safety goals. The fundamental principles of Pay for Performance are (1) common performance measures for providers (usually represent a balance of patient satisfaction, prevention, and chronic care management) and (2) significant health plan financial payments based on that performance, with each plan independently deciding the source, amount, and payment method for its incentive program.

Payback method The payback period determines the number of years it will take for the cash inflows from each project to pay back the initial investment.

Payback period The time in which a project saves enough money to pay for itself. To determine the payback period, a comparison between total old system (project) costs and total new system (project) costs (including investment) is made. The difference between new and old costs is calculated on a year-by-year (cumulative) basis. When the difference between old costs and new costs reaches zero, the payback period has been reached.

Payer The party who is financially responsible for the reimbursement of the health care costs.

Pearson correlation coefficient A statistic used to assess the direction and degree of relationship between two continuous variables. The direction of the relationship between two continuous variables can be either positive or negative.

Peer-reviewed journal A journal with articles that have been extensively reviewed by peers within the specific research area. Peers have provided comments and feedback to the authors to incorporate into their revision of the article before publication.

Pen-based device A device used to capture and enter data into computer systems that has built-in communications and organizer software and can be carried in the pocket.

Per case A fixed payment system.

Per diem Established payment for a day's worth of services.

Percentage of occupancy (*See* Inpatient bed occupancy rate.)

Performance appraisal A systematic method for observing, evaluating, documenting, and giving feedback to employees about their performance.

Performance assessment An assessment that involves a formal periodic review of performance measurement results. Sometimes called evaluation, appraisal, or rating.

Performance measure A generic term used to describe a particular value or characteristic designated to measure input, output, outcome, efficiency, or effectiveness.

Performance measurement A strategic process used to assess accomplishment of goals and objectives. The process of performance measurement involves review of many different performance measures or indicators.

Performance ratios Ratios that evaluate the use of resources to achieve a goal based on data from the statement of revenues and expenses.

Period prevalence rate Refers to evaluating a health condition over a *period of time*, such as 1 year.

Personal data assistant (PDA) A device available for point-of-service input; travels with caregiver; can be wireless. Also known as pocket devices.

Personal health record (PHR) An electronic or paper record of health information compiled and maintained by the patient. The PHR is not a part of the health record that is compiled by health care provider's legal health record.

PERT network The acronym for Program Evaluation Review Technique; diagram that illustrates the dependency relation of several projects leading to a larger nonroutine goal (e.g., building project); tool used to plan and coordinate the smaller projects and accomplish the larger goal; used to give likely completion times.

Phishing A type of security threat that uses e-mail messages that appear to come from a legitimate business or organization. These e-mail messages request personal information, such as an account number, and contain a link to a Web site to submit the information.

Physical system design Specifies all the characteristics that are necessary so that the logical design can be implemented, including details about the design of hardware, software, databases, communications, and procedures and controls.

Physician advisory Physicians who participate in the utilization management process by reviewing hospitalized patients whose conditions do not meet criteria for remaining in the hospital. This provides a type of peer review.

Picture archiving and communication system (PACS) Provides rapid access to digitized film images, such as for radiology applications, and can help eliminate the cost of film processing and storage.

Pie chart Used to represent the relative frequency of categories or intervals within a sample. A pie chart is constructed by drawing a circle, 360 degrees, and dividing that circle into sections that correspond to the relative frequency in each category.

Pilot testing Testing a survey with a small sample of the potential recipients. Recipients go through the survey as if they are going to answer the questions and provide feedback on any changes or additions to the survey. Once the feedback is received by the research team, the survey should be changed to meet the feedback received where applicable.

Plaintiff The party that initiates the lawsuit.

Pleading When the defendant files an answer to the complaint from the plaintiff. In this answer, the defendant denies or otherwise responds to the plaintiff's claims.

Point of care system A system by which data are captured at the place where the care is provided. For example, a bedside terminal system that is located where the patient is receiving care, such as the bedside.

Point of service A type of managed care plan that combines characteristics of both the HMO and the PPO. Members of a POS plan do not make a choice about which system to use until the point at which the service is being used.

Point prevalence rate Refers to evaluating a health condition at a specific point in time. Therefore, each study participant is assessed only *once* at *one point* in time, although the actual point prevalence study may take months or years to conduct.

Point system A job evaluation method that analyzes key elements of the job and assigns point values to these factors of the basis of predetermined descriptive standards or criteria.

Pointer In computer science a pointer is a data type whose value refers directly to (points to) another value stored elsewhere in the computer.

Point-to-point Refers to the method of connection between two endpoints, usually host computers. The term point-to-point telecommunications is used to refer to wireless data communications for Internet or Voice over IP via radio frequencies.

Policies The guides that managers use to make decision. Policies translate the mission statement and corporate objectives into practical and easily understood terms.

Polyhierarchy An arrangement that is necessary to support different users and uses of the same terminology.

Population-based cancer registry A registry that collects data for a defined geographic area. There are three types of population based registries: incidence only, cancer control, and research.

Postoperative death rate A cause-specific death rate that expresses the number of deaths that may have resulted from surgical complications. The number of patients who die within 10 days of surgery is divided by the number of patients who underwent surgery for the period.

Postoperative infection rate A rate used by the health care facility to determine which infections occur after surgery and are probably due to the surgical procedure.

Potentially compensable event (PCE) An adverse occurrence, usually involving a patient, that could result in a financial obligation for the health care organization.

Power The ability of one person A to influence another person B to do something he or she would otherwise not decide to do.

Power of attorney The legally recognized authority to act and make decisions on behalf of another party.

Practitioner An individual who is licensed or certified to deliver care to patients.

Practitioner profiles Profiles used to integrate information compiled from performance improvement activities into the credentialing process. A practitioner's profile provides a concise summary of information crucial to objective credentialing of professional staff.

Precedent The rulings of similar previous cases. By referring to similar cases that have been decided in the past and applying the same principles, courts generally arrive at the same ruling in the current case as in similar previous cases.

Preempt or preemption Override.

Pre-existing condition A disease, injury, or condition identified as having occurred before a specific date.

Preferred provider organization (PPO) A network of physicians and or health care organizations that enter into an agreement with payers or employers to provide health care services on a discounted fee schedule in turn for increased patient volume. Patients are encouraged to use these providers by having a lower deductible, copayment, and coinsurance for services given by these providers.

Preponderance of evidence "More likely than not" when weighing whether something is true or not true when the evidence supports the case by 51%.

Prevalence The number of *existing* cases of disease

Prevalence rate The number of existing cases of a disease in a specified time period divided by the population at that time. The quotient is then multiplied by a constant, such as 1000 or 100,000. Prevalence rates are determined to examine the frequency of specific types of disease.

Prevalence study A type of descriptive study that examines the distribution of disease or health characteristics in population at one point in time. This study is used to generate hypotheses. (*See* Cross-sectional study.)

Preventive discipline A disciplinary approach that encourages understanding of the rationale for and compliance with policies, standards, and rules so that significant violations of policy are avoided.

Primary care The care provided at the point of first contact (encounter) with the health care provider in an ambulatory care setting; the care is continuous and comprehensive. Primary care encompasses preventive care (comprehensive care) and acute care.

Primary data The information contained in the actual patient record.

Primary key In database design a primary key is a value that can be used to identify a unique row in a table. Attributes are associated with the primary key. In a relational model of data, a primary key is a key chosen as the main method of uniquely identifying a tuple in a relation. A tuple represents some object and its associated data. A key is a constraint which requires that critical information about the object not be duplicated.

Primary patient record The record that is used by health care practitioners while providing patient care services to review patient data or document their own observations, actions, or instructions.

Privacy The right of individuals to control disclosure of their personal information.

Privilege delineation The process of determining the specific procedures and services a physician or other professional is permitted to perform under the jurisdiction of the health care organization. The applicant formally requests specific privileges, and any award of privileges must be supported with documentation of training, education, and other evidence of qualification or competence.

Privileged communication Statements made to attorneys, priests, physicians, spouses, or others in a legally recognized position of trust. The confidentiality of these statements is generally protected by law from being revealed, even in court.

Procedures The guides and plans for action. The step-by-step instructions for accomplishing a specific task or job.

Productive time The time during which a worker is present and working.

Productive unit of work An item produced that meets established levels of quality.

Productivity Process for converting the resources of an organization (labor, capital, materials, and technology) into products and/or services that meet the organization's goals.

Productivity standards Tools used to specify the expected performance and to measure actual performance. Also known as work standards.

Profession A profession is an occupation that requires extensive training and the study and mastery of specialized knowledge and skill and usually has a professional association, ethical code, and process of certification or licensing.

Profit The amount of money (cash) actually received from the payer (patient or insurance company) less the actual cost to do the service, assuming that the cost is less than the cash received.

Progressive discipline A process used in response to employee misconduct, in which there is a planned sequence of managerial responses of increasing severity to correct continuing violations of policy. Progressive discipline gives the employee subject to the disciplinary process several opportunities to correct the offensive behavior before the final irrevocable step of termination is invoked.

Project A unit of work to acquire or build, and implement a computer system (software, hardware, and all infrastructure) with a definitive start date, targeted stop date, steps, milestones, and outcome.

Project management Group of people with expertise in a variety of functions led by a project manager who work to accomplish a single goal.

Promulgated Formally made public, most frequently used in relationship to the act of formally, publicly declaring new statutory or administrative law when it receives final approval.

Proprietary Private, for profit, or investor-owned (hospitals).

Proprietary system A system that uses only equipment designed and manufactured by a certain vendor.

Prospective payment A method of reimbursement based on payment rates that are established in advance and reflect an average of what a service should cost.

Prospective payment system (PPS) A reimbursement program where the amount of payment is determined in advance of services rendered. Rates are established annually by the Centers for Medicare and Medicaid Services.

Prospective study A type of study that determines whether the characteristic or suspected risk factor truly preceded the disease or health condition. The prospective study design is the best method for determining the magnitude of risk in the population with the characteristic or suspected risk factor. Also referred to as a cohort or incident study.

Protected group A group, such as women or minorities, that is protected from discrimination under Equal Employment Opportunity laws.

Protected health information Under the HIPAA privacy rule patient health information that could be used to identify an individual and should be kept confidential.

Protocols Computer-based communication protocols are specifications or algorithms for how data are to be exchanged. Protocols may also be used to describe the expected or recommended course of treatment for a particular health condition.

Prototype A draft that is developed to provide a preliminary model or early version.

Provider Any entity that provides health care services to patients, including health care organizations (hospitals, clinics) and health care professionals.

Proximate cause That which, in a sequence unbroken by intervening causes, produced injury, and with which the injury would not have occurred; in other words, the primary or substantial cause of an injury. Whether an action or omission is the proximate cause of an injury is sometimes a difficult question involved in negligence/malpractice litigation.

Proximity chart Matrix that provides information useful in work space design; shows the desirability of having work areas close to or far apart from one another.

Proxy server A form of firewall that intercepts all messages entering and leaving the network so that the network address is hidden.

Public health Focuses on the threats to the overall health of a community based on population-based health data analysis, as opposed to medical health care, which focuses on the treatment of the individual.

Public key One of the most popular forms of encryption. A public key is a key that the user gives to anyone he or she wants to receive the message. Web servers often have a public key available to the requester of a Web document.

Purge The process of cleaning out or ridding patient records of certain items not important to ongoing patient care to conserve file space. Items are either moved to an alternative storage site or converted to another medium, such as microforms or optical disks to be filmed.

Qualitative record analysis A review of the patient record that assesses how well a standard is being met. Typically requires training and judgment on the part of the assessor, frequently used to assess documentation standards.

Qualitative research A type of descriptive study design that is used when little is known about a specific topic. Qualitative research provides richer information than cannot be obtained from quantitative-based studies alone. Qualitative research is most appropriate to use when one is examining attitudes, feelings, perceptions, or relationships.

Quality improvement Initiatives or efforts to improve the quality of health care and customer satisfaction.

Quality improvement organizations Organizations contracted by CMS (Centers for Medicare and Medicaid Services) at the state level to direct and oversee nationwide health care performance measurement and improvement initiatives.

Quantitative record analysis A review of the patient record to assess whether an item of required documentation is present or absent. This analysis may also apply time requirements to the expectation of required documentation.

Qui tam Whistleblower-based prosecutions.

Random sample A sample in which every member of the population has the same chance of being included in the sample and the selection of one member has no effect on selection of another member.

Range The difference between the highest and lowest values of a set of numbers; a way to measure dispersion.

Rapid cycle improvement (RCI) A performance improvement model that uses an accelerated method (usually less than 4 to 6 weeks per improvement cycle) to collect and analyze data and to make informed changes on the basis of that analysis. This is then followed by another improvement cycle to evaluate the success of the change. RCI relies on small process changes and immediate, careful measurement of the effect of these changes.

Rate The number of individuals with a specific characteristic divided by the total number of individuals, or alternatively the number of times an event did occur compared with the number of times it *could* have occurred.

Ratio analysis The management process of formulating judgments and decisions from the relationship between the numbers represented on two reports: the balance sheet and the statement of revenues and expenses. (*See* Financial analysis.)

Reasonable accommodation Adjustments made to the workplace to accommodate an employee's disability that allow the employee to perform the essential job functions without causing undue hardship to the employer.

"Reasonable man" standard If a claim involves simple (not professional) negligence such as in a personal injury suit, the jury uses the "reasonable man" standard to evaluate the defendant parties' conduct in light of the jury's own general experience and background.

Recognized redundancy Terms with the same meaning are treated as synonyms and are represented by the same identifying code.

Record tracking A method of tracking the current location of a patient record.

Recruitment pool A maintained list of potential applicants who are presumably qualified and willing to perform one or more target positions in the organization.

Reduction ratio Indicates the amount by which an image has been reduced in size. A standard ratio for patient records is 24×, or 24 to 1, meaning that the image is 1/24 the size of the original.

Redundant array of independent disks (RAID) Describes a data storage scheme using multiple hard drives to share or replicate data among drives.

Re-engineering Fundamental rethinking and radical redesign of business processes to achieve dramatic improvements in performance, such as cost, quality, service, and speed; management theory in which the way business is done is radically re-evaluated to achieve dramatic performance improvement.

Reference date The date the registry began accessioning cases.

Regional health information organizations (RHIOs) Organizations that are working together to develop means of sharing health information for patient care and other uses, typically within a geographic area. Various models exist including models where the information stays with its originator and is accessed as authorized and models that centralize data and control access as authorized. RHIOs are part of the development of a national health information infrastructure.

Registered health information administrator (RHIA) A credential offered by AHIMA to individuals who pass a certification examination and successfully meet the academic requirements of a CAHIIM-accredited health information management program at the baccalaureate degree level or have a certificate of completion from a CAHIIM-accredited health information management program plus a baccalaureate degree from a regionally accredited college or university. The RHIA functions in the managerial areas of health services and information systems and the uses of health-related data for planning, delivering, and evaluating health care.

Registered health information technician (RHIT) A credential offered by AHIMA to individuals who pass a certification examination and successfully meet the academic requirements of a CAHIIM-accredited health information management program at the associate degree level. The RHIT typically functions in the technical areas of health data collection, analysis and monitoring and often specializes in coding diagnoses and procedures for reimbursement and research purposes.

Registered record librarian (RRL) A credential first offered to individuals in 1933 when the American Association of Medical Record Librarians (now known as AHIMA) formed a Board of Registration to set standards for its members.

Registration (1) For the purpose of professional recognition entails entering on an official list an individual who has been certified as eligible by set qualifications of an organization or agency. (2) The process of gathering information from an individual to assist in providing care. This information consists of administrative data and pertinent clinical data. The data are entered into a computer system that is used to track registration for services, outpatient, emergency, admission to inpatient care, transfers within the care system, and discharge from care.

Regression analysis Analysis used to learn to what extent one or more explanatory variables can predict an outcome variable.

Regulation Dictates of government agencies charged with enforcing and implementing legislation in a particular area; these dictates are designed to carry out the intent of the law.

Rehabilitation The processes of treatment and education that lead the disabled person to the achievement of maximum independence and function and a personal sense of well-being.

Reimbursement formula The agreement between the third-party payers and the providers concerning what will be paid for and how much will be paid to the provider.

Relational model The most popular database model. Designed around the concept that all data are stored in tables with relationships between the tables. A relationship is created by sharing a common data element; for example, if two tables have a patient identifier, patient identifier relates those tables. Developed by E. F. Codd in 1970.

Relative humidity The percentage of moisture in the air.

Relative risk An estimate of risk found by using the odds ratio in an epidemiologic study.

Reliability Refers to consistency between users of a given instrument or method.

Reliable A term used to describe a measure that is stable, showing consistent results over time and among different users of the measure. A reliable measure has low levels of random error.

Replacement charts Charts used in human resource planning that present a visual representation of who is available to fill projected vacant positions. Replacement charts usually identify individual incumbents, the most likely (or all potential) replacements, and summary measures of performance and promotion potential.

Report cards Published reports that reflect provider or health plan performance on critical indicators of cost, clinical outcomes, and consumer satisfaction.

Request for information (RFI) Solicits general information from vendors about their products. The RFI may state in general terms what the facility is looking for in system functionality. Vendors then respond with information about their product lines and their experience in the marketplace and provide copies of their annual reports.

Request for proposal A document that details all required system functionality, including functional, technical, training, and implementation requirements. The document is distributed to a selected number of vendors, who are invited to respond to the proposal.

Requisition An acknowledgment that someone has taken a record and intends to return it.

Res ipsa loquitur "The Thing Speaks for Itself" doctrine applied to cases where the defendant had exclusive control of the thing that caused the harm and where the harm ordinarily could not have occurred without negligent conduct.

Research question Asks a question to be answered and identifies the goal of the research.

Resident A patient who resides in a long-term care facility.

Respite care A type of short-term care that allows caregivers time off while continuing the care of the patient. Respite care is often provided to caregivers of terminally ill patients or severely disabled children or adults.

Respondeat superior "Let the master answer." Under this doctrine, health care organizations must take reasonable steps to supervise the actions of their employees and professional staff (including medical staff). Organizations can be held liable for damages when their employees fail to perform their duties adequately.

Response rate The rate of individuals who respond (in a survey).

Restraint of trade Contracts or agreements that tend to or are designed to eliminate or stifle competition, create a monopoly, artificially maintain prices, or otherwise hamper or obstruct the course of trade and commerce. When the medical or professional staff credentialing process interferes with a physician's or health professional's ability to pursue his or her profession.

Results reporting Applications designed to retrieve diagnostic test and treatment results from feeder systems such as laboratory, radiology, and other departmental settings such as transcription and present them directly on inquiry to the care provider. Results reporting usually includes a graphical user interface (GUI) for viewing laboratory results, ECG results, and other reports using graphics displays such as flow sheets.

Retention period The amount of time a health care organization keeps patient records. The retention period varies depending on federal and state regulations and organization needs.

Retrospective payment system A payment method in which the charges for the health care services is determined after the health care was provided. The actual amount paid may be based on fee for service or on the usual, customary, and reasonable charges.

Retrospective review A review that occurs after care has been rendered. A retrospective review can provide valuable information about patterns of undesirable practices that can be used to improve future performance.

Retrospective study (*See* Case-control study.)

Return on investment (ROI) The money earned from investment at a certain interest rate.

Revenue Money earned from the services provided (in a health care organization).

Right of privacy A constitutionally recognized right to be left alone, to make decisions about one's own body, and to control one's own information. Right of privacy is an important constitutional right for the health care industry.

Risk Any event or situation that could potentially result in injury to an individual or financial loss to the health care organization.

Risk factors Factors that may increase the risk for development of a disease. Also referred to as exposure characteristics.

Roll microfilm A continuous film strip, similar in appearance to movie film that holds several thousand document pages, depending on the reduction ratio used when the documents were filmed. Because roll microfilm cannot be updated, it is usually a choice only for extremely old records, records of deceased patients that will never need updating, or as an archival copy of records maintained in microfilm jackets.

Rolling budget method A budgeting method that requires management to prepare a budget for a period of time and add to the end of that period another month when a month is consumed.

Root cause analysis A systematic investigation process that occurs after a complication or adverse event that resulted in a patient injury caused by medical management rather than by the underlying disease or condition of the patient.

Run chart A chart used to provide a visual method of monitoring trends over time. A run chart can illustrate performance trends and standards of evaluation over a long time period.

Sample size In a study, the number of subjects included in the sample.

Sampling error The principle that the characteristics of a sample are not identical to the characteristics of the population from which the sample is drawn.

Satellite clinic An ambulatory care facility that is not located on the campus of the main hospital. Satellite clinics are established in areas that are convenient to the patients, such as places of employment, or in areas that are closer to a specific patient population.

Satisfactory assurance For a subpoena duces tecum for health information to be valid under the HIPAA privacy rule, reasonable efforts must be made by the party seeking information to ensure that the individual who is the subject of the protected health information has been given notice of the request or that the party seeking the information has made reasonable efforts to secure a qualified protective order that meets the requirements of the HIPAA privacy rule.

Scanner A device that converts the images on paper into digital images. Dot patterns (bitmaps) are created in the same pattern as the dots in the paper image.

Scenario A "story," narrative description or simulation that represents an actual situation. Also referred to as a use case.

Script-based systems An alternative form of structured text, script-based systems combine key words and scripts. Scanning for key words invokes a particular script. The script itself then serves as a building block for the remainder of the text-processing event and may act as a template that specifies necessary components and the properties required.

Secondary care Care by a specialist, usually through referral from the primary care physician.

Secondary data The information that is generated from the patient record.

Secondary patient record A subset that is derived from the primary record and contains selected data elements.

Security of health information HIPAA and good business practices require that health care organizations implement administrative, technical, and physical safeguards to protect the confidentiality, integrity, and appropriate availability of health information maintained in either paper or electronic format. HIPAA's focus is on protected health information in electronic format.

Selection process Involves a sequence of activities that should result in the hiring of a well-qualified employee to fill the target position.

Self-appraisal A method of employee performance evaluation that requires an employee to reflect on his or her performance for the period, identify strengths and weaknesses, and identify accomplishments and obstacles to progress before the formal performance appraisal review.

Self-pay A payment method in which the patient pays the health care provider directly. Also referred to as out-of-pocket pay or direct pay.

Semantic content The meaning of the message.

Semantic interoperability The most sophisticated level of interoperability, incorporating the semantic content of the message. At this level, data received from another system can be displayed, interpreted, and manipulated as if it were generated locally.

Sensitivity A measure of validity, sensitivity is the percentage of all true cases correctly identified.

Sentinel event A term used to describe serious patient incidents that should have a root cause analysis (a systematic investigation as to what, how and why something happened). Examples of sentinel events include abduction of a baby from the newborn nursery and amputation of the wrong body part.

Serial numbering A numbering system in which a patient receives a number for each encounter at the facility. The patient could have multiple numbers, all of which require entry onto the manual index card or maintenance in the computerized database.

Serial-unit numbering A numbering method in which numbers are assigned serially to patients, but as each new encounter takes place, all the former records are brought forward to the most recently assigned record number and filed as a unit.

Servlet A program that executes itself on the Web server and handles multiple requests simultaneously. Servlets reside on the server side and function by having the user's request run directly on the Web server to generate dynamic HTML pages. This technology is generally used to provide interactive Web sites that interface to databases or other data sources.

Sexual harassment A form of gender discrimination that can produce a number of negative effects in the workplace including decreased productivity, increased worker stress and illness, higher turnover and absenteeism, lower morale, interference with team building, additional recruitment and training costs, and potential legal liabilities.

Simultaneous equations method An allocation method that permits multiple allocations to occur through sophisticated mathematical software and the use of simultaneous mathematical equations. This method, also known as the algebraic or multiple apportionment method, may require 10 to 12 different distributions of costs.

Six Sigma A performance improvement approach that aims to eliminate defects. Under this approach, results that fail to meet performance standards are called "defects," typically reported as defects per million opportunities. Six Sigma is the performance level attained when a process yields only 3.4 defects per million opportunities. The goal is to achieve an almost perfect level of quality by eliminating these defects.

Slander Oral defamation of character that tends to damage the defamed person's reputation in the eyes of the community.

Sliding scale fee The cost of health care is based on the patient's ability to pay.

Software The set of instructions required to operate computers and their applications. Software includes programs that are sets of instructions that direct actual computer operating functions, called the operating system, and sets of instructions used to accomplish various types of business processes, known as application software.

Solo practices Physicians who are self-employed and legally the sole owners of their practices.

Specific aims Briefly describes a project's goals or objectives.

Specificity A measure of validity, specificity is the percentage of all true noncases correctly identified.

Staff hour Sixty minutes of time during which an employee is working on a task or a particular function and being paid for that work.

Staffing table A tool used in human resource planning that provides a graphic representation of job titles and anticipated position vacancies.

Stage In reference to cancer, the stage is the extent of the spread of the disease.

Stakeholder In relationship to a computer project any individual who has a stake or real interest in the project and its implementation, regardless of department, position, or functional role in the company.

Standard deviation The square root of variance. Represented by the symbol σ.

Standard of care The generally accepted standards of care (for each profession), determined by referring to current standards published by the relevant specialty society and the professional literature. Sometimes referring to accreditation and licensing standards determines it.

Standardization movement In the early 1900s physicians in the United States decided to upgrade and standardize medical education and the practice of medicine and surgery. They also decided that it would be important to standardize the clinical records. This general effort is referred to as the "standardization movement" in health care.

Standardized mortality ratio (SMR) An indirect method of age adjustment.

Stare decisis "Let the decision stand." A legal principle that courts should decide similar cases similarly. In other words, cases that have similar facts and questions should ordinarily be decided the same way.

Statement of revenues and expenses A financial report of the expected or earned income and the associated expenses for an accounting period. This financial report may also be referred to as the income statement and can be described by the following equation: Revenue − Expense = Net income.

Statistical analysis A process performed to select specific data items from medical records for clinical and administrative decision making. Uses of statistical analysis range from billing and case-mix analysis to selection of cases for quality review. (*See* Abstracting.)

Statistical process control Quality control method using statistics to detect variations from acceptable levels of quality.

Statistics budget Budget based on historical data regarding the volume and type of health care services provided, data about the community, and future projection of need for health care services. All available data are used to estimate types and volumes of health care services needed for the projected budget period.

Statute A law enacted by Congress or state legislatures.

Statute of limitations A law that requires a claim to be filed within a certain period of time; otherwise the claim will not be heard by a court. Statutes of limitations are designed to encourage the timely filing of claims, when evidence is fresh and witnesses are likely to be available. In most states the statute of limitations begins at the time of the event or (in a health care case) at the age of majority if the patient was treated as a minor.

Step-down method A common allocation method in which the indirect department that receives the least amount of service from other indirect departments and provides the most service to other departments has its costs allocated first.

Store and forward Data are initially gathered and then sent at another time.

Strategic control Final stage of strategic management; process that includes (1) establishment of standards (objectives), (2) measurement of performance, (3) evaluation of organizational performance against the standards, and (4) taking corrective action, if necessary.

Strategic human resource planning A proactive human resource management activity in which managers must continually forecast and coordinate the supply of qualified human resources with the predicted demand on the basis of workflow cycles in health information services. This strategic approach to planning anticipates and prepares for future staffing needs.

Strategic implementation The third step in the strategic management process; based on the operational strategies that have been developed.

Stratified random sample A random sample that's obtained by dividing a population into groups (strata) and taking random samples from each stratum. Stratified random sampling is done to ensure that the sample is representative of the population.

Subpoena A written court order that requires someone to come before the court to testify.

Subpoena duces tecum A written court order that requires someone to come before the court and to bring certain records or documents named in that order.

Surveillance The collection, collation, analysis, and dissemination of data.

Survey design A type of descriptive study in which the research focuses on collecting data with a survey instrument such as a questionnaire or interview guide.

Swing beds Designated hospital beds that have the flexibility of serving as acute care or post acute care long-term beds.

Symbology The way the lines and spaces in a bar code are arranged.

Syndromic surveillance system A public health surveillance system that can detect patterns of disease in a population and that is designed to recognize outbreaks on the basis of the symptoms and signs of infection.

System Series of elements tat are interrelated according to a plan for achieving a well defined goal.

System analysis and design The activities related to specifying the details of a new system. Typically, this includes making decisions about the logical and physical design of the system.

System development life cycle The process used to identify, investigate, design, select, and implement information systems. The system development life cycle consists of five principal phases: Initiation phase, analysis phase, design phase, implementation phase, and evaluation phase.

System testing Often called user acceptance testing. For electronic health record applications, information systems staff set up a "test database" that consists of the full system features and functions complete with dummy patients supplied by users. This test database is isolated from the "production" database and made available to selected users who add fake data and then test the system's features and functionality. Performance is measured against test plan criteria established earlier.

Systematic sampling A sampling method in which the researcher must first decide what fraction or proportion of the population is to be sampled. If a researcher decided to sample one tenth of the population, the researcher would first randomly choose a starting point on a list of the population and then select every tenth record beginning with the designated starting point.

Systems flowchart Depicts the flow of data through all or part of the system, the various operations that take place within the system, and the files that are used to produce various reports or documents.

Tags Used to define or describe the text that is contained in them.

Task lighting Light fixtures that are built into the furniture or workstations to illuminate specific work areas; especially important in an open office design. Also referred to as accent lighting.

Task-ambient lighting Combination of general light with light directed to the work surface.

Tax Equity and Fiscal Responsibility Act (TEFRA) A law enacted in 1983 that brought prospective pricing to health care and enhanced the value of the patient record because it became the key document for supporting and determining reimbursements to hospitals.

Template A pattern used in computer-based patient records to capture data in a structured manner; it may contain both text and data objects.

Terminal Connected to information systems and used to enter and retrieve information.

Terminal digit filing A filing method based on a patient identification number that is divided into three parts. The number is read from left to right for identification purposes and from right to left (from the terminal end) for terminal digit filing purposes.

Terminology The usage and study of terms. The labeling or designating of concepts particular to one or more subject fields through the research and analysis of terms in context, for the purpose of documenting and promoting correct usage.

Tertiary care The care provided at facilities with advanced technologies and specialized intensive care units, such as teaching institutions and university medical centers.

Test statistic Measures the size of the difference or relationship observed in the sample.

Tests of significance Used to determine whether observed differences between groups or relationships between variables in the sample being studied are likely to be due to chance and sampling error or reflect true differences or relationships in the population of interest.

Text processing The computerized processing of natural language.

The Joint Commission A private entity whose primary function is to develop and assess standards of performance by health care organizations. The organization's goal is to improve the quality of health care. Recent initiatives include data collection and dissemination regarding sentinel events and treatment for certain types of health problems. This organization changed its name from the Joint Commission for the Accreditation of Healthcare Organizations (JCAHO) to The Joint Commission (TJC) in 2007.

Thick client A device that requires a substantial amount of memory and disk space to perform functions that the application may require. Thick clients are devices that might include a desktop PC or a workstation.

Thin A term used in reference to clinical records, especially paper records, to indicate that a portion of the record has been removed and stored in a secondary location. Records that are active for a long period of time such as nursing home records can become unwieldy. An organization develops a policy and procedure to thin records in an orderly and agreed on manner.

Thin client A device that has minimal or no disk space; it loads its software and data from a server and then uploads any data it produces back to the server. Thin clients are devices that vary from a laptop computer to a hand-held network instrument.

Third-party payer Private insurance companies, managed care organizations (MCOs), and fiscal intermediaries (FIs) that process claims for Medicare and Medicaid.

Three tier A type of client-server architecture that has three components: user interface, application server, and database server. The user interface is the software that runs on the user or client machine, and it can be customized to the needs of the client. The application server processes the data. The logic behind the database queries is hidden from the user.

Threshold The minimum acceptable quality on the basis of the organization's historical performance.

Time value of money A basic concept of money management that says that it is more beneficial to receive a dollar today than to receive it 1 year from now. A dollar received today can be invested and gain interest for 1 year longer than a dollar received 1 year from now.

Token ring When transmissions travel from one computer to another until they reach their final destination, allowing a single computer to be added to or disconnected from the network without affecting the rest of the computers on the local area network.

Topography Site or location of a neoplasm.

Tort In private law, tort refers to an action where one party alleges that another party's wrongful conduct has caused him or her harm. The party bringing the action to court seeks compensation for that harm.

Training manual Materials that teach concepts that serve as background to hands-on exercises that teach system functionality and outcomes.

Transactional leadership Those behaviors associated with the more routine and continuous exchanges of effort and commitment between managers and employees in carrying out the business of the organization and sustaining effective working relationships.

Transfer notice A notice that a record has been forwarded to another location. Transfer notices that make their way to the file area should be given a higher priority than the retrieval of records. Filing the transfer notices first ensures that the most current location for every record is known before retrieval is attempted.

Transformational leadership The visionary, motivational, and charismatic aspects of leadership. The transformational leader is able to articulate a vision of the organization's future, to convince followers that they have a stake in the achievement of that vision, and to achieve commitment to change (personal and organizational) as not only inevitable but also beneficial both to the organization and to the employee's self-interest.

Trauma center An emergency care center that is specially staffed and equipped to handle trauma patients; most trauma centers are equipped with an air transport system.

Triage The process of sorting out patients in the emergency department to determine the urgency and priority for care and to determine the appropriate source of care. Triage promotes efficiency and effectiveness in the management of the diverse patient group arriving in the emergency department.

TRICARE (formerly CHAMPUS) A health insurance program provided by the Department of Defense for active and retired military personnel and their dependents.

Trip frequency chart Matrix that represents the number of times employees interact with one another in a specified period of time; used in designing a work space.

Turnover ratios Ratios that use data from the balance sheet and the statement of revenues and expenses to measure an organization's ability to generate net operating revenue in relation to its various assets. Also referred to as activity ratios.

Two-factor authentication Authentication protocol that requires two forms of authentication to access the system (token plus a password). Also referred to as strong authentication.

Two-tier A type of client-server architecture that was developed in the early 1990s in which most of the processing occurs on the server. It reduces network traffic by providing a query response rather than total file transfer. The user interface is located on the user's desktop, and the database management application and data tables are stored on a database server.

Undue hardship Any action that would require significant difficulty or expense when considered in light of the nature and cost of the accommodation in relation to the size, resources, technology, and structures of the employer's operation.

Uninterruptable power supply (UPS) A battery that keeps the system running during a power failure and protects it from the power surges associated with power outages.

Unique identifier A number that is assigned to link patients to their records. This number is used on all record forms and views to collect all patient data in the correct record or to be accessed by computer database query.

Unit numbering system A numbering system in which each patient receives an identification number at the first encounter and retains that number throughout all contacts with the facility.

Unit record A type of patient record that's created under the unit numbering system. Each patient receives an identification number at the first encounter and retains that number throughout all contacts with the facility, allowing for the same folder to be used for all encounters and filed in one location in the file.

Use case A scenario, "story," or description that represents an actual situation.

User A user in computing context is one who uses a computer system. Users typically have an account (a user account), a username and a password.

User's manual A complete textural documentation of the system that includes all system features and functionality, complete rationale behind use of particular features, complete picture of system usage within organization or user environment, solutions to potential problems with usage, sources of help for users, and so forth.

Usual, customary, and reasonable charges The physician's usual charge for the service, the amount that physicians in the area usually charge for the same service, and whether the amount charged is reasonable for the service provided.

Utilization review The process of evaluating the efficiency and appropriateness of health care services according to predetermined criteria.

Valid The degree to which all items in the measure relate to the performance being measured; extent to which all relevant aspects of performance are covered; and extent to which the measure appears to measure what it is intended to measure.

Validity Assesses relevance, completeness, accuracy, and correctness. Validity measures how well a data collection instrument, laboratory test, medical record abstract, or other data source measures what it should measure.

Value chain Process or linked processes that support customers and contribute to the organization's overall goals and business objectives.

Values The fundamental beliefs or truths that the organization adheres to.

Values clarification The idea that reflecting on and understanding our own value commitments and priorities is an essential process as a precondition for ethically responsive decision making and leadership.

Variance Measures the deviations of the values from the mean. Variance is computed by squaring each deviation from the mean, summing the deviations, and then dividing their sum by one less than n, the sample size.

Variance report A document that reflects the budget that was prepared and approved and shows the actual results on at least a monthly basis.

Vertical integration Network of health care organizations that provide or arrange to provide a continuum of services to a population; the network assumes the clinical and fiscal responsibility for the outcomes and health status of the population.

View In a computer system a view is a particular way of looking at the data in a database. The view organizes the data visible on the computer screen in a way that meets the needs of a user. Different users may need different views of data from the same database. Different views do not affect the physical organization of the database.

Vision View of the future that management believes is optimum for the organization and is communicated throughout the organization.

Vital statistics Data collected for vital events in our lives, such as births and adoptions, marriages and divorces, and deaths, including fetal deaths.

Vocabulary A set of terms and their corresponding definitions. Used to represent concepts and to communicate these concepts.

Voice recognition The computer capability to understand human speech. Voice recognition allows practitioners to talk directly to devices and record findings.

Weighted mean An overall mean (average) for a total sample when separate means are reported for different subdivisions of the sample.

Whistleblower An individual who goes outside regulatory bodies in an organization to raise a problem rather than reporting a suspected unlawful activity internally.

Whole service When facilities or individuals are paid for all services rendered at the rate the facility or individual charges with no discount applied.

Wide area network (WAN) Used for extensive, geographically larger environments. Wide area networks are often used for computer systems connecting separate institutions.

Wi-Fi A type of network that enables computers and other hand-held devices to communicate with the Internet and other network servers without being physically connected to the network. Also referred to as wireless.

Wireless A type of network (popular in health care) that enables computers and other hand-held devices to communicate with the Internet and other network servers without being physically connected to the network. (*See* Wi-Fi.)

Work breakdown structures Divides the project into major objectives, partitions each objective into activities, further divides the activities into sub-activities and creates work packages that must be done to complete the project.

Work sampling Method of measuring work that collects data about the work being performed on randomly selected time of observations

Work simplification Organized approach to determine how to accomplish a task with less effort, in less time, or at a lower cost while maintaining or improving the quality of the outcome.

Workforce The authorized employees of an organization as used in the HIPAA Privacy Rule.

Workstation A PC or other device that is connected to an information system. A workstation is used to connect directly with the database in the system and to access and receive information from the system directly. A workstation is well suited for applications that require more memory and disk storage than a desktop PC, and usually functions as part of a hospital network. Also, a collection of desks or work surfaces, equipment, storage facilities, and chairs shaped by technology, the tasks to be performed, and various human needs.

Write once read many (WORM) A type of laser technology that stores the data in a permanent capacity and does not allow the user to alter the documents. The document is written once and can be read as many times as necessary from the disk. WORM technology is preferred for health information storage because data cannot be misfiled, accidentally erased, or altered.

Zero-based budget A type of budgeting approach that requires management to complete a program assessment and define consequences if specific programs are terminated or reduced.

Index

Page numbers followed by f indicate figures; t, tables; b, boxes.

A

AAFP (American Academy of Family Physicians), 483
AAMT (American Association for Medical Transcription), 102, 122
Abbreviated Injury Scale (AIS), 484
Abbreviation(s), in patient records, 113-114, 116
Abbreviation list, 113
ABC (Alternative Billing Codes), 209t
Abdomen, physical examination of, 108t
Abrupt changeover, 337, 364
Abstracting
  with electronic document management, 258
  of medical records, 124, 183
  for registry, 475
    cancer, 477, 478f
Abuse, financial aspects of, 660-661, 661b
AcademyHealth, 74t
Accent lighting, 645
Acceptance, of electronic health record system, 193
Acceptance and testing, 352
Access and retention, 218-265
  automated, 243-247
    client server technology in, 246-247
    communications in, 246
    computer-assisted coding tools in, 245-246
    document imaging devices in, 245
    hardware for, 243
    input, output, and storage devices for, 243, 243t-244t
    pen-based devices for, 244-245
    radiofrequency identification for, 245
    terminals and workstations for, 244
    voice recognition in, 245
  of image-based records, 247-264
    electronic document management for, 255-264, 269t
    micrographics for, 247-255, 248t, 249t, 251t, 253t
  key concepts in, 264-265
  of paper-based records, 220-243
    disaster recovery in, 242-243
    filing equipment for, 221-223, 222t, 223f
    filing methods in, 223-226, 224b, 225b, 226t
    legal health record definition in, 242
    master patient index in, 226-231, 227f-231f, 232b-233b
    record identification in, 220-221, 221t
    record management issues with, 234-236, 235b
    record tracking in, 237-240, 237f, 238b, 239b
    retention in, 240-242
    space management in, 223, 224t
Access controls, 295-296, 296t
Access management, in revenue cycle, 655-656
Access time, 257
Accessibility, of data, 144, 144t
Accessioning, 476
Accounting
  accrual basis, 671-672
  cash basis, 671
  financial, 669-672, 671t

Accounting (*Continued*)
  fundamental principles of, 669-671
  managerial, 661-662
  patient, in revenue cycle, 657
Accounting principles, generally accepted, 650, 653
Accounting rate of return, 679-680
Accounts receivable, 672
Accounts receivable turnover ratio (AR days ratio), 675
Accreditation, 439, 14015
  advantages of, 14
  defined, 14, 52, 439
  of educational programs, 52
  institutional, 562
  patient record and, 46
Accreditation Council on Graduate Medical Education, 32
Accredited Record Technician (ART), 51
Accrediting agencies, 14-15, 439
  data collection standards of, 100
  use of health data by, 96
Accrual basis accounting, 671-672
Accuracy
  of data, 144, 144t
  of documentation, 178
  of system performance, 333, 334t
ACIP (Advisory Committee on Immunization Practices), 483
Acknowledgment of Health Information Portability and Accountability Act privacy notice, 104
Acknowledgment of patient rights, 104-105
Acoustics, in workstation design, 645
ACS (American College of Surgeons)
  on cancer registries, 475, 476
  history of, 6b, 7b, 46
  Minimum Standards of, 6, 6b, 7b, 46
ACSCOT (American College of Surgeons Committee on Trauma), 484
Action steps, 662
Action-entry segment, of decision table, 620, 622f
Actions segment, of decision table, 620, 622f
Active case ascertainment surveillance systems, 479
Active records, 254
Activities, in PERT network, 633
Activity list, 608, 609f
Activity ratio, 674-675
Activity sequence, in project planning, 631
Acute care, 16, 16t
  data needs for, 129-130
Acute care facility, 20
ADA. *See* Americans with Disabilities Act (ADA).
Adaptive strategies, 628–629
Addendum(a), to patient records, 189, 513-514
ADEA (Age Discrimination in Employment Act), 544, 563t, 565-566
Adjusted hospital autopsy rate, 378, 379t
Administration for Children and Families, 11
Administration on Aging (AoA), 11
Administrative agencies, rules and regulations of, 505
Administrative and diagnostic summary, on patient record, 149

Administrative applications, 283-284, 283t
Administrative coding, 201
Administrative data, on patient record, 147t
Administrative decision making, ethical aspects of, 553b
Administrative forms, 103t, 104-105
Administrative safeguards, 294, 294t
Administrative Simplification amendment, 512
Administrative terminologies, 201-204
Administrative uses
  of electronic health records, 164
  of health information, 522
Administrators, use of health data by, 95
Admissibility, as evidence, 514-515, 529
Admission, 163
  discharge, and transfer (ADT) application, 156, 163, 280, 283-284, 283t
  ordering and documentation at, 163
Admission event review, 185f
Admission note, 109
Admitting, in revenue cycle, 655-656
Adolescent immunization status, 693
Adoption, access to health records with, 525
ADT (admission, discharge, and transfer) application, 156, 163, 280, 283-284, 283t
Adult day care services, 29
Advance directives, 13, 105, 532
Advanced registered nurse practitioners (ARNPs), 102
Adverse events, 457
Advertising, for job openings, 580
Advisory Committee on Immunization Practices (ACIP), 483
Advocacy, by AHIMA, 95
Affinity diagrams, 450, 450f, 455f
Affirmative action programs, 562-563
Against medical advice (AMA), 108
Age discrimination, 565-566
Age Discrimination in Employment Act (ADEA), 544, 563t, 565-566
Age distribution, of workforce, 560-561
Age-adjusted death rate, 377, 377t
Agency for Healthcare Research and Quality (AHRQ)
  establishment of, 8b, 11
  focus of, 11
  on health information technology, 67, 71t
  on patient safety, 458, 458t
  on performance measurement, 441, 443
Agency for Toxic Substances and Disease Registry, 11
Aggregate data, 94, 96, 168, 443
Aggregate information system life cycle, of organization, 312
Aging workforce, 544, 560-561, 565-566
AHA (American Hospital Association), 5-6, 46, 439
AHIC (American Health Information Community), 70, 71t, 166, 216
AHIMA. *See* American Health Information Management Association (AHIMA).
AHRQ. *See* Agency for Healthcare Research and Quality (AHRQ).
AICPA (American Institute of Certified Public Accountants), 661, 669, 674
Aide, 30

Aims, of research, 408
Air conditioning, in workstation design, 643-644
Air pollution, 644
Air quality, in workstation design, 644
AIS (Abbreviated Injury Scale), 484
AJCC (American Joint Committee on Cancer), 477
Alcohol abuse, confidentiality of records of, 516-517, 518, 520f
Alerting system, automated, 286-287
Algebraic method, of cost allocation, 669
Alias, in data dictionary, 318f, 319, 319f
Alias names
    for celebrities, 527
    in master patient index, 227, 227f-228f
Alias term, 145
All Kids Count, 74t
All Patient DRGs (AP-DRGs), 203
All Patient Refined DRGs (APR-DRGs), 203
Allergy data, standardization of, 212
Allied health professionals, 33-34
ALOS (average length of stay), 382-383, 383t, 431, 432t
α, 393
Alphabetical filing, 224, 224b, 225b
Alphabetical identification, for paper-based records, 220
Alteration, of records, 512
Alternative Billing Codes (ABC), 209t
Alternative care settings, patient records in, 127
Alternative dispute resolution, 506
Alternative hypothesis, 392-393
Alternative medicine, 29
AMA (American Medical Association), 5, 15, 46
AMA (against medical advice), 108
Ambient lighting, 645
Ambulatory care, 17-18
    data needs for, 130-134, 135f
    shift toward, 130
Ambulatory Care Quality Alliance, 73, 74t
Ambulatory deficiency analysis, 134, 135f
Ambulatory surgery centers, 18
AMDIS (Association of Medical Directors of Information Systems), 75t
Amendment(s)
    to document, 189
    to electronic health information, 175t
    of patient record, 513-514
Amenities, in care, 442
American Academy of Family Physicians (AAFP), 483
American Academy of Pediatrics, 456
American Association for Medical Transcription (AAMT), 102, 122
American Association of Medical Record Librarians, 49
American College of Medical Informatics, 686
American College of Surgeons (ACS)
    on cancer registries, 475, 476
    history of, 6b, 7b, 46
    Minimum Standards of, 6, 6b, 7b, 46
American College of Surgeons Committee on Trauma (ACSCOT), 484
American Health Care Association's Quality Award, 439
American Health Information Community (AHIC), 70, 71t, 166, 216
American Health Information Management Association (AHIMA), 56-58, 74t
    on accreditation, 15
    Code of Ethics of, 58, 58b, 549, 552
    communication in, 57-58
    on corporate compliance, 510

American Health Information Management Association (AHIMA) (Continued)
    data collection standards of, 101
    on electronic medical records, 74t
    Foundation of Research and Education in Health Information Management of, 58, 73t, 537, 685
    on fraud and abuse, 661
    history of, 49–50
    on ICD-10-CM, 202
    on legal health record, 157-161, 160t-161t
    as legal resource, 537
    mission and role of, 44, 74t
    on personal health record, 95, 162
    structure of, 56–57, 56b, 57f
    on transition to electronic health records, 685
    on vision for future, 690
American Hospital Association (AHA), 5-6, 46, 439
American Institute of Certified Public Accountants (AICPA), 661, 669, 674
American Joint Committee on Cancer (AJCC), 477
American Medical Association (AMA), 5, 15, 46
American Medical Informatics Association (AMIA), 75t, 102, 686-688
American Medical Record Association, 49
American National Standards Institute (ANSI), 39, 74t, 174t, 215
American National Standards Institute (ANSI) 837 electronic remittance advice, 659
American National Standards Institute (ANSI) 837 health care claim, 657
American Nurses Association (ANA), 207
American Nurses Association (ANA) Quality Indicators, 102
American Nursing Informatics Association, 75t
American Osteopathic Association (AOA), 14, 15
American plan of office design, 641
American Society for Testing and Materials (ASTM), 78, 145-149, 157
American Society of Anesthesiologists, 456
Americans with Disabilities Act (ADA), 565
    accessibility requirements of, 600-601
    and equal opportunity, 564
    key points of, 505, 563t, 565
    and work space design, 640
AMIA (American Medical Informatics Association), 75t, 102, 686-688
ANA (American Nurses Association), 207
ANA (American Nurses Association) Quality Indicators, 102
Analysis document, 330-331
Analysis of data, in research proposal, 409, 410
Analysis of variance (ANOVA), one-way, 394-396
Analysis phase, of system development, 306-307
Analytic study, 415t, 421-426
    case-control or retrospective, 421-424, 423f, 424t, 427t-428t
    historical-prospective, 426, 426f, 427t-428t
    prospective, cohort, or incidence, 424-425, 425t, 426-428t
Ancillary services, 18
Anesthesia death rate, 374t, 375
Anesthesia report, 110
Anesthesiology, 23t
ANOVA (analysis of variance), one-way, 394-396
ANSI (American National Standards Institute), 39, 74t, 174t, 215
ANSI (American National Standards Institute) 837 electronic remittance advice, 659

ANSI (American National Standards Institute) 837 health care claim, 657
Antepartum record, 110-111
Antitrust claims, 505, 510
Antitrust liability, 534
AoA (Administration on Aging), 11
AOA (American Osteopathic Association), 14, 15
AP-DRGs (All Patient DRGs), 203
Apgar score, 111
Appeals, 506
Appellate court, 507
Appendix, of research proposal, 411
Applets, 291
Application gateway, 297
Application server, 279, 280
Application service providers (ASPs), 299
Application software, 275
Appointments, scheduled, 149
APR-DRGs (All Patient Refined DRGs), 203
Aptitude tests, 582
AR days ratio (accounts receivable turnover ratio), 675
Arbitration, 506
Arbitrator, 594
Arden syntax, 287
ARLNA (Association of Record Librarians of North America), 49
ARNPs (advanced registered nurse practitioners), 102
ARPAnet, 288
ART (Accredited Record Technician), 51
Ascension number, 285
Ascertainment bias, 415
Ascertainment surveillance systems
    active case, 479
    passive case, 479-481
ASCR (Association of Specialists in Cleaning and Restoration International), 242
ASPs (application service providers), 299
Assault and battery, 508
Assembly language, 275
Assets, 672
Assistant, 30
Assisted living, 28
Associate administrator, 22
Associate degree
    in health information management, 52
    in nursing, 33t
Association of Medical Directors of Information Systems (AMDIS), 75t
Association of Record Librarians of North America (ARLNA), 49
Association of Specialists in Cleaning and Restoration International (ASCR), 242
Asthma, use of appropriate medications for, 692
ASTM (American Society for Testing and Materials), 78, 145-149, 157
Asynchronous transfer mode (ATM), 278-279
Atlas, 384
Attorneys, disclosure of health information to, 522-523
Attributes, 322, 495
At-will employment, 590-591
Audiology, 27
Audit logs, standards for, 175t
Authentication
    defined, 294
    of records, 114, 124, 175t, 178, 514
        electronic health, 189-190
    strong, 295
    tools for, 294-296, 296t
    two-factor, 295

Authorization(s)
for disclosure of patient information, 515, 518, 519f, 520f
for internal use of records, 517, 518, 522
Automated alert alarm, 286-287
Automated data access and retention, 243-247
client server technology in, 246-247
communications in, 246
computer-assisted coding tools in, 245-246
document imaging devices in, 245
hardware for, 243
input, output, and storage devices for, 243, 243t-244t
pen-based devices for, 244-245
radiofrequency identification for, 245
terminals and workstations for, 244
voice recognition in, 245
Automated record-tracking systems, 238-240, 238b, 239b
Automation assessment, for business plan, 666-667
Autopsy, disclosure of health information for, 523-524
Autopsy rates, 378-379, 379t
Average daily inpatient census, 382, 382t
Average length of stay (ALOS), 382-383, 383t, 431, 432t
Axillae, physical examination of, 108t

B

Baccalaureate degree
in health information management, 52
in nursing (BSN), 33t
Backup(s)
of master patient index, 230
at remote location, 242-243
in system development, 309f
Bailiff, 507
Balance sheet, 672, 672f
Balanced Budget Act (BBA), 293, 510
Baldrige Healthcare Criteria for Performance Excellence, 439
Baldrige National Quality Award, 439
Ballot boxes, on forms, 117-119
Bandwidth, 292
Bar chart, 452, 452f, 455f
Bar code(s), 287–288
in electronic document management, 256
and patient safety, 700
in record-tracking system, 238-239, 240
Bar code devices, 239, 256
Bar code readers, 239, 256
Bar code scanners, 239, 256
Bar graph, 386, 387f, 388f
Bargaining units, 569
Barnett, Octo, 272
BARS (behaviorally anchored rating scales), 587, 587f
Baseline data, 362
Basic interoperability, 214
Battery, 508
BBA (Balanced Budget Act), 293, 510
BCBS (Blue Cross and Blue Shield of America), 34
Bed count, 20
Bed occupancy day, 382t
Bed size, 20
Bed turnover rate, 383, 383t
Behavioral health, data needs for, 142-143
Behavioral health services, 20
Behavioral Health Standards Manual, 142
Behaviorally anchored rating scales (BARS), 587, 587f

Benchmarking
comparative, 447
competitive (performance), 446-447
internal, 446
in performance assessment, 446-447, 446f
in productivity program, 613
sample values for, 366, 367t-368t
Beneficence, 550
Beneficiary(ies), 35b, 37
Benefit, 35b
Benefit period, 35b
Benefits Improvement and Protection Act (BIPA), 293
Benefits realization, 338-339
Best evidence rule, 514
β, 393
Between-groups degrees of freedom (dfb), 395
BFOQ (bona fide occupational qualification), 566
Biases, 414-415
that affect performance appraisal, 589
Bibliography, 407
BICS (Brigham Integrated Computing System), 176
Bicycle helmets, 695
Bill of Rights, 505
Billing consent form, 522, 523f
Biometric devices, for security, 295
Bioterrorism, 486
BIPA (Benefits Improvement and Protection Act), 293
Birth and development, in system life cycle, 310
Birth certificate, 105, 372-373
Birth defects
classification of, 481
major, 481
Birth Defects Monitoring Program, 481
Birth Defects Prevention Act, 479
Birth defects registries, 479-481
Birth history, 111
Blinded study, 427
Blood vessels, physical examination of, 108t
BLS (Bureau of Labor Statistics), 641
Blue Cross and Blue Shield of America (BCBS), 34
Board of directors (BOD), 21-22
of AHIMA, 56
Board of governors, 21-22
Board of Inquiry, 568-569
Board of Registration, 53
Board of trustees, 21-22
Body, of form, 117
Boeing Company, 166
Bona fide occupational qualification (BFOQ), 566
Book of Knowledge, 58
Borders, on forms, 119
Boundary, of system, 624
Boxes, on forms, 117-119
Brailer, David, 166, 200
Brainstorming, 450, 455f
Breach
of confidentiality, 509
of contract, 509-510, 536
in negligence or malpractice case, 530
Break glass policy, 294
Break-even analysis, 339-340, 340t
Breasts
physical examination of, 108t
in review of systems, 106t
Bridges to Excellence, 75t
Brigham and Women's Hospital
computerized physician order entry at, 688-689
electronic health record system of, 176

Brigham Integrated Computing System (BICS), 176
Browsers, 289
BSN (baccalaureate degree in nursing), 33t
Budget(s), 662-665
as control, 664
defined, 662
flexible, 664
master, 663
operating, 663
rolling, 663-664
staffing (salary), 664, 665t
statistics, 662-663
and variance reports, 664-665, 665t, 666t
zero-based, 664
Budget development, 663
in research proposal, 411
Budget periods, 663-664
Budgeting
participatory approach to, 663
for staff, 664, 665t
Bulletin of the Association of Record Librarians of North America, 49
Burden of proof, 530
Bureau of Labor Statistics (BLS), 641
Burn hospitals, 20
Burton, Harold H., 6
Bush, George W., 48, 166, 684
"Business" analyst, 308
Business associate agreement, 516
Business data, 360
Business logic layer, 314, 314f
Business plan, 665-668, 666b, 667f
Business process re-engineering, 636-637, 637b
Business Roundtable, The, 76t
Business rules
electronic health record system and, 187, 187b, 280
in request for proposal, 345, 347f
Bylaws, 22

C

CA (certificate authority), 297
CAAHEP (Commission on Accreditation of Allied Health Education Programs), 15
CAAHEP (Council on Accreditation of Allied Health Educational Programs), 52
caBIG (Cancer Biomedical Informatics Grid), 72t
Cache memory, 257-258
Cafeteria benefit plans, 558
CAH (critical access hospital), 19
CAHIM (Commission on Accreditation for Health Informatics and Information Management Education), 15, 52, 57
California HealthCare Foundation, 75t
CAM (complementary and alternative medicine), 29
CAMBHC (*Comprehensive Accreditation Manual for Behavioral Health Care*), 142
CAMHC (*Comprehensive Accreditation Manual for Home Care*), 137
CAMLTC (*Comprehensive Accreditation Manual for Long Term Care*), 134
Canadian Hospital Association, 46
Cancer abstract, 477, 478f
Cancer Biomedical Informatics Grid (caBIG), 72t
Cancer committee, 478
Cancer control registries, 476, 477
Cancer hospitals, 20
Cancer registrar profession, 479
Cancer registries, 475-479
abstracting for, 477, 478f

Cancer registries (*Continued*)
  coding for, 477
  hospital, 475, 476
  population-based, 475-477
  quality management of, 478-479, 480f
  staging in, 477
  use of, 479
Cancer Registries Amendment Act, 476
Cancer staging, 477
CAP (College of American Pathologists), 69-70, 204
Capital decisions, 675-680, 677f-678f, 679t
Capital expenditure(s), 675-676
Capital expenditure approval form, 676, 677f-678f
Capital expenditure committee, 675-678
Capital expense decisions, 675-680, 677f-678f, 679t
Capital planning, 675-680, 677f-678f, 679t
Capital request(s), 675-676
Capital request evaluation process, 676-678, 677f-678f
Capitalization ratio, 674, 675
Capitation method, 34, 35-36, 660
CAR (computer-assisted retrieval), of microfilm, 248, 248t, 249t
Carbon copies, 119
Card(s), for security, 295
Cardiology, 23t
Cardiovascular disease, 695
Cardiovascular surgery, 23t
Cardiovascular system
  physical examination of, 108t
  in review of systems, 106t
Care
  acute, 16, 16t
  ambulatory, 17-18
  components of, 442
  continuum of, 16-17, 16t
  defined, 5
  end-of-life, 16t
  episodes of, 16
  home, 27
  hospice, 16t, 28-29, 29t
  long-term, 16t, 28
  palliative, 28
  preventive, 16, 16t
  primary, 16, 16t
  rehabilitative, 16t
  respite, 16t, 29
  secondary, 16
  specialist, 16t
  subacute, 27
  tertiary, 16-17
  that meets professional standards, 529-531
Career counseling, 599
Career planning, 599-600, 600b
Career plateaus, 600
CARF (Commission on Accreditation of Rehabilitation Facilities), 14
Carpal tunnel syndrome (CTS), 641
Cascading style sheets (CSS), 282
Case(s), 408, 422, 474
Case definitions, 474
Case eligibility, 476
Case finding, 416, 474-475
Case law, 505–506, 506b
Case management, 36
  in revenue cycle, 656
  in utilization management, 465
Case management record, 112
Case managers, 36
  use of health data by, 96
Case mix analysis, 494, 660

CASE (computer-aided software engineering) programs, 307
Case studies, 421
CASE (computer-aided systems engineering) tools, 324, 324b
Case-control study, 421-424, 423f, 424t, 427t-428t
Cash basis accounting, 671
Cash flow, statement of, 672-674, 673f
Catchment area, 17
Categorical data, 384, 384t
Category, in data dictionary, 496
Catholic hospitals, 20
Causal factors, 459
Cause-and-effect diagrams, 451-452, 451f, 455f
CBA (cost-benefit analysis)
  of electronic document management, 260-261
  of electronic health record system, 193
  for system evaluation, 339-341, 340t, 341t
CC (chief complaint), 106t
CCA (Certified Coding Associate), 53-54
CCC (Clinical Care Classification), 209t
CCHIT (Certification Commission for Health Information Technology), 74t, 216
CCOW (Clinical Context Object Workgroup), 295
CCR (Continuity of Care Record), 145, 175t, 700-701
CCS (Certified Coding Specialist), 53-54
CCS (Clinical Classification Software), 485
CCS-P (Certified Coding Specialist–Physician Based), 53-54
CDA (Clinical Document Architecture), 175t
CDC (Centers for Disease Control and Prevention), 11, 72t, 100, 443
CDM (charge description master), 655, 655t
CDSS (clinical decision support system), 39, 286-287
Cedars-Sinai Medical Center, computerized physician order entry at, 689
Celebrities, release of information to media on, 526-527
Censoring, of survival time, 429
Census day, 382t
Census statistics, 381-382, 381t-382t
Center for Health Information Technology, 75t
Center for Health Transformation, 75t
Centers for Disease Control and Prevention (CDC), 11, 72t, 100, 443
Centers for Medicare and Medicaid Services (CMS), 11-12, 505
  collaboration with, 67
  and Conditions of Participation, 11-12
  on cost control, 650-651
  on e-prescribing, 71t-72t
  on fraud and abuse, 660
  on performance management, 438-439, 443
Central processing unit (CPU), 274
Central tendency, measures of, 388-391
Central tendency error, 589
Centralized files, 223, 224t
CEO (chief executive officer), 22
Certificate authority (CA), 297
Certificate of need, 652
Certification
  by Centers for Medicare and Medicaid Services, 12
  defined, 12, 53
  maintenance of, 54-55
  professional, 52–54
Certification Commission for Health Information Technology (CCHIT), 74t, 216

Certified Coding Associate (CCA), 53-54
Certified Coding Professional (CPC), 54
Certified Coding Specialist (CCS), 53-54
Certified Coding Specialist–Physician Based (CCS-P), 53-54
Certified in Healthcare Privacy (CHP), 54
Certified Medical Transcriptionist (CMT), 54
Certified nurse midwife, 33
Certified nursing assistants (CNAs), 25
Certified Professional Health Quality (CPHQ), 54
Certified Professional in Electronic Health Records (CPER), 54
Certified Professional in Health Information Management Systems (CPHIMS), 54
Certified Professional in Health Information Technology (CPHIT), 54
Certified registered nurse anesthetist, 33
Certified Tumor Registrar (CTR), 54, 479
Certifying agencies, use of health data by, 96
CEUs (continuing education units), 54-55
CFO (chief financial officer), 22-23
CGI (common gateway interface) program, 289-290, 290f
Chair, 642-643
CHAMPUS (Civilian Health and Medical Program for the Uniformed Services), 38
Change management, 627-637
  project management as, 629-636, 632b, 633f, 635f
  re-engineering as, 636-637, 637b
  strategic management as, 627-629, 628f
CHAP (Community Health Accreditation Program), 14
Charge(s), in patient record, 149
Charge capture, in revenue cycle, 656-657, 656b
Charge description master (CDM), 655, 655t
Charge master, 655, 655t
Charitable immunity, doctrine of, 505-506, 506b
Chart of accounts, 671
Chart order, 114
ChartMaxx, 262-264
CHCs (community health centers), 17
"Cheat sheets," 365
Check boxes
  on forms, 117-119
  on Web page, 283
Checklists
  for evaluation criteria, 351
  for performance appraisal, 588, 589f
Checksheet, 444
Checksum, 288
CHI (Consolidated Health Informatics), 67t, 69, 212-213, 213t-214t
Chief complaint (CC), 106t
Chief executive officer (CEO), 22
Chief financial officer (CFO), 22-23
Chief information officer (CIO), 22, 129
Chief operating officer (COO), 22
Chief technology officer (CTO), 129
Child abuse, reporting of, 511
Child nodes, 315
Child safety seats, 695
CHIME (College of Healthcare Information Management Executives), 75t
Chi-square test, 397-398, 397t
CHP (Certified in Healthcare Privacy), 54
Cigarette smoking, 695
CIO (chief information officer), 22, 129
Circuit courts, 506
CIS (commercial information system) vendor-neutral design, of terminology, 211
Citations, 407

City hospitals, 20
Civil rights, 562-564
Civil Rights Act, 562, 563, 563t
Civilian Health and Medical Program for the
    Uniformed Services (CHAMPUS), 38
Claim(s), 35b
    clean, 657
Claim denial management, 657-659
Claim forms, 657, 658f
Claims data, 487-488
Claims management, 461
Claims processing, 657, 658f
Clarification feedback exercise, 360-361
Classification, defined, 201
Classification systems, 170, 201
Clayton Act, 534
Clear window approach, 491-492
Clerk of the court, 507
CLIA (Clinical Laboratory Improvement
    Amendment), 654
Client(s)
    adult day care, 29
    defined, 5
Client record. See Patient record(s).
Client server technology, 246-247
Client-server platforms, 279-280
Clinical applications, 284-287, 284t, 287t
Clinical Care Classification (CCC), 209t
Clinical case definition, 474
Clinical Classification Software (CCS),
    485
Clinical Context Object Workgroup (CCOW),
    295
Clinical course, on patient record, 149
Clinical data, on patient record, 147t
Clinical data management
    continuing education units in, 55
    international, 691
Clinical data repositories, 167, 169-170
Clinical decision support, 494
Clinical decision support system (CDSS), 39,
    286-287
Clinical Document Architecture (CDA), 175t
Clinical Document Type Definitions, 175t
Clinical forms, 103t, 105-109, 106t-108t
Clinical foundations, continuing education
    units in, 55
Clinical groupings, 491
Clinical guidelines, 194
Clinical imaging, documentation via, 182
Clinical Laboratory Improvement Amendment
    (CLIA), 654
Clinical laboratory scientist, 31t
Clinical laboratory services, 25-26
Clinical laboratory technician, 31t
Clinical nurse specialist, 25
Clinical order, 148
Clinical practice guidelines, 441
Clinical privileges, 23
Clinical record. See Patient record(s).
Clinical résumé, 109
Clinical terminologies, 204-208, 205f, 206f, 209t
Clinical trial, 426-427, 427t-428t
Close, of form, 117
Closed Claims Project, 456
Closed-loop solutions, in digital information
    convergence, 699
Close-ended questions, 418
CMS. See Centers for Medicare and Medicaid
    Services (CMS).
CMS 1500 claim form, 657, 658f
CMT (Certified Medical Transcriptionist), 54
CNAs (Certified nursing assistants), 25
COBOL, 275

COBRA (Consolidated Omnibus Budget
    Reconciliation Act), 8b, 13
CoC (Commission on Cancer), 476, 477
COC (Council on Certification), 53, 57
Codd, E. F., 276
Code(s)
    controlled vocabulary as, 170
    defined, 201
    of ethics, 58, 58b, 549, 552, 661
    universal product, 239
Code 39, 288
Code 128, 288
Code set, 201
Coded data, 170
Coder(s), 53-54
Coder/decoder (CODEC), 293
CODES (Crash Outcomes Data Evaluation
    System), 486
Coding, 183, 201
    cancer registry, 477
    in data dictionary, 495-496
    with electronic document management, 258
    outcomes and, 490-491, 492
    in revenue cycle, 656-657, 656b
Coding systems, 170
Coding tools, computer-assisted, 245-246
Coding validity, 412, 413f
Coefficient of variation (CV), 392
Cohort studies, 424-425, 425t-428t
Coinsurance, 34
COLD (computer output to laser disk), 257
Collaboration
    for change, 688-690
    defined, 356
    multidisciplinary, 701
    requirement(s) for, 356-362
        expectations in, 359
        knowledge as, 361-362
        personal commitment as, 357
        policy setting in, 358-359
        respect as, 358
        trust as, 357-358
        understanding in, 360-361
        vocabulary in, 359-360
Collaboration principle, 356, 357
Collection follow-up, 657-659
Collective bargaining, 568
College of American Pathologists (CAP), 69-70,
    204
College of Healthcare Information
    Management Executives (CHIME), 75t
Color
    in screen display, 332
    in workstation design, 646
Color coding
    of file folders, 234
    of outguides, 237
Colorado Connecting Communities: Health
    Information Collaborative, 85t
Colorado Health Information Exchange, 86t
Column total, 397, 397t
Column variable, 397, 397t
COM (computer output microfiche), 248-249
Commercial information system (CIS) vendor-
    neutral design, of terminology, 211
Commercial storage, of inactive records, 235
Commission on Accreditation for Health
    Informatics and Information
    Management Education (CAHIM), 15,
    52, 57
Commission on Accreditation of Allied Health
    Education Programs (CAAHEP), 15
Commission on Accreditation of Rehabilitation
    Facilities (CARF), 14

Commission on Cancer (CoC), 476, 477
Commission on Professional Hospital Activities
    (CPHA), 272
Commission on Systemic Interoperability, 70,
    72t
Commitment, personal, 357
Committee on Allied Health Education and
    Accreditation, 8b
Common gateway interface (CGI) program,
    289-290, 290f
Common law, 505-506, 506b
Common Procedural Terminology (CPT), 201,
    203
Communicable disease conditions, reportable,
    696, 696b
Communication
    confidential, 509
    privileged, 509
Communication links, 163
Communications technology, 246
Communities of Practice (CoP), 58
Community building, 550
Community Health Accreditation Program
    (CHAP), 14
Community health centers (CHCs), 17
Community Health Services and Facilities Act,
    7b, 17
Community Quality Index Study, 486
Community trial, 426-427, 427t-428t
Community-acquired infection rate, 380, 380t,
    381
Community-based care, 18
Comorbidity, 485, 491
Comorbidity rate, 380, 380t, 381
Comparable worth doctrine, 567
Comparative benchmarking, 447
Comparative data, in performance assessment,
    446-447, 446f
Compensation management, 567, 595-598,
    596f
Competence testing, 336
Competitive benchmarking, 446-447
Complaint, 507
Complaint procedure, 592, 594-595
Complementary and alternative medicine
    (CAM), 29
Complementary medicine, 29
Completeness, of documentation, 178
Completion, of electronic health records,
    189-190
Compliance Certification Process, 74t
Compliance program, 510
Complication rate, 379, 380, 380t
Component state associations (CSAs), 56
Compounding effect, 676
Comprehensive Accreditation Manual for
    Behavioral Health Care (CAMBHC),
    142
Comprehensive Accreditation Manual for Home
    Care (CAMHC), 137
Comprehensive Accreditation Manual for Long
    Term Care (CAMLTC), 134
Comprehensive initial assessment, for
    behavioral health, 143
Comprehensiveness, of data, 144, 144t
Compressible units, 222t, 223, 223f
Compression ratio, 293
Computer(s)
    disposal of, 296
    in health care, history of, 271-273
    lighting and, 645
    network, 274
    personal, 274
    in workstation design, 643

Computer applications, 283-287
  administrative, 283-284, 283t
  clinical, 284-287, 284t, 287t
Computer downtime, 192b
Computer hardware, 274
Computer monitor, in workstation design, 643
Computer output microfiche (COM), 248-249
Computer output microfilm, 244t
Computer output to laser disk (COLD), 257
Computer security, 293-299
  administrative safeguards for, 294, 294t
  authentication tools for, 294-296, 296t
  external controls for, 296-299, 298f
  HIPAA on, 293-294, 294t
  physical, 294, 294t, 296
  reporting capabilities for, 296
  technical safeguards for, 294, 294t
Computer simulations, for system evaluation,
    343
Computer software, 275-277, 276f
  malicious, 297-298
Computer views, design and control of, 115-
    117, 120-122, 120f, 121f, 280-283
Computer virus, 297-298
Computer worm, 298
Computer-aided software engineering (CASE)
    programs, 307
Computer-aided systems engineering (CASE)
    tools, 324, 324b
Computer-assisted coding tools, 245-246
Computer-assisted retrieval (CAR), of
    microfilm, 248, 248t, 249t
Computer-based patient record (CPR), 155
Computer-Based Patient Record Institute, 8b,
    48
Computerized Patient Record System (CPRS),
    207
Computerized physician/provider order entry
    (CPOE), 285, 286
  benefits of, 80, 286
  decision support in, 163
  in electronic health record systems, 156
  viewpoint on, 688–689
Computer-stored ambulatory record systems
    (COSTAR), 272
Concept, *vs.* detail, 360
Concept permanence, of terminology, 210
Conception orientation, of terminology,
    209-210
Concurrent review, in utilization management,
    463-465, 464f
Condition-entry segment, of decision table,
    620, 622f
Conditions of Participation (COP), 11-12, 47,
    438
Conditions of response, in request for proposal,
    345
Conditions segment, of decision table, 620, 622f
Conference room, 638
Confidence interval, 398-399
Confidential communication, 509
Confidentiality. *See also* Privacy.
  breach of, 509
  of credentials files and quality profiles,
    535-536
  duty to maintain, 515-517
  with electronic document management,
    259-260
  with electronic health record systems, 40,
    172, 178
  in international health information
    management, 691
  mandatory reporting requirements and,
    511-512

Confidentiality *(Continued)*
  nondisclosure agreement for, 533, 533f
  of patient records, 515-517, 566-567
  of registry information, 475
  work space design for, 639, 645
Confidentiality obligations, in contracts, 537
Confidentiality of Alcohol and Drug Abuse
    Records, 516-517, 518, 520f
Confounding variables, 415
Congress, in health information infrastructure,
    73
Connecting Communities for Better Health
    Program, 73
Connecting for Health, 73, 75t, 166
Connecting Maine, 86t
Consent
  and assault and battery, 508
  informed
    duty to obtain, 531-532
    waiver of, 532
  to release information, 104
  to special procedures, 105
  to treatment, 104
Consistency, of data, 144, 144t
Consolidated Health Informatics (CHI), 67t,
    69, 212-213, 213t-214t
Consolidated Omnibus Budget Reconciliation
    Act (COBRA), 8b, 13
Constitutional law, 504-505
Constraints, in system, 624-625
Consultation report, 109
Consumers
  in performance management, 440
  use of data by, 486
Contact scanner, 239
Contemporaneous documentation, 512
Content
  semantic, 214
  of terminology, 208-209
Content and Structure of Electronic Health
    Records, 175t
Content Guide for the Electronic Health
    Record, 146, 146t, 147t
Context representation, of terminology, 210
Contingency approach, to leadership, 546
Contingency table, 397-398, 397t
Continuing education, 54-55, 55b
Continuing education units (CEUs), 54-55
Continuing record reviews, 128
Continuity of Care Record (CCR), 145, 175t,
    700-701
Continuous data, 385, 385t
Continuous quality improvement, 128
Continuous variables, 384
Continuum of care, 16-17, 16t
Contract(s)
  breach of, 509-510, 536
  components of, 536-537
  implied, and employee termination, 590-591
  review of, 537, 538f
Contract actions, 504
Contract liability, 536-537, 538f
Contract negotiation, 352
Contract services, 29–30
Contracted amount, 34
Contracting, in revenue cycle, 653-654
Contractual disputes, 509-510
Contractual information, in request for
    proposal, 349
Control(s), 408, 422
  budget as, 664
  in system, 624-625
Control charts, 453-454, 453f, 454b, 455f
Controlled vocabulary, 170

Controls and security design, 331
Conversion, of files, 235-236, 235b
COO (chief operating officer), 22
Cooperative health information system, 271
Cooperative processing, 246-247
CoP (Communities of Practice), 58
COP (Conditions of Participation), 11-12, 47,
    438
Copayments, 35b, 37
Copying and pasting, 182, 182b
Core health data elements, 100, 101t
Core measures, 486-487
Core values, 550, 552
Cornell Medical Center, microfilm system of,
    255
Coroner, disclosure of health information to,
    523-524
Corporate compliance plans, 510
"Corporate information factory," 16, 167f
Corporate negligence, 508
Corporate person index (CPI), 232b
Correction, of electronic health records,
    188-189.189b
Correlation analysis, 454, 454f
Correlation coefficient *(r)*, 396, 413-414, 454
Corruption, 298
Cost allocations, 668–669, 670f
Cost analysis, for microfilm, 250-254, 251t, 253t
Cost containment, with electronic health
    records, 168
Cost estimates, in project planning, 631
Cost reduction, and human resource
    management, 559-560
COSTAR (computer-stored ambulatory record
    systems), 272
Cost-benefit analysis (CBA)
  of electronic document management, 260-261
  of electronic health record system, 193
  for system evaluation, 339-341, 340t, 341t
Cost-effectiveness analysis, 341-342
Cost-efficiency, and human resource
    management, 559
Council on Accreditation of Allied Health
    Educational Programs (CAAHEP), 52
Council on Certification (COC), 53, 57
Counseling, employee, 592
County hospitals, 20
Court decisions, 505-506, 506b
Court order, 504, 527, 528-529
Court procedures, 507
Court reporter, 507
Court system, 506-507
Coverage, 35b
Covered entity(ies), 511, 516
CPC (Certified Coding Professional), 54
CPER (Certified Professional in Electronic
    Health Records), 54
CPHA (Commission on Professional Hospital
    Activities), 272
CPHIMS (Certified Professional in Health
    Information Management Systems), 54
CPHIT (Certified Professional in Health
    Information Technology), 54
CPHQ (Certified Professional Health Quality),
    54
CPI (corporate person index), 232b
CPOE. *See* Computerized physician/provider
    order entry (CPOE).
CPR (computer-based patient record), 155
CPRS (Computerized Patient Record System),
    207
CPT (Common Procedural Terminology), 201,
    203
CPT (Current Procedural Terminology), 170

CPU (central processing unit), 274
Crash Outcomes Data Evaluation System (CODES), 486
Credential(s)
 for coding specialists, 53-54
 verification of, 467-468
Credentialing, 466-468
 antitrust claims involving, 510
 defined, 466
 external requirements for, 467
 legal aspects of, 534-535
 objective of, 466
Credentialing program, components of, 467-468, 469f
Credentials committee, 535
Credentials files
 accessibility of, 535-536
 material in, 534-535
Credentials registry, 468
Credentials verification organizations (CVOs), 468
Criminal activity, 510
Criminal law, 504
Critical access hospital (CAH), 19
Critical activities, in project planning, 631
Critical incident method, 587
Critical path, 631, 633-634
Crossing the Quality Chasm, 166, 438
Cross-reference, 220, 232b
Cross-sectional study, 415-417, 416f, 417t, 427t-428t
Cruzan v. Missouri, 8b, 13
Cryotechnologist, 31t
CSAs (component state associations), 56
CSS (cascading style sheets), 282
CTI (cumulative trauma disorder), 641
CTO (chief technology officer), 129
CTR (Certified Tumor Registrar), 54, 479
CTS (carpal tunnel syndrome), 641
Cullen, Charles, 510
Cultural assessment, 143
Cultural tool kits, 561b
Culture, organizational, 569-570, 570b
Cumulative trauma disorder (CTI), 641
Currency, of data, 144, 144t
Current Procedural Terminology (CPT), 170
Current ratio, 674
Custodial facility, 28
CV (coefficient of variation), 392
CVOs (credentials verification organizations), 468

D
Daily inpatient census, 382t
Damages, in negligence or malpractice case, 530
DAP format, 115
Darling v. Charleston Community Memorial Hospital, 506, 506b
DARPA (U.S. Defense Department Advanced Research Project Agency), 288
Data
 accessibility of, 144, 144t
 accuracy of, 123, 144, 144t
 aggregate, 94, 96, 168, 443
 baseline, 362
 coded, 170
 comprehensiveness of, 144, 144t
 consistency of, 144, 144t
 continuous, 385, 385t
 currency of, 144, 144t
 defined, 44, 97
 deidentified, 523
 discrete, 385, 385t

Data (Continued)
 in electronic health record systems, 168-169, 169f
 granularity of, 144, 144t
 and health, 486
 integrity of, 144t, 145
 interval, 384-385
 nominal (categorical, qualitative, named), 384, 384t
 ordinal (ranked), 384, 385t
 in patient record, 44-45
 precision of, 144t, 145
 primary, 474
 ratio, 385
 relevance of, 144t, 145
 secondary, 474
 timeliness of, 144t, 145
 types of, 384-385, 384t, 385t
 uses of, 474
Data access and retention. See Access and retention.
Data access layer, 314, 314f
Data analysis
 in epidemiology, 431-433, 432t-434t
 for process improvement, 452-454, 452f-455f, 454b
 in research, 409, 410
 in systems analysis and design, 625
 in work simplification, 618
Data broker, 485
Data collection
 abbreviations and symbols in, 113-114
 administrative forms for, 103t, 104-105
 ancillary forms for, 104t
 authentication in, 114
 basic principles of, 102-115
 for business plan, 666, 666b
 clinical forms for, 103t, 105-109, 106t-108t
 cost-effectiveness of, 97
 design and control of forms and views for, 115-122, 118f, 120f, 121f
 documentation guidelines for, 113-114, 113t
 documentation responsibilities in, 102
 format types for, 114-115, 115t
 general documentation forms and views for, 102-113, 103t-104t
 key concepts for, 150
 for neonatal data, 103t, 111
 nursing forms for, 103t, 111-113
 for obstetrical data, 103t, 110-111
 operative forms for, 103t, 110
 with paper-based records, 114
 patient identification in, 104
 for performance measurement, 444, 445f
 purpose of, 97
 in research proposal, 409-410, 410f
 standards for, 98-102, 99f, 99t, 101t
 in systems analysis and design, 625
 user needs and, 102
 in work simplification, 615-618, 616f-621f, 618b
Data compression, 292-293
Data definition, 144, 144t, 309f, 493
Data dictionary, 495-499
 cataloging standards for, 497-499
 in computerized provider order entry systems, 286
 criteria for data element inclusion in, 497
 defined, 315t, 318
 definitions related to, 495-496, 495t
 development of, 318-319, 318f-321f, 497, 498b
 importance of, 319-321
 meta-content of, 496-497

Data dictionary (Continued)
 in project management, 309f
 purpose of, 496
 scope of, 496
Data display, 385-386, 386b, 387f-390f
Data elements
 core, 100, 101t
 in data dictionary, 318, 318f, 497
 defined, 495
 in electronic health records, 168, 169, 169t
Data Elements for Emergency Department Systems (DEEDS), 99t, 133
Data exchange standards, with electronic health record systems, 173, 173f, 174t
Data flow(s), 315-316, 316t
Data flow diagrams (DFDs), 315-318, 315t, 316t, 317f
Data interface standards, 169
Data management technology, 299-302, 300f, 301t
Data mapping, 321-322
Data mart, 299-301, 301t
Data migration, 365
Data mining, 299, 301, 492
Data modeling, 301-302, 309f, 315t
 for health care, 146
 in system analysis, 315t
Data needs, 129-143
 for acute care, 129-130
 for ambulatory care, 130-134, 135f
 for behavioral health, 142-143
 for home health care, 137-141, 139f-141f
 for hospice, 141-142
 for long-term care, 134-136, 136t
 for rehabilitation, 137
Data organization, for process improvement, 450-452, 451f, 452f
Data presentation, 385-386
 formats for, 384t, 385t, 386, 387f-390f
 guidelines for, 386b
 overview of, 372
 for process improvement, 452-454, 452f-455f, 454b
 role of health information management professional in, 372
Data quality
 characteristics of, 143-145, 144t
 clinical staff activities related to, 128
 defined, 143-144
 facility structure that encourages, 128-129
 methods to ensure, 122-126, 124t, 125f
 monitoring and solutions for, 126-129
Data quality council, 129
Data quality management (DQM), 143-144
Data repository, 299, 300f
Data requirements, in electronic health record systems, 168-169, 169f
Data security, with electronic health record systems, 172, 178
Data sets, overview of, 99, 99t
Data sheet, 444, 445f
Data standard(s), 211-216, 213t-214t
 development and selection of, 214-215
Data standardization, interoperability and, 213-214
Data stores, 315-316, 316t
Data tables, 239-240
Data types, 169, 169t
Data warehouses, 167, 169-170
 outcomes, 491, 492
Database(s), 146, 276
 patient safety, 456-458, 458t
Database design, 331, 363
Database management system (DBMS), 276

Database model(s), 276-277, 276f
Database retrieval, with electronic document management, 260
Database server, 279
Database software, for electronic document management, 258
Day outlier, 660
Days of revenue in patient accounts receivable ratio, 674-675
Days of stay, 382t
DBMS (database management system), 276
DCE (Distributed Computing Environment), 493-494
Death certificate, 105, 372-373
Death rate
    age adjusted, 377, 377t
    anesthesia, 374t, 375
    fetal, 374t, 376
    gross, 374, 374t
    infant, 374t, 376
    maternal, 374t, 376
    neonatal, 374t, 376
    net, 374t, 375
    postoperative, 374t, 375-376
Death registries, 481
Decentralized files, 223, 224t
Decimal, in data dictionary, 496
Decision grid, 619–620, 621f
Decision making, health data in, 96-97
Decision matrix, 619-620, 621f
Decision support system (DSS), 39, 164, 165f, 284, 313
Decision table, 620, 622f
Decision tree, 620, 622f
Decline, in system life cycle, 310
Decomposition diagrams, in system analysis, 315, 315t
Deductible, 35b, 37
DEEDS (Data Elements for Emergency Department Systems), 99t, 133
Deemed status, 12, 14
Defamation of character, 509
Defendants, 507
Deficiency slip, 125, 125f
Definition
    data, 144, 144t
    in data dictionary, 496
Degrees of freedom
    between-groups, 395
    within-groups, 395
Deidentified data, 523
Delaware Health Information Network, 85t
Deletion, of document, 189
Delinquent medical records, 124, 124t, 126
Deliverables, 308
Delivery terms, 352
Demand, key indicators of, 573
Demilitarized zone (DMZ), 291-292
Demographic changes, in workforce, 560-561
Demographic data, 104
    on patient record, 146
Demographic level, of master patient index, 226
Demonstrations, in purchasing process, 351
Denial of service (DOS) attack, 298
Denominator, 373
Dental history, 148
Department of Health and Human Services (DHHS), 10-12, 505
    data collection by, 98-99, 99f
    on health goals, 9
    and health information technology, 66, 67-73, 68f
    history of, 8b
    organization of, 10-12, 10f

Department of Health and Human Services (DHHS) (Continued)
    Workgroup on Electronic Data Interchange of, 8b, 38
Department of Health, Education, and Welfare (HEW), 7b, 8b, 10
Department of Justice, 505
Department of Veterans Affairs (VA), 207, 212
Department of Veterans Affairs (VA) medical centers, 19
Departmental health information system, 271, 272-273
Departmental objectives, for budget planning, 667-668
Dependent practitioner, 30
Dependent variables, 406
Deployment coordinator, 308
Depositions, 507
Depreciation, 678
Dermatology, 23t
Description, in data dictionary, 318, 318f, 319, 319f
Descriptive statistics, 388-392
Descriptive study, 415-421, 415t
    cross-sectional or prevalence, 415-417, 416f, 417t, 427t-428t
    qualitative, 419-421
    survey, 417-419, 419f-422f
Design phase, of system development, 307, 310
Designated record set (DRS), 162-163, 511
Desk, 642
Destruction, of records, 241
Destruction letter, 241
Detail, concept vs., 360
Deterministic search, 232b
Developer, 308
Developing countries, needs of, 691
Development lead, 308
Device capture, documentation via, 181-182
dfb (between-groups degrees of freedom), 395
DFDs (data flow diagrams), 315-318, 315t, 316t, 317f
dfw (within-groups degrees of freedom), 395
DHHS. See Department of Health and Human Services (DHHS).
Diabetes registries, 482
Diagnosis bias, 415
Diagnosis-related groups (DRGs), 37, 203, 651, 659-660
Diagnostic and Statistical Manual of Mental Disorders (DSM), 202-203
Diagnostic radiology services, 25
Diagnostic tests, 148
Dialogue boxes, 332
DICOM, 173, 173f, 174t
Dictation, 122, 164, 180-181
"Dictionaries," 239-240
Dietary services, 25
Differentiation, of neoplasms, 477
Digital certificate, 297
Digital dashboards, 700
Digital imaging, in electronic document management, 258
Digital Imaging Communications in Medicine, 69
Digital information convergence, 699-702
Diploma, in nursing, 33t
Direct care functions, 157, 158f, 159f
Direct cost(s), of electronic document management, 261
Direct cost departments, 668
Direct input, documentation via, 181
Direct patient care, disclosure for, 518-521
Direct pay, 34

Directional strategies, 627, 628, 629
Director of finance, 22-23
Disability(ies)
    defined, 565
    protecting rights of persons with, 564-565, 565b
    and work space design, 640
Disaster recovery, 242-243, 294
Discharge
    of employee, 590-592, 590b, 591f, 593-594
    Uniform Hospital Discharge Data Set for, 99t, 102, 130
Discharge and interval summary, 109
Discharge days, 382t
Discharge plan, 113
Discharge planning, in utilization management, 465
Disciplinary actions, 592-594
Disciplinary checklist, 591f
Disclaimer, in request for proposal, 344
Disclosure
    in accounting, 671
    of health information, 517-529
        for administrative purposes, 522
        to attorneys, 522-523
        authorization for, 518, 519f, 520f
        for direct patient care, 518-521
        for educational purposes, 521
        in emergency, 518
        to family
            in cases of incompetence or incapacity, 524
            of emancipated minor or adult, 524
            of minor, 524
        to law enforcement personnel and agencies, 523-524
        to new physician or facility, 518-521
        to news media, 526-527
        to outsourcing firms, 526
        ownership and, 517
        to patient, 511, 524-525
        patient-directed, 525
        for payment purposes, 522, 523f
        for performance management and patient safety, 521
        pursuant to legal process, 527-529, 528f
        and redisclosure, 518, 525-526
        for research, 521-522
        resources on, 517-518
        security measures to prevent unauthorized, 529
Disclosure logs, standards for, 175t
Discounted payback period, 340-341, 341t
Discounting, 676
Discovery process, 507
Discrete data, 385, 385t
Discrete time period approach, 491
Discrete variables, 384
Discrimination, 562-566
Disk drive, for data input and output, 244t
Diskette, for data input and output, 244t
Disparate impact, 564
Disparate treatment, 564
Dispersion, measures of, 391-392
Disposition
    in acute care, 130
    in ambulatory care, 132
    of encounter or episode, 149
Distributed Computing Environment (DCE), 493-494
Distributions, 446
Diversity management, 560, 561, 561b
Diversity of jurisdiction cases, 506
DMAIC, 449

DME (durable medical equipment), 37
DMZ (demilitarized zone), 291-292
DNS (Doctor of Science in Nursing), 33t
DO (doctor of osteopathic medicine), 32
Docket number, 527
Doctor of medicine (MD), 32
Doctor of osteopathic medicine (DO), 32
Doctor of philosophy (PhD), in nursing, 33t
Doctor of Science in Nursing (DNS), 33t
Doctor's Office Quality Information
    Technology initiative, 71
Document(s), standards for, 175t
Document digitizing, 181
Document imaging, 181
Document imaging devices, 245
Document review, in system analysis, 330
Document titles, 188
Document type definition (DTD), 290
Document windows, 332
Documentation
    abbreviations and symbols in, 113-114
    accuracy of, 178
    authentication of, 114, 178
    business rules for, 187
    contemporaneous, 512
    format types for, 114-115, 115t
    forms for, 102-113, 103t-104t
        administrative, 103t, 104-105
        clinical, 103t, 105-109, 106t-108t
        neonatal, 103t, 111
        nursing, 103t, 111-113
        obstetrical, 103t, 110-111
        operative, 103t, 109-110
    guidelines for, 113-114, 113t
    integrity of, 178
    legibility of, 177
    methods of, 180-182
    on-line, 163-164
    with paper-based records, 114
    of patient identification, 104
    principles of, 177-178
    privacy, confidentiality, and security of, 178
    responsibility for, 102
    timeliness of, 178
    unique patient identification in, 177
Documentation analysis, 183
Domain, 495, 496
"Domain" expert, 308
Domiciliary facility, 28
Donabedian, Avedis, 441-442, 442t
DOS (denial of service) attack, 298
Double blind study, 427
Double-barreled questions, 328
Double-distribution method, of cost allocation,
    668
Double-entry method, in accounting, 671-672
Downsizing, 559-560
DQM (data quality management), 143-144
Draft standard for trial use (DSTU), 156-157,
    158f, 159f, 175t
DRGs (diagnosis-related groups), 37, 203, 651,
    659-660
DRS (designated record set), 162-163, 511
Drucker, Peter, 588
Drug abuse, confidentiality of records of, 516-
    517, 518, 520f
Drug terminologies, 207
DSM (Diagnostic and Statistical Manual of
    Mental Disorders), 202-203
DSS (decision support system), 39, 164, 165f,
    284, 313
DSTU (draft standard for trial use), 156-157,
    158f, 159f, 175t
DTD (document type definition), 290

Due process, 505
Duplicate medical record numbers, 230f,
    232b-233b
Duplication equipment, for microfilm, 250
Durable medical equipment (DME), 37
Durable power of attorney for health care, 532
Duration of inpatient hospitalization, 382t
Duty(ies)
    to maintain confidentiality, 515-517
    to maintain health information, 511-512
    in negligence or malpractice case, 530
    to obtain informed consent, 531-532
    to patients in general, 511
    to provide care that meets professional
        standards, 529-531
    to provide safe environment for patients and
        visitors, 532-533
    to retain health information, 512-515, 513f
    to supervise actions of employees and
        professional staff, 533-536, 533f

E
EAPs (Employee Assistance Programs), 572,
    592
Ears
    physical examination of, 108t
    in review of systems, 106t
EBM (evidence-based medicine), 31, 441
Economy forces and trends, and human
    resource management, 559-560
ED (emergency department), 26
EDI (electronic data interchange), 129, 256-257
EDM. See Electronic document management
    (EDM).
Education
    of electronic health record users, 193
    in international health information
        management, 691
Education programs, in health education
    management, 51-52
Educational purposes, disclosure of health
    information for, 521
Educators, use of health data by, 96
EEOC (Equal Employment Opportunity
    Commission), 562, 566
Effect size, 400
Effectiveness, 441
Efficiency, 333, 334t, 441
e-health (electronic health), 29, 48
eHealth Foundation, 83
e-health (electronic health) information
    management (e-HIM), 15, 44, 49-50,
    50b
eHealth Initiative, 73, 76t
e-HIM (electronic health information
    management), 15, 44, 49-50, 50b
EHRs. See Electronic health record(s) (EHRs).
EHR-S. See Electronic health record system(s)
    (EHR-S).
EISs (executive information systems), 284
Elam v. College Park Hospital, 534
Elderly, disclosure of health information to
    family of, 524
Electrocardiographic reports, 112
Electroconvulsive therapy, 143
Electronic data exchange, 38-39
Electronic data interchange (EDI), 129, 256-257
Electronic document management (EDM),
    255-264, 269t
    applications of, 262-264
    benefits and advantages of, 258-260, 259t
    components of, 255-258
    defined, 255
    electronic health records and, 255

Electronic document management (EDM)
    (Continued)
    evaluating system requirements for, 260-262
    implementation strategies for, 262
    legal considerations with, 262
Electronic health (e-health), 29, 48
Electronic health (e-health) information
    management (e-HIM), 15, 44, 49-50,
    50b
Electronic health record(s) (EHRs), 39, 155-156
    administrative uses of, 164
    amendments to, 175t
    ASTM E1384 Content Guide for, 146, 146t,
        147t
    ASTM standards for, 145
    characteristics of data quality of, 143-145,
        144t
    completion and authentication of, 189-190
    copying and pasting in, 182, 182b
    correction of, 188-189, 189b
    in decision support systems, 164, 165f
    defined, 155
    and electronic document management, 255
    evolution of, 48
    international use of, 690-691
    interoperability of, 684-686
    key concepts with, 40
    maintenance of, 188-189, 189b
    major segments of, 146-149
    outcomes and, 488-489, 489f, 490f
    patient access to, 700
    printing of, 190
    and results management, 163
    standardization of, 186-187
    standards development and, 156-157, 158f,
        159f
    storage and retention of, 182
    templates for, 188
    thinning of, 183
    titles of, 188
    users of, 356, 356t
    versioning of, 187-188, 188b
    vocabularies and, 170-171
Electronic health record system(s) (EHR-S),
    152-195
    acceptance of, 193
    barriers to, 171-173, 173f, 174t-175t, 194
    and business rules, 187, 187b
    capabilities of, 164-165
    challenges to health information
        professionals with, 190-195
    changes in business processes due to,
        177-190
    components of, 156, 157f
    confidentiality and security of, 40, 172
    cost containment and return on investment
        with, 168
    cost of, 171
    cost-benefit analysis of, 193
    data requirements in, 168-169, 169f
    defined, 66
    functions of, 156
        and patient record development, 163-165,
            165f
    improved health information with, 166-167,
        167f
    industry forces that advance adoption of,
        165-168, 167f
    in information systems master plans,
        193-194
    infrastructure requirements for, 171
    introducing components of, 194
    issues to address in move to, 177-190
    laws related to, 172

Electronic health record system(s) (EHR-S) (Continued)
leadership for, 194-195
legal frameworks for, 194
migration to, 173-177, 190, 191b-192b
and patient safety, 165-166
and policies, 186-187, 187b
technical infrastructure of, 168
vendors for, 164-165, 173-176
Electronic health record system(s) (EHR-S) Functional Model, 215
Electronic medical records (EMRs), 39
Electronic patient record (EPR) system, 262-264
Electronic prescribing (e-prescribing), 71, 71t-72t, 688
Electronic remittance advice (ERA), 659
Electronic signatures, 175t, 178
legal aspects of, 514
Elixhauser, Anne, 485
Elixhauser Comorbidity Measurement, 485
Emancipated minor, disclosure of health information to family of, 524
Emergency
disclosure of health information in, 518
informed consent in, 532
Emergency department (ED), 26
Emergency Department Systems, Data Elements for, 99t, 133
Emergency medical technician, 31t
Emergency Medical Treatment and Active Labor Act (EMTALA), 8b, 13, 511
Emergency record, for ambulatory care, 133-134
Emergency services, 26
Emotional distress, intentional infliction of, 509
Emotional intelligence, 554b
Employee(s)
as client of human resource management system, 571-572
duty to supervise actions of, 533-536, 533f
Employee Assistance Programs (EAPs), 572, 592
Employee compensation, 567, 595-598, 596f
Employee counseling and referral, 592
Employee development, 598-600, 599b, 600b
Employee discipline, 592-594
Employee expectations, changing work environment and, 584
Employee handbooks, 578-579
Employee health, 566
safety, and well-being, 600-601
Employee identification, verification of, 529
Employee performance, adverse outcomes of, 590-592, 590b, 591f
Employee ranking, for performance appraisal, 586
Employee retention, 583-584
Employee Retirement Income Security Act (ERISA), 567
Employee selection, 580-583
Employee selection tests, 581-582
Employee service record, 141, 141f
Employee termination, 590-592, 590b, 591f, 593-594
Employers, use of health data by, 96
Employment at will, 590-591
EMRs (electronic medical records), 39
EMTALA (Emergency Medical Treatment and Active Labor Act), 8b, 13, 511
Encapsulation, 277
Encoding, 201
Encounter(s)
defined, 133

Encounter(s) (Continued)
and folder size, 234
on patient record, 147t, 149
in primary care, 16
Encounter data, core elements of, 101t
Encounter record, for ambulatory care, 133
Encryption, 297
End tab configuration, 234
Endocrine system, in review of systems, 107t
Endocrinology, 23t
End-of-life care, 16t
End-user training, 335-336
Enrollment data, core elements of, 101t
Enterprise profile, in request for proposal, 344-345
Enterprise-wide health information system, 271
Entity(ies)
in accounting, 670
in data dictionary, 495
in system analysis, 322, 322f
Entity-relationship diagrams (ERDs), 315t, 322-324, 322f, 323f
Entry type, in data dictionary, 319, 319f
Environmental analysis
external, 627
internal, 627
Environmental basic(s), 356-362
expectations in, 359
knowledge as, 361-362
personal commitment as, 357
policy setting in, 358-359
respect as, 358
shared, 357-359
trust as, 357-358
understanding in, 360-361
unshared, 359-362
vocabulary in, 359-360
Environmental considerations, in workstation design, 643-646, 645b
Environmental influences, and human resource management, 557-561, 561b
Environmental Protection Agency (EPA), 69, 644
EOB (explanation of benefits), 659
Epidemiologic case definitions, 474
Epidemiologic study design, 415-429, 415t
analytic, 415t, 421-426
case-control or retrospective, 421-424, 423f, 424t, 427t-428t
historical-prospective, 426, 426f, 427t-428t
prospective, cohort, or incidence, 424-425, 425t, 426-428t
descriptive, 415-421, 415t
cross-sectional or prevalence, 415-417, 416f, 417t, 427t-428t
qualitative, 419-421
survey, 417-419, 419f-422f
experimental, 415t, 426-429, 427t-428t, 430f
Epidemiologists, use of health data by, 96
Epidemiology
biases in, 414-415
defined, 404
experimental, 415t, 426-429, 427t-428t, 430f
outcome studies and, 430-434, 432t-434t
overview of, 404
reliability in, 412-414
role of health information management professional in, 404-405
sensitivity and specificity in, 412, 412t
validity in, 411-412
coding, 412, 413f
web sites on, 435
EPIINFO, 420

Episode(s)
of care, 16
in outcome systems, 491-492
on patient record, 149
Episode level, of master patient index, 226
Episodic groupers, 491-492
EPR (electronic patient record) system, 262-264
e-prescribing (electronic prescribing), 71, 71t-72t, 688
Equal employment opportunity, 562-564
Equal Employment Opportunity Act, 562
Equal Employment Opportunity Commission (EEOC), 562, 566
Equal Pay Act, 567
Equipment, in system development, 309
Equity, 672, 672f
ERA (electronic remittance advice), 659
ERDs (entity-relationship diagram), 315t, 322-324, 322f, 323f
Ergonomics, 641-642
ERISA (Employee Retirement Income Security Act), 567
Error(s), on electronic health records, 188-189,189b
ESC (Evidence and Standards Compliance), 183
Essential functions, 578t
Essential services, 24-27
Ethernet, 278
Ethical decision making
administrative, 553b
power and, 551
Ethical principles, 58, 58b
Ethics
code of, 58, 58b, 549, 552, 661
in human resources management, 551-552
of leadership, 549–550, 554b
normative, 549
of the ordinary, 550-551
Etiology, 476
Evaluation criteria, in purchasing process, 349-351, 350f, 350t, 351t
Evaluation phase, of system development, 307, 337-343
Event(s), in PERT network, 633
Event engine, 176
Evidence, 507
admissibility as, 514-515, 529
health information as, 514-515
preponderance of, 530
secondary, 514-515
Evidence and Standards Compliance (ESC), 183
Evidence-based medicine (EBM), 31, 441
Ex officio members, 21
Exchange time, 257
Exclusion, 35b
Executive committee, 23
Executive information systems (EISs), 284
Executive vice president, 22
Expectations, 359
Expenses, fixed vs. variable, 663
Experimental epidemiology, 415t, 426-429, 427t-428t, 430f
Experimental research, for system evaluation, 342-343
Experimental study, 415t, 426-429, 427t-428t, 430f
Expert system, 287
Explanation of benefits (EOB), 659
Explosion diagrams, 317
Exposure characteristics, 421-422
Exposure to hazardous substances, 148
Express powers, 504-505
Extensible markup language (XML), 171, 290-291

External controls
    for security, 296-299
    in system, 624-625
External entity, 315-316, 316t
External environmental analysis, 627
External forces, continuing education units in, 55
External health information system, 271
Extinction, termination by, 632
Extranet, 291-292
Extremities, in review of systems, 107t
Eyes
    physical examination of, 108t
    in review of systems, 106t

F

F ratio, 395, 396
Facilities, in system development, 309
Facility closure, record retention after, 241-242
Factor comparison, 597
Failure mode and effects analysis (FMEA), 460
Fair Labor Standards Act (FLSA), 563t, 567
Fairness, 550
Faith-based hospitals, 20
False imprisonment, 508-509
False negatives (FN), 412
False positives (FP), 232, 412
Falsification, of records, 512
Family, disclosure of health information to
    in cases of incompetence or incapacity, 524
    of emancipated minor or adult, 524
    of minor, 524
Family and Medical Leave Act (FMLA), 558, 563t, 567
Family history (FH), 106t, 148
Family medicine, 23t
FASB (Financial Accounting Standards Board), 669
Favoritism, 589
FDA (Food and Drug Administration), 11, 207, 456-457, 505
FDDI (fiber-distributed data interface), 278
Federal Administrative Procedure Act, 505
Federal Advisory Committee Act, 70
Federal courts, 506
Federal data collection, standards for, 98-99, 99f
Federal False Claims Act, 510
Federal information and data sets, 99, 99t
Federal initiatives, 67, 67t-68t
Federal involvement, in health information technology, 67-73, 67t-68t, 68f, 71t-77t
Federal Mediation and Conciliation Service (FMCS), 568
Federal oversight agencies, 438-439
Federal question cases, 506
Federal Register, 438, 440, 505, 537, 660
Federal Regulations on Alcohol and Drug Abuse, 527
Federal regulatory agencies and organizations, 9-12, 10f
    that affect human resource management, 563t
Federal regulatory context, and human resources development, 544
Federal statutes and regulations, 505
    on record retention, 240
    that affect human resource management, 563t
Federal Trade Commission, 505
Federal Trade Commission Act, 534
Federally owned hospitals, 19, 19f
Federation Licensing Examination (FLEX), 32
Fee schedule, 655, 655t
Feedback, in system, 624

Fee-for-service, 34, 47
Fellow of the American Health Information Management Association, 56
Fellowship program, 55-56
Fetal death certificates, 372-373
Fetal death rates, 374t, 376
FH (family history), 106t, 148
FI (fiscal intermediary), 35b, 37
Fiber-distributed data interface (FDDI), 278
Field, 495
Field test, 326
File(s), centralized and decentralized, 223, 224t
File and database design, 331
File conversion, 235-236, 235b
File folders, 234
File guides
    for alphabetical filing, 224
    for straight numerical filing, 225
    for terminal digit filing, 225-226
File server, 246
    for electronic document management, 256
Filing, in workstation design, 643
Filing cabinets, 222, 222t
Filing equipment, 221-223, 222t, 223f
Filing methods, 223-226
    alphabetical, 224, 224b, 225b
    straight numerical, 224-225, 226t
    terminal digit, 225-226, 226t
Finance committee, 22-23
Financial accountability, 660, 661b
Financial accountant, 671, 671t
Financial accounting, 669-672, 671t
Financial Accounting Standards Board (FASB), 669
Financial analysis, 674-675
Financial data, 104
    ratios to evaluate, 674-675
Financial decisions, setting priorities for, 661-662
Financial department, 23
Financial elements, on patient record, 147
Financial management, 648-681
    budgets in, 662-665, 665t, 666t
    business plan in, 665-668, 666b, 667f
    capital expense and investment decisions in, 675-680, 677f-678f, 679t
    cost allocations in, 668-669, 670f
    financial accounting in, 669-672, 671t
    financial reports in, 672-674, 672f, 673f
    of fraud and abuse compliance, 660-661, 661b
    historical perspective on, 650-652, 651f, 652b
    implementation process in, 680
    managerial accounting in, 661-662
    ratios to evaluate financial data in, 674-675
    resources on, 681
    of revenue cycle, 652-660, 654f
        back-end activities in, 657-660
        case mix analysis in, 660
        charge master in, 655, 655t
        claims processing in, 657, 658f
        coding in, 656-657, 656b
        collection and claim denial in, 657-659
        contracting in, 653-654
        front-end activities in, 653-657
        licensure and provider enrollment in, 654-655
        patient accounting in, 657
        patient encounter in, 656
        payment processing in, 659
        registration and admitting in, 655-656
        reimbursement analysis in, 659-660, 659t
        utilization management in, 656

Financial management *(Continued)*
    role of health information management professional in, 680-681
    seeking alternatives in, 680
    setting priorities for financial decisions in, 661-662
    variance reports in, 664-665, 665t, 666t
Financial manager, 671, 671t
Financial reports, 672-674, 672f, 673f
Financial summary, for electronic document management, 261-262
Financing
    of health care, 34-38, 35b
    of Medicare, 35b, 37
    in request for proposal, 349
Firewalls, 296-297
Firing, of employee, 590-592, 590b, 591f, 593-594
Fiscal affairs director, 22-23
Fiscal intermediary (FI), 35b, 37
Fiscal periods, 672
Fiscal year, 672
Fishbone diagrams, 451-452, 451f, 455f
Fixed expenses, 663
Fixed payment system, 659-660
FLEX (Federation Licensing Examination), 32
Flex time, 558
Flexible budget, 664
Flexner, Abraham, 6, 7b
Flexner Report, 6, 7b
Floor stock, 26
Flow process chart, 616-617, 616f, 617f
Flowchart(s)
    guidelines for constructing, 618, 618b
    layout, 618, 621
    operation or procedure, 618, 619f
    in performance improvement, 450-451, 451f, 455f
    symbols in, 618, 620f
    systems, 618, 618f
    in work simplification, 617-618
FLSA (Fair Labor Standards Act), 563t, 567
FMCS (Federal Mediation and Conciliation Service), 568
FMEA (failure mode and effects analysis), 460
FMLA (Family and Medical Leave Act), 558, 563t, 567
FN (false negatives), 412
Focus groups, 420-421
Focused review, 444
Focused review form, 185f
FOIA (Freedom of Information Act), 516
Follow-up
    for ambulatory care, 132
    in registry, 475
Follow-up plan, 112-113
Fonts, for forms, 117
Food and Drug Administration (FDA), 11, 207, 456-457, 505
Food, Drug, and Cosmetic Act, 9
Footer, of form, 117
Force field analysis, 452, 452f, 455f
Forced distribution, 586
Forced-choice methods, for performance appraisal, 588
FORE (Foundation of Research and Education in Health Information Management), 58, 73t, 537, 685
Forecasting, in human resource management, 573-576, 574b, 575f, 576f
Formal definitions, of terminology, 210
Formal organizational infrastructure, 626-627
Forms committee, 187
Forms review, in system analysis, 330

Forms team, 116
Formulary, 26
For-profit hospitals, 20
FORTRAN, 275
Foundation of Research and Education in Health Information Management (FORE), 58, 73t, 537, 685
FP (false positives), 232, 412
Frames, on Web page, 283
Franklin, Benjamin, 45
Fraud, 509
    financial aspects of, 660-661, 661b
Freedom of Information Act (FOIA), 516
Free-standing medical centers, 17
Freezer drying, of wet records, 242
Frequency distribution, 384t, 385t, 386, 397t
Frequency polygon, 386, 389f
Functional analyst, 308
Functional interoperability, 214
Functional models, 215
Functional primitives, 315
Functional specifications, in request for proposal, 345-348, 346f-348f
Functional strategies, 629
Fund balance, 672, 672f

G

GAAP (generally accepted accounting principles), 650, 653
Gantt chart, 631, 634, 635f
Gantt, Henry, 634
Gartner Research Group on Information Technology, 165
GASB (Government Accounting Standards Board), 669
Gastroenterology, 23t
Gastrointestinal system, in review of systems, 106t
Gatekeeper, 16, 36
GDSS (group decision support software), 330
Gender discrimination, 564, 567
General condition, physical examination of, 108t
General hospital, 20
General system life cycle, 310, 311f
Generalist, 32
Generalizability, 421
Generally accepted accounting principles (GAAP), 650, 653
Genitoreproductive system, in review of systems, 107t
Genitourinary system, physical examination of, 108t
4GL programming languages, 276
Glasgow Coma Scale, 484
Global positioning system (GPS) technology, 699
"Go live," 365–366
Goal(s)
    organizational, 662
    in PERT network, 632
    of research, 408
Goal setting, for performance appraisal, 587-588, 588f
Goal statement, in project planning, 630
Going concern, 670
Good Health Study, 431-434, 432t-434t
Governing board, 21-22
Governing body, 21-22
Government, as payer, 36-38
Government Accounting Standards Board (GASB), 669
Governmental agencies, use of health data by, 96

Governmental data collection, standards for, 98-99, 99f
Government-owned hospitals, 19-20, 19f
GPS (global positioning system) technology, 699
Grading, of cancer, 477
Gradual phase-in of applications, 337, 364
Grand total, 397, 397t
Granularity(ies)
    of data, 144, 144t, 300
    of terminology, 210
Graphic rating scales, for performance appraisal, 585, 586-587, 586f
Graphic sheet, 111-112
Graphical user interface (GUI), 120, 121f, 258, 285, 494
Greater Cincinnati Public Health InformationLinks Project, 87t
"Green building" design, 601
Grievance procedure, 592, 594-595
Griggs v. Duke Power, 582
Griswold v. Connecticut, 505
Gross autopsy rate, 378, 379t
Gross death rate, 374, 374t
Grounded champions, 357
Group analysis and design, in system analysis, 330
Group decision support software (GDSS), 330
Group model HMO, 36
Group practice, 17
Growth and maturity, in system life cycle, 310
GUI (graphical user interface), 120, 121f, 258, 285, 494
Gynecology, 24t

H

Halo effect, 582, 589
Hammonds v. Aetna Casualty and Surety Co., 510, 536
Hand-held computers, for data access, 243t, 244-245
"Handicapped," 564-565
Handwriting, documentation via, 180
Hardware, for data access and retention, 243
Harm
    defined, 460
    in negligence or malpractice case, 530
Harvard Medical System, 457
Hazard(s), 566
Hazardous substances, exposure to, 148
HCFA (Health Care Financing Administration), 11, 650-651
HCPCS (Healthcare Common Procedure Coding System), 132, 203
Head
    physical examination of, 108t
    in review of systems, 106t
Header, of form, 117
Health
    data and, 486
    defined, 5
    determinants of, 405
    of employees, 600-601
Health Alert Network, 67t
Health and Human Services (HHS) Data Council, 98
Health care
    financing of, 34-38, 35b
    health information technology in, 66
    in nineteenth century, 5-6
    twentieth-century reforms in, 6-8, 6b-8b
    in twenty-first century, 8-9, 545
Health care administrators, use of health data by, 95

Health Care Amendments, 568-569
Health care costs, factors driving, 652, 652b
Health care delivery systems, 16-30
    adult day care services in, 29
    ambulatory care in, 17-18
    complementary and alternative medicine in, 29
    continuum of care in, 16-17, 16t
    contract services in, 29-30
    e-health in, 29
    expenditure for, 684
    home care in, 27
    hospice care in, 28-29, 29t
    hospitals in, 18–27
        bed size of, 20
        clinical classification of, 20
        composition and structure of, 21-22
        essential services of, 24-27
        health information management in, 27
        leadership of, 22-23
        length of stay at, 20
        medical staff of, 23, 23t-24t
        organization of, 20-21, 20f
        ownership of, 19-20, 19f
        patients of, 20
    integrated, 30
    long-term care facilities in, 28
    mobile diagnostic services in, 29
    respite care in, 29
    subacute care in, 27
Health care expenditures, total, 8
Health care facilities
    licensure of, 12-13, 13t, 46
    organization of, 20-21, 21f
Health Care Financing Administration (HCFA), 11, 650-651
Health care fraud, 660-661, 661b
Health care information standards, with electronic health record systems, 172-173, 173f, 174t-175t
Health care operations, 517
    use of health information for, 522
Health care practitioners, use of health data by, 95
Health care professional(s), 30-34, 31t
    allied health, 33-34
    attributes of, 30
    nurses as, 32-33, 33t
    physician assistant as, 32
    physicians as, 31-32
Health care provider(s)
    defined, 5, 95
    use of health data by, 95
Health care quality, key dimensions of, 438
Health Care Quality Improvement Act, 534
Health care reform, and human resource management, 559
Health care services
    defined, 5
    payment for, 34-38, 35b
        historical perspective on, 650-652, 651f, 652b
Health care systems
    evolution of, 5-9
    future issues for, 39-40
Health care team, 30-34, 31t
Health data
    core elements of, 100, 101t
    in decision making, 96-97
    essential, 94, 94b
    in patient record, 44-45
    users and uses of, 95-96, 95f
Health data standards, 211-216, 213t-214t
    development and selection of, 214-215

Health disparities, elimination of, 405
Health expenditures, historical perspective on, 650-651, 651f
Health Grades, 486
Health indicators, 405
Health informatics
  defined, 166
  electronic health records in, 166
Health information
  disclosure of, 517-529
    for administrative purposes, 522
    to attorneys, 522-523
    authorization for, 518, 519f, 520f
    for direct patient care, 518-521
    for educational purposes, 521
    in emergency, 518
    to family
      in cases of incompetence or incapacity, 524
      of emancipated minor or adult, 524
      of minor, 524
    to law enforcement personnel and agencies, 523-524
    to news media, 526-527
    to outsourcing firms, 526
    ownership and, 517
    to patient, 511, 524-525
    patient-directed, 525
    for payment purposes, 522, 523f
    for performance management and patient safety, 521
    pursuant to legal process, 527-529, 528f
    and redisclosure, 525-526
    for research, 521-522
    resources on, 517-518
    security measures to prevent unauthorized, 529
  duty to maintain, 511-512
  duty to retain, 512-515, 513f
  as evidence, 514-515
  individually identifiable, 515-516
  internal uses of, 517, 518, 522
  ownership of, 517
  in patient record, 44-45
  protected, 515-516
  security of, 512, 529
  technology in, 38-39
Health information administrator, 31t
Health information exchange (HIE), 83-88, 83t-87t
  national network for, 215-216
Health information infrastructure, 64-90
  background of, 64-65
  emerging networks in, 81-88, 83t-87t
  federal involvement in, 67-73, 67t-68t, 68f, 71t-77t
  key concepts on, 88-90
  private sector in, 73
  role of health information management in, 88, 89t
Health information management (HIM)
  defined, 50
  international, 690-692
  re-engineering and, 637
  role of, 88, 89t
Health Information Management Compliance Program, 510
Health information management (HIM) department, virtual, 190-195
Health information management (HIM) profession, 44
  code of ethics of, 58, 58b
  education programs for, 51-52
  evolution of, 49-56, 50b

Health information management (HIM) profession (Continued)
  fellowship program in, 56-57
  future of, 59
  job opportunities in, 51
  key concepts on, 59-60
  maintenance of certification and lifelong learning for, 56-57, 57b
  professional certification in, 52-54
  roles and competencies in, 50, 50b
  in transition, 685
Health information management (HIM) professional
  in financial management, 680-681
  in system development, 308
Health information management system, 270-271
Health information networks
  emerging, 81-88
  financial issues with, 87
  organization and governance issues with, 84
  privacy, security, and confidentiality issues with, 87
  technical issues with, 84-87
Health information services (HIS), systems approach to, 555, 556f
Health information systems (HISs)
  components of, 271
  as emerging discipline, 273
  evolution of, 271-273
  expenditures for, 270
  hierarchy of, 271, 272f
  levels of, 273
  scope of, 271
Health information systems (HIS) committee, 129
Health information technology (HIT)
  adoption of
    goals for, 78
    obstacles to, 79-81, 81t-82t
  applications of, 78t
  compelling reasons to implement, 73-79, 78t-80t
  cost savings of, 80, 81
  defined, 66n
  federal involvement in, 67-73, 67t-68t, 68f, 71t-77t
  in health care, 66
  and patient record, 47-48
  potential benefits of, 78-79, 79t, 80, 80t
Health information technology (HIT) federal initiatives, 67, 67t-68t
Health information technology (HIT) Portfolio, 70
Health Information Technology Promotion Act (HITPA), 202
Health Information Technology Standards Panel (HITSP), 213
Health insurance, 34, 35b
  and patient record, 46-47
Health Insurance for the Aged, 7, 7b
Health Insurance Portability and Accountability Act (HIPAA), 8b, 13-14, 59
  on access to records, 525
  on data collection, 98, 104
  on designated record set, 162
  on health information technology, 66, 69
  on improper billing practices, 510
  as legal resource, 537
  on privacy, 515, 517, 518, 519f, 527, 566-567
  on provider enrollment, 655
  on security, 293-294, 294t, 512, 529
Health Level Seven (HL 7), 39, 69, 156, 215
Health Level Seven (HL 7) Functional Model, 215

Health maintenance organizations (HMOs), 35-36, 660
Health occupations, regulatory mechanisms of, 15
Health Outcomes Institute (HOI), 490
Health Personnel Shortage Areas (HPSAs), 293
Health Plan Employer Data and Information Set (HEDIS), 14-15, 100, 439, 488, 692-693
Health policy, and human resource management, 558-559
Health record(s). See Patient record(s).
  legal, 157-161, 160t-161t, 242
Health record review, 183-184, 185f, 186f
Health Resources and Services Administration (HRSA), 11
Health services research, 485
Health-based risk adjustment, 485
HealthBridge, 87t
Healthcare Common Procedure Coding System (HCPCS), 132, 203
Healthcare Information and Management Systems Society (HIMSS), 76t, 102
Healthcare Integrity and Protection Data Bank (HIPDB), 468
Healthy Communities 2000, 9
Healthy People 2000, 9
Healthy People 2010, 9, 405
Hearsay rule, 514
Heating, ventilating, and air conditioning (HVAC) systems, in workstation design, 643-644
HEDIS (Health Plan Employer Data and Information Set), 14-15, 100, 439, 488, 692-693
Hematologic system, in review of systems, 107t
Hematology, 24t
HEW (Department of Health, Education, and Welfare), 7b, 8b, 10
HHS (Health and Human Services) Data Council, 98
HIE (health information exchange), 83-88, 83t-87t
  national network for, 215-216
Hierarchical database, 277
Hierarchical organization, 20-21, 21f
Hierarchical structure, of systems, 623
Hierarchy chart, in system analysis, 315, 316f
Hierarchy of needs, 571
High-volume film scanners, 254
Hill, Lister, 6
Hill-Burton Act, 6, 7b
HIM. See Health information management (HIM).
HIMSS (Healthcare Information and Management Systems Society), data collection standards of, 76t, 102
HIPAA. See Health Insurance Portability and Accountability Act (HIPAA).
HIPDB (Healthcare Integrity and Protection Data Bank), 468
Hippocratic Oath, 515, 550
Hire-from-within policy, 580
HIS(s). See Health information systems (HISs).
Hispanics, in workforce, 544-545
Histograms, 386, 388f, 452, 455f
Historical-prospective study, 426, 426f, 427t-428t
History and physical examination (H&P) report, 105-107, 106t-108t
  for acute care, 130
History of present illness (HPI), 106t, 149
HIT. See Health information technology (HIT).

HITPA (Health Information Technology Promotion Act), 202
HITSP (Health Information Technology Standards Panel), 213
HIV (human immunodeficiency virus), and internal disclosure of health information, 517
HL 7 (Health Level Seven), 39, 69, 156, 215
HL 7 (Health Level Seven) Functional Model, 215
HMOs (health maintenance organizations), 35-36, 660
HOD (House of Delegates), of AHIMA, 56
HOI (Health Outcomes Institute), 490
Hold harmless clauses, 536
Home care, 27
Home health agencies, 137
Home health aides, 25
Home health care, 27
    data needs for, 137-141, 139f-141f
    defined, 137
Home health care documentation flowchart, 138, 139f-140f
Honesty, 550
Horizontal organization, 30
Hospice, 16t, 28-29, 29t
    data needs for, 141-142
Hospital(s), 18-27
    bed size of, 20
    city, 20
    classification of, 18-21, 19f
        clinical, 20
    composition and structure of, 21-22
    county, 20
    critical access, 19
    defined, 18
    essential services of, 24-27
    evolution of, 6
    faith-based, 20
    for-profit (proprietary, private, investor-owned), 20
    general, 20
    health information management in, 27
    leadership of, 22-23
    length of stay at, 20
    medical staff of, 23, 23t-24t
    not-for-profit (voluntary), 20
    organization of, 20-21, 20f
    ownership of, 19-20, 19f
    patients of, 20
    psychiatric, 20
    rehabilitation and chronic disease, 20
    specialty, 20
    state, 20
Hospital administrator, 22
Hospital ambulatory care, 18
Hospital cancer registries, 475, 476
Hospital formulary, 26
Hospital inpatients, 20
Hospital insurance, Medicare, 37
Hospital patients, 20
Hospital Standardization Movement, 59
Hospital Standardization Program, 6-7, 7b, 446
Hospital Survey and Construction Act, 6, 7b
Hospital-wide health information system, 271
House of Delegates (HOD), of AHIMA, 56
H&P (history and physical examination) report, 105-107, 106t-108t
    for acute care, 130
HPI (history of present illness), 106t, 149
HPSAs (Health Personnel Shortage Areas), 293
HRM. See Human resource management (HRM).
HRSA (Health Resources and Services Administration), 11

HSQ, 490
HSQ-12, 490
HTML (hypertext markup language), 170, 289-290, 290f
HTTP (Hypertext Transfer Protocol), 289
Huff, Stan, 206
Human Gene Nomenclature, 69
Human immunodeficiency virus (HIV), and internal disclosure of health information, 517
Human resource audit, 576
Human resource management (HRM), 542-602
    adverse outcomes of employee performance in, 590-592, 590b, 591f
    aging workforce in, 544-545, 560-561, 565-566
    compensation management in, 567, 595-598, 596f
    current challenges in, 544-546
    employee as client of, 571-572
    employee assistance programs in, 572
    employee counseling and discipline in, 592-594
    employee expectations in, 584
    employee handbooks in, 578-579
    employee health, safety, and well-being in, 600-601
    employee retention in, 583-584
    employee selection in, 580-583
    environmental influences and, 557-561, 561b
    equal employment opportunity in, 562-564
    ethical aspects of, 550-552, 553b
    future issues in, 601
    grievance process in, 594-595
    information systems and, 570-571
    job analysis and design in, 576-578, 577f
    job description in, 558, 578, 578t
    key concepts in, 601-602
    labor unions in, 545, 567-569, 568b-570b
    leadership and, 546-550, 547f, 548f, 553b-555b, 572b-573b
    legal and regulatory requirements affecting, 561-569, 563t, 565b, 568b-570b
    organizational culture and, 569-570, 570b
    orientation in, 584
    performance appraisal in, 584-590, 586f-589f
    planning and forecasting for, 573-576, 574b, 575f, 576f
    recruitment in, 579-580
    role in health care organization of, 571, 571f
    systems perspective on, 552-557, 556f, 557f
    training and development in, 598-600, 599b, 600b
Human subjects, in research proposal, 410
Humidity, in workstation design, 644
HVAC (heating, ventilating, and air conditioning) systems, in workstation design, 643-644
Hybrid records, 48, 160, 161t, 178, 179
Hypertext links, 282
Hypertext markup language (HTML), 170, 289-290, 290f
Hypertext Transfer Protocol (HTTP), 289
Hyphenated names, in master patient index, 227
Hypothesis, 392-393, 406

I

IBM Medical Information Systems Program, 272
ICCS (International Classification of Clinical Services), 491
ICD, International Classification of Disease (ICD). See International Classification of Disease (ICD).

ICNP (International Classification of Nursing Practice), 209t
Icons, 332
ICUs (intensive care units), virtual, 699
IDDM (insulin-dependent diabetes mellitus), 482
Idea-generating techniques, for process improvement, 450, 450f
Identification of products and services, 352
Identity management, 163, 179-180
IDS (integrated delivery systems), 30
IEEE (Institute of Electrical and Electronics Engineers), 69
IEEE (Institute of Electrical and Electronics Engineers) Standards Association, 174t
IETF (Internet Engineering Task Force), 288
IFHRO (International Federation of Health Records Organizations), 690
IHS (Indian Health Service), 11
IIHI (individually identifiable health information), 515-516
Illegal aliens, 566
Image-based records, access and retention of, 247-264
    electronic document management for, 255-264, 269t
    micrographics for, 247-255, 248t, 249t, 251t, 253t
Imaging reports, 112
Immigration Reform and Control Act (IRCA), 566
Immunization record, 148
Immunization registries, 483
Immunization status, of adolescents, 693
Implant registries, 482-483
Implanted devices, 699, 701
Implementation phase, of system development, 307, 310, 335-337
Implementation plan, for electronic document management, 262
Implementation process, in financial management, 680
Implementation readiness, 363-366
Implementation strategies, for electronic document management, 262
Implied contract, and employee termination, 590-591
Implied covenant of good faith and fair dealing, and employee termination, 591
Implied powers, 505
Imprisonment, false, 508-509
Improper billing practices, 510
In Confidence, 529
Inactive records, 225, 234-235, 254
Incapacitation, 298
    disclosure of health information to family in cases of, 524
    durable power of attorney for health care in case of, 532
Incidence, 380t, 381, 484
Incidence rate (IR), 381, 425
Incidence study, 424-425, 425t-428t
Incidence-only cancer registries, 476
Incident cases, 409
Incident reports, 455-456, 456t, 457f
    confidentiality of, 516
    in legal cases, 530-531
Inclusion, termination by, 632
Income statement, 672, 673f
Incompetence, disclosure of health information to family in cases of, 524
Indemnification clauses, 536
Independent contractor clauses, 536
Independent living facility, 28

Independent practice association (IPA), 36
Independent practitioner, 30
Independent samples *t* test, 394
Independent Study Program for the Health
    Information Technician (ISP for HITs),
    51
Independent variables, 406
Index, in electronic document management,
    256
Indian Health Service (IHS), 11
Indiana Health Information Exchange Project,
    206
Indiana University, Regenstrief Institute at, 85t
Indicators, 441
Indigent, defined, 7
Indirect cost(s), of electronic document
    management, 261
Indirect cost departments, 668
Indirect pay, 34
Individually identifiable health information
    (IIHI), 515-516
Individuals chart, 454, 454b
Individuals with Disabilities Education Act, 564
Industry development, and human resource
    management, 558-559
Infant death rate, 374t, 376
Infectious disease, 24t
Inference(s), 392
Inferential statistics, 392
Informal organization, 626-627
Informaticians, workforce needs for, 687
Informatics training programs, 687-688
Informatics work group (IWG), 497b
Information
    defined, 97, 169
    in electronic health record systems, 169
    in patient record, 44-45
    release of, 184
    ways of gathering, 325-329
        document and forms review as, 329
        group analysis and design as, 329
        interviews as, 325-327
        observation as, 328-329, 328f
        questionnaires as, 327-328
Information Access Privilege, 175t
Information dissemination, 492-493, 493t
Information infrastructure functions, 158f
Information resources management committee,
    129
Information services or systems (I/S), 356
Information system(s), and human resource
    management, 570-571
Information system development life cycle,
    313-314, 314f
Information system fluctuation, 311-312, 311f
Information system life cycle, 310-311, 311f
    in organization, 311-312, 311f
    aggregate, 312
Information systems master plans, electronic
    health record system in, 193-194
Information warehouses, 167, 169-170, 300f
InformationLinks, 76t
Informed consent
    duty to obtain, 531-532
    waiver of, 532
Infrastructure, standards for, 175t
Initiation phase, of system development, 306
Injury, defined, 460
Injury Severity Scale, 484
Inland Northwest Health Services, 85t
Inpatient(s)
    defined, 5
    hospital, 20
Inpatient bed count, 382t

Inpatient bed occupancy rate, 382, 383t
Inpatient day, 382t
Inpatient service day, 382t
Input
    measuring, 611
    of system, 624
Input design, 331, 332
Input devices, 333
    for data access and retention, 243,
        243t-244t
Input processes, goals of, 332
Input-output cycle, of system, 624-625
In-service training and development, 598-599
Installation requirements, in request for
    proposal, 348-349
Institute for Safe Medication Practices, 456
Institute of Electrical and Electronics Engineers
    (IEEE), 69
Institute of Electrical and Electronics Engineers
    (IEEE) Standards Association, 174t
Institute of Medicine (IOM), 7-8, 39, 438, 457
Institutional accreditation, 562
Institutional Review Board (IRB)
    application to, 409, 410
    approval by, 521-522
Instructions
    on forms, 117
    on user interface, 282
Insulin-dependent diabetes mellitus (IDDM),
    482
Insurance, 34, 35b
Insurance companies
    disclosure of health information to, 522,
        523f, 526
    historical perspective on, 650-652
Insurance coverage
    lack of, 652
    primary and secondary, 657
Integrated delivery systems (IDS), 30
Integrated medical record, 115
Integrating Information–Improving the
    Exchange Project, 86t
Integration, termination by, 632
Integration testing, 337
Integrity
    of data, 144t, 145
    of documentation, 178
    of system, 624
Intensity of service/severity of illness (IS/SI)
    criteria, 463
Intensive care units (ICUs), virtual, 699
Intentional torts, 508–509
Interdisciplinary patient care plan, 107, 138,
    142-143
Interest inventories, 582
Interface(s), 333
Interface engine, 280, 280f
Intermediate appellate court, 507
Internal benchmarking, 446
Internal controls, in system, 624
Internal environmental analysis, 627
Internal medicine, 24t
Internal Revenue Service (IRS), 505, 654
International Classification of Clinical Services
    (ICCS), 491
International Classification of Disease (ICD), 57,
    201-203
International Classification of Diseases for
    Oncology (ICD-O), 203
*International Classification of Diseases for
    Oncology,* Third Edition (ICD-O-3),
    477
International Classification of Diseases, Ninth
    Revision (ICD-9), 201-202

International Classification of Diseases, Ninth
    Revision, *Clinical Modification* (ICD-9-
    CM), 170, 174t, 202
International Classification of Diseases, Tenth
    Revision (ICD-10), 202
International Classification of Diseases, Tenth
    Revision, *Clinical Modification* (ICD-10-
    CM), 202
International Classification of Diseases, Tenth
    Revision, *Procedural Coding System*
    (ICD-10-PCS), 202
International Classification of Nursing Practice
    (ICNP), 209t
International Computer Driving License
    Foundation, 687
International Federation of Health Records
    Organizations (IFHRO), 690
International health information management,
    690-692
International Implant Registry, 482
International Medical Informatics Association,
    686
International Organization for Standardization
    (ISO), 211
International Union Against Cancer, 477
Internet, 288-292
    in data access, 244
    in electronic health record systems, 156
    fundamentals of, 289
    in literature search, 406-407
Internet Engineering Task Force (IETF), 288
Internet protocol (IP), 289
Internet security, 297, 298f
Internet Society, 288
Internet tools, 289-292, 290f
Interobserver reliability, 413
Interoperability
    basic, 214
    and data standardization, 213-214
    with electronic health record systems, 172-
        173, 173f, 174t-175t, 213-214, 684-686
    functional, 214
    semantic, 214
Interpersonal domains, of care, 442
InterQual, 463
Interrogatories, 507
Interval data, 328, 384-385
Interval estimation, 398-399
Interview(s)
    focus group, 420-421
    selection, 582-583
    in system analysis, 325-327
Interviewer bias, 415-416
Intradepartmental health information system,
    271
Intranet, 291
Intraobserver reliability, 413
Intraorganizational outcomes teams, 488
Introduction, on form, 117
Intuitive decisions, 554b
Invasion of privacy, 509
Investment decisions, 675-680, 677f-678f, 679t
Investor-owned hospitals, 20
IOM (Institute of Medicine), 7-8, 39, 438, 457
IP (Internet protocol), 289
IPA (independent practice association), 36
IR (incidence rate), 381, 425
IRB (Institutional Review Board)
    application to, 409, 410
    approval by, 521–522
IRCA (Immigration Reform and Control Act),
    566
IRS (Internal Revenue Service), 505, 654
I/S (information services or systems), 356

"is-a" relationship, 205, 206f, 210
ISO (International Organization for Standardization), 211
ISP for HITs (Independent Study Program for the Health Information Technician), 51
IS/SI (intensity of service/severity of illness) criteria, 463
Iterative design, 363
"Itineraries," 141, 141f
IWG (informatics work group), 497b

J

Jacket microfilm, 247-248, 248t, 249t
JAD (joint application design), 330
James W. Ashton Ambulatory Care Center, 239-240
JAVA, 291
JCAH (Joint Commission on Accreditation of Hospitals), 7, 7b, 46
JCAHO. See Joint Commission on Accreditation of Healthcare Organizations (JCAHO).
Job analysis, 576-578, 577f
Job applicants, 579-583
Job application, 581
Job descriptions, 558, 578, 578t
Job evaluation, 596-598, 596f
Job grading, 578t, 597
Job interview, 582-583
Job opening, 579
Job performance standards, 578
Job postings, 580
Job ranking, 596-597
Job requirements, 579
Job sharing, 558
Job specifications, 578t
Job status, 578t
Job summary, 578t
Joint application design (JAD), 330
Joint Commission on Accreditation of Healthcare Organizations (JCAHO), 7, 7b, 14
  on accreditation, 46, 562
  on credentialing, 467
  data collection standards of, 100, 128-129
  and human resource management, 563t
  international division of, 692
  on patient safety, 454-455
  on performance management, 439, 446, 486-487
  record deficiency standards of, 122-124, 124t
Joint Commission on Accreditation of Hospitals (JCAH), 7, 7b, 46
Joint requirement planning (JRP), in system analysis, 330
Journal of the American Health Information Management Association, 57
Judgment non obstante verdicto (judgment n.o.v.), 507
Jukebox, in electronic document management, 257
Jurisdiction, 506
  diversity of, 506
Jury, 507
Justice, 550

K

Kaiser Permanente, 36
Kansas City Health Exchange, 86t
Kansas Immunization Registry, 86t
Kaplan-Meier product limit method, 429, 430f
Kerr-Mills Medical Assistance Program, 7, 7b
Key indicators of demand, 573

Key words, 170
  for literature search, 406
Keyboard(s)
  for data input and output, 243t
  for electronic document management, 256
  in workstation design, 642, 643
Knowledge, 44
  in collaboration, 361-362
  defined, 169
  in electronic health record systems, 169
Knowledge base, 287
Kotter, John, 553b
Krause, Donald, 553b
Kurten Medical Group, microfilm system of, 254-255

L

Label, in data dictionary, 318, 318f, 319, 319f
Labor and delivery record, 111
Labor Management Relations Act, 563t, 568
Labor Management Reporting and Disclosure Act, 563t, 568
Labor unions, 545, 567-569, 568b-570b
  grievance procedure with, 594
Laboratory Logical Observation Identifier Name Codes, 69
Laboratory reports, 112
LANs (local area networks), 246, 278
  and outcomes research, 494
Lateral filing cabinets, 222
Law(s), 504
  case, 505-506, 506b
  common, 505-506, 506b
  constitutional, 504-505
  criminal, 504
  private, 504
  public, 504
  sources of, 504-506, 506b
Law enforcement personnel and agencies, disclosure of health information to, 523-524
Layoffs, 591-592
Layout flowchart, 618, 621
Leadership, 546-550
  case studies on, 553b-555b, 572b-573b
  challenges for, 554b
  contingency approach to, 546
  ethics of, 549-550, 554b
  of hospital, 22-23
  and human resources management, 546
  relational nature of, 546-548, 547f, 548f
  servant, 551
  transactional, 548
  transformational, 548-549, 554b
  translational, 549
  visionary, 554b
Leadership development, 549, 553b
Leadership grid, 546, 547f
Leadership style, relationships and, 546-548, 547f, 548f
Leadership theory, overview of, 546
Lean thinking, 449
Leapfrog Group, 76t, 166, 440
Leavitt, Mike, 70, 71t
Ledgers, for record keeping, 45
Legacy systems, 321
Legal analysis, of patient records, 127
Legal case, disclosure of health information in, 527-529, 528f
Legal considerations
  with electronic document management, 262
  with microfilm, 250
Legal context, of public health, 696, 696b
Legal document, patient record as, 45

Legal elements, on patient record, 146
Legal frameworks, for electronic health record systems, 194
Legal guardian, disclosure of health information to, 524
Legal health record (LHR), 157-161, 160t-161t, 242
Legal issues
  antitrust claims as, 510
  contractual disputes as, 509-510
  crimes and corporate compliance as, 510
  importance of, 504
  intentional torts as, 508-509
  key concepts on, 537-539
  malpractice and negligence as, 507-508
  noncompliance with statues, rules, and regulations as, 510
  products liability as, 509
  with telemedicine, 293
Legal obligations and risks, 511-537
  contract liability issues as, 536-537, 538f
  disclosure of health information as, 517-529
    for administrative purposes, 522
    to attorneys, 522-523
    authorization for, 518, 519f, 520f
    for direct patient care, 518-521
    for educational purposes, 521
    to family
      in cases of incompetence or incapacity, 524
      of emancipated minor or adult, 524
      of minor, 524
    to law enforcement personnel and agencies, 523-524
    to news media, 526-527
    to outsourcing firms, 526
    ownership and, 517
    to patient, 511, 524-525
    patient-directed, 525
    for payment purposes, 522, 523f
    for performance management and patient safety, 521
    pursuant to legal process, 527-529, 528f
    and redisclosure, 525-526
    for research, 521-522
    resources on, 517-518
    security measures to prevent unauthorized, 529
  duties to patients in general as, 511
  duty to maintain confidentiality as, 515-517
  duty to maintain health information as, 511-512
  duty to obtain informed consent as, 531-532
  duty to provide care that meets professional standards as, 529-531
  duty to provide safe environment for patients and visitors as, 532-533
  duty to retain health information as, 512-515, 513f
  duty to supervise actions of employees and professional staff as, 533-536, 533f
  for employee health, safety, and well-being, 600-601
  internal uses of health information as, 517, 518, 522
Legal requirements, affecting human resource management, 561-569, 563t, 565b, 568b-570b
Legal resources, for health information management professionals, 537
Legal system, 506-510
  case law in, 507-510

Legal system (Continued)
  courts in, 506-507
  fundamentals of, 504
  sources of law in, 504-506, 506b
  use of health data in, 96
Legibility, of documentation, 177
Legislation, on health care delivery, 13-14
Length, in data dictionary, 496
Length of stay, 20, 382t, 383
  average, 382-383, 383t, 431, 432t
Leniency bias, 589
Lethality assessment, 143
Level of care, 26
Level of significance, 393
LHR (legal health record), 157-161, 160t-161t, 242
Liabilities, 672
Libel, 509
License grant, 352
Licensed independent practitioner (LIP), 102, 107
Licensed practical nurse (LPN), 25, 33t
Licensed vocational nurse (LVN), 33t
Licensing agencies, use of health data by, 96
Licensure
  of health care facilities, 12-13, 13t, 46
  of health information management professionals, 52-53
  of physicians, 32, 467
  of practitioners, 15
  in revenue cycle, 654-655
Life care centers, 28
Life domains, 488
Life expectancy, 8-9
Lifelong learning, 54-55, 55b
Life-table analysis, 427-429, 430f
Light pen, 239
Lighting, in workstation design, 644-645
Likert scale, for evaluation criteria, 349-351, 350f
Line(s), on forms, 117-119
Line graphs, 386, 387f, 452-453, 455f
Linkage strategies, 629
LIP (licensed independent practitioner), 102, 107
Liquidity ratio, 674
Literature referenced, in research proposal, 410-411
Literature review, 406-407, 407f, 408
Literature search, 406-407
Living arrangements, 131
Living will, 532
Local area networks (LANs), 246, 278
  and outcomes research, 494
Local-state-federal model, 697f
Logical data model, 496
Logical name, in data dictionary, 496
Logical Observation Identifiers Names and Codes (LOINC), 170, 174t, 205-207, 209t
Logical system design, 331
Longitudinal patient record, 98
Long-term care, 16t, 28
  data needs for, 134-136, 136t
Long-term care facilities, 20, 28
Long-term debt/total assets ratio, 675
Look-up tables, 277
Loss prevention, 461
Loss reduction, 461
Lossless compression ratio, 293
Lossy compression ratio, 293
Louisiana Health Information Exchange, 86t
LPN (licensed practical nurse), 25, 33t
Lungs, physical examination of, 108t

LVN (licensed vocational nurse), 33t
Lymphatics, physical examination of, 108t

M

M programming language, 275
MACDP (Metropolitan Atlanta Congenital Defects Program), 481
MacEachern, Malcolm, 49
Machine language, 275
Macy Foundation, 688
Magnetic disk, 256-257
Magnetic storage, secure, 257
Magnification ratio, 250
Mainframe machines, 274
  for data access and retention, 243
Major birth defects, 481
Malicious software (malware) protection, 297-298
Malpractice, 507-508, 530
Mammography, 25
Managed care, 35-36, 545
  and cost control, 652
  earliest forms of, 6
  and human resource management, 559
Managed care organizations (MCOs), 35-36
Management by objectives (MBO), 587-588
Management development, continuing education units in, 55
Management information system committee, 129
Managerial accountant, 671, 671t
Managerial accounting, 661-662
Managerial finance officer, 671, 671t
Managerial grid, 546, 547f
Mandatory reporting requirements, 511-512
Manual for Staging of Cancer, 477
Manual record-tracking systems, 237-238, 237f
Many-to-many relation, 322
Mapping, 208
Margins, on forms, 119
Market entry strategies, 629
Marketing, use of health information for, 522
Markle Foundation, 73, 75t, 166
MA-SHARE, 85t
Maslow, Abraham, 571
Masqueraders, 298
Massachusetts General Hospital Utility Multi-Programming System (MUMPS), 275
Massachusetts Health Data Consortium, 85t
Master(s), of forms, 119
Master budget, 663
Master charge list, 655, 655t
Master patient index (MPI), 226-231
  alias names in, 227, 227f-228f
  alphabetical identification vs., 220
  backup of, 230
  case study of, 232b-233b
  content of, 226-227
  correction of, 179
  creation of, 227-231, 229f-230f
  hyphenated names in, 227
  importance of, 104, 122
  merging of, 231, 232b
  with numerical identification, 220
  prefix names in, 227
  registration and, 163
  sample screen for, 120f, 228, 228f
  validity of, 228-230, 231f
Master's degree, in health information management, 52
Matching, in research study design, 423
Matching concept, in accounting, 670, 671
Materials, in system development, 309
Maternal death rate, 374t, 376

Mathematical simulations, for system evaluation, 343
Matrix, 451, 455f
Matrix organization, 21
MBO (management by objectives), 587-588
MCAT (Medical College Admission Test), 32
MCOs (managed care organizations), 35-36
MD (doctor of medicine), 32
MDS (minimum data set), 114, 129
Mean, 389-390
Mean square between groups (MSB), 395
Mean square within groups (MSW), 395
Measures of central tendency, 388-391
Measures of dispersion, 391-392
Media
  disclosure of health information to, 526-527
  use of health data by, 96
Median, 390-391
Mediation, 506
Medibase, Inc., 232b-233b
Medicaid, 7, 7b, 36, 38, 47
Medical Assistance Program, 7, 7b, 38
Medical assistant, 31t
Medical centers, free-standing, 17
Medical College Admission Test (MCAT), 32
Medical errors, 8, 438, 684
Medical Errors Reporting Program, 456
Medical examination, pre-employment, 583
Medical examiner, disclosure of health information to, 523-524
Medical executive committee, 535
Medical history, 105, 106t-107t, 148
Medical imaging department, 25
Medical informatics, 273, 686-688
Medical Information Bureau (MIB), 526
Medical information system, 271
Medical Information Systems Program, 272
Medical insurance, Medicare, 37
Medical laboratory technician, 31t
Medical logic modules (MLMs), 287
Medical necessity, 462
Medical Outcomes Trust, 490
Medical Products Reporting Program, 457
Medical record. See Patient record(s).
Medical record committee, 128
Medical record numbers, duplicate, 230f, 232b-233b
Medical record technicians, 51
Medical records department, 27
Medical specialties, 23, 23t-24t
Medical staff, 23, 23t-24t
  credentialing process for, 534-535
  duty to supervise actions of, 533-536, 533f
Medical staff coordinator, 535-536
Medical Subject Headings (MeSH), 208
Medical technologist, 31t
Medical transcription, 122, 180-181
MedicAlert Foundation, 482
Medically indigent, 38
Medicare, 36-37
  electronic prescriptions for, 71, 71t, 72t
  history of, 7, 7b
  and patient record, 47
  reimbursement by, 650
Medicare abuse, 660-661, 661b
Medicare Advantage, 37
Medicare fraud, 660-661, 661b
Medicare Modernization Act (MMA), 37, 70
Medicare Prescription Drug, Improvement, and Modernization Act, 37
Medicare Prescription Drug Plan, 37
Medication errors, 456
Medication profile, 148-149
Medication Safety Alert, 456

Medication sheet, 112
MEDLINE, 406, 407
MedPlus, 262-264
MedWatch, 457
Memorial Hospital Enterprise System, 262-264
Mendenhall, Stan, 491
Mental distress, intentional infliction of, 509
Mental Health Council of America (MHCA), 490
Mental health records, patient access to, 525
Mental institutions, foundation of, 6
Mental status, physical examination of, 108t
Menus, 332
Merging, of master patient index, 231, 232b
Meritor Savings v. Vinson, 564
Mesa County Public Health Information Exchange Project, 86t
MeSH (Medical Subject Headings), 208
Messaging standards, 174t
Metadata, 495
Methodology, of research study, 408, 409-410, 410f
Methods improvement, 614-623
   data analysis in, 618
   data collection in, 615-618, 616f-621f, 618b
   defined, 614-615
   formulating alternative solutions in, 618-619
   implementation and evaluation of, 622-623, 623b
   objectives of, 615
   philosophy of, 615
   problem identification in, 615
   selecting improved method in, 619-620, 621f, 622f
   steps in, 615
Metropolitan Atlanta Congenital Defects Program (MACDP), 481
MFDs (multifunctional devices), for electronic document management, 255
MHCA (Mental Health Council of America), 490
MIB (Medical Information Bureau), 526
Michigan Electronic Medical Record Initiative, 76t
Microcomputers, 274
   for data access and retention, 243
Microfiche, 248
   computer output, 248-249
   for data input and output, 244t
Microfilm, 247-255
   applications of, 254-255
   cost analysis of, 250-254, 251t, 253t
   for data input and output, 244t
   equipment for, 249-250
   as evidence, 515
   jacket, 247-248, 248t, 249t
   legal considerations with, 250
   processing of
      contracted service bureaus for, 252-254, 253t
      in-house, 250-252
   roll, 247, 248, 248t, 249t
Microfilm cabinet, 249-250
Microfilm cameras, 250-252
Microfilm jackets, 247-248, 248t, 249t
Microfilm reader, 250
Microforms, 247-249, 248t, 249t
Micrographics, 247-255
   applications of, 254-255
   cost analysis of, 250-254, 251t, 253t
   defined, 247
   equipment for, 249-250
   formats for, 247-249, 248t, 249t
   legal considerations with, 250

Middleware, 280
Midlevel practitioner, 30
Migration
   data, 365
   to electronic health record system, 173-176, 190, 191b-192b
Miller, Dale, 529
Milliman, 463
Miniaturized cathode ray tubes, for data input and output, 243t
Minicomputers, 274
   for data access and retention, 243
Minimum data set (MDS), 114, 129
Minimum Data Set for Nursing Home Resident Assessment and Care Screening, 134-136
"Minimum necessary" principle, 517
Minimum Standards, 6, 6b, 7b
Minors
   disclosure of health information to family of, 524
   informed consent of, 531
Mirroring backup server, 258
Mishap databases, 457
Mission, organizational, 628, 662
Misuse, 298
MLMs (medical logic modules), 287
MMA (Medicare Modernization Act), 37, 70
Mobile diagnostic services, 29
"Mock screen" technique, 363
Mode, 391
Money, time value of, 676
Morbidity, 26
Morbidity rates, 379-381, 380t
Morphology, of neoplasms, 477
Mortality, 26
Mortality rate(s), 373-378
   factors influencing, 377
   fetal, 374t, 376
   infant, 374t, 376
   maternal, 374t, 376
   neonatal, 374t, 376
   using and examining, 376-378, 377t, 378t
Motion to quash, 528
Motivation, 614
Motor vehicle crashes, 695
Motorized revolving units, 222t, 223
Mouth
   physical examination of, 108t
   in review of systems, 106t
Movement diagrams, 618, 621
MPI (master patient index), 226-231
MSB (mean square between groups), 395
MSW (mean square within groups), 395
Multicultural workforce, 560
Multidisciplinary collaboration, 701
Multifunction workstations, 643
Multifunctional devices (MFDs), for electronic document management, 255
Multimedia capacity, 168, 245
Multipart forms, 119
Multiple consistent views, in terminology, 210
Multiple granularities, of terminology, 210
Multiple-apportionment method, of cost allocation, 669
Multiple-copy forms, 117
Multispecialty group, 17
MUMPS (Massachusetts General Hospital Utility Multi-Programming System), 275
Musculoskeletal system
   physical examination of, 108t
   in review of systems, 107t
Music, in workstation design, 646

Myers, Grace Whiting, 49
MyPHR, 95

N
NAACCR (North American Association of Central Cancer Registries), 479
Name normalization, 233b
Named data, 384, 384t
NANDA (North American Nursing Diagnosis Association), 209t
National Alliance for Health Information Technology, 76t
National Association of Health Data Organizations, 76t
National Board of Medical Examiners (NBME), 32
National Cancer Act, 475
National Cancer Data Base (NCDB), 479
National Cancer Institute, 72t
National Cancer Registrars Association, Inc. (NCRA), 477, 479
National Center for Complementary and Alternative Medicine, 29
National Center for Emergency Medicine Informatics, 76t
National Center for Health Statistics (NCHS), 98–99, 372, 373
National Center for Injury Prevention and Control (NCIPC), 132–133
National Committee for Quality Assurance (NCQA), 14–15, 76t
   on credentialing, 467, 654
   data collection standards of, 100
   on outcomes data, 488
   on performance management, 439
   on utilization management, 463
National Committee on Vital and Health Statistics (NCVHS), 72t, 98, 99, 202, 213
National Coordinator for Health Information Technology, 48
National Council for Prescription Drug Programs (NCPDP), 69, 173, 174t
National Drug Codes (NDCs), 207, 288
National Drug File Reference Terminology (NDF-RT), 69, 207
National Electronic Disease Surveillance System (NEDSS), 68t, 100
National Electronics Manufacturers Association, 174t
National Guidelines Clearinghouse, 441
National Health Care Survey, 381
National Health Information Infrastructure (NHII), 39, 64-90
   background of, 64-65
   emerging networks in, 81-88, 83t-87t
   federal involvement in, 67-73, 67t-68t, 68f, 71t-77t
   key concepts on, 88-90
   private sector in, 73
National Health Information Infrastructure Network (NHIN). *See* National Health Information Infrastructure (NHII).
National Immunization Program (NIP), 68t
National Institute for Occupational Safety and Health (NIOSH), 641
National Institute of Standards and Technology (NIST), 439
National Institutes of Health (NIH), 11, 72t
National Labor Relations Act (NLRA), 563t, 567-568
National Labor Relations Board (NLRB), 568, 569
National League for Nursing Accrediting Commission, Inc. (NLNAC), 15

National Organ Transplant Act (NOTA), 483
National Patient Safety Goals, 454-455
National Practitioner Data Bank (NPDB), 468, 534
National Provider Identifier (NPI), 655
National quality awards, 439
National Quality Forum (NQF), 440-441
National Residency Matching Program, 32
National Resource Center (NRC), 70, 71t
National Trauma Data Bank (NTDB), 484
National Vaccine Advisory Committee (NVAC), 483
Natural language processing, 170
NBME (National Board of Medical Examiners), 32
NCDB (National Cancer Data Base), 479
NCHS (National Center for Health Statistics), 98-99, 372, 373
NCIPC (National Center for Injury Prevention and Control), 132-133
NCPDP (National Council for Prescription Drug Programs), 69, 173, 174t
NCQA. See National Committee for Quality Assurance (NCQA).
NCR (no-carbon-required) forms, 117, 119
NCRA (National Cancer Registrars Association, Inc.), 477, 479
NCVHS (National Committee on Vital and Health Statistics), 72t, 98, 99, 202, 213
NDCs (National Drug Codes), 207, 288
NDF-RT (National Drug File Reference Terminology), 69, 207
NEC (Not Elsewhere Classified) terms, 210
Neck
    physical examination of, 108t
    in review of systems, 106t
NEDSS (National Electronic Disease Surveillance System), 68t, 100
Needs, hierarchy of, 571
Needs assessment, 599, 599b
Negligence, 507-508, 530
Neonatal data, 103t, 111
Neonatal death rate, 374t, 376
Neonatal identification, 111
Neonatal physical examination, 111
Neonate progress notes, 111
Neonates, in master patient record, 230f
Nephrology, 24t
Net, 675
Net autopsy rate, 378, 379t
Net days of revenue in patient accounts receivable ratio, 675
Net death rate, 374t, 375
Net operating revenue, 675
Net present value, 678-679, 679t, 680
Network(s)
    local area, 246, 278
    wide area, 246, 278
    wired vs. wireless, 278-279, 279t
Network computer, 274
Network database, 277
Network technology, 277-280, 279t
Network type HMO, 36
Neurological system, physical examination of, 108t
Neurology, 24t
Neurosurgery, 24t
New York Hospital–Cornell Medical Center, microfilm system of, 255
Newborns. See Neonates.
News media
    disclosure of health information to, 526-527
    use of health data by, 96
NGT (nominal group technique), 450, 455f

NHII. See National Health Information Infrastructure (NHII).
NHIN (National Health Information Infrastructure Network). See National Health Information Infrastructure (NHII).
NIC (Nursing Interventions Classification), 207, 209t
NIDDM (non–insulin-dependent diabetes mellitus), 482
Niemi, Wayne, 634
NIH (National Institutes of Health), 11, 72t
NIOSH (National Institute for Occupational Safety and Health), 641
NIP (National Immunization Program), 68t
NIST (National Institute of Standards and Technology), 439
NLNAC (National League for Nursing Accrediting Commission, Inc.), 15
NLRA (National Labor Relations Act), 563t, 567-568
NLRB (National Labor Relations Board), 568, 569
NMDS (Nursing Minimum Data Set), 102, 209t
NMMDS (Nursing Management Minimum Data Set), 102, 209t
NOC (Nursing Outcomes Classification), 207-208, 209t
No-carbon-required (NCR) forms, 117, 119
Node, 315
Nomenclature, defined, 201
Nominal data, 327, 384, 384t
Nominal group technique (NGT), 450, 455f
Noncaregiving group, 30
Noncompliance, with statutes, rules, and regulations, 510
Noncontact scanners, 239
Nondisclosure agreement, 533, 533f
Non–government-owned hospitals, 19f, 20
Non–insulin-dependent diabetes mellitus (NIDDM), 482
Nonmaleficence, 550
Nonoperating revenues, 653
Nonrepudiation, 178
Nonresponse bias, 415
Non–revenue-generating departments, 668
Nonsemantic concept identifier, of terminology, 210
Nonvoting members, of board of trustees, 21
Normative ethics, 549
North American Association of Central Cancer Registries (NAACCR), 479
North American Nursing Diagnosis Association (NANDA), 209t
North Carolina Healthcare Information and Communications Alliance, 85t
Nose
    physical examination of, 108t
    in review of systems, 106t
Nosocomial infection, 415
Nosocomial infection rate, 379, 380-381, 380t
Not Elsewhere Classified (NEC) terms, 210
NOTA (National Organ Transplant Act), 483
Not-for-profit hospitals, 20
Notifiable conditions, 696, 696b
Notification clauses, 536
NP (Nurse Practitioner), 33
NPDB (National Practitioner Data Bank), 468, 534
NPI (National Provider Identifier), 655
NQF (National Quality Forum), 440-441
NRC (National Resource Center), 70, 71t
NTDB (National Trauma Data Bank), 484
Nuclear medicine, 25

Nuclear medicine technologist, 31t
Null hypothesis, 392-393
Numbering systems, 221, 221t
Numerator, 373
Numerical filing, straight, 224-225, 226t
Numerical identification, for paper-based records, 220-221, 221t
Nurse(s), 32-33, 33t
Nurse anesthetist, certified registered, 33
Nurse director, 24-25
Nurse executive, 24-25
Nurse manager, 25
Nurse midwife, certified, 33
Nurse Practitioner (NP), 33
Nurse vice-president, 24-25
Nurses aides, 25
Nurses' notes, 111
Nursing, 32-33, 33t
Nursing assistants, 25
Nursing care, 24-25
Nursing care models, 33
Nursing care standards, 33
Nursing facility, 28
Nursing forms, 103t, 111-113
Nursing Home Reform Act, 8b
Nursing informatics, 686-688
Nursing Interventions Classification (NIC), 207, 209t
Nursing Management Minimum Data Set (NMMDS), 102, 209t
Nursing Minimum Data Set (NMDS), 102, 209t
Nursing notes, 111
Nursing Outcomes Classification (NOC), 207-208, 209t
Nursing Practice Act, 15
Nursing specialties, 33
Nursing terminologies, 207-208, 209t
Nutrition services, 25
NVAC (National Vaccine Advisory Committee), 483

O

OASIS (Outcome and Assessment Information Set), 99t, 137-138
Object, 277
Objectives
    organizational, 662
    in project planning, 630
    of research, 408
Objectivity, in accounting, 670-671
Object-oriented database, 277
Observation
    participant, 419-420
    in system analysis, 328-329, 328f
Observation patient, 18
Observation unit, 18
Obsolescence
    of employees, 600
    of system, 310, 312-313
Obstetrical data, 103t, 110-111
Obstetrics, 24t
Occupancy percentage, 382, 383t
Occupancy rate, 382, 383t
Occupational Safety and Health Act (OSHA), 8b, 12, 563t, 566
    on air quality, 644
    and work space design, 221, 600, 640, 641
Occupational Safety and Health Administration (OSHA), 12
Occupational therapist, 31t
Occupational therapy, 26-27
Occupational therapy assistant, 31t
Occurrence reports, in legal cases, 530-531
OCR (optical character recognition), 256

Odds ratio, 423-424
Odiorne, George, 588
OFCCP (Office of Federal Contract Compliance Program), 562
Office design. *See* Work space design; Workstation design.
    American plan of, 641
Office for Rural Health Policy, 67
Office for the Advancement of Telehealth, 67, 72t
Office landscaping, 641
Office of Federal Contract Compliance Program (OFCCP), 562
Office of the Inspector General (OIG), 11, 510, 661
Office of the National Coordinator for Health Information Technology (ONCHIT), 72t-74t
    creation of, 66, 270
    on health care fraud, 661
    on health information exchange, 215-216
    on vision for health care information infrastructure, 48, 166
Office space, guidelines for allocating, 643, 644b
Offsetting revenues, of electronic document management, 261
OIG (Office of the Inspector General), 11, 510, 661
Older Americans Act, 7b
O'Leary, Dennis S., 692
Omaha System, 208, 209t
Omnibus Budget Reconciliation Act, 8b, 13
ONCHIT. *See* Office of the National Coordinator for Health Information Technology (ONCHIT).
Oncology, 24t
One-to-many relation, 322, 322f
One-to-one relation, 322
One-way analysis of variance, 394-396
On-line documentation, 163-164
On-line questionnaire, 328
On-line survey, 418, 419f-422f
On-line system interface, for data collection, 120-121, 121f
Open architecture, 258, 260
Open office design plan, 644
Open systems, 258, 260
    and outcomes research, 493
Open Systems Foundation (OSF), 493
Open-ended questions, 418
Open-shelf files, 222t, 223, 223f
Operating budgets, 663
Operating margin ratio, 675
Operating revenue(s), 653
    net, 675
Operating system, 275
Operation(s), projects *vs.*, 356, 356t
Operation flowchart, 618, 619f
Operational management, 604-647
    of individual work processes (micro level), 606-623
        of productivity, 611-614, 612f, 614f
        work distribution chart in, 606-611, 608f-610f
        work division in, 606, 607f, 607t
        work simplification or methods improvement in, 614-623, 616f-622f, 623b
    at organization-wide level (change management), 627-637
        project management for, 629-636, 632b, 633f, 635f
        re-engineering for, 636-637, 637b
        strategic management for, 627-629, 628f

Operational management (*Continued*)
    at systems and organizational level (midlevel), 623-627, 624f
        work space design in, 637-641, 638f, 639f
        workstation design in, 641-646, 644b, 645b
Operational strategies, 629
Operation/maintenance activity, of information system life cycle, 310
Operative forms, 103t, 110
Operative report, 110
Ophthalmology, 24t
Opportunity costs, 676
Optical character recognition (OCR), 256
Optical disk, for data input and output, 244t
Optical disk platters, in electronic document management, 257
OPTN (Organ Procurement and Transplantation Network), 483, 484
Oral warning, 593
Order(s), practitioner's, 107-109, 148
Order entry, 163, 176, 285-286
Order management systems, 285-286
Order templates, 176
Orderlies, 25
Ordinal data, 327, 384, 385t
Organ Procurement and Transplantation Network (OPTN), 483, 484
Organ transplant registries, 483-484
Organization(s)
    formal *vs.* informal, 626-627
    of hospitals, 20-21, 21f
    information system life cycles in, 311-312, 311f
        aggregate, 312
Organization chart, 626
Organizational culture, 569-570, 570b
Organizational structure, 626-627
Orientation, 584
Orthopedics, 24t
OSF (Open Systems Foundation), 493
OSHA. *See* Occupational Safety and Health Act (OSHA).
Osteopathic medicine, 14
Otorhinolaryngology, 24t
Outcards, 237
Outcome(s), 441, 487-494
    and coding issues, 490-491, 492
    defined, 487
    and electronic health record, 488-489, 489f, 490f
Outcome analysis, use of data in, 486
Outcome and Assessment Information Set (OASIS), 99t, 137-138
Outcome indicators, 489-490
Outcome measures, 430-431, 442, 442t, 489-490
Outcome studies, 430-434, 432t-434t
Outcome systems, desirable, 491-494, 493t
Outcomes data
    and information systems, 488
    uses of, 488
Outcomes Data Conversion Utilities, 490
Outcomes data warehouse, 491, 492
Outcomes research, 487-488, 487f
Outguides, 237-238
Out-of-pocket pay, 34, 35b
Outpatient, defined, 5
Outpatient care, data needs for, 130-134, 135f
Outpatient departments, 18
Outpatient surgery departments, 18
Outpatient surgical review, 186f
Output, 441
    measuring, 611-613, 612f
    of system, 624
Output design, 331, 332

Output devices, for data access and retention, 243, 243t-244t
Output processes, 332
Outside contractors, disclosure of health information to, 526
Outsourcing, 29-30
Outsourcing firms, disclosure of health information to, 526
Overtime compensation, 567
Owners, 307

P
P value, 393, 396
PA (physician assistant), 32
Packet filter, 297
PACS (picture archiving and communication system), 255
Pages per minute (PPM), 256
Pairing rule, 233b
PAiRS (Provider Access to Immunization Registry Securely), 85t
Palliative care, 28
Pandemics, 544
Paper, for forms, 119
Paper forms, design and production of, 115-119, 118f
Paper-based records, 114
    access and retention of, 220-243
        disaster recovery in, 242-243
        filing equipment for, 221-223, 222t, 223f
        filing methods in, 223–226, 224b, 225b, 226t
        legal health record definition in, 242
        master patient index in, 226-231, 227f-231f, 232b-233b
        record identification in, 220-221, 221t
        record management issues with, 234-236, 235b
        record tracking in, 237-240, 237f, 238b, 239b
        retention in, 240-242
        space management in, 223, 224t
    drawbacks of, 167-168
    storage and transfer of, 178-179
Parallel work division, 606, 607f, 607t
Paramedic, 31t
Parent(s), disclosure of health information to, 524
Parent node, 315
Pareto chart, 453, 453f, 455f
Pareto diagram, 386, 390f
Participant observation, 419-420
Participating provider, 653-654
Participatory approach, to budgeting, 663
Partitions, in workstation design, 643
Partners Healthcare System
    computerized physician order entry at, 688-689
    electronic health record system of, 176
Partnership, 17
Passive case ascertainment surveillance systems, 479-481
Password(s), 294-295
Password aging, 295
Password history file, 295
Past medical history (PMH), 106t
Pathology report, 110
Pathology services, 25-26
Patient(s)
    access to medical records by, 511, 524-525
    defined, 5
    duties to, 511
    hospital, 20
    unidentified, 229f
    use of health data by, 95

Patient accounting, in revenue cycle, 657
Patient advocacy, 440
Patient and family teaching and participation record, 112-113
"Patient Antidumping Law," 8b, 13
Patient assessment, 24
"Patient at a glance," 176
Patient care, disclosure for, 518-521
Patient Care Data Set (PCDS), 209t
Patient care plan, interdisciplinary, 107, 138, 142–143
Patient care record. *See* Patient record(s).
Patient care technicians, 25
Patient centered care, 9
Patient Data Validity and Correction Tracking Form, 231f
Patient day, 382t
Patient encounter, in revenue cycle, 656
Patient health record. *See* Patient record(s).
Patient identification, 104, 177
Patient identity management, 179-180
Patient medical history, 148
Patient medical record information (PMRI), 213
Patient name, incorrect, 229f
Patient record(s), 154-155
  abbreviations in, 113-114, 116
  addenda to, 513-514
  administrative use of, 522
  with adoption, 525
  alteration of, 512
  in alternative care settings, 127
  amendment of, 513-514
  authentication of, 114, 124, 175t, 178, 514
  authorization for disclosure of, 518, 519f, 520f
  authorization to make entries in, 180
  of celebrities, 526-527
  confidentiality of, 515-517, 566-567
  content structure of, 146, 147t
  continuing reviews of, 128
  defined, 97
  delinquent, 124, 124t, 126
  duty to maintain, 511-512
  duty to retain, 512-515, 513f
  educational use of, 521
  electronic .*See* Electronic health record(s) (EHRs).
  error correction in, 512-513, 513f
  as evidence, 514-515
  evolution of, 45-48
  falsification of, 512
  flow and processing of, 122, 123f
  hybrid, 48, 160, 161t, 178, 179
  incomplete, 124-126, 124t, 125f
  legal analysis of, 127
  longitudinal, 98
  major segments on, 146-149
  overview of, 97-98
  ownership of, 517
  patient access to, 511, 524-525
  and patient safety, 521
  in performance management, 521
  primary, 97
  quality of
    clinical staff activities related to, 128
    facility structure that encourages, 128-129
    methods to ensure, 122-126, 124t, 125f
    monitoring and solutions for, 126-129
  quantitative analysis of, 124, 126-127
  research use of, 521-522
  retrieval of prior, 180
  review of, 183-184, 185f, 186f
  secondary, 98

Patient record(s) (*Continued*)
  as source of health data and information, 44-45
  unauthorized access to, 529
  unique roles of, 97
Patient record development, electronic health record system functions and, 163-165, 165f
Patient record form(s), 102-113, 103t-104t
  administrative, 103t, 104-105
  clinical, 103t, 105-109, 106t-108t
  design and control of, 115-122, 118f, 120f, 121f
  instructions on, 117
  needs of users and, 116
  neonatal, 103t, 111
  nursing, 103t, 111-113
  obstetrical, 103t, 110-111
  operative, 103t, 109-110
  purpose of, 116
  selection and sequencing of items on, 116
  simplification of, 117
  template for, 116-117
  terminology and abbreviations on, 116
Patient registration, 163
Patient rights, acknowledgment of, 104, 440
Patient safety, 454-460
  databases for, 456-458, 458t
  disclosure of health information for, 521
  electronic health records and, 165-166
  improvement of, 458-460
  integration for, 700
  measurement of, 455-456, 456t, 457f
Patient safety indicators (PSI), 458, 458t
Patient Safety Institute, 77t
Patient safety report, 456t, 457f
Patient Self-Determination Act (PSDA), 8b, 13, 105, 532
Patient-directed disclosure, of health information, 525
Pay for Performance, 440, 486
Payback method, 680
Payback period, 340, 340t
  discounted, 340-341, 341t
  for microfilm, 250
Payer, 5, 35b
Payer contracts, 653-654
Payment, for health care services, 34-38, 35b
  historical perspective on, 650-652, 651f, 652b
Payment processing, in revenue cycle, 659
Payment purposes, disclosure of health information for, 522, 523f
PC(s) (personal computers), 274
PC workstations, for data access, 243t, 244
PCAOB (Public Company Accounting Oversight Board), 660
PCDS (Patient Care Data Set), 209t
PCE (potentially compensable event), 461
PCS (Procedural Coding System), 202
PDAs (personal digital assistants), 243t, 274
PDCA (Plan-Do-Check-Ask) method, 447, 447f
Pearson correlation coefficient, 396
Peaslee, Gregory, 572b-573b
Pediatric hospitals, 20
Pediatric Perioperative Cardiac Arrest Registry, 456
Pediatrics, 24t
Peer review records, confidentiality of, 516
Peer reviewed journals, 407
Peete v. Blackwell, 508
Pen-based devices, for data access, 244-245
Per case payment system, 659-660
Per diem payments, 651
Percentage(s), 373, 373t, 374t
  of occupancy, 382, 383t

Performance appraisal, 584-590
  implementation of, 589-590
  information systems for, 571
  measurement, judgment, and communication in, 585
  methods of, 586-589, 586f-589f
  of organization, 444-447, 446f
  rater biases that affect, 589
Performance assessment, 444-447, 446f
Performance benchmarking, 446-447
Performance evaluation, 444-447, 446f
Performance goals, 446
Performance improvement, 447-454, 462t
  continuing education units in, 55
  models of, 447-449, 447f, 448f
  tools for, 449-454, 450f-455f, 454b
Performance improvement plans, 587-588, 588f
Performance improvement program, 613-614, 614f
Performance management, 436-470
  big picture and key players in, 438-441
  credentialing in, 466-468, 469f
  disclosure of health information for, 521
  key concepts of, 468-470
  patient safety in, 454–460
    databases for, 456-458, 458t
    improvement of, 458-460
    measurement of, 455-456, 456t, 457f
  performance assessment in, 444-447, 446f
  performance improvement in, 447-454, 462t
    models of, 447-449, 447f, 448f
    tools for, 449-454, 450f-455f, 454b
  performance measurement in, 441-444, 442t, 443f, 443t, 445f
  risk management in, 460-461, 462t
  role of managers in, 468
  use of data in, 486-487
  utilization management in, 462-466, 462t, 464f, 466f
Performance measure(s), 441-444, 442t, 443f, 443t, 445f
Performance measurement, 441-444, 442t, 443f, 443t, 445f
Performance measurement reports, 445-446
Performance monitoring, 614
Performance rating, 444-447, 446f
Performance ratio, 674, 675
Performance standards, 611-613, 612f
Performance targets, 446
Period prevalence, 416, 416f
Perioperative Nursing Data Set (PNDS), 209t
Peripheral vascular system, in review of systems, 107t
Perna v. Pirozzi, 508n
Personal commitment, 357
Personal computers (PCs), 274
Personal data, core elements of, 101t
Personal digital assistants (PDAs), 243t, 274
Personal health information (PHI), 567
Personal health records (PHRs), 9, 95, 161-162, 162t
Personal identification number (PIN), 295
Personal interview, 582-583
Personal prejudice, 589
Personal space, 641
Person-time denominator, 429
Perspective in Health Information Management, 57
PERT (Program Evaluation Review Technique) network, 631, 632–634, 633f
Pew Commission, 545
Pharmaceutical services, 26
Pharmacy consultation, for long-term care, 136
PhD (doctor of philosophy), in nursing, 33t

PHI (personal health information), 567
PHI (protected health information), 515-516
PHIN (Public Health Information Network), 72t, 77t
Phishing, 298
Phonetic file, 233b
Photographs, in health record, 182
PHRs (personal health records), 9, 95, 161-162, 162t
PHS (Public Health Service) Commissioned Corps, 11
Physical building, of form, 119
Physical examination, 107, 108t, 148
    neonatal, 111
    pre-employment, 583
Physical name, in data dictionary, 496
Physical rehabilitation services, 26-27
Physical security, 294, 294t, 296
Physical system design, 331
Physical therapist, 31t
Physical therapy, 26
Physician(s), 31-32
    credentialing of, 534-535
Physician advisors, 466
Physician assistant (PA), 32
Physician practice(s), 17
Physician Practice Connections, 76t
Physician's orders, 107-109, 148
"Pick list," 285-286
Picture archiving and communication system (PACS), 255
Pie chart, 386, 388f
Pilot testing, of survey, 418
PIN (personal identification number), 295
PITAC (President's Information Technology Advisory Committee), 48
Pixels per inch (PPI), 255
Place of study, 409
Plaintiff, 507
Plan-Do-Check-Ask (PDCA) method, 447, 447f
Planetary camera, 252
Planners, use of health data by, 96
Planning, human resource, 573-576, 574b, 575f, 576f
Plastic and reconstructive surgery, 24t
Playscript format, 637
PMH (past medical history), 106t
PMRI (patient medical record information), 213
PNDS (Perioperative Nursing Data Set), 209t
Point prevalence, 416, 416f
Point system, 597
Point to point interface, 280
Pointer, 277
Point-of-care clinical information systems, 38
Point-of-care systems, 287, 287t
Point-of-enrollment plan, 36
Point-of-service information systems, 38
Point-of-service (POS) plan, 36
Police officers, disclosure of health information to, 523
Policy(ies), 35b
    electronic health record system and, 186-187, 187b, 193
    in re-engineering, 636
    standards for, 175t
Policy developers, use of health data by, 96
Policy setting, in collaboration, 358-359
Polyhierarchy, of terminology, 210
POMR (problem-oriented medical record), 114-115, 115t
Population, defined, 613
Population under study, 409
Population-based cancer registries, 475-477
Population-based data, 692-693

POS (point-of-service) plan, 36
Positioning strategies, 629
Postanesthesia note, 110
Postman, Neil, 688
Postmortem examination, disclosure of health information for, 523-524
Postoperative death rate, 374t, 375-376
Postoperative diagnosis, 110
Postoperative infection rate, 379-380, 380t, 381
Postpartum record, 111
Potentially compensable event (PCE), 461
Power(s), 400
    defined, 551
    and ethical decision making, 551
    express, 504-505
    implied, 505
Power of attorney, 524
    durable, 532
Power supply, uninterruptible, 258
PPI (pixels per inch), 255
PPM (pages per minute), 256
PPOs (preferred provider organizations), 36
PPS (prospective payment systems), 37, 47, 651
Practice Act, 15
Practitioner(s)
    state licensure of, 15
    use of health data by, 95
Practitioner profiles, 468, 469f
Practitioner's orders, 107-109, 148
Preanesthesia note, 110
Precedent, 505
Precision, of data, 144t, 145
Pre-employment medical examination, 583
Pre-emption, 515
Pre-existing condition, 35b
Preferred provider organizations (PPOs), 36
Prefix names, in master patient index, 227
Pregnancy Discrimination Act, 564
Preliminary research, 408
Premium, 35b
Prenatal record, 110-111
Preoperative diagnosis, 110
Preponderance of evidence, 530
Present value, 341, 676
    net, 678-679, 679t, 680
Presentation layer, 314, 314f
President, of hospital, 22
President's Information Technology Advisory Committee (PITAC), 48
Pressure sores, in long-term care, 136t
Prevalence, 380t, 381
    period, 416, 416f
    point, 416, 416f
Prevalence rate, 381, 415-416
Prevalence study, 415-417, 416f, 417t, 427t-428t
Prevarication bias, 416
Preventive care, 16, 16t
Preventive discipline, 594
Price and payments, 352
Primary care, 16, 16t
Primary Care Health Information Technology Strategy project, 87t
Primary care provider, 37
Primary data, 474
Primary insurance coverage, 657
Primary key, 276
Primary patient record, 97
Printers
    for data input and output, 244t
    for electronic document management, 258
    in workstation design, 643
Printing
    of electronic health records, 190
    of forms, 119

Privacy. See also Confidentiality.
    with electronic health record systems, 172, 178
    of information, 566-567
    in international health information management, 691
    invasion of, 509
    right of, 505
    in workstation design, 639, 645
Privacy Act, 516
Privacy and Security, continuing education units in, 55
Privacy and Security Solutions, 74t
Privacy Rule, 13
Privacy standards, 519f
Private duty nurse, 25
Private hospitals, 20
Private law, 504
Private offices, 641
Private practice, 17
Private sector, in health information infrastructure, 73, 74t-77t
Privilege(s), denial of, 534
Privilege delineation, 467
Privileged communication, 509
Proactive risk assessment, 459-460
Probabilistic algorithms, 232b, 233b
Probability, 393
Probationary employment, 583
Problem analysis, 313-314, 314f
Problem Classification Scheme, 208
Problem identification, in work simplification, 615
Problem list
    for ambulatory care, 133
    on patient record, 147
Problem solving, 362
Problem statement, in project planning, 630
Problem-oriented medical record (POMR), 114-115, 115t
Procedural Coding System (PCS), 202
Procedure(s)
    with electronic health record system, 193
    in implementation readiness, 363-364
    on patient record, 149
    in re-engineering, 636-637, 637b
    in research proposal, 409-410
    in system, 624
Procedure flowchart, 618, 619f
Procedure manual, 637
Process(es), 315-318, 316t
    defined, 179
    in implementation readiness, 363-364
    re-engineering of, 194
    understanding of, 361
Process description, in data dictionary, 319f
Process measures, 442, 442t
Process modeling, 315-318, 315t, 362-363
"Process owner," 363
Processing, in system, 624
Processing design, 331
Product line management, 21
Productive time, 666
Productive unit of work, 611
Productivity, 611-614, 612f, 614f
    application of systems model to, 571f
    defined, 611
    increasing, 613
Productivity enhancement, and human resource management, 559
Productivity improvement program, 613-614, 614f
Productivity program, implementation of, 613-614, 614f

Productivity standards, 611-613, 612f
Products liability, 509
Professional certification, 52-54
Professional negligence, 507-508
Professional organizations, data collection standards of, 100-102
Professional recruiters, 579
Professional service departments, 18
Professional staff, 23, 23t-24t
    credentialing of, 466-468, 469f
    duty to supervise actions of, 533-536, 533f
Professional standards, duty to provide care that meets, 529-531
Profit, 671
Program assessment, for business plan, 666-667
Program Evaluation Review Technique (PERT) network, 631, 632-634, 633f
Program generators, 276
Programming languages, 275-276
Progress notes, 109, 149
    for home health care, 140-141
    neonate, 111
Progressive discipline, 592, 593-594
Project(s)
    characteristics of, 629-630
    in data dictionary, 318f, 319, 319f
    defined, 356, 630
    vs. operations, 356, 356t
Project activities, 308-309, 630-631
Project budget, 309
Project control, 631-632, 632b
Project deliverables, 308
Project evaluation, 366
Project implementation, 631-632, 632b
Project leadership, 631-632, 632b
Project management, 308-310, 629-636
    characteristics of, 630
    defined, 629
    information technology applications to, 634-636
    software for, 634-636
    work breakdown in, 309, 309t
Project manager, 307-310, 631-632, 632b
Project organization, 631
Project plan, 308, 630-631
Project planning, 630-634, 632b, 633f, 635f
Project proposal, 631
Project schedule, 309
Project scope, 308
Project team, 309, 631
Project termination, 632
Project tools, 632-634, 633f, 635f
Promotion-from-within policy, 580
Promulgation, of data sets, 99
Property and valuables list, 105
Proportions, 373, 373t
Proprietary hospitals, 20
Proprietary system, 258, 260
Prospective payment systems (PPS), 37, 47, 651
Prospective reimbursement, 37
Prospective review, in utilization management, 463
Prospective study, 424-425, 425t-428t
Protected group, 564
Protected health information (PHI), 515-516
Protocols, 194
    for network communication, 278-279, 279t
Prototype, 307, 334-335
Provider(s)
    defined, 5, 95
    use of health data by, 95
Provider Access to Immunization Registry Securely (PAiRS), 85t
Provider data, on patient record, 147

Provider enrollment, in revenue cycle, 654-655
Provisional employment, 583
Proximate cause, 530
Proximity chart, 638-639, 639f
Proxy server, 297
PSDA (Patient Self-Determination Act), 8b, 13, 105, 532
Pseudonyms, in master patient index, 227, 227f-228f
PSI (patient safety indicators), 458, 458t
Psychiatric disorders, in review of systems, 107t
Psychiatric history and diagnosis report, 143
Psychiatric hospital, 20
Psychiatry, 24t
Psychometric tests, 582
Public accountability, 440
Public Company Accounting Oversight Board (PCAOB), 660
Public figures, release of information to media on, 526-527
Public health, 12, 692-699
    cooperation in, 696-699, 697f
    core functions in, 693-694, 693b, 694f, 698b
    goals of, 692, 693
    and improving health, 695
    information needs in, 693-694
    integrated information system for, 695-696
    legal context of, 696, 696b
    and medical care, 692
    population-based data in, 692-693
    reportable conditions in, 696, 696b
    use of data in, 486
    use of health data in, 96
Public Health Data Standards Consortium, 77t
Public Health Emergency Preparedness and Response Program, 67t
Public Health Informatics Institute, 77t
Public Health Informatics Standards Consortium, 164
Public Health Information Network (PHIN), 72t, 77t
Public health problems, 695
Public health programs, 694-695
Public Health Service (PHS) Commissioned Corps, 11
Public key, 297
Public law, 504
Public policy exception, and employee termination, 591
PublicHealth Statistical System, 87t
Pulmonary medicine, 24t
Purchasers, in performance management, 439-440
Purchasing process, 343-352
    analyzing system requirements in, 344
    demonstrations in, 351
    development of system specifications in, 344
    evaluation criteria in, 349-351, 350f, 350t, 351t
    request for information in, 343
    request for proposal in, 343
        conditions of response in, 345
        contractual information, references, and other materials in, 349
        development of, 344-349
        disclaimer and table of contents of, 344, 345f
        distribution of, 349
        enterprise profile in, 344-345
        functional specifications in, 345-348, 346f-348f
        installation and training requirements in, 348-349
        overview of, 344

Purchasing process (Continued)
        planning steps before preparation of, 344
        system costs and financing arrangements in, 349
        technical requirements in, 348
        time table in, 344, 345f
        vendor profile in, 349
    site visits in, 351-352
    system selection and contract negotiation in, 352
Pure Food and Drug Act, 9
Purging, of health records, 183, 237
Purposes, of research, 408

Q
QI (quality improvement)
    goals of, 441
    re-engineering and, 637
QI (quality improvement) study, of patient records, 126-127
QIOs (Quality Improvement Organizations), 12, 70-71, 438
Qualitative analysis, of patient records, 127
Qualitative data, 384, 384t
Qualitative research, 419-421
    for system evaluation, 342
Quality, defined, 143
Quality assessment, of patient records, 126-127
Quality assurance, patient record and, 45
Quality assurance coordinator, 308
Quality awards, 439
Quality control
    of birth defects registry data, 481
    in registry, 475
Quality improvement (QI)
    goals of, 441
    re-engineering and, 637
Quality Improvement Organizations (QIOs), 12, 70-71, 438
Quality improvement (QI) study, of patient records, 126-127
Quality management
    of cancer program and registry data, 478-479, 480f
    disclosure of health information for, 521
Quality of care, duty to provide, 529-531
Quality of care committees, use of health data by, 96
Quality profiles, 535
    accessibility of, 535-536
Quantitative analysis, of patient records, 124, 126-127
Quest for Quality Prize, 439
Question(s)
    double-barreled, 328
    open-ended vs. close-ended, 418
    research, 406
    structured and unstructured, 326, 418
Questionnaires, in system analysis, 327-328
Qui tam prosecutions, 510
Quick Medical Reference, 39

R
r (correlation coefficient), 396, 413-414, 454
R^2 (R-squared), 396
RA (remittance advice), 659
Race norming, 563
Radiation therapy, 25
Radiation therapy reports, 112
Radio buttons, on Web page, 283
Radiofrequency identification device (RFID), 245, 288, 700
Radiographer, 31t
Radiology, 24t

Radiology department, 25
Radiology reports, 112
RAID (redundant array of independent disks), 257
Random sample, 399
Random selection, 422-423, 613
Range, 391
Ranked data, 384, 385t
Rapid cycle improvement (RCI), 447-448
Rate(s), 373, 373t
  autopsy, 378-379, 379t
  morbidity, 379-381, 380t
  mortality, 373-378, 374t, 377t, 378t
Rate of return, accounting, 679-680
Rater biases, that affect performance appraisal, 589
Ratio(s), 373, 373t
  to evaluate financial data, 674-675
Ratio analysis, 674-675
Ratio data, 328, 385
RBAC (role-based access control), 295-296, 296t
RBRVS (resource-based relative value scale), 37, 652
RCI (rapid cycle improvement), 447-448
Reasonable accommodation, 565, 565b
"Reasonable man" standard, 530, 532
Reassignment, of document, 189
Recall bias, 415
Recency effect, 589
Reception area, 638
Recognized redundancy, of terminology, 211
Record(s)
  active, 254
  defined, 44, 495
  destruction of, 241
  inactive, 225, 234-235, 254
  unit, 221
Record content review, 124-126, 124t, 125f
Record identification, for paper-based records, 220-221, 221t
Record requests, 669, 670f
Record retention, 240-242, 512-515, 513f
Record retrieval, 237-238
  with electronic document management, 258-259, 259t
Record tracking, 237-240
  automated, 238-240, 238b, 239b
  manual, 237-238, 237f
Recovery room record, 110
Recovery services, in system development, 309f
Recruitment, 579-580
Recruitment pool, 579
Redisclosure, of health information, 518, 525-526
Reduction ratio, 247
Redundant array of independent disks (RAID), 257
Re-engineering, 194, 636-637, 637b
Reference(s)
  in credentials file, 535
  in data dictionary, 496-497
  in request for proposal, 349
Reference checks, 581
Reference date, 476
Reference list, 407
Reference manual, 364-365, 365t
Referral form, for long-term care, 136
Refresh, 233b
Reg-ADT (registration–admission, discharge, and transfer) application, 156, 163
Regenstrief Institute, 85t
Regenstrief LOINC Mapping Assistant (RELMA), 206

Regional health information organizations (RHIOs), 82, 83-84, 85t-86t
Registered Health Information Administrator (RHIA), 53
Registered Health Information Technologist (RHIT), 53
Registered nurse (RN), 25
Registered record librarian (RRL), 49
Registration
  of health information management professionals, 53
  patient, 163
  in revenue cycle, 655-656
Registration application, 156, 163
Registration record, 104, 105
Registration–admission, discharge, and transfer (Reg-ADT) application, 156, 163
Registry(ies), 474–484
  abstracting in, 475
  birth defects, 479-481
  cancer, 475-479, 478f, 480f
  case definition and eligibility in, 474
  case finding in, 474-475
  confidentiality of, 475
  death, 481
  defined, 474
  diabetes, 482
  immunization, 483
  implant, 482-483
  organ transplant, 483-484
  overview of, 474–475
  quality control in, 475
  trauma, 484
Registry Operations and Data Standards (ROADS), 477
Regression analysis, 396-397
Regression equation, 396-397
Regulations, 504
  of administrative agencies, 505
  noncompliance with, 510
Regulatory agencies and organizations, 9-15
  for accreditation, 14-15
  federal, 9-12, 10f
  for health occupations, 15
  state, 12-13, 13t
Regulatory requirements, affecting human resource management, 561-569, 563t, 565b, 568b-570b
Rehabilitation
  data needs for, 137
  defined, 14
Rehabilitation Act, 564
Rehabilitation and chronic disease hospital, 20
Rehabilitation services, 26-27
Rehabilitative care, 16t
Reimbursement, 34, 35b
  historical perspective on, 650-652
  under Medicaid, 38
  under Medicare, 37
  patient record and, 44-45, 46-47
  prospective, 37
Reimbursement analysis, in revenue cycle, 659-660, 659t
Reimbursement contracts, in revenue cycle, 653-654
Reimbursement formula, 34
Reject "Not Elsewhere Classified" characteristic, 210
Relation(s), 322, 322f
Relational database, 276-277, 276f
Relationships, and leadership style, 546-548, 547f, 548f
Relative humidity, in workstation design, 644
Relative risk (RR), 423-424, 425

Relative value unit (RVU), 652
Release of information, 184
Release-of-information vendors, disclosure of health information to, 526
Relevance, of data, 144t, 145
Reliability, 412-414
  of performance measures, 444
RELMA (Regenstrief LOINC Mapping Assistant), 206
Remedies and liabilities, 352
Remittance advice (RA), 659
Removal, of document, 189
Repetitive strain (or stress) injuries (RSIs), 641
Replacement charts, 575, 575f
Report cards, 440
Reportable communicable disease conditions, 696, 696b
Reportable patient incidents, 455, 456t
Reporting capabilities, 296
Reprimand, 593
Reproduction equipment, for microfilm, 250
Request for information (RFI), 343-344
Request for proposal (RFP), 343
  conditions of response in, 345
  contractual information, references, and other materials in, 349
  development of, 344-349
  disclaimer and table of contents of, 344, 345f
  distribution of, 349
  enterprise profile in, 344-345
  functional specifications in, 345-348, 346f-348f
  installation and training requirements in, 348-349
  overview of, 344
  planning steps before preparation of, 344
  system costs and financing arrangements in, 349
  technical requirements in, 348
  time table in, 344, 345f
  vendor profile in, 349
Requisitions, 237, 237f
Res ipsa loquitur, 530
Research, 402-435
  biases in, 414-415
  computer software in, 429-430
  cyclical nature of, 405f
  disclosure of health information for, 521-522
  overview of, 404
  preliminary, 408
  qualitative, 419-421
  reliability in, 412-414
  role of health information management professional in, 404-405
  sensitivity and specificity in, 412, 412t
  survey, 417-419, 419f-422f
  use of data in, 485
  validity in, 411-412
    coding, 412, 413f
  web sites on, 435
Research plan, 408-411, 410f
Research proposal, 406-411
  appendix of, 411
  budget in, 411
  hypothesis and research questions in, 406
  methodology in, 408, 409-410, 410f
  research plan in, 408-411, 410f
  review of literature in, 406-407, 407f
Research question, 406
Research study design, 415-429, 415t
  analytic, 415t, 421-426
    case-control or retrospective, 421-424, 423f, 424t, 427t-428t
    historical-prospective, 426, 426f, 427t-428t

Research study design *(Continued)*
 prospective, cohort, or incidence, 424-425, 425t, 426-428t
 descriptive, 415-421, 415t
  cross-sectional or prevalence, 415-417, 416f, 417t, 427t-428t
  qualitative, 419-421
  survey, 417-419, 419f–422f
 experimental, 415t, 426-429, 427t-428t, 430f
Researchers
 data collection standards of, 102
 use of health data by, 96
Research-oriented cancer registries, 476-477
Residency, 32
Resident, defined, 5
Resident record. *See* Patient record(s).
Residential facility, 28
Resource(s), in project planning, 630
Resource allocation, 309
Resource tug-of-war, 358
Resource-based relative value scale (RBRVS), 37, 652
Respect, 358, 550
Respiratory care services, 27
Respiratory system, in review of systems, 106t
Respite care, 16t, 29
Respondeat superior, 507-508, 533
Response rate
 for survey, 418
 in system performance, 333, 334t
Responsive pleading, 507
Rest breaks, 642
Restoration specialist, 242
Restraint
 of psychiatric patients, 143
 of trade, 534
Results management, 163
Results reporting applications, 285
Résumé(s), 581
 clinical, 109
Retention, of health records, 182
Retention period, 234
Retention schedule, 241
Retiree, 233b
Retirement, 592
Retraction, of document, 189
Retrieval workstation, in electronic document management, 257
Retrospective payment system, 34
Retrospective record completion, 124-126, 125f
Retrospective review, in utilization management, 465, 466f
Retrospective study, 421-424, 423f, 424t, 427t-428t
Return on investment (ROI), 340-341, 341t
 with electronic health records, 168
Revenue(s)
 nonoperating, 653
 offsetting, of electronic document management, 261
 operating, 653
 net, 675
Revenue cycle, 652-660, 654f
 back-end activities in, 657-660
 case mix analysis in, 660
 charge master in, 655, 655t
 claims processing in, 657, 658f
 coding in, 656-657, 656b
 collection and claim denial in, 657-659
 contracting in, 653-654
 front-end activities in, 653-657
 licensure and provider enrollment in, 654-655
 patient accounting in, 657

Revenue cycle *(Continued)*
 patient encounter in, 656
 payment processing in, 659
 registration and admitting in, 655-656
 reimbursement analysis in, 659-660, 659t
 utilization management in, 656
Revenue-generating departments, 668
Reverse discrimination, 563
Review of literature, 406-407, 407f, 408
Review of systems (ROS), 106t-107t
Rewritable magneto-optical platters, 257
RFI (request for information), 343-344
RFID (radiofrequency identification device), 245, 288, 700
RFP. *See* Request for proposal (RFP).
RHIA (Registered Health Information Administrator), 53
RHIOs (regional health information organizations), 82, 83-84, 85t-86t
RHIT (Registered Health Information Technologist), 53
Rhode Island: State and Regional Demonstrations in Health Information Technology, 85t
Rider, 35b
Right(s)
 constitutional, 505
 of privacy, 505
 to refuse treatment, 532
Risk
 defined, 460
 relative, 423-424, 425
Risk factors, 422
Risk management, 460-461, 462t
Risk Management Incident Collaborative, 457
RN (registered nurse), 25
Roadmap to Electronic Connectivity, 73
ROADS *(Registry Operations and Data Standards),* 477
Robert Wood Johnson (RWJ) Foundation, 73, 74t, 77t, 84, 86t-87t
ROI (return on investment), 340-341, 341t
 with electronic health records, 168
Role-based access control (RBAC), 295-296, 296t
Roll microfilm, 247, 248, 248t, 249t
Rolling budget method, 663-664
Root cause analysis, 458, 459
ROS (review of systems), 106t-107t
Rotary camera, 252
Routing slip, 237f
Row total, 397, 397t
Row variable, 397, 397t
RR (relative risk), 423-424, 425
RRL (registered record librarian), 49
RSI (repetitive strain or stress injuries), 641
R-squared (R^2), 396
Rule(s)
 of administrative agencies, 505
 on forms, 117
 noncompliance with, 510
Rule v. Lutheran Hospitals and Homes Society of America, 534
Run charts, 452-453, 455f
RVU (relative value unit), 652
RWJ (Robert Wood Johnson) Foundation, 73, 74t, 77t, 84, 86t-87t
RxNORM, 69

S
s^2 (variance), 391-392
 one-way analysis of, 394-396
Safe environment, duty to provide, 532-533, 562

Safe Medical Devices Act, 482, 505
Safety
 of employees, 600-601
 patient, 454-460
  databases for, 456-458, 458t
  disclosure of health information for, 521
  electronic health records and, 165-166
  improvement of, 455, 458-460
  integration for, 700
  measurement of, 455-456, 456t, 457f
 and work space design, 640-641
 workplace, 566
Safran, Charles, 687
Salary budget, 664, 665t
Salary surveys, 598
Sample
 defined, 613
 random, 399
Sample size, 399-400
Sampling, 399-400
Sampling error, 392
Sampling variability, 415
SANs (storage area networks), 257
Santa Barbara County Care Data Exchange, 85t
Sarbanes-Oxley Act, 660
Satellite clinics, 18
"Satisfactory assurance," 527
Scanner(s)
 bar code, 239
 for data input and output, 243t
 for electronic document management, 255-256
SCD (Steering Committee of Databases to Support Clinical Nursing Practice), 207
Scenarios, 326, 331, 351
Scheduled appointments, 149
SCHIP (State Children's Health Insurance Program), 38
Scoring, 233b
 of evaluation criteria, 349-351, 350f
Screen design, 115-117, 119-122, 120f, 280-283
 general principles of, 116-117, 282-283
 importance of, 281
 interface elements in, 120-121, 121f, 332-333
 team for, 115-116, 281-282
Screen space, 282-283
Script-based systems, 170
SDOs (standards development organizations), 214, 215
Seal of authenticity, 297
Seclusion, of psychiatric patients, 143
Secondary care, 16
Secondary data, 474
Secondary evidence, 514-515
Secondary insurance coverage, 657
Secondary patient record, 98
Secure magnetic storage, in electronic document management, 257
Secure socket layer (SSL), 297, 298f
Securing Health Access and Records Exchange (SHARE), 86t
Security
 computer, 293-299
  administrative safeguards for, 294, 294t
  authentication tools for, 294-296, 296t
  external controls for, 296-299, 298f
  HIPAA on, 293-294, 294t
  physical, 294, 294t, 296
  reporting capabilities for, 296
  technical safeguards for, 294, 294t
 with electronic document management, 259-260
 with electronic health record systems, 40, 172, 178

Security *(Continued)*
   of health information, 512, 529
   in international health information
     management, 691
   and outcomes research, 493-494
   with paper-based records, 234
   to prevent unauthorized access, 529
   in system development, 309f
Security design, 331
Security reports, 296
Security rules, 13-14, 293-294
Security Standards for the Protection of
   Electronic Protected Information, 293
"Seed" screens, 363
SEER (Surveillance, Epidemiology, and End
   Results) Program, 475
Selection bias, 415
Selection interview, 582-583
Selection process, 580-583
Self Instructional Manual for Tumor Registrars,
   477
Self-appraisal, 588
Self-care management, 700
Self-insured companies, 34
Self-paced training modules, 336
Self-pay, 34
Self-pay balances, collection of, 658-659
Semantic content, 214
Semantic interoperability, 214
Sensitivity, 412, 412t
Sensors, for data input and output, 244t
Sentinel events, 456, 459
Serial numbering, 221, 221t
Serial work division, 606, 607f, 607t
Serial-unit numbering, 221, 221t
Servant leadership, 551
Server, proxy, 297
Server-side scripting, 291
Service, 550
Service(s), on patient record, 147t
Service agreement, 138
Service set identifier (SSID), 278
Servlet, 291
Severity of illness scores, 384
Sexual harassment, 564
SF-12, 490
SF-36, 490
SGML (standard generalized markup
   language), 170, 290
SH (social history), 106t
SHARE (Securing Health Access and Records
   Exchange), 86t
Shared workstations, 643
Shelving, in workstation design, 643
Sherman Act, 534
Shewhart, Walter A., 453-454
Shibumi, 555b
Shift workers, work space design for, 639
Short-term care facility, 20
S-HTTP, 289
Sibling nodes, 315
Signature(s)
   electronic, 175t, 178
     legal aspects of, 514
   on records, 114
Signature stamps, 114
Significance
   level of, 393
   of research, 408-409
   tests of, 392-398, 397t
Simple ranking, 586
Simulation, 460
Simultaneous-equations method, of cost
   allocation, 669

Single blind study, 427
Single sign-on technology, 295
Sinuses, physical examination of, 108t
SIP (surgical infection prevention) project, 443,
   443t
Site preparation, 336
Site visits, in purchasing process, 351-352
Situational analysis, 627-628
Six Sigma, 448-449, 448f
Skilled nursing facility, 28
Skills inventory, 576
Skin
   physical examination of, 108t
   in review of systems, 106t
Slander, 509
Sliding scale fee, 17, 34
SMR (standardized mortality ratio), 377-378,
   377t, 378t
SNO(s) (subnetwork organizations), 82-83
SNODENT *(Systematized Nomenclature of
   Dentistry),* 205
SNOMED *(Systematized Nomenclature of
   Medicine),* 170, 174t, 201, 204-205, 205f,
   206f
SNOMED CT *(Systematized Nomenclature of
   Medicine–Clinical Terms),* 204, 205, 208,
   209t
SNOMED RT *(Systematized Nomenclature of
   Medicine–Reference Terminology),* 204-
   205
SNOP (Systematized Nomenclature of
   Pathology), 204
SOAP format, 114–115, 115t
Social history (SH), 106t
Social needs, of employees, 641
Social Security Act, 7, 7b
Social Security Administration (SSA), 12
Social service(s), 27
Social service record, 112
Software, 275-277, 276f
   malicious, 297-298
   project management, 634-636
   in research, 429-430
Software contract, 352
Solo practices, 17
Solutions architect, 308
Sound, in workstation design, 645-646, 645b
Source-oriented medical record, 114
SOW (Statement of Work), 438-439
Space allocation, 643, 644b
Space management, with paper-based records,
   223, 224t
Space planning
   for alphabetical filing, 224, 225b
   for straight numerical filing, 225
   for terminal digit filing, 226
Space requirements, in system design, 336
SPC (statistical process control), 453-454
Special care units, forms for, 112
Special committees, 22
Specialist care, 16t
Specialty(ies), 32
Specialty clinics, 18
Specialty hospital, 20
Specific aims, of research, 408
"Specification for Continuity of Care (E2369-
   05)", 78
Specificity, 412, 412t
Speech, documentation via, 180-181
Speech pathologists, 27
Speech privacy, in workstation design, 645
Speech recognition software, 180
Speech therapy, 27
Spyware, 298

SQL (structured query language), 277
SSA (Social Security Administration), 12
SSB (sum of squares between groups), 395
SSID (service set identifier), 278
SSL (secure socket layer), 297, 298f
SSW (sum of squares within groups), 395
Stable monetary unit, in accounting, 670
Stacked bar graph, 386, 388f
Staff, budgeting for, 664, 665t
Staff development, 599
Staff hour, 611
Staff members, duty to supervise actions of,
   533–536, 533f
Staff model HMO, 36
Staff nurse, 25
Staffing budget, 664, 665t
Staffing information, for business plan, 666
Staffing plan, 573–576, 574b, 575f, 576f
Staffing table, 576, 576f
Staging, of cancer, 477
Stakeholders, 307, 356, 356t
Standard(s)
   cataloging of, 497-499
   defined, 211
   health data, 211-216, 213t-214t
     development and selection of, 214-215
Standard deviation *(s),* 391-392
Standard generalized markup language
   (SGML), 170, 290
Standard of care, in negligence or malpractice
   case, 530
Standardization, of electronic health records,
   186–187
Standardized mortality ratio (SMR), 377–378,
   377t, 378t
Standards development organizations (SDOs),
   214, 215
*Standards for Health Information Management
   Education,* 52
Standards Harmonization Project, 74t
Standing committees, 22
Stare decisis, 505
Start character, 288
Startup, 337
State Children's Health Insurance Program
   (SCHIP), 38
State courts, 506–507
State Health Departments, 12–13, 13t
State health information networks, 84, 85t–86t
State hospitals, 20
State licensure, of practitioners, 15
State regulatory agencies and organizations,
   12-13, 13t
State statutes and regulations, 505
   on record retention, 240-241
State supreme courts, 507
Statement of cash flow, 672-674, 673f
Statement of revenues and expenses, 672, 673f
Statement of Work (SOW), 438-439
Statistic(s), 370-400
   census, 381-382, 381t-382t
   descriptive, 388-391
   health care, 372-383
     autopsy rates as, 378-379, 379t
     census, 381-382, 381t-382t
     morbidity rates as, 379-381, 380t
     mortality rates as, 373-378, 374t, 377t, 378t
     rates, ratios, proportions, and percentages
       as, 373, 373t, 374t
     vital, 372-373
   inferential, 392
   overview of, 372
   role of health information management
     professional in, 372

Statistic(s) *(Continued)*
   test, 393
   vital, 372-373
Statistical analysis, of medical records, 124
Statistical measures and tests, 388-400
   descriptive statistics as, 388-392
   inferential statistics as, 392
   interval estimation as, 398-399
   sampling and sample size as, 399-400
   tests of significance as, 392-398, 397t
Statistical process control (SPC), 453-454
Statistics budget, 662-663
Status, work space design and, 641
Statute(s), 504
   federal and state, 505
   of limitations, 241, 512, 529-530
   noncompliance with, 510
Steelcase Study II, 643
Steering Committee of Databases to Support
   Clinical Nursing Practice (SCD), 207
Step-and-repeat camera, 252
Step-down method, of cost allocation, 668
Stereotyping, 589
Stop character, 288
Stopwatch studies, in productivity program,
   613
Storage
   of health records, 182
   of inactive records, 234-235
   of microforms, 249-250
   of paper-based records, 178-179, 234
   of patient records, 221-223, 222t, 223f, 234
Storage area networks (SANs), 257
Storage devices, for electronic health records,
   243
Storage space, in workstation design, 643
Store and forward technology, 292
"Stove pipes," 695
Straight numerical filing, 224-225, 226t
Straight-line depreciation, 678
Strategic control, 629
Strategic human resource planning, 573
Strategic implementation, 629
Strategic management, 627-629, 628f
Strategic planning, use of data in, 486
Strategy(ies)
   adaptive, 628-629
   directional, 627, 628, 629
   functional, 629
   linkage, 629
   market entry, 629
   operational, 629
   positioning, 629
Strategy formulation, 628-629
Stratified random sample, 399
Street normalization, 233b
Strictness bias, 589
Strike notice, 568
Strong authentication, 295
Structure measures, 442, 442t
Structured query language (SQL), 277
Structured questions, 326, 418
Structured text, 164, 170
Subacute care, 27
Subcultures, organizational, 570
Subject matter expert, 308
Subnetwork organizations (SNOs), 82-83
Subpoena, 527-529, 528f
   ad testificandum, 527
   duces tecum, 527, 528f
Subscriber, 35b
Subspecialties, 32
Substance Abuse and Mental Health Services
   Administration, 11

Substance Registry System, 69
Suicide concerns, 143
Sum of squares between groups (SSB), 395
Sum of squares within groups (SSW), 395
Summarizing, of numbers, 446
Summary Staging Guide, 477
Supervisory coaching, 584
Supervisory relationships, 578t
Support and maintenance, 352
Supporting staff, 30
Supportive functions, 158f
Supreme Court, 506
Surgeon general, 11
Surgical infection prevention (SIP) project, 443,
   443t
Surgicenters, 18
Surveillance, 474
Surveillance, Epidemiology, and End Results
   (SEER) Program, 475
Surveillance systems, 486
Survey(s), in system analysis, 327-328
Survey methods, for system evaluation, 342
Survey research, 417-419, 419f-422f
Survival bias, 415
Survival time, 429, 430f
Survivor, 232b, 233b
Suspension, 593
Swing beds, 28
Symbol(s), in documentation, 113-114
Symbology, of bar code, 239, 288
Syndromic surveillance, 271, 486, 696
Synthesis methods, in productivity program,
   613
System(s)
   boundary or integrity of, 624
   defined, 179, 623, 624f
   determining need for, 625
   hierarchical structure of, 623
   input-output cycle of, 624-625
   unity of purpose of, 624
   well-designed, 625
System analysis, 306-307, 314-331
   investigative strategies for, 324-330
      document and forms review as, 330
      group analysis and design as, 330
      interviews as, 325-327
      observation as, 328-329, 328f
      questionnaires as, 327-328
   in operational management, 623-626, 624f
   tools and aids for, 314-324, 315t
      computer-aided systems engineering, 324,
         324b
      data dictionary as, 315t, 318-321, 318f-
         321f
      data flow diagrams as, 315-318, 315t, 316t,
         317f
      data mapping as, 321-322
      data modeling as, 315t
      decomposition diagrams as, 315, 315t
      entity-relationship diagrams as, 315t, 322-
         324, 322f, 323f
      hierarchy chart as, 315, 316f
      process modeling as, 315-318, 315t
System analysis document, 330-331
System conversion, 337, 363-366
System costs, in request for proposal, 349
System design, 306, 307, 331-334
   logical, 331
   in operational management, 625-626
   physical, 331
   principles of, 332-334, 334t
System development
   players involved in, 307-308
   principles for, 313

System development life cycle, 306-307,
   313-314, 314f
System diagram, for electronic document
   management, 261
System evaluation, 307, 337-343, 366
   benchmarks for, 366, 367t-368t
   benefits realization for, 338-339
   cost-benefit analysis for, 339-341, 340t, 341t
   cost-effectiveness analysis for, 341-342
   experimental research methods for, 342-343
   mathematical and computer simulations for,
      343
   qualitative research for, 342
   questions for, 342
   survey methods for, 342
System file conversion, 235-236, 235b
System implementation, 307, 310, 335-337
System initiation, 306
System life cycle(s), 310-313, 356-357
   general, 310, 311f
   information, 310-311, 311f
      in organization, 311-312, 311f
      aggregate, 312
System obsolescence, 310, 312-313
System performance, 333-334, 334t
System requirements, 344
System selection, 352
System specifications, 344
System startup, 337, 363-366
System summary, for electronic document
   management, 261
System testing, 307, 336-337, 365
Systematic sampling, 399
Systematized Nomenclature of Dentistry
   (SNODENT), 205
Systematized Nomenclature of Medicine
   (SNOMED), 170, 174t, 201, 204-205,
   205f, 206f
*Systematized Nomenclature of Medicine–Clinical
   Terms* (SNOMED CT), 204, 205,
   208, 209t
*Systematized Nomenclature of
   Medicine–Reference Terminology*
   (SNOMED RT), 204-205
Systematized Nomenclature of Pathology
   (SNOP), 204
Systems approach, to health information
   services, 555, 556f
Systems flowchart, 618, 618f
Systems model
   for human resource management, 556-557,
      557f
   in operational management, 623-624, 624f
Systems perspective, on human resource
   management, 552-557, 556f, 557f

T
Tab(s), 332
Table, 495, 495t
Table of contents, of request for proposal, 344,
   345f
Taconic Health Information Network and
   Community, 85t
Taft-Hartley Act, 563t, 568
Tags, 290-291
"Take call," 17
Target audience, in system analysis, 325
Targeted advertising, for job openings, 580
Task forces, 22
Task lighting, 645
Task list, 606-608, 608f
Task-ambient lighting, 645
Tax Equity and Fiscal Responsibility Act
   (TEFRA), 8b, 37, 651

TCP/IP (transmission control protocol/Internet protocol), 278, 280, 289
TDS (Technicon Data System), 272
Team development, 554b
Technical domains, of care, 442
Technical infrastructure, of electronic health record systems, 168
Technical requirements, in request for proposal, 348
Technical safeguards, 294, 294t
Technician, 30
Technicon Data System (TDS), 272
Technological change, and human resource management, 558
Technologist, 30
Technology
  continuing education units in, 55
  defined, 555
  in health information, 38–39
  and human resource management, 555
  and patient record, 47–48
Technology Informatics Guiding Educational Reform (TIGER), 689-690
Technology infrastructure, for electronic health record system, 193
Technology-enabled processes, 78t
TEFRA (Tax Equity and Fiscal Responsibility Act), 8b, 37, 651
Telecommuting oversight, 699
Telehealth, 72t, 186, 292
Telemedicine, 292-293, 699
Telemonitoring, 186
Telenursing, 699
Telepharmacy, 699
Telephone, in workstation design, 643
Telesage, 490
Temperature control, in workstation design, 643-644
Templates
  design and control of, 115-117, 119-122, 120f, 121f
  for documentation, 164
  for electronic health records, 188
  order, 176
  for patient record forms, 116-117
  for point-of-care system, 287
Tendinitis, 641
Tennessee Health Network project, 87t
Tennessee–Volunteer eHealth Initiative, 86t
Term, of contract, 352
Terminal(s), 274
  for data access, 243t, 244
Terminal digit filing, 225-226, 226t
Termination
  of contract, 352
  of employment, 590-592, 590b, 591f, 593-594
  project, 632
Termination clauses, 536
Terminology(ies)
  administrative, 201-204
  characteristics of, 208-211
  clinical, 204-208, 205f, 206f, 209t
  commercial information system vendor-neutral, 211
  Common Procedural, 201, 203
  concept orientation of, 209-210
  concept permanence of, 210
  content of, 208-209
  context representation in, 210
  copyright and license of, 211
  defined, 201
  drug, 207
  formal definitions of, 210
  graceful evolution of, 210-211

Terminology(ies) (Continued)
  multiple consistent views in, 210
  multiple granularities in, 210
  nonsemantic concept identifier of, 210
  nursing, 207-208, 209t
  polyhierarchy of, 210
  recognized redundancy of, 211
  reject "not elsewhere classified" in, 210
  scalable infrastructure and process control of, 211
  scientific validity of, 211
  self-sustaining, 211
  standards for, 174t
  well-maintained, 211
Territoriality, 641
Territory courts, 506-507
Tertiary care, 16-17
Test(s)
  employee selection, 581-582
  of significance, 392-398, 397t
Test database, 365
Test phases, 336-337
Test scripts, 336
Test statistic, 393
Testifying, 529
Text processing, 170
Therapeutic outcomes monitoring, 701
"Therapeutic privilege," 532
Therapeutic services reports, 112
Therapist, 30
Therapy(ies), on patient record, 149
Thick clients, 274
Thin clients, 274
Thinning, of health records, 183, 237
Third-party payers, 34, 35b, 651
  use of health data by, 95-96
Thoracic surgery, 24t
Thorax, physical examination of, 108t
360-degree evaluation, 585
Three-tier architecture, 279
Threshold, 444
Throat
  physical examination of, 108t
  in review of systems, 106t
TIGER (Technology Informatics Guiding Educational Reform), 689-690
Time estimates, in project planning, 631
Time frame, of research study, 409
Time ladder, 611, 612f
Time table, in request for proposal, 344, 345f
Time value of money, 676
Time-boxing, 335
Timeline tag, 358
Timeliness
  of data, 144t, 145
  of documentation, 178
Title(s), of documents, 188
Title III, 7b
Title VII, 562, 563t
Title XVIII, 7, 7b, 12
Title XIX, 7, 7b
TN (true negatives), 412
TNM system, 477
To Err Is Human, 8, 166, 438, 689
Tobacco-related illnesses, 695
Token(s), for security, 295
Token ring, 278
Top tab configuration, 234
Topography, of neoplasms, 477
Tort(s), intentional, 508-509
Tort actions, 504
Tort law, and employee termination, 590
Total infection rate, 380, 380t, 381
Total inpatient days of stay, 382t

Total length of stay, 382t
Total situational awareness, 701
TP (true positives), 412
Tracking systems
  automated, 238-240, 238b, 239b
  manual, 237-238, 237f
Traffic patterns, 638, 638f
Trainers, 308, 336, 364
  use of health data by, 96
Training
  for electronic health record system, 364-365, 365f
  of employees, 598-600, 599b, 600b
  user, 307, 335-336
Training manual, 363-364, 364t
Training program, 599-600, 599b, 600b
Training requirements, in request for proposal, 349
Transaction and Code Set Regulations, 38-39
Transactional leadership, 548
Transcription, 122, 180-181
Transfer, of paper-based records, 178-179
Transfer form, for long-term care, 136
Transfer notice, 237, 237f
Transformational leadership, 548-549, 554b
Translational leadership, 549
Transmission control protocol/Internet protocol (TCP/IP), 278, 280, 289
Trauma center, 26
Trauma registries, 484
Treatment, right to refuse, 532
Treatment plans, 148
Trends, in business plan, 666
Triage, 26
Trial courts, 506-507
Tricare, 38
"Trigger" words, 245
Trip frequency chart, 638, 638f
Triple blind study, 427
Trojan horses, 298
True negatives (TN), 412
True positives (TP), 412
Trust, 357-358
Tumor Registry Software Checklist, 479, 480f
Turnover ratio, 674-675
Two-factor authentication, 295
Two-tier architecture, 279
Type, in data dictionary, 496
Type I error, 393
Type II error, 393
Type styles, for forms, 117

U
UACDS (Uniform Ambulatory Care Data Set), 99t, 131-132
UB-04 (Uniform Billing Code of 2004) claim form, 657, 658f
UB-92 (Uniform Billing Code of 1992) claim form, 657
UHDDS (Uniform Hospital Discharge Data Set), 99t, 102, 130
UM. See Utilization management (UM).
UMLS (Unified Medical Language System), 174t, 208
Unauthorized access, to patient records, 529
Understanding
  in collaboration, 360-361
  of process, 361
Undue hardship, 565
UNet, 484
Unfair labor practices, 568, 568b
Unidentified patients, 229f
Unified Medical Language System (UMLS), 174t, 208

Uniform Ambulatory Care Data Set (UACDS), 99t, 131-132
Uniform Billing Code of 1992 (UB-92) claim form, 657
Uniform Billing Code of 2004 (UB-04) claim form, 657, 658f
Uniform Hospital Discharge Data Set (UHDDS), 99t, 102, 130
Uninterruptible power supply (UPS), 258
Union(s), 545, 567-569, 568b-570b
    grievance procedure with, 594
Union benefits, 569, 569b
Union organizing, 569, 570b
Unique identifier, 104
Unique patient identification, 177
Unique personal identifiers (UPINs), 150
Unit assembly work division, 606, 607f, 607t
Unit number, duplicate, 230f, 232b-233b
Unit numbering system, 221, 221t
Unit record, 221
Unit testing, 336
United Network for Organ Sharing (UNOS), 483, 484
United States Pharmacopeia, 456
Unity of purpose, of system, 624
"Universal" chart order, 114
Universal product codes (UPCs), 239
University of Iowa Hospitals and Clinics, 240
University of Texas, James W. Ashton Ambulatory Care Center at, 239-240
UNIX, 275
Unknowns, in understanding of process, 361
UNOS (United Network for Organ Sharing), 483, 484
Unstructured questions, 326, 418
Unstructured text, 164, 170
Unwritten organization, 626-627
UPCs (universal product codes), 239
UPINs (unique personal identifiers), 150
UPS (uninterruptible power supply), 258
UR. See Utilization review (UR).
URAC (Utilization Review Accreditation Commission), 463
Urgent care centers, 18
Urinary system, in review of systems, 106t
Urology, 24t
U.S. Court of Appeals, 506
U.S. Defense Department Advanced Research Project Agency (DARPA), 288
U.S. district courts, 506
U.S. Supreme Court, 506
Use cases, 326, 331, 345, 346f, 351
User, 356
"User acceptance test," 365
User access, 294-296, 296t
User input, in system analysis, 325-329
User interface, 279
    design and control of, 115-117, 119-122, 120f, 121f, 280-283
User interface team, 281-282
User manual, 364-365, 365t
User perspective, value of, 356
User preparation, 335-336
User processes and procedures, in implementation readiness, 363-364
User training, 307, 335-336
Usual, customary, and reasonable charges, 34
Utah Health Information Network, 86t
Utility windows, 332
Utilization management (UM), 36, 462-466
    external requirements for, 462-463
    goal of, 462
    plan and program structure for, 465-466

Utilization management (UM) (Continued)
    program components for, 463-465, 464f, 466f
    in revenue cycle, 656
Utilization managers, use of health data by, 96
Utilization review (UR), 36
    concurrent, 463-465, 464f
    prospective, 463
    retrospective, 465, 466f
Utilization Review Accreditation Commission (URAC), 463

V
VA (Veterans Administration), 207, 212
VA (Department of Veterans Affairs) medical centers, 19
Vaccine Adverse Event Reporting System, 457
Vacuum freezer drying, of wet records, 242
Vagueness, 360
Validity, 411-412
    coding, 412, 413f
    of master patient index, 228-230, 231f
    of performance measures, 444
Value(s)
    in data dictionary, 495-496
    organizational, 628
Value benchmarks, 366, 367t-368t
Value chain, 449
Values clarification, 551
Values/meaning, in data dictionary, 318-319, 318f-321f
Variable(s)
    confounding, 415
    discrete vs. continuous, 384
    independent or dependent, 406
Variable expenses, 663
Variance (s^2), 391-392
    one-way analysis of, 394-396
Variance reports, 664-665, 665t, 666t
Variation, coefficient of, 392
Vendor(s)
    for electronic document management, 260, 262
    for electronic health record systems, 164-165, 173-176
Vendor profile, in request for proposal, 349
Versioning, 187-188, 188b
Vertical filing cabinets, 222
Vertical forms guide, 118f
Vertical integration, 30
Veterans Administration (VA), 207, 212
Veterans Administration (VA) medical centers, 19
Veterans Health Administration, 457
Veterans Integrated Service Networks, 19
Vice president, of hospital, 22
Vietnam Era Veterans' Readjustment Assistance Act, 563t
View(s), 146
    multiple consistent, in terminology, 210
View design, 115-117, 119-122, 120f, 280-283
    general principles of, 116-117, 282-283
    importance of, 281
    interface elements in, 120-121, 121f, 332-333
    team for, 115-116, 281-282
View identification, 121
Views team, 115-116
Virtual intensive care units, 699
Virtual Private Network (VPN), 291-292
Virus, computer, 297-298
Visible Analyst Workbench, 319
Vision, organizational, 628
Visionary leadership, 554b
Visit level, of master patient index, 226
Visit summary, 164

VistA system, 207, 212
Vital records, 105
Vital signs
    graphic sheet for, 111-112
    physical examination of, 108t
Vital statistics, 372-373
Vocabulary(ies)
    in collaboration, 359-360
    defined, 201
    and electronic health record, 170-171
Vocabulary blockade, 359-360
Vocational Rehabilitation Act, 600, 640
Voice recognition, 244t, 245, 274-275
Voice response, for data input and output, 244t
Volume testing, 337
Voluntary hospitals, 20
VPN (Virtual Private Network), 291-292

W
W3 (World Wide Web Consortium), 288-289
Wage and Hour Law, 567
Wage and salary surveys, 598
Wagner Act, 563t, 567-568
WAN(s) (wide area networks), 246, 278
    and outcomes research, 494
Wand(s), 239
    for data input and output, 243t
    in electronic document management, 256
Warning, 593
Warranties, 352
Washington State Public Health Improvement Plan, 695
Water damage, 242
Web pages, guidelines for designing, 282-283
Web-based survey, 418, 419f-422f
Weed, Lawrence L., 114-115
Weight, in long-term care, 136t
Weighted mean, 389-390
Weighted scores, 349-351, 350f
Weighting scale, 349-351, 350f
Well-being, of employees, 600-601
WEP (wired equivalent privacy) system, 278
Wet records, 242
Whistleblowers, 510
WHO (World Health Organization), 691, 692
Whole service cost, 651
Wide area networks (WANs), 246, 278
    and outcomes research, 494
Wi-Fi (wireless) network, 278-279, 279t
Wi-Fi–protected access (WPA), 278
Windows, 332
Windows-style interfaces, 120-121
Wired equivalent privacy (WEP) system, 278
Wired health care system, 684-686
Wireless (Wi-Fi) network, 278-279, 279t
Within-groups degrees of freedom (dfw), 395
Witness fee, 527
Women, in workforce, 557-558, 560
Women's center, 17
Women's hospitals, 20
Work activities, in project implementation, 631
Work breakdown structure, 309, 309t, 630-631
Work distribution chart, 606-611, 608f-610f
Work division, 606, 607f, 607t
Work flow, 637-638
Work sampling, 611-613
Work simplification, 614-623
    data analysis in, 618
    data collection in, 615-618, 616f-621f, 618b
    defined, 614-615
    formulating alternative solutions in, 618-619
    implementation and evaluation of, 622-623, 623b
    objectives of, 615

Work simplification (*Continued*)
philosophy of, 615
problem identification in, 615
selecting improved method in, 619-620, 621f, 622f
steps in, 615
Work space, sharing of, 639
Work space design, 637-641
confidentiality of work in, 639
employees' personal needs in, 639-640
flexibility for future needs in, 639-640
functioned performed in work space in, 638-639, 639f
sharing of work space in, 639
traffic patterns in, 638, 638f
work flow in, 637-638
Work standards, 611-613, 612f
Work surface, 642
Work-based relative value unit, 652
Workers' compensation, 38

Workforce, 521
age distribution of, 560-561
aging, 544, 560-561, 565-566
demographic changes in, 560-561
diversity in, 560, 561, 561b
"externalization" of, 584
Hispanics in, 544-545
multicultural, 560
women in, 557-558, 560
Workgroup on Electronic Data Interchange, 8b, 38
Working conditions, 578t
Workplace safety, 566
Workstation(s), 274
components of, 642-643
for data access, 243t, 244
defined, 642
shared or multifunction, 643
Workstation design, 641-646
environmental considerations in, 643-646, 645b

Workstation design (*Continued*)
ergonomics in, 641-642
space standards and guidelines for, 643, 644b
World Health Organization (WHO), 691, 692
World Wide Web Consortium (W3), 288-289
Worm, computer, 298
WPA (Wi-Fi–protected access), 278
Write once read many (WORM) technology, 257
Written warning, 593
Wrongful discharge, 590
Wrongful discharge defense, 591, 591f

X

XML (extensible markup language), 171, 290-291

Z

Zero-based budget, 664